Color Plate. *A* and *B,* A view through a flexible fiberoptic endoscope of esophagitis in a 2-year-old female Kerry Blue Terrier. Note the large hemorrhagic areas. A biopsy specimen obtained during the endoscopy examination confirmed an esophagitis. The patient developed clinical signs 4 days after a routine ovohysterectomy. *C,* An endoscopic examination of a 14-year-old neutered male Siamese revealed numerous nodular growths that were present in the caudal pharynx and diffusely involved the entire proximal one-third of the esophagus. This is a view through a flexible endoscope of one of the nodules. A biopsy specimen of a nodule was obtained through the endoscope. The histological diagnosis was squamous cell carcinoma. *D,* A view through a flexible endoscope of the esophagus of a 14-year-old canine that was presented for dysphagia and odynophagia. The raised white areas are abnormal. A biopsy specimen was obtained with a Quinton Multi-purpose Suction Biopsy Tube (note the red punched-out area). A definitive diagnosis of carcinoma was made from the specimen obtained. *E,* A view of a bone esophageal foreign body in the esophagus as seen through a flexible endoscope. The bone is located just cranial to the cardia of the stomach. Insufflation of the esophagus increased its internal diameter. *F,* View through a flexible endoscope of the hernia-like ring in a patient with an esophageal epiphrenic diverticulum. The diverticulum is on the right side of the picture. The cardia is just to the left of the hernia ring. *G,* View through a flexible endoscope looking into the diverticular pouch. Note the hernia ring in the upper right hand corner. *H,* A view through a flexible endoscope of an extraluminal stricture. Note that the stricture is composed of normal mucosa, which is indicative of a periesophageal mass causing the stricture. This patient had a history of regurgitating for 2 months prior to presentation. Surgery revealed a mass totally encircling the esophagus. Histologically the mass was a fibrosarcoma. *I,* View through a flexible endoscope demonstrating an intraluminal esophageal stricture. *J,* View through a flexible endoscope of an intraluminal esophageal stricture. Note the hemorrhagic areas around the stricture. The white area is fibrous connective tissue. *K,* Normal colonic mucosa as viewed through a flexible fiberoptic colonoscope. The mucosa appears creamy pink or pink and reflects light uniformly. Blood vessels are usually apparent in the submucosa; failure to see these vessels is a reliable sign of colonic disease and suggests the presence of inflammation, congestion, or edema. *L,* Colon of a dog with chronic idiopathic colitis as viewed through a colonoscope. No submucosal blood vessels are visible; the mucosa reflects light abnormally, and several large erythematous areas can be seen. These areas bled readily when rubbed with the tip of the colonoscope. *M,* Endoscopic appearance of whipworm-induced colitis. The mucosa reflects light unevenly (bright areas), indicating excessive mucus secretion. There are several areas of obvious mucosal hemorrhage, and a whipworm can be seen attached to the mucosa. Numerous other whipworms were found throughout the proximal colon. The patient, an 11-year-old mixed-breed dog, had a 6-month history of intermittent bloody diarrhea. Repeated fecal examinations had failed to reveal parasitic ova. Appropriate anthelmintic treatment in conjunction with sulfasalazine brought about an almost immediate cessation of signs. Whipworm infection would not have been confirmed without endoscopy. *N,* Endoscopic picture of the colon of a 2-year-old female boxer with histolytic ulcerative colitis. Changes in the colon wall are much more extensive than those seen in chronic idiopathic colitis. Areas of extensive hemorrhage and desquamated epithelium (*yellow material*) are obvious. No submucosal blood vessels are visible, and the mucosa reflects light unevenly, indicating excessive mucus secretion.

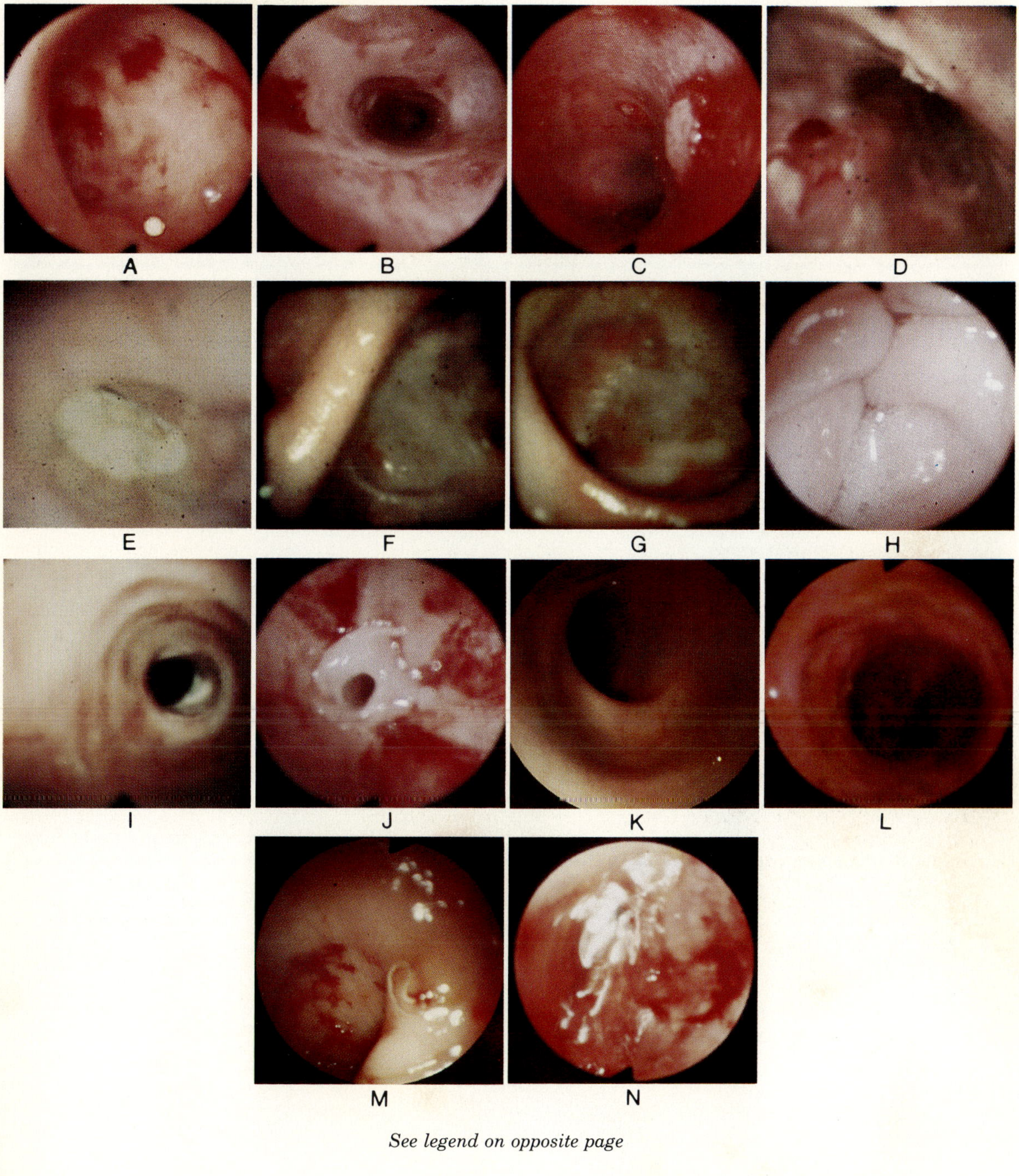

See legend on opposite page

AAHA®

AMERICAN ANIMAL HOSPITAL ASSOCIATION

1986

W. B. SAUNDERS COMPANY

Philadelphia London Toronto Mexico City Rio de Janeiro Sydney Tokyo Hong Kong

CANINE AND FELINE

GASTROENTEROLOGY

Edited by

BRENT D. JONES, D.V.M.

Associate Professor
Department of Veterinary Medicine and Surgery
College of Veterinary Medicine
University of Missouri
Columbia, Missouri

Associate Editor

WILLIAM D. LISKA, D.V.M.

Diplomate, American College of Veterinary Surgeons
Research Instructor, Department of Orthopedics
Baylor College of Medicine
Referral Surgery Practitioner
Westbury Animal Hospital, Inc., Houston, Texas

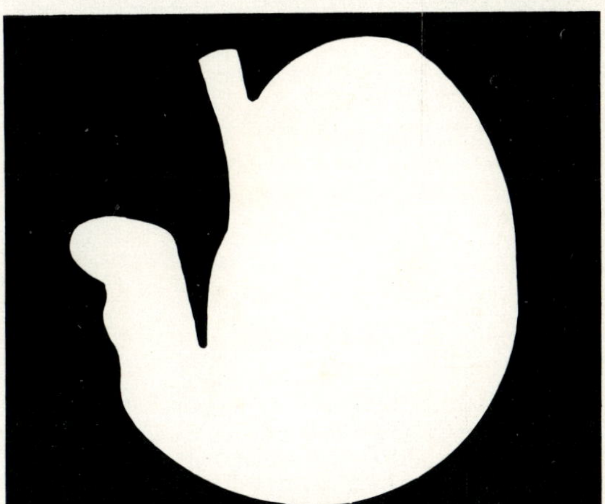

with 20 Contributors

W. B. Saunders Company: West Washington Square
Philadelphia, PA 19105

Library of Congress Cataloging-in-Publication Data

Main entry under title:

Canine and feline gastroenterology.

At head of title: AAHA, American Animal Hospital Association.

Includes index.

1. Dogs—Diseases. 2. Cats—Diseases. 3. Veterinary gastroenterology. I. Jones, Brent D. II. American Animal Hospital Association.

SF991.C22 1986 636.7′089633 85–27866

ISBN 0–7216–5206–9

Designer: Karen O'Keefe
Production Manager: Bill Preston
Manuscript Editor: Susan Short
Illustration Coordinator: Walter Verbitski

Canine and Feline Gastroenterology ISBN 0–7216–5206–9

Last digit is the print number: 9 8 7 6 5 4 3 2 1

This book is dedicated to:

1) The contributors; for it is their work
2) My parents, Zeno W. Jones and Helen M. Jones; although they are deceased, they are still very much alive in my mind and in my heart. I thank God for allowing them to be my parents, and I thank them for giving me a firm foundation from which to grow.
3) My children, who were conceived and born while this project was conceived and born; Clark Lafferty Jones (06/15/82), and Tyler Douglas Jones (04/05/84). Although they are still young, they have taught me a lot about life. I love them dearly.
4) My best friend and wife, Patricia Lafferty Jones. I am thankful we are able to spend our lives together.

Contributors

Everett Aronson, D.V.M.
Diplomate, American College of Veterinary Radiology; Assistant Professor of Radiology, Department of Veterinary Medicine and Surgery, College of Veterinary Medicine, University of Missouri; Head of Radiology, Veterinary Medicine Teaching Hospital, College of Veterinary Medicine, University of Missouri, Columbia, Missouri.
Radiology of the Gastrointestinal System

C. W. Betts, D.V.M.
Diplomate, American College of Veterinary Surgeons; Professor of Surgery, School of Veterinary Medicine, North Carolina State University; Staff Surgeon, Veterinary Teaching Hospital, School of Veterinary Medicine, North Carolina State University, Raleigh, North Carolina.
Surgery of the Large Bowel

M. Joseph Bojrab, D.V.M., M.S., Ph.D.
Diplomate, American College of Veterinary Surgeons; Professor and Head, Department of Veterinary Medicine and Surgery, College of Veterinary Medicine, University of Missouri; Head of Surgery, Veterinary Medicine Teaching Hospital, College of Veterinary Medicine, University of Missouri, Columbia, Missouri.
Surgery of the Small Intestine

Colin F. Burrows, B. Vet. Med., Ph.D., M.R.C.V.S.
Associate Professor of Medicine, College of Veterinary Medicine, University of Florida, Gainesville, Florida.
Diseases of the Colon

Colin B. Carrig, B.V.Sc., Ph.D.
Professor, Virginia-Maryland Regional College of Veterinary Medicine, Virginia Polytechnic Institute and University of Maryland; Staff Radiologist, Veterinary Medicine Teaching Hospital, Virginia-Maryland Regional College of Veterinary Medicine, Virginia Polytechnic Institute and University of Maryland, Blacksburg, Virginia.
Radiology of the Gastrointestinal System

Jonathan N. Chambers, D.V.M.
Diplomate, American College of Veterinary Surgeons; Associate Professor of Surgery, College of Veterinary Medicine, University of Georgia, Athens, Georgia.
Surgical Diseases of the Anorectum

Robert M. Corwin, D.V.M., Ph.D.
Professor, Department of Veterinary Parasitology, College of Veterinary Medicine, University of Missouri, Columbia, Missouri.
Gastrointestinal Parasitism of the Dog and Cat

William D. DeHoff, D.V.M., M.S.
Diplomate, American College of Veterinary Surgeons; Professor, Department of Veterinary Clinical Sciences, College of Veterinary Medicine, The Ohio State University; Attending Senior Clinician, Veterinary Teaching Hospital, College of Veterinary Medicine, The Ohio State University, Columbus, Ohio.
Surgery of the Stomach

A. R. Dillon, D.V.M., M.S.
Diplomate, American College of Veterinary Internal Medicine; Associate Professor, Department of Small Animal Surgery and Medicine, Scott-Ritchey Research Program, School of Veterinary Medicine, Auburn University, Auburn, Alabama.
The Oral Cavity

Frederick H. Drazner, B.V.Sc., D.V.M.
Diplomate, American College of Veterinary Internal Medicine; Chief of Staff, Animal Specialty Services of Cook County; Director of Services, Wright Animal Hospital, Des Plaines, Illinois; Consultant, Immunologic Diagnostic Services, Chicago, Illinois.
Diseases of the Pancreas

Bernard F. Feldman, D.V.M., Ph.D.
Associate Professor of Clinical Pathology, Department of Clinical Pathology, School of Veterinary Medicine, University of California; Chief, Department of Bone Marrow Cytology and Chief, Hemolysis Laboratory, Veterinary Medical Teaching Hospital, School of Veterinary Medicine, University of California, Davis, California.
Medical Diseases of the Small Intestine

Robert T. Franklin, D.V.M.
Assistant Professor, Department of Veterinary Internal Medicine, Western College of Veterinary Medicine, University of Saskatchewan; Veterinary Teaching Hospital, Western College of Veterinary Medicine, University of Saskatchewan, Saskatoon, Saskatchewan, Canada.
Medical Diseases of the Small Intestine

Sara E. Green, M.S.
Assistant Instructor for Labs, Department of Veterinary Parasitology, College of Veterinary Medicine, University of Missouri, Columbia, Missouri.
Gastrointestinal Parasitism of the Dog and Cat

R. E. Hoffer, D.V.M., M.S.
Diplomate, American College of Veterinary Surgeons; Soft Tissue Surgical Consultant, Salt Lake City, Utah.
Primary Esophageal Neuromuscular Diseases
Surgery of the Esophagus

Brent D. Jones, D.V.M.
Associate Professor, Department of Veterinary Medicine and Surgery, College of Veterinary Medicine, University of Missouri; Staff Gastroenterologist, Veterinary Medicine Teaching Hospital, College of Veterinary Medicine, University of Missouri, Columbia, Missouri.
Medical Aspects of Esophageal Disease
Medical Diseases of the Small Intestine

Jimmy C. Lattimer, M.S., D.V.M.
Diplomate, American College of Veterinary Radiology; Assistant Professor of Radiology, Department of Veterinary Medicine and Surgery, College of Veterinary Medicine, University of Missouri, Columbia, Missouri.
Radiology of the Gastrointestinal System

William A. Rogers, D.V.M.
Diplomate, American College of Veterinary Internal Medicine; Adjunct Professor, College of Veterinary Medicine, The Ohio State University; Specialty Practice, Internal Medicine, Cincinnati, Ohio.
Diseases of the Liver

Philip Roudebush, D.V.M.
Diplomate, American College of Veterinary Internal Medicine; Associate Professor, College of Veterinary Medicine, Mississippi State University, Mississippi State, Mississippi.
Medical Aspects of Esophageal Disease

David C. Twedt, D.V.M.
Diplomate, American College of Veterinary Internal Medicine; Associate Professor, Department of Clinical Sciences, College of Veterinary Medicine and Biomedical Sciences, Colorado State University; Attending Senior Clinician of Small Animal Medicine, Veterinary Teaching Hospital, College of Veterinary Medicine and Biomedical Sciences, Colorado State University, Fort Collins, Colorado.
Medical Diseases of the Stomach

Richard W. Vaughan, B.S., D.V.M.
Associate Veterinarian, Southwest Animal Hospital, Jefferson City, Missouri.
Medical Aspects of Esophageal Disease

Wayne E. Wingfield, D.V.M., M.S.
Diplomate, American College of Veterinary Surgeons; Professor of Medicine, Department of Clinical Sciences, College of Veterinary Medicine and Biomedical Sciences, Colorado State University; Chief, Emergency Medicine and Intensive Care, Veterinary Teaching Hospital, Colorado State University, Fort Collins, Colorado.
Medical Diseases of the Stomach

Preface

The purpose of this textbook is to provide the practicing veterinarian and the veterinary student with a practical but comprehensive reference on canine and feline gastroenterology. To make it a practical textbook, various unique aspects have been incorporated. This textbook includes both medicine and surgery chapters. When possible, dosages of drugs have been stated in the text, and the brand name and manufacturer's name and address have been supplied. Radiology and parasitology chapters have also been included. It has been organized in a way in which information can be easily retrieved. Ideally, it will be found to be an easy and enjoyable text to read.

Gastroenterology is just emerging (as it rightfully should) as a specialty in veterinary medicine. It is indeed encouraging to the author to see so many practitioners, interns, and residents demonstrate a "special interest" in gastroenterology. It is truly an exciting area (I feel it is the most exciting area) in veterinary medicine. I hope that this text will encourage even more interest in a fascinating and challenging field.

Comments and criticism are welcome. The best judges of a textbook are its readers. Perfection is elusive and can be obtained only after critical analysis of what has been accomplished.

BRENT D. JONES

Acknowledgements

First of all, I am grateful to the contributors to this book for their professional expertise, and their cheerful willingness to share their knowledge and to meet (usually) the deadlines. An editor is like a football coach. He is the organizer, and may be the mastermind, but it is the players who make the touchdowns and win the games. This book really represents the contributors' accomplishments.

Second, I appreciate the contribution that Dr. Bill Liska, my associate editor, has made to this textbook. His dedication and hard work are unparalleled. He truly should be recognized for the work that he has put into this project. I especially appreciated his patience while he was trying to teach me surgery.

In addition to the contributors and Dr. Liska, many other people helped with this venture: Drs. Richard Vaughn, Linda Garrison, and Al Jergens for their editorial assistance and proofreading, and Linda Salmon, Brenda Stafford, and Barbara Drechsel of our Secretarial Services for some of the typing and technical aspects of the project. Our students, interns, and residents were the biggest source of stimuli. They, along with my colleagues at the Veterinary Teaching Hospital, have been a constant source of encouragement. The support given to me from my Department Chairman, Dr. James Creed, is also appreciated.

I want to thank the devoted "pros" at the W. B. Saunders Company—specifically John Dyson, Bill Preston, Susan Colaiezzi-Short, Karen O'Keefe, and Walter Verbitski, who were extremely helpful. With individuals such as these, it is no wonder that W. B. Saunders is a "first class company."

I am grateful to the American Animal Hospital Association for the support they have given me. The Executive Committee, and Drs. Andy Hudson and Shirley Gilbert in particular, have been very helpful and very patient.

Last, but not least, I would like to thank my wife Pat for her constant encouragement and her editorial assistance. Pat's ability to spell is very much appreciated.

BRENT D. JONES

Contents

CHAPTER

1

The Oral Cavity

A. R. DILLON

The oral cavity is routinely examined in small animal practice; however, the extent of pathology found is related to the examiner's attention to detail and knowlege of normal anatomy. Subtle oral disease is often overlooked during a routine physical examination, when the mouth is opened only "to catch a passing glance at the tonsils."

Examination of the oral cavity of the dog or cat does not usually necessitate sedation. However, in cases when resistance is encountered, chemical restraint is mandatory. During the routine physical examination of a dog, the head is tilted upward and gentle pressure applied to the lips posterior to the upper canine teeth. By placing the thumb of the left hand in the roof of the mouth and placing the third finger of the right hand on the mandibular incisors, the examiner can use the first finger of the right hand to explore the oral cavity. A gauze sponge aids in grasping and manipulating the tongue. A cat's mouth is easily opened using the same technique if the head is tilted back at a more acute angle. If an animal demonstrates oral problems or extreme resistance to examination of the oral cavity, sedation or anesthesia is appropriate.

The routine oral examination should rule out common problems. Congenital anomalies, such as cleft palate, should be identified on the initial examination of the neonate. Teeth should be counted in puppies and kittens as well as in adult animals. Early detection of retained deciduous teeth and impacted teeth is paramount to ensure a normal occlusal pattern. The occlusal pattern should always be examined regardless of the age of the animal. Abnormal wearing of the teeth may be a clue to problems that are not obvious on physical examination. The client should be made aware of the problems associated with malocclusion and the possibility of pulp necrosis from excessive wearing. The gingiva, particularly the gingival margins, should be examined. Hyperemic and edematous areas should be investigated with a dental probe for subgingival calculus. Supragingival and subgingival calculis should be shown to the client and recorded in the medical record.

The complaint of halitosis can usually be resolved in the diagnosis of periodontal disease and calculi. However, stomatitis, oral neoplasia, rhinitis, or upper respiratory disease can be the origin of the odor. A careful examination for the cause usually necessitates the use of anesthesia. Exfoliative cytological studies, culture, radiology, and biopsy may be required for a definitive diagnosis. Self-inflicted trauma must be separated from the primary lesion.

Masses within the mouth should be considered malignant until proven otherwise. Therefore, suspicious lesions should be carefully examined for size, consistency, location, and depth of involvement. Radiographs, fine-needle aspiration biopsy, and surgical biopsy will aid in the diagnosis.

DEVELOPMENT AND RETENTION

Normal Tooth Development

The first indication of a tooth in the fetus is an invagination of oral ectoderm known as the dental lamina. From this, the tooth bud forms and develops into a cap-shaped dome over an area of mesoderm, the dental papilla, that becomes the dentin and pulp tissue. The enamel covering is formed from the ectoderm and determines the shape and size of the root and crown portions (Fig. 1–1). Cementum and periodontal fibers that attach the tooth to the alveolar bone are

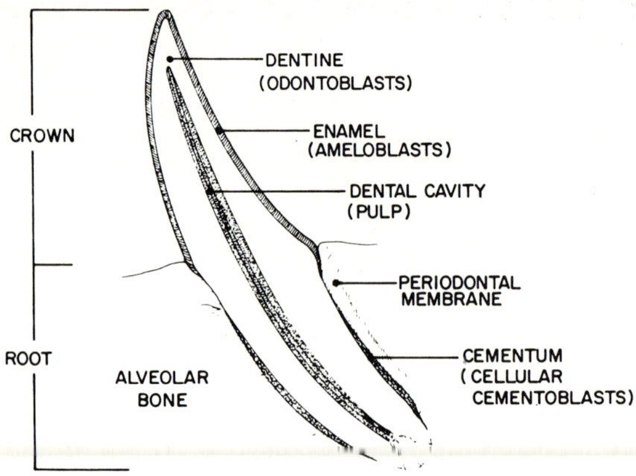

Figure 1–1. The structural components of the normal canine tooth. The associated cell types are in parentheses.

formed from the dental sac, which is of mesodermal origin.

The dental pulp, which contains blood vessels and nerves, furnishes nourishment to the tooth, produces dentin through the odontoblastic process, and registers pain from heat, cold, chemical, or traumatic stimuli. The pulp is continuous with the periodontal ligaments through multiple foramina at the apex of each root.[55]

Dentin, the bulk of the tooth, is a slightly compressible, highly elastic lining tissue. Collagen and water compose the organic matter content (30%), and the apatite, which is the mineral matrix of the dentin, makes up the inorganic portion (70%) (Table 1–1). The high sensitivity to pain of dentin possibly can be explained as a change in surface tension or in electrical charge. When penetration of the enamel occurs, caries spread rapidly through dentin. Enamel is permeable to iodine, calcium, and water.[104]

Eruption of Teeth

Dogs are born edentulous, with eruption of deciduous teeth beginning at two to four weeks of age.[1,2] The eruption time varies with the individual. Generally, central and intermediate incisors and canine teeth appear at 4 weeks, corner incisors at 5 to 6 weeks, and molars at 4 to 8 weeks. The eruption process can be as short as 10 days. Eruption of teeth in larger breeds usually occurs a few days before it does that in smaller breeds. On the average, the latest that teeth begin to emerge is on the 35th day, with variation due to breed. By 8 weeks the eruption process should be complete (Tab. 1–2).

Almost all deciduous teeth resemble their permanent functional successors except in their smaller size and pointed cusps. The second deciduous molar is very similar to the permanent upper carnassial tooth, and the third deciduous molar is similar to the permanent first upper molar. Lower incisors should occlude posterior to the upper incisors. Centric occlusion of the deciduous molars does not occur because the lower second and third molars are lingual to the upper teeth (Fig. 1–2). During the initial dental examination, a careful inspection for difficult eruption of deciduous teeth should be included. A longitudinal incision into the gum over an unerupted tooth generally facilitates eruption.

Resorptive processes start as soon as the deciduous tooth has erupted. Histological and radiographic studies have demonstrated similar processes in humans and dogs. Even-

Table 1–1. THE CHEMICAL CONTENT OF TEETH

Tooth Component	Substances H_2O (%)	Organic Matter (%)	Ash* (%)
Enamel	2.3	1.7	96
Dentin	13.2	17.5	69.3
Cementum and compact bone	32	22	46

*100 gm of ash contains 35 gm calcium, 17 gm phosphorus, 3 gm CO_2, and small amounts of other elements.

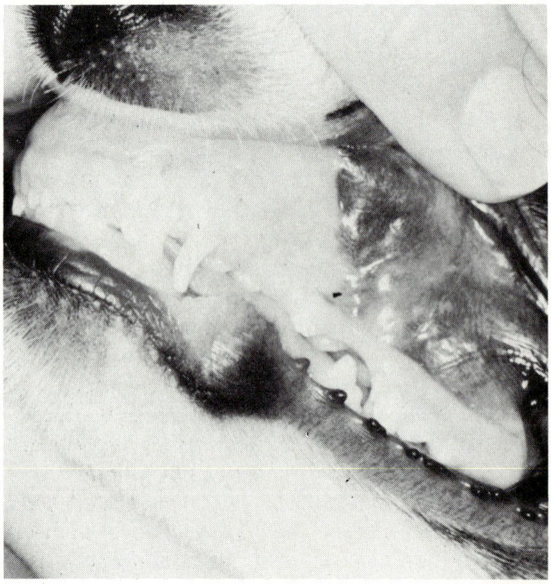

Figure 1–2. The normal deciduous teeth resemble their permanent successors except that no occlusion of the upper and lower molars occurs.

Table 1–2. DENTAL FORMULA OF DOGS AND CATS*

	Dog	Cat
Deciduous dentition	2(I3/3, C1/1,P3/3) = 28	2(I3/3, C1/1, P3/2) = 26
Permanent dentition	2(I3/3, C1/1, P4/4, M2/3) = 42	2(I3/3, C1/1, P3/2, M1/1) = 30

*I = incisor, C = canine, P = premolar, and M = molar.

tually, most of the dentin and the crown are removed, leaving only an enamel cap by the time the permanent teeth begin erupting. The deciduous tooth is often shed before the successor erupts. As with deciduous teeth, the permanent teeth of larger breeds of dogs begin erupting before those in smaller breeds (Tab. 1–3). Incisors are first to erupt, premolars and canines are next, and molars are last (Figs. 1–3 to 1–5).

In the cat, eruption of deciduous teeth starts at 2 weeks and is usually complete at 7 weeks of age. The permanent teeth erupt between 3 and 6 months of age.[12] Anodontia in the cat has been reported.[44]

Retention of Teeth

The pathology involved in retention of deciduous teeth is not totally understood. Failure of the periodontal membrane to detach from the tooth is a possible cause.[28] In response to the pressure exerted by the erupting permanent tooth, osteoclasts progressively resorb the cementum and dentin of the deciduous root. If the deciduous roots are not in the direct path of the erupting permanent tooth, then they may escape resorption. This unsuccessful resorption of deciduous roots is primarily a mechanical failure, since the normal position of the permanent incisors is not directly beneath the deciduous incisors, and the permanent canines generally are rostral (anterior) to the deciduous canines.

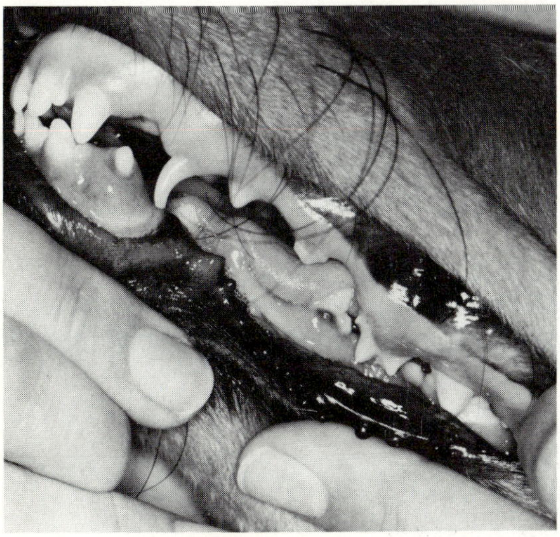

Figure 1–3. The permanent incisor and lower canine teeth and the deciduous premolar and upper canine teeth are visible in this 4-month-old dog.

Sequelae to retention of deciduous teeth are varied. Malocclusion of the permanent teeth is of primary concern. The maintenance of deciduous teeth even for 2 or 3 weeks can cause permanent displacement. The displacement of one tooth may cause overcrowding of the entire arcade. The maxillary canine tooth tends to erupt rostral to the retained deciduous canine (Fig. 1–6). Retention of lower deciduous canine teeth forces the lower permanent canines forward, and the lower incisors either crowd and rotate or move forward to form an abnormal scissor bite.[97] The maxillary incisors tend to erupt lingual to the deciduous incisors, and anterior crossbite with ventral deviation of the incisive bone usually follows if a sufficient deviation of eruption position has occurred (Fig. 1–7). Trauma to the roof of the mouth occurs when the lower canine is retained and the permanent canine erupts lingual to it. The lower incisors erupt lingual to the deciduous ones, and retention causes overcrowding with rotation and staggering. Food entrapment is common in overcrowded teeth, leading to periodontal damage, gingivitis, and premature loss of teeth.[104]

There should be no waiting period to see

Table 1–3. AVERAGE TIME OF ERUPTION OF PERMANENT TEETH

Tooth	Time of Eruption
Incisors	2–5 months
Canines	5–6 months
Premolars	
1st	5–6 months
2nd	6 months
3rd	6 months
4th	4–5 months
Molars	
1st	5–6 months
2nd	6–7 months
3rd	6–7 months

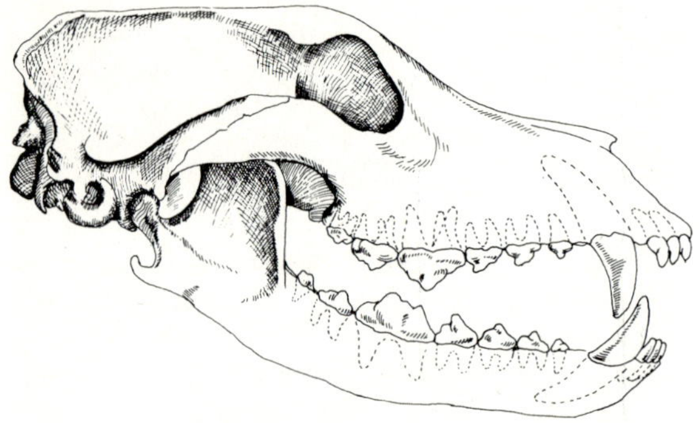

Figure 1–4. This hemisection of a canine skull shows the relationship of the normal permanent dentition.

if retained deciduous teeth will "fall out" naturally. A good rule of thumb is that two teeth of the same type should never be in the same place in the mouth at the same time. To prevent abnormal positioning of permanent teeth, retained deciduous teeth should be extracted at the time the permanent teeth are through the gingival surface or at 6 to 7 months. Care should be taken to avoid damaging the underlying permanent tooth bud. A dental elevator is used to loosen the gum around the neck of the tooth, and the root is separated from its alveolar attachment. Forceps may be used to lift the tooth out. Drainage aids healing, or if considerable tissue damage has occurred, systemic administration of antibiotics for 72 hours is indicated. Removal of the entire root is desirable, but if it is not possible, the remaining deciduous root is usually reabsorbed or sloughed off as a sequestrum. Fractured deciduous teeth should be extracted if more than 7 to 10 days elapse before anticipated natural exfoliation.

DEVELOPMENTAL PROBLEMS

Normal Occlusion

Sequential dental examination is important, especially in the pure-bred pet. Malocclusion should be identified as early as possible. Although the uncoordinated growth pattern of the oral bone structures generally is of genetic origin, developmental factors may be synergistic or antagonistic with the phenotypic expression of the traits. The mandible is smaller than the maxilla at birth in the dog and cat. The mandible grows rostrally faster than the maxilla. Although the maxillary teeth overlap the mandibular teeth, the mature mandibular arch is larger than the maxillary arch. Interdigitation of the deciduous teeth may regulate growth of the jaw. The removal of deciduous incisor teeth or canine teeth that seem to be inhibiting the forward growth of an obviously shorter mandible is recommended at 10 to 12 weeks of age. The occlusal position of the lower canines and the lower fourth premolars should be used to evaluate occlusion.[97] In the normal bite of the dog and cat, the maxillary incisors overlap the mandibular incisors, the mandibular canine teeth articulate rostral to the maxillary canine teeth, and the mandibular premolars close the interproximal space rostral to their maxillary counterparts (see Fig. 1–4). The widest part of the maxillary arch is at the fourth premolar level, and the widest part of mandibular arch is at the third molar level. Thus, the maxillary and mandibular premolars have no occlusal contact. However, owing to repeated selective breeding, the normal pattern has been distorted into an arrangement that is aesthet-

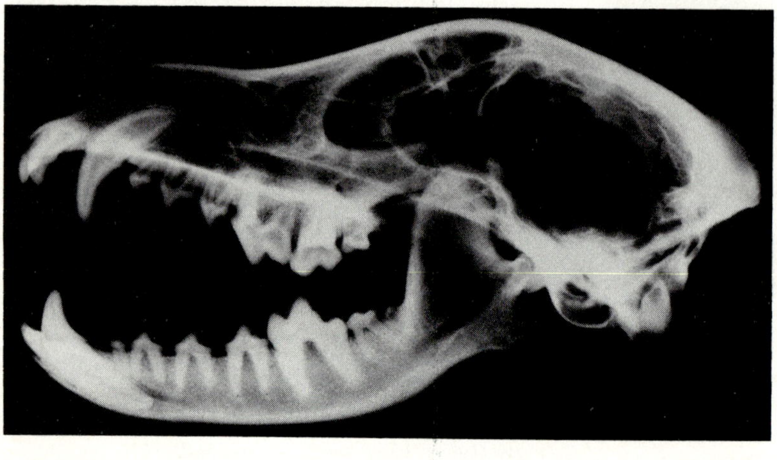

Figure 1–5. The normal permanent dentition is radiographically outlined on a lateral view of the skull.

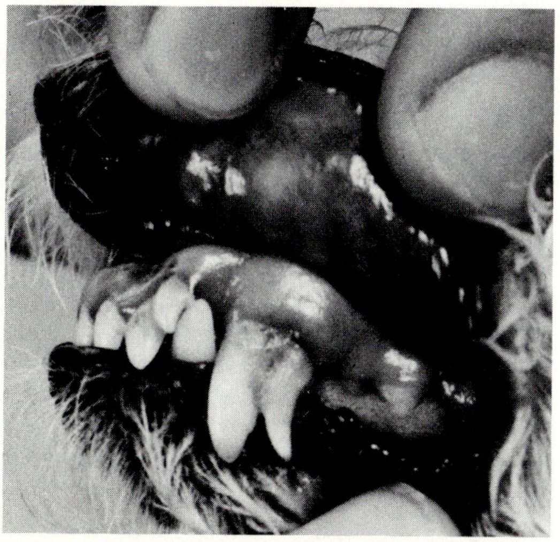

Figure 1–6. The retention of deciduous teeth, the maxillary canine erupts rostral to the deciduous canine.

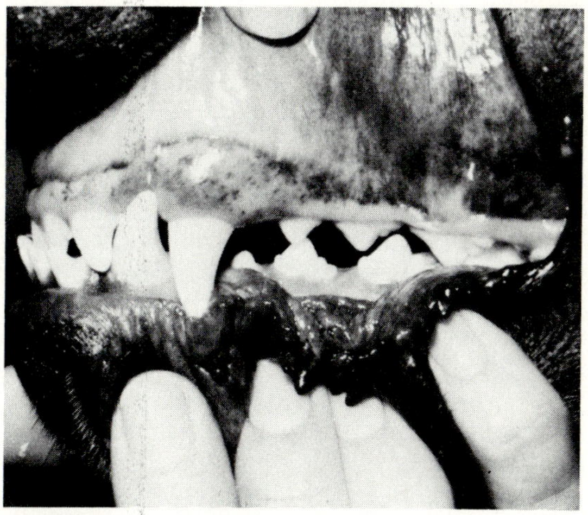

Figure 1–8. The normal relationship between the canine teeth and the premolar teeth combined with the malocclusion of the incisors is characteristic of anterior crossbite.

ically pleasing to owners. Especially in small breeds, selective breeding alters the size of the mouth more quickly than it alters the size and shape of the teeth.

Malocclusion

Confusion of terminology has resulted in broad definitions of variations of jaw length in veterinary medicine. When the mandibular incisors contact or are rostral to the maxillary incisors, the occlusion is termed *prognathism* (undershot). When the mandibular incisors are caudal to and do not contact the maxillary incisors, the occlusion is termed *retrognathism* (overshot). These conditions are often normal in certain breeds; for example, boxers are prognathic and collies are retrognathic.

Anterior crossbite is considered to be a developmental problem, although the genetic influence is difficult to determine. The defect can be misdiagnosed as prognathism. Anterior crossbite may be distinguished because the lower canines and the lower four premolars are in proper occlusion with the upper arcade, and only the lower incisors are lacking proper occlusion (Fig. 1–8). The maxillary incisors generally receive the majority of the trauma, resulting in wearing and blunting of the teeth. If anterior cross-

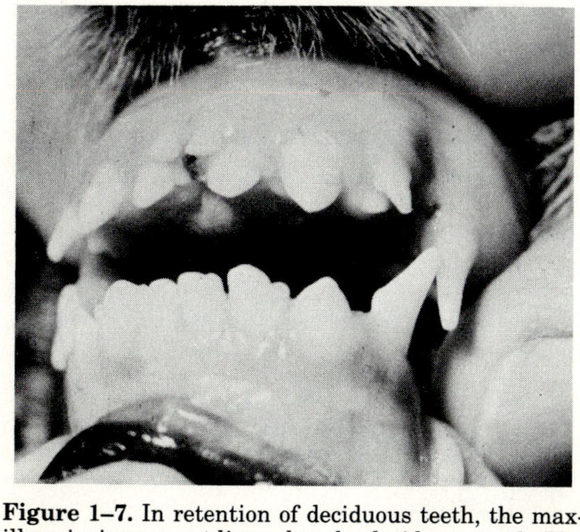

Figure 1–7. In retention of deciduous teeth, the maxillary incisors erupt lingual to the deciduous teeth. The central and lateral deciduous incisors have been retained.

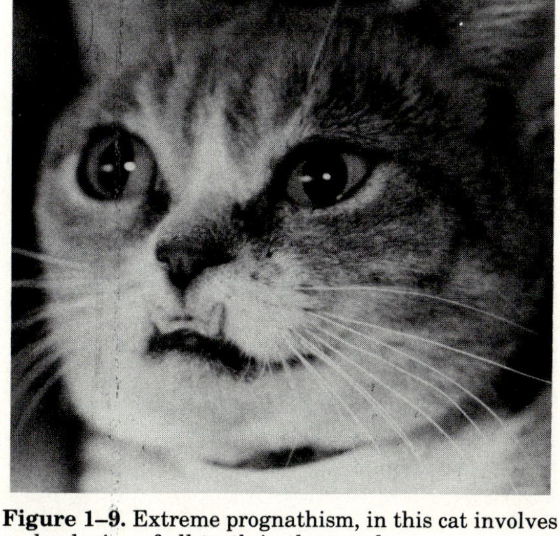

Figure 1–9. Extreme prognathism, in this cat involves malocclusion of all teeth in the arcade.

bite is diagnosed early, orthodontic movement may correct the anomaly.[97]

If the canine teeth interdigitate correctly, terior crossbite is more likely traumatic in origin. If the mandibular canine teeth strongly contact the maxillary lateral incisors or displace the lateral incisor rostrally (anteriorly), then a degree of prognathism exists (Fig. 1–9). If the mandibular third premolar is displaced from the normal position, pointing between the maxillary third and fourth premolars, the problems are more likely genetic rather than traumatic or developmental in origin. Whether a congenital defect is inherited cannot be accurately determined in most cases.

A unique form of prognathism is generally not expressed until the permanent dentition is in place and the animal is 7 to 10 months old. During this particular growth phase, the mandible lengthens more than the maxilla, and the occlusal pattern may be rapidly altered.[97]

Treatment

Orthodontic brackets, which attach directly on the enamel of teeth by use of new dental material, preclude the need for complicated bands and brackets. An increase in the number of pet owners who can afford and will request orthodontic correction of their pets' teeth can be anticipated. Correction of malocclusion in an animal to meet specifications for show or breeding purposes is indicated only if medically warranted or if the problem is obviously acquired. Notification of the American Kennel Club of major orthodonic therapy is indicated in dogs that are used for show and breeding purposes. Careful evaluation of local factors (e.g., retained deciduous teeth, ectopic eruption) and history (e.g., trauma, orthopedic jaw procedures)[22] have to be correlated with physical and radiographic findings in the assessment of malocclusion.

Abnormal Permanent Dentition

Close inspection of the mouth at 9 to 12 months is essential to prevent future problems with permanent teeth. In rotation of the corner incisors that occurs in brachycephalic breeds,[49] these teeth become positioned anterior to the canine teeth and behind the intermediate incisors, which may be lingual to the other incisors. The corner incisors should be extracted to give adequate space to the remaining incisors and to prevent impaction and abscess formation. In brachycephalic breeds, the second and third premolars may be rotated and impacted, and the roots may be exposed on the buccal surface of the tooth. The premolar with the greater impaction should be extracted.

Anodontia, a condition in which one or more teeth are absent, is generally considered to be inheritable, especially if several teeth are absent in one area or the same tooth is absent on both sides of the dental arcade. A deciduous tooth may be present and a permanent replacement tooth missing, but the reverse situation is rare.

Improper germination may lead to splitting of the tooth bud to form two teeth, resulting in rotation or crowding. A unique condition called dens in dente is caused by an enfolding of the enamel, dentin, and pulp within the tooth bud, which exposes the dentin at tooth eruption. Endodontic procedures will generally save the normal portion of the tooth. If endodontic procedures are not performed, abscesses commonly arise.

If the cartilaginous attachment at the mandibular symphysis fails to mature, the central incisors have no supporting alveolar bone. Sequelae to this condition may be periodontal disease, drifting of the incisors, and separation of the mandible. If periodontal disease develops, removal of affected teeth may be necessary to prevent osteomyelitis and destruction of the mandibular symphysis, which would result in a chronic malunion.

MICROBIOLOGY

The mouth supports a concentrated and varied microbiological population, which is distinct from the microbial flora of the nearby areas of the nares, nasopharynx, and oropharynx. In early life, the main focus of bacteria is the dorsum of the tongue. With eruption of the teeth, distinctive biotas begin to colonize on tooth surfaces, about the gingival sulcus, and on the crowns of teeth, forming dental plaque. Dental plaque averages 2×10^{12} bacteria per gram, which is similar to the number in a bacterial colony on solid medium.[104] Accumulation and mineralization of gingival plaques form dental calculi. Within the first days of life, a predominantly streptococcal flora (90%) is established. Other bacteria develop as the an-

Table 1–4. NORMAL CANINE ORAL FLORA*

Aerobic Bacteria	Incidence (%)
Streptococcus	82
Staphylococcus	60
Actinomyces	14
Escherichia coli	22
Corynebacterium	26
Pasteurella	22
Caryophanon	20
Mycoplasma	83
Antinobacter	10
Moraxella	40
Neisseria	20
Enterobacter	2
Bacillus	12

*Reprinted with permission from Saphir DA, Carter GR: Gingival flora of the dog with special reference to bacteria associated with bites. J Clin Microbiol 3:344, 1976.

imal matures. Some species, such as spirochetes and *Bacteroides,* whose habitat is the gingival sulcus, are not present until the eruption of teeth. Some gram-positive organisms may precipitate the formation of dental caries. Though bacteria may invade the oral soft tissue, infection is rarely established because there is local resistance. The oral flora has great potential virulence when introduced into other tissues such as in bite wounds.[102] The gross number of microorganisms and, later, the proportions of certain organisms have an effect on the nature and severity of gingival inflammation.[27, 88, 113, 114]

The indigenous microbial population of the mouth (Table 1–4) is maintained and exogenous organisms are suppressed.[104] Exogenous mouth infections are rare; clinical infections by endogenous organisms occur when one group becomes dominant or in immunosuppressed individuals.

DISEASE OF THE PULP

The pulp can be defined as dental soft tissue that is composed of blood vessels, nerves, and connective tissue (see Fig. 1–1). The pulp supplies nutrients and sensory information to the dentin and has no role in maintaining the stability of the tooth in the alveolar socket. Because the vessels enter through the multiple apical foramina and because the pulp is "walled off" in a mineral shell, infections and trauma rapidly affect the pulp. Damage to the pulp may occur through direct exposure of the pulp to the oral cavity, extension of periodontal disease to the apex of the tooth, or trauma.

Fractures and caries may result in exposure of the pulp to the oral flora. Exposure of the pulp of one or more teeth occurs in 10 per cent of dogs.[49] Necrosis of the pulp, evidenced by a dark discoloration, indicates a chronic condition. Any exposure of the pulp for 12 hours is an indication for endodontic therapy. Brown or tan dentin around exposed pulp indicates that repair of the tooth by the formation of secondary dentin over the receding pulp has occurred. This condition is commonly noted in the canines and incisors of an older dog or a dog with a history of constant wear of the teeth through chewing on foreign objects[49] (Fig. 1–10). These teeth usually remain viable, but the clients should be alerted to watch for color changes or painful prehension. A red or pink color can be interpreted as recent pulp exposure, and pulp death can be anticipated in 6 to 12 months.[99]

Trauma may result in pulpal hemorrhage, as indicated by a pink translucent color of the crown. Pulpal hemorrhage predisposes to pulpal necrosis, and endodontic therapy is indicated to prevent periapical abscesses. Fracture lines in the anterior teeth may be seen coursing in any direction in the enamel. Fractures usually run from rostral to distal on either the labial or lingual tooth surface. The lines may be difficult to see unless observed carefully with reflected light or transillumination. If crown fractures are transverse or oblique with no damage to the alveolus or the pulp cavity, the tooth should be left *in situ.* Longitudinal

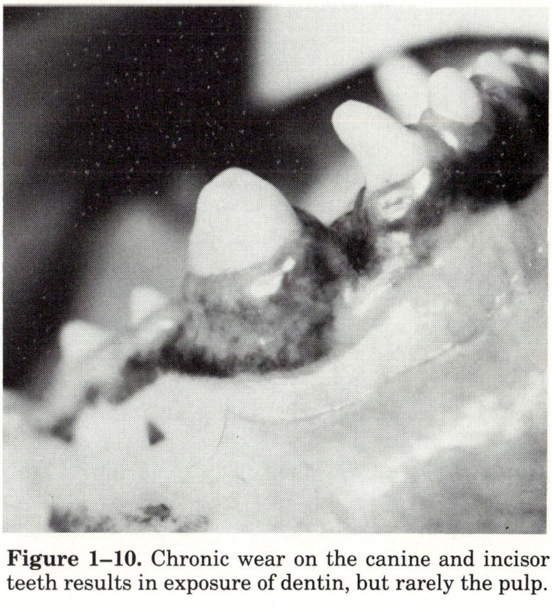

Figure 1–10. Chronic wear on the canine and incisor teeth results in exposure of dentin, but rarely the pulp.

fractures with damage or exposure of the pulp cavity require either repair or extraction. Fractures below the gum line are uncommon except those caused iatrogenically during extraction. Radiography is indicated to determine whether a fracture is present below the gum line or excessive mobility is due to weakening of the periodontal ligaments.

Invasion of apical tissue from periodontal disease is uncommon in the dog and cat, but its occurrence may induce pulpal necrosis. Generally, periapical abscesses are secondary to pulp disease rather than being the inciting pathological factor. When periodontal disease has induced an apical abscess and pulpal necrosis, endodontic therapy or extraction is recommended.[94, 99]

With necrosis of pulp material, bacteria invade the root canal and rapidly spread through the pulp, eventually causing a periapical abscess. Root resorption due to necrosis of the periodontal ligaments and alveolar bone may eventually result in loss of the tooth. Pain may be observed intermittently. As the condition progresses, the dog may hold its head to one side, have altered eating habits, lose weight, and paw at the mouth. Sensitivity is particularly noticeable following eating or drinking. Radiographic signs of a periapical abscess may include distention of the periodontal membrane, sclerosis, cyst formation or radiolucency at the apex, or osteomyelitis. Fistulas occurring with apical abscesses are rare except when associated with the upper fourth premolar.

CARIES

Microbial activity is responsible for the initiation of enamel caries. Cariogenic bacteria of plaque induce acidogenic demineralization of enamel. Thus, soft food diets high in fermentable carbohydrates would seem to predispose the pet to caries. Caries are initiated on enamel surface areas where plaque stagnates and oral microbial flora finds an environment for colonization and metabolism of carbohydrates to form organic acids. These acids demineralize enamel and alter the permeability of deeper structures. Remineralization of enamel is the only natural route of defense (Fig. 1–11).

The frequency of dentin caries is not consistently reported in the dog and cat.[104] Twenty per cent of total teeth lost in the cat can be traced to dental decay, compared with 10 per cent or less in the dog. This finding is contradicted by the failure of experimental models to induce caries[76] and by the low incidence of caries in other reports.[49] Like enamel caries, dentin caries is a plaque-dependent infectious disease. Plaque generates acid, which penetrates and demineralizes the dentin. Proteolytic degeneration of the matrix develops. Progress of caries through dentin is faster than through enamel, and in increased susceptibility in the dog and cat can be expected on exposed root surfaces.[5] Lesions often start at the enamel-cementum junction in the gingival sulcus. The cementum recedes after exposure to the oral environment, leaving the dentin exposed.[104] The dentin has a tubular structure, permitting rapid passage of infection; a higher organic content than enamel, permitting more rapid diffusion of acids; and smaller apatite crystals, allowing faster acid demineralization. A combination of dentinal resorption, lysis, and infection of pulp tissues results in a weak tooth that is susceptible to periapical abscesses, trauma, and fractures at or below the gum line (Fig. 1–12). Rarely can such a tooth be extracted in one piece, and broken roots can remain nidi for osteomyelitis.

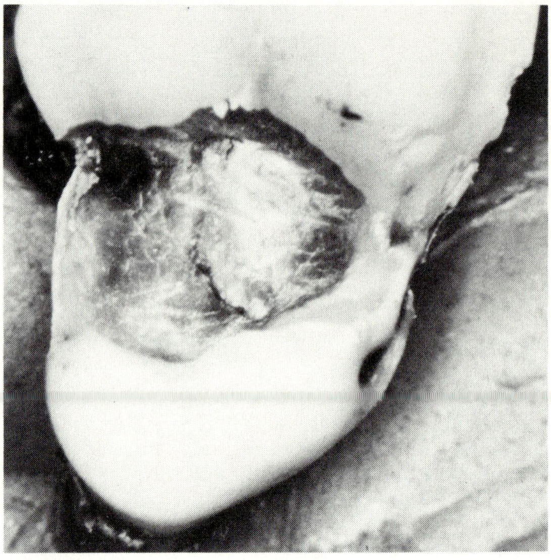

Figure 1–11. Caries are the result of acid demineralization of the tooth by bacterial metabolism of carbohydrates.

Early detection of caries may prevent loss of teeth by permitting restoration.[99] Avoiding introduction of bacteria during restoration at the gingival margin is important. A gingivectomy may be needed to identify the

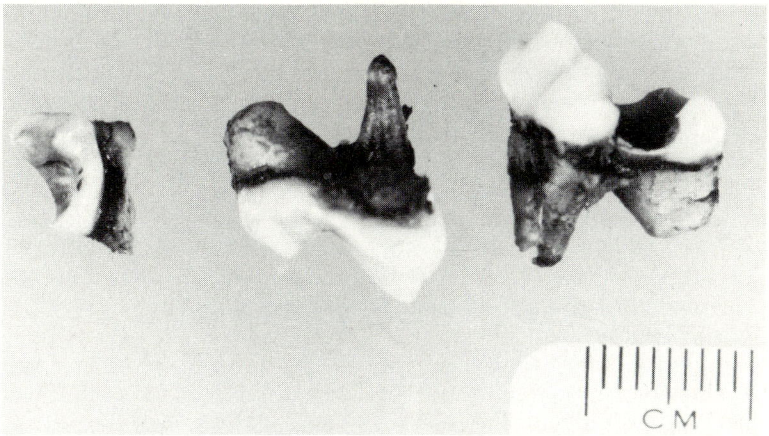

Figure 1–12. Caries result in tooth resorption, lysis, fractures, and abscesses.

caries. If these cavities are located in interproximal areas, the amount of gingival tissue that must be removed makes restoration impractical. If the degree of tooth damage is severe, careful extraction is necessary. Involvement of more than one tooth is common, and the client should be advised of this predisposition. Because of the location of the caries, the patient may be presented with what appears to be simple periodontal disease. In the susceptible animal three to ten teeth can be affected at the same time. A mistaken diagnosis of severe gingivitis with involvement of the periodontal ligaments resulting in loss of teeth is often noted.

Prophylaxis in susceptible animals would include decreasing gingival plaque formation and bacterial concentrations through daily oral hygiene at home, i.e., diet, chewing exercises, cleaning of the teeth, and avoiding soft, high carbohydrate diets.

ENAMEL LESIONS

Enamel hypoplasia from disruption of enamel formation *in utero* or the neonate is usually caused by canine distemper virus.[40] The lesions can be confused with caries. On rare occasions, the enamel hypoplasia will expose dentin, ultimately causing pulpal disease. The defects can be corrected by resin restoration.

The administration of tetracycline during tooth development results in bonding of the drug with calcium in the enamel and dentin.[11] The orange or brown discoloration is permanent. Tetracycline, and presumably the newer generation of tetracycline derivatives, should not be given to a pregnant animal or to neonates less than 6 months of age. Staining of teeth can occur with the use of iron supplements in young dogs and can result in darker teeth. Bleaching with baking soda will correct this discoloration.

Periodontium

THE NORMAL PERIODONTIUM

The periodontium (Fig. 1–13) is composed of four tissues: the gingiva, the periodontal ligament, the cementum, and the alveolar process.

The gingiva is the oral mucous membrane

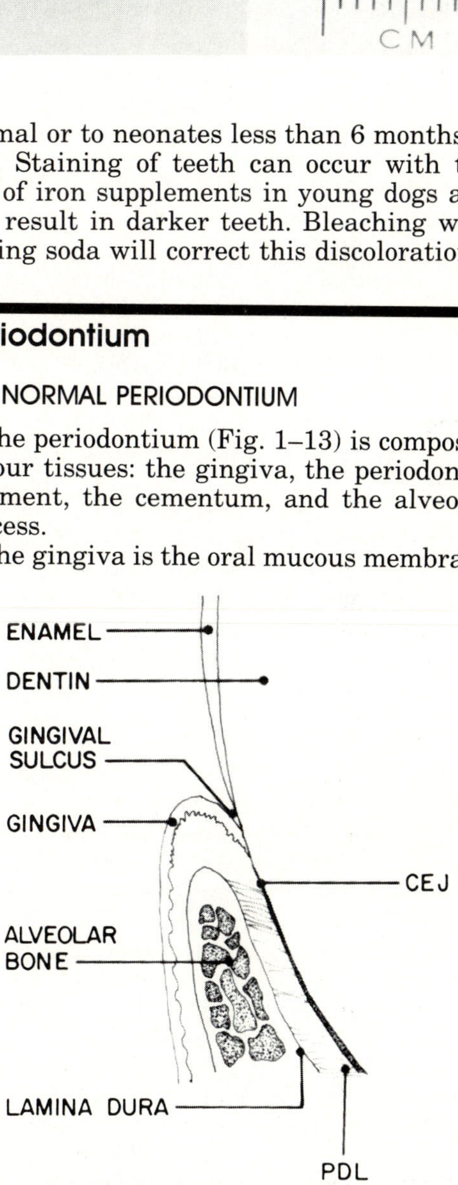

Figure 1–13. A sulcus is formed where the gingiva attaches to the tooth, usually at the cementum-enamel junction (CEJ). The periodontal ligament (PDL) attaches the cementum to the alveolar bone.

and consists of two layers: surface epithelium and lamina propria. The surface epithelium is of stratified squamous type. Only the masticatory mucosa and specialized mucosa of the tongue are keratinized. The lamina propria of the gingiva consists of several fiber groups. The basic function of the gingiva fiber apparatus is to maintain the free gingiva in close approximation to the tooth. The blood supply to the gingiva is derived mainly from the supra-periosteal branches of the lingual and buccinator arteries. The gingival sulcus (approximately 1 to 3 mm) is the area from the epithelial attachment of the gingiva root surface to the top of the gingival margin. The gingival attachment is generally the cementum-enamel junction. The thin edge of the gingiva that lies against the enamel is the important sulcus area where most periodontal disease originates (Fig. 1–13).

The periodontal ligament is the connective tissue that surrounds the root of the tooth, attaches to alveolar bone, and serves as a shock absorber. The ligament is continuous with the connective tissue of the gingiva and communicates with the marrow space of the alveolar bone through the lamina dura. This communication is important in periodontal disease. The periodontal ligament essentially has no elastic fibers; however, part of this ligament is embedded in bone and cementum via Sharpey's fibers. Initially, the attachment between gingiva and tooth is like a basement membrane between the enamel of the erupting tooth and the oral epithelium. The metabolic activity of these fiber bundles is greater on the alveolar bone side than on the cementum bone side, with a greater number of individual fibers and a greater collagen turnover rate being present on the alveolar bone side. The normal periodontal ligament is wider at the cementum-enamel junction and apical areas than at the midroot area. These factors aid in the development of subgingival pockets. Innervation of the periodontal ligament is through unmyelinated sensory fibers whose proprioceptive functions are important for normal mastication. Because of the anatomy and metabolism of the fibers, tension on the periodontal ligament, such as occurs during orthodontic movement, will result in bone apposition, whereas prolonged compression of the periodontal ligaments will result in bone resorption. Changes in the length of the periodontal ligaments occur before osseous changes develop.[104]

The cementum is modified osseous tissue that attaches the periodontal ligament to the dentin of the tooth root. As is common in most osseous structures, cementum has the vital capacity to repair and regenerate. The functions of the cementum can be summarized as (1) attachment of the periodontal ligament fibers to the tooth, (2) compensation by apposition for coronapical loss of tooth length due to occlusal wear, which occurs in animals with continuous eruption, (3) repair of horizontal root fractures, and (4) regulation of the width of the periodontal ligaments relative to alveolar bone. The cementum-enamel junction has not been thoroughly investigated in dogs or cats; however, as is noted in other animals, the cementum and enamel may fail to meet or may overlap in various combinations in some individuals. If the cementum and enamel do not meet, the dentin is exposed to the oral environment at the epithelial attachment of the gingiva. Although the cementum has the ability to repair itself, if it is exposed to the oral cavity recession will be induced and the dentin will be exposed.

The alveolar process is the portion of the maxilla and mandible that forms and supports the sockets containing the teeth. The alveolar process is dependent upon the tooth for its formation and existence. The portion of the alveolar bone that appears radiographically as an opaque line paralleling the tooth is called the lamina dura. Other parts of the alveolar process include the area in which the periodontal ligament fibers are embedded and the supporting alveolar bone, consisting of both cortical compact bone and cancellous bone, which gives strength to the socket. Bone is perhaps the least stable of all of the periodontal tissues, and bone that is resorbed is seldom replaced by osseous tissue. Where bone is covered by vascularized connective tissue, it is extremely sensitive to pressure and tension. As stated previously, because bone is more metabolically active than cementum, pressure on teeth results in bone resorption, and tension on periodontal ligaments results in bone apposition.

LOOSE TEETH

The problem of increased tooth mobility was seen in 75 per cent of dogs studied at random[49] and can be classified in two etiological categories: traumatic and pathological. The fate of a tooth is not totally dependent on its degree of mobility. The incisors, because of their small conical roots, may have some normal mobility. Initially, movement can be due to intra-alveolar changes confined to the socket and is associated with redistribution of the fluids, interstitial contents, and fibers. A secondary stage can involve progressive deformation of the alveolar bone. Therefore, bone loss is not the sole cause of tooth mobility, and the degree of mobility does not necessarily correspond with the amount of bone loss. In the loss of apical periodontal attachments or the absence of severe weakening in them, a correlation can be found between bone loss and tooth mobility but only after more than half of the bone surrounding the tooth has been lost (Fig. 1–14). Therefore, recurrent gingivitis resulting in receding of the gingival margin and bone and exposure of the root is not an absolute indication for the extraction of the tooth. Proper dental hygiene, prevention of occlusal forces, and prevention of excessive mobility would facilitate periodontal ligament reattachment. Local etiological factors of pocket formation and periodontitis are discussed later in this chapter. Careful examination of malpositioned loose teeth is important. Extraction of an improperly aligned tooth may result in decreased mobility, and correction of the pathological condition in the occlusal tooth. Clinically,

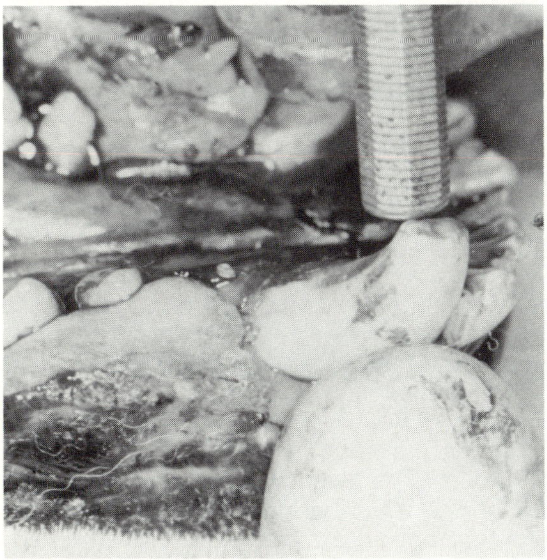

Figure 1–14. Tooth mobility is properly assessed by pressing with an instrument on one side of a tooth and with a finger on the other side.

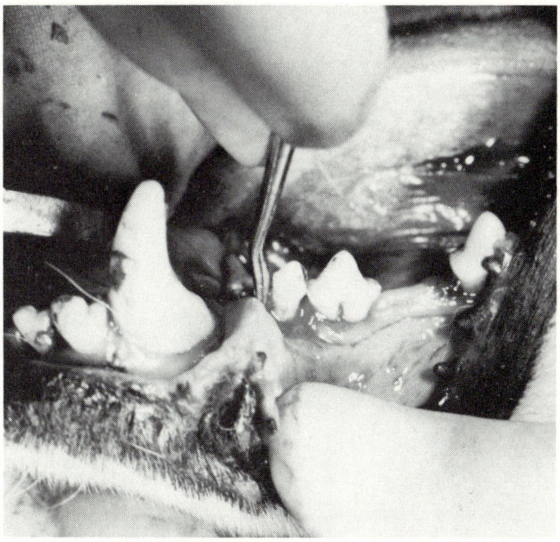

Figure 1–15. Although recession of the gingiva can occur in periodontitis, the tooth mobility is reversible since it was caused by inflammation rather than the loss of supporting alveolar bone.

tooth mobility is most often due to the loss of attachment apparatus as a result of periodontal disease (Fig. 1–15).

In a trauma case in which a tooth has been totally dislodged, immediate replacement of the tooth in the socket is important. A maximum of 30 minutes has been used as a guide in humans. Adequate splinting of the tooth is essential for attachment. Endodontic therapy should be performed before or after most teeth are replaced unless large apical foramina are present to prevent pulpal necrosis. If the periodontal ligaments are devitalized, the tooth may reattach by ankylosis of the alveolar bone and cementum. However, even after successful initial reattachment, the root may be resorbed by osteoclasts from the alveolar bone.

Treatment

Splinting is based on the concept that teeth bound together create a multi-rooted unit that increases the total area of root resistance. Altering the center of rotation provides a greater resistance especially to rostral-distal forces. Temporary measures are beneficial in the acute trauma case when extreme mobility of several teeth is noted. External splints are easy to apply, and a measure as simple as placing a stainless steel wire around the crown of affected teeth or across the arcade is advantageous. Wire extending techniques have included acrylic resins, metal bands attached through brack-

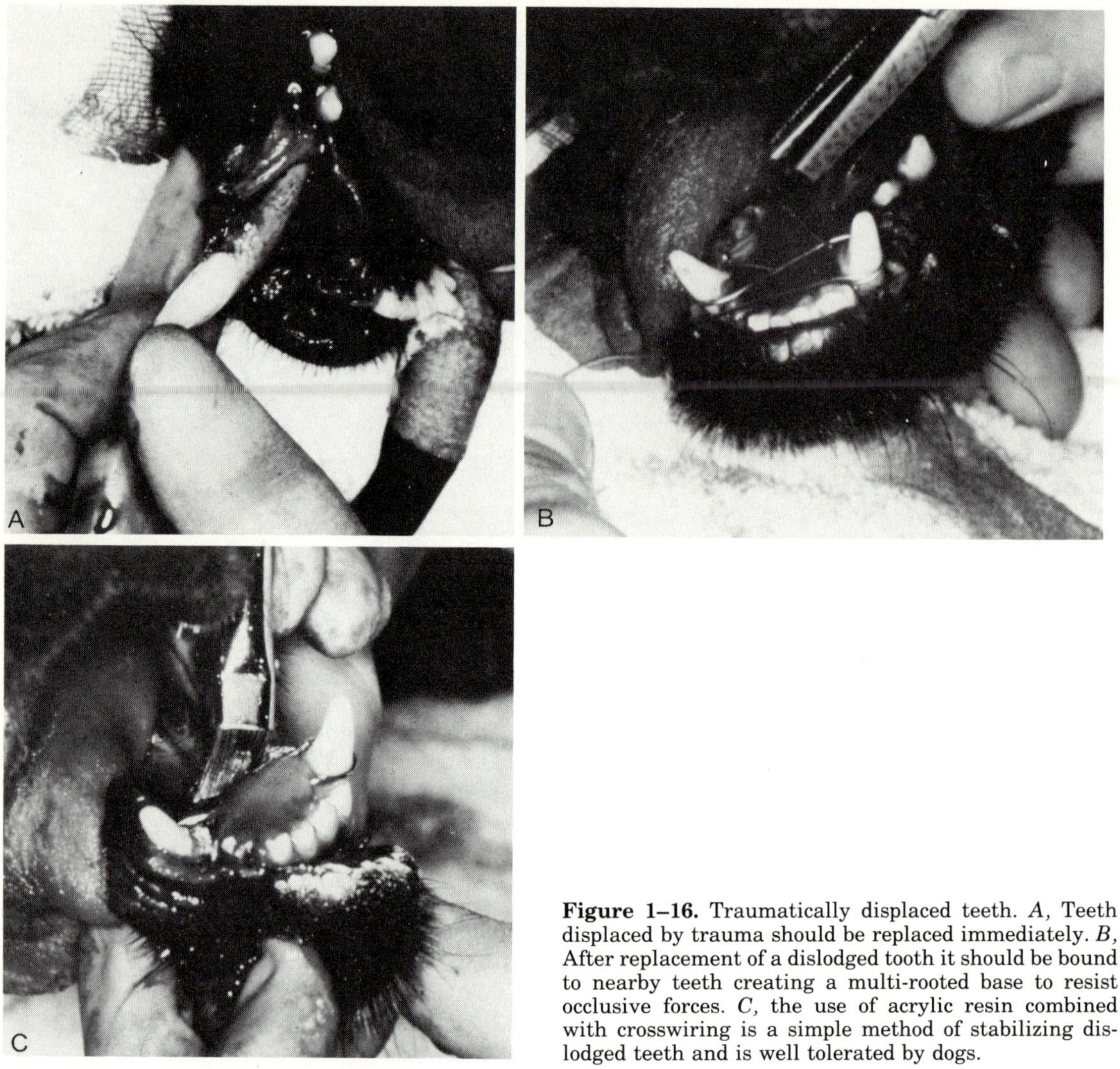

Figure 1–16. Traumatically displaced teeth. *A*, Teeth displaced by trauma should be replaced immediately. *B*, After replacement of a dislodged tooth it should be bound to nearby teeth creating a multi-rooted base to resist occlusive forces. *C*, the use of acrylic resin combined with crosswiring is a simple method of stabilizing dislodged teeth and is well tolerated by dogs.

ets or buttons, and permanent procedures involving wire passed through amalgam-filled holes in the teeth. The wide variety of composites (mixed pastes, mixed powders and liquids, and ultraviolet light–activated pastes) have made bonding and splinting available and easy for veterinarians. Although the length of time necessary for reattachment is variable, after gingival flap surgery in humans, 10 to 14 days are needed before initial reattachment occurs.[104] Full maturation of collagen and complete renewal of gingival reattachment may take a minimum of 5 to 6 weeks. Devices applied too tightly or malaligned may cause excessive mobility after splints are removed. In trauma cases involving the canines or incisors, a period of 3 weeks before removal seems to be adequate (Fig. 1–16).

PERIODONTAL DISEASE

Periodontal disease is the most common problem of the oral cavity. Since the gingiva, periodontal ligament, and alveolar bone can be involved, diseases include gingivitis, periodontitis, periapical abscesses, and osteomyelitis.[46, 49, 53, 64] Although gingivitis is the most common form of periodontal disease, one study found loss of bone (periodontitis) in 53 per cent of dogs and 14 per cent of cats.[49]

The clinical syndromes seem to be a progression of the same process, and the severity of the lesion is often not recognized on the basis of clinical findings. Although the amount of plaque and calculus often correlates with the severity, this relationship is not absolute.[46, 49] Genetic predisposition (e.g., poodles have a higher incidence of the disease) and soft diets appear to be the most consistent positive correlations to periodontal disease.[42, 43, 49, 103]

Chronic nonresponsive gingivitis in cats may be caused by feline leukemia virus and upper respiratory viruses.[81] Cats with chronic gingivitis or stomatitis should always be tested for feline leukemia virus. Chronic gingivitis has been seen in purebred cats, suggesting an inheritable pattern.[38, 47] Gingival hypertrophy has been experimentally induced in cats by the administration of phenytoin.[84]

Since periodontal disease is common, the periodontium should receive a thorough examination. The signs most predictive of periodontal disease include (1) Color changes; (2) Swelling, enlargement or cratering of the marginal and papillary gingivae; (3) Bleeding on gentle probing; and (4) Periodontal pockets (Fig. 1–17). Of the more predictive signs, the first two can be detected visually. A probe can be used to check for the latter two signs. Probing of the rostral surface of the teeth and the interproximal areas usually reveals the most severe disease.

Less predictive signs, including recession of gingival margins, tooth mobility, and bone loss, may be related to other diseases or may follow resolution of periodontal disease.

Dental deposits can be classified as plaque, supragingival calculus, and subgingival calculus. Plaque is a concentrated bacterial aggregation that is lightly adherent and constantly growing. Composed mostly of bacteria, the plaque induces gingival changes that are initially reversible (gingivitis). As new plaque forms, gram-positive cocci are overgrown by the gram-negative

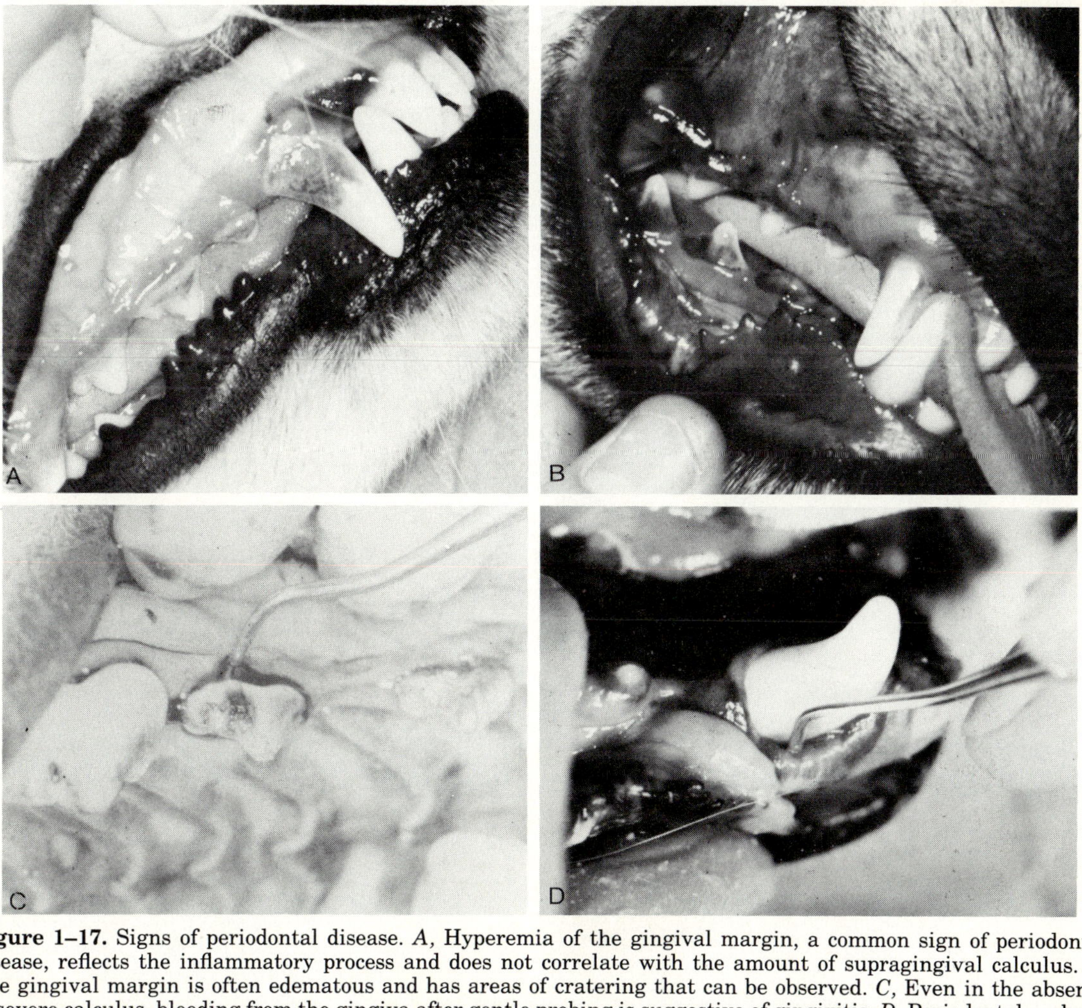

Figure 1–17. Signs of periodontal disease. *A*, Hyperemia of the gingival margin, a common sign of periodontal disease, reflects the inflammatory process and does not correlate with the amount of supragingival calculus. *B*, The gingival margin is often edematous and has areas of cratering that can be observed. *C*, Even in the absence of severe calculus, bleeding from the gingiva after gentle probing is suggestive of gingivitis. *D*, Periodontal pockets, which are more common in humans than dogs and cats, are deep sulci in which the normal gingival-tooth attachments have been destroyed.

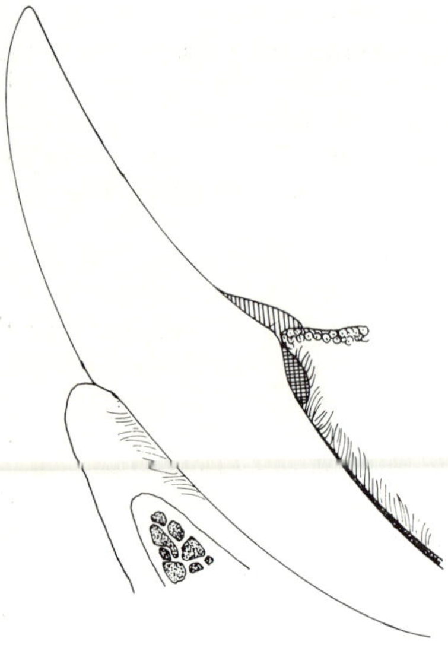

Figure 1–18. Calculi can be either supragingival (above the gum) or subgingival (below the gingival margin in the sulcus).

flora. The predominating organisms in the dog are gram-negative anaerobes. Calculus is mineralized plaque. Supragingival calculi are usually creamy white or yellow and can be stained. Subgingival calculi are formed in the gingival sulcus and are hard. Because the pathogenic potential of plaque lies in the organism and not mechanical irritation, the beneficial effects of simple mechanical removal of calculus are temporary (Fig. 1–18).

Etiology

The initial inflammation may be related to the increase in bacterial numbers rather than a change in bacterial flora.[120] As the bacteria proliferate, the metabolic products increase, exposing the connective tissue to antigens (Fig. 1–19). The subgingival bacterial population can change in 2 weeks as motile, gram-negative, rod-shaped, anaerobic organisms predominate.[51, 113, 114, 120] There is a higher proportion of gram-positive bacteria supragingivally than subgingivally.[51] Beagles with gingivitis and periodontitis had supragingival and subgingival plaque caused primarily by anaerobes.[113, 114] The gram-negative organisms *Fusobacterium nucleatum* and *Bacteroides melaninogenicus asaccharolyticus* predominate.[113] The latter organism was found more commonly in the plaque of dogs with periodontitis than of those with gingivitis and may influence the course of the inflammation. Dogs with more

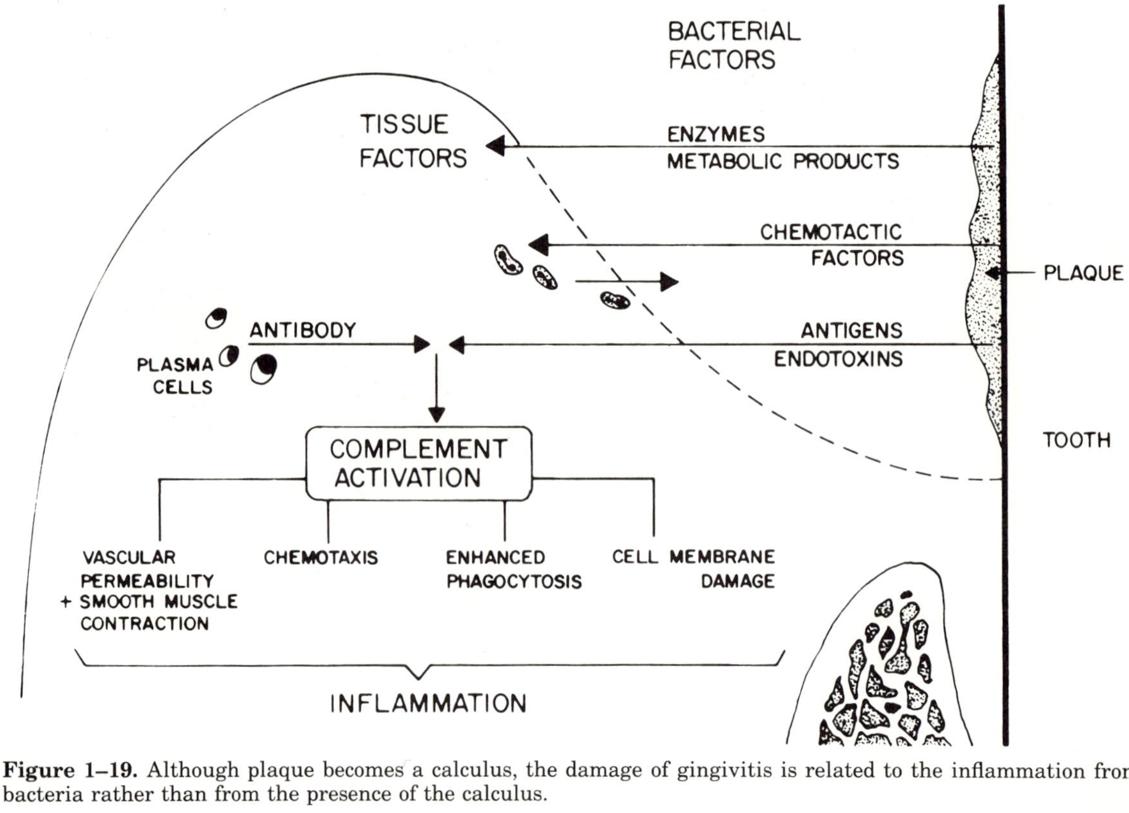

Figure 1–19. Although plaque becomes a calculus, the damage of gingivitis is related to the inflammation from bacteria rather than from the presence of the calculus.

severe disease (periodontitis) have a higher proportion of gram-negative bacteria in the subgingival areas than do dogs with gingivitis. Actinomyces is more common in plaque of dogs with periodontitis than with gingivitis.

The insult results in vasculitis of the marginal gingiva, transudation of fluid, and migration of neutrophils into the gingival sulcus. As gingivitis progresses, lymphocytes, macrophages and, especially, plasma cells infiltrate. In the dog, periodontitis is the sequela to gingivitis and results in ulceration of the subgingival epithelium, degradation of the collagen of the periodontal gingiva, and resorption of marginal alveolar bone. The pattern of bone resorption follows the vascular pathways through the alveolar bone. As the inflammation continues, the predominant infiltrates are lymphocytes, plasma cells, and neutrophils, and partial resorption of the root may occur.[21, 53, 54, 64, 77, 83, 85, 87, 88, 110] The resultant destruction of supporting tissues, compounded by inappropriate repair of connective tissue and bone, causes apical migration of the epithelial attachments,[51] the formation of gingival pockets, and mobility of teeth.

The body's attempt to eliminate the infection, and even the tooth if necessary, is mediated primarily by neutrophils responding to chemotactic factors, which are produced by both the host and the bacteria. The neutrophils line the gingival sulcus, forming a barrier between the subgingival bacteria and the gingiva.[51] Thus, the gingiva becomes a battleground where both the host and bacteria are damaged by the neutrophils. The argument for the protective role of neutrophils is reinforced by the theory that some subgingival bacteria can impair neutrophil function and by the high incidence of gingivitis in hosts with diseases that affect neutrophilic function (e.g., cyclic neutropenia, granulocytopenia, diabetes mellitus, Down's syndrome, and periodontosis).[51, 88]

Although IgA probably regulates normal bacterial colonization, B-cells and plasma cells are more numerous in severe periodontitis; antibody production is polyclonal and is not specific for subgingival bacterial antigens. In localized human periodontitis, some hosts have specific antibody titers to subgingival bacteria.[88] Thus, in severe disease with lymphocyte mitogenic transformation, the non-specific response includes the production of lymphokines, which with neutrophils may play the major role in immunological tissue destruction.[88] Lymphotoxins may be chemotactic for neutrophils and toxic to fibroblasts and may enhance osteoclast-mediated bone resorption.[55, 88]

Clinical Course

Subclinical or minor clinical periodontal disease can occur over a 3 to 5 year period before the onset of obvious signs. The first signs usually are unnoticed by the owner, and by the time they are observed, irreparable damage may have occurred. A change in eating habits or halitosis may be noticed first. Inflammation of the gingival margins, calculus, increased areas of food entrapment, and minor changes in the gingival contour precede the stages of purulent infection, gum recession, pyorrhea, loose teeth, pain with chewing, depression, and weight loss. Because the disease progresses slowly in the final stages, the owner may associate the depression and weight loss with old age.

The progression of periodontal disease in young dogs is primarily characterized by gingivitis, whereas in older dogs, bone loss is the common sequela. Bone loss primarily occurs on the buccal surface of the arcade rather than interdentally as in humans. The loss on the buccal surface results in the early involvement of the bifurcation and trifurcation areas of multirooted teeth (Fig. 1–20). These changes occur earlier in the maxilla than in the mandible. The histopathologic signs of canine periodontal disease are similar to those described for human periodontal disease and the beagle is a suitable model for a study of periodontal disease.[64] Normally, a few scattered cells—primarily plasma cells and leuko-

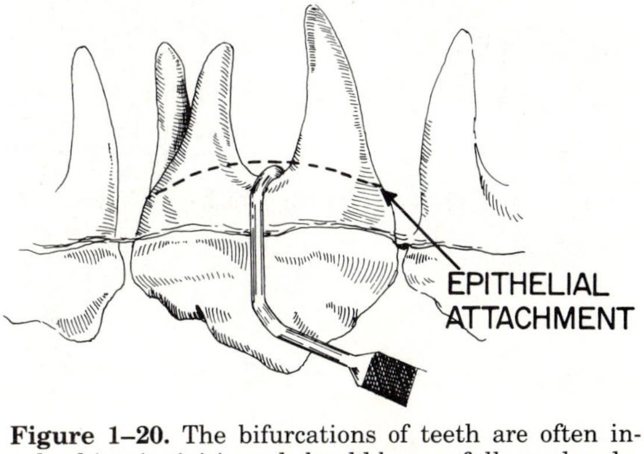

Figure 1–20. The bifurcations of teeth are often involved in gingivitis and should be carefully explored.

cytes—can be observed beneath the sulcular and junctional epithelium. With the presence of periodontal disease, the population of inflammatory cells greatly increases. Plasma cells, a few small lymphocytes, and large numbers of leukocytes are found within the sulcular epithelium, the coronal part of the junctional epithelium, and the gingival crevice. Proliferative response by the junctional epithelium causes the formation of rete ridges into the underlying connective tissue. The migration and accumulation of polymorphonuclear leukocytes into the crevice are the result of chemotactic factors released from bacterial deposits on the tooth surface.

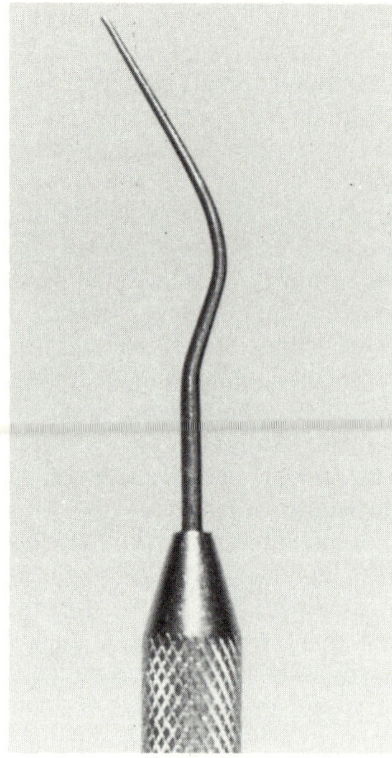

Figure 1–22. The dental probe is used for examination and measurement of the gingival sulcus.

Gross Stages of Gingivitis

There are six gross stages of gingivitis (1) insult caused by plaque, (2) hyperemia of capillaries, (3) inflammatory response (exudation), (4) destruction of irritant, (5) limitation of inflammation and proliferation of connective tissue, and (6) repair.

The enlarged gingiva can be edematous, because of hypertrophy and proliferation in the acute stages, or fibrotic, because of hyperplasia in the chronic stages. The area most likely to be inflamed, the margins and papillae, should be compared to the rest of the attached gingiva in order to judge color changes. Hyperplasia, interproximal cratering, and retraction of gingival margins are chronic morphological changes. In the "breakdown" phase of inflammation, the tissues are engorged with fluid, soft, edematous, and non-resilient. An instrument, such as a probe, pressed slightly against the tissue and then removed leaves a momentary indentation or pit. In fibrosis, the gingiva has a firm, leathery consistency (Fig. 1–21).

In the careful examination of chronic gingivitis the best instrument for detecting the presence or absence of periodontal pockets is the probe (Fig. 1–22). The bifurcations should be carefully explored. Persistent in-

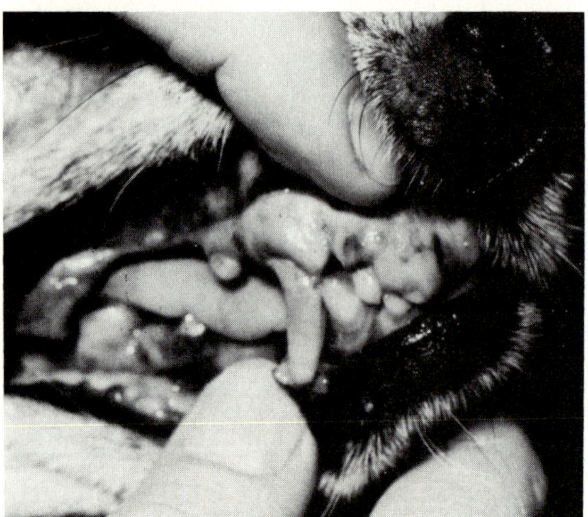

Figure 1–21. Chronic periodontal disease results in retraction and fibrosis of the gingiva, loss of alveolar bone, and a "long of tooth" appearance.

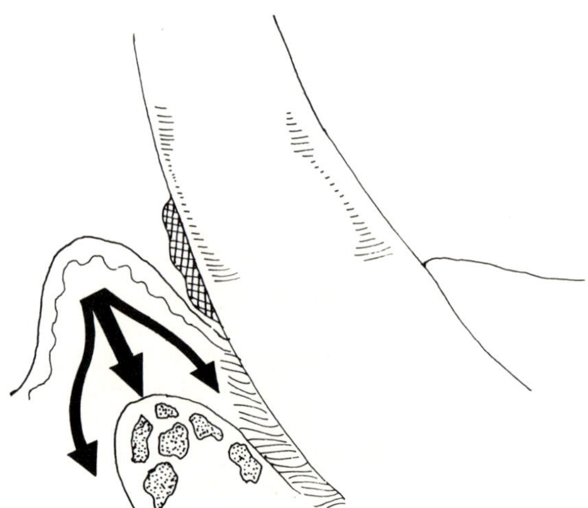

Figure 1–23. In chronic periodontitis, inflammation may involve the periodontal ligament, the alveolar bone, or the attached gingiva.

flammation at the gingival margin and loss of the attachment apparatus cause a deepening of the sulcus, producing a periodontal pocket (Fig. 1–23). As the pocket deepens, the supporting structures are lost. The pocket and periodontitis are, thus, the *sine qua non* of periodontal disease. Identification and elimination of the periodontal pocket will help preclude tooth mobility and premature loss of teeth.

Even though pocket depth is recorded as the distance from the marginal gingiva to the base of the pocket, the more important consideration is the gingival recession plus pocket depth, i.e., the distance from the cementum-enamel junction to the bottom of the sulcus. A periodontal probe should be of small diameter so that it can penetrate the depth of the sulcus. Only mild sedation may be necessary for examination. The probe (see Fig. 1–22) should be calibrated for measurement for future reference; this type of probe is available in a double-ended combination with other instruments. Usually, the probe can be inserted into the pocket. However, calculus may block the probe and feel hard. The pocket bottom is soft tissue, not bone. The force used in probing should be similar to that which would produce blanching when pressing the probe against the back of a finger. Interproximal areas are important regions to probe. Sulcular bleeding in response to gentle probing is one of the most reliable indications of periodontal inflammation (see Fig. 1–17*C*). If neither pockets nor bleeding is evident, even in the presence of calculi, significant inflammation is probably not present.

Therapy

Since bacteria are the primary cause of periodontal disease, scaling and polishing are the initial steps in the treatment of gingivitis. The readily visible supragingival calculus can be removed either by hand scaling or by using an ultrasonic instrument. Improper cleaning can induce more damage than the disease. Because of the vibration, the heat of the instrument, and the size of its cleaning tip, ultrasonic instrument is not recommended to remove subgingival calculus. Although supragingival calculus is most noticeable, the subgingival calculus is more important to the health of the patient. Subgingival calculus can be located in three ways.

1. Drying the tissue and directing a stream of air into the sulcus will retract the gingival tissue away from the tooth and will provide the examiner with direct vision of the subgingival tissues.
2. Passing an explorer or the working end of a scaler vertically and subgingivally along the root surface will allow the examiner to feel the irregular calculus.
3. Examining the marginal surface of the gingiva often will permit the examiner to see the localized edematous areas or the darkening caused by subgingival calculus.

Clinical Technique for Scaling. The scaler is primarily used to remove supragingival calculus. The scaler is effective in removal of subgingival calculus but a curette is often more efficient. The curette is a sharp instrument that can remove calculus and plane exposed root surfaces. The removal of subgingival calculus depends largely on the examiner's sense of touch. Scalers and curettes *must be sharpened frequently*.

With ultrasonic cleaning instruments, vibration disrupts the attachment of calculus to the tooth. A shower of bacteria will be produced, and the operator should always wear a surgical mask to prevent inhalation of bacteria (Fig. 1–24). Although ultrasonic scaling has become widely accepted, care must be taken when using the instrument because of the possibility of burning gingi-

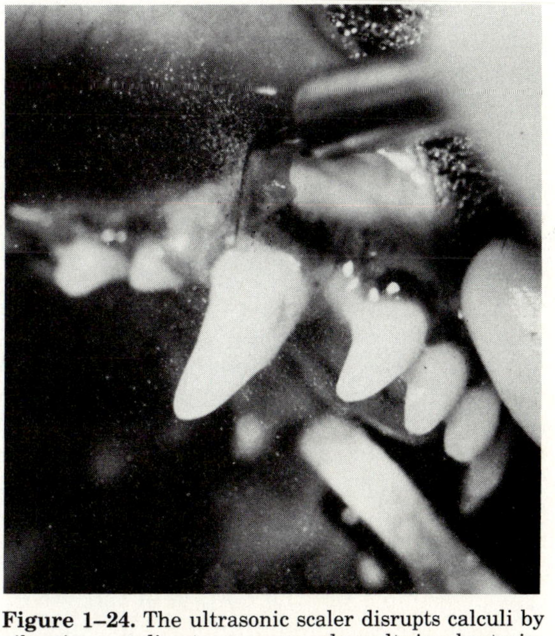

Figure 1–24. The ultrasonic scaler disrupts calculi by vibration, not direct pressure, and results in a bacteria-laden mist.

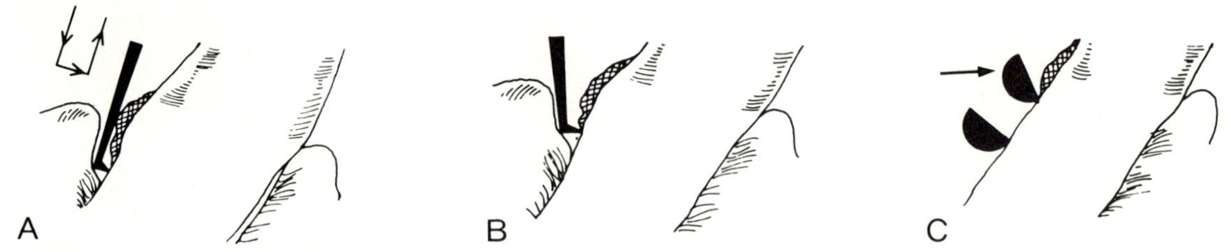

Figure 1–25. *A,* A scaling instrument should be inserted into the sulcus to the apical limit, then a coronal movement should be used to remove calculi. *B,* The root should not be gouged unnecessarily. *C,* The cutting plane of a curette is incorrectly applied in the upper example *(arrow)*, but is correctly applied in lower example.

val tissue, etching the enamel, and irritating the pulp tissue with heat. Many ultrasonic instruments vibrate at 25,000 to 28,000 cycles per second, and a lack of water for 1 to 2 seconds produces damaging heat. Less than one gram of force should be applied to the tooth, since the vibration and not the amount of force loosens the calculus. Ultrasonic units are not effective in removing stains, and they leave a rough surface that will encourage new plaque formation within 24 hours if it is not planed.[33]

Subgingival calculus must be removed carefully and thoroughly. The use of the ultrasonic unit is not recommended below the gingival margin unless extreme care and respect for tissues are maintained. Instrument vibration makes tactile sensation extremely limited; therefore injury from overzealous pressure applied to sensitive tissue is a common sequela. Although supragingival calculi are often the primary complaint of the owner, the most important step of the cleaning operation for the animal's health is removing subgingival calculus. The normal depth of the gingival sulcus, which is determined by the dental probe, is approximately 1 to 3 mm. Inflammation and edema of the gingival crest may swell the gingival tissues and cause the appearance of a deepened gingival sulcus without the actual recession of the underlying periodontal ligaments and subgingival tissues. Dental pockets may appear at the bifurcation of the tooth roots; therefore careful probing of this area is necessary. Although bacterial plaque may extend to the bottom of the subgingival sulcus, it is unusual for the calculus to develop at the very bottom of the sulcus (see Figs. 1–18 and 1–23). Therefore, once the probe or scaler has found the depth of the sulcus, most of the movements with the instruments are in a gingival direction from the bottom of the sulcus. The area of the cementum-enamel junction normally has a rough texture, and a slight bulge may be felt even if this area is free from calculus. When the depth of the gingival sulcus has been reached, the use of a pulling motion with the instrument held at a 40° to 25° angle to the tooth is advocated. Repeated pulling strokes will pull the calculus out of the gingival sulcus (Fig. 1–25). Because of the ease with which a sharp instrument may damage the gingiva at the depth of the sulcus, pushing strokes are not recommended. Sharp instruments are essential; use of dull instruments are a waste of time, traumatic to the patient, and a source of frustration for the operator. When a deep periodontal pocket has been identified and removal of the calculus has been performed, the root of the tooth must be smoothed. Small curettes are the best instruments for

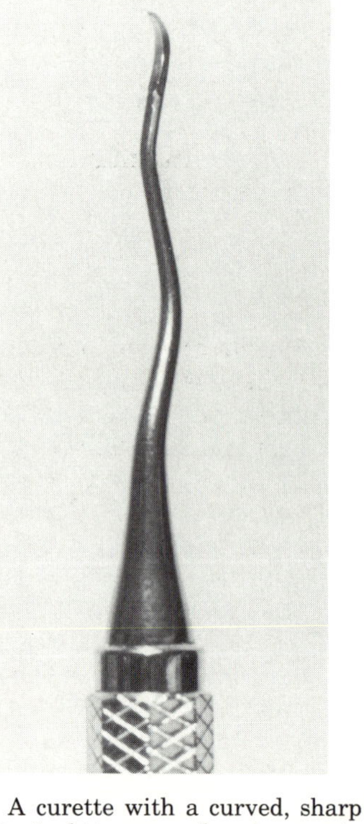

Figure 1–26. A curette with a curved, sharp hook is ideal for subgingival tissues and root cementum.

root planing and débridement of soft tissue (Fig. 1–26). By moving the instrument in various directions, the operator smoothes the root cementum and eliminates small indentations from the scaling (see Fig. 1–25). By directing the cutting edges of the curette toward the soft tissue, the operator removes the damaged epithelial lining of

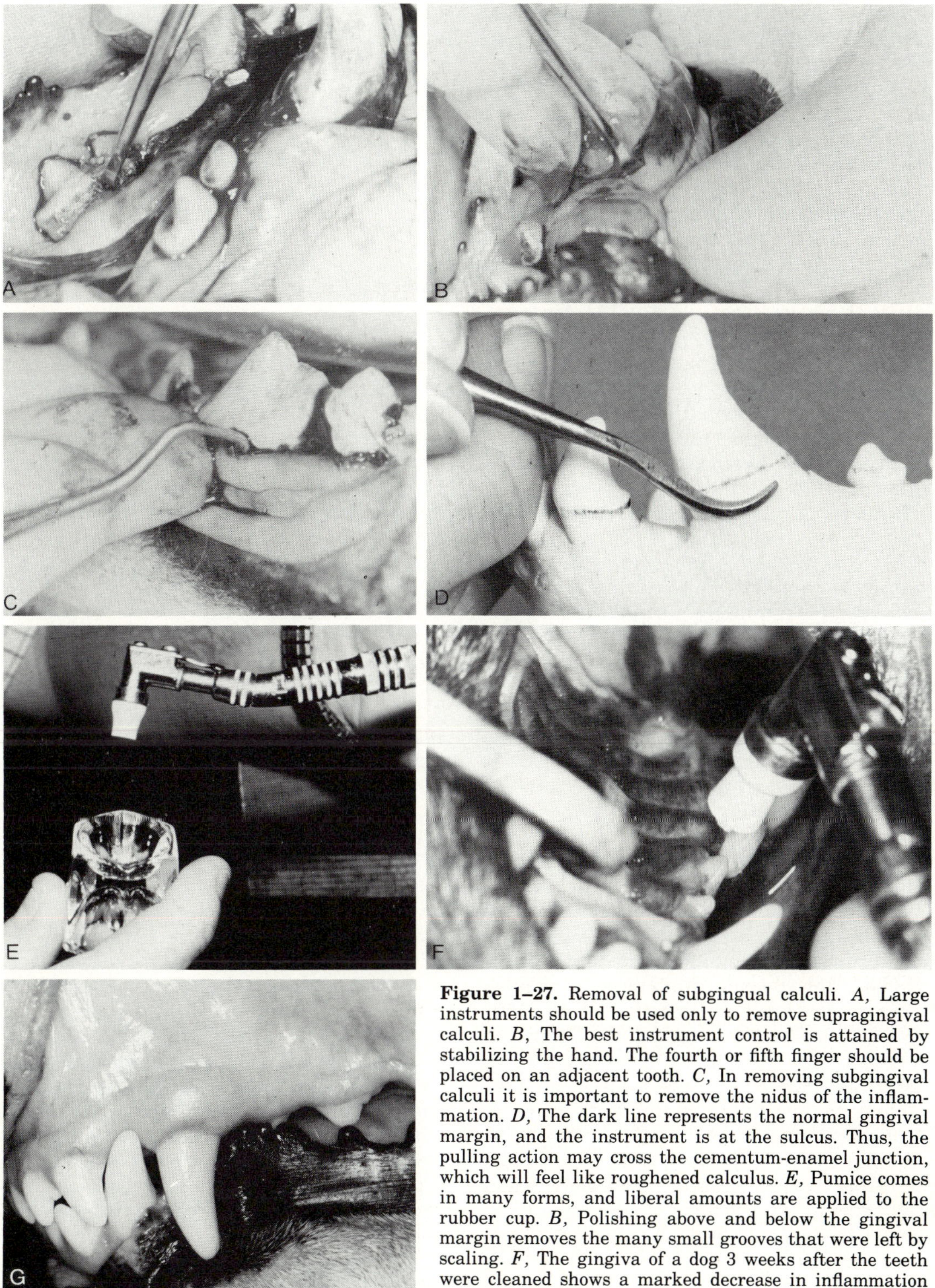

Figure 1–27. Removal of subgingual calculi. *A,* Large instruments should be used only to remove supragingival calculi. *B,* The best instrument control is attained by stabilizing the hand. The fourth or fifth finger should be placed on an adjacent tooth. *C,* In removing subgingival calculi it is important to remove the nidus of the inflammation. *D,* The dark line represents the normal gingival margin, and the instrument is at the sulcus. Thus, the pulling action may cross the cementum-enamel junction, which will feel like roughened calculus. *E,* Pumice comes in many forms, and liberal amounts are applied to the rubber cup. *B,* Polishing above and below the gingival margin removes the many small grooves that were left by scaling. *F,* The gingiva of a dog 3 weeks after the teeth were cleaned shows a marked decrease in inflammation (See Fig. 1–17B.)

the pocket, inducing re-epithelialization. If the pocket appears to be suprabony or intrabony in nature, more extensive curettage is necessary for re-epithelialization to be successful. Simply scaling supragingival calculus does both the patient and client an injustice (Fig. 1–27; see Fig. 1–19).

After all teeth have been scaled, the remaining plaque should be removed by polishing. Rubber cups or brushes can be used with a dental handpiece or a small, variable-speed hand drill, which is commercially available in hobby shops. The pumice should be mixed with water into a fine consistency (see Fig. 1–27*D*). In the dog and cat, medium-grit pumice is usually adequate. The rubber cups will flatten out when placed against the tooth (see Fig. 1–27*E*). By running the drill at slow rate and carefully directing the rubber cup, the surface of the tooth beneath the gingival margin and the crown can be polished. Proper elimination of subgingival plaques and calculus is essential to decrease the loss of gingiva, periodontal ligament, and alveolar bone.[33]

After proper scaling, tissue repair occurs in the following sequence: (1) epithelial migration, 1 to 2 days; (2) epithelial coverage, 4 days; (3) complete epithelial coverage, 6 to 10 days; (4) clinically normal gingiva, 10 days; and (5) complete repair, 14 to 21 days (see Fig. 1–27*F*). However, if substantial bony defects are present, epithelial regeneration outgrows bone repair, and bony defects are replaced by epithelial tissue.

Surgical Correction. If the gingival tissue does not return to normal after careful scaling and polishing, surgical removal of periodontal pockets and gingivectomy are indicated.[55] Removal of this soft tissue wall reduces the amount of food and bacteria that is held in contact with the periodontium. A periodontal probe will measure the pocket depth before gingivectomy. The depth of the periodontium pocket increases normally with age. The gingival incision is at a 45° angle away from the tooth. The point of interest is the bottom of the pocket (Fig. 1–28). All exposed root is planed smooth, and four to five applications of tincture of benzoin and myrrh are used for protection of the cut surface. Although the use of electrocutting surgery units reduces hemorrhage during gingivectomy, electrocautery is not considered a necessity, and improper use of the unit may damage other adjacent tissue. Following gingivectomy, the dog

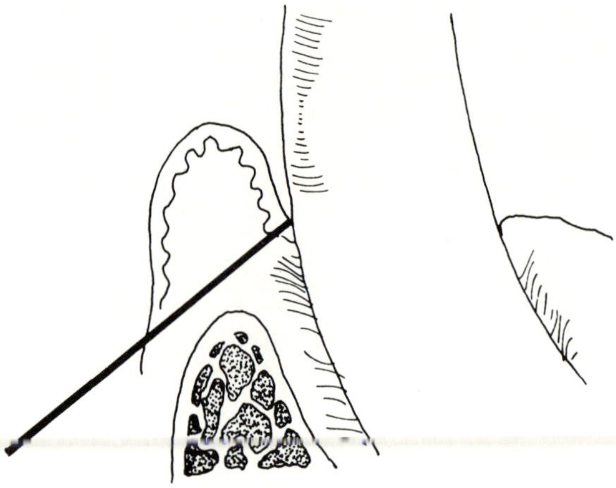

Figure 1–28. A gingivectomy is used to decrease the depth of the sulcus.

should return to normal eating habits within a few days, with total healing in 2 to 4 weeks. The client should be warned that this procedure is very unattractive but is necessary to prevent future loss of teeth. Owing to the nature of periodontal disease, many teeth are frequently involved, and large areas of gingiva are removed.

A mandibular frenulectomy may be performed when the frenulum enhances development of periodontal disease around the mandibular canine teeth. A flaccid frenulum may cause increased food entrapment and may make cleaning the area more difficult. The procedure involves removal of the frenulum on the buccal surface of the mandible. Antibiotics and soft diet are required for 5 days postoperatively.

Complications

For 15 to 20 minutes after eating, scaling, or extraction, oral bacteria can be cultured from the peripheral blood of dogs with periodontal disease.[13] Obviously, oral pathogens and toxic products have access to the systemic circulation; in the normal animal, the septicemias are transient.[108] A correlation has been found between periodontal disease and bacterial endocarditis in humans and some laboratory animals and has been suggested in the dog.[123] Digestive and urinary complications have also been incriminated,[100] but controlled studies have failed to show definite correlation between periodontal disease and organ malfunction.

The use of antibiotics in periodontal therapy is a well-established clinical practice.

Because of the vascularity and inflammation commonly encountered, bactericidal antibiotics are usually indicated, and initiation of therapy 12 hours preoperatively is recommended. The frequency of bacteremia after dental procedures would discourage combining dental and complicated surgical procedures. Topical antibiotics for periodontal disease are of questionable efficacy. Cautery agents and teeth whiteners, usually acidic compounds, may damage the gingiva.

Prevention

In addition to bacteria, several other factors predispose to periodontal disease. Incorrect and abusive procedures including careless technique in hand scaling, ultrasonic scaling, and home oral hygiene may cause early separation of the periodontal ligament. After such procedures, a temporary improvement is often followed by rapid exacerbation of the condition. Heredity influences gingival morphology, tooth formation, tooth placement, and individual resistance to bacteria.[19, 21, 33, 51, 78, 103] When beagles were maintained under identical conditions and diets, the severity of the periodontal condition varied considerably.[64] Confinement, stress, malnutrition, and soft foods add to the problem. Dogs with food constantly available are more likely to have problems because periodontal repair is delayed.[19, 42, 43]

Successful therapy depends on regular and thorough home care; without it, relief is brief despite the efforts of the veterinarian.[105] The use of chemicals such as hydrogen peroxide and baking soda is of questionable efficacy and may be detrimental if the substances are subsequently swallowed regularly. Chlorhexidine gluconate* applied to the teeth and gingiva aids in the treatment of gingivitis,[79] but the results are transient; gingivitis returns after the drug is discontinued, and staining of the teeth can occur.[61] The use of systemic antibiotics may be beneficial in severe periodontitis. In chronic unresponsive periodontitis, metronidazole† (30 mg/kg orally, once a day for 5 to 7 days) may be successful.[60]

Daily brushing of an affected dog's teeth is extremely important.[33, 100] A short, small toothbrush is most effective. All plaque material should be removed from the teeth and the surrounding tissues. Areas of special interest would be the interproximal areas of the teeth, exposed roots in the area of the bifurcation of molars, and the deep gingival sulcus of the canine teeth. In addition to removing debris, this procedure stimulates blood circulation, augmenting the formation of gingival attachments. Non-detergent toothpaste should be used. Most tooth pastes used by humans are not recommended because they have a detergent base. It has been determined experimentally that bacterial plaque not removed once every 48 hours is calcified into hard deposits that cannot be removed by brushing.[35] Most dogs will tolerate brushing after a period of familiarization (2 weeks), but if they will not, cleaning of debris from the tooth surfaces with a soft rag is helpful. In this procedure, emphasis should be placed on the gingival margins.

Demonstration of proper technique is required if a veterinarian expects the client to utilize this procedure. The simple statement that the dog's teeth should be brushed will not sufficiently motivate the client. The brushing technique is essentially the same as the proper technique for humans. The easiest way to reach the molar area is by holding the brush at a 75° angle while cleaning the inside and outside surfaces of these teeth. The anterior arcade is best cleaned by using circular brush strokes with emphasis placed at the gingival margin. Dog biscuits, vinyl chew toys, and dry dog foods exercise the teeth and gums and have been advocated as aids in reducing plaque formation. Although oral hygiene may decrease supragingival calculi formation on the exposed root tooth surface, in the predisposed dog it may not prevent formation of bacterial plaque and calculus in the gingival sulcus. Chewing exercises stimulate the flow of alkaline salivary secretions, which may neutralize some of the acid-producing capacity of the bacteria. Since the carbohydrate content of the diet is considered to limit the number and distribution of oral bacteria, carbohydrate-containing substances and especially sweet snacks should be avoided in the predisposed animal. Mouth washes and breath cleaners are of questionable effectiveness in decreasing bacterial concentration. Most dogs will not tolerate the foaming sensation these products cause,

*Hibiclens, Stuart Pharmaceuticals, Wilmington, DE.

†Flagyl Tablets, Searle Laboratories, Chicago, IL. Metronidazole Oral Tablets, Henry Schein, Inc., Port Washington, NY.

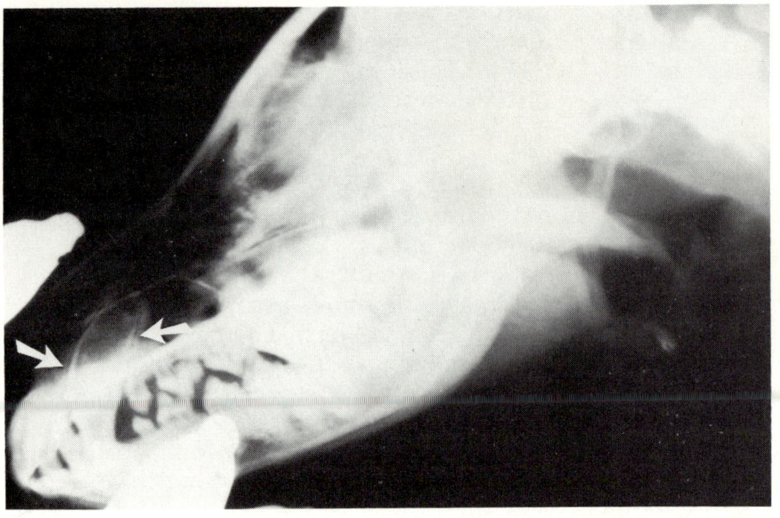

Figure 1–29. A periapical abscess may cause tooth lysis without manifesting clinical signs. The arrows are at the lamina dura.

and swallowing of these mixtures may produce untoward effects.

The oral hygiene program should be initiated with a clean set of teeth and an adequate demonstration of proper procedures. If the client is extremely conscientious, oral irrigation, which is accomplished with an electric Water Pik, a water pistol, or a syringe, can be advocated. Irrigation will help dislodge plaque from subgingival areas and will promote better oral hygiene.

Periapical Disease

Periapical disease is a common condition in the dog. Often it is unnoticed until irreparable damage has occurred. The first indication of disease is usually pain on chewing. This characteristically slow and insidious condition can be present in any tooth but is most common in the canine and carnassial teeth; eventual destruction and loss may take up to 5 years (Fig. 1–29). On radiographic evaluation, a radiolucent area at the root apex indicates periapical infection.

Most periapical disease originates as an extension of inflammation and necrosis of the pulp cavity rather than an extension of periodontal disease. Bacteria may gain access to the pulp cavity after tooth lysis from periodontal disease, tooth fracture, or trauma. Cysts and tumors can also cause periapical disease. Owing to the rich vascular supply at the tooth root apex, septi-

Table 1–5. NUMBER OF ROOTS ON DOGS' TEETH

Tooth	No. of Roots
Upper	
Incisor, canine	1 each
1st premolar	1
2nd, 3rd premolar	2 each
4th premolar, 1st, 2nd molar	3 each
Lower	
Incisor, canine	1 each
1st premolar	1
2nd, 3rd, 4th premolar, 1st molar	2 each
2nd molar	1

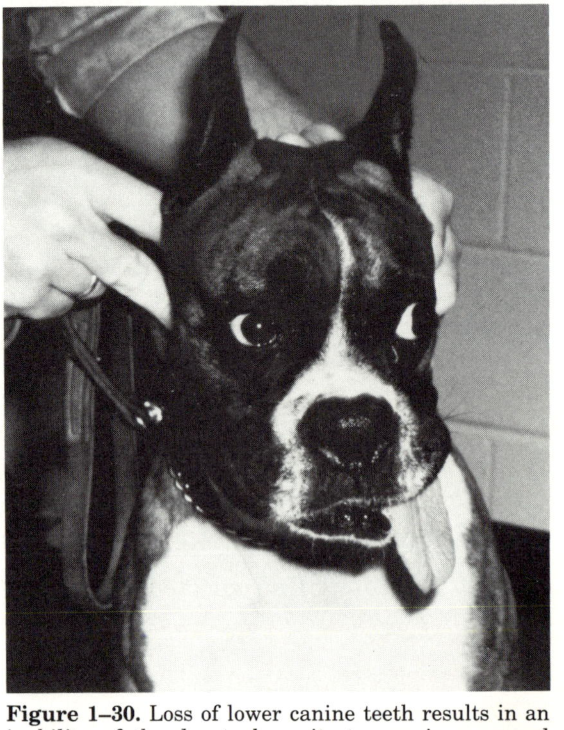

Figure 1–30. Loss of lower canine teeth results in an inability of the dog to keep its tongue in a normal position; (therefore, removal of the lower canine teeth as a treatment for periapical disease should be avoided.

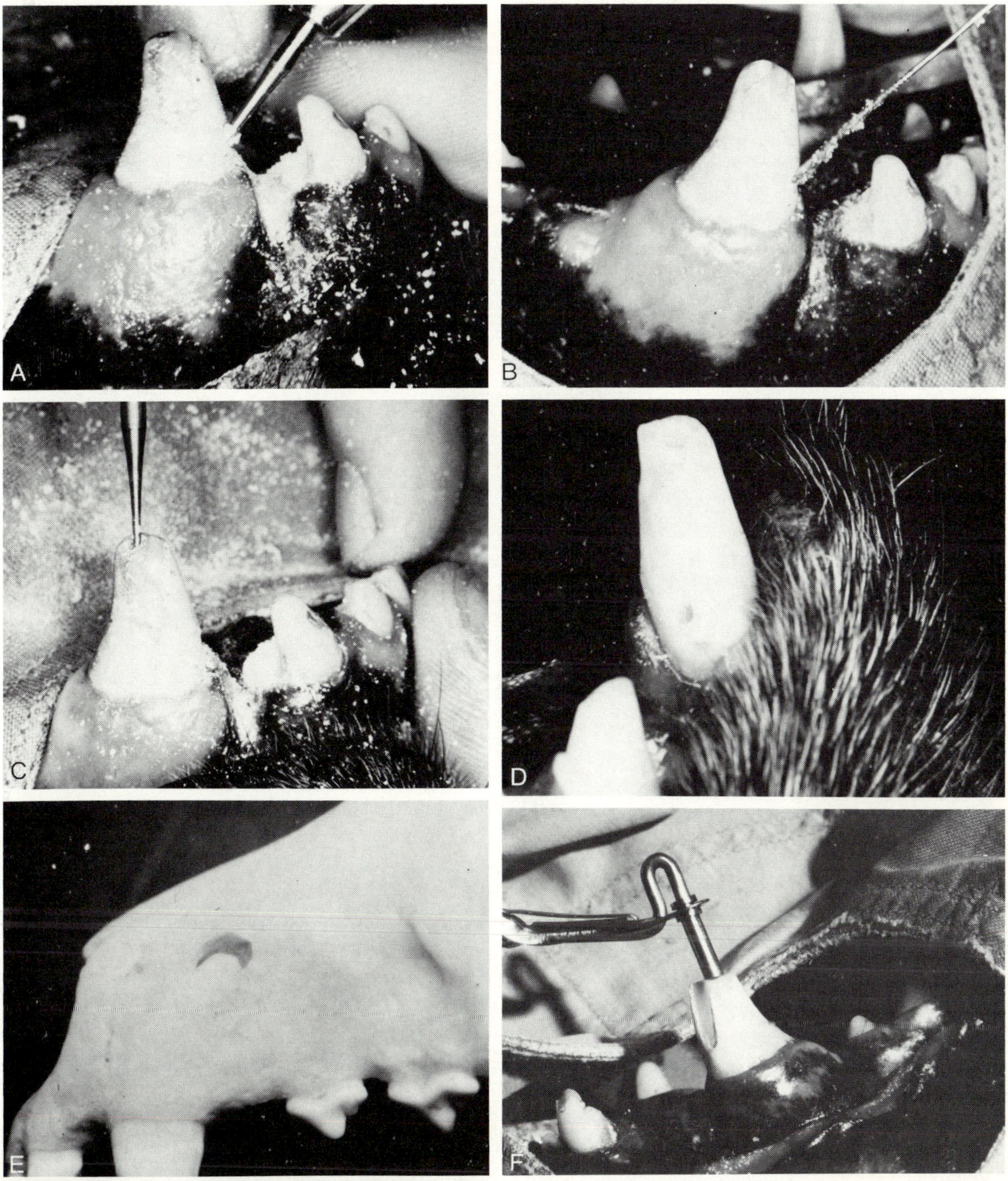

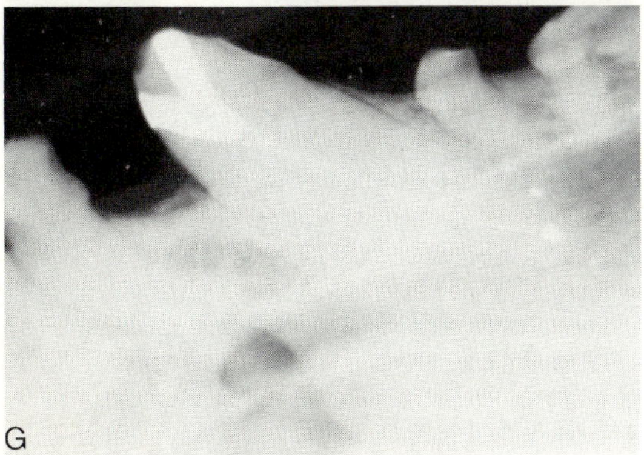

Figure 1–31. Endodontic therapy of the canine teeth for pulp necrosis or periapical abscesses. *A,* an entry just above the gingival margin is necessary to allow straight access to the major part of the curved pulp cavity. *B,* After the enamel and dentin have been penetrated, 40-mm dental files are used to remove the pulp material. *C,* A second approach to the curved pulp cavity is made through the point of the crown. *D,* The largest dental file possible should be used to clean both approaches. *E,* The apex of the maxillary canine tooth is exposed by incising the gingiva, reflecting the periosteum, and removing the bone. Access to the pulp cavity is possible after the apex is removed. *F,* The pulp cavity is cleaned, dried, and packed with gutta-percha or another sealant, and then all access holes are closed with amalgam. *G,* The final result of endodontic therapy is a cleaned, sealed root canal in which the tooth is securely held by the periodontal ligaments.

cemia may localize and, in rare situations, manifest as periapical disease. The apex of a dog's tooth has many foramina.[55] Variation of root involvement determines which external signs are manifested (Table 1–5).[28]

Endodontic therapy has been reviewed; it represents an alternative to extraction (Fig. 1–30).[94, 97–100] The objective of the procedure is to remove the infected pulp and to seal the root canal; it is not difficult to perform (Fig. 1–31).

CARNASSIAL ABSCESS

Abscess of the upper fourth premolar is the most widely recognized form of periapical disease. An external draining fistula located ventral to the eye is the classic sign, but it is not a common presenting complaint. The lesion may be a small, hard swelling with subcutaneous cellulitis or a persistent or recurring fistula 2 to 3 cm below the nasal canthus of the eyelid.[45] When pus collects between the skin and bone, there is often osteolysis of the maxilla (Fig. 1–32). A controversy exists as to which root is most often involved, the single large caudal root or the rostral buccal root (Fig. 1–33).[45] Both can cause the characteristic bulging and fistulous tract ventral to the eye. Draining may also occur into the conjunctival sac. If the lingual root is involved, a unilateral chronic epistaxis can occur. Fistulous tracts from lower carnassial (first molar) tooth abscess, which drain through the skin, are not common but do occur.

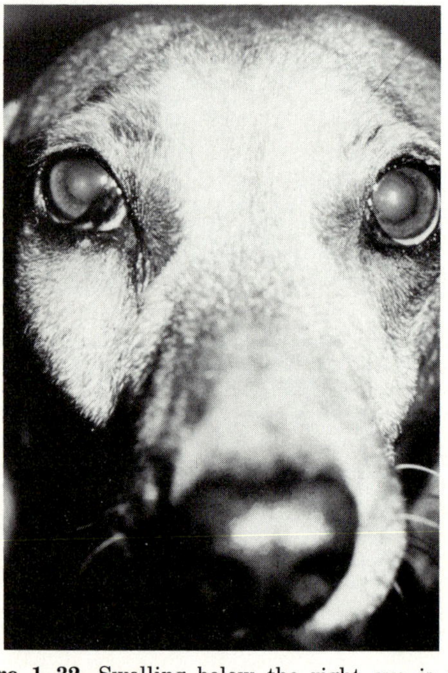

Figure 1–32. Swelling below the right eye is from osteomyelitis and an abscess of the carnassial tooth.

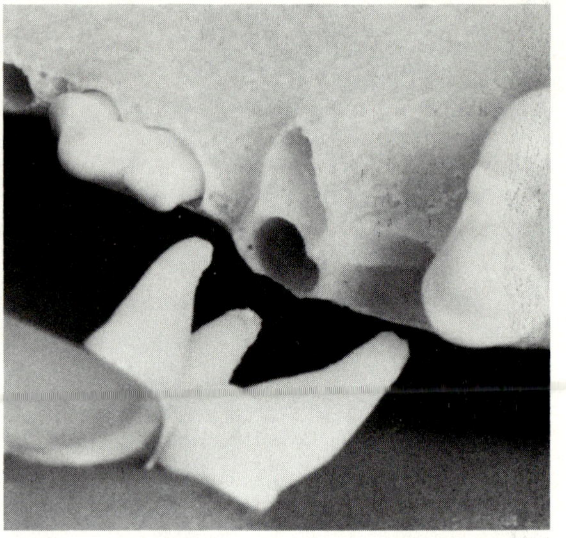

Figure 1–33. The upper fourth premolar tooth, characteristically, has three roots.

Extraction of the infected tooth is the primary treatment for periapical disease. However, if chronic infection and fistulous formation do not exist, removal of the tooth is not always necessary. If the root is firm in the alveolus and the periodontal ligaments are intact, an apicoectomy can be performed to save the tooth (see Fig. 1–31). In humans, a resolved chronic lesion can form new cementum and bone to anchor the tooth. Extraction of the carnassial tooth does not usually require splitting of the tooth. Several methods of tooth extraction are possible.

1. The gingiva is elevated from the tooth. All surfaces of the alveolus are elevated from the tooth. Dental forceps are then used to lift and rotate the tooth from its deeper attachment (Fig. 1–34). The tooth should not be pulled from the alveolus.

2. The single posterior tooth root is separated from the anterior pair by using a blade to split the tooth to the gum line. The final splitting is performed with a tooth splitter, and the separate roots are elevated and removed.[28]

3. In alveolar resection, the gum is incised vertically between the anterior and posterior roots and reflected from the tooth. With a mallet and chisel, the lateral aspect of the alveolus is removed. A ¼ inch chisel or root elevator is driven between the roots

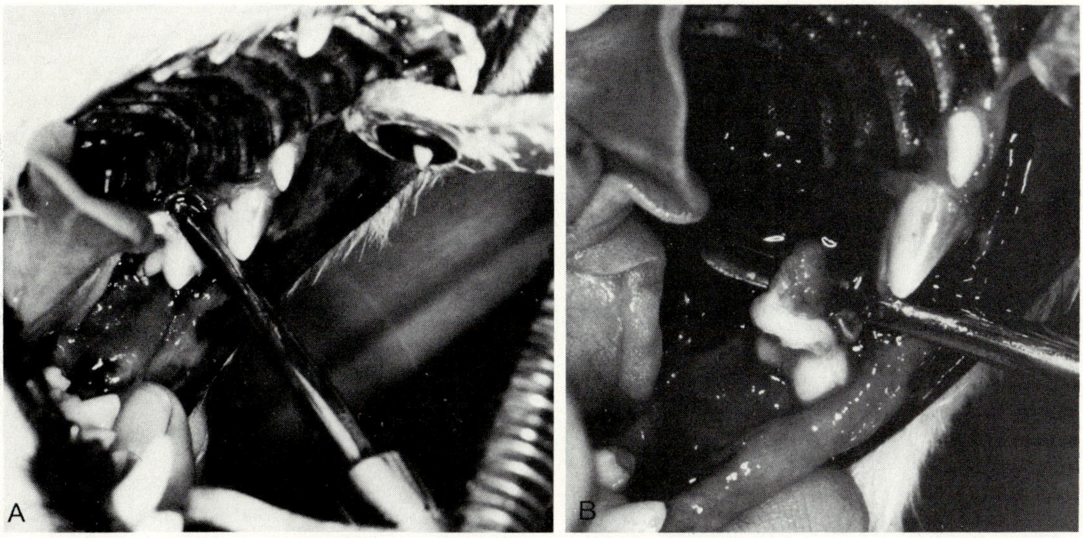

Figure 1–34. The removal of a diseased carnassial tooth. *A,* The periodontal ligaments surrounding the roots are carefully dissected with a small dental elevator. *B,* Only after the roots have been carefully separated from the alveolar bone can the carnassial tooth be elevated and removed without splitting.

and manipulated to loosen them from the periodontal membrane. The tooth is removed with non-crushing molar forceps, and the cut edges of the gum line sutured with gut.

4. A high-speed drill is used to cut a hole between the roots. A needle containing a cutting wire is then passed through the hole. The tooth is sawed from the gingival surface, elevated, and removed.

5. A dental drill with a diamond disk in the handpiece is used to split the tooth roots to the gum line. The distal root is elevated and removed first. If difficulty is encountered in removing the two anterior roots together, they can also be halved with the drill.

Before closure in any of the preceding techniques, good drainage should be established. The entire abscessed alveolus should be curetted by hand or with a high-speed drill. If the lingual root is draining into the sinus, a Steinmann's pin driven into the medial alveolus to penetrate the sinus will establish drainage.[28] If a fistula is present, a seton soaked in a suitable ointment (e.g., mild tincture of iodine) may be passed through it to aid in drainage. With good drainage through the alveolus, the fistula may be closed by routine surgical procedure[45] or it may be allowed to heal as an open wound.

Osteomyelitis, endocarditis, and suppurative arthritis may occur following oral surgery.[28, 123] When possible, the patient should receive broad-spectrum antibiotics such as ampicillin for 24 to 48 hours preoperatively and for 3 days postoperatively.

OSTEOMYELITIS

Osteomyelitis is commonly encountered in the old patient with chronic periodontal disease. Generally it occurs in the patient who has lost teeth either naturally or by extraction. Sequestered roots of lost teeth can often be seen radiographically. When these roots are noted concomitant with osteomyelitis and substantial loss of bone, extraction and curettage are inadvisable until osteomyelitis is controlled. Individual cases must be studied carefully as to the danger of an iatrogenically fractured mandible versus continued osteomyelitis.

Firm, non-painful, unilateral swelling of gingival tissue is a primary complaint in actinomycosis. The gingival margin may be normal.[24] Filamentous organisms can be obtained by fine-needle aspiration biopsy of the gingiva. Anaerobic incubation of the aspirate is required to culture *Actinomyces* spp. Long-term ampicillin therapy is usually effective.

Stomatitis

The oral mucosa is aided in its function as an important protective barrier by abundant vasculature and lymphoreticular tissue. Inflammation of oral structures, e.g., stomatitis, glossitis, gingivitis, and pharyngitis, is a non-specific sign of an abnormal host-environment relationship. The etiology can be internal (genetic, immunological, nutritional, hormonal, or systemic) or external (traumatic, toxic, viral, bacterial, or fungal).

The protection of the oral mucosa is augmented by local immunological activity and by the immunosecretory products of the salivary glands. In response to injury, the oral mucosa rapidly heals, and in most species, healing proceeds more rapidly than in comparable lesions in the skin.[81] Potentially harmful agents are in constant contact with the mucosal barrier. Thus, endogenous infectious stomatitis is rare and occurs when one group of organisms becomes dominant or when host defense mechanisms are depressed. Frequency, duration, and intensity of exposure to the harmful agent determine both the severity of lesion and the host's response.

DIAGNOSIS

A complete history should be supplemented with dietary and environmental information (Table 1–6). Primary lesions, concomitant diseases, and self-inflicted lesions must be differentiated. The diagnostic approach depends on the severity of the lesions and the response to initial medical therapy. Since oral lesions regardless of their cause often appear similar, careful attention to the details of the history and physical examination are important. Skin disease may be associated with oral mucosal disease and the skin should be carefully examined with emphasis on the mucocutaneous junctions, e.g., the eyes, anus, prepuce, and vagina.[81] Sedation is often needed for a thorough oral examination. The normal oral mucosa is pink except in areas of pigmentation. Red coloration indicates inflammation, hemoconcentration, or vasodilation. The surface should be smooth and glistening. Changes in pigmentation may provide a clue to the chronicity or location of healed lesions. The saliva often becomes thick and tenacious in oral disease and may obscure the pathology. Pink saliva inicates oral ulceration. In patients with severe or chronic lesions, laboratory tests should include a complete blood count, blood urea nitrogen (BUN) concentration, urinalysis, blood glucose level (if the animal is polydipsic or polyuric), platelet count, and clotting time. Lesions of adjacent tissues (lips, nares, pharynx), regional lymph nodes, and salivary glands should be examined to help determine possible etiologies. Additional diagnostic testing includes

Table 1–6. DIAGNOSIS OF CHRONIC STOMATITIS

Initial data base	CBC
	Serum chemistries
	Urinalysis
	Fecal flotation
	Knott's test
	Feline leukemia virus–cats
Oral cavity examination	Scraping of multiple lesions for microscopic examination
	Impression smears–stains
	Biopsies of edges of transition areas (normal-abnormal junction)
	Immunofluorescent testing–biopsies in Michel's solution
If there is cutaneous involvement	Skin scraping
	Bacterial culture
	Fungal culture
	Direct microscopic examination
	Biopsy
If autoimmune cause is suspected	Antinuclear antibody
	LE cell test
	Serum electrophoresis
	Direct immunofluorescent testing of tissue
If immunodysfunction is suspected	CBC
	Serum electrophoresis
	Immunoelectrophoresis
	Radial immunodiffusion
	Nitroblue tetrazolium dye test
	Lymphocyte blastogenesis transformation
If neoplasia/proliferation is suspected	Radiographs–mouth, thorax
	Fine-needle biopsy–lesion, lymph nodes
	Surgical biopsy

Table 1–7. CAUSES OF STOMATITIS*

Physical agents
Foreign body (plant material, bones, porcupine quills)
External trauma (fight wounds, automobile accidents)
Electrical burns
Radiation therapy
Chemical agents
Strong Alkalis (lye)
Petroleum distillates
Acids
Heavy metals
Others
Biological agents
Bacterial diseases
Fungal infections
Viral diseases
Metabolic diseases
Diabetes mellitus
Uremia
Nutritional deficiencies
Blood dyscrasias and reticuloendothelial diseases
Allergic and toxic drug reactions
Autoimmune diseases
Immunodysfunction
Neoplastic diseases
Idiopathic

*Adapted with permission from MacDonald JM: Stomatitis. Vet Clin North Am (Small Anim Pract) 13:415, 1983.

cytological examination, surgical biopsy, culture, fungal titers, immunological tests for autoimmune or immune deficiencies, and FeLV tests in cats.

Stomatitis, inflammation of the oral mucosa, is a clinical term that rarely denotes disease of a specific etiology (Table 1–7). Erosions and ulcers are common, non-specific indicators of mucosal damage that occurs faster than repair. Tumors, masses, and nodules suggest infiltrative diseases, but not always neoplasia. Vesicles and bullae in the oral cavity are rare but if they are encountered, an examination of all mucocutaneous junctions should be initiated. An occurrence of these inflammations may be attributed to autoimmune disease. Accumulation of debris on the surface of the mucosa may indicate necrosis or rapid proliferation of mucosal epithelium.

INFECTIOUS STOMATITIS

Bacteria, fungi, and viruses are the primary causes of stomatitis. Their role as secondary or opportunistic invaders is often neglected. The transient response of noninfectious stomatitis to antibiotic therapy reflects the effect of bacterial overgrowth.

Acute Necrotizing Ulcerative Gingivitis (Vincent's Stomatitis)

Spirochetes and fusiform bacilli are normal inhabitants of the oral cavity.[102] Owing to the acute onset of clinical signs, it has been generally assumed that another agent or factor is responsible for initiation of Vincent's stomatitis. Elevation of corticosteroid activity by stress or steroid therapy may be involved. *Bacteriodes melaninogenicus* has been studied experimentally, and is suspected of being the primary causitive organism. Severe necrosis of mucous membranes, with periodontal invasion resulting in apical abscesses, has been observed. Halitosis, pain, anorexia, and copious salivation are commonly encountered.[67, 119] The mucous membranes denude easily upon examination, and gingival bleeding is common (Fig. 1–35). Exfoliative cytological examination will demonstate an abundance of organisms but is non-specific, since normal animals can have the organisms. Isolation of spirochetes is difficult; any procedure must depend upon the ability of motile spirochetes to penetrate culture media and migrate away from the remainder of the oral microorganisms.

Local and systemic ampicillin (20 mg/kg) therapy for 2 to 3 weeks may be necessary for recovery. Recurrences are not uncommon, if therapy is not properly administered. Topical ampicillin should be applied

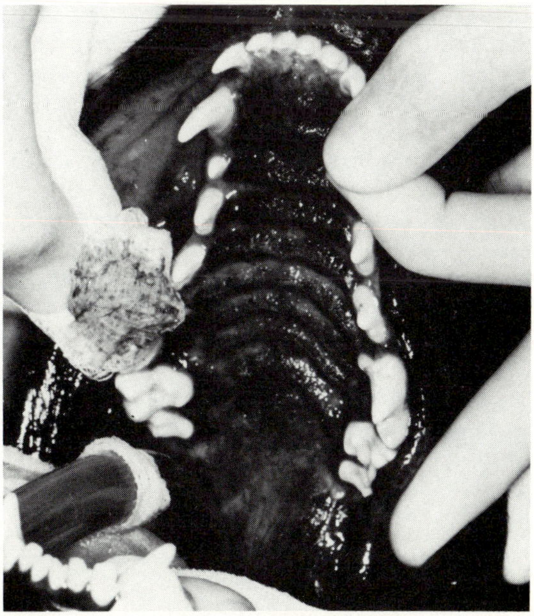

Figure 1–35. The severity of stomatitis may not be evident until surface epithelium and debris are removed. Note the back of the hard palate.

orally in solution or spray 3 to 4 times daily. Oxygenating mouth rinses (3 per cent hydrogen peroxide in equal volume with water) are helpful. If severe necrosis is present, débridement by mechanical and chemical (2 to 5 per cent silver nitrate) means is necessary. Soft food is provided to prevent further trauma and to ensure adequate caloric intake. The degree of communicability of Vincent's stomatitis has not been determined in the dog and cat.

Fungal Infections

Stomatitis of fungal etiology is uncommon in dogs and cats. Overgrowth of *Candida albicans* (thrush) is characterized by creamy white patches in the mouth. The adjacent mucosa is usually erythematous. Scraping the lesions creates a raw, bleeding surface. The tongue and palate are commonly affected. Pain, ropy salivation, and anorexia are often present. Although this fungus can be normally found in the mouth, overgrowth occurs when the oral flora is disturbed, e.g., by debilitating or acute illness, antibiotic therapy, or decreased host resistance. Concomitant candidiasis of the gastrointestinal tract rarely occurs. The diagnosis is based on the clinical examination, exfoliative cytological examination, culture, and a biopsy revealing hyphae of candida invading epithelium (PAS stain). A change from budding form to mycelial form is an indication of pathogenicity. Treatment is not uniformly successful. Specific antifungal therapy consists of nystatin* (100,000 units orally 3 times daily). Nystatin powder† or mystecin–F‡ suspensions that are painted on the mucous membrane have been successful. One per cent aqueous gentian violet solution (staining is unattractive to clients), 2 per cent solution of potassium permanganate mouth wash, and 0.2 per cent chlorhexidine§ have been advocated as oral flushes or to be painted on 4 times a day.[81] Ketoconazole‖ has not been evaluated for candidal stomatitis but has been effective in yeast infections in humans. A recommended dosage in the dog is 10 mg/kg 3 times daily or 30 mg/kg once a day.[81]

Other mycotic diseases that can infect the oral cavity include sporotrichosis, blastomycosis, histoplasmosis, cryptococcosis, and coccidioidomycosis.

Viral Diseases

Feline rhinotracheitis virus (FRV) and feline calicivirus (FCV) can cause oral lesions. Lingual ulcers are primarily on the tip of the tongue. The hard palate, lips, external nares, and foot pads can also be affected, and these ulcers are more severe in FCV than FRV. Feline leukemia virus has been associated with chronic recurring stomatitis, presumably because of immune (T–lymphocyte) suppression.

Canine distemper and feline parvovirus can cause stomatitis, although these viruses typically affect other organs. Viral oral papillomatosis is discussed under oral tumors.

STOMATITIS DUE TO PHYSICAL AGENTS

Foreign bodies may traumatize the oral mucosa. The animal is presented in various phases of recovery with secondary bacterial infection and scar tissue camouflaging the foreign body. Careful examination under sedation is often necessary. Removal of bones, wood splinters, hooks, or needles usually effects a cure. Intermittent problems due to migrating grass awns or porcupine quills may be eliminated only by careful dissection of scar tissue.

Trauma to the tongue and lips is common, and secondary bacterial infections may complicate the original lesion. Oral necrosis from electrical burns is seen in young animals that chew through the insulation of electrical cords. Seizures, pulmonary edema, and cardiac arrhythmias are complications of electrical shock injuries.

Stomatitis from ingestion of caustic or corrosive substances is uncommon but requires immediate, liberal lavage of the mouth with copious amounts of water. Strong alkali (lye), acids, phenol, and petroleum distillate are frequently ingested. Vinegar or lemon juice may be used to counteract contact with alkaline substances. Sodium bicarbonate may be used for contact with acids. Usually, neutralization is not effective because of the delay from time of

---

*Mycostatin Oral Tablets, E.R. Squibb & Sons, Inc., Princeton, NJ.

†Mycostatin Topical Powder, E.R. Squibb & Sons, Inc., Princeton, NJ.

‡Mysteclin–F Syrup, E. R. Squibb & Sons, Inc., Princeton, NJ.

§Hibiclens, Stuart Pharmaceuticals, Wilmington, DE.

‖Nizoral Tablets, Janssen Pharmaceutica, Inc., Piscataway, NJ.

exposure to presentation. Chronic exposure to chemicals, especially pesticides, in the environment may cause severe glossitis, which is common in dogs in agricultural settings. Symptomatic care includes prophylaxis of secondary bacterial infection, cleaning and occasional débridement of the oral cavity, and a soft diet to ensure adequate caloric intake.

STOMATITIS DUE TO SYSTEMIC FACTORS

Stomatitis may be an indication of systemic disease. Lesions heal rapidly after the underlying problem is corrected. Uremia, diabetes mellitus, vitamin deficiency, heavy-metal poisoning, blood dyscrasias, and immune-mediated diseases can cause oral lesions (Fig. 1–36).[8, 29] Oral lesions in humans occur when the diet is deficient in thiamine, riboflavin, niacin, pyridoxine, cyanocobalamin, folic acid, biotin, ascorbic acid, vitamin A, vitamin D, iron, or zinc.[8, 29] Niacin deficiency (black tongue) is no longer seen clinically.[35] Thallium is the classic heavy-metal cause of oral ulcers. Petechiation of the mucosa or bleeding of the gums can be seen in blood dyscrasia (e.g., warfarin poisoning, thrombocytopenia, disseminated intravascular coagulation). Silver-gray collies affected with cyclic neutropenia may develop a recurrent stomatitis.[25] A proliferative ulcerating stomatitis has been noted in Siberian huskies.[80, 89]

Many ulcerative and inflammatory lesions of the mouth are early lesions of malignancy or autoimmune diseases. After underlying systemic causes have been ruled out, a biopsy is indicated in cases that are not responding to conventional therapy. Owing to secondary bacterial infections, the neoplastic and autoimmune diseases may transiently respond to antibiotic therapy.

STOMATITIS IN AUTOIMMUNE DISORDERS

In autoimmune disease it is unusual for oral lesions to occur without involvement of the skin, especially other mucocutaneous junctions (eyes, anus, vagina, prepuce). Circulating autoantibodies to intercellular epidermal antigens cause acantholysis and intraepidermal bullae (pemphigus complex) or epidermal bullae (bullous pemphigoid). In the pemphigus complex, pemphigus vulgaris usually causes transient buccal mucosal lesions but rarely causes vesicles. Pemphigus foliaceus is an exfoliative dermatitis that rarely affects the oral cavity. Bullous pemphigoid affects the oral cavity in about 50 per cent of cases, and will cause vesicles and bullae.

Autoimmune diseases affecting the mouth must be differentiated from allergic drug reaction and toxic epidermal necrolysis. Severe ulceration of the tongue and secondary stomatitis may appear prior to cutaneous lesions.

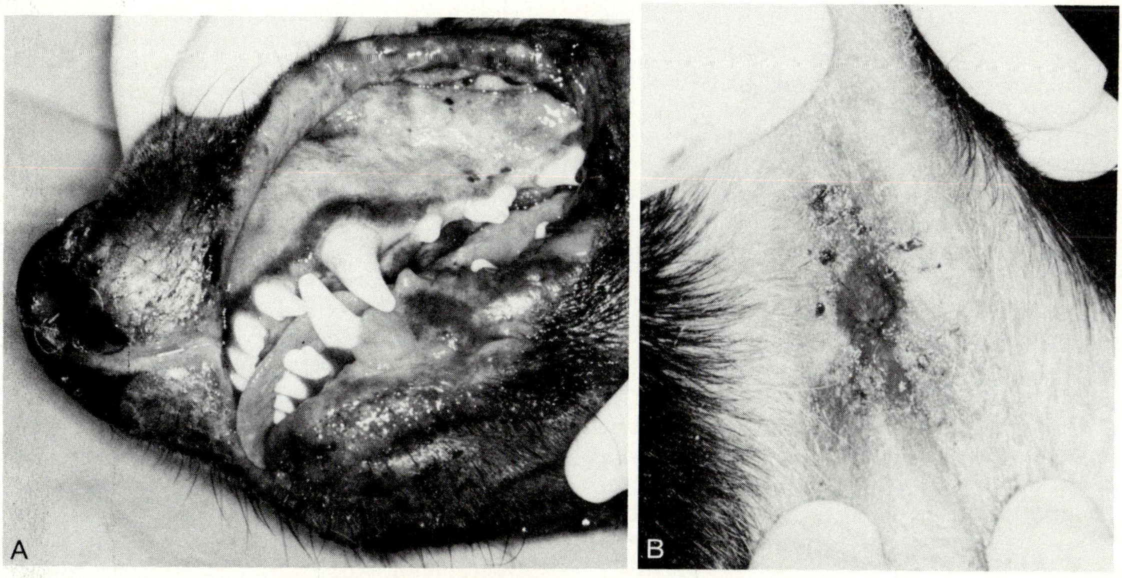

Figure 1–36. *A*, Severe stomatitis may seem to spread along the lip margins and nose. *B*, Involvement of other mucocutaneous junctions such as the anus indicates a systemic disease. Histopathological examination indicated pemphius vulgaris.

Pemphigus Complex

Pemphigus is a group of chronic blistering diseases of unknown etiology characterized by the direction of tissue-bound autoantibodies against intercellular epidermal antigens. Histological evidence of acantholysis with resulting intraepidermal cleft formation is a prerequisite of the diagnosis. There are two types of pemphigus, each having a variant form.[52, 81] Pemphigus vulgaris (PVU) is the most severe type; it is characterized by ulceration of the mucous membranes, mucocutaneous junctions, and skin. Involvement of a singular cutaneous region is unusual, and the buccal mucosa contains lesions in over 90 per cent of the cases. Vesicles or bullae rarely appear, and when observed, they are transient. Diagnosis is made via history, physical examination, histopathological study, and direct immunofluorescent testing. A rare and more benign variant of pemphigus vulgaris is pemphigus vegetans (PVE), which rarely causes oral lesions.[10, 18]

Pemphigus Foliaceus. Pemphigus foliaceus (PF) is an exfoliative dermatitis in which oral lesions are less commonly observed. Cutaneous lesions include erythema, edema, ulcers, erosions, crusting, and scaling. Since the pathological lesion occurs at the subcorneal or superficial epidermal level, a pustular eruption may be observed. The lesions often have a predilection for the facial region. Oral lesions are usually in the form of erosions or ulcers. Diagnostic procedures are the same as those for pemphigus vulgaris. Pemphigus erythematosus (PE), which is either an early stage of pemphigus foliaceus or a different form of the disease, has similar lesions that are restricted to the head and neck. Positive antinuclear antibody titers are detected in some cases of *PE*.

Bullous Pemphigoid (BP). Bullous pemphigoid is clinically similar to pemphigus and is characterized by autoantibodies that are directed toward basement membrane zone antigens.[74] Clinical signs include mucocutaneous blistering and ulceration. Oral cavity involvement, although not as common as in pemphigus vulgaris, is seen in at least 50 per cent of the cases. True vesicles or bullae are more commonly observed with this disease than with the pemphigus complex. Lesions present on the oral mucosa may consist of hemorrhagic (blood filled) vesicles and, therefore, may be confused with petechiation suggestive of a hemostatic disorder. Ruptured vesicles become ulcers with secondary bacterial stomatitis.

Co-existing cutaneous involvement is almost always present. Diagnosis of bullous pemphigoid by biopsy requires histological demonstration of the characteristic lesions of subepidermal bullae. Detection of immunoglobulin, with or without complement, at the basement membrane zone may be accomplished by direct immunofluorescent testing of affected skin or mucosa.[10, 52, 74]

Lupus Erythematosus

Systemic Lupus Erythematosus. Oral or nasopharyngeal ulceration is included in the preliminary criteria for the diagnosis of systemic lupus erythematosus (SLE) in humans.[8, 29] SLE is a disease affecting many systems and with a wide variation of clinical signs, including polyarthritis, anemia, glomerulonephritis, and dermatitis. Cutaneous manifestations of SLE are diverse and observed in 30 to 40 per cent of affected dogs and in 80 per cent of affected humans.[29] Lesions may include an erythematous, macular rash, vesicobullous eruptions, urticaria, ulceration, alopecia, seborrheic disorders, purpura, photosensitization, leukoderma, and scarring. A predilection for the facial region exists. Concurrent oral disease is usually in the form of erosions and ulcers particularly of the tongue, hypoglossal region, and the soft palate. Mucocutaneous lesions are indistinguishable from those of other autoimmune disorders.[106]

Traditional immunological tests for the disease include the LE cell test and the antinuclear antibody (ANA) test. The antinuclear antibody test is generally considered superior to the LE cell test because it is more frequently positive in dogs with lupus, a positive result is more consistently present (LE cell test results are often transitory), and the test results are less affected by glucocorticoid therapy.[81] Neither the LE cell test nor the ANA test is consistently positive in all lupus cases; false negative results occur when corticosteroid therapy has been given, and false positive results occur in inflammatory disease. The lupus band test, which should not be confused with the LE cell test, is direct immunofluorescent testing of the skin and the demonstration of linear deposits (lupus bands) of immunoglobulin (IgG) and complement in the area of the dermal-epidermal junction. Because systemic lupus erythematosus attacks many organ systems, other available immunological tests including rheumatoid factor, antiglobulin (Coomb's test), antithyroid antibody, and serum electrophoresis may need to be done.[81, 106]

Discoid Lupus Erythematosus. Discoid lupus erythematosus (DLE), in both humans and dogs, is a less severe form of lupus erythematosus that involves only the skin and possibly the oral cavity.[29, 50] LE cell test and antinuclear antibody test results are often negative. The incidence of DLE in humans is higher than that of SLE. The appearance of the lesions can be triggered by a number of factors, the most common being sunlight. Oral ulceration and stomatitis are counterparts of the disease but they are not found consistently. Diagnosis is made through histological examination and immunological and hematological testing.

Therapy

Treatment of autoimmune diseases may utilize immunosuppressive drugs such as glucocorticoids and cancer chemotherapeutic agents. Chrysotherapy with various gold salt preparations is an alternative to the use of immunosuppressive drugs in the treatment of pemphigus foliaceus. Immunostimulants (levamisole)* have been effective in some cases with demonstrable immunosuppression.[86] D–1–α–tocopherol acetate (Vitamin E) has been used in the treatment of lupus (primarily DLE) with variable results.[81]

Animals with oral mucosal disease (stomatitis and ulceration) are often placed on immunosuppressive glucocorticoid therapy after a cursory examination. An initial clinical response to therapy is interpreted as a diagnosis of pemphigus, particularly if any concurrent dermatitis is present. This approach is potentially dangerous if the wrong diagnosis is made, if for example the toxic condition is epidermal necrolysis secondary to bacteremia.[81] Appropriate diagnostic information should be collected before glucocorticoid or other immunosuppressive therapy is administered, rather than after it fails. Regardless of the preferred treatment of the specific autoimmune disease, a necessary prerequisite to therapy is a definitive diagnosis.

*Levasole, Pitman-Moore, Inc., Washington Crossing, NJ.

STOMATITIS DUE TO IMMUNODYSFUNCTION

Inadequate immunological response of the mucosal barrier (immunodysfunction, immunological dysfunction) may result in changes in the microbial population and subsequent development of mucosal disease. Immunodysfunction, involving either the specific (lymphocytic) or non-specific (phagocytic) immune system, can be classified as either congenital versus acquired or primary versus secondary. On the basis of speculation about the cause-and-effect relationship in specific disease states, it is believed that acquired immunodysfunctions occur most frequently in the dog.[81] The immune system (usually cell mediated immunity) is too often incriminated, without proof, as the cause of a particular disease when, in fact, the immunodysfunction is an effect of the disease. On the basis of observations of diseases such as generalized demodicosis in the dog, silver-gray collie syndrome, canine distemper virus infection, and feline leukemia virus, it is believed that immunodysfunction occurs in certain disease states. In chronic, recurrent stomatitis the animal's immunological status should be considered.[5, 35, 47, 52] However, dogs with generalized demodicosis and depressed T-cell function as determined by *in vitro* testing rarely have co-existing stomatitis.[81] Dogs with certain autoimmune disorders for which there are no adequate T-lymphocyte function tests, such as systemic lupus erythematosus, pemphigus vulgaris, and pemphigus foliaceus,[81] could exhibit oral ulceration or stomatitis because of the direct effect of the immunocompromise or conversely because of reduced immunomodulation of B-cells, which allows the development of autoantibody to tissue antigen. The cause-and-effect relationship needs further evaluation.

Routine clinicopathological findings that support a diagnosis of immunoincompetence include persistent lymphopenia ($<$ 1000/mm^3), hypoglobulinemia ($<$ 2.5 gm/dl), decreased beta or gamma globulin fractions on serum protein electrophoresis, and failure to develop a neutrophilic leukocytosis in the presence of an infection. Depressed humoral immunity is uncommon and, if suspected, should be pursued by more accurate assessment of immunoglobulin content in serum, since only an estimated 30 to 60 per cent of the beta and gamma fractions are immunoglobulins. Immunoelectrophoresis

(IEF) and radial immunodiffusion (RID) offer more precise qualitative and quantitative information.[81]

Impairment of cell-mediated immunity (CMI) is the most commonly encountered immunodysfunction in the dog. Association of stomatitis with depressed CMI is exemplified in cats with feline leukemia virus infection.[5] In animals with chronic, recurrent stomatitis CMI should be appraised if possible. Cell-mediated immunity function testing *(in vitro)* by mitogen-stimulated lymphocyte transformation assays is very sensitive. Test results are influenced by many factors, and the test must be individually standardized for most animal species. A low response can be the cause of the disease or the result of the disease.

Although allergic reactions rarely involve tissues of the mouth, drugs can potentially cause cutaneous and mucosal reactions. Drug-related eruptions may result from an allergy to the compounds, direct toxicity, or other unexplained mechanisms. Allergic eruptions may appear immediately or months to years after drug use.

In humans a period of 5 to 21 days of therapy, following the sensitizing exposure, elapses before an eruption appears. Re-exposure may result in a reaction within minutes to several days. Confirmation of a drug allergy is rare in the dog, although suggestive histories can be associated with the presence of cutaneous and oral lesions.[81]

Toxic Epidermal Necrolysis

Toxic epidermal necrolysis (TEN, Lyell's disease) is a rare, severe mucocutaneous disease of dogs and cats.[105] Although many causes have been associated with TEN, 50 per cent of human cases are caused by drug administration, 25 per cent are associated with underlying systemic disease, and the remaining 25 per cent are idiopathic in origin. Oral disease is most commonly observed as an ulceration of the mucous membranes, particularly the tongue. Secondary stomatitis may ensue. The cutaneous lesions may not be present at the initial clinical examination. Erythemic macules, with the rare formation of vesicles, develop into well-demarcated areas of devitalized skin surrounded by epidermal collarettes, that progress to large, ulcerative areas. A prominent feature is painfulness to touch. Diagnosis is made on the basis of history, physical examination, and skin biopsy. The finding of full-thickness of coagulation necrosis of the epidermis with minimal inflammatory infiltrate in the dermis in biopsy specimens of early lesions is characteristic of TEN. Treatment includes removal of the underlying cause, supportive care, and prophylactic antibiotics. Corticosteroids may be started early in the disease, but after ulceration occurs they may retard re-epithelialization.[81]

Idiopathic Stomatitis

Many cases of stomatitis are presented with non-specific lesions, and frequently, secondary complications. Despite a comprehensive diagnostic plan, no diagnosis of these lesions can be determined.

Feline Glossopharyngitis

Glossopharyngitis (ulcers of the posterior oral cavity) is observed in the cat (Fig. 1–37). The ulcers usually are observed caudal to the last molars at the angle of the junction of the upper and lower arcades. The condition may be a manifestation of feline eosinophilic complex. The clinical appearance and size are variable, but usually the ulcers are 0.25 to 1 cm in diameter with a granulomatous appearance. Culture of the area does not reveal a significant pathogen. A mixture of chronic inflammation with invasion of eosinophils and plasma cells is noted histopathologically. The cat may be presented with anorexia and weight loss as the only signs. Although these lesions can occur in cats without underlying disease, they have been associated with chronic calicivirus and feline leukemia virus infections (Fig. 1–38C). Systemic and topical antibiotics are usually ineffective. Vigorous cautery, both mechanical and chemical, combined with steroid therapy seems to be the treatment of choice, but total cure of the problem is uncommon. Mechanical débridement can be followed by cautery with silver nitrate. Systemic antibiotics, topical penicillin, and hydrogen peroxide mouth lavage are used for 1 week. Prednisolone (0.5 mg/kg) is instituted on the fifth day and administered on an alternate-day basis for 2 weeks. The lesions may decrease in size and the cat may become clinically normal for 4 to 6 months. Rarely does the lesion totally disappear without recurrence.

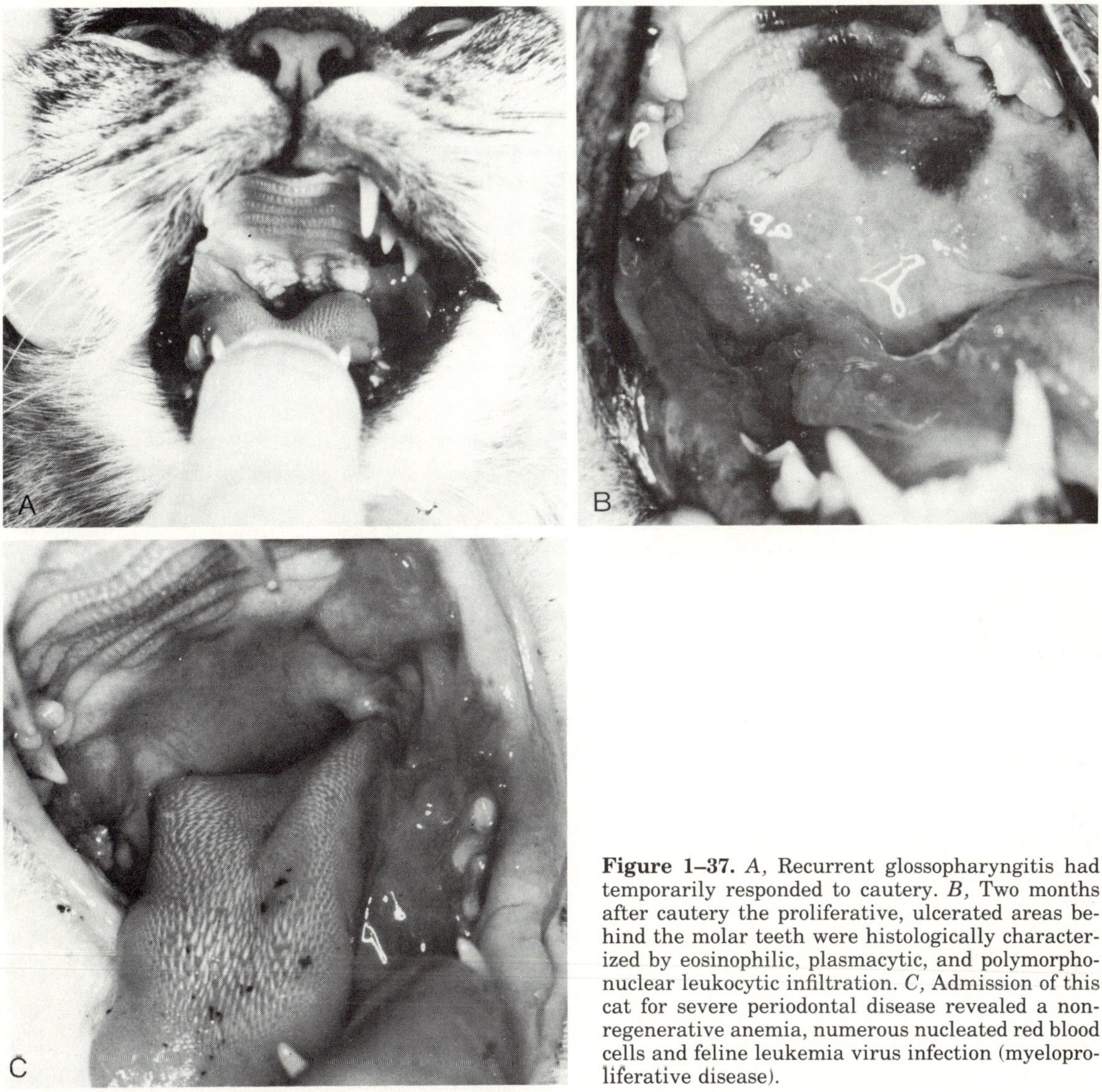

Figure 1–37. *A*, Recurrent glossopharyngitis had temporarily responded to cautery. *B*, Two months after cautery the proliferative, ulcerated areas behind the molar teeth were histologically characterized by eosinophilic, plasmacytic, and polymorphonuclear leukocytic infiltration. *C*, Admission of this cat for severe periodontal disease revealed a nonregenerative anemia, numerous nucleated red blood cells and feline leukemia virus infection (myeloproliferative disease).

Eosinophilic Granuloma

Eosinophilic granuloma complex of the cat exists in three forms, each with characteristic morphological and histological features (Fig. 1–38).[51, 107] The eosinophilic ulcer is typically observed either unilaterally or bilaterally on the upper lip where the canine teeth contact the arcade. Eosinophilic plaques are usually found on the ventral abdomen but may occur anywhere on the skin as well as in the oral cavity. The linear granuloma classically appears on the caudal aspect of either one or both rear legs but may be on the lip as well as the oral cavity. More than one form of the feline eosinophilic granuloma complex may be seen on the same animal. The eosinophilic plaque most consistently has both tissue and peripheral eosinophilia. Diagnosis is made through histological examination of tissue. Treatment of choice is systemic glucocorticoids with or without intralesional steroid injections. Megestrol acetate* (5 mg every other day for 10 to 14 doses) has been used successfully. Beta-radiation has also been proven effective.[35]

Proliferative eosinophilic lesions on the tongue or in the oral cavity occur in young Siberian huskies.[80, 89] A hereditary influence may be present. The stomatitis, a mixture

*Pallace, Bristol Laboratories, Syracuse, NY. Megace Tablets, Mead Johnson, Pharmaceutical Division, Evansville, IN.

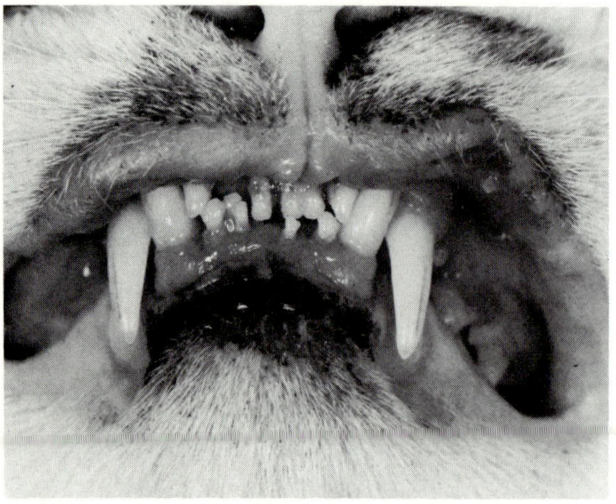

Figure 1–38. The lesions of eosinophilic granuloma on the lips were accompanied by a lesion on a rear leg.

of proliferation and erosion, may be localized or generalized and results in halitosis. Histological examination of the proliferative lesions reveals a well-demarcated area of degenerating collagen surrounded by monocytoid inflammatory cells. An eosinophilic infiltrate is observed in the surrounding tissue. Impression smears will also demonstrate the eosinophilic component of the inflammatory reaction. Initial response to the use of systemic glucocorticoids is dramatic but relapses do occur.

Lymphoplasmacytic Stomatitis

In lymphoplasmacytic stomatitis the oral mucosa is very hyperemic, with focal ulceration and diphtheritic membranes. Excessive salivation, halitosis, and painful mastication are common. An abnormal population of microorganisms can be demonstrated by direct microscopic examination of mucosal scrapings and by bacteriological culture.[51] The principle histological feature of this condition is the intensive, superficial infiltration of plasma cells and lymphocytes, suggesting an immunological mechanism. Ulcerated areas may reveal a polymorphic infiltrate that contains neutrophils. A depressed response of lymphocytes to phytomitogens has been observed on *in vitro* stimulation assays. The results of other immunological tests, including antinuclear antibody titer, LE cell test, and direct immunofluorescent testing of biopsy tissue specimens, are negative. Response to systemic glucocorticoid therapy is usually good, although initial improvement is noted with antimicrobial therapy when bacteria contributes to the stomatitis.[51]

SYMPTOMATIC THERAPY OF STOMATITIS

A specific etiology of simple stomatitis cannot be determined in many cases (Fig. 1–39). Culture often reveals the normal mixed flora of the mouth; therefore, antibiotic sensitivity is unreliable. In these cases symptomatic therapy is often efficacious. A gauze sponge can be used for mechanical débridement of the mucosal surface. Hydrogen peroxide (3 per cent) will help clean affected areas. Chemical cautery with a 5 to 10 per cent silver nitrate solution is useful where the underlying mucosa is ulcerated and necrotic. Collection of the silver nitrate in the pharyngeal area should be avoided, or edema of the larynx may result. Cautery may have to be repeated in 5 days. Penicillin should be instilled into the mouth three times daily. Systemic penicillin therapy is indicated for 3 weeks. Soft

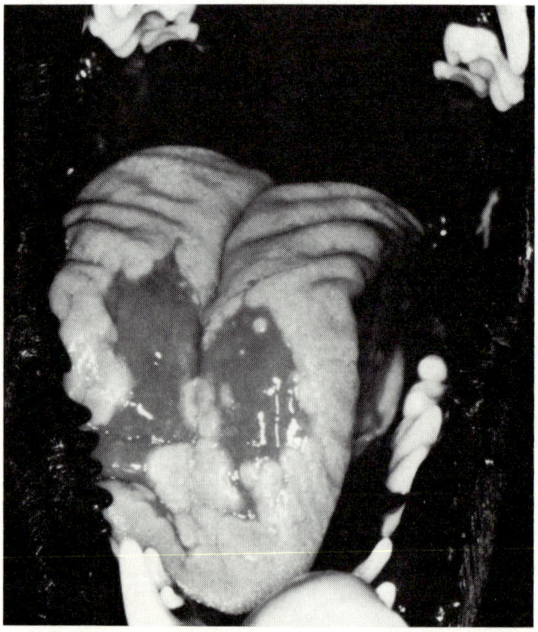

Figure 1–39. Ulcerative glossitis of unknown etiology healed after symptomatic therapy.

food and analgesics may be needed for several days following vigorous cautery.

Palate

The anterior two-thirds of the palate is hard (bony) and the posterior one-third is soft. The palatal mucosa on the oral side is keratinized, stratified, squamous epithelium that is highly sensitive to stimuli. The soft palate is suspended from the posterior edge of the hard palate as a movable fibromuscular fold. The mucous membrane encloses muscle fibers and an aponeurosis.

During the first trimester of development, the primitive, fetal palate separates the nasal sac from the oral cavity. The union of the medial nasal process with the lateral nasal processes and maxillary processes forms the primary palate. The mesodermal nasal septum is continuous with the premaxillary portions of the palate. Fusion of the palatine shelves results in the disappearance of the intervening ectoderm, which accounts for the formation of the median raphe that is visible in the midline of the hard palate. Caudally, where union with the nasal septum does not occur, no ossification arises, so the palate is soft in this region.

Owing to the developmental anatomy, a high degree of variability exists in the cleft palate–cleft lip complex. With cleft lip, incomplete development of the mesoderm of the medial palatine process results in absorption of the overlying ectoderm. The cleft lip is usually a unilateral defect in the lip or in the floor of the nostril. Careful examination may reveal extension of the defect into the foramen. Cleft lips are infrequently encountered in conjunction with cleft palates (Fig. 1–40).

Lack of growth of the lateral palatine processes can result in offset palatal rugae on the roof of the mouth, incomplete fusion of the soft palate, or a complete oronasal fistula through a cleft palate.

The developmental defect may be congenital or hereditary in etiology. The genetic pattern is a simple recessive trait. Excessive corticosteroid therapy, griseofulvin, metabolic abnormalities, and severe stress have also been incriminated.[35] Although minor mucosal or soft palate pathology is compatible with life, neutering or euthanasia is recommended for affected animals in order to decrease the incidence of the trait in the gene pool. In severe defects the lesion prohibits the formation of negative pressure between the tongue and palate that is necessary in nursing. Tube feeding is the most effective method of offering supplemental nutrients. A temporary prosthesis made of acrylic resins has been used to allow an animal to grow and the tissue to develop prior to surgery (Fig. 1–41). Surgical repair should not be attempted until the animal is 6 to 8 weeks of age. Multiple surgical procedures may be necessary for complete restoration of hard palate defects (Fig. 1–42).

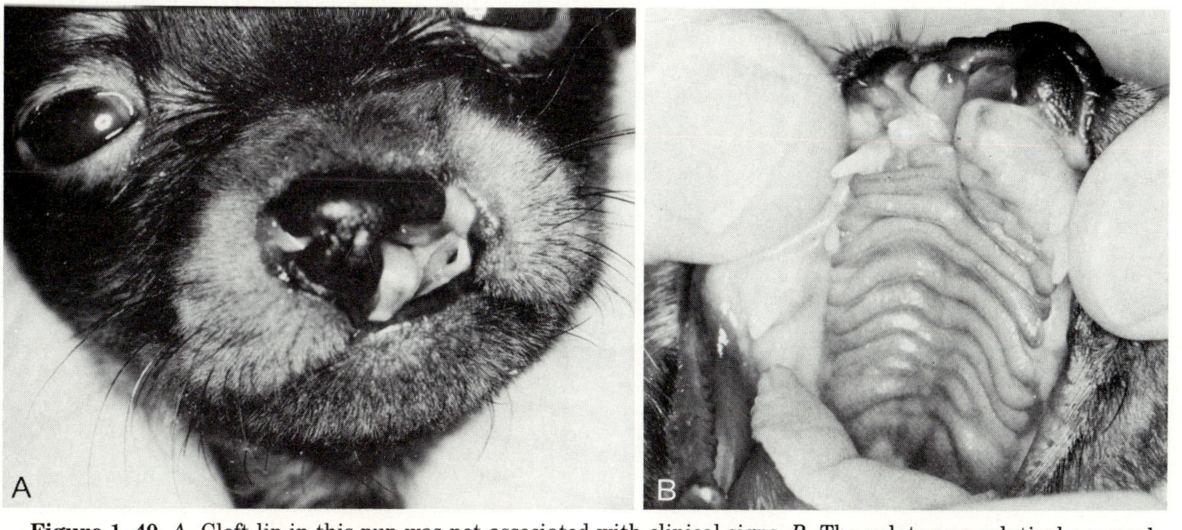

Figure 1–40. *A*, Cleft lip in this pup was not associated with clinical signs. *B*, The palate was relatively normal.

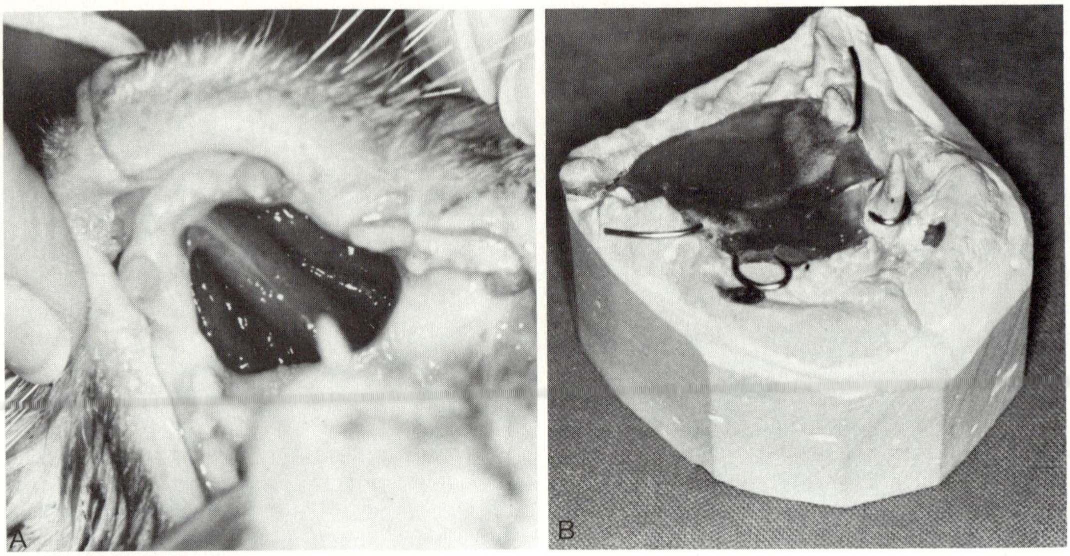

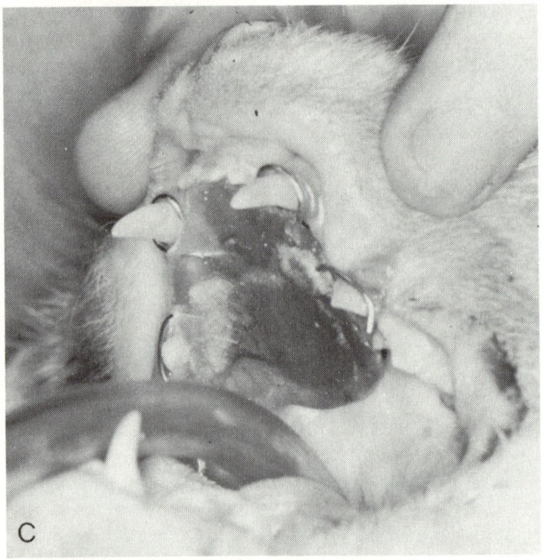

Figure 1–41. *A*, Necrosis of the hard palate in this cat was a consequence of chewing an electrical cord. *B*, Because of the total absence of the hard palate, an acrylic prothesis was made from an oral impression. *C*, The acrylic prothesis temporarily corrected the palate defect.

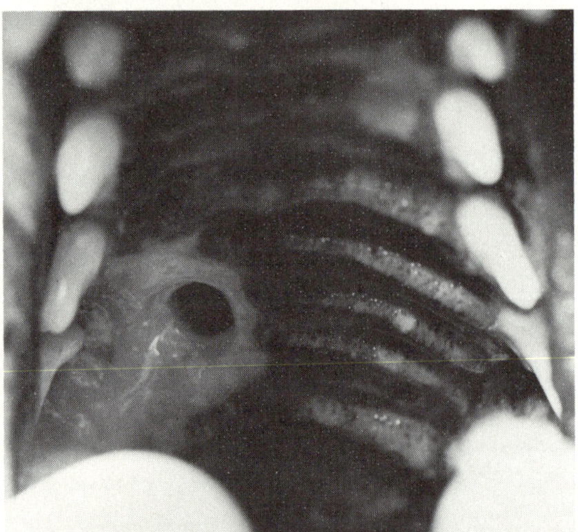

Figure 1–42. Oronasal fistulas of traumatic origin are surgically correctable.

Tonsils

ANATOMY

The paired tonsils lie in the tonsillar fossa in the lateral wall of the oropharynx. They can be located caudal to the palatoglossal arch and ventral to the soft palate. Although the tonsils are elongated, they can be divided into a small submucosal portion and a larger protruding portion.

The physiological function of the tonsils is not completely understood. However, since the palatine tonsils consist primarily of lymphoreticular tissue, they are presumed to be part of the body's defense system. The lack of a well-defined afferent lymphatic system poses questions about their function. The medial retropharyngeal lymph nodes receive the efferent lymphatics from the tonsils. In addition to the palatine tonsil, other lymphatic tissue scattered in the mucous membranes of the pharynx is observed as elevated plaque.[87]

EXAMINATION

The tonsils should be closely examined if disease is suspected. Observation of phlegm in the pharyngeal area should not be used to diagnose tonsillitis. With the tongue pulled forward, the palatine tonsils normally appear as pink, elongated structures in the pharynx. A fold of mucous membrane forms a pocket at the base of the tonsil that can be gently grasped; the minor portion is

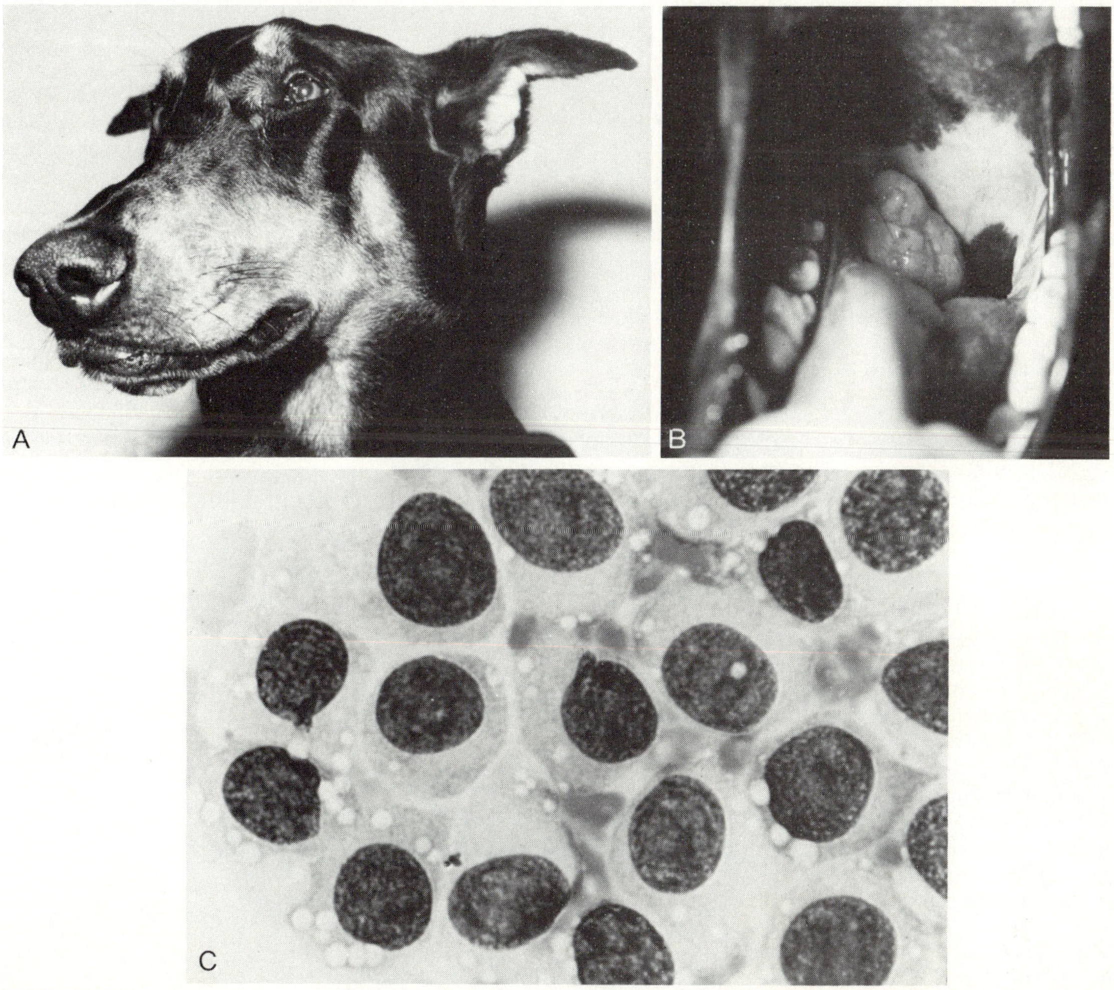

Figure 1–43. *A,* Causes of swelling in the submandibular area of a 7-month-old Doberman pinscher include salivary gland disease, lymphadenopathy, abscess formation, cellulitis, foreign body cysts, and neoplasia. *B,* Oral examination revealed unilateral tonsillar enlargement. *C,* Needle aspiration biopsy of the submandibular lymph node and tonsil recovered a specimen with round, neoplastic cells typical of a transmissible venereal tumor, which responded to vincristine therapy.

then drawn forward and appears caudally as a bulge in the mucosa. Ventral pressure on the base of the tongue will prolapse the tonsils from the crypt.

Depending on the animal's age and breed, the tonsils differ greatly in size, shape, and percentage of tonsil within the crypt. The physical size and shape of the tonsils often have no correlation with the pathological condition. Observation of the tonsils protruding from the crypts is not sufficient evidence to support a diagnosis of tonsillitis. Color is considered to be the best criterion of the inflammatory status of the tonsils. Acutely inflamed tonsils appear red and edematous. The surrounding mucosa and other oral lymphatics may appear inflamed, and the tonsils may not be protruding from the crypt. Under close observation, petechial hemorrhage may be seen on the surface. In subacute inflammation a mottled appearance may represent necrotic foci, small abscesses, or areas of resolution. The inflamed tonsils are soft, and friable, and they bleed easily when manipulated.[28, 35]

Most disease of the tonsils is bilateral. Unilateral involvement dictates close observation for neoplastic conditions, tonsillar cysts, foreign bodies, or localized pharyngeal abscesses (Fig. 1–43).[35]

PRIMARY TONSILLITIS

Primary tonsillitis denotes the lack of any predisposing factors for the inflammation. Small-breed dogs are the most commonly affected. Primary tonsillitis in dogs over 1 year is uncommon. Anorexia, lethargy, dysphagia, coughing, retching, and pyrexia may be the presenting complaints. The absence of tonsillar swelling does not preclude the diagnosis of tonsillitis, especially in cats. Pharyngitis may be noted. Clinical improvement, observed with systemic antibiotic therapy, generally precedes resolution of the inflammatory process, and tonsillar swelling may continue to be present. Recurrence is common, with exacerbations lasting several days. Tonsillectomy is rarely required in chronic primary tonsillitis unless the tonsillar enlargement significantly obstructs the pharynx or the dog is in poor health between acute exacerbations. Most dogs can be treated medically and appear to "outgrow" this problem. In chronic tonsillitis predisposing factors must be carefully ruled out.

SECONDARY TONSILLITIS

The inflammatory process of secondary tonsillitis can be attributed to systemic or local predisposing factors. The presence of tonsillitis does not indicate the site of primary pathology and should not be used as a "catch-all" diagnosis. Any chronic irritation or inflammatory process of the oral cavity or pharynx (e.g., abscesses, gingivitis, chronic oral foreign body, chronic vomiting, or regurgitation) may induce a lymphoreticular tonsillar reaction. The gagging, regurgitation, and vomiting of foam described by owners in cases of tonsillitis necessitates differentiation of megaesophagus, pylorospasm, cricopharyngeal achalasia, chronic

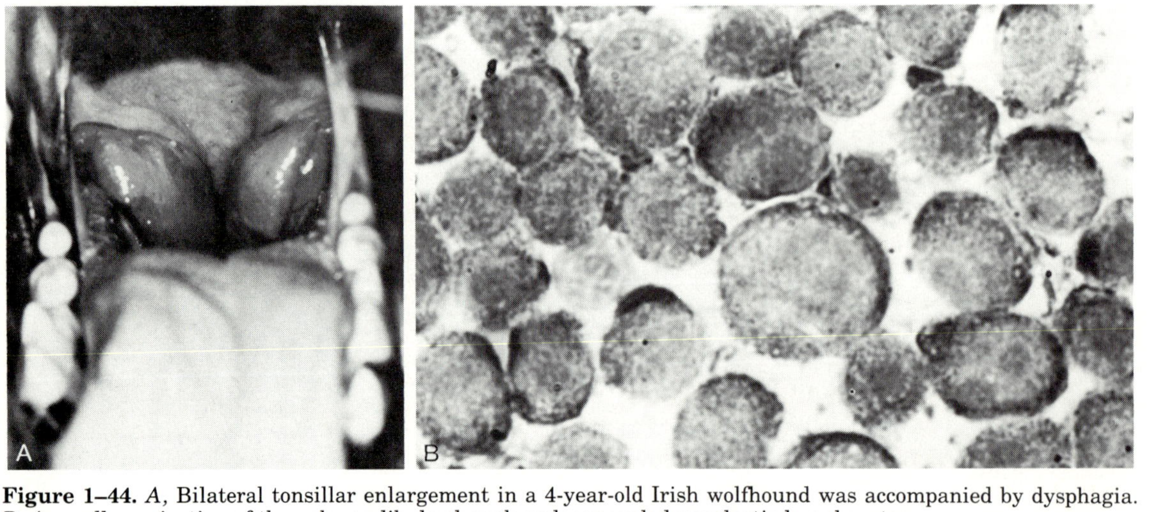

Figure 1–44. *A*, Bilateral tonsillar enlargement in a 4-year-old Irish wolfhound was accompanied by dysphagia. *B*, A needle aspiration of the submandibular lymph nodes revealed neoplastic lymphocytes.

productive cough, retropharyngeal abscesses, and foreign bodies.[28, 35]

Medical treatment of tonsillitis using systemic broad-spectrum antibiotics, supportive care, and occasionally analgesics is generally rewarding. Culture of inflamed tonsils may produce streptococci (beta-hemolytic), coliform bacteria, and normal oral flora. Tonsillectomy is usually not needed in the acute inflammatory stage.[28, 35]

Gross tonsillar enlargement may cause dysphagia in breeds that have a narrow oropharynx, such as cocker spaniels, and dyspnea in brachycephalic breeds that are predisposed to upper airway disease. Primary metastatic neoplasia should always be suspected in chronic tonsillitis. The predilection for squamous cell carcinomas to metastasize to regional lymph nodes and to be locally invasive dictates early diagnosis if extirpation is to be successful. Unlike squamous cell carcinomas, which are most commonly unilateral, lymphosarcoma usually occurs bilaterally, with enlargement of the retropharyngeal lymph nodes (Fig. 1–44).[17]

Oral and Pharyngeal Tumors

Oropharyngeal tumors, commonly encountered problems in clinical practice, compose 6.6 per cent of all neoplasms in dogs,[91] with 50 per cent occurring in dogs over 10 years old.[91, 118] German shepherds and cocker spaniels are breeds that are predisposed to oral neoplasia.[118] Excluding epulis and viral papilloma, 97 per cent of all oral and pharyngeal tumors are malignant. Oral tumors constitute 6.7 per cent of feline cancers; there is a greater incidence in animals over 10 years. Sixty-eight per cent of all feline oral tumors are malignant, and compared with other domestic cats, the Siamese has one-third the expected rate of occurrence.[15–17, 91]

Malignant melanoma, squamous cell carcinoma, and fibrosarcoma are the three most common oral neoplasms of the dog.[91, 118] Squamous cell carcinoma and fibrosarcoma are the most common neoplasms in the cat.[15–17] The areas most commonly involved in oropharyngeal neoplasms are the gingivae and the tonsils.[91, 118] The clinical signs are variable, depending on the size, nature, and duration of the tumor. Dysphagia and reluctance to eat are often the primary complaints. Pain is uncommon except when ulceration or bony involvement is present. Other signs include hypersalivation or drooling, a fetid odor from the mouth, hemorrhage, and loss of teeth. When swelling of the face or mouth is present, tumors must be differentiated from scar tissue, diseases of the salivary glands, abscesses, and encapsulated foreign bodies.[15–17]

Diagnosis is based on physical examination, exfoliative cytological studies, radiology, and histopathological studies. Exfoliative cytology or fine-needle biopsy aspirates may be diagnostic. Cytoplasmic granules of the malignant melanoma, if present, are classic (Fig. 1–45). Several areas should be carefully selected for scraping or biopsy so that neoplastic tissue rather than associated chronic inflammatory tissue is exfoliated. When the tumor can be totally removed,

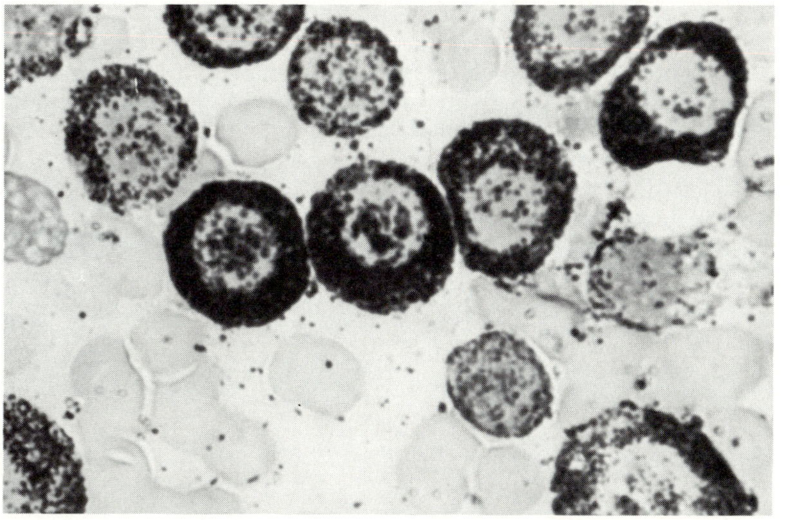

Figure 1–45. Melanoma can usually be diagnosed by cytological examination.

excisional biopsy is an excellent technique. Since malignant melanomas are common in the dog, incisional biopsy of this type of tumor is contraindicated. Before treatment is discussed with the client, thorough examination for metastasis to regional lymph nodes and lungs should be performed. Careful staging of oral tumors is important for predicting therapy, prognosis, and survival. If total resection is performed, the animal should be examined physically and radiographically for metastatic lesions every 3 months for the first year and biannually thereafter.

Radiation therapy is often a valuable therapeutic tool for oral and pharyngeal tumors. True cures are rare, but long periods of regression may occur. The radiosensitivity of tumors should be considered before an animal is referred for this treatment. A definitive diagnosis must be made before radiotherapy is instituted. At the present time, chemotherapeutic agents are not commonly used for oropharyngeal neoplasms. Most malignant oropharyngeal tumors metastasize via the lymphatics; rostral areas drain to the mandibular lymph nodes, which then drain with the lymphatics of the oral cavity and the pharynx into the lateral and medial pharyngeal lymph nodes.[87] Metastasis to the contralateral lymph nodes is not uncommon. Fibrosarcoma and osteosarcoma metastasize via the blood stream rather than through the lymphatics.

The prognosis for malignant oropharyngeal tumors is poor because most are characterized by early invasion of soft and bony tissues. With or without regional lymph node involvement or distant metastasis, a surgical cure is unlikely. Regional node metastasis is a poor prognostic sign, and rapid recurrence usually follows extirpation of the affected nodes. In spite of the poor prognosis, affected dogs and cats should be first diagnosed and then treated when possible. The client should not be automatically presented with euthanasia as the only option. Long-term remission and palliation have been observed in correctly managed oral neoplasias. The key to correct management of oral neoplasia starts with a definitive diagnosis.

ORAL PAPILLOMATOSIS

Papilloma is a common benign tumor caused by papillomavirus. Commonly occurring in young dogs with a mean age of 1 year, it reportedly may spread through kennels and dog colonies with an incubation period of approximately 1 month. Cats are considered nonsusceptible. The cauliflower-like growths begin as smooth cream-colored elevations, which later become rough and gray. Histologically, a thick squamous epithelium is noted covering branching cords of dermal papillae. The oral mucosa and commissures of the lips are most commonly affected, and involvement of deeper structures is uncommon. The number and size of lesions are variable. Although diagnosis is usually based on physical examination, a biopsy may be required on the very early lesions, which are not classic, or on the hyperpigmented, contracted lesion that forms during regression (6 to 12 weeks). Therapy is generally unnecessary because the lesion regresses spontaneously. Treatments include: (1) wart vaccine administered every 7 days until remission, (2) sodium bismuth tartrate applied topically, (3) cyclophosphamide*, 2 to 4 mg/kg once daily for 9 to 14 days with complete remission in 3 weeks.

Surgical excision of warts will produce hemorrhage. Excision may be a means of stimulating regression and eliminating confluent pedunculated masses, which impair prehension. The client should be advised as to its viral etiology and possible communicability to other dogs. Although the long-term prognosis is excellent and lifetime immunity generally follows recovery, repeated reoccurrences of the tumor and weight loss from impaired prehension may occur before permanent immunity develops.

EPULIDES

Epulis, the most common benign oral neoplasm, arises from the connective tissues of the periodontal membranes.[41] This origin differentiates epulides from odontogenic tumors.[38, 41] The three types of epulides are fibromatous, ossifying, and acanthomatous. The fibromatous epulis originates from periodontal ligament stroma. The ossifying epulis contains an osteoid matrix in the fibromatous stroma. The acanthomatous epulis contains sheets and cords of epithelial cells within the stroma. Acanthomatous epulides are differentiated from odontogenic tumors

*Cytoxan, Mead Johnson, Pharmaceutical Division, Evansville, IN.

by the absence of dental structures and enamel inclusions.[41] The confusion surrounding the differentiation of acanthomatous epulides from one odontogenic tumor, the ameloblastoma, has led to the recommendation that the term "adamantinoma," which was used to describe both of the tumors,[38] be omitted from descriptive terminology and classification.[38, 39, 41, 93]

The exact cause of epulis is unknown, but chronic inflammation and irritation has been considered to be the inciting factor. Affected dogs are generally over 6 years old, and multiple epulides were reported in 30 per cent of boxers over 5 years.[28] Although these tumors may have a very malignant gross appearance and occur in the location common for squamous cell carcinomas, they are generally solitary and non-invasive, except for the acanthomatous epulis, which invades bone (Fig. 1–46). Ulceration and bleeding are common, especially if the tumor has been manipulated. The teeth in the gingival margins may be displaced and mobile.

Therapy includes surgical removal, extraction of adjacent teeth, radiation,[117] hyperthermia, or cryotherapy.[93] Since all three types of tumors will recur if not successfully managed, evidence of bony involvement necessitates curettage, mandibulectomy, or partial maxillectomy.[93] Radiation therapy is very effective in treating epulides and is recommended after partial resection or recurrence of the tumors.[93, 117]

ODONTOGENIC TUMORS

The odontogenic tumor is rare in the dog;[59] it arises from the dental laminar epithelium (tissue that contains enamel inclusions, dental pulp, or dental structures), and deserves separate notation only because of a confusion in terminology (see "Epulides").[38] Odontogenic tumors have been classified as ameloblastomas, keratinizing ameloblastomas, ameloblastic fibrodontomas, compound odontomas, and complex odontomas.[38] The confusion arises because another system of classifying odontogenic tumors exists, terming them ameloblastomas (adamantinomas), calcifying epithelial odontogenic tumors, ameloblastic fibromas, odontoameloblastomas, complex odontomas, compound odontomas, myxomas, and primary intraosseous carcinomas.[59]

Ameloblastomas, the most common odontogenic tumor of dogs, must be differentiated from other tumors that have abundant epithelial cells, such as squamous cell carcinoma and acanthomatous epulis. Although these tumors grossly appear as gingival soft tissue tumors, osteolytic and osteoblastic reactions around loose or absent teeth are noted radiographically.[93]

Because the origin of the tumor is in bone, radical surgical excision (mandibulectomy or partial maxillectomy) offers the best chance for a cure, although intense cryotherapy may be effective. Confusion over classification of reported cases (ameloblas-

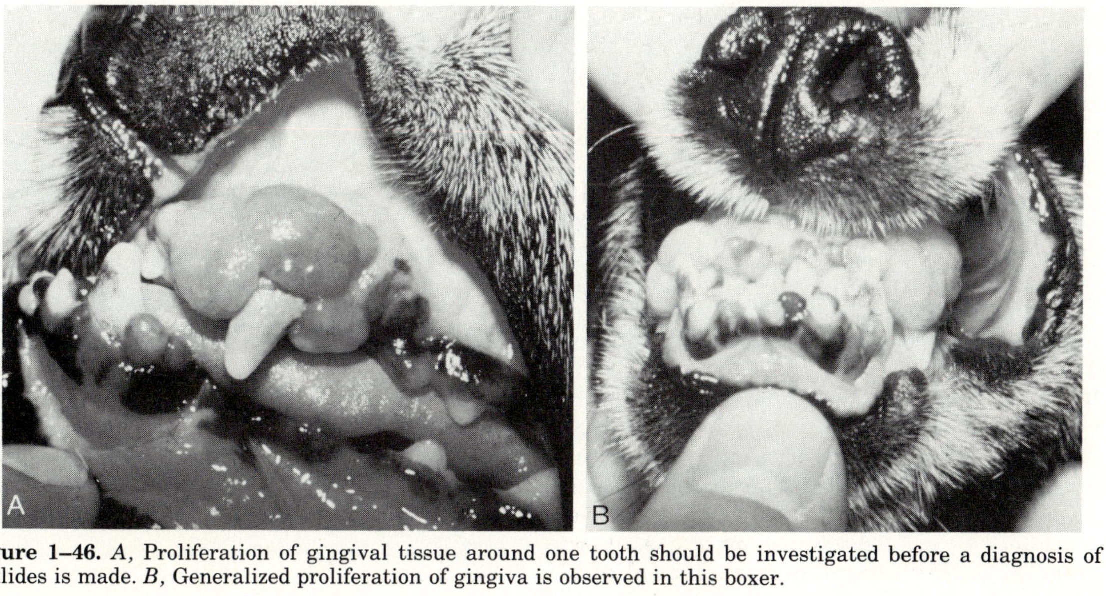

Figure 1–46. *A*, Proliferation of gingival tissue around one tooth should be investigated before a diagnosis of epulides is made. *B*, Generalized proliferation of gingiva is observed in this boxer.

tomas vs. acanthomatous epulides) has led many workers to question the good results reported with radiation therapy.[41, 75, 93]

MALIGNANT MELANOMA

Although it is a common canine oral malignancy,[91] malignant melanoma is extremely rare in the cat.[16] The tumor, which is more common in the male than in the female dog,[118] originates from melanocytes in the mucosal epithelium or the gingival stroma.[38] The average age of occurrence is 10 years.[118] The tumor is located in the following areas, listed in decreasing order of incidence: gingival tissues, mucosa, the palate, and sublingual areas.[122] Local invasion may loosen teeth. The gross appearance of malignant melanoma is variable and influenced by the amount of melanin produced.[122] Visualization of a rapidly growing, firm, ulcerated, non-pigmented (amelanotic) tumor does not preclude the diagnosis of melanoma. Owing to high incidence, a diagnosis of melanoma should always be considered if an oral tumor is present. Metastasis is often present before the primary oral tumor is detected. Sites for metastasis are regional lymph nodes, lungs, and, occasionally, abdominal viscera.[30, 118] Involved lymph nodes may be normal in size. Melanomas grow rapidly and will invade soft tissue and bone. Bone invasion was present radiographically in 8 of 14 cases, and 44 of 54 cases had metastasis beyond regional lymph nodes at necropsy.[118]

Diagnosis by fine-needle aspiration biopsy of the tumor is the best approach. It is a non-invasive technique and is highly diagnostic. An incisional biopsy has no advantages over an excisional biopsy. The classic pattern of dark, melanin pigments within the cytoplasm is not present, especially in the amelanotic state. In contrast, fine-needle aspiration biopsy of regional lymph nodes can produce a black fluid resembling motor oil because of the high production of melanin pigments. Nuclear pleomorphism and mitotic figures are commonly observed during cytological examination (see Fig. 1–46*B*). Metastasis occurs early, and the client should be advised of the poor prognosis. Tumor staging is conducted prior to client education and therapy. Treatment by surgical excision, radiation, cryotherapy, chemotherapy, and immunotherapy has been attempted.[4, 58, 93] Since radical surgical excision is often not possible and recurrence (20 of 23 cases) at the site is common,[118] mandibulectomies and partial maxillectomies have been recommended.[93] Electrocautery and cryotherapy combined with wide surgical excision may be effective in removing local neoplastic cells. The rationale for cryotherapy is the ability of this treatment to kill neoplastic cells in bone without removing the bony matrix, which should serve as an autograft.[122]

Although radiation therapy is considered to be only palliative, temporary remission and even cures have been reported with its use.[4] Chemotherapy with doxorubicin hydrochloride* and dacarbazine† and immunotherapy using Bacille Calmette Guerin‡ have been suggested but their effectiveness has not been proven.[93]

SQUAMOUS CELL CARCINOMA

Squamous cell carcinomas (SCC) are common in both dogs and cats.[91] The two most common sites in the dog are the gingiva and tonsils.[118] Gingival SCC is a grayish-white, nodular mass similar in appearance to granulomatous, ulcerated, or infected areas. (Fig. 1–47). Although local invasion is common, there is no osseous involvement initially. Despite radiographic evidence of osteolysis later in the disease (77 per cent),[118] metas-

---

*Adriamycin, Adria Laboratories, Inc., Dublin, OH.
†DTIC-Dome, Miles Pharmaceuticals, West Haven, CT.
‡BCG Vaccine, Glaxo, Inc., Ft. Lauderdale, FL.

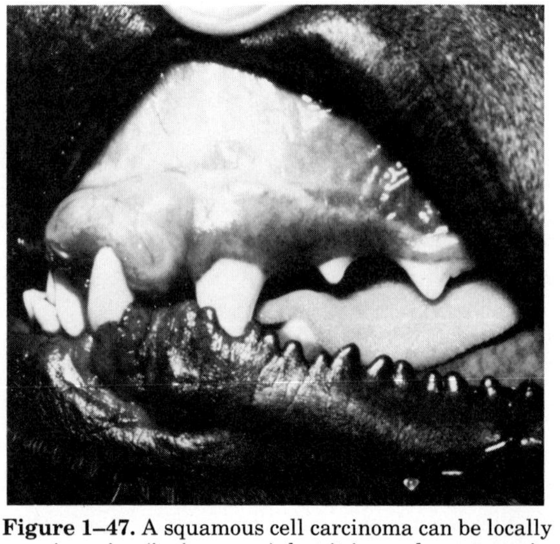

Figure 1–47. A squamous cell carcinoma can be locally very invasive (incisor area), but it is rarely metastatic.

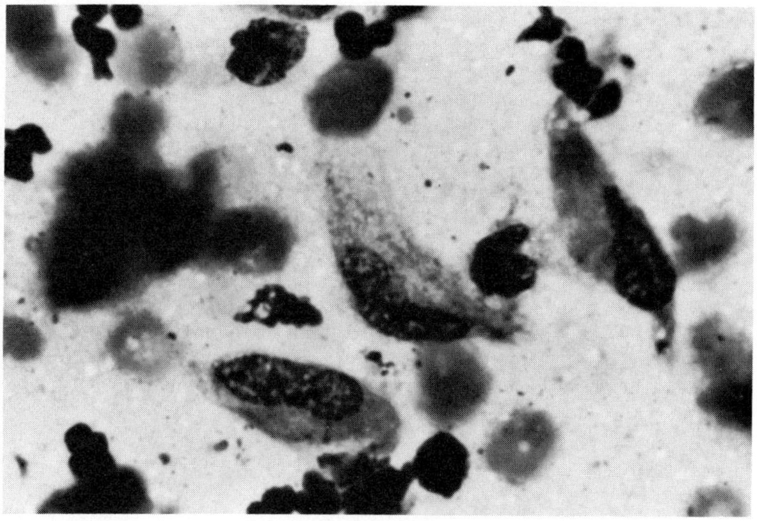

Figure 1–48. Spindle-shaped cells that were retrieved from an oral mass are characteristic of fibrosarcoma, but their presence does not confirm the diagnosis.

tasis to regional lymph nodes is rare (10 per cent).[93] Tonsillar SCCs are usually unilateral, diffuse, uniform firm masses. Metastasis to regional lymph nodes is common and may be the presenting sign.

In the cat, the gingiva and the tongue are most commonly involved.[17, 28, 91] Initially, the neoplasia may appear as any other feline oral ulcer, but it is not responsive to therapy. Impression smears and fine-needle aspiration biopsy are rarely productive, and positive diagnosis usually requires histopathological examination.

Tonsillar SCCs must be differentiated from tonsillitis and lymphosarcoma, which usually involve the tonsils and mandibular lymph nodes bilaterally. As with any other oral neoplasms, tumor staging through palpation, biopsy, blood chemistry measurements and radiographs is indicated before therapy is begun. Wide excision combined with radiation therapy has been recommended as a treatment of choice. The gingival SCCs can be highly invasive but are slow to metastasize. The more rostral the tumor, the better the prognosis.[93] However, the tonsillar SCCs should be considered already metastasized to the regional lymph nodes. A poor prognosis must be offered in canine tonsillar SCC. Because of the highly invasive nature of the tumor and the rapid metastasis, cats with squamous cell carcinomas have a poor prognosis.

Because gingival SCCs rarely metastasize, radiation therapy is often palliative, although the local tissue destruction can be severe. Cisplatin* chemotherapy has reportedly provided a transient, mild response.[93] Removal of regional lymph nodes is recommended if metastasis occurs.[93]

*Plantinol, Bristol Laboratories, Syracuse, NY.

FIBROSARCOMA

Fibrosarcoma is more common in large breeds of dogs, especially the German shepherd, and is found more commonly in males rather than females.[91, 93, 118] Grossly, fibrosarcomas are initially noted on the maxillary gingiva along the dental arcade especially between the canine and the fourth premolar or the hard palate.[122] The firm, fleshy color and slow growth of the tumor make it difficult to differentiate from

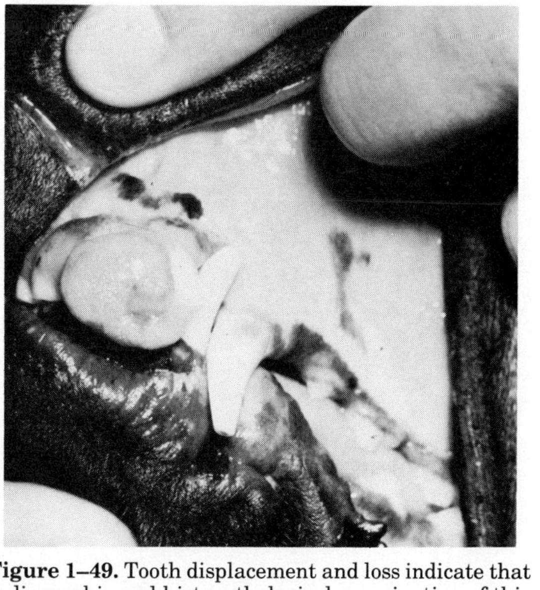

Figure 1–49. Tooth displacement and loss indicate that radiographic and histopathological examination of this tumor is necessary.

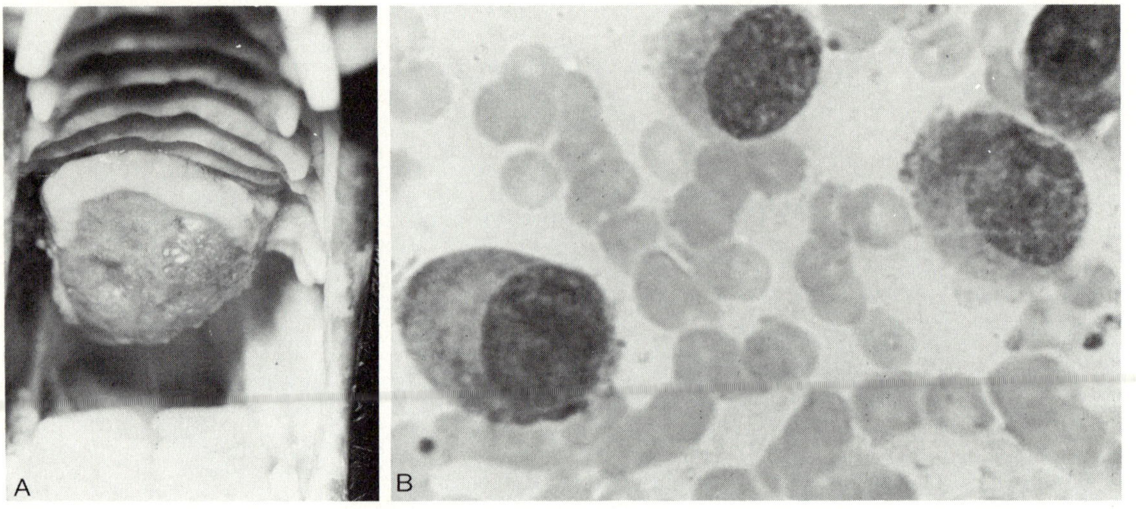

Figure 1–50. *A*, Radiography indicated that this mass on the hard palate was invading the bone. *B*, The cytologic diagnosis of osteogenic sarcoma was confirmed by histopathological examination.

chronic scar tissue or gingival hyperplasia. Infiltration of soft tissue and bone with ulcerations and secondary infections may be noted.

The histological typing of this tumor is controversial. The "true" fibrosarcoma is generally considered to be a circumscribed, infiltrating tumor composed of collagen and reticular fibers with spindle-shaped or stellate tumor cells that are irregularly arranged. Another type, defined as a neurofibrosarcoma, is composed of spindle-shaped cells arranged in interlacing bundles in a herringbone pattern. Regardless of the tumor type, the prognosis is poor because of local invasiveness and common recurrence.[118]

Excisional or fine-needle aspiration biopsy is usually diagnostic (Fig. 1–48). Excision of the tumor is the treatment of choice. Extensive local infiltration often prevents removal of the tumor, bony involvement is common, and metastases were noted in about one-third of cases at necropsy.[118] Although fibrosarcomas are weakly radiosensitive, radiation therapy can provide palliation for 6 months to 1 year.[4, 116] Chemotherapy and immunotherapy have not been successful.[122]

OTHER OROPHARYNGEAL TUMORS

Other oropharyngeal tumors, which do not commonly occur, are malignant lymphosarcoma, adenocarcinoma, odontogenic tu-

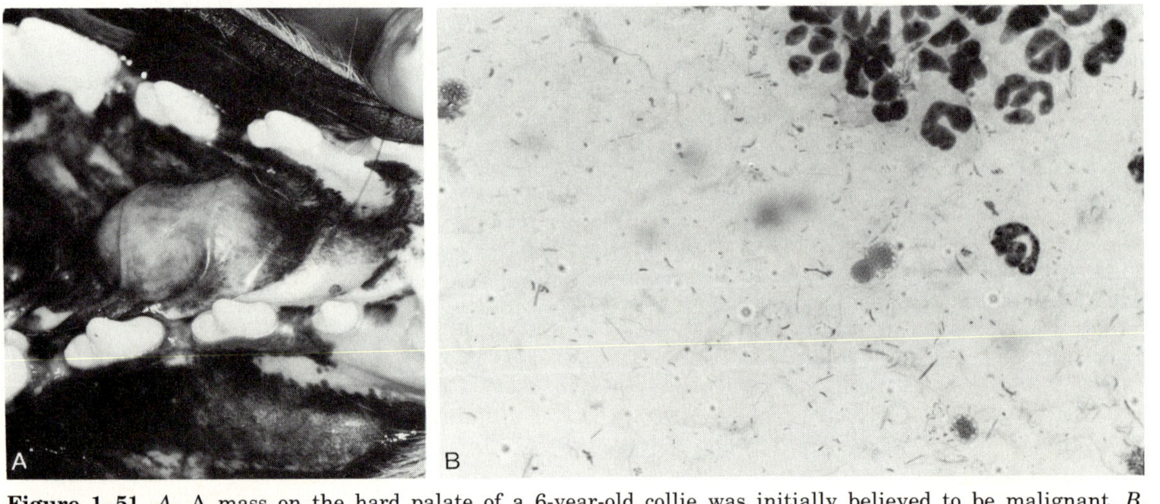

Figure 1–51. *A*, A mass on the hard palate of a 6-year-old collie was initially believed to be malignant. *B*, Cytological examination of the oral mass revealed purulent inflammation and bacteria.

mor (Fig. 1–49), transmissible venereal tumor, basal cell carcinoma, and mast cell tumor.[118, 122] Osteosarcomas generally arise from the mandible or maxilla and rapidly metastasize to the lungs. A common site for this tumor is the hard palate (Fig. 1–50). Adenocarcinomas generally arise from the salivary glands and occur more commonly in cats than dogs. Adenocarcinoma of the nasal cavity may penetrate the hard palate and produce an oronasal fistula. Uniquely, these are very invasive tumors that rarely metastasize. Basal cell carcinomas involving the lip, are more common in older cats. Although they are not an intra-oral tumors, invasion of the oral cavity may be present. These tumors generally respond well to excision, and recurrence is uncommon. Compared with their incidence on the skin, mast cell tumors are uncommon in the mouth. Involvement of the oral mucosa of the upper lip is most commonly found in boxers, bull terriers, and bulldogs. Wide surgical excision is difficult, and recurrence is very common. Any tumor involving the nasal cavity may invade the oral cavity (Fig. 1–51). Therefore, careful examination of the nasal cavity and turbinates is important in any radiographic examination of problems.

Prehensile Dysfunction

Anorexia may be related to an inability to open the jaws or to pain on opening the mouth. The differential diagnosis should include retrobulbar abscess, abscess of the zygomatic gland, oral foreign bodies, inflammatory myositis, myofascitis, fractures of the mandible or maxilla, dislocation or arthritis of the temporomandibular joint, cranial mandibular osteoarthropathy, and trauma to soft tissue or periosteum. Pain on opening the mouth concomitant with pyrexia and exophthalmos is an indication for examination for retrobulbar abscess, either secondary to a penetrating foreign body or due to sialadenitis of the zygomatic salivary gland. Careful examination under sedation may demonstrate inflammation of the oral tissue posterior to the last upper molar, with a focal area of inflammation or edema (Fig. 1–52). Draining the abscess through an incision in this area combined with 14 days of systemic antibiotics is an effective treatment. Adequate drainage is important.

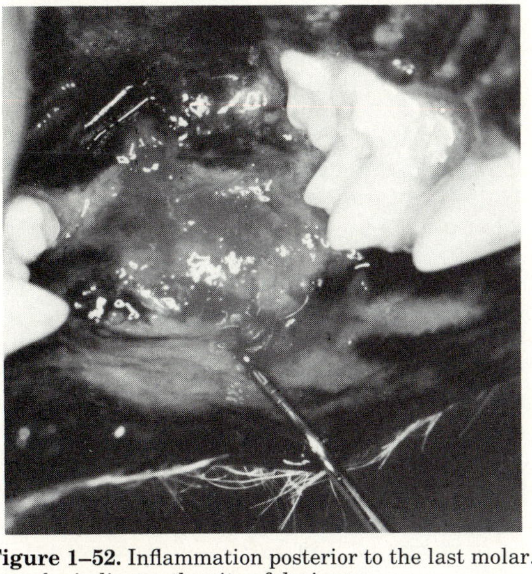

Figure 1–52. Inflammation posterior to the last molar. A probe indicates the site of drainage.

Other conditions may manifest with pyrexia that is due to pain and inflammation. Eosinophilic myositis occurs in larger breeds of dogs such as the German shepherd, and extreme pain is a classic sign in the acute syndrome. Pain is absent when fibrosis is a sequela to repeated bouts. Bilaterally symmetrical swelling of the masseter, temporalis, and pterygoid muscles is the clinical appearance, although other skeletal musculature may also be involved. Exophthalmos may lead to exposure keratitis. An absolute eosinophilia may be present, but a normal hemogram does not preclude the diagnosis of eosinophilic myositis. Electromyographic studies demonstrate positive sharp waves with fibrillation potentials. Muscle biopsy is necessary for a definitive diagnosis of eosinophilic myositis. Histologically, mononuclear cells, hemorrhage, and muscle fiber necrosis are noted. Treatment is supportive therapy and corticosteroids to allow the animal to maintain an adequate caloric intake until mastication is normal. Inability to open the mouth occurs in recurrent or chronic cases in which atrophy and fibrosis have resulted. This condition may be unilateral and must be differentiated from acute trauma. Electromyographic studies after acute trauma are generally normal; however, if atrophy is severe or if fibrosis has occurred, a decrease in insertion potential is noted. Included in the differential diagnosis should be denervation atrophy, and an electromyographical examination 7 to 10 days after the insult will reveal denervation changes such as fibrillation potentials. In acute trauma, corticosteroid therapy, rest, tube feeding, or feeding through an esophagostomy tube is indicated.

Myofascitis has been noted in several young dogs that exhibited extreme pain. As in any myositic condition, fibrosis may restrict opening of the mouth. Generally in myofascitis, a mild or moderate attack is noted at 8 to 12 months of age and may last from several days to 2 weeks. The attacks occur with regular frequency until the animals are 1½ to 2 years old. The symptoms are responsive to corticosteroid therapy. As the dog matures, the attacks decrease in intensity and duration until the animal becomes asymptomatic. Repeated attacks that are not treated or that are overlooked may result in permanent fibrosis.

Regardless of the etiology of myositis, atrophy of the musculature of the head and masseter muscles are common sequelae. Common presenting signs include weight loss, the observation that the dog is chewing bones with its front teeth only, or the inability to open the mouth wide enough to eat or catch a ball or a stick. Any breed of dog may be affected. Partial or complete inability to open the mouth even under general anesthesia indicates myositis. This condition may be unilateral or bilateral. Unilateral disuse atrophy has been noted with inflammation and fibrosis present on the other side. Electromyographically, the abnormal side demonstrates increased insertional activity, positive sharp waves, fibrillation potentials, and myopathic potentials. Later, large muscles may have decreased insertional potentials or electrical silence, which is indicative of fibrosis. Several muscle biopsies are needed to demonstrate the pathological condition, which is a mixture of fibrosis, lymphocytic infiltration, and adipose tissue deposition. When severe myositis is found, the client should be informed of a poor prognosis. Mechanical methods for opening the mouth and trying to break down fibrotic tissue are not recommended. The resulting trauma and muscle tearing may only aggravate the fibrosis. Corticosteroids and emphasis on jaw exercise by the dog are important. The client should be encouragd to make the dog chew in an effort to decrease the atrophy and keep the fibrosis at a minimum. Inability to open the mouth as a sequela always indicates a poor prognosis.

Fractures of the mandible or temporomandibular joint often induce pain on manipulation of the jaws. Crepitation localized to the temporomandibular joint on opening of the jaw may be noted only after anesthesia. Radiographs are necessary to differentiate fractures from luxation.[115] Myositis and inability to open the mouth must be differentiated from masseter muscle atrophy secondary to arthritis of the temporomandibular joint. Temporomandibular luxation, in the absence of any fractures, is reduced with the aid of a 1.5 cm piece of wood placed between the last molars on the affected side. The wood should be used as a fulcrum while the mandibular symphysis and nose are pushed together, elevating the temporomandibular joint into reduction.[70,112] It should be emphasized that this technique is performed only in the confirmed absence of fractures of the oral structures. Luxation of the mandible with locking of the coronoid process lateral to the zygomatic arch can occur in the dog when the mouth is opened fully.[95]

Craniomandibular osteoarthropathy may manifest as an inability to open the mouth. This periosteal exostosis is classically observed in young West Highland white and Scottish terriers. Although other breeds are affected, the age, breed, and clinical presentation make diagnosis obvious. Although it is generally considered to be a self-limiting disease, supportive therapy is often needed to maintain proper nutrition. An esophagostomy tube is rarely needed.

Other conditions that may manifest with pain on opening the jaws include oral foreign bodies, acute stomatitis, and insect bites of the oral mucous membranes. If adequate examination cannot be performed, general anesthesia or sedation is indicated to facilitate a thorough oral examination.

Swelling below the eye is commonly associated with some conditions of the upper fourth premolar. (See Figs. 1–32 and 1–33.) This syndrome can be produced by a variety of other causes, and simple removal of the upper fourth premolar does not always effect a cure.[62] When the buccal roots of the upper fourth premolar are affected, the condition generally causes alveolar periostitis with drainage through the buccal cortical bone. When the lingual roots of the upper fourth premolar, the distal roots of the third premolar, or the mesial root of the first molar are involved, drainage is frequently through the maxillary sinus and may produce swelling but rarely fistular drainage. The maxillary sinus is the lateral diverticulum of the nasal fossa, which lies transversely near the rostral roots of the upper carnassial tooth. The maxillary sinus may become infected from several non-dental causes. Involvement of the zygomatic salivary gland and abscesses of soft tissues may produce a swelling in the same area.[28] Furthermore, swelling below the eye can be associated with abscesses and fistulae of the nasolacrimal system.[35] When swelling is noted, a careful examination of the teeth, periodontal tissue, and glands in this area is required. Special care should be used to check for periodontal pockets at the area of bifurcation of the upper fourth premolar. Drainage may be induced by directing a pin or probe into the sinus from between the buccal root of the fourth premolar. Long-term systemic antibiotic therapy is indicated, and bactericidal antibiotics should be instilled into the sinus.

Salivary Glands

FUNCTION

The role of saliva is complex and often overlooked. The functions of saliva include:

1. Digesting. Alpha amylase breaks down the alpha 1–4 linkage of starch. This role is not as important in digestion as in the liquefaction and removal of retained starch from the mouth.
2. Cleansing. Saliva, which is composed primarily of water, literally washes exposed tooth surfaces.
3. Destroying bacteria. Specific and non-specific factors that affect the bacterial flora, such as lysozymes, salivary agglutinating factors, antibodies, and leukocytes, are present in saliva.
4. Buffering. The pH of saliva contributes to the bicarbonate pool of the body and buffers the ingesta.
5. Lubricating. The passage of food to the stomach is aided by lubrication by the saliva.
6. Maturing teeth. The enamel surfaces of the newly erupted teeth are more permeable to ionic penetration than they are several months after eruption. The exchange of minerals between saliva and tooth surfaces results in increased surface hardening and decreased permeability.

The salivary glands of the dog and cat can be divided into two types, mucous and serous, on the basis of the consistency of their secretions. The triangular parotid salivary gland, the only serous gland, is multi-lobed. Connective tissue firmly attaches it to the cranial and caudal portions of the ear canal. The superficial temporal and maxillary arteries are associated with it medially. The palpebral, the auriculotemporal, and the dorsal and the ventral buccal nerves emerge from the cranial border of the gland. The smaller and more loosely attached parotid lymph node is easily distinguished from the gland. The parotid duct exits the gland as one or two radicles, which unite to course across the buccal surface of the masseter muscle between branches of the facial nerve, and enter the mouth as the parotid papilla on the oral surface opposite the upper fourth premolar. Accessory parotid glands (about 1 cm in diameter) may enter the duct anywhere along its surface.

The mandibular, sublingual, and zygomatic salivary glands are mixed glands that secrete both mucous and serous fluids. The mandibular gland is a large gland surrounded by a capsule; and it is deeper than and ventral to the parotid gland. It lies between the maxillary and facial veins, caudal and ventral to the parotid gland. The mandibular duct courses dorsal to the digastricus along the floor of the mouth and opens with the sublingual duct into the sublingual caruncle on the frenulum. The caudal portion of the sublingual gland is enclosed within the same fibrous capsule as the mandibular salivary gland. The cranial portion of the sublingual gland is a loose collection of lobules that course with the mandibular and sublingual ducts. The polystomatic portion of the sublingual gland consists of multiple radicles that open directly into the floor of the oral cavity. The zygomatic gland lies on the ventrocaudal floor of the orbit within a connective tissue capsule medial to the zygomatic arch. The gland is deep to the mucous membranes of the roof of the mouth just posterior to the last upper molar tooth. The duct opens in the buccal cavity through a papilla opposite the last upper molar.

Many other smaller glands are embedded within the oral mucosa and empty directly into the oral cavity via short ducts. These small papilla may be observed paralleling the lower dental arcade. The sympathetic innervation of the salivary glands, accompanies the arterial branches; the parasympathetic innervation is via the facial and glossopharyngeal nerves.[28, 55, 72, 73]

Only the parotid and mandibular glands can normally be palpated. Fine-needle aspiration biopsy can readily differentiate questionable masses.

DISEASES OF SALIVARY GLANDS

Common signs of salivary gland disease include drooling or sialozemia. The signs are generally related to oral lesions, dysphagia , or excessive parasympathetic stimulation. Excessive drooling has been reported with parotid gland hyperplasia and hypersialosis[6, 56] and with mandibular gland infarction.[68, 69] Xerostomia is rarely encountered, since simultaneous impairment of all salivary glands would be unusual. Decreased saliva production has been encountered following extensive radiation therapy for oral or nasal tumors. Sialadenitis is rare in the dog and cat, except when it occurs in association with infection of the zygomatic salivary gland. Deviation of the eye may be noted if the zygomatic glands are enlarged. Exudate is infrequently observed in infection of salivary glands. Abscess of the zygomatic salivary gland may cause exophthalmos, pyrexia, and pain on manipulation of the jaws. Thus, the condition mimics retrobulbar abscess. An abscessed gland may be drained into the oral cavity posterior to the last upper molar, through a hole in the mucous membranes.[70–73]

Salivary Mucocele

A salivary mucocele is a collection of saliva in tissue. The mucocele is not lined with epithelium, and thus, the term "cyst" is not appropriate. Because the secretions of glands are not entirely mucous, the terms sialoceles and salivary pseudocysts are advocated. Mucocele formation most commonly involves the sublingual and mandibular glands. The differential diagnosis should include abscesses, foreign bodies, lymph node involvement (e.g., benign hyperplasia, primary neoplasm, or metastatic neoplasm), and tumors of the skin, thyroid gland, carotid body, or branchial cyst.[71]

The pathophysiology is related to blockage of the duct or rupture of the gland, which results in extravasation of saliva into the connective tissues. Causes include lacerations, bites, blunt trauma, surgical and dental procedures in the area of the glands or ducts, and abscesses of the upper fourth premolar, especially if the parotid gland is involved. The saliva may gravitate to the sublingual area, intermandibular space, cervical area, mediastinum, or, uncommonly, the parapharyngeal area. Swelling may develop acutely, but sialocele is generally a slowly developing, fluctuant sac. Occurrence of the sialocele beneath the mucosa of the oral cavity is termed a ranula. The saliva appears to be non-irritating, since the wall of the sialocele is generally thin. Well-vascularized connective tissue is present especially in cases that have been unsuccessfully treated.

The cause of the sialocele is rarely discovered, and the duct of the gland is usually patent. Rarely, a sublingual foreign body or abscess may be identified. Blunt trauma rupturing the connective tissue capsule of the gland may be an etiological factor. Any age, breed, or sex of dog can be affected,

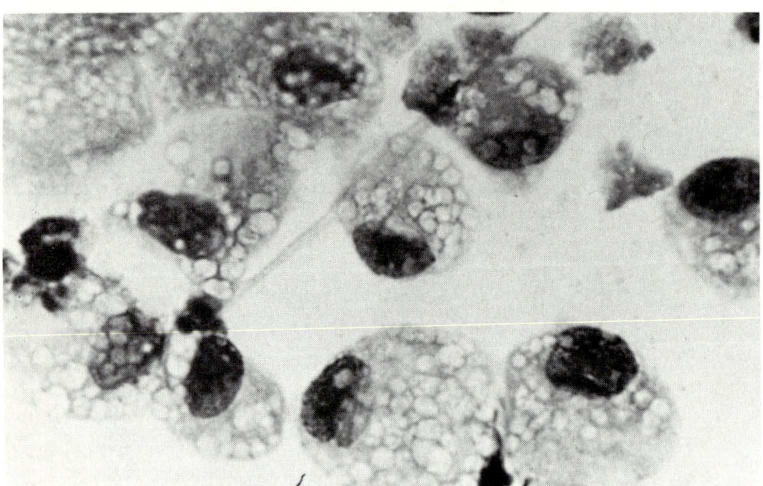

Figure 1–53. A specimen obtained by aspiration biopsy of a normal salivary gland will help differentiate types of masses.

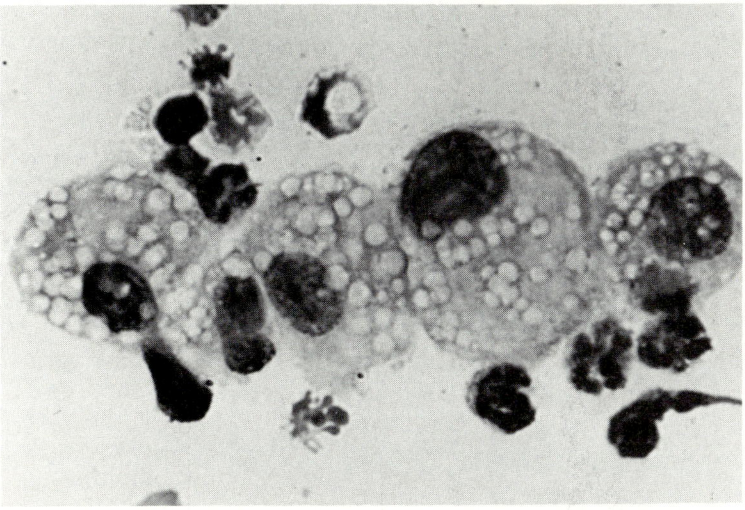

Figure 1–54. Cytological examination of swellings from salivary mucoceles will reveal polymorphonuclear leukocytes and red blood cells with saliva.

although the poodle and German shepherd are reported as having an increased incidence.[55–57, 70–73]

The diagnosis of sialocele is not always obvious. In chronic cases, needle aspiration will yield a viscous, mucoid fluid with small calculi. The fluid is generally clear or brown, but hemorrhage and exudate will develop after excessive manipulation or infection. Cytological evaluation is helpful in identification of salivary tissue (Fig. 1–53). Function tests for the production of saliva and chemical tests of the fluid are not discriminatory. The presence of calculi can be confused with the presence of granulomas of bacterial origin. Calculi of sialoceles are composed of non-degenerative neutrophils (Fig. 1 54). The injection of water-soluble contrast medium through the ducts may help to identify the affected gland, but a careful physical examination provides more reliable information.[55]

A sialocele in the pharyngeal area may produce dysphagia or dyspnea and may mimic diffuse cellulitis. A mandibular mucocele rarely may have an acute onset and be painful. The insidious onset of a nonpainful mass is more common (Fig. 1–55). Early swelling is usually ipsilateral. The fluid may be gently compressed back around the affected gland. Localization of the side and gland affected is more difficult in chronic cases and in cases in which prior surgical drainage has been attempted. Contrast sialography may be indicated if the affected gland cannot be identified. Lancing and probing of the cyst to explore possible tracts is not recommended, since this procedure ruptures the cyst and complicates surgery.[71]

TREATMENT

Various treatments of sialoceles have been advocated, such as aspiration biopsy, marsupialization, and excision.[28, 55–57, 70–73]

Aspiration of the fluid generally gives only temporary relief. The mucoceles usually reappear, unless scarring of the affected duct or gland or atrophy of the secretory capacity of the gland has occurred. The sial-

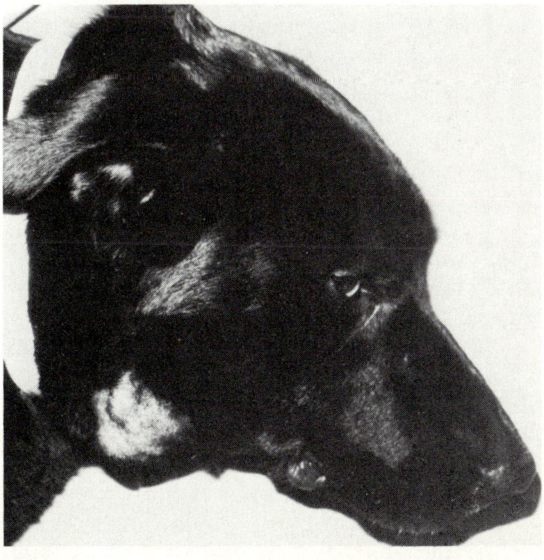

Figure 1–55. In a long-haired or an obese dog, a salivary mucocele can be an incidental finding on routine physical. The hair was clipped for needle aspiration biopsy.

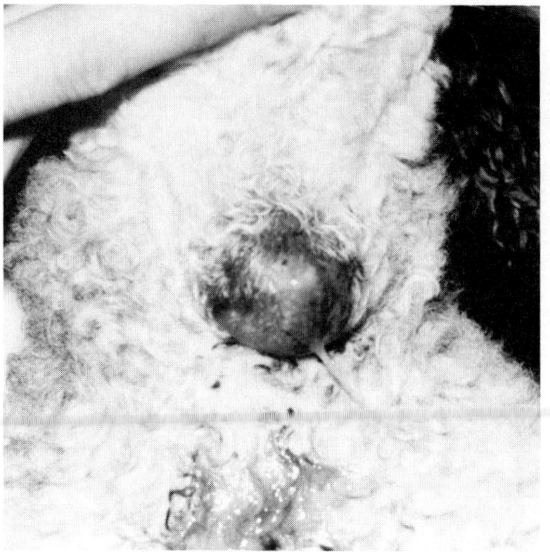

Figure. 1–56. Marsupialization of cervical mucoceles will provide an esthetically unpleasing cure.

ocele will require repeated aspiration at 3 to 4 month intervals; however, sialoceles can recur as soon as 1 week after aspiration. If aspiration is performed, as in geriatric patients, the client must be advised of the potential for self-inflicted trauma, dysphagia, and dyspnea. Aspiration is an important emergency procedure in the dyspneic animal with a pharyngeal mass and will help differentiate sialoceles from retropharyngeal lymph nodes, abscesses, masses of the thyroid gland, and brachial cleft cysts.

Marsupialization, or creation of a fistula from the cyst to the body surface, has been used with varying degrees of success. Removal of an elliptical portion of the wall of a ranula will allow direct drainage of saliva into the oral cavity. Rarely is the fistula permanent. In the absence of an epithelial lining, no advantage is gained by suturing the inner lining of the sialocele to the oral mucosa. Marsupialization of cervical sialoceles should not be attempted, since the pouch may become infected and is unsightly (Fig. 1–56).

Total excision of the affected gland and drainage of the mucocele provides the only permanent therapy. Although the sublingual gland is most commonly affected, the close apposition and common course of the ducts dictate the removal of both the mandibular and sublingual glands. The surgical technique has been described.[48] Dissection of the non-epithelial lined mucocele is unnecessary. Portions of the salivary gland not removed but isolated by surgery may lead to recurrence. Penrose drains will aid drainage of the postoperative fluctuant swelling, which is indicative of the presence of serum and blood in the soft tissue dead spaces. If sialoceles reappear, sialography may locate residual glandular tissue or the involvement of a different salivary gland. The prognosis after surgery is good, if the operation is performed correctly. Surgical trauma to the hypoglossal nerves can cause transient dysphagia. The lingual branches of the facial and glossopharyngeal nerves may also be damaged.

Salivary cysts are rare in the cat. Surgical correction by removal of the mandibular and sublingual salivary glands is successful. Swellings in the mandibular area are more commonly related to cellulitis or abscesses. Aspiration or needle biopsy will confirm the diagnosis.[55]

ACKNOWLEDGEMENT. The author wishes to thank individuals in the departments of Radiology, Small Animal Medicine & Surgery, and Learning Resources for their aid in the preparation of illustrations and this manuscript.

References

1. Andrews AH: A case of partial anodontia in a dog. Vet Rec 90:144, 1972.
2. Arnall L: Some aspects of dental development in the dog. Some common variations in the dentitions. J Small Anim Pract 2:195, 1961.
3. Attstrom R, Laurel AB, Lahsson U, Sjoholm A: Complement factors in gingival crevice material from healthy and inflamed gingiva in humans. J Periodont Res 10:19, 1975.
4. Bank WC, Morris E: Results of radiation treatment of naturally occurring animal tumors. J Am Vet Med Assoc 166:1063, 1975.
5. Barrett RE, Post JE, Schultz RD: Chronic relapsing stomatitis in a cat associated with feline leukemic virus infection. Feline Pract 5:34, 1975.
6. Bedford PGC: Unilateral parotid hypersialation in a dachshund. Vet Rec 107:557, 1980.
7. Bedford PGC: A repair technique for dental abrasion in the dog. Vet Rec 101:327, 1977.
8. Beitman R, Frost SS, Roth JLA: Oral manifestations of gastrointestinal disease. Dig Dis Sci 26:741, 1981.
9. Bell AF: Dental disease in the dog. J Small Anim Pract 6:421, 1965.
10. Bennett D, Lauder JM, Kirkham D: Bullous autoimmune skin disease in dog. 1. Clinical and pathological assessment. 2. Immunopathological assessment. Vet Rec 106:497, 523, 1980.
11. Bennett L, Law D: Incorporation of tetracycline in developing dog enamel and dentin. J Dent Res 44:788, 1965.

12. Berman E: The time and pattern of eruption of the permanent teeth of the cat. Lab Anim Sci 24:929, 1974.
13. Black AP, Crichlow AM, and Saunders JR: Bacteremia during ultrasonic teeth cleaning and extraction in the dog. J Am Anim Hosp Assoc 16:611, 1980.
14. Brewer WD, Turrel JM: Radiotherapy and hyperthermia in the treatment of fibrosarcomas in the dog. J Am Vet Med Assoc 181:146, 1982.
15. Brodey RS: The biological behavior of canine oral and pharyngeal neoplasms. J Small Anim Pract 11:45, 1970.
16. Brodey, RS: Canine and feline neoplasia. Adv Vet Sci Comp Med 14:309, 1970.
17. Brodey RS: A clinical and pathologic study of 130 neoplasms of the mouth and pharynx of the dog. Am J Vet Res 27:787, 1960.
18. Brown NO, Hurvitz AI: A mucocutaneous disease in cat resembling human pemphigus. J Am Anim Hosp Assoc 15:25, 1979.
19. Burwasser P, Hill IJ: The effect of hard and soft diets on the gingival tissues of dogs. J Dent Res 18:389, 1939.
20. Buyukmihci N, Rubin LF, Harvey CE: Exophthalmos secondary to zygomatic adenocarcinoma in a dog. J Am Vet Med Assoc 167:162, 1975.
21. Carlson J, Egelberg J: Local effect of diet on plaque formation and development of gingivitis in dogs. 2. Effect of high carbohydrate versus high protein-fat diets. Odont Rev 16:42, 1965.
22. Cechner PE: Malocclusion in the dog caused by intramedullary pin fixation of mandibular fractures: Two case reports. J Am Anim Hosp Assoc 16:79, 1980.
23. Chandler EA: Mumps in the dog. Vet Rec 96:365, 1975.
24. Chastain CB: Actinomycotic periodontitis. J Am Anim Hosp Assoc 13:65, 1977.
25. Cheville NF: The gray collie syndrome. J Am Vet Med Assoc 152:6, 1968.
26. Cianco SG: Chemotherapeutics in periodontics. Dent Clin North Am 24:813, 1980.
27. Clagett JA, Page RC: Insoluble immune complexes and chronic periodontal disease in man and the dog. Arch Oral Biol 23:153, 1978.
28. Clifford DH, Clark JJ: Mouth, lips and tongue. *In* Archibald J (ed): *Canine Surgery*. American Veterinary Publications Inc., Santa Barbara, 1965.
29. Cohen L: Ulcerative lesions of the oral cavity. Int J Dermatol 19:362, 1980.
30. Conrad FG: Treatment of malignant melanoma. Arch Surg 104:587, 1972.
31. Craig RG, O'Brien WJ, Powere JM: *Dental Materials: Properties & Manipulation,* 2nd ed. C. V. Mosby Company, St. Louis, 1979.
32. Davis RM, Jensen SG, Rindon-Schitt C, Loe JJ: The effect of topical chlorhexidine on the bacterial colonization of the teeth and gingiva. J Periodon Res 5:96, 1970.
33. Dietrich U: Dental care: Prophylaxis and therapy. Canine Pract 3:44, 1976.
34. DeYoung DW, Kealy JK, Khige JP: Attempts to produce salivary cysts in the dog. Am J Vet Res 39:185, 1978.
35. Dillon AR: The oral cavity. *In* Kirk RW (ed): *Current Veterinary Therapy VII*. W. B. Saunders Company, Philadelphia, 855, 1980.
36. Dorn CR, Priester WA: Epidemiologic analysis of oral and pharyngeal cancer in dogs, cats, horses and cattle. J Am Vet Med Assoc 169:1202, 1976.
37. Douglas AW, Kelly DF: Calcinosis circumscripta of the tongue. J Small Anim Pract 7:441, 1966.
38. Dubielzig RR: Proliferative dental and gingival diseases of dogs and cats. J Am Anim Hosp Assoc 18:577, 1982.
39. Dubielzig RR, et al: The nomenclature of periodontal epulides in dogs. Vet Pathol 19:596, 1982.
40. Dubielzig RR: The effect of canine distemper virus on ameloblastic layer of the developing tooth. Vet Pathol 16:268, 1979.
41. Dubielzig RR, Goldschmidt MT, and Brodey RS: The nomenclature of periodontal epulides in dogs. Vet Pathol 16:209, 1979.
42. Egelberg J: Local effect of diet on plaque formation and development of gingivitis in dogs. I. Effect of hard and soft diets. Ondont Rev 16:31, 1965.
43. Egelberg J: Local effect of diet on plaque formation and development of gingivitis in dogs. III. Effect of frequency of meals and tube feeding. Odont Rev 16:50, 1965.
44. Elzay RP, Hughes RD: Anodontia in a cat. J Am Vet Med Assoc 154:667, 1969.
45. Firth LK: Dental care. *In* Kirk RW (ed): *Current Veterinary Therapy VI,* W. B. Saunders Company, Philadelphia, 718, 1974.
46. Gad F: Periodontal disease in dogs. I. Clinical investigation. J Periodont Res 3:268, 1968.
47. Gaskell RM, Gruffydd-Jones TJ: Intractable feline stomatitis. Vet Ann 17:195, 1975.
48. Glen JB: Canine salivary mucoceles: Results of sialographic examination and surgical treatment of 50 cases. J Small Anim Pract 13:515, 1972.
49. Golden A, Harvey CE, Stoller NH: A survey of oral health in small animals. J Am Anim Hosp Assoc 187:891, 1982.
50. Griffin CE, Stannard AA, Irke PJ: Canine discoid lupus erythematosus. Vet Immunol Immunopathol 1:79, 1969.
51. Grove TK: Periodontal disease. Comp Cont Ed 4:564, 1982.
52. Halliwell REW: Skin diseases associated with autoimmunity. Vet Clin North Am (Small Anim Pract) 9:57, 1979.
53. Hamp SE: Prevalence of periodontal disease in the dog. I. Clinical and roentgenographical observations. (Abst) L.A.D.R. 119, 1975.
54. Hamp SE, Lindhe J, Loe H: Long-term effect of chlorhexidine on developing gingivitis in the beagle dog. J Periodont Res 8:63, 1973.
55. Harvey CE, O'Brien JA, Rossman L, and Stoller NH: Oral, dental, pharyngeal and salivary gland disease. *In* Ettinger SJ (ed). *Textbook of Veterinary Internal Medicine,* 2nd ed. W. B. Saunders Company, Philadelphia, 1982.
56. Harvey CE: Hypersialosis and parotid gland enlargement in a dog. J Small Anim Pract 22:19, 1981.
57. Harvey CE: Parotid salivary duct rupture and fistula in the dog and cat. J Small Anim Pract 18:163, 1977.
58. Harvey JH: Prognostic criteria for dogs with oral melanoma. J Am Vet Med Assoc 178:580, 1981.
59. Head, KW: Tumors of the upper alimentary tract. Bull WHO 53:145, 1976.
60. Heigl L, Lindhe J: The effect of metronidazole on the development of plaque and gingivitis in the beagle dog. J Clin Periodont 6:197, 1979.
61. Hill PS, Davies RM: The effect of chlorhexidine gel on tooth deposits in beagle dog. J Small Anim Prac 13:207, 1972.

62. Holmberg DC: Abscessation of the mandibular carnassial tooth in the dog. J Am Vet Med Assoc 15:347, 1979.
63. Howard DR, Merkley DR, Lammerding JJ, et al: Primary cleft palate (harelip) and closure repair in puppies. J Am Anim Hosp Assoc 12:636, 1976.
64. Hull PS, Soames JV, Davies RM: Periodontal disease in a beagle dog colony. J Comp Pathol 84:143, 1974.
65. Humphreys GU: Dropped jaw in dogs. Vet Rec 95:222, 1974.
66. Jennings PB, Lewis GE, Grumrine HH, et al: Glossitis of military working dogs in Vietnam: Experimental production of tongue lesions. Am J Vet Res 35:1295, 1974.
67. Kaplan ML, Jeffcoat MK: Acute necrotizing ulcerative gingivitis. Canine Prac 5:35, 1978.
68. Kelly DF, Lucke VM, Denny HR, Lane JG: Histology of salivary gland infarction in the dog. Vet Pathol 16:438, 1979.
69. Kelly DF, Lucke VM, Lane JG, et al: Salivary gland necrosis in dogs. Vet Rec 104:268, 1979.
70. Knecht CD, Schiller AG: Acquired lesions of the mandible. *In* Archibald J (ed): *Canine Surgery*. American Veterinary Publications Inc., Santa Barbara, 1974.
71. Knecht CD, Phares J: Characterization of dogs with salivary cyst. J Am Vet Med Assoc 158:5, 1971.
72. Knecht CD: Treatment of diseases of the zygomatic salivary gland. J Am Vet Med Assoc 6:1, 1970.
73. Knecht CD, Slusher R, Guibor E: Zygomatic salivary cyst in a dog. J Am Vet Med Assoc 155:4, 1969.
74. Kunkle G, Goldschmidt MH: Bullous pemphigoid in a dog. A case report with immunofluorescent findings. J Am Anim Hosp Assoc 14:52, 1978.
75. Langham RF: X-ray therapy of selected odontogenic neoplasms in the dog. J Am Vet Med Assoc 170:820, 1977.
76. Lewis TM: Resistance of dogs to dental caries: A two-year study. J Dent Res 44:1254, 1965.
77. Lindhe J, Hamp SE, Löe H: Plaque-induced periodontal disease in beagle dogs: A 4-year clinical, roentgenographical and histometrical study. J Peridont Res 10:235, 1975.
78. Lindhe J, Hamp SE, Löe H: Experimental periodontitis in the beagle dog. J Periodont Res 8:1, 1973.
79. Lindhe J, Hamp SE, Löe H, Schott R: Influence of topical application of chlorhexidine on chronic gingivitis and gingival wound healing in the dog. Scand J Dent Res 78:471, 1970.
80. Madewell BR, Stannard AA, Pulley LT, and Nelson VG: Oral eosinophilic granuloma in Siberian husky dogs. J Am Vet Med Assoc 177:701, 1980.
81. MacDonald JM: Stomatitis. Vet Clin North Am (Small Anim Pract) 13:3, 415, 1983.
82. Matsson L, Attstrom R: Development of experimental gingivitis in the juvenile and adult beagle dog. Test of a model for comparative studies. J Clin Periodon 6:186, 1979.
83. Matsson L, Attstrom R: Histologic characteristics of experimental gingivitis in the juvenile and adult beagle dog. J Clin Periodon 6:334, 1979.
84. Nuki K, Cooper S: The role of inflammation in the pathogenesis of gingival enlargement during the administration of diphenylhydantoin sodium in cats. J Periodont Res 7:102, 1972.
85. Nyman S, Lindhe J, Ericsson L: The effect of progressive tooth mobility on destructive periodontitis in the dog. J Clin Periodontol 5:213, 1978.
86. Olson JA, Nelms DC, Silverman S, Spitler LE: Levamisole: A new treatment for recurrent aphthous stomatitis. Oral Surg 41:588, 1976.
87. Ossoff RH, Bytell DE, Hast MH, Sisson GA: Lymphatics of the floor of the mouth and periosteum: Anatomical studies with possible clinical correlations. Otolaryngol Head Neck Surg 88:625, 1980.
88. Page RC, Schroeder HE: Current status of the host response in chronic marginal periodontitis. J Periodontol 52:477, 1981.
89. Potter KA, Tucker RD, Carpenter JL: Oral eosinophilic granuloma of Siberian huskies. J Am Vet Med Assoc 16:595, 1980.
90. Prescott CW: Ranula in the dog: A surgical treatment. Aust Vet J 44:382, 1968.
91. Priester WA, McKay FW: The occurrence of tumors in domestic animals. Natl Cancer Inst Monogr 54:1, 1980.
92. Ramfjord SP: The periodontal disease index (PDI). J Periodontol 38:602, 1967.
93. Richardson RC, Jones MA, Elliott GS: Oral neoplasma in the dog: A diagnostic and therapeutic dilemma. Comp Cont Ed 5:441, 1983.
94. Ridgway RL, Zielke DR: Nonsurgical endodontic technique for dogs. J Am Vet Med Assoc 174:82, 1979.
95. Robins GM, Grandage J: Temporomandibular joint dysplasia and open mouth jaw locking in the dog. J Am Vet Med Assoc 171:1072, 1977.
96. Robins GM: Dropped jaw—mandibular neuropraxia in the dog. J Small Anim Pract 17:753, 1976.
97. Ross DC: Occlusion in the dog. Southwest Vet 28:247, 1975.
98. Ross DC: Dental diagnostic and therapeutic techniques. J Am Vet Med Assoc 16:1462, 1972.
99. Ross DC, Myers J: Endodontic therapy for canine teeth in the dog. J Am Vet Med Assoc 157:1713, 1970.
100. Ross DL: Veterinary Dentistry. *In* Ettinger SJ (ed): *Textbook of Veterinary Internal Medicine*. W. B. Saunders Company, Philadelphia, 1975.
101. Ruben MP, McCoy J, Person P, Cohen DW: Effects of soft dietary consistency and protein deprivation on the periodontium of the dog. A preliminary report. Oral Surg 15:1061, 1962.
102. Saphir DA, Carter GR: Gingival flora of the dog with special reference to bacteria associated with bites. J Clin Microbiol 3:344, 1976.
103. Saxe R, Greene JC, Vermillion JR: Debris, calculus and periodontal disease in the beagle dog. Periodontics 5:217, 1967.
104. Schneck GW: Caries in the dog. J Am Vet Med Assoc 150:1142, 1967.
105. Scott DW, Halliwell REW, Goldschmidt MH: Toxic epidermal necrolysis in two dogs and a cat. J Am Anim Hosp Assoc 15:271, 1979.
106. Scott DW: Immunologic skin disorders in the dog and cat. Vet Clin North Am (Small Anim Pract) 8:641, 1978.
107. Scott DW: Observations on the eosinophilic granuloma complex in cats. J Am Anim Hosp Assoc 11:261, 1975.
108. Silver JG, Martin L, McBride BC: Recovery and clearance rates of oral microorganisms following experimental bacteremias in the dog. Arch Oral Biol 20:675, 1975.
109. Skrentary TT: Preliminary study of the inheri-

tance of missing teeth in the dog. Wien tierarzl Mschr 51:231, 1964.
110. Soames V, Entwisle N, Davies M: The progression of gingivitis to periodontitis in the beagle dog: Histologic and morphometric investigation. J Periodontol 47:435, 1976.
111. Sorensen WF, Löe H, Ramfjord SO: Periodontal disease in the beagle dog. J Periodont Res 15:380, 1980.
112. Stewart WC, Baker GJ, Lee R: Temporomandibular subluxation in the dog. A case report. J Small Anim Pract 16:345, 1975.
113. Syed SA, Sywanberg M, Sytanberg G: The predominant cultivable dental plaque flora of beagle dogs with periodontitis. J Clin Periodontol 8:15, 1981.
114. Syed SA, Sywanberg M, Sytanberg G: The predominant cultivable dental plaque flora of beagle dogs with gingivitis. J Periodont Res 15:123, 1980.
115. Ticer JW, Spencer DP: Injury of the feline temporomandibular joint: Radiographic signs. J Am Vet Radiol Soc 19:146, 1978.
116. Thrall DE: Orthovoltage radiotherapy of oral fibrosarcomas in dogs. J Am Vet Med Assoc 179:159, 1981.
117. Thrall DE, Goldschmidt MH, Biery DN: Malignant tumor formation at the site of previously irradiated acanthomatous epulides in four dogs. J Am Vet Med Assoc 178:127, 1981.
118. Todoroff RJ, Brodey RS: Oral and pharyngeal neoplasia in the dog: A retrospective study of 361 cases. J Am Vet Med Assoc 175:567, 1979.
119. van Campen GJ: The occurrence of acute necrotizing ulcerative gingivitis in a beagle dog colony. (Abst) L.A.D.R. 12, 1977.
120. Van Palenstein Helderman WH: Mictobial etiology of periodontal disease. J Clin Periodontal 8:261, 1981.
121. Voelker FA, Stedham MA, Robinson FR: Glossitis of military working dogs in South Vietnam: Histopathologic observations. Am J Vet Res 36:683, 1975.
122. Withrow SJ: Oral and pharyngeal tumors. Proc 9th Ann Vet Surg Forum, Chicago, Il., 186, 1981.
123. Withrow J: Dental extraction as a probable cause of septicemia in dog. J Am Vet Med Assoc 15:345, 1979.
124. Zymet C: Periapical rarefaction associated with canine dental caries. J Am Vet Med Assoc 152:483, 1968.

CHAPTER

2

Medical Aspects of Esophageal Disease

PHILIP ROUDEBUSH
BRENT D. JONES
RICHARD W. VAUGHAN

The esophagus is the tubular, muscular organ that functions to transmit a bolus of material from the pharynx to the stomach. Because the esophagus is strictly an organ of transport, esophageal disease relates to impairment of only this transport function and not of digestive or absorptive processes. Even though the esophagus may be considered a relatively simple organ, we know less about the pathophysiology of esophageal diseases than about that of any other organs in the body. For this reason, treating the diseases that affect the esophagus is a therapeutic challenge.

The purpose of this chapter is to review several diseases of the esophagus and their medical therapy. A section on physiology is also included in the hope that practitioners will more completely understand the pathophysiology of esophageal diseases. Discussions of the neuromuscular diseases of the esophagus and surgical therapy of esophageal diseases are contained in chapters three and four.

Anatomy

The esophagus has three portions: the cervical portion, which extends from the pharynx to the thoracic inlet; the thoracic portion, which extends from the thoracic inlet to the diaphragm; and the abdominal portion, which extends from the diaphragm to the stomach.

The esophagus consists of four coats. The outer coat is adventitia. There is no true serosal layer of esophagus. The muscular coat in the dog consists of two oblique layers of striated muscle fibers. The proximal portion of the cat esophagus consists of striated muscle with smooth muscle in the distal one-third. The striated muscle consists of two layers that are oblique in the proximal portion and become spiral in the distal portion. They gradually form a distinct inner, circular layer and an outer, longitudinal layer. The muscle fibers transition from striated muscle to smooth muscle occurs gradually. The amount of smooth muscle increases distally until the final 2 to 3 cm of the esophagus where all of the muscle fibers are smooth.

The submucosal coat loosely connects the mucous and muscular coats. It allows the inelastic mucosa to be thrown into longitudinal folds when the esophagus is contracted. In the cat these folds are very prominent and produce a herringbone appearance. This is obvious when the mucosa is viewed through an endoscope or even looking at a feline esophagram. The submucosal coat contains blood vessels, nerves, and mucous glands.

The mucosa is composed of a superficially cornified stratified squamous epithelium that contains openings for the ducts of the esophageal mucous glands. The mucous glands are present over the entire length of the esophagus in the dog, but only at the pharyngoesophageal junction in the cat.

In dogs, the arteries to the cervical portion of the esophagus arise from the cranial and caudal thyroid arteries. The cranial two-thirds of the thoracic portion of the esophagus receives its blood supply from the esophageal portion of the bronchoesophageal artery. The remaining portion of the esophagus is supplied by branches of the aorta, dorsal intercostal artery, and left gastric artery. The veins that drain the esophagus are, essentially, satellites of the arteries that supply it. Lymph is drained into the medial retropharyngeal, deep cervical, cranial mediastinal, bronchial, portal, splenic, and gastric lymph nodes.

The cervical portion of the esophagus is supplied with motor fibers from the pharyngoesophageal and recurrent laryngeal nerves. It is generally believed that the recurrent laryngeal nerves provide the sensory and motor nerve supply to the cranial thoracic part of the esophagus as far caudal as the heart. The dorsal and ventral vagi supply the esophagus caudal to the heart. Cells of the myenteric plexus are found between the internal and external muscle layers.

Physiology

Deglutition is a sequential, complex, coordinated action that transports food and liquid from the oral cavity to the stomach. It has been divided into three phases: oropharyngeal, esophageal, and gastroesophageal.[59] The oropharyngeal phase has been subdivided into three stages: oral, pharyngeal, and cricopharyngeal (pharyngoesophageal).[49, 59]

The oropharyngeal phase begins with the formation of a bolus in the mouth and ends as the bolus passes through the cricopharyngeal area.[59] After the food is prehended, the oral stage is initiated. Prehension and the oral stage are voluntary actions. During the oral stage, food is organized into a bolus and pushed aborally to the base of the tongue. The bolus then elicits a complex, rapid, well-coordinated series of reflexes, which make up the next two involuntary stages. The pharyngeal stage consists of peristaltic contractions of the pharynx and propulsion of the bolus from the base of the tongue into the laryngopharynx. The cricopharyngeal stage involves relaxation of the upper esophageal sphincter (cricopharyngeal muscle and subjacent esophageal circular muscles) and passage of the bolus into the cranial esophagus. Following the passage of the bolus, the upper esophageal sphincter contracts to close the upper esophagus and to initiate the esophageal phase of swallowing. The relaxation of the high-pressure cricopharyngeal zone must be coordinated with pharyngeal peristalsis so that the bolus will pass without delay into the esophagus.[59] The cricopharyngeus is an involuntary, striated muscle that is indirectly controlled by the voluntary initiation of a swallow.

The cricopharyngeus muscle and subjacent esophageal circular muscles serve as the functional upper esophageal sphincter. The cricopharyngeus is not in continuous resting activity (tonic), but is phasic. The muscle tone is linked with the respiratory cycle as well as with deglutition. The pressure is highest during preglutition inspiration.

The esophageal phase of deglutition begins with the arrival of the bolus in the cranial esophagus. This phase encompasses the passage of the bolus from the cranial esophagus to the gastroesophageal junction. Watrous and Suter[59] describe four sequences of events that might occur during the esophageal phase.

1. A swallow is followed immediately by an esophageal peristaltic wave, which progresses uninterrupted to the gastroesophageal junction (primary peristalsis).
2. The bolus remains in the proximal esophagus until a second or third swallow occurs, then a peristaltic wave carries the combined boluses to the gastroesophageal junction (primary peristalsis).
3. A bolus temporarily pauses in the proximal esophagus, then a stimulated peristaltic wave carries it to the gastroesophageal junction (secondary peristalsis).
4. Several boluses accumulate in the proximal esophagus, then a stimulated peristaltic wave carries them to the gastroesophageal junction (secondary peristalsis).

During respiration, small areas along the esophageal wall make longitudinal, oscillatory movements in rhythm with respiration. This passive movement is caused by motion of the diaphragm. Esophageal movement during peristalsis is more dynamic and involves active contraction of both the circular and longitudinal esophageal musculature.[9]

In the cat, esophageal peristalsis not only is caudal migration of a band of contracting circular muscle fibers, but also is represented by the coordinated sequential contraction of bands of longitudinal and circular muscle fibers.[56] Longitudinal peristaltic contraction causes the esophagus to engulf the bolus, to shorten and thereby decrease the length of bolus travel, to pull the bolus toward the stomach, and to contribute to the mechanism by which the lower esophageal sphincter opens.[9] Contraction of the circular band of muscles not only serves to push a bolus toward the stomach, but also may function to seal the esophageal lumen, thus preventing proximal escape of a bolus.[11]

Esophageal function in the dog differs somewhat from that in the cat and also in humans, in that the dog esophagus has no distinct longitudinal and circular bands of muscle. As stated earlier, the canine esophagus consists of two oblique layers of striated muscle that are arranged in a spiral or helical formation. Esophageal movement during peristalsis in the dog resembles the process in the cat and man but must be investigated further.[51, 59]

A second peristaltic wave (secondary peristalsis) is initiated by the direct stimulation of the esophageal wall by a bolus. Progression of primary or secondary peristaltic contractions depends on the presence, size, and location of the bolus in the esophagus. A primary peristaltic contraction is entirely bolus-dependent only in its course through the cervical esophagus. In the absence of a bolus, peristalsis in the esophagus does not follow the act of swallowing.[27] In the thoracic esophagus, the contractions are facilitated by, but do not depend on a bolus.[25] Thus, two mechanisms are involved in the regulation of esophageal contraction: a central regulatory mechanism (swallowing center) in the brain stem and afferent nerve impulses that originate in the esophagus in the presence of a bolus.[25]

The lower esophageal sphincter (LES) is not a true anatomical sphincter, but rather a physiological high-pressure zone. This zone is found in the most distal portion of the esophagus and separates the esophagus from the stomach. Lower esophageal sphincter is the functional term used for this region, whereas gastroesophageal junction (GEJ) is the anatomical term used by many authors.[59] The nature of this "sphincter" has been one of great speculation and research. In cats, markers labeling the LES and GEJ slide orally through the hiatus, during longitudinal peristaltic shortening. This transient physiological herniation of a small portion of the stomach normally occurs during esophageal peristalsis.[9] During peristalsis, the LES relaxes and allows the bolus to pass into the stomach (gastroesophageal phase). A prevalent misunderstanding is that LES relaxation and opening are synonymous. Lower esophageal sphincter relaxation and opening are related but distinct events. Lower esophageal sphincter opening is a passive mechanical event affected by the force of an oncoming bolus, whereas sphincter relaxation occurs as an active reflex process mediated neurologically.[9] The average canine LES begins to relax several seconds before the esophageal pressure wave has peaked in the distal esophagus. Even if the LES opens and closes normally, synchronization of LES with the esophageal wave is still required for normal passage of a bolus.[16]

The gastroesophageal junction is the only known area of the gastrointestinal tract where luminal structures having opposite cavitary pressures are in continuity.[8] Mechanical factors and intrinsic LES tone serve as the major control mechanisms to prevent reflux of gastric contents. Whatever external force or positive pressure is applied to the stomach is also exerted on the terminal abdominal esophagus, so no pressure gradient occurs between the stomach and thoracic esophagus.[22, 59] Other mechanical factors that prevent gastroesophageal reflux include: interdigitating gastric rugal folds, focal thickening of the distal esophageal muscular coat, oblique implantation of the distal esophagus into the stomach, and the flap-like cardiac incisura, which is pushed against the GEJ by the enlarging gastric fundus.[59] Gastrin and other gastrointestinal hormones at pharmacological doses appear to increase LES tone. Whether these hormones function when released physiologically during normal food ingestion to increase LES tone is still speculative.[23] Resting intrinsic LES tone is thought to be a part of the distal esophageal muscle.[7] This muscle maintains normal strength of closure and resists stretch. Length-tension curves indicate that the distal esophagus is maximally efficient when in the closed position.[1] If this is so, minimal muscle tension will maintain an effective strength of closure.[21, 22]

Clinical Signs

The clinical signs of esophageal disease may be quite obvious or very subtle. The degree of esophageal involvement, location of the problem, chronicity, and presence of secondary problems will influence the amount and severity of clinical signs. Either signs will be attributable to alimentary tract disease, or to secondary complications, such as aspiration pneumonia, which may be mistaken for the primary problem.

Signs of esophageal disease include: regurgitation through the mouth or the nares, dysphagia, odynophagia, repeated swallowing movements, and copious salivation or drooling. A common misconception is that esophageal disease causes regurgitation only immediately after eating; regurgitation may occur during and shortly after eating or may be delayed for several hours. Differentiating regurgitation from vomiting is important in distinguishing esophageal from lower gastrointestinal disease. Characteristics of vomiting include expulsion of digested and bile-stained food and retching with involuntary abdominal contractions. Gastric contents are often highly acidic and the pH of vomited material may be tested. However, vomiting often involves the reflux of bicarbonate-rich fluid into the stomach from the duodenum, which buffers the gastric acid. The vomited material may then have a neutral or near-neutral pH. Regurgitation involves less forceful casting-up of tubular, bile-free, undigested food. Regurgitation may involve only foam or liquid and, as stated previously, may or may not be directly related to ingestion of food. Mucoid secretions mixed with the undigested food will usually have a pH 6.5 to 7.0.[20] Copious salivation may also be a confusing sign. It may be a major sign of esophageal diseases, such as a foreign body or it may be part of the nausea which may accompany vomiting.

Signs of esophageal disease may also be attributable only to the respiratory system. Mucopurulent nasal discharge, dyspnea, or moist coughing will often accompany esophageal disease because of the high incidence of aspiration of ingesta. Coughing and dyspnea associated with aspiration pneumonia will accompany esophageal signs or often will be the only complaint of the owner.

All of these signs may be intermittent and prolonged, or acute and progressive, depending on the disease process. Anorexia and weight loss or a voracious appetite may accompany esophageal disease. Anorexia and dysphagia usually occur with esophageal foreign bodies or perforations. Young animals with congenital megaesophagus might have a voracious appetite accompanied by regurgitation and weight loss. Other signs include cervical cellulitis or a draining fistulous tract secondary to esophageal perforation by a foreign body. Repeated attempts at swallowing that occur with extension, flexion, or twisting of the head and neck are also hallmarks of esophageal disease. Rarely, diarrhea has been associated with other clinical signs of esophageal disease. In summary, the major clinical signs of esophageal disease are: regurgitation, dysphagia, coughing, and dyspnea.

History

As in the treatment of any medical problem, it is imperative that a complete and careful history be taken. The owner's primary complaint may be attributable to the primary esophageal signs or may reflect a secondary aspiration pneumonia. Historical details should include the exact onset and course of the problems, the type of dysphagia, and its relationship to ingestion of food. Information regarding the ability of the animal to retain liquids, soft food, or solid food may be helpful. If the animal shows signs in adulthood, the owner should be questioned regarding its possible exposure to caustic agents, foreign bodies, and traumatic incidents, previous neurological problems, prior surgery, or anesthesia. Recurrent pharyngitis or tonsillitis of unknown etiology should be explored historically for other signs of esophageal disease. The clinical signs associated with congenital problems, such as vascular ring anomalies and cricopharyngeal achalasia, will be manifested in an animal that is still nursing or recently weaned to solid food. Acute onset of signs in either a young or older animal often is consistent with the presence of a foreign body. Chronic or slowly progressive regurgitation is more suggestive of gastroesophageal reflux or a developing esophageal stricture.

Physical Examination

Physical examination of patients with esophageal problems is often unrewarding but is helpful when specific abnormalities are noted. Frequently, special diagnostic

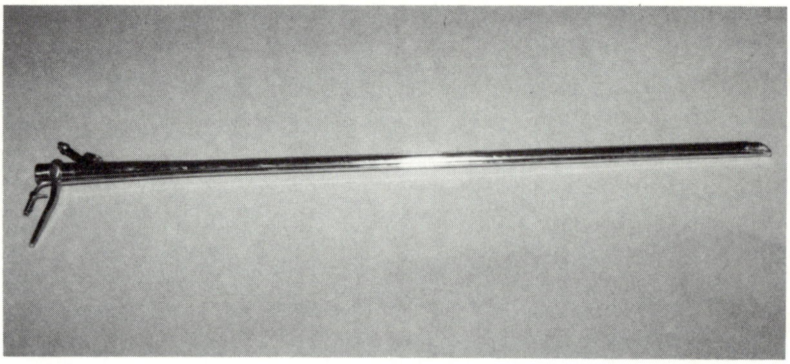

Figure 2–1. A rigid endoscope that may be used for esophagoscopy.

techniques are needed to further evaluate esophageal changes in addition to those found on physical examination.

The physical condition of the animal may vary from normal to emaciated, depending on the severity of the disease process. Chronic regurgitation or vomiting may produce chronic tonsillitis, pharyngitis, or nasal discharge. Occasionally, rancid halitosis is present. Copious salivation may be present but needs to be differentiated from salivation that occurs with oral disease, nausea, and vomiting. Abdominal palpation is usually normal. Fever and depression are usually present only when an infection exists concurrently with a foreign body, cellulitis, or aspiration pneumonia. Observations and careful palpation of the cervical and thoracic inlet region may be helpful. A dilated cervical esophagus may be visualized or palpated, especially when examined during respiration.

Coarse crackles (moist rales), associated with aspiration pneumonia or fluid movement in the dilated esophagus, may produce abnormal thoracic sounds on auscultation. Auscultation of the cervical esophagus and the thoracic inlet may be helpful. Watching the animal eat is often a valuable adjunct to physical examination. The type of dysphagia and regurgitation is easily observed.

The differentiation of various esophageal diseases depends on subtle differences in history and physical examination, especially in the character, duration, and time intervals between ingestion, dysphagia, regurgitation, and respiratory signs. Definitive diagnosis and differentiation of esophageal diseases depend on radiographic techniques (i.e., contrast studies and cinefluorography), endoscopy, biopsy, and occasionally manometry, electromyography, and exploratory surgery.[20, 22]

Diagnostic Techniques

Radiography is an essential and invaluable technique in the diagnosis of esophageal disorders. It is discussed in greater detail in Chapter 14.

Endoscopy (esophagoscopy) with either

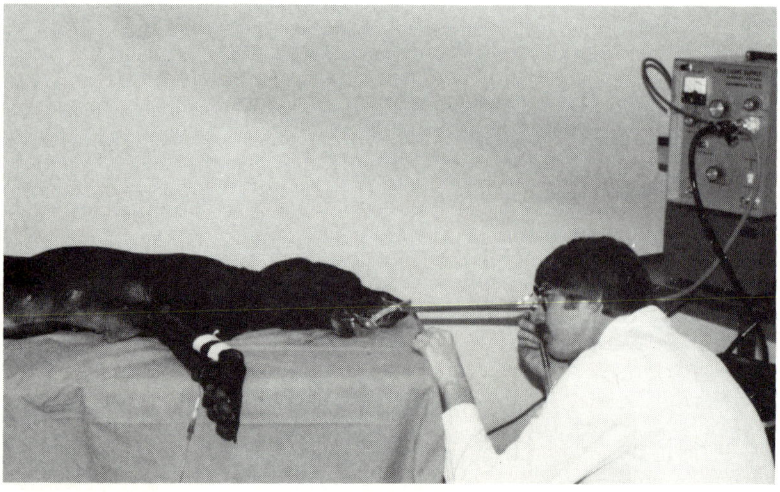

Figure 2–2. The use of a rigid endoscope for esophagoscopy.

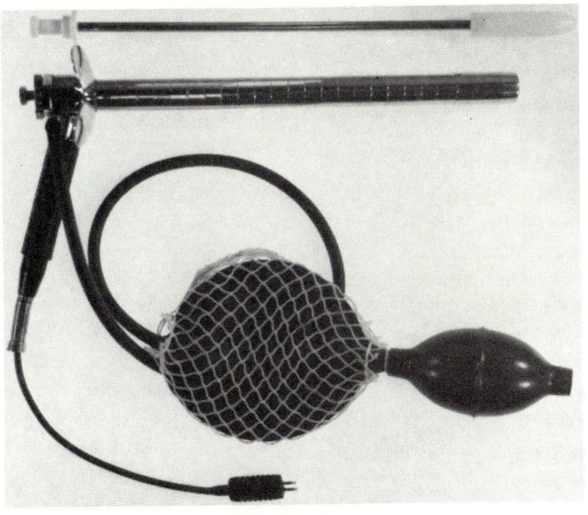

Figure 2–3

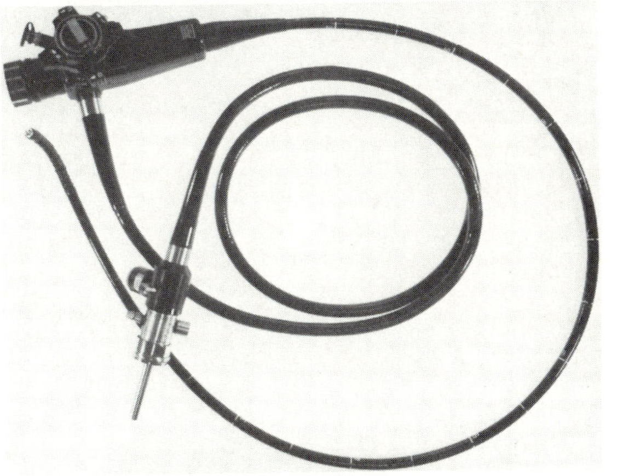

Figure 2–4

Figure 2–3. A human sigmoidoscope. This instrument can be used quite effectively as a rigid esophagoscope.

Figure 2–4. A flexible endoscope that may be used for esophagoscopy. This is an Olympus Model G.I.F.-P2 Esophagogastroduodenoscope (Olympus Corporation, New Hyde Park, NY).

rigid or flexible fiberoptic instruments is an increasingly important tool in evaluation of esophageal diseases. Esophagoscopy with a rigid endoscope has been used for many years in both veterinary and human medicine (Figs. 2–1 to 2–3). Recently, however, fiberoptic esophagoscopy has replaced rigid endoscopy in human medicine (Figs. 2–4 and 2–5). Fiberoptic endoscopy is just beginning to become popular as a diagnostic tool in veterinary medicine.

The advantage of endoscopy over the other methods of evaluating esophageal diseases is that one is able to visualize the esophagus and any of its lesions with a noninvasive procedure. Most endoscopes are equipped with a biopsy channel, which enables tissue specimens (biopsy, brush cytology, impression smears) to be obtained for a more definitive diagnosis. Most foreign bodies can be removed via endoscopy. The technique will be discussed completely later in this chapter. The major disadvantage is that the procedure requires a light plane of anesthesia. The reader is referred to other texts for detailed information and techniques of endoscopy.[26, 38, 63]

Esophageal biopsy specimens may be obtained by three methods. The easiest method is to use alligator forceps through either the rigid or the flexible endoscope (Figs. 2–6 to 2–9). Surgical excisional biopsy may also be utilized. Another convenient method of esophageal biopsy is to use suction biopsy equipment.[28] The authors are currently using the Multi-purpose Suction Biopsy Tube.* It is a versatile instrument that can be used

*Multi-purpose Suction Biopsy Tube, Quinton Instrument Company, Seattle, WA.

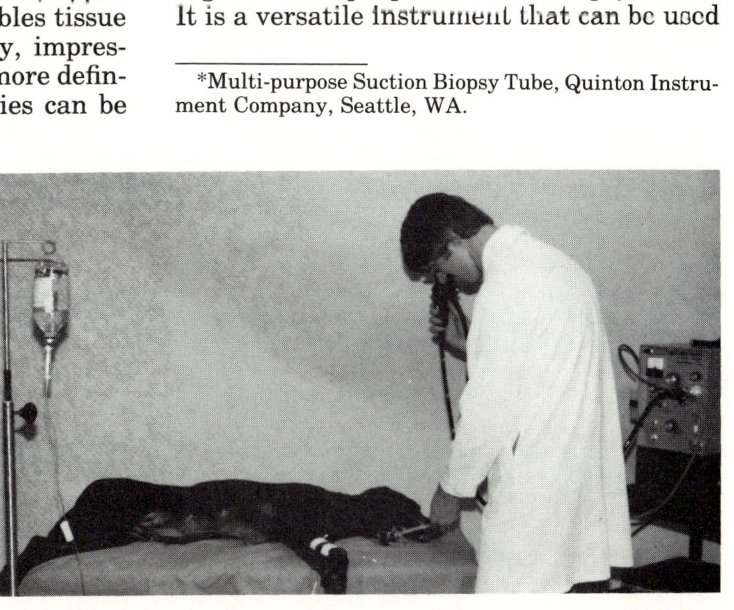

Figure 2–5. The use of a flexible endoscope (Olympus G.I.F.-P2 esophagogastroduodenoscope with Olympus CLS light source) for esophagoscopy.

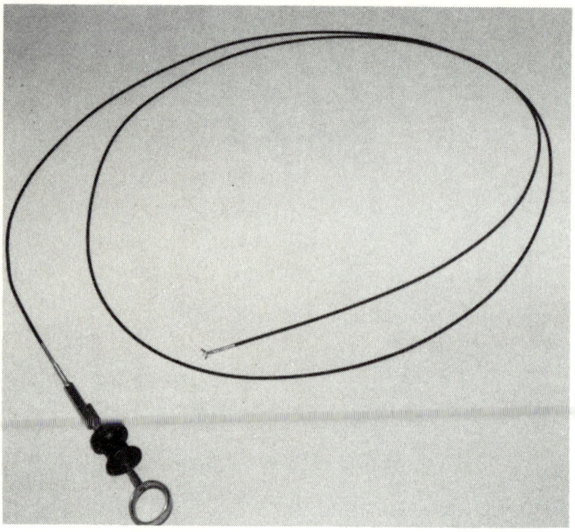

Figure 2–6. A flexible alligator forceps biopsy instrument, which may be passed through the biopsy channel of a flexible endoscope.

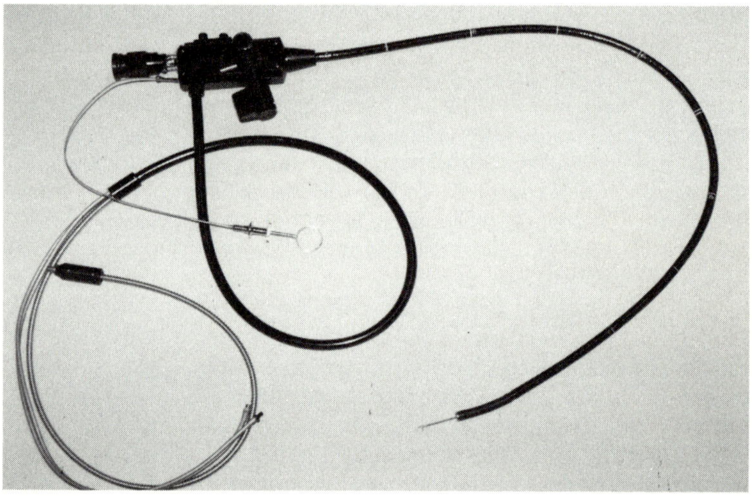

Figure 2–7. A flexible alligator forceps biopsy instrument passing through the biopsy channel of the A.C.M.I. Model F7 flexible endoscope.

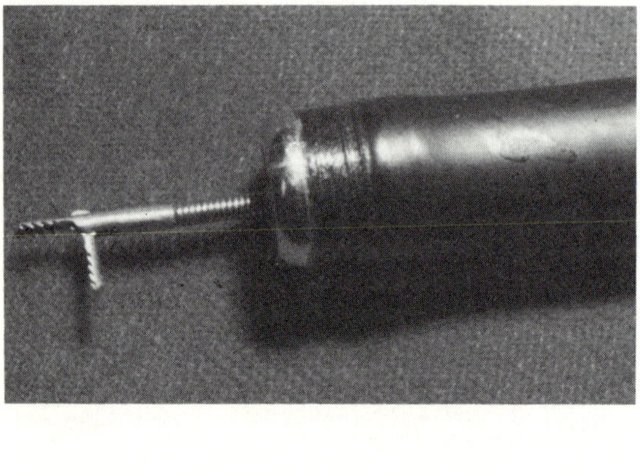

Figure 2–8. The tip of the flexible alligator forceps biopsy instrument emerging from the biopsy channel of the A.C.M.I. Model F7 flexible endoscope.

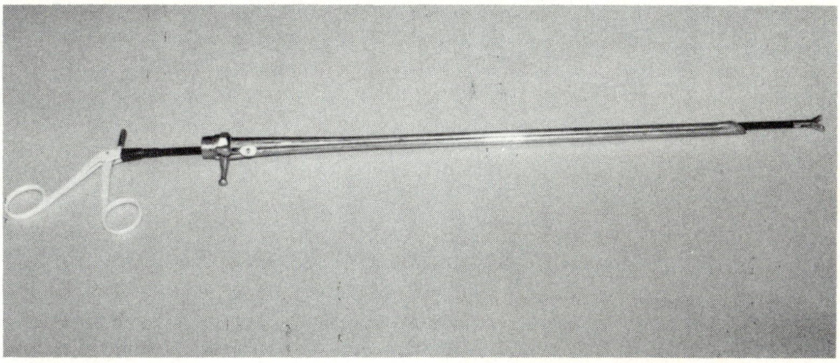

Figure 2–9. A rigid alligator forceps biopsy instrument is passed through a rigid endoscope.

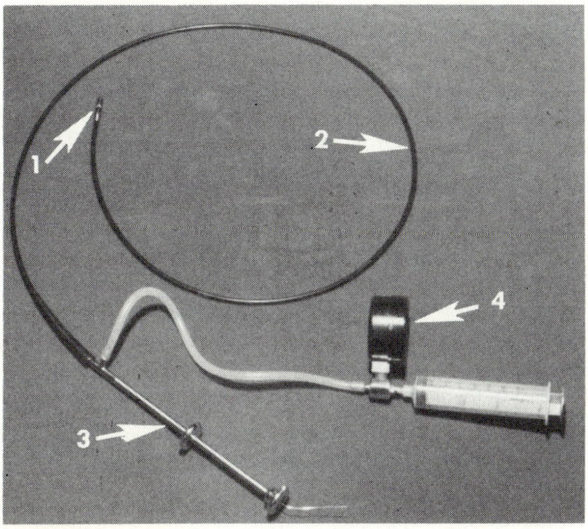

Figure 2–10. The Multi-Purpose Suction Biopsy tube manufactured by Quinton Instruments. Note the following sections of the instrument: *1,* biopsy capsule; *2,* flexible black tube that connects the biopsy capsule to the operating handle; *3,* stationary handle with pull wire that operates the biopsy knife; *4,* vacuum gauge with syringe and white connecting tube.

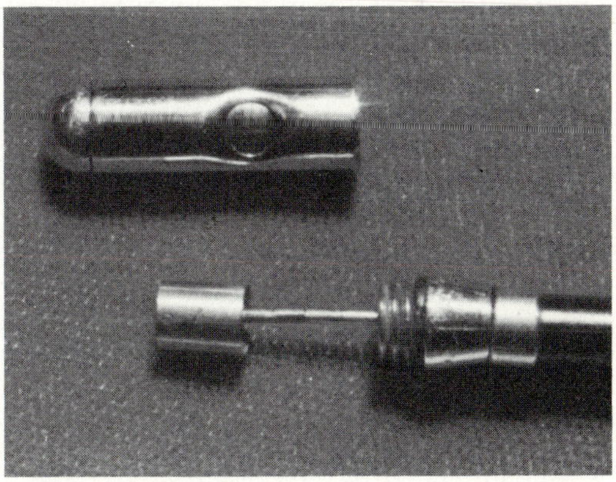

Figure 2–11. Cylindrical biopsy knife and a single aperture capsule.

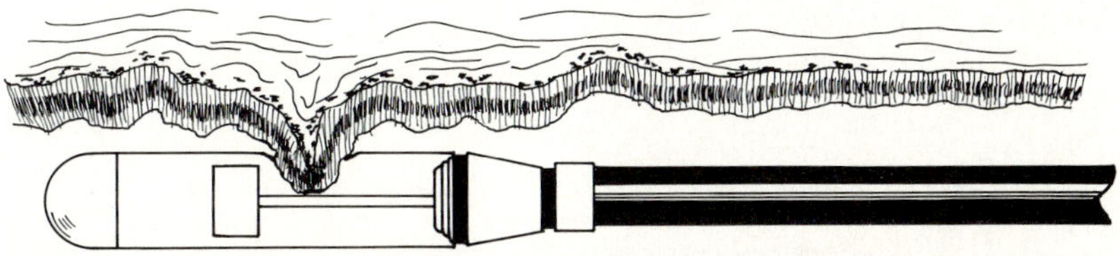

Figure 2–12. The suction of mucosa into the capsule. The cylindrical knife will be retracted to obtain the biopsy specimen.

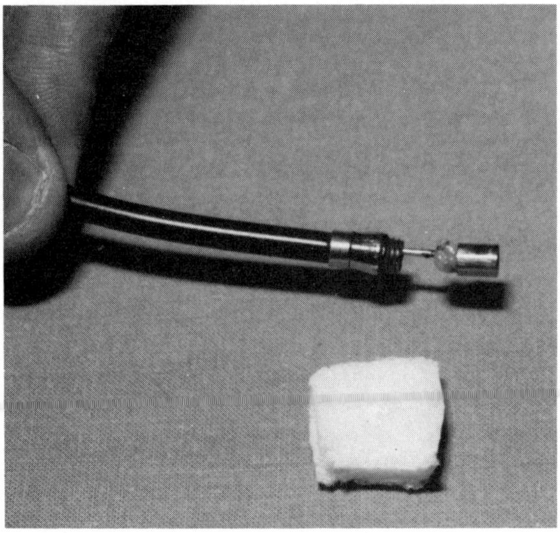

Figure 2–13. Quinton Multi-purpose Suction Biopsy Tube with the capsule opened to remove the biopsy specimen.

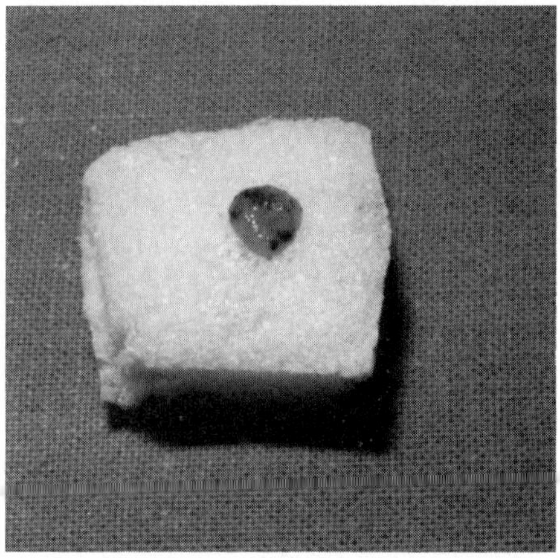

Figure 2–14. The esophageal biopsy specimen is laid flat on a piece of Gelfoam before it is placed in formalin. This enables the pathologist to properly orient the tissue and obtain cuts at right (90°) angles to the tissue. (Gelfoam, The Upjohn Company, Kalamazoo, MI.)

to obtain biopsy material from many different areas. The instrument consists of the following sections: a cylindrical knife, which fits snugly into a capsule with a single or multiple aperture(s), a flexible tube, which connects the biopsy capsule to the operating handle, a stationary handle with pull wire, which operates the biopsy knife, and a vacuum gauge (Figs. 2–10 and 2–11). The instrument is assembled and passed down the area of interest with the capsule aperture closed. When the capsule is in the region from which the specimen is to be obtained, the aperture is opened, negative pressure is produced, and the desired tissue is pulled into the capsule (Fig. 2–12). The desired pressure is maintained by manipulating the pressure gauge. A satisfactory pressure is ten to fifteen mm/Hg. While maintaining suction, the operator excises the biopsy specimen by pulling the knife firmly but gently closed with the handle, to ensure complete excision and to enable severed vessels to retract. The instrument is then removed, and the capsule opened to remove the biopsy specimen (Fig. 2–13). The authors have found this technique to be very successful in obtaining suitable biopsy specimens from the small intestine, colon, rectum, vagina, and esophagus.

No matter which method is used to obtain a gastrointestinal biopsy specimen, one should lay or pin the specimen flat on a piece of thin cardboard, tongue depressor, or foam* before placing it in the formalin solution (Fig. 2–14). This maneuver will enable the pathologist to orient the tissue properly and to obtain cuts at right (90°) angles to the tissues. Impression smears should also be obtained before the tissue is placed in formalin.

Intraluminal esophageal manometry is a useful clinical and investigative method for the evaluation of esophageal pressure and motor function.[16] It is currently being utilized extensively in human medicine and on research animals but is used on a limited basis in clinical veterinary medicine at this time.

Esophageal Diseases

VASCULAR RING ANOMALIES

Vascular ring anomalies are congenital malformations of the great vessel system

*Gelfoam, the Upjohn Company, Kalamazoo, MI.

Figure 2–15. *A,* The embryonic aortic arches and dorsal aortas before they are transformed. In the embryo the first aortic arches regress before the sixth arches form. *B,* The canine aortic arches and dorsal aortas after transformation. The regressed portions are outlined by the dashed areas. One must remember that the ventral aortas unite to form the heart. *C,* The normal arterial arrangement in adult dogs. The left subclavian artery shifts up the aortic arch as the heart moves caudally during development.

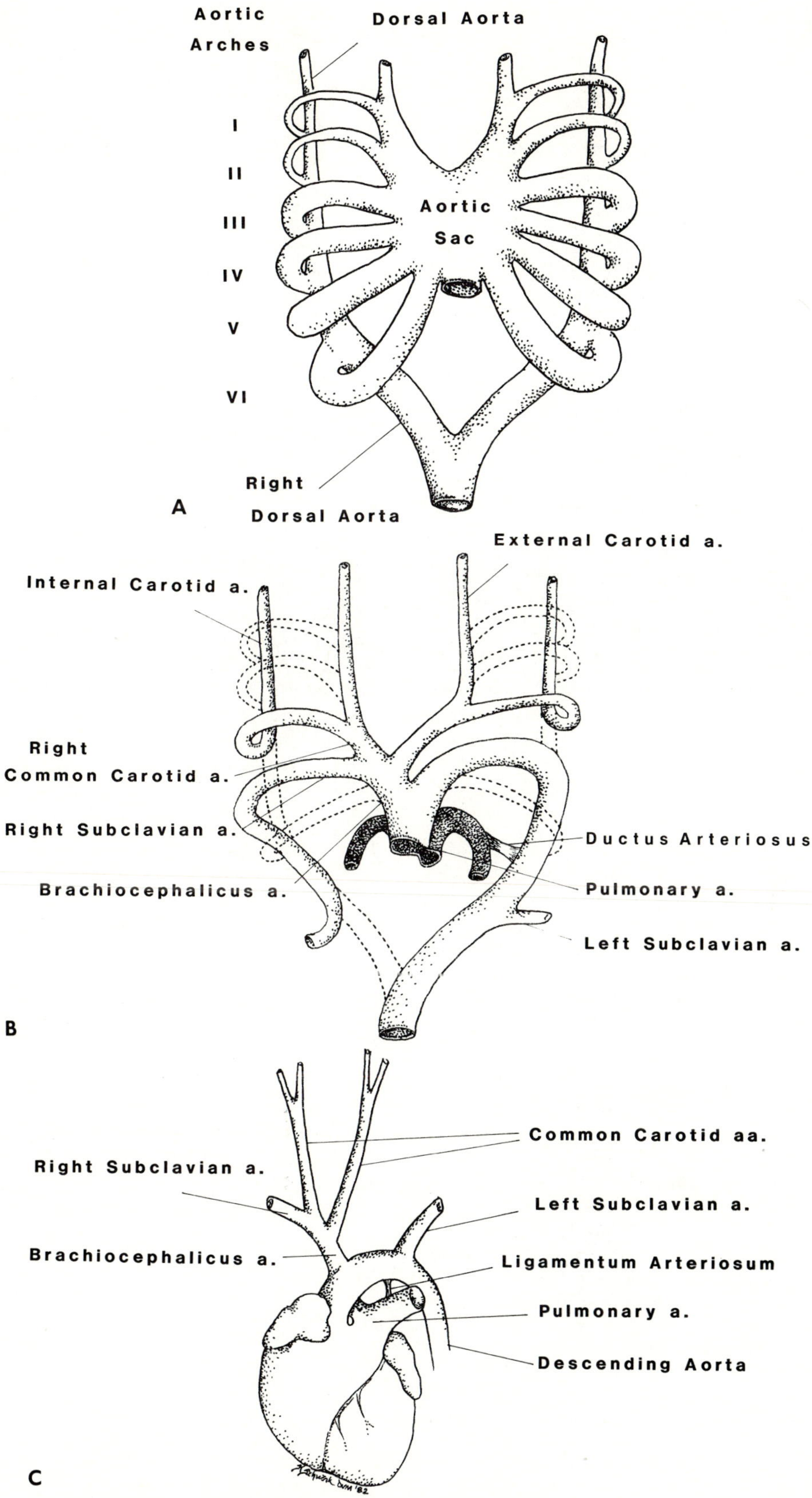

Figure 2–15. *See legend on opposite page*

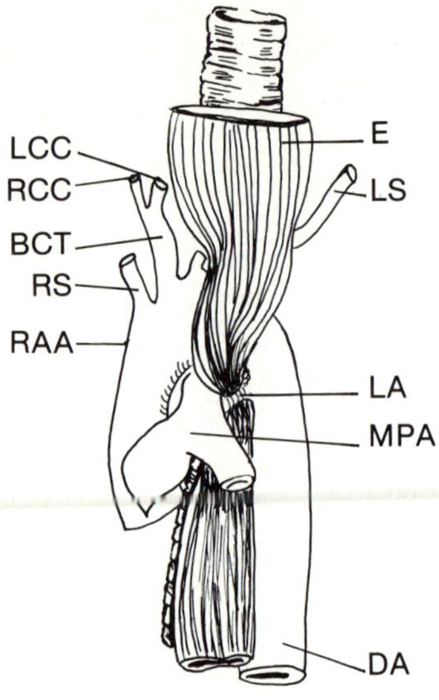

Figure 2–16. The vascular ring caused by a persistent right aortic arch. *E,* esophagus; *LS,* left subclavian artery; *LA,* ligamentum arteriosum; *MPA,* main pulmonary artery; *DA,* descending aorta; *RAA,* right aortic arch; *RS,* right subclavian artery; *BCT,* bicarotid trunk; *RCC,* right common carotid artery; *LCC,* left common carotid artery.

that interfere with esophageal function. These anomalies produce an esophageal stenosis at the base of the heart and affect the trachea or cardiovascular system only rarely.

The functional integrity of the esophagus is subject to the normal embryological development of the great vessels at the base of the heart.[33] Therefore, the normal embryological development of the heart and great vessels will be reviewed briefly. At different times during early embryonic life, six ancestral branchial arches form a series of six vascular arches that connect the primitive paired ventral aortas with the paired dorsal aortas (Fig. 2–15). The paired ventral aortas unite caudally to form the primordial heart. The paired dorsal aortas fuse caudally to form the descending aorta. The first, second, and fifth pairs of aortic arches are transient and involute early in development. The third pair forms the internal carotid arteries; the right fourth arch forms the right subclavian and brachiocephalic arteries; and the left fourth arch normally forms the aortic arch. The left sixth arch forms the ductus arteriosus, which connects the fetal pulmonary artery and the aorta in utero. This arrangement causes the arch of the aorta, the ductus arteriosus, and the pulmonary artery all to lie on the left side of the esophagus where they encounter no esophageal interference. This relationship does not occur in vascular anomalies, and the esophagus becomes entrapped in a "vascular ring."

The most common vascular anomaly in the canine is the persistent right aortic arch.[13] In this developmental anomaly, the embryonic right fourth arch, instead of the left fourth arch, persists as the functional aorta. This arrangement causes the esophagus to be encircled on the right by the aortic arch, ventrally by the base of the heart and pulmonary artery, and on the left by the ductus arteriosus or ligamentum arteriosum, which passes dorsally (Figs. 2–16 and 2–17). Other vascular anomalies which occur much less frequently are a double aortic arch, anomalous origin of the subclavian or intercostal arteries, or an aberrant patent ductus arteriosus associated with the left or right aortic arches. Vascular rings do

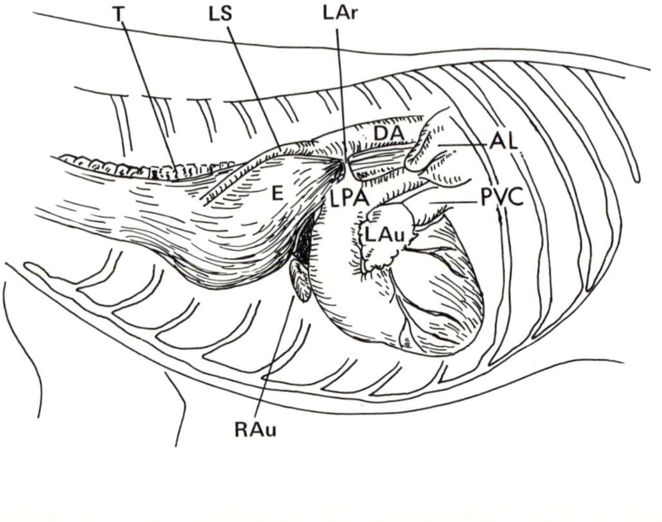

Figure 2–17. The vascular ring caused by a persistent right aortic arch. *T,* trachea; *LS,* left subclavian artery; *LAr,* ligamentum arteriosum, *DA,* descending aorta; *ALA,* left cranial lung lobe; *PCV,* posterior vena cava; *LAu,* left auricle; *LPA,* left pulmonary artery; *E,* esophagus; *RAu,* right auricle.

occur in cats but are rare. Irish setters, Boston terriers, and German shepherds are the most commonly affected canine breeds.[34, 40]

Signs produced by these anomalies result from esophageal entrapment and stenosis with subsequent precordial esophageal dilation.[4] At the time of weaning to solid food, young dogs suffer from persistent regurgitation. Regurgitation is associated with eating in the early stages of the disease but will occur at variable times after eating as the precordial dilation develops. The food-filled esophagus may be palpated at the thoracic inlet. Affected puppies are usually malnourished and weak. Auscultation usually reveals coarse crackles due to aspiration pneumonia, although cardiac sounds are normal. The diagnosis of a vascular ring anomaly can be confirmed by positive contrast radiology. (See Chapter 14).

Surgery is the treatment of choice and should be done early. Prognosis is guarded pending full postoperative recovery because of several complicating factors. Complications are common because of the initial malnourished and weakened state of the animal and concurrent aspiration pneumonia. Most patients will show clinical improvement if they survive the immediate postoperative period. Another complicating factor is permanent esophageal dilation despite surgical correction of the stenosis. This occurs if the esophagus develops sacculations or an extensive dilation that fills the anterior mediastinum. A final possible complication is a dilation of the esophagus caudal to the vascular ring, a condition which probably represents neuromuscular disease of the esophagus in conjunction with the vascular ring anomaly and represents a much poorer prognosis. The surgical treatment of vascular ring amomalies will be covered in Chapter 4.

Vascular compression of the esophagus has also been described in English bulldogs.[62] Clinical signs of recurrent regurgitation and aspiration pneumonia occur in bulldogs less than 2 years of age. An esophagram will reveal an abrupt ventral deviation of the esophagus at the level of the first or second rib. Two patients underwent thoracotomy, which revealed compression of the esophagus by the left subclavian artery and brachiocephalic artery.[62] Transection and anastomosis of the left subclavian artery relieved the clinical signs. This type of vascular compression of the esophagus should be considered in young brachycephalic dogs with signs of esophageal disease.

ESOPHAGITIS

Primary acute esophagitis is rare and usually occurs because of trauma or ingestion of caustic agents. Esophagitis is usually a secondary complication of another esophageal disease. It can be mild and transient, in which case only the esophageal mucosa is involved. Clinical signs are mild or nonexistent, and the esophageal mucosa heals quickly without significant fibrosis. Esophagitis with significant muscularis involvement is comparatively uncommon but can lead to severe ulceration with subsequent perforation, fibrotic stenosis, or chronic inflammation. Clinical signs in these cases are much more severe. Experimental esophagitis in dogs results in severely disordered motor activity, thus re-emphasizing that sensory information originating in the esophagus is important in reinforcing primary peristalsis.[51] Chronic inflammatory esophagitis with secondary papilloma formation has been described in one cat.[60]

Reflux esophagitis is a separate clinical entity that is associated with hiatal hernias and other periesophageal diseases occurring near the LES, such as abscesses or metastatic neoplasms. Reflux esophagitis that occurs when a pharyngostomy tube is placed into the gastric lumen has been demonstrated experimentally. Experimentally, reflux esophagitis has been demonstrated that occurs when the pharyngostomy tube is placed on the gastric lumen.[32] Erosions and ulcerations of the esophageal epithelium can also occur because of the presence of the tube in the esophageal lumen.[32] Reflux esophagitis may also occur as a postoperative complication leading to esophageal stricture (Fig. 2–18). The complex of gastric acid, pepsin, bile salts, and proteolytic pancreatic enzymes appears to be a potent combination for causing esophageal mucosal damage. The extent and severity of reflux esophagitis depends on the potency and volume of refluxed material, the "dwell time" the noxious material remains in the body of the esophagus, the resistance of esophageal tissue to injury, and the competency of the anti-reflux mechanisms.[10]

The clinical signs of esophagitis are regurgitation and dysphagia. The diagnosis of esophagitis is often difficult. It is not uncom-

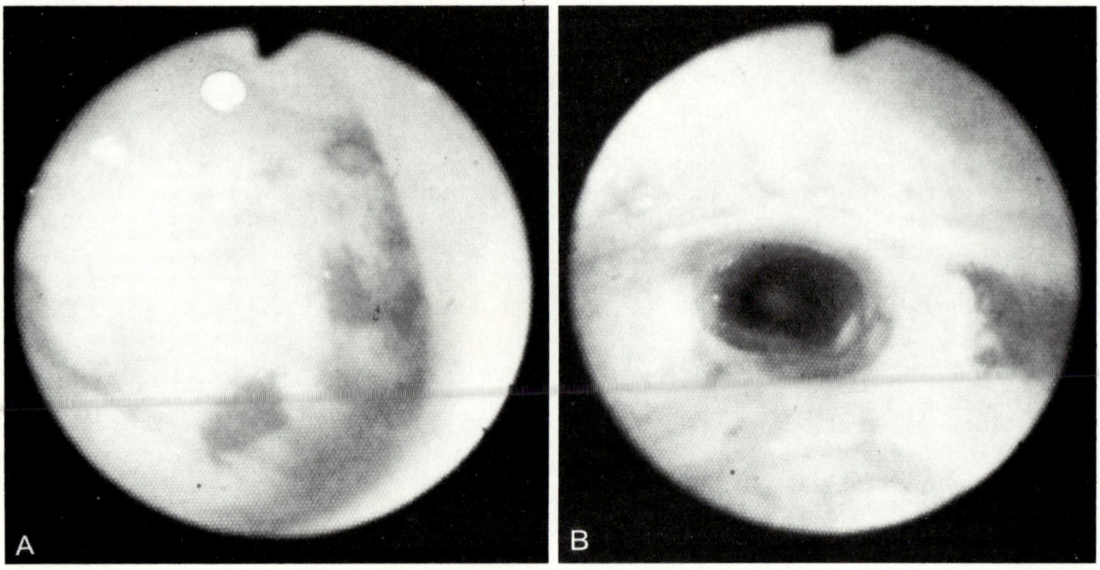

Figure 2–18. *A* and *B*, Views through a flexible fiberoptic endoscope of esophagitis in a 2-year-old female Kerry Blue Terrier. Note the large hemorrhagic areas. A biopsy specimen otained during the endoscopy examination confirmed an esophagitis. The patient developed clinical signs four days after a routine ovarohysterectomy. See Color Plate.

mon for the esophagram to be normal. A diagnosis of esophagitis is suspected on visualization of the esophageal mucosa (usually through an endoscope) and is confirmed by histopathology. The biopsy specimen can be obtained during the endoscopic evaluation or obtained surgically.

Treatment of esophagitis should be aimed at the initial, underlying esophageal problem. Forms of symptomatic relief include esophageal rest; frequent, small feedings of soft, bland food; antibiotics; liquid antacid gels; and local anesthetics (lidocaine gel*). Bethanecol† may be used to diminish or abolish the symptoms of esophagitis. The proposed mechanism of its action is to increase LES pressure by reducing gastroesophageal reflux, improve esophageal acid clearance by stimulating secondary peristalsis, and to increase gastric emptying.[10] In dogs, these beneficial effects may be limited because the esophagus consists primarily of striated muscle. Dosage is adjusted to clinical response but can begin at 2.5 to 10.0 mg every 8 hours orally to dogs and cats.

Reflux esophagitis is treated by reducing the amount of gastric acid refluxed into the esophagus. Antacids have historically been used for this purpose; however, since the antacids leave the stomach rapidly, they must be given frequently (about every hour) to achieve maximum results.[44, 52] Another drug that has been shown to be of benefit in humans with reflux esophagitis is cimetidine.* It is an H_2 blocker and therefore reduces gastric acid output. It has no effect on the LES. Cimetidine has been used by the authors in a few canine cases with success. The oral dosage in the canine is 5 to 10 mg/kg 4 times daily. To prevent reflux esophagitis, pharyngostomy tubes should not be passed into the gastric lumen. A short tube that terminates at the anterior or midthoracic esophagus is ideal. Soft tubing should be utilized to minimize the mechanical trauma to the esophageal epithelium.

*Xylocain Viscous, Astra Pharmaceutical Products, Worcester, MA.

†Urecholine, Merck Sharp & Dohme, West Point, PA.

ESOPHAGEAL NEOPLASIA

Primary and secondary neoplasms of the canine and feline esophagus are rare. In the canine the following primary neoplasms have been described: squamous cell carcinoma, osteosarcoma, fibrosarcoma, undifferentiated carcinomas, and leiomyomas.[37, 45, 55] Feline primary esophageal neoplasms are reported to be carcinomas.[57]

The most common esophageal neoplasms are fibrosarcomas or osteosarcomas arising secondarily to the formation of granulomas caused by the parasite *Spirocerca lupi*.[24, 48] These esophageal tumors are common in

*Tagamet, Smith Kline & French Lab Co., Carolina, P.R.

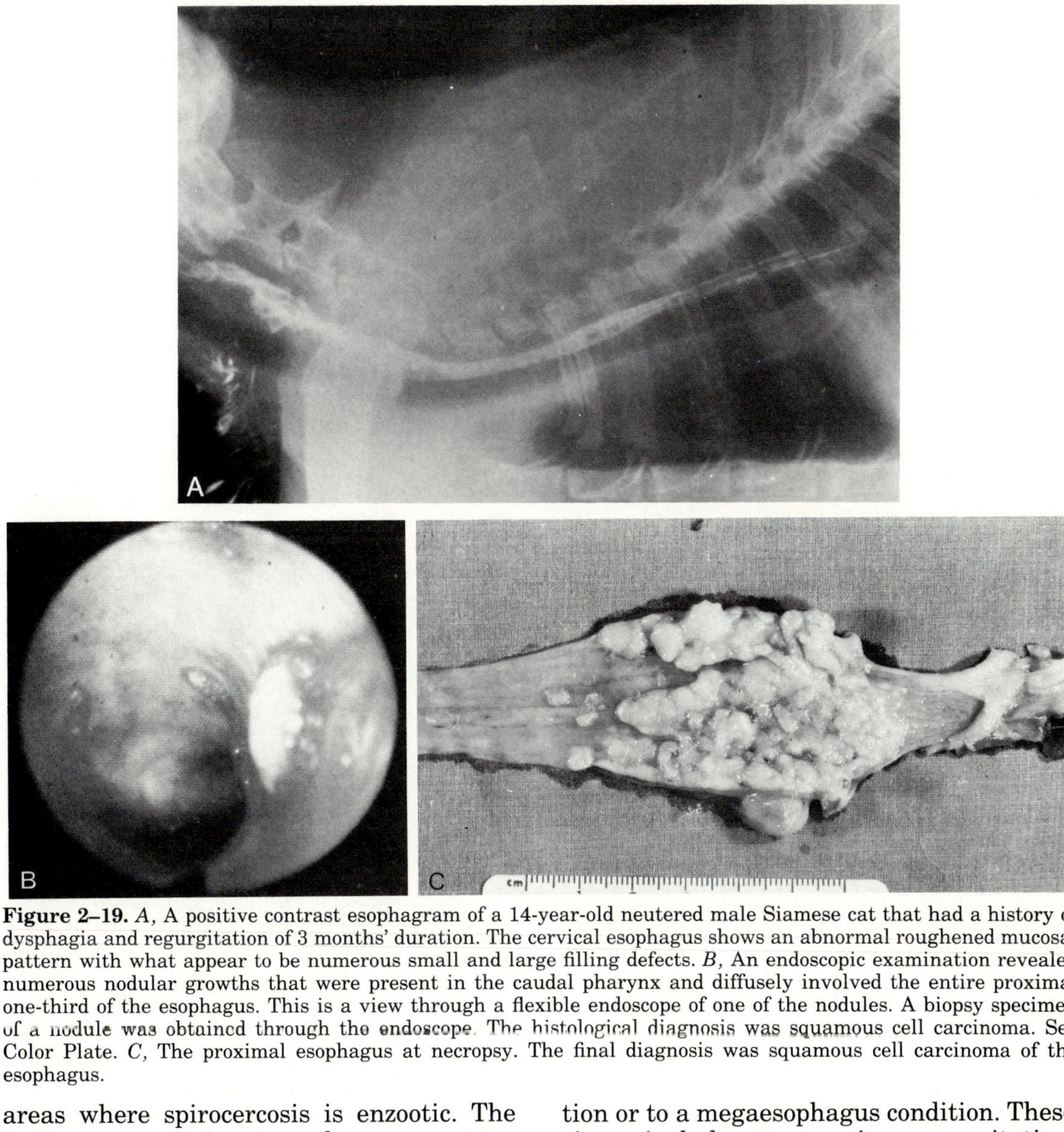

Figure 2–19. *A,* A positive contrast esophagram of a 14-year-old neutered male Siamese cat that had a history of dysphagia and regurgitation of 3 months' duration. The cervical esophagus shows an abnormal roughened mucosal pattern with what appear to be numerous small and large filling defects. *B,* An endoscopic examination revealed numerous nodular growths that were present in the caudal pharynx and diffusely involved the entire proximal one-third of the esophagus. This is a view through a flexible endoscope of one of the nodules. A biopsy specimen of a nodule was obtained through the endoscope. The histological diagnosis was squamous cell carcinoma. See Color Plate. *C,* The proximal esophagus at necropsy. The final diagnosis was squamous cell carcinoma of the esophagus.

areas where spirocercosis is enzootic. The lesions metastasize to pulmonary parenchyma and other tissues. Several cases have been described with hypertrophic pulmonary osteopathy secondary to the esophageal lesions.[50, 54] The life cycle of *Spirocerca lupi* and control of the organism are covered in greater detail in Chapter 15.

Secondary metastatic neoplasms to the esophagus are diagnosed more often than primary esophageal tumors but are still uncommon. Reported metastatic tumors to the esophagus include: bronchogenic carcinoma, gastric carcinoma, thyroid medullary carcinoma, and, in the authors' experience, mammary adenocarcinoma and squamous cell carcinoma.[17, 45]

Clinical signs of esophageal neoplasia are attributable to a slowly developing obstruction or to a megaesophagus condition. These signs include: progressive regurgitation, usually associated with eating, dysphagia, weight loss, and debilitation. Primary or metastatic esophageal tumors usually occur in dogs and cats over 6 to 8 years old. Diagnosis is made by radiography, esophagoscopy, and biopsy (Figs. 2–19 and 2–20). Surgical excision and tissue reconstruction may be successful for treatment of localized lesions.

ESOPHAGEAL FOREIGN BODIES

Despite the distensibility of the normal esophagus, partial or complete obstruction due to the presence of foreign bodies is common in both the dog and cat. Indiscriminate eating habits and inadequate masti-

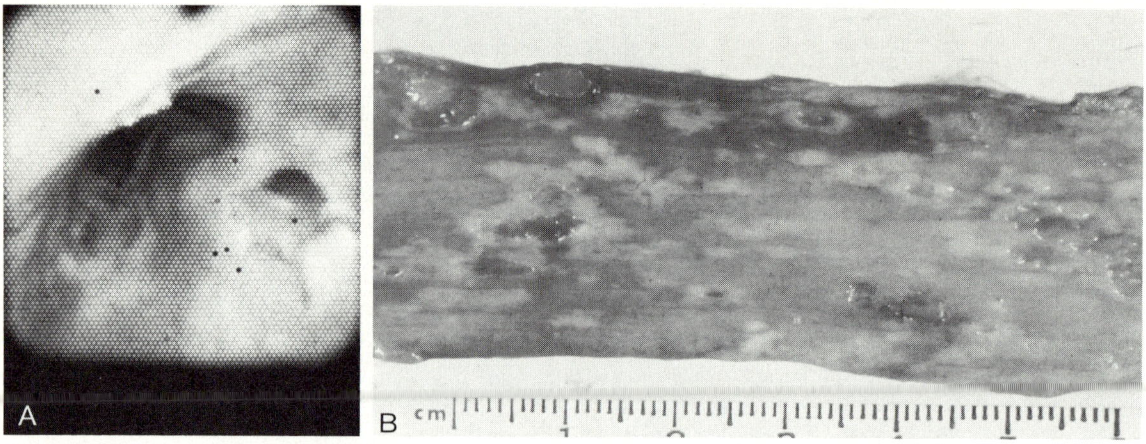

Figure 2–20. *A,* A view through a flexible endoscope of an esophagus of a 14-year-old canine that was presented for dysphagia and odynophagia. The raised white areas are abnormal. A biopsy specimen was obtained with a Quinton Multi-purpose Suction Biopsy Tube (note the red punched-out area). A definitive diagnosis of carcinoma was made from the specimen obtained. See Color Plate. *B,* The gross appearance of the same esophagus. Note the raised white areas that were visible through the endoscope.

cation contribute to canine problems with esophageal foreign bodies. Cats are usually more fastidious but acquire foreign bodies because of their hunting or playing behavior. Common types of esophageal foreign bodies are steak, chicken, or pork chop bones, wood, string, fish hooks, needles, and other metal objects. In the authors' experience bones are the most common foreign bodies encountered.

Anatomically, the esophagus has several narrow areas where swallowed foreign bodies tend to lodge. These are the cranial esophageal sphincter; the thoracic inlet, where adjacent soft tissues impede esophageal dilation; the heart base area, where the aorta moves the esophagus to the right; and the distal esophageal hiatal region.[46] Most foreign bodies are found in the thoracic esophagus, although a large percentage also occurs in the cervical esophageal region.

Diagnosis is often aided by the history of ingestion of a foreign body. Most esophageal foreign bodies are found in animals 2 to 3 years old or younger. Clinical signs are related to either partial or complete obstruction of the esophagus. Acute signs include: regurgitation associated with eating, painful dysphagia, ptyalism, persistent gulping, and anorexia. Chronic signs include: depression, weight loss, and other signs of complications. Foreign bodies located in the thoracic esophagus are usually associated with a higher incidence of complications than are those in the cervical esophagus.[46] Complications include: a perforated esophagus, pleuritis, mediastinitis, pyothorax, mucosal lacerations, esophageal stricture, diverticula, and severe esophagitis. The extent of esophageal damage is a function of the size, shape, and type of foreign body, as well as the length of time it is in contact with the mucosa.[22] The management of esophageal foreign bodies must be considered an emergency situation, since the incidence of complications increases with the duration of the disease process. Diagnostic procedures consist of careful physical examination, including a thorough oral examination, radiography, and esophagoscopy (Fig. 2–21).

In most cases of esophageal foreign bodies, it is advisable to use esophagoscopy. This procedure not only allows visualization of the foreign body, but also affords valuable

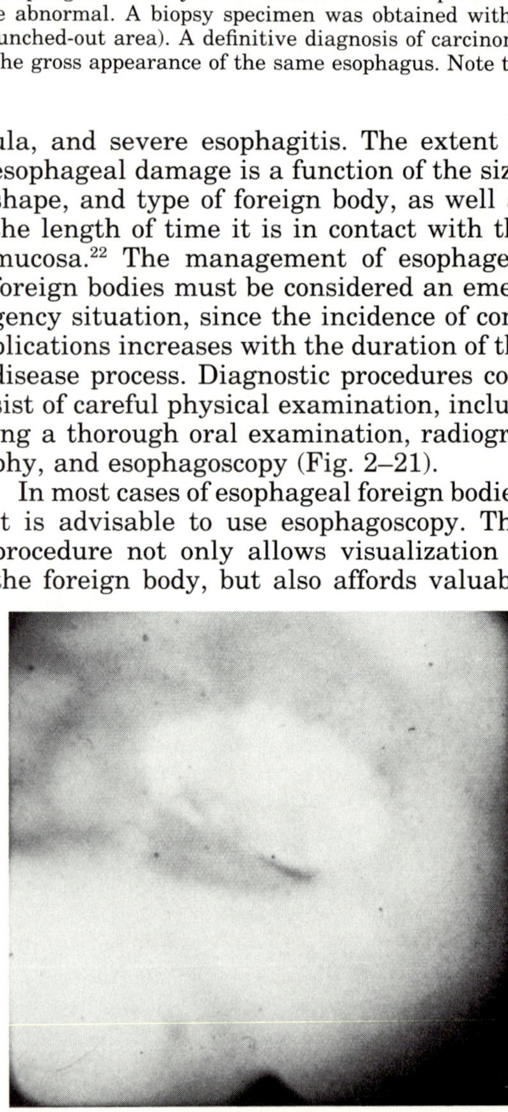

Figure 2–21. A bone esophageal foreign body in the esophagus as seen through a flexible endoscope. The bone is located just cranial to the cardia of the stomach. Insufflation of the esophagus increased its internal diameter. See Color Plate.

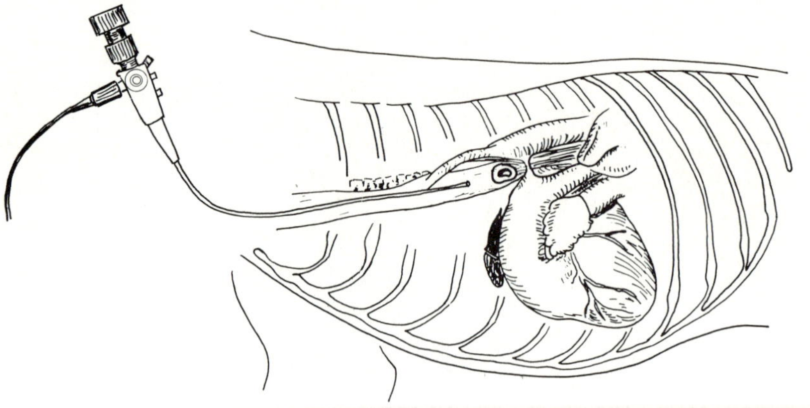

Figure 2–22. The use of a flexible endoscope to visualize a bone foreign body lodged at the base of the heart.

information in determining the extent of esophageal damage.[46] Esophagoscopy can often be utilized successfully to remove the foreign object.

In cases of suspected esophageal foreign body, the authors initially pass a flexible endoscope into the cavity to visualize the foreign body and to inspect for any esophageal damage (Fig. 2–22). If the foreign body is small, it can frequently be removed by passing flexible four-prong grasping forceps* through the endoscope, grasping the foreign body, and pulling it retrograde (Fig. 2–23). If the foreign body is too large for the flexible grasping forceps, rigid grasping forceps may be passed, in conjunction with a flexible endoscope, (Figs. 2–24 and 2–25). Once the foreign body is grasped, it and the endoscope can be pulled retrograde through the mouth. Frequently, the foreign body becomes dislodged from the grasper as it passes through the cranial esophageal sphincter. Usually, the foreign body can be easily retrieved by grasping it with large surgical forceps through the cranial esophageal sphincter. If flexible endoscopes are not available, rigid endoscopes work quite nicely (Figs. 2–26 to 2–28).

If the foreign body cannot be removed in a retrograde manner, the second procedure of choice is to push the foreign body into the stomach. Care should be utilized because of the distal esophageal deviation at the gastroesophageal junction. In the stomach, foreign bodies may be passed to the intestine and digested, excreted, or removed by gastrotomy. Most bone foreign bodies are digested by the acid in the stomach and then are eliminated in the feces in 7 to 10 days. A series of abdominal radiographs should be

*Grasping forceps, Microvasive, Inc., Belmont, MS.

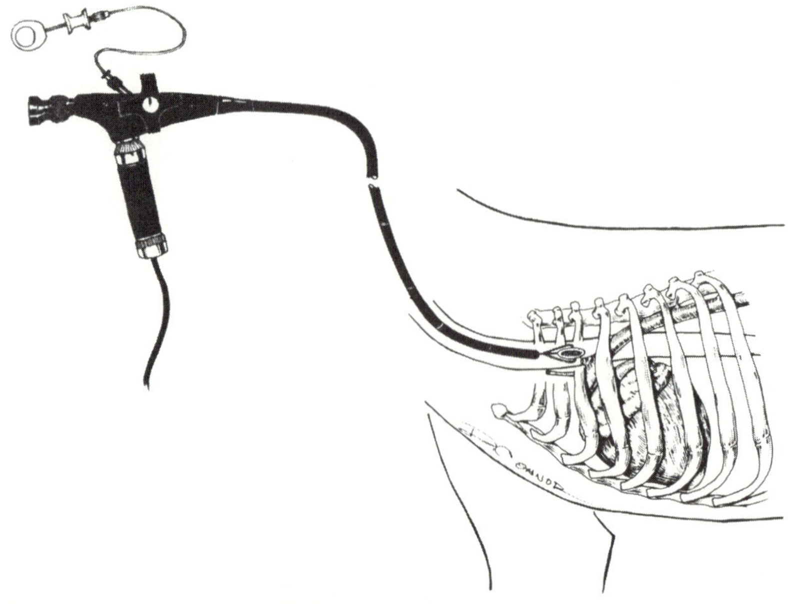

Figure 2–23. The use of a flexible endoscope with a four prong grasping forceps being passed through the operating channel. The grasping forceps is grasping the bone foreign body. Small foreign bodies can then be removed by pulling the endoscope and grasping forceps retrograde through the mouth.

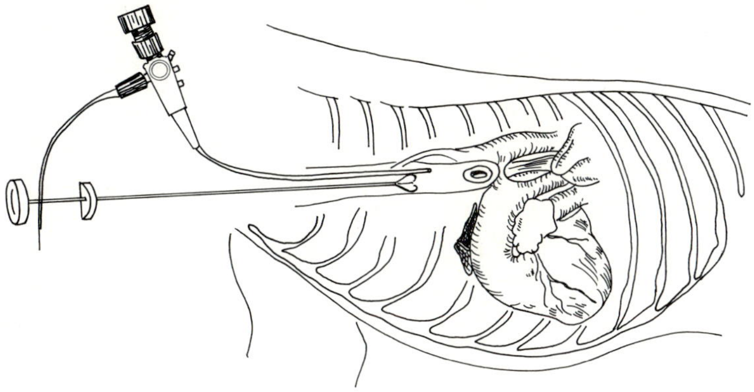

Figure 2–24. The use of rigid grasping forceps being passed along side the flexible endoscope to grasp the bone foreign body. The foreign body can easily be grasped as one visually observes the grasping forceps and foreign body through the endoscope.

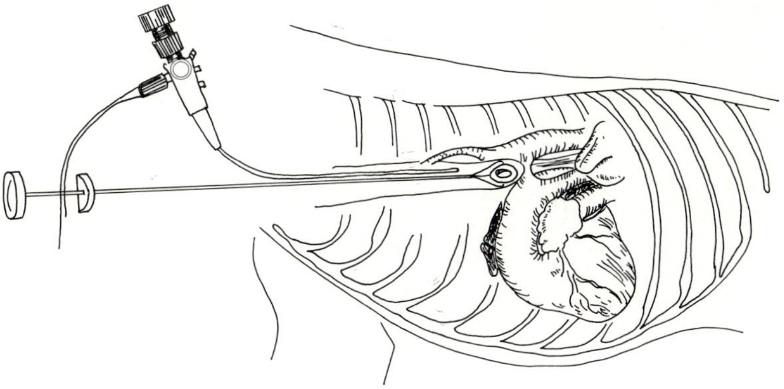

Figure 2–25. The grasping forceps and flexible endoscope in place. These two instruments are then both pulled retrograde to extract the foreign body from the esophagus.

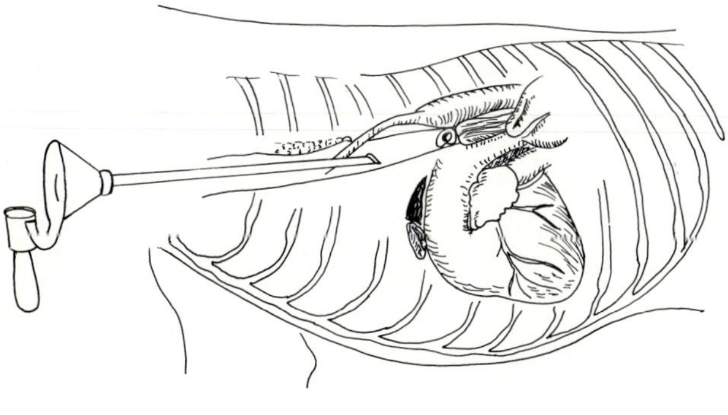

Figure 2–26. Use of a rigid endoscope to visualize a bone foreign body lodged at the base of the heart. A human sigmoidoscope (Fig. 2–3) can sometimes be used as a rigid endoscope.

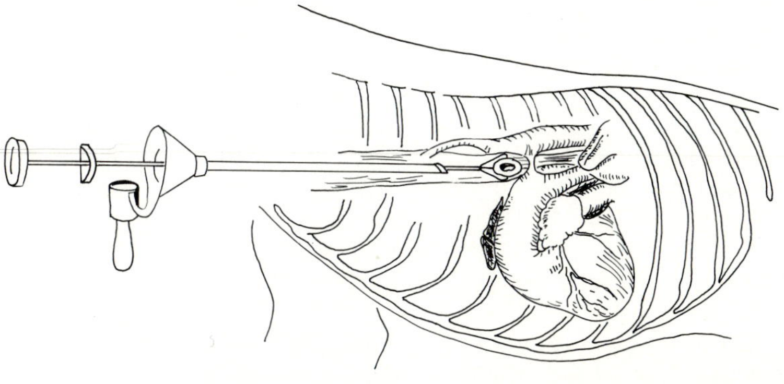

Figure 2–27. Grasping forceps passing through the rigid endoscope to grasp the bone esophageal foreign body.

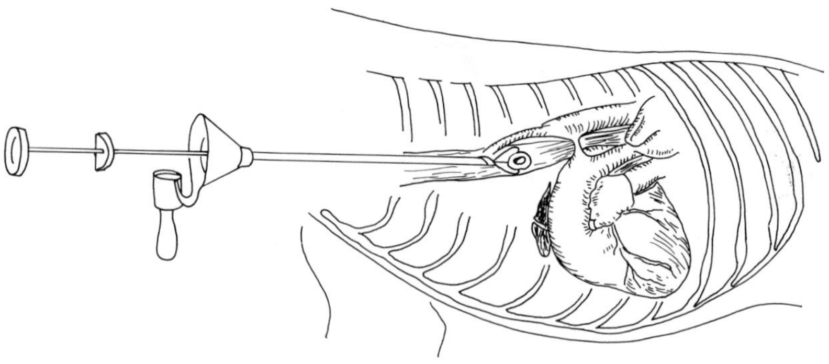

Figure 2–28. Grasping forceps and rigid endoscope being pulled retrograde to remove the bone foreign body. Note that the foreign body is pulled snug against the rigid endoscope to facilitate removal as the endoscope dilates the esophagus as it is pulled retrograde.

taken to confirm that the foreign body has indeed left the stomach and to make sure that it does not cause an obstruction further distally in the gastrointestinal tract.

The authors have used a combination of surgery and endoscopy to remove embedded fish hooks. The surgeon can cut off the end of the hook, and then the hook can be removed via endoscopy. By using this method the surgeon can avoid making an incision into the esophagus.

After the foreign body has been removed (either retrograde or into the stomach), an assessment of the esophageal damage should be made. The esophageal mucosa should be visually examined by passing an endoscope through the length of the esophagus. Usually, the degree of mucosal disease present is directly proportional to the duration of the foreign body in the esophagus. Erythema and mild ulceration at the site of entrapment are common. Special attention should be given to any evidence of tears, lacerations, or perforations of the esophageal wall. Thoracic radiographs should be taken after the removal of all esophageal foreign bodies, as a pneumothorax or a pneumomediastinum may be present if the esophagus was perforated.

In the authors' experience, mild tears, lacerations, and ulcerations will heal with the symptomatic treatment described for esophagitis. Esophageal lacerations and perforations have also reportedly been treated conservatively with pharyngostomy tubes, chest drainage, and supportive management.[2,46] The use of pharyngostomy tubes will allow the oral alimentation of an animal while resting the esophagus. Disadvantages of the use of pharyngostomy tubes are continuing irritation of the esophagus from the tube, and maintaining an open gastroesophageal sphincter with the possible reflux of gastric contents.[32] Large esophageal rents and signs of mediastinitis or other thoracic cavity involvement demand surgical exploration.

ESOPHAGEAL DIVERTICULA

Esophageal diverticula of any type are rarely documented in the veterinary literature. Research findings concerning the pathophysiology of diverticula formation are not available for animals and are extrapolated from human literature. In humans, esophageal diverticula have been classified according to their location and mode of development.

The areas of the esophagus most commonly involved are the area cranial to the thoracic inlet and the area just cranial to the diaphragm (epiphrenic). The human abnormality, pharyngoesophageal (Zenker's) diverticulum, has not been reported in domestic animals.

Diverticula can also be categorized as congenital or acquired. Causes of congenital diverticula are highly speculative and have been attributed to abnormal separation of tracheal and esophageal embryonic buds, development of eccentric vacuoles in the formation of the esophageal lumen, and congenital weakness of the esophageal wall.[31] Congenital diverticula have been reported only at the thoracic inlet.[3,53] Periodic diverticularization of the esophagus at the thoracic inlet is considered by some authors to be within normal limits for the English bulldog.[62] In the authors' experience, only 10 to 15 per cent of all dogs with congenital diverticula develop clinical signs. Developmental redundancy of the esophagus at the thoracic inlet may cause transient regurgitation in young dogs or may be detected as a coincidental finding during evaluation of vomiting or regurgitation problems.

Acquired diverticula can be further subdivided into the traction and pulsion vari-

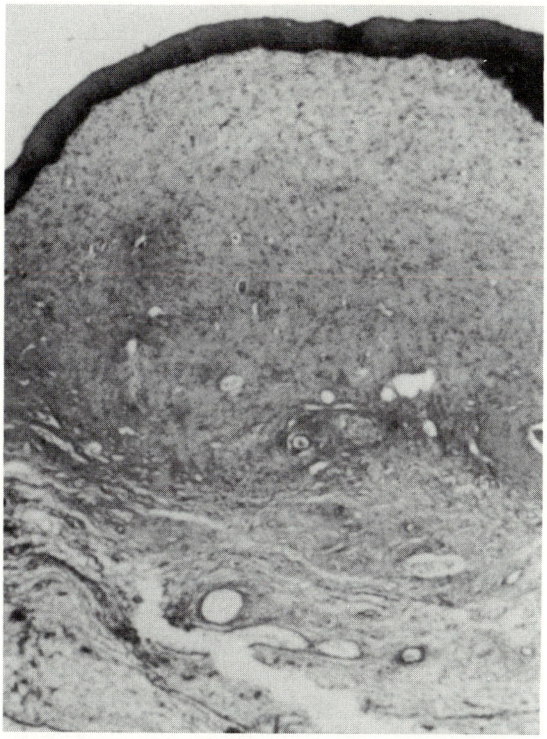

Figure 2–29. Photomicrograph of a section from the wall of a true pulsion diverticulum. A normal layer of stratified squamous epithelium, which was well keratinized in the luminal surface, rested on a sheet of connective tissue. The connective tissue on which the stratified squamous epithelium rested was composed of relatively immature collagen fibers. No muscle bundles and no muscle fibers were in any part of the tissue. This arrangement contrasts with that in a traction diverticulum, which consists of all layers of the esophagus (adventitia, muscle, submucosa, and stratified squamous mucosa).

eties. Traction diverticula have not been reported in the veterinary literature. In humans, they occur primarily in the midesophageal area. Their development is thought to be associated with a past inflammatory process involving the trachea, bronchi, or hilar lymph nodes. This inflammatory process leads to the production of fibrous tissue, which causes an outward traction of the esophageal wall. Traction diverticula rarely cause problems, because the wide neck of the diverticulum affords little chance of ingested material's becoming entrapped.[31]

Pulsion diverticula are true diverticula, in most cases. By definition, a diverticulum is "a circumscribed pouch or sac of variable size created by herniation of the mucous membrane lining through a defect in the muscular coat of a tubular organ."[31a] Pulsion diverticula can form cranial to any stenosed or diseased esophageal segment. Increased esophageal intraluminal pressure, along with food accumulation and deep esophageal inflammation can lead to mucosal herniation. The wall of a pulsion diverticulum generally consists of only esophageal epithelium and connective tissue (Fig. 2–29), whereas the traction diverticulum consists of all layers of the esophagus (adventitia, muscle, submucosa, stratified squamous mucosa). Predisposing factors in pulsion diverticula run the entire gamut of esophageal disease. These factors include: esophagitis, esophageal stenosis, cricopharyngeal achalasia, vascular ring anomalies, foreign bodies, megaesophagus, hiatal hernia, myas-

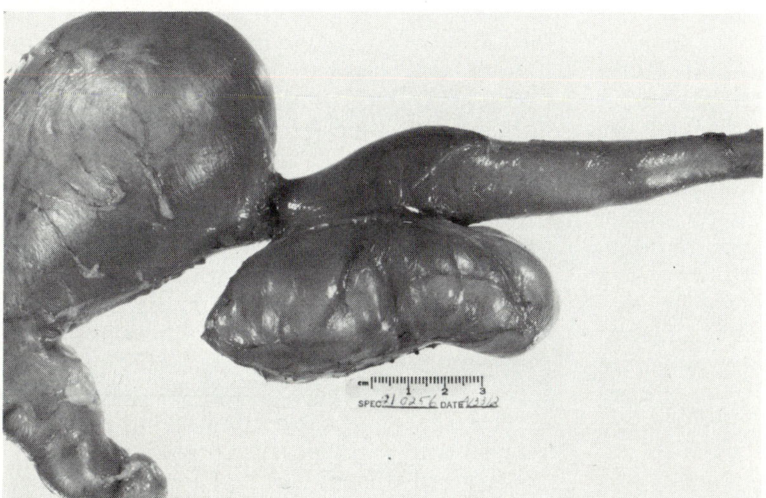

Figure 2–30. A large epiphrenic diverticulum is readily visualized in this necropsy specimen.

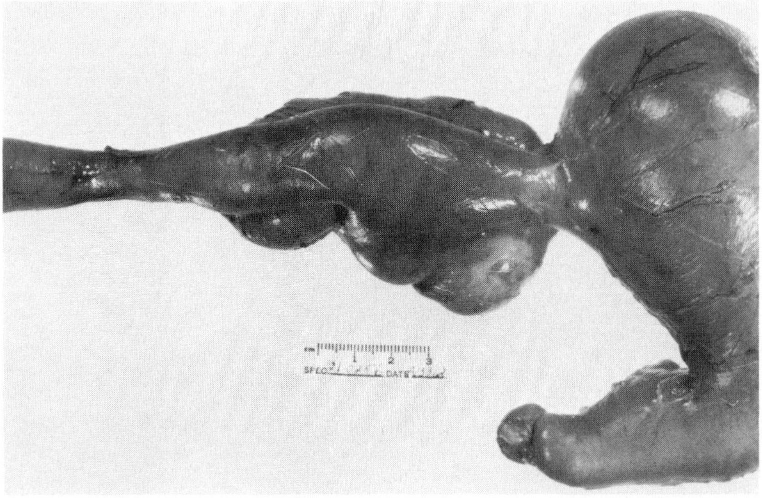

Figure 2–31. A large epiphrenic diverticulum.

thenia gravis, and other disorders of neuromuscular function. Acquired pulsion diverticula usually occur in the distal esophagus (epiphrenic) but rarely at the thoracic inlet (Figs. 2–30 and 2–31).[14, 17, 31, 42] It must be emphasized that the underlying etiology of diverticula should be fully investigated. Conservative therapy or surgical resection of a diverticulum may be unsuccessful if the signs and the diverticulum are the result of some other esophageal disorder.[31]

Once the diverticulum is formed, it has the potential of causing several complications including: impaction of ingested material with partial esophageal obstruction, chronic esophagitis and mucosal ulceration, peridiverticulitis with associated painful adhesions, and rupture of the diverticular wall with resultant mediastinitis or tracheoesophageal fistula.

Clinical signs of esophageal diverticula are distress or gagging soon after eating, postprandial regurgitation, intermittent anorexia and listlessness, fever, pain on abdominal palpation, reluctance to move, and incoordination or ataxia after eating. Further diagnostic techniques to differentiate diverticula from other causes of esophageal disease include: esophagography, fluoroscopy, and endoscopy. Esophagoscopy will show a hernia-like outpocketing from the esophageal lumen (Figs. 2–32 to 2–36).

Small diverticula with no other associated esophageal lesions may be treated conservatively by using a soft, bland diet, feeding the animal in a standing position, and administering plenty of liquids to wash out the diverticulum.[31] Symptomatic epiphrenic diverticula require surgical excision and reconstruction of the esophageal wall (see Chapter 4). Underlying causes must be treated appropriately.

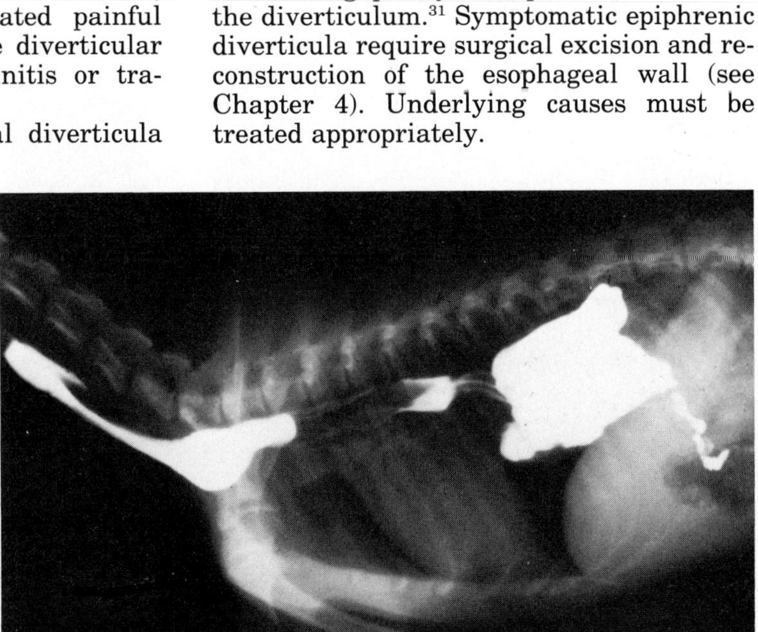

Figure 2–32. Lateral view of a positive-contrast esophagram demonstrating the large epiphrenic diverticulum shown in Figures 2–30 and 2–31.

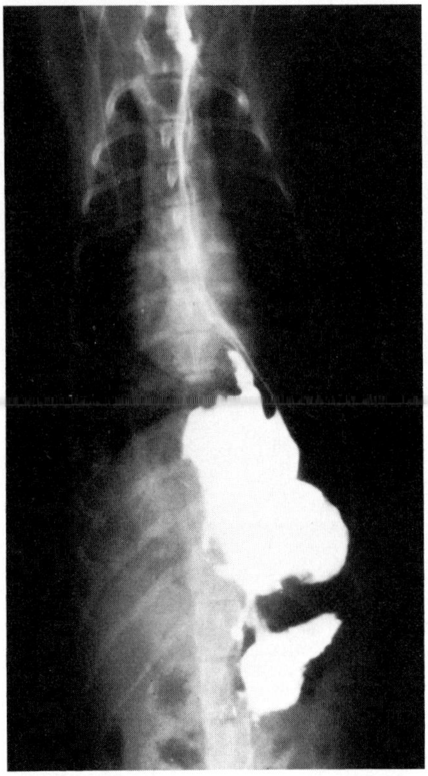

Figure 2–33. Ventrodorsal view of a positive contrast esophagram demonstrating a large epiphrenic diverticulum. This should not be confused with a gastric herniation into the thoracic cavity because the stomach is in its normal position.

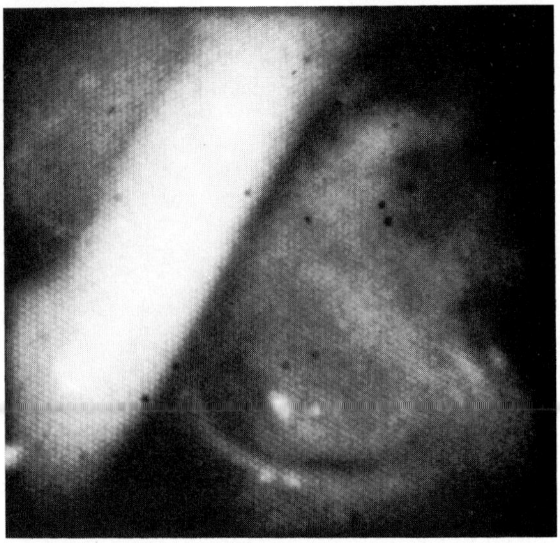

Figure 2–34. View through a flexible endoscope of the hernia-like ring in a patient with an esophageal epiphrenic diverticulum. The diverticulum is on the right side of the picture. The cardia is just to the left of the hernia ring. See Color Plate.

ESOPHAGEAL STRICTURES

Esophageal strictures can result from either extraluminal sources such as periesophageal masses or, more commonly, from intraluminal lesions of the esophagus.

Lesions in the tissues surrounding the esophagus have the potential to mechanically obstruct normal deglutition and cause secondary esophageal stricture. These periesophageal masses will cause clinical signs such as dysphagia, regurgitation, and debilitation due to external pressure and obstruction without actually invading the esophagus. Dilation of the esophagus cranial to such a lesion often occurs. Clinical signs other than those associated with the esophagus may be present, depending on the nature of the mass. Periesophageal masses include: cervical neoplasms (thyroid tumors), abscesses in the cervical region (foreign body) or anterior thoracic region (nocardiosis), lymphosarcoma or undifferentiated sarcoma involving the anterior mediastinum, extreme hilar lymphadenopathy, heart base tumors, and primary or secondary pulmonary neoplasms.[17] Radiographic studies with or without contrast material usually illustrate the obstructive lesion. Esophagoscopy will reveal a stricture with no mucosal involvement unless the periesophageal mass has invaded the esophageal lumen (Fig. 2–37). Treatment is aimed at the cause of the mass lesion.

Intraluminal stricture is a common sequela to esophageal surgery, to the ingestion of foreign bodies, ingestion of caustic materials, external trauma to the cervical or thoracic esophagus, or esophagitis of various

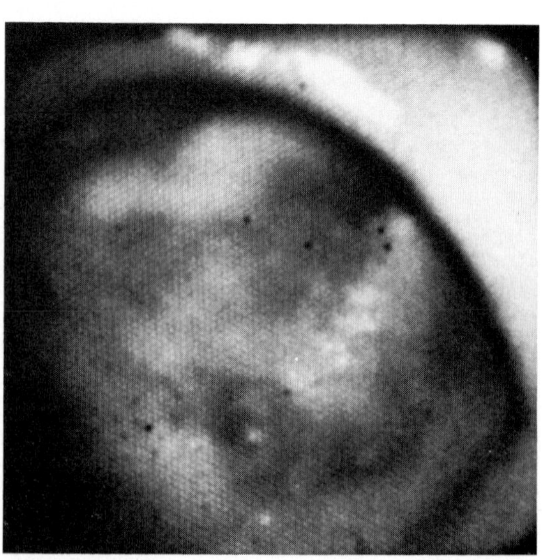

Figure 2–35. View through a flexible endoscope looking into the diverticulum pouch. Note the hernia ring in the upper right corner. See Color Plate.

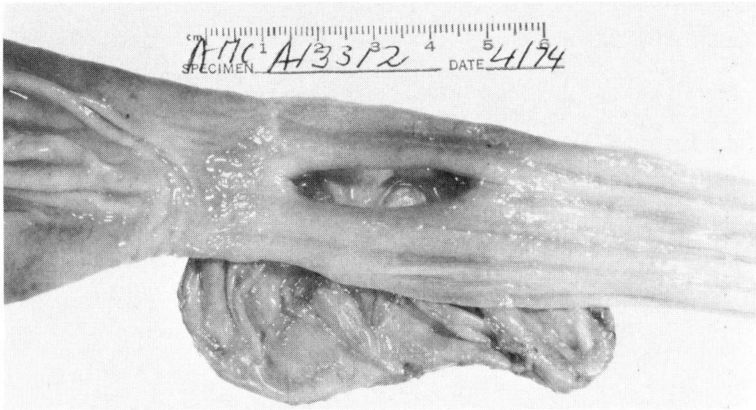

Figure 2–36. Necropsy specimen demonstrating the epiphrenic diverticulum and the characteristic hernia-like outpocketing from the esophageal lumen. This is the same patient as in Figures 2–34 and 2–35. Note how the endoscopy findings correlate with the necropsy findings.

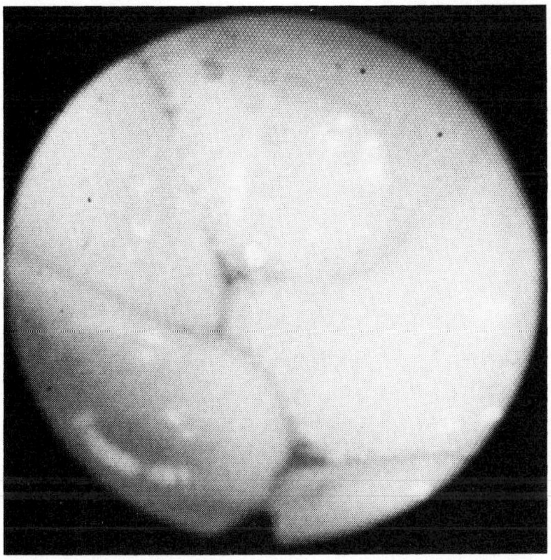

Figure 2–37. A view through a flexible endoscope of an extraluminal stricture. Note that the stricture is composed of normal mucosa, which is indicative of a periesophageal mass causing the stricture. This patient had a history of regurgitating for 2 months prior to presentation. Surgery revealed a mass totally encircling the esophagus. Histologically the mass was a fibrosarcoma. See Color Plate.

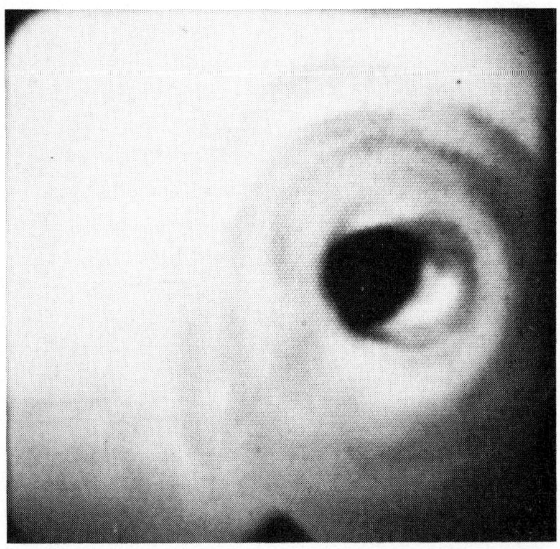

Figure 2–38. View through a flexible endoscope demonstrating an intraluminal esophageal stricture. See Color Plate.

causes. One case of esophageal stricture in the cat was caused by an acute viral infection, which led to extensive esophageal desquamation and erosion.[5] In the authors' experience, esophageal stricture most commonly results from the previous presence of an esophageal foreign body.

The esophageal mucosa has extensive recuperative powers. Superficial mucosal inflammation will produce a transient, mild, segmental narrowing of the esophagus but will not precipitate stricture formation. Severe inflammation or damage that involves the deeper esophageal submucosa and muscularis is needed to produce fibrotic changes and stricture. The location of the stricture and the amount of luminal obstruction will determine the severity of clinical signs.

The signs of esophageal stricture are similar to those of obstructing foreign bodies or neoplasms. A previously normal animal will develop gradually increasing dysphagia and regurgitation, particularly with solid food. Liquids are well tolerated until late in the course of the disease. Initially, regurgitation usually occurs soon after eating. In a chronic stricture, in which there is dilation of the esophagus cranial to the stricture, regurgitation may not be related to eating. Diagnosis is based on a history of previous trauma or foreign body, positive contrast radiographic studies of the esophagus, and esophagoscopy (Figs. 2–38 and 2–39).

A separate clinical entity termed iatrogenic esophageal stricture has recently been described in both dogs and cats.[19, 41, 61] The stricture develops after routine, elective surgical procedures such as ovariohysterectomy. The patients have no previous history of dysphagia or regurgitation but develop a severe esophageal stricture several days or weeks postoperatively. The stricture most commonly develops near the thoracic inlet but may occur anywhere along the esophagus. Various etiologies have been considered, but the exact cause is still not understood. These strictures probably result from reflux of highly acidic gastric contents during routine surgery. This acidic fluid pools in the region of the esophagus from the thoracic inlet to the base of the heart, causing a caustic reflux esophagitis. Factors during the operation that might encourage reflux and pooling of gastric contents are airway occlusion, increased intra-abdominal pressure, lateral or dorsal recumbency with the head lowered, and loss of the secondary peristaltic contractions during anesthesia. These strictures are perplexing to the veterinarian and damaging to the animals and produce a severe strain on client relations.

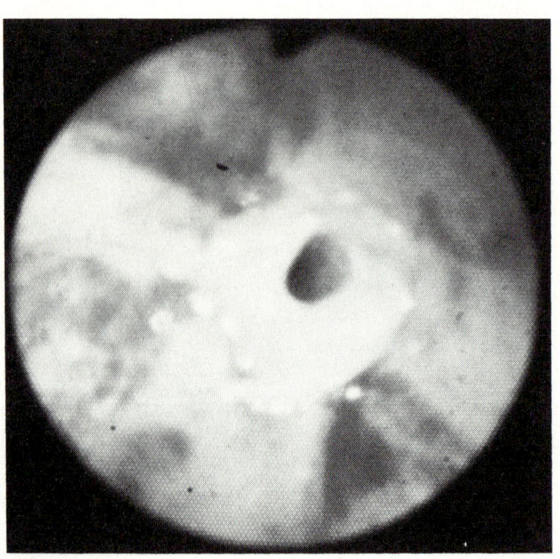

Figure 2–39. View through a flexible endoscope of an intraluminal esophageal stricture. Note the hemorrhagic areas around the stricture. The white tissue is fibrous connective tissue. See Color Plate.

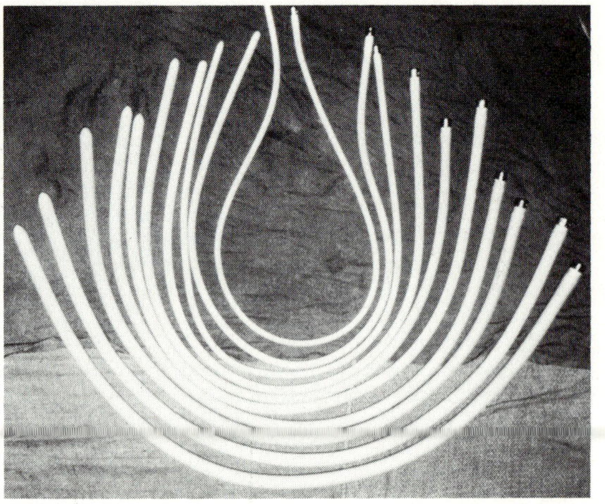

Figure 2–40. A complete set of mercury-filled esophageal bougies.

Therapy of esophageal strictures can be approached from either a medical or surgical aspect, depending on the extent and number of strictures. Experimental work is being done with various scar tissue inhibiting compounds, which can be given during acute esophageal disease to inhibit stricture formation.[47] These compounds are not yet being used in clinical practice and are of no value once the stricture is diagnosed. The best medical approach is the utilization of bougienage to mechanically dilate the esophagus at the stricture site. In the authors' experience, tapered, mercury-filled esophageal bougies, which come in a series of graded diameters, work very well (Fig. 2–40). The animal is anesthetized, and the smallest, well-lubricated bougie is introduced through the full length of the esophagus. This process is repeated with each bougie of progressively increasing diameter to mechanically dilate the stricture site. With experience and the proper bougies, the procedure is accomplished quickly and easily. A full set of esophageal bougies can usually be borrowed from a local human hospital or are available through a surgical supply company.* The bougienage procedure may need to be repeated every few months to alleviate signs of obstruction. Intralesional corticosteroid injections or prolonged use of oral corticosteroids following bougienage have been reported to reduce the number of times that bougienage must be repeated in an individual patient.[20, 39] A dosage of oral prednisolone at 1 mg/kg for 3 to 4 weeks after bougienage is recommended.[39] Surgical intervention with either esophageal resection and anastomosis or esophagoplasty may be utilized in persistent cases. The authors have routinely placed a pharyngostomy tube into the esophagus beyond the stricture site. As stated earlier, it is best not to have the pharyngostomy tube extend into the stomach. The authors leave the tube in place approximately 10 days and use a tube that is about the same diameter as the patient's trachea. It is believed that the use of a pharyngostomy tube reduces the incidence of restricturing after dilation or surgery.

SECONDARY NEUROMUSCULAR DISEASES

A variety of systemic diseases may also involve the esophagus. Most of the conditions are neuromuscular abnormalities, and dysphagia or regurgitation may be clinical problems. In a few individuals, esophageal signs may be the initial or only clinical problem.

Myasthenia Gravis

Animals with myasthenia gravis may be found to have esophageal dilation. There are two forms of the disease, congenital and acquired. In congenital myasthenia gravis, a deficiency of acetylcholine receptors on the postsynaptic membrane exists.[6] It is thought that the acquired disease may be an immune-mediated disorder at the motor endplates, since immune complexes have been demonstrated on the endplates, and circulating antibody to the acetylcholine receptors has been found.[6] Signs of megaesophagus have not been reported in myasthenia gravis of congenital origin.[6] Patients are usually presented with weakness, which is exacerbated on exercise, increased dysphonia and dysphagia, along with an increasing frequency of regurgitation. It was once thought that megaesophagus occurred only in cases of canine myasthenia gravis, but it has also been seen in cats.[36] Since this is a disorder at the motor endplates of skeletal muscle, the dilation occurs in the proximal two-thirds of the feline esophagus, whereas the entire length of the canine esophagus is affected.

The diagnosis in suspected cases of myasthenia gravis is made by intravenous injection of 0.1 to 0.5 mg edrophonium chloride.* Affected patients will usually show a dramatic return to normal coordination and activity that lasts only a few moments. There is no change in the esophageal condition during these moments. Once a diagnosis is made, the animals may be treated with neostigmine methylsulfate† at a dosage of 0.5 mg/kg given three times a day for the rest of the animal's life. The neostigmine methylsulfate should also be combined with prednisolone (usually 2 mg/kg) to suppress the immune reaction. Over time, the dosage of neostigmine methylsulfate can usually be slowly decreased and the animal placed on alternate day therapy of prednisolone. Some animals may even respond to the point of not requiring medication, but regression does occur and should be watched for. It must be noted that the esophageal damage is usually permanent and does not respond to therapy;[36] therefore, special care such as feeding the animal in an upright position may be necessary.

Polymyositis

A condition that may manifest signs similar to those of myasthenia gravis is polymyositis; a distinction between the conditions must be made because their treat-

*Esophageal bougies and dilator sets, Pilling Company, Fort Washington, PA.

*Tensilon, Roche Laboratories, Nutley, NJ.
†Prostigmin, Roche Laboratories, Nutley, NJ.

ments differ. Many of the causes of polymyositis are inflammatory or degenerative in origin. Inflammatory non-infectious polymyositis has been reported to be associated with megaesophagus.[29] The dog is usually presented with the complaint that it is weakened after periods of exercise and may or may not have an associated pain or stiffness. Spinal reflexes are normal. There may also be a non-painful loss of muscle mass. The progression of signs may vary from hours to months.

The diagnosis of polymyositis is made through the use of serum chemistry measurements, electromyographic (EMG) studies, serum electrophoresis, and histology. In polymyositis, the muscle enzymes—creatinine phosphokinase (CPK), lactate dehydrogenase (LDH), and aspartate aminotransferase (AST/SGOT)—are elevated. Patients with mild disease may show no change in the EMG or may have positive waves and fibrillation potentials on the tracing.[6] The more severe cases will have bizarre high-frequency discharges.[6] It is possible for there to be a hypergammaglobulinemia and positive results of an antinuclear antibody (ANA) test with this disease.[6] Confirmation of the diagnosis of polymyositis is provided by a histological evaluation of the muscle tissue that reveals a mononuclear interstitial inflammation with muscle fiber necrosis.

A reducing dosage regimen of prednisolone has been recommended for dogs with inflammatory muscle disease.[29] Initially, these dogs may be given 0.25 to 0.5 mg/kg three times a day; this dosage should be reduced over 7 to 10 days. Some dogs may not need any further medication after this period, whereas others may require lifelong alternate day therapy.[29] Although esophageal function can return to normal, the prognosis is guarded to poor in animals with severe damage to the esophageal and laryngeal musculature.

Systemic Lupus Erythematosus

Megaesophagus may be seen with systemic lupus erythematosus (SLE).[30] The diagnosis of the polymyositis condition of SLE is made on the basis of elevated concentrations of serum muscle enzymes (CPK, LDH, AST) and EMG studies showing polyphasic small motor unit potentials, fibrillation potentials, positive sharp waves, increased insertional activities, and bizarre, high-frequency repetitive discharges.[30] The use of LE cell preparations and ANA tests help to arrive at a diagnosis of SLE. Therapy is aimed at immunosuppression with corticosteroids. Some animals may not respond to steroids; therefore stronger drugs such as azathioprine* and cyclophosphamide† may be required. Remission may occur in some cases, but recurrence of the disease can be expected.

Other Secondary Neuromuscular Diseases

Pearson has reported megaesophagus occurring simultaneously with pylorospasm in cats.[43] The significance of the esophageal dilation is unknown in these cases, since the clinical signs were more closely associated with the pylorospasm and did not persist after a pyloromyotomy was performed.[43] These animals had a history of poor condition with a projectile vomitus. Radiology revealed reduced gastric emptying and a dilated esophagus. Pearson suggests the possibility of a heritable condition or conditions, since a high proportion of patients were Siamese cats.[43]

Metastatic neoplastic invasion of the esophagus may result in disrupted motor activity.[45] In one study, metastatic tumors were three times more common than primary neoplastic conditions of the esophagus.[45] Survey radiographs, contrast studies, fluoroscopy, and endoscopy are useful, but a definitive diagnosis is usually dependent on histopathological studies.

Neoplastic conditions, trauma, and surgery may cause damage to the vagus nerve. Should this damage be bilateral, esophageal dilation may occur. To further localize the lesion, laryngeal paralysis will occur simultaneously when the injury is above the recurrent laryngeal nerve. Canine giant axonal neuropathy has been reported to cause megaesophagus in dogs.[12] It is suspected of causing a demyelination of the vagus nerve.[12] The neuropathy involves both central and peripheral nerves.

A demyelinating neuritis of the vagus nerves can occur in thallium toxicosis.[65] This neuritis, as with the conditions listed above,

*Imuran, Burroughs Wellcome; Research Triangle Park, NC.

†Cytoxin, Mead Johnson Pharmaceutical, Evansville, IN.

will lead to dilation of the esophagus. Although thallium is not much used as a rodenticide today, it affects a number of organs and tissues. Mature animals seem to be more sensitive than younger ones. Clinical signs are reflected in many body systems including the gastrointestinal tract, respiratory system, nervous system, and skin. As the duration of exposure lengthens, the involvement of other previously unaffected systems occurs. With chronicity, brick-red gums, cutaneous erythema, and alopecia are evident. The dilation is evident in a canine esophagus, which has skeletal muscle, whereas a human esophagus is of smooth muscle and megaesophagus is not a feature of demyelinating neuritis.

Megaesophagus can develop in any shock-like condition, particularly hypoadrenocorticism (Addison's disease).[15] If Addison's is the cause of shock, the signs disappear with shock therapy and corticosteroids.

Other disease conditions to which megaesophagus is reported to be secondary are glycogen storage–like disease, chronic cholinesterase inhibition,[18] hypothyroidism, chronic lead toxicosis,[64] trypanosomiasis,[35] trauma,[56] and cachexia.[58] Some of these conditions are not well described in the literature.

References

1. Biancani P, Goyal RIC, Phillips A, et al: Mechanics of sphincter Action: Studies on the lower esophageal sphincter. J Clin Invest 52:2973, 1973.
2. Bohning RH, DeHoff WD, McElhinney A, et al: Pharyngostomy for maintenance of the anorectic animal. J Am Vet Med Assoc 156:611, 1970.
3. Bone WJ: What is your diagnosis? Thoracic inlet diverticulum. J Am Vet Med Assoc 155:549, 1969.
4. Clifford DM, Malek R: Diseases of the canine esophagus due to prenatal influence. Am J Dig Dis 14:578, 1969.
5. Clifford DM, Soifer FK, Freeman RG: Stricture and dilatation of the esophagus in the cat. J Am Vet Med Assoc 156:1007, 1970.
6. Chrisman CL, Averill DR: Diseases of peripheral nerves and muscles. *In* Ettinger SJ (ed). *Textbook of Veterinary Internal Medicine.* 2nd ed, Philadelphia, W. B. Saunders Company, 608, 1983.
7. Cohen S: Motor disorders of the esophagus. N Engl J Med 301:184, 1979.
8. Cohen S, Harris LC: The lower esophageal sphincter. Gastroenterology 63:1006, 1972.
9. Dodds WJ: Current concepts of esophageal motor function: Clinical implications for radiology. Am J Roentgenol 128:549, 1977.
10. Dodds WJ, Hogan WJ, Nulter WN: Reflux esophagitis. Am J Dig Dis 21:49, 1976.
11. Dodds WJ, Stewart ET, Hodges D, et al: Movement of the feline esophagus associated with respiration and peristalsis. J Clin Invest 52:1, 1973.
12. Duncan ID, Griffiths IR: Canine giant axonal neuropathy. Vet Rec 101:438, 1977.
13. Ettinger SJ, Suter PF: Diseases of the great vessels. *In* Ettinger SJ (ed): *Textbook of Veterinary Internal Medicine.* Philadelphia, W. B. Saunders Company, 980, 1975.
14. Faulkner RT, Caywood D, Wallace LS, Johnson GR: Epiphrenic esophageal diverticulectomy in a dog: A case report and review. J Am Anim Hosp Assoc 17:77, 1981.
15. Feldman EC, Tyrrell JB: Hypoadrenocorticism. Vet Clin North Am 7:555, 1977.
16. Gaynor F, Hoffer RE, Nichols MF, et al: Physiologic features of the canine esophagus: Effects of tranquilization on esophageal motility. Am J Vet Res 41:727, 1980.
17. Guffy, MM: Esophageal disorders, in Ettinger, SJ (ed): *Textbook of Veterinary Internal Medicine.* Philadelphia, W. B. Saunders Company, 1098, 1975.
18. Harris LD, Ashworth WD, Ingelfinger FJ: Esophageal aperistalsis and achalasia produced in dogs by prolonged cholinesterase inhibition. J Clin Invest 39:1744, 1960.
19. Harvey CE: Iatrogenic esophageal stricture in the dog. J Am Vet Med Assoc 166:1100 1975.
20. Harvey CE, O'Brien JA: Esophageal diseases and disorders. Proc Am Anim Hosp Assoc 155, 1975.
21. Hoffer RE: Surgical esophageal diseases. *In* Bojrab MJ (ed): *Pathophysiology in Small Animal Surgery.* Philadelphia, Lea & Febiger, 90, 1981.
22. Hoffer RE: Diseases of the esophagus. *In* Kirk RW (ed): *Current Veterinary Therapy VI.* Philadelphia, W. B. Saunders Company, 931, 1977.
23. Hollenbeck JI, Maher JW, Wickbom G, et al: The effect of feeding on the canine lower esophageal sphincter. J Surg Res 18:497, 1975.
24. Ivoghli B: Esophageal sarcomas associated with canine spirocercosis. Vet Med/Sm Anim Clin 73:47, 1978.
25. Janssens J, Valembois S, Vantrappen G, et al: Is the primary peristaltic contraction of the canine esophagus bolus-dependent? Gastroenterology 65:241, 1973.
26. Jones BD: The use of fiberoptic endoscopy in veterinary medicine. Proc Am Anim Med Hosp Assoc 45:241, 1978.
27. Jordan PM, Langhi EM: Relationship between size of bolus and cat of swallowing in esophageal peristalsis in dogs. Proc Soc Exp Biol Med 137:868, 1971.
28. Kasper JB, Chiapella AM: Gastrointestinal biopsy techniques. *In* Kirk RW (ed): *Current Veterinary Therapy VII.* Philadelphia, W. B. Saunders Company, 962, 1980.
29. Kornegay JN, Gorgacz, EJ, Dawe DL, et al: Polymyositis in dogs. J Am Vet Med Assoc 176:431, 1980.
30. Krum SH, Cardinet GH, Anderson BL, Holliday TA: Polymyositis and polyarthritis associated with systemic lupus erythematosus in a dog. J Am Vet Med Assoc 170:61, 1977.
31. Lantz GC, Bojrab MJ, Jones BD: Epiphrenic esophageal diverticulectomy. J Am Anim Hosp Assoc, 12:629, 1976.

31a. *Dorland's Illustrated Medical Dictionary.* 26th ed, Philadelphia, W. B. Saunders Company, 1981.

32. Lantz GC, Cantwell HD, Vleet, JF: Pharyngostomy tube induced esophagitis in the dog: An experimental study. J Am Anim Hosp Assoc 19:207, 1983.

33. Lawson DD, Pirie HM: Conditions of the canine esophagus II. Vascular rings, achalasia, tumors and periesophageal lesions. J Small Anim Pract 7:117, 1966.
34. Leipold HW: Nature and causes of congenital defects of dogs. Vet Clin North Am 8:47, 1977.
35. Marsden PD, Hagstrom JWC: Experimental *Trypanosoma cruzi* infection in beagle puppies. The effect of variations in the dose and source of infection trypanosomes and the routes of inoculation on the course of the infection. Trans R Soc Trop Med Hyg 62:816, 1968.
36. Mason KV: A case of myasthenia gravis in a cat. J Small Anim Pract 17:467, 1976.
37. McCaw D, Pratt M, Walshaw R: Squamous cell carcinoma of the esophagus in a dog. J Am Anim Hosp Assoc 16:561, 1980.
38. O'Brien JA: Esophagoscopy. Vet Clin North Am 2:99, 1972.
39. O'Brien JA, Harvey CE, Brodey RS: The esophagus. *In* Anderson NV (ed): *Veterinary Gastroenterology*. Philadelphia, Lea & Febiger, 372, 1980.
40. Patterson DV: Epidemiologic and genetic studies of congenital heart disease in the dog. Circ Res 23:171, 1968.
41. Pearson H, Darke PG, Gibbs C, et al: Reflux esophagitis and stricture formation after anesthesia: A review of seven cases in dogs and cats. J Small Anim Pract 19:507, 1978.
42. Pearson H, Gibbs C, Kelly DV: Esophageal diverticulum formation in the dog. J Small Anim Pract 19:341, 1978.
43. Pearson H, Gaskell CH, Gibbs C, Waterman A: Pyloric and esophageal dysfunction in the cat. J Small Anim Pract 15:487, 1974.
44. Pope CE: Gastroesophageal reflux disease (reflux esophagus). *In* Sleisenger MO, and Fordtran JS (eds): *Gastrointestinal Disease*. Philadelphia, W. B. Saunders Company, 568, 1978.
45. Ridgway RL, Suter PF: Clinical and radiographic signs in primary and metastatic esophageal neoplasms of the dog. J Am Vet Med Assoc 174:700, 1979.
46. Ryan WW, Greene RW: The conservative management of esophageal foreign bodies and their complications: A review of 66 cases in dogs and cats. J Am Anim Hosp Assoc 11:243, 1975.
47. Saedi S, Nyhus LM, Gabrys BF: Pharmocological prevention of esophageal stricture. Am Surg 39:465, 1973.
48. Seibold HR, Bailey WS, Hoerlein BF, et al: Observations on the possible relations of malignant esophageal tumors and *Spirocerca lupi* lesions in the dog. Am J Vet Res 16:5, 1955.
49. Shelton GD: Swallowing disorders in the dog. Comp Cont Ed 4:607, 1982.
50. Silvadas CG, Nau MK, Rajan A: Neoplastic changes associated with esophageal spirocerca tumor in a dog. Indian Vet J 43:195, 1966.
51. Strombeck DR: Pathophysiology of esophageal motility disorders. Vet Clin North Am 8:229, 1978.
52. Strombeck DR: *Acute Gastritis in Small Animal Gastroenterology*. Davis, CA Stongate, 98, 1979.
53. Thrall DE: The esophagus. *In* Gillette EL, Thrall DE and Lebel JL (eds): *Carlson's Veterinary Radiology*. 3rd ed. Philadelphia, Lea & Febiger, 254, 1977.
54. Thrasher JP, Barrett RB, Tyler DE: Osteogenic sarcoma of the canine esophagus. Vet Med/Sm Anim Clin 63:333, 1963.
55. Turnwald GH, Smallwood JE, Helman RG: Esophageal osteosarcoma in a dog. J Am Vet Med Assoc 174:1009, 1979.
56. Ueda M, Schlegel JF, Code CF: Electric and motor activity of innervated and vagally denervated feline esophagus. Am J Dig Dis 17:1075, 1972.
57. Vernon FF, Roudebush P: Primary esophageal carcinoma in a cat. J Am Anim Hosp Assoc 16:547, 1980.
58. Watrous BJ: Esophageal disease. *In* Ettinger SJ (ed): *Textbook of Veterinary Internal Medicine*. 2nd ed, Philadelphia, W. B. Saunders Company, 1191, 1983.
59. Watrous BJ, Suter PF: Normal swallowing in the dog: A cineradiographic study. Vet Radiol 20:99, 1979.
60. Wilkinson GT: Chronic papillomatous esophagitis in a young cat. Vet Rec 87:355, 1970.
61. Wilson GP: Ulcerative esophagitis and esophageal stricture. J Am Anim Hosp Assoc 13:180, 1977.
62. Woods CB, Rawlings C, Barber D, et al: Esophageal deviations in four English bulldogs. J Am Vet Med Assoc 172:934, 1978.
63. Zimmer JF: Gastrointestinal fiberoptic endoscopy. *In* Kirk RW (ed): *Current Veterinary Therapy VII*. Philadelphia, W. B. Saunders Company, 954, 1980.
64. Zook BC: The pathologic anatomy of lead poisoning in dogs. Vet Pathol 9:310, 1972.
65. Zook BC, Gilmore CE: Thallium poisoning in dogs. J Am Vet Med Assoc 151:206, 1967.

CHAPTER

3

Primary Esophageal Neuromuscular Diseases

R. E. HOFFER

Neuromuscular diseases of the esophagus may be divided into primary diseases and secondary diseases. Conditions such as myasthenia gravis, Addison's disease, polymyositis, scleroderma, and systemic lupus erythematosus produce esophageal neuromuscular dysfunction secondarily and are discussed in Chapter 2.

Primary neuromuscular diseases of the esophagus include hiatal hernia with reflux, gastroesophageal intussusception, oropharyngeal dysphagia, and idiopathic megaesophagus-achalasia syndrome. These diseases are characterized by non-synchronous passage of a bolus from the mouth to the stomach, which occurs because of faulty peristalsis, failure of the sphincters to relax or contract, or an improper propulsion or misdirection of a bolus.

Primary neuromuscular diseases of the esophagus are uncommon; idiopathic megaesophagus syndrome is most often diagnosed. In one study, 79 dogs out of a total population of 41,154 were affected with this problem.[15] Primary neuromuscular disease is less commonly reported in the cat than in the dog.[3, 6, 26]

The normal esophageal swallowing complex may be measured manometrically in the dog. This measurement is made with a triple lumen catheter with measurement ports at three separate points located 5 centimeters apart. Each lumen is connected to a transducer that measures the pressure changes within the esophagus. The transducers convert the pressure changes to an electrical impulse, which is then recorded on a chart. To measure pressures, the catheter is placed so that the three ports are in the mid-esophagus. An induced swallow produces a measurable peristaltic pressure wave (Fig. 3–1). The catheter is then advanced so the distal port is in the stomach,

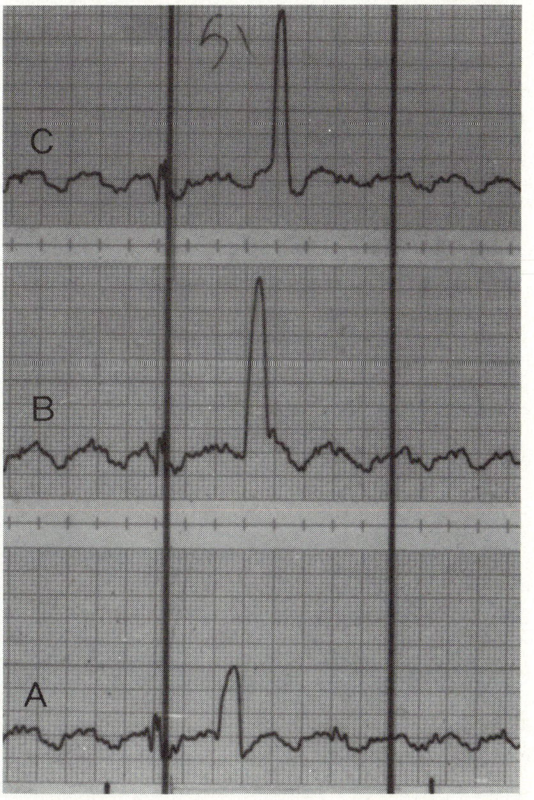

Figure 3–1. A normal esophageal swallowing complex is recorded in the mid-esophagus. Note that the waves are progressive; the bottom, *A*, being closest to the mouth and the top wave, *B*, the farthest away. The wave progression rate is 100.7 cm/s in the middle portion of the esophagus.[11]

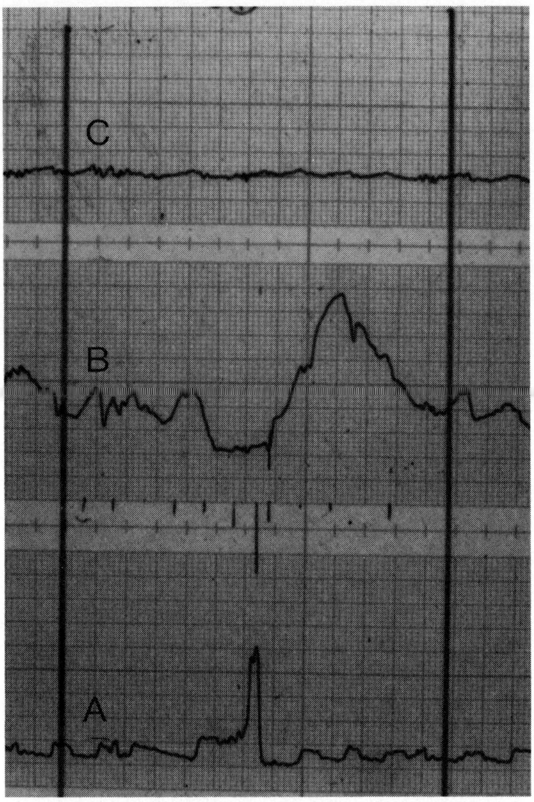

Figure 3–2. A normal esophageal swallowing complex. *A*, Pressure in the distal esophagus; *B*, the LES; *C*, pressure in the stomach. Note that the LES was relaxed before the esophageal high pressure, represented by a bolus, reached it. The LES contracted after the bolus had passed through it.

the middle port in the lower esophageal sphincter (LES), and the proximal port in the distal esophagus. A swallow is induced and the pressure changes at these areas are recorded (Fig. 3–2).

The passage of a peristaltic contraction through the body of the esophagus, the interaction of the esophagus with the LES, and the passage of a bolus from the mouth through the body of the esophagus are synchronous functions. Interference with this synchronous function, by elimination of progressive peristaltic contraction of the esophageal body, by interference with the interaction of the LES and esophageal body, or by interruption of the progress of a bolus from the mouth through the cricopharyngeal sphincter, results in esophageal disease.[11, 17, 19] The type of interruption or the location of the interference will determine the clinical entity. The concept of synchronous function of the esophagus and LES is the key to understanding esophageal neuromuscular diseases and their therapy.[2, 10, 11, 19]

Oropharyngeal Disorders

Suter and Watrous[37] described in detail nine cases of oropharyngeal dysphagia in dogs, utilizing cineradiographic analysis with contrast material. This condition has not been reported in cats. They demonstrated that oropharyngeal swallowing disorders have multiple sites of origin. Not all conditions should be considered cricopharyngeal achalasia, and diseases should be classified according to where they occur in the normal swallowing pattern.[33]

The normal oropharyngeal phase of swallowing can be divided into three stages: oral, pharyngeal, and cricopharyngeal.[38] The oral stage includes prehension of food and collection of the bolus at the base of the tongue (Fig. 3–3*A*). The pharyngeal stage occurs when the bolus is propelled from base of the tongue to the cricopharyngeal passage (Fig. 3–3*B*). The cricopharyngeal stage encompasses relaxation of the cricopharyngeal sphincter, passage of the bolus into the esophagus, closure of the sphincter, and relaxation of the pharyngeal muscles (Fig. 3–3*C*).[33, 37, 38]

Oral stage dysphagias appear to result from damage to various motor and sensory tracts and peripheral nerves. Branches of cranial nerves V, IX, and X furnish sensory innervation for swallowing, and cranial nerves V, VII, IX, X, XI, and XII—via the nucleus ambiguus and the respiratory centers—deliver motor innervation.[28]

CLINICAL SIGNS

Clinical signs of oral stage dysphagia can vary but include: difficulty in prehension of food and lapping of water, extreme chewing or chomping, excessive salivation, and decreased or absent gag reflex. Evidence of denervation of the tongue may exist, and food may drop from the animal's mouth or may be trapped in the buccal cavity.[33, 37] The cineradiographic features of oral dysphagia are reduction in tongue movement, absence of plunger action of the tongue, and deficient bolus accumulation. Additionally, there is retention of contrast material in the oropharynx.[37]

Clinical signs of pharyngeal stage dys-

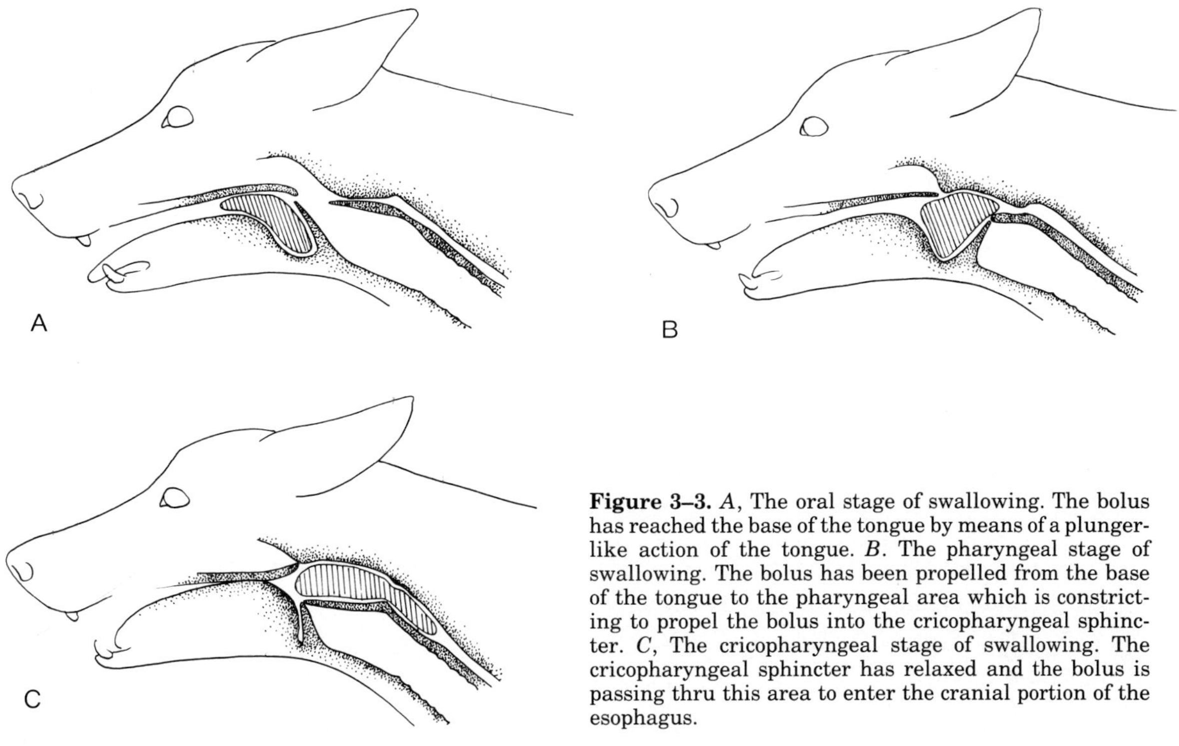

Figure 3–3. *A*, The oral stage of swallowing. The bolus has reached the base of the tongue by means of a plunger-like action of the tongue. *B*. The pharyngeal stage of swallowing. The bolus has been propelled from the base of the tongue to the pharyngeal area which is constricting to propel the bolus into the cricopharyngeal sphincter. *C*, The cricopharyngeal stage of swallowing. The cricopharyngeal sphincter has relaxed and the bolus is passing thru this area to enter the cranial portion of the esophagus.

phagias are less consistent and more difficult to localize.[33, 37] The most common signs are coughing with repeated unsuccessful attempts to swallow and aspiration pneumonia. Often the dog will spit out masticated food, or food will be misdirected into the nasopharynx, causing the dog to regurgitate food 2 to 12 hours after ingestion.[37] Cineradiographic signs are more diagnostic than the clinical signs; the major signs are residual gas and contrast medium in the pharynx with normal cricopharyngeal sphincter function, slow initiation and progress of pharyngeal peristaltic contractions, retention of contrast medium in the oropharynx, pharynx, and piriform recesses, and inhalation of contrast medium into the larynx.[37]

The accepted definition of cricopharyngeal achalasia is failure of the cricopharyngeus muscle to relax and thus to permit a bolus to enter the esophagus.[12, 14, 27, 31] The study by Suter and Watrous demonstrated other swallowing problems similar to cricopharyngeal achalasia that must be differentiated from it.[37] Clinical signs of cricopharyngeal phase dysphagias will vary, depending on whether or not there is an absolute failure of the cricopharyngeal sphincter to relax or whether there is incoordination between cricopharyngeal sphincter relaxation and pharyngeal contraction; both are forms of cricopharyngeal stage dysphagias.[33, 37] Cricopharyngeal stage and pharyngeal stage dysphagias are similar in their clinical manifestations, with signs of laryngotracheal aspiration and unsuccessful attempts to swallow present in both.[33, 37] Cricopharyngeal and pharyngeal dysphagias must be differentiated by means of cineradiographic studies. If there is incomplete relaxation of the cricopharyngeal sphincter, cricopharyngeal dysphagias usually show a dorsal indentation of the bolus as it passes through the sphincter. If there is incoordination of sphincter and pharynx, the bolus will be misdirected into the nasopharynx.[33, 37]

TREATMENT

Differentiation between the stages of dysphagia is important because the recommended treatment for cricopharyngeal achalasia is cricopharyngeal myotomy.[12, 27, 29, 34] One case of oral and one case of oropharyngeal dysphagia that were made worse by cricopharyngeal myotomy have been documented.[37] Oropharyngeal and pharyngeal stage dysphagias should be managed by treating any underlying medical illness, feeding the animal food of a consistency different from what it usually eats, and feeding the animal in an elevated position. The placement of a pharyngostomy tube or feeding via a stomach tube positioned by the owner before feeding may be considered.[33] Other techniques of value are feeding by means of a esophagostomy or gastrostomy. If conservative therapy is not helpful and the client does not wish to maintain the dog by feeding by means of esophagostomy or gastrostomy, cricopharyngeal myotomy might be considered as a salvage procedure. Even though, in one study, this procedure aggravated the disease process in two of nine cases of oropharyngeal swallowing disorders,[37] more data are needed before its effect on pharyngeal stage dysphagia can be completely evaluated. The client should be made aware that cricopharyngeal myotomy may make the animal's condition worse.

Acquired Achalasia and Idiopathic Megaesophagus

Acquired achalasia (AA) and idiopathic megaesophagus (IME) are two separate disease entities characterized by failure of progressive esophageal peristaltic contractions and asynchronous esophageal function with the LES.[17, 19, 22] These two diseases represent distinct clinical entities, each with a well-defined series of clinical signs and pathophysiological changes. The use of this terminology is not intended to, nor does it have to, coincide with the terminology used to describe a disease that occurs in humans. Acquired megaesophagus does not apply to a distinct disease, since it can occur as a sign of the primary diseases mentioned earlier. Much of the confusion in the literature regarding esophageal disease is caused by the use of terminology relating to the function of the lower esophageal sphincter (LES). Certain authors contend that acquired achalasia does not exist in the dog.[9, 30, 33] Other investigators believe that it does.[5, 8, 20, 21, 22] The concept of asynchronous function of the esophagus and the LES best describes the functional abnormalities noted with AA and IME. Investigators have judged the sphincters normal in dogs with both conditions on the basis of measurements of sphincter resting pressure.[9, 29, 33] However, sphincter function is too complex to be judged solely on the basis of resting pressure measurements. Esophageal and LES function involve the temporal relationship between resting, relaxation, and contracting pressures.[11] Thus, even if the LES relaxes when a swallow is induced, if there is no peristaltic contraction to move the bolus, the sphincter will be closed by the time gravity moves the bolus down the esophagus, and it will not easily enter the stomach.[11, 18] Also, if a bolus is at the sphincter and the sphincter is open only for a short length of time, the bolus will not be able to enter the stomach. Therefore, when esophageal neuromuscular disease is evaluated the clinician cannot base decisions on the esophageal resting pressure or use this criterion to say function is normal. Canine acquired achalasia and idiopathic megaesophagus have their own signs and pathophysiological changes that do not necessarily reflect a human disease counterpart.

Idiopathic megaesophagus (IME) is noticed in young dogs, usually at weaning. It is characterized by esophageal dilation and lack of progressive peristalsis. Synchronous function of the LES and esophagus has failed, although the LES may relax in response to a swallow.[9, 30] One-third of the

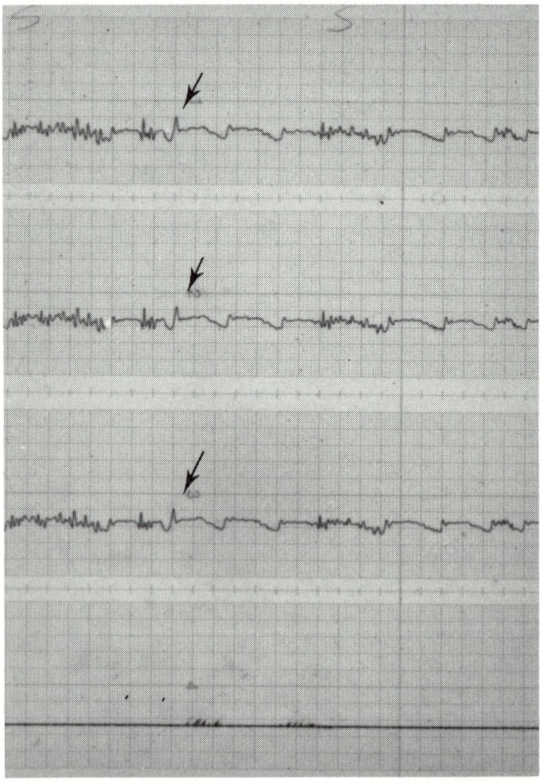

Figure 3–4. Manometric tracing in a dog with IME. A swallow has been induced. Note that the changes in esophageal pressure (*arrow*) are of low amplitude and are not progressive.

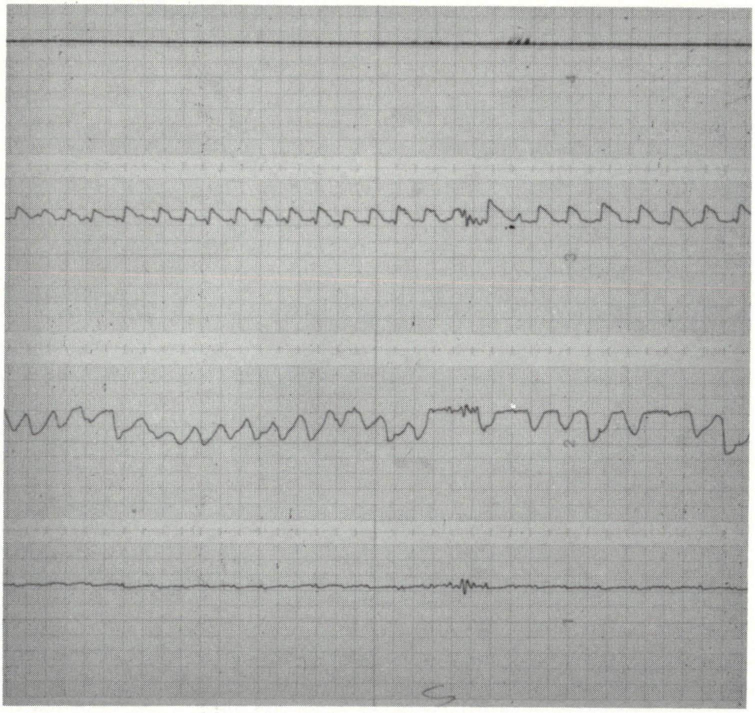

Figure 3–5. Manometric tracing in a dog with IME. A swallow has been induced. There is no esophageal peristaltic wave as in Figure 3–2A, nor is there a marked change of resting or contracting LES pressure, as is noted in Figure 3–2.

affected animals, in the author's experience, will spontaneously recover from the disease by the time they are mature. Feeding the affected animals in an elevated position aids in their recovery.[35]

Figures 3–4 and 3–5 demonstrate the lack of progressive peristalsis and synchronous function between the LES and the esophagus in a dog with IME. Although there is some alteration of sphincter functon in IME, it is minimal, and there is no esophageal wave to propel the bolus through the sphincter. The bolus is moved by gravity alone.

The author has observed that as a dog with IME spontaneously recovers, the esophageal function gradually returns to normal. During the recovery period, manometric pressure patterns and wave forms vary from a complete disease pattern to a normal function pattern. Radiographically, progressive peristalsis and synchronous LES/esophageal function return to a recovered IME patient. Fluoroscopic studies obtained during the recovery phase may show one of many types of esophageal function; this can be confusing unless the clinician remembers that there is a possibility of variations.

Acquired achalasia (AA) occurs in the mature dog without a history of esophageal problems as a puppy. The disease is characterized by esophageal dilation, lack of progressive peristalsis, and asynchronous function of the LES and esophagus.[17, 20, 21] Animals with acquired achalasia do not spontaneously recover or regain normal esophageal function.

CLINICAL SIGNS

Clinical signs of IME and AA are similar; in both, chronic regurgitation is the primary complaint. Usually, the animal is thin to emaciated and has inhalation pneumonia. Often, a bulging of the cervical esophagus is noted on physical examination. The diagnosis is made by a fluoroscopic barium swallow demonstrating esophageal dilation, lack of progressive peristalsis, and asynchronous function of the LES and esophagus. Radiography, without fluoroscopy that shows the esophageal dilation, should engender a high index of suspicion; however, demonstration of the functional defects requires a barium study.

One can differentiate IME from AA according to the age of onset of the disease. A young dog or a dog with signs of disease as a young dog has IME. A mature dog with a history of esophageal regurgitation is most likely to have non-responding IME. Acquired achalasia should be suspected in a mature dog that has no previous history of esophageal disease.

The lack of synchronous function between the esophagus and the LES in IME and AA may be neurogenic in origin, although myogenic and humoral factors have been suggested as causes in humans.[16] Some investigators feel that the defect is central in origin.[4,5] Others believe that the defects involve the afferent innervation of the esophagus.[13,35] It has also been proposed that an increased sensitivity to endogenous gastrin is responsible for the defect.[16] Diament and co-workers suggest that IME is the result of failure of developmental maturity of innervation of esophageal musculature, since some dogs do recover when mature.[9]

TREATMENT

The treatment of AA is controversial. One study of 79 dogs suggested that surgical treatment was not as effective as non-surgical treatment; however, treatment results were not separated according to disease.[15] In one study, the conditions of three out of four dogs with AA that were operated on improved (75%), five out of seven dogs that were treated conservatively either died or were euthanized because of the disease, and two dogs that were treated conservatively showed no improvement.[19] The surgical treatment of choice is the modified Heller procedure, which will be described in Chapter 4. This procedure does not eliminate the esophageal and sphincter dysfunction or return esophageal and sphincter function to normal. It does, however, lower the resting pressure of the LES so that the esophagus will empty with a lower intraluminal pressure, thereby preventing regurgitation.[18,19] It is often necessary to feed these dogs in an upright position to aid esophageal emptying.[19]

Dogs with idiopathic megaesophagus have been reported to recover spontaneously from the neuromuscular disease.[9,36] In the author's experience, one third of the patients with IME recover with treatment by at least 1 year of age. The disease is best treated by feeding the dog a slurry in an elevated position and having the animal remain elevated for 10 minutes postprandially.[15,19,35] The dog should be fed two to three times a day to reduce the volume of food at each feeding. Close observation of the dog is necessary, since almost 100 per cent of patients develop inhalation pneumonia. In six cases of IME that the author followed for 2 years, four patients did not recover and died of inhalation pneumonia within 1 to 2 years. Immediate therapy of the clinician's choice should be started at the first sign of inhalation pneumonia.

MEGAESOPHAGUS IN CATS

Megaesophagus has been reported in cats.[3,6] The condition manifested as described in dogs with IME, and the lesions were similar. Clifford proposed a hereditary predisposition for IME and suggested that a modified Heller procedure might be helpful, although only one cat has been successfully treated by surgery.[6]

Pearson and associates reported on a series of eight cases in which megaesophagus was associated with pyloric dysfunction in cats.[25] They suggested that the presence of a functional disturbance at two sites in the alimentary canal indicated that autonomic nervous system dysfunction was the more likely cause of the disease than specific organ lesions. Cats with problems involving megaesophagus and pyloric dysfunction were presented with persistent vomiting of a projectile nature or dyspnea. In cats with mild esophageal dilation in association with pyloric dysfunction, regression of symptoms followed pyloromyotomy. If gross esophageal dilation was present, symptoms persisted after pyloromyotomy. The relationship between esophageal dilation and pyloromyotomy is not completely understood and must be further investigated.

Disorders of the Lower Esophageal Sphincter

Diseases involving only lower esophageal sphincter (LES) function are uncommon. The conditions that have been reported are hiatal hernia with reflux esophagitis[2,10,14,28,30] and gastroesophageal intussusception.[1,10,23,26,32] Hiatal hernia is the result of a defect of the phrenoesophageal ligament that allows displacement of the LES forward of the diaphragm. Gastric contents reflux through the incompetent LES into the esophagus, where they may produce esophagitis.[2,10,14,24,28,30] Signs of a hiatal hernia usually result from esophagitis due

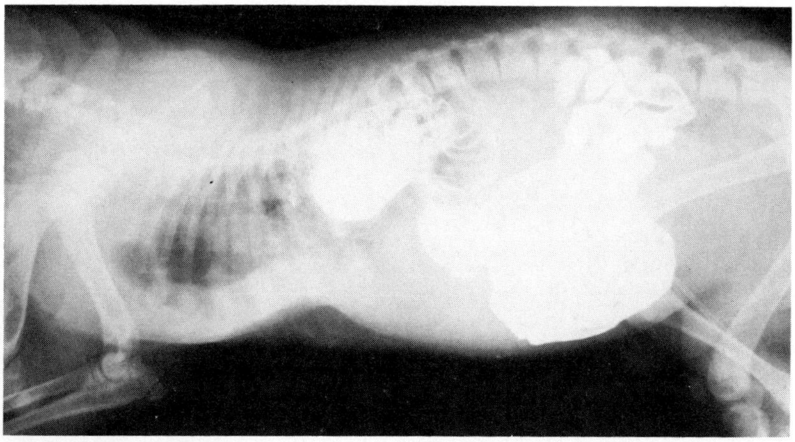

Figure 3–6. A barium swallow reveals a fixed hiatal hernia. The cardiac portion of the stomach and part of the fundus of the stomach are cranial to the diaphragm.

to the refluxed gastric contents. Signs include chronic gagging and retching, regurgitation of bloody mucus, drooling, dysphagia, and weight loss.[12,24] Diagnosis requires a high index of suspicion followed by a careful barium swallow performed under fluoroscopic observation. The hernia may be a sliding type hernia,[10] which moves in and out of its normal position, or a fixed hernia,[2] which remains out of position (Fig. 3–6). However, the amount of stomach that protrudes through the esophageal hiatus determines the radiographic appearance. Usually, external abdominal pressure is necessary to demonstrate a sliding hiatal hernia.

Treatment of reflux esophagitis is outlined in Chapter 2. The hiatal hernia may be repaired surgically.[2,10] If excessive reflux occurs, the LES may be surgically strengthened by a Nissen gastric fundoplication procedure.[24]

Gastroesophageal Intussusception

Gastroesophageal intussusception involves invagination of the stomach into the esophagus (Fig. 3–7).[1,10,23,26,32] The etiology of this condition is not known, but an incompetent LES must be suspected.[10,21]

Gastroesophageal intussusception generally occurs in young dogs; an 11-month-old dog is the oldest animal in which the condition has been reported. A dog will be presented with acute dyspnea, impending shock, and a history of acute vomiting. An epiphrenic mass is visualized radiographically (Fig. 3–7). The acute signs and radiographic appearance of the epiphrenic mass are the keys to the diagnosis.

Treatment is surgical reduction of the intussusception and a gastropexy. However, most affected animals are presented in such

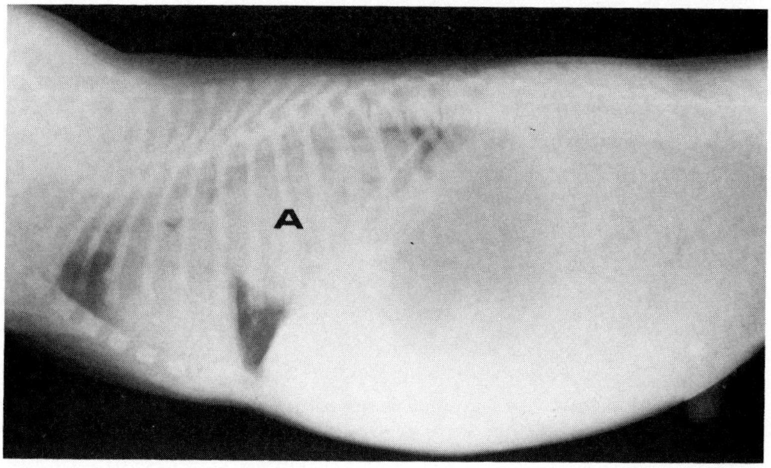

Figure 3–7. Gastroesophageal intussusception. An epiphrenic mass in the invaginated portion of the stomach, (*A*). The remaining portion of the stomach is distended with gas.

poor condition that they are unable to survive surgery and generally die in shock, often before surgery can be initiated.

References

1. Alcantara P: The clinical diagnosis of oesophageal invagination of the stomach of the dog. J S Afr Vet Med Assoc 42:2, 1971.
2. Alexander JW, Hoffer RE, MacDonald JM, et al: Hiatal hernia in the dog. J Am Anim Hosp Assoc 6:793, 1975.
3. Burke TJ, Froehlich PS, Chambers JN: Congenital esophageal disease in two kittens. Fel Pract 8:18, 1978.
4. Casella RR, Ellis FH, Brown JT Jr: Fine structure changes in achalasia of the esophagus. Am J Pathol 46:467, 1965.
5. Clifford DH, Pirsch JG, Maildin ML: Comparison of motor nuclei of the vagus nerve in dogs with and without esophageal achalasia. Proc Soc Exper Biol Med 142:878, 1973.
6. Clifford DH, Soifer FK, Wilson CF, et al: Congenital achalasia of the esophagus in 4 cats of common ancestry. J Am Vet Med Assoc 158:1554, 1971.
7. Clifford DH, Soifer FK, Freeman RG: Stricture and dilatation of the esophagus in the cat. J Am Vet Med Assoc 156:1007, 1970.
8. Clifford DH, Gyorkey F: Myenteric ganglial cells in dogs with and without achalasia of the esophagus. J Am Vet Med Assoc 150:205, 1967.
9. Diamant N, Szczepanski M, Mui H: Manometric characteristics of idiopathic megaesophagus in the dog: An unsuitable animal. Gastroenterology 65:216, 1973.
10. Gaskell CO, Gibbs C, Pearson H: Sliding hiatus hernia with reflux esophagitis in two dogs. J Small Anim Pract 15:503, 1974.
11. Gaynor F, Hoffer RE, Nichols MF, et al: Physiologic features of the canine esophagus: Effects of tranquilization on esophageal motility. Am J Vet Res 41:727, 1980.
12. Gourley IN, Leighton RL: Surgical treatment for cricopharyngeal achalasia in the dog. Pract Vet 44:11, 1972.
13. Gray GW: Acute experiment on neuroeffector function in canine esophageal achalasia. Am J Vet Res 35:1075, 1974.
14. Harvey CE, O'Brien JA: Esophageal diseases and disorders. Proc Am Anim Hosp Assoc 42:155–161, 1975.
15. Harvey CE, O'Brien JA, Durie VR, et al: Megaesophagus in the dog: A clinical survey of 79 cases. J Am Vet Med Assoc 165:443, 1974.
16. Henderson RD: *Motor Disorders of the Esophagus.* Williams and Wilkins Company, Baltimore, 1976.
17. Hoffer RE: Surgical esophageal diseases. *In* Bojrab MJ (ed): *Pathophysiology in Small Animal Surgery.* Lea & Febiger, Philadelphia, p. 90, 1981.
18. Hoffer RE, MacCoy DM, Gaynor F, et al: Physiologic features of the canine esophagus: Effect of modified Heller's esophagomyotomy. Am J Vet Res 41:723, 1980.
19. Hoffer RE, MacCoy DM, Quick CB, et al: Management of acquired achalasia in dogs. J Am Vet Med Assoc 175:814, 1979.
20. Hoffer RE: Diseases of the esophagus. *In* Kirk RW (ed): *Current Veterinary Therapy VI.* W. B. Saunders Company, Philadelphia, p. 931, 1977.
21. Hoffer RE, Valdez-Dapena A, Baue AE: A comparative study of naturally occurring canine achalasia. AMA Arch Surg 95:83, 1967.
22. Hoffer RE: Unpublished data.
23. Klopfer U, Heller ED: Invagination of the stomach into the esophagus in a dog. Vet Med Small Anim Clin 66:820, 1971.
24. Krupp S, Rossetti M: Surgical treatment of hiatal hernia by fundoplication and gastropexy. Ann Surg 164:927, 1966.
25. Pearson JC, Gaskell CG, Waterman A: Pyloric and esophageal dysfunction in the cat. J Small Anim Pract 15:487, 1974.
26. Pollock S, Rhodes WH: Gastroesophageal intussusception in an Afghan hound: A case report. Am Vet Rad Soc XI:5, 1970.
27. Quick CG, Hankes G, Womer R, Kueven K: Cricopharyngeal achalasia. Auburn Vet Surg 90:1977.
28. Robotham GR: What is your diagnosis; hiatal hernia. J Am Vet Med Assoc 170:1425, 1977.
29. Rogers WA, Fenner WR, Sherding RG: Electromyographic and esophagomanometric finding in clinically normal dogs and in dogs with idiopathic megaesophagus. J Am Vet Med Assoc 174:181, 1979.
30. Rogers WA, Donovan EF: Peptic esophagitis in a dog. J Am Vet Med Assoc 163:462, 1973.
31. Rosin E, Hanlon GF: Canine cricopharyngeal achalasia. J Am Vet Med Assoc 160:1496, 1972.
32. Roth JLA: Achalasia and other disorders of the esophagus. *In* Bockus JL (ed): *Gastroenterology.* W. B. Saunders Company, Philadelphia, p. 191, 1974.
33. Shelton GD: Swallowing disorders in the dog. Comp Cont Educ 7:607, 1982.
34. Sokolovsky V: Cricopharyngeal achalasia in a dog. J Am Vet Med Assoc 150:281, 1967.
35. Sokolovsky V: Achalasia and paralysis of the canine esophagus. J Am Vet Med Assoc 160:943, 1972.
36. Strombeck RR, Troya L: Evaluation of lower motor neuron function in two dogs with megaesophagus. J Am Vet Med Assoc 169:411, 1976.
37. Suter PF, Watrous BJ: Oropharyngeal dysphagias in the dog. A cinefluorographic analysis of experimentally induced and spontaneously occurring swallowing disorders. Vet Radiol 21:24, 1980.
38. Watrous BJ, Suter PF: Normal swallowing in the dog. A cineradiographic study. Vet Radiol 20:99, 1979.

CHAPTER

4

Surgery of the Esophagus

R. E. HOFFER

Four basic surgical techniques, either singly or in combination, are utilized when the clinician performs any esophageal surgical procedure in dogs or cats.[2,6,12,16,17,18] The techniques are: (1) esophagotomy or laceration repair, (2) resection and anastomosis, (3) esophagoplasty, and (4) esophagomyotomy. Esophageal surgery requires attention to detail and good basic surgical techniques, such as good hemostasis, atraumatic handling of tissues, accurate suture placement, and knot security. In addition, special technical considerations apply specifically to surgery of the esophagus.

General Principles

The esophagus lacks a serosal covering, which the intestine has. The lack of serosa requires perfect apposition of esophageal tissue, especially the mucosa, so that a fibrin seal can form at the suture line. The mucosa has excellent strength for suturing.[6] Since there is no omentum to seal the suture line secondarily, good apposition is even more important.[6,16]

Tension on the suture line and the constant motion of the esophagus contribute to potential complications of esophageal surgery. Excess tension is probably the single most important reason for dehiscence of the suture line and stricture of an esophageal anastomosis. Mobilization of the esophagus to reduce tension will aid healing of the incision. Various techniques have been developed to reinforce and to seal an esophageal suture line.[3,4,9,10,11,15]

The suture technique of choice for the esophagus is a two-layer interrupted closure. The first layer apposes the mucosa and submucosa; the second layer apposes the muscularis.[6,16] The type of suture material to be used is left to the discretion of the surgeon. The literature suggests that meticulous suture pattern and closure are more important to esophageal healing than the type of material used. The author prefers a non-absorbable suture material for the mucosa and submucosa and an absorbable material for the muscularis. This technique is successful,[6] although two-layer closure using silk has also been reported to be successful.[16]

The most common complication of esophageal surgery is leakage along the suture line, which results in dehiscence and infection. In the thorax, leakage will result in mediastinitis and pleuritis.[2,4,6,12] In both clinical and experimental literature, postoperative stricture of the esophagus, unassociated with wound breakdown, is almost nonexistent.

The number of complications that occur after esophageal surgery is inversely related to the skill and experience of the surgeon. The following basic principles must be adhered to:[2,4,6,12,16,18] (1) minimize tension along the suture line, (2) accurately appose mucosa and submucosa and muscularis, (3) meticulously place suture patterns, and (4) use atraumatic technique. Esophagotomy and esophagomyotomy procedures can successfully be performed by an experienced small animal surgeon who is familiar with the anatomy. Resection and anastomosis procedures carry a much greater complication rate and require special technical skill, as well as familiarity with uncommon techniques. If the need for these techniques is anticipated, it is sometimes best to refer the patient to a specialist in small animal surgery.

Surgical Procedures

ESOPHAGOTOMY (Fig. 4–1)

An esophagotomy is performed to expose the esophageal lumen for exploration or to remove a foreign object. The location of the problem determines the approach used. The esophagus cranial to the third rib is approached via a ventral midline cervical incision between the strap muscles of the neck. Additional exposure of the cranial thoracic esophagus is obtained by splitting the first three sternebrae. Caudal to the third rib, a right thoracotomy is performed over the site of the object or lesion. An exception occurs in a right aortic arch vascular anomaly. In this instance, the approach is through a left thoracotomy because the great vessels lie to the right of the esophagus and obstruct the surgeon's vision when a right thoracotomy is performed.

The esophagus is approached carefully. Adhesions, if present, are carefully dissected away. Hemorrhage must be controlled so that the surgical site is clearly visualized. Structures such as the vena cava and aorta must be avoided or retracted. The lung is reflected caudally. After exposing the esophageal lesion, the surgeon must evaluate the viability and blood supply of the esophagus to determine whether the tissues will survive. If a sharp foreign body such as a fish-

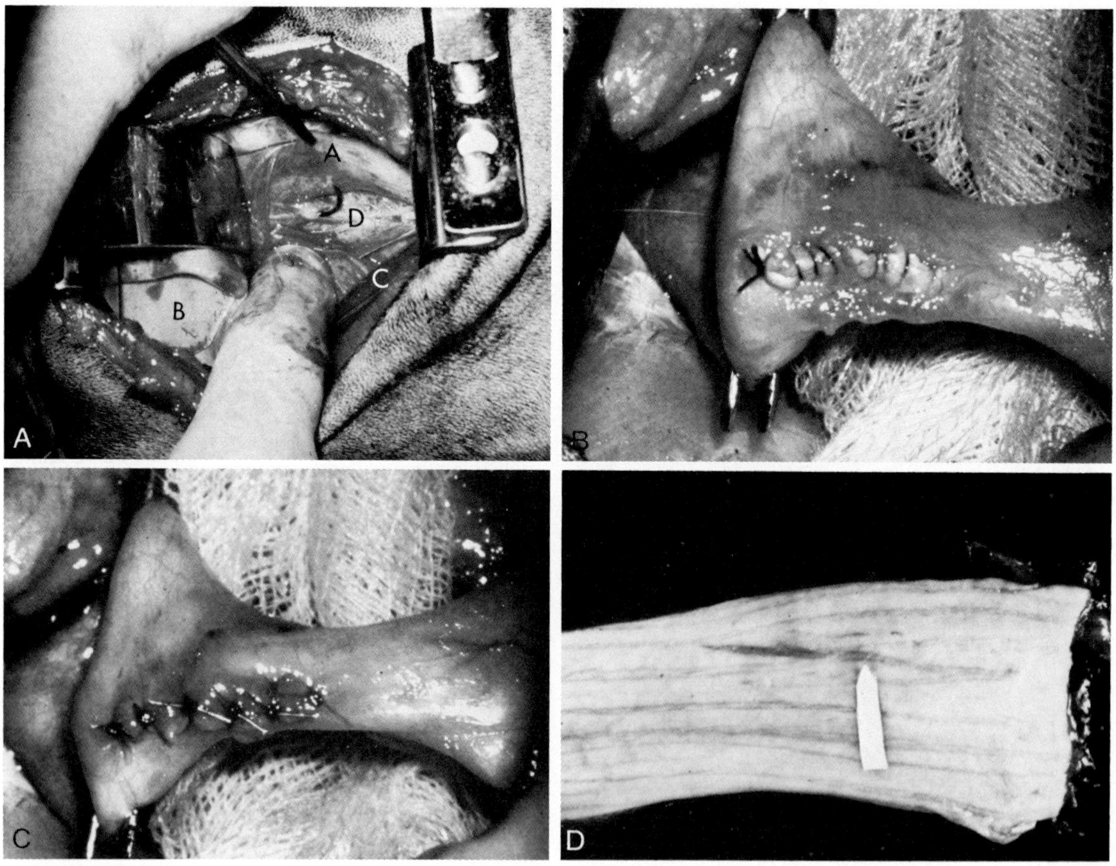

Figure 4–1. *A*, A right thoracotomy has been done. The esophagus (A) is visualized. Note that the tip of the hook has penetrated into deeper tissue (D). The lung (B) has been reflected ventrally to expose the vena cava. Note that the cranial vena cava (C) in its normal position would be very susceptible to damage when the foreign body is being manipulated. The esophagus will be mobilized.

B, The mucosa and submucosa have been sutured with a simple continuous pattern of non-absorbable material. The suture is started past one end of the mucosal incision and finished past the other end.

C, The muscularis has been sutured with a simple interrupted pattern of absorbable material. The mucosal-submucosal suture line has been completely covered by the muscularis closure.

D, The esophagotomy site has healed. The non-absorbable sutures were sloughed off into the esophageal lumen by the normal healing process of the mucosa and submucosa. Note that the incision site is being covered by the mucosa.

hook or needle is identified, it is immobilized so it does not damage contiguous structures such as the vena cava, aorta, and pulmonary vessels.

The esophagus is dissected free from the mediastinum and vagus nerves and is packed off. Atraumatic intestinal clamps are placed cranial and caudal to the lesion. A lateral, longitudinal incision is made in the esophagus to remove a foreign body or to inspect the lumen. The incision in the esophageal muscularis extends slightly cranial and caudal to the mucosal incision. If there is a foreign body obstruction, the incision is made in the dilated portion of the esophagus cranial to the obstructing object.

The esophageal mucosa is approximated with a simple continuous pattern of 4/0 to 5/0 non-absorbable suture material using a swaged taper needle. The pattern is started at one end of the incision with the knot inside the lumen and is continued to the other end. The needle penetrates both mucosa and submucosa. It is important to place even tension along the suture line. The ends of the suture line are meticulously closed. The suture line is checked for leaks by injecting sterile saline into the esophageal lumen under pressure. Leaks are closed with a simple interrupted pattern of 5/0 suture material.

Simple interrupted sutures of 3/0 absorbable material are used to approximate the esophageal muscularis. It is important that the muscle closure cover both ends of the mucosal suture line. The esophagus is replaced in the normal position. The mediastinum is not approximated.

ESOPHAGEAL RESECTION AND ANASTOMOSIS (Fig. 4–2)

Esophageal resection is performed only when no other method of repair will correct the lesion. The lack of serosa, constant motion, and incisional tension result in a guarded prognosis, at best, for any esophageal anastomosis. The key to success in this procedure is to minimize tension by removing as little esophagus as possible. When more than 2 cm is resected, tension is present. When larger segments of the esophagus are involved in a disease process, e.g., neoplasia or necrosis (see later discussion), surgical techniques such as grafting are necessary.

Atraumatic clamps are placed on the esophagus cranial and caudal to the section to be resected. The surgical site is packed off, and the esophagus is resected between the clamps. Stay sutures are placed through the mucosa-submucosa dorsally and ventrally. If necessary, clamps may be removed and umbilical tape tension used to control esophageal spillage.

Traction is placed on the esophageal stay sutures to approximate the cut edges of the mucosa. The esophageal mucosa-submucosa is apposed with a simple interrupted pattern of 4/0 non-absorbable sutures with the knots tied inside the lumen. The suture pattern is started within the lumen on the far side of the esophagus and continued toward the stay sutures. The far side of the esophagus is sutured until the corners are turned. The sutures are placed 2 mm apart and 3 mm from the cut edge. The suture pattern is carried from the middle of the far side of the esophagus past the stay sutures dorsally and ventrally. The near side of the esophagus is sutured until only one or two sutures are needed to close the lumen. The last two sutures are preplaced and tied. The last suture may be placed as an ordinary simple interrupted suture with the knot on the outside. Atraumatic clamps are applied to the esophagus, and the lumen of the esophagus is distended with sterile saline and examined for leaks. Leaks are closed with simple interrupted sutures. After all mucosal leaks are sealed, the esophageal muscularis is approximated with a simple interrupted pattern of 3/0 absorbable sutures.

The primary complication of an esophageal resection and anastomosis is leakage. Leakage will usually manifest itself between the third and fifth postoperative days. If there is concern about the esophageal suture line, partial circular myotomy may be performed;[1, 10] or sections of lung,[11] pericardium,[8] omentum,[4] diaphragm,[15] sternothyroideus muscle,[9] or intercostal muscle[3] may be utilized to reinforce the closure and to reduce tension.

A feeding gastrostomy tube should be utilized to support the dog that is in poor preoperative nutritional condition, in order to allow immediate alimentation of the patient. This is particularly important with thoracic esophageal resection and anastomosis because of the severe consequences of pleuritis resulting from esophageal leakage within the thorax. If leakage occurs in the cervical region, drainage to the outside will prevent mediastinitis and allow an esophageal fistula to form. A fistula will usually spontaneously close, but it may be closed surgically after the rest of the esophagus

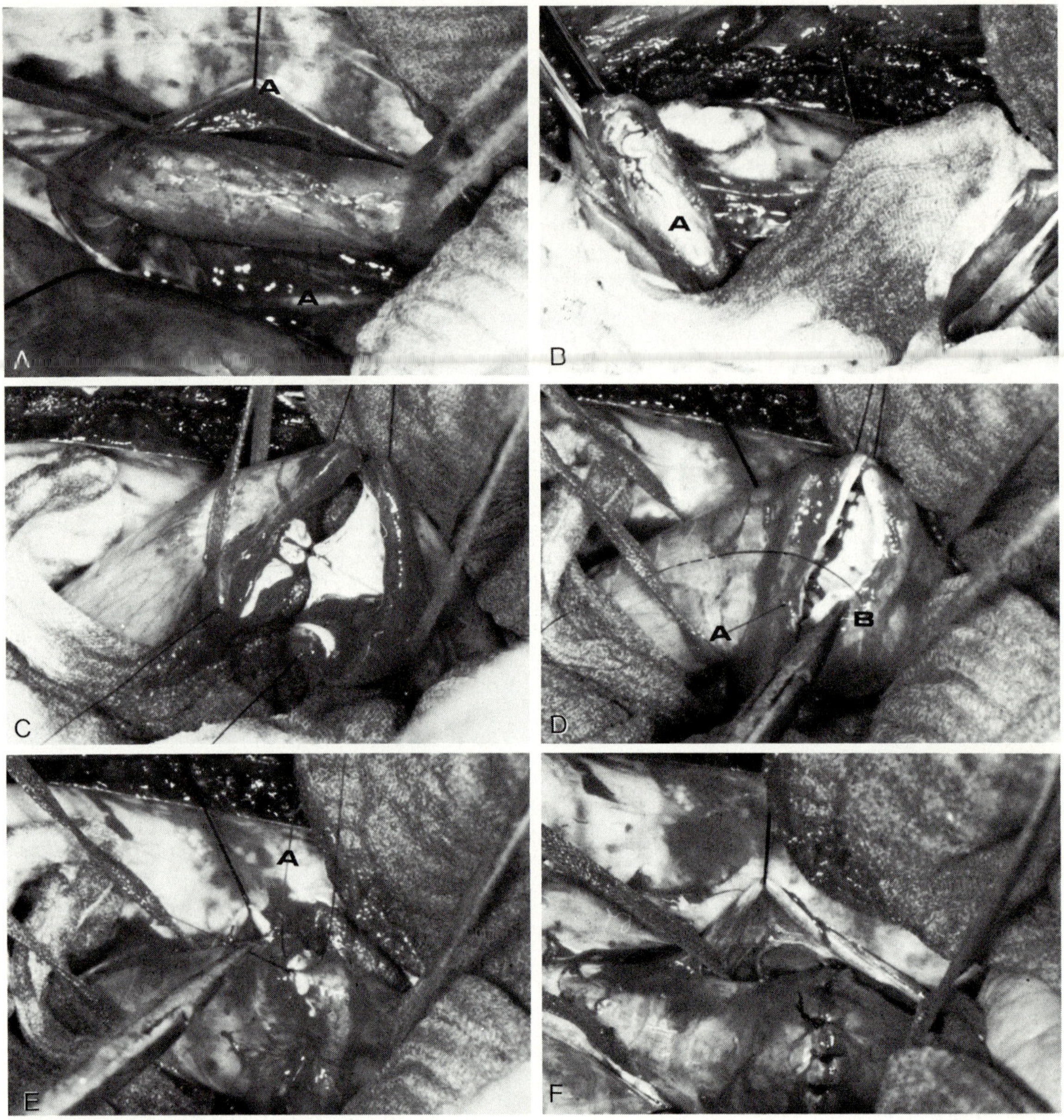

Figure 4–2. *A*, The distal esophagus has been exposed by a right ninth thoracotomy. The mediastinum and the vagus nerves (A) have been reflected.

B, Two centimeters of esophagus have been resected between the atraumatic clamps. The clamps are too close to the resection site to permit suturing. They will be replaced with umbilical tape after stay sutures and the first mucosal-submucosal suture are placed. Additional cranial and caudal dissection of the esophagus would allow more esophageal mobilization, and the clamps then could be placed further away from the resected ends of the esophagus. The mucosa, (*A*), is easily visualized following esophageal resection.

C, The atraumatic clamps have been replaced with umbilical tape. Stay sutures have been placed at 6 and 12 o'clock. The first suture has been placed, knotted in the lumen, in the middle of the far side of the esophagus. The suture pattern is continued toward 12 and 6 o'clock alternately until it has passed the stay sutures at both sides.

D, The esophageal mucosa is being sutured. The suture is started inside the lumen and carried to the outside on the left (A). The needle has been placed from the outside of the mucosa into the lumen on the right (B). The suture is pulled into the lumen and tied, placing the knot in the esophageal lumen.

E, The last two sutures have been preplaced through the esophageal mucosa as a simple interrupted suture with the knot on the outside. The last suture (A) will be tied, the lumen pressurized with saline, and any leaks closed with a simple interrupted suture with the knot outside the lumen.

F, The esophageal muscularis has been apposed with simple interrupted sutures of 3/0 absorbable material. Note that the mucosal suture line is completely covered.

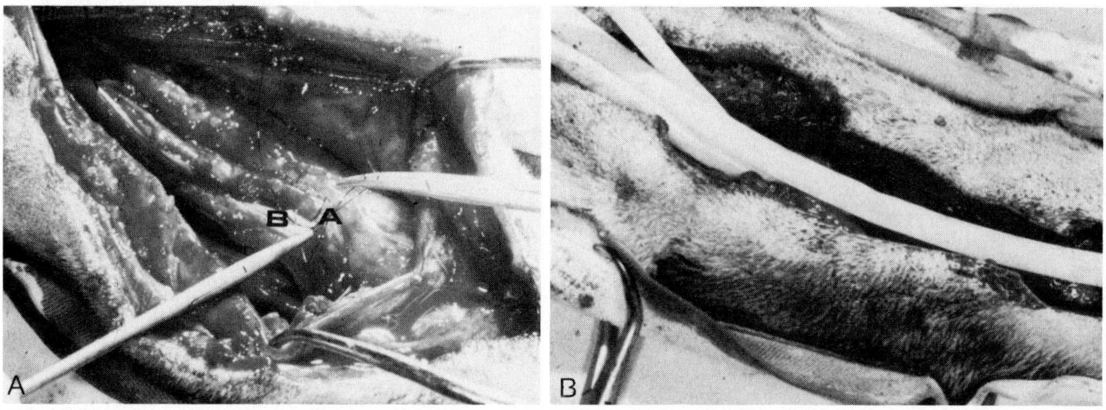

Figure 4–3. *A*, A lacerated cervical esophagus. The laceration is being closed utilizing the same technique as that described for esophageal resection and anastomosis. Note that the knot (B) will be in the lumen. It is important to close both ends of the laceration (A). The muscularis will be closed as previously described.

B, Penrose drains have been placed in the incision. The drains will ensure that there is no spread of infection into the mediastinum through the cervical fascial planes.

has healed. The presence of a small fistula usually does not create a nutritional problem.

Postoperative stricture after resection and anastomosis is more likely if there is tension on the suture line.

ESOPHAGEAL LACERATION AND PERFORATION (Fig. 4–3)

Esophageal perforation or laceration may occur after ingestion of a sharp object, secondarily to foreign body pressure necrosis, iatrogenically following surgery or esophagoscopy, or as the result of external trauma such as a bite or gunshot wound. Perforation or laceration of the thoracic esophagus is difficult to manage because of the accompanying pleuritis and mediastinitis. An acute esophageal perforation may be sealed by the lung or mediastinum to avoid pleuritis and mediastinitis.

Laceration is more common in the cervical than in the thoracic esophagus because of its accessibility. Lesions of the cervical esophagus often manifest as cervical cellulitis or abscess. The esophagus should be evaluated whenever a cervical abscess is present. Treatment depends upon the condition of the patient and the type of lesion. If infection is present, the area should be opened, drained, lavaged with saline, and treated until the acute infection is under control. This treatment will greatly reduce the chance of mediastinitis by extension through cervical fascial planes. After the acute infection is under control, the esophageal defect should be debrided and closed using the suture pattern described for esophageal anastomosis. Penrose drains should be used to drain the area postoperatively. If the defect is too large to close primarily, patch grafting techniques should be utilized.[7] The drains should be removed after the seventh postoperative day. If there is a leak, the drains will permit an esophageal fistula to form rather than allow infection to descend into the chest.

ESOPHAGOPLASTY (Fig. 4–4)

Esophagoplasty is utilized to widen a narrow esophageal stricture or stenotic area. The procedure converts a longitudinal incision into a horizontal closure. A longitudinal incision is made through the stenotic area. The length of the longitudinal incision is determined by the length of esophagus that can be mobilized to relieve tension on the suture line. If there is excess tension on the suture line, the risks of leakage, dehiscence, and restricture are increased. The length of the longitudinal incision is usually equivalent to the length of esophagus that can be resected.

The esophagus is approached, and the stenotic area mobilized. Traction stay sutures or atraumatic clamps are placed on either side of the stenotic area, and the esophagus is longitudinally incised between them. A simple interrupted suture of 5/0 non-absorbable material is placed at the cranial and caudal ends of the longitudinal incision. The suture is placed so that the knot is inside the lumen and penetrates only the mucosa and submucosa. This center suture is tied, converting the longitudinal incision into a horizontal closure. While this

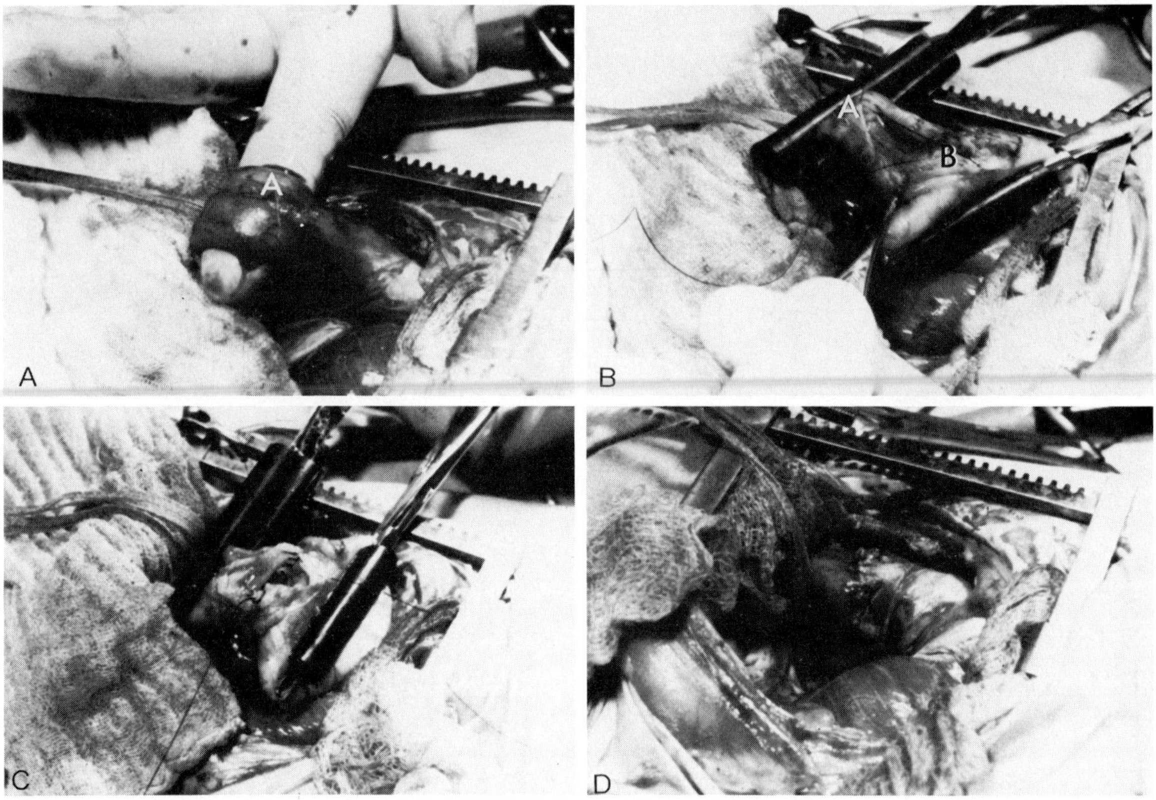

Figure 4–4. *A*, A stenotic area (A) of the esophagus has been mobilized and isolated. Umbilical tape is being utilized to apply cranial traction to the esophagus.

B, Rubber-shod atraumatic clamps have been placed across the proximal esophagus and the portion of the cardia of the stomach has been covered by the phrenoesophageal ligament, which has not been incised. A suture of 5/0 non-absorbable material has been placed at the cranial end (A) and caudal end (B) of the mucosal-submucosal incision. The suture has been placed so that the knot will be inside the esophageal lumen.

C, The center suture has been tied, and the far side of the mucosal-submucosal incision closed. A suture has been placed in the near side of the horizontal closure, and traction is applied to it to allow placement of the rest of the sutures. The last two or three sutures are preplaced.

D, The muscularis has been closed with 3/0 absorbable material using a simple interrupted suture pattern. The esophagus is returned to the thorax; the mediastinum is not closed.

Figure 4–5. *A*, A ninth left thoracotomy has been performed. The esophagus (A) is seen with the mediastinum containing the vagus nerves. The phrenoesophageal ligament (B) as it reflects off the diaphragm (C) is also shown.

B, The phrenoesophageal ligament (A) has been picked up prior to its incision. Note how the ligament reflects off the diaphragm onto the esophagus.

C, The phrenoesophageal ligament has been incised. The cardia of the stomach (A) is protruding through the incision. The phrenoesophageal ligament (B) is reflected onto the esophagus.

D, The phrenoesophageal ligament is being incised where it blends with the esophageal muscularis (A).

E, The phrenoesophageal ligament has been completely incised. The reflection of the ligament onto the esophagus (A) and the esophagogastric junction is demonstrated. (B) The cardia of the stomach (C) is completely exposed.

F, The esophageal muscularis (A) has been incised by exposing the submucosa (B) of the esophagus. This incision is begun 1 to 2 cm cranial to the point (C) at which the phrenoesophageal ligament blends, with the esophageal muscularis.

G, The esophageal incision is continued caudally by means of scissor dissection in order to develop the tissue plane. The oblique fibers of the stomach (A) will be incised. Care must be taken not to perforate the mucosa. The tissue planes in the area are difficult to develop, and good hemostasis control is necessary.

H, The muscular incision of the esophagus, (A), and cardia, (B), is completed. A sponge will be utilized to remove any muscularis fibers that are left at the surgical site.

I, A non-absorbable suture has been placed from the cranial end of the esophageal incision (A) through the center of the diaphragmatic incision (B). This area is more easily identified if two stay sutures (C&D) are placed on either side of the phrenoesophageal incision. When the center suture (A&B) is tied, the incised esophagogastric junction will be replaced in the abdomen.

J, The phrenoesophageal ligament is completely closed using simple interrupted, non-absorbable sutures. This procedure reconstructs the esophageal hiatus and the functional physiological lower esophageal sphincter. This reconstruction, if not done properly, can result in the development of a hiatal hernia or a diaphragmatic hernia.

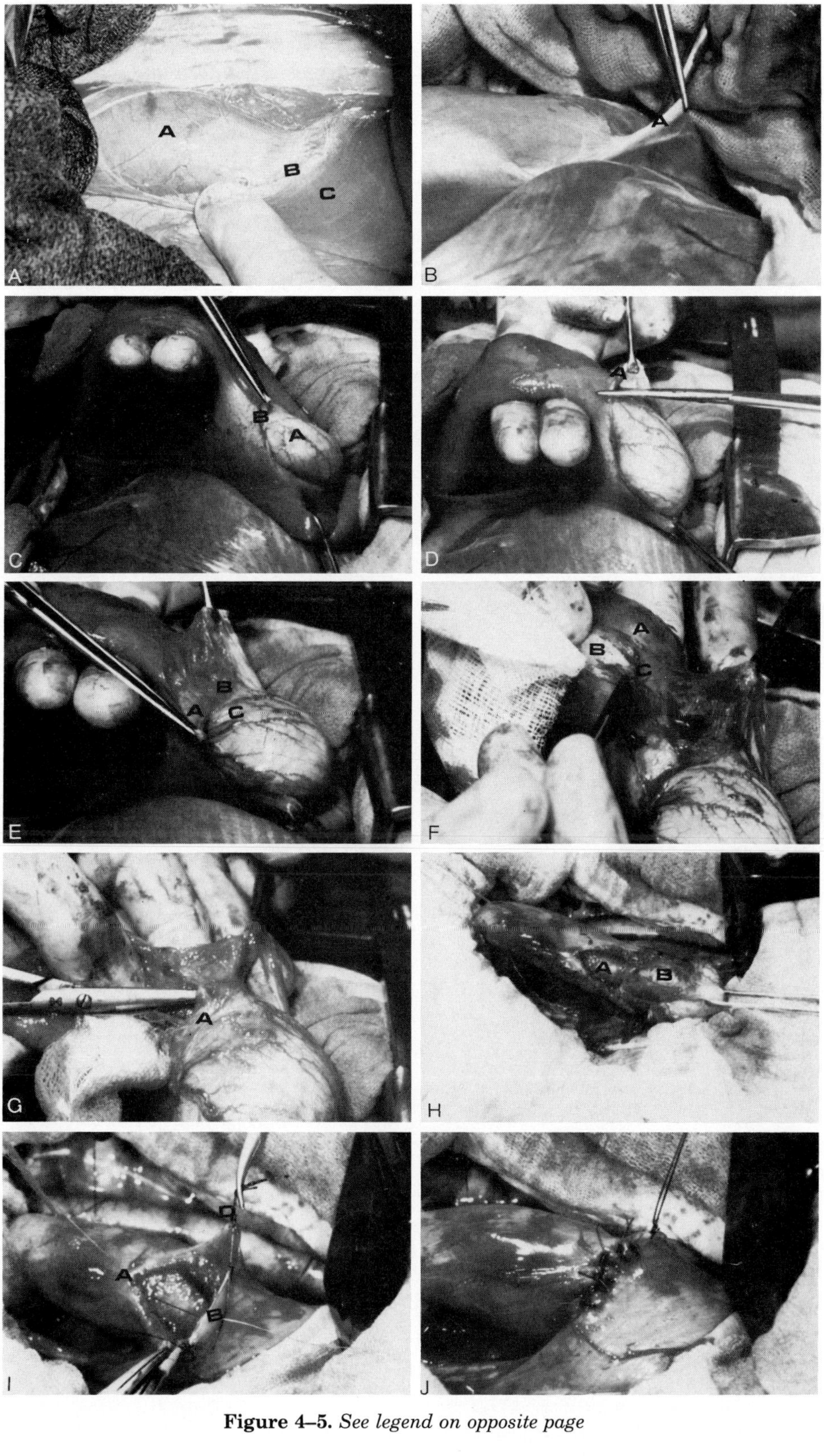

Figure 4–5. *See legend on opposite page*

suture is being tied, the clamps are approximated to relieve tension on the suture line. The next two sutures are placed on the ends of the incision. Gentle traction applied to these sutures will make closure of the incision easier. The remaining mucosa and submucosa are closed with the knot-in-the-lumen technique described for resection and anastomosis. The esophageal muscularis is closed over the mucosal suture line with simple interrupted 3/0 absorbable sutures.

EXCISION OF ESOPHAGEAL DIVERTICULA

The surgical excision of an esophageal diverticulum depends upon the type, size, and location of the lesion.[14] If the diverticulum is solitary, resection of the pouch and closure of the resulting defect in the esophagus employ the same technique as that described for esophageal anastomosis. A stenotic area may be produced if an excessive amount of the circumference of the normal esophageal wall is removed. If bilateral diverticula are present, it is best to resect and anastomose the entire segment of esophagus containing them. Extreme care must be taken to avoid removal of a long segment of esophagus. If there is any question, at the time of diagnosis, as to how much normal esophageal tissue is to be removed, the clinician should consider consulting with a surgical specialist.

MODIFIED HELLER PROCEDURE (Fig. 4–5)

The modified Heller procedure, or esophagomyotomy, may be used as an adjunct to the management of acquired achalasia in the dog. Its purpose is to reduce the functional obstruction produced by the asynchronous function of the esophagus and lower esophageal sphincter (LES) and to allow the esophagus to empty more easily.[5] The procedure is not a cure for esophageal neuromuscular dysfunction; the asynchronous function of the esophagus remains.

The esophagus is approached via a left ninth thoracotomy. The vagus nerve, within the mediastinal covering of the esophagus, is visualized and dissected from the distal esophagus. The phrenoesophageal ligament is incised, exposing the cardia of the stomach. The incision is carried cranially along the esophagus. When the phrenoesophageal ligament has been opened to its full extent, a good portion of the cardia of the stomach is exposed, as well as the esophagus.

The esophageal muscularis is incised down to, but not through, the esophageal submucosa. The incision is continued onto the cardia of the stomach through the oblique fibers of the cardia. The total extent of the esophageal myotomy is about 4 cm. Scissors are used to incise the oblique muscle of the cardia of the stomach. Care must be taken not to perforate the esophageal or gastric mucosa. After the esophageal musculature, as well as the oblique fibers of the stomach, has been incised, the submucosa is clearly visualized. The defect is checked for leaks at this time. If a leak is present, it is safer to convert the procedure to a cardioplasty than to try to suture the mucosal defect. The technique is similar to that described for an esophagoplasty.

In continuing the modified Heller procedure, the cardia of the stomach is replaced caudal to the diaphragm and the phrenoesophageal ligament is sutured. A suture of 3/0 non-absorbable material is placed from the corner of the cranial aspect of the esophageal muscularis incision to the mid-point of the diaphragmatic defect. This suture will appose the esophageal muscularis to the diaphragm and the phrenoesophageal ligament, placing the incised muscularis of the esophagus into the abdomen. The esophageal muscularis and phrenoesophageal ligament are sutured to the diaphragm. This procedure effectively restores an abdominal esophageal segment, and the closure effectively reconstructs the esophageal hiatus.

Prior to closure, the chest is lavaged and a chest tube is placed. The dog is not permitted food and water for 24 hours and then is started on a soft diet. Dietary adjustments are necessary following the modified Heller procedure. Feeding the animal a slurry while it is in an elevated position is necessary. The client may experiment with different diets and different methods of feeding until a suitable one is found. The dilated portion of the esophagus remains and usually lacks primary peristalsis. The diet must be carefully managed for life, since the aperistaltic segment of the esophagus does not usually regain function.

It should be remembered that the modified Heller procedure is not curative. Its function is to help a dog with an unmanageable problem and to help it retain its desirability as a pet.

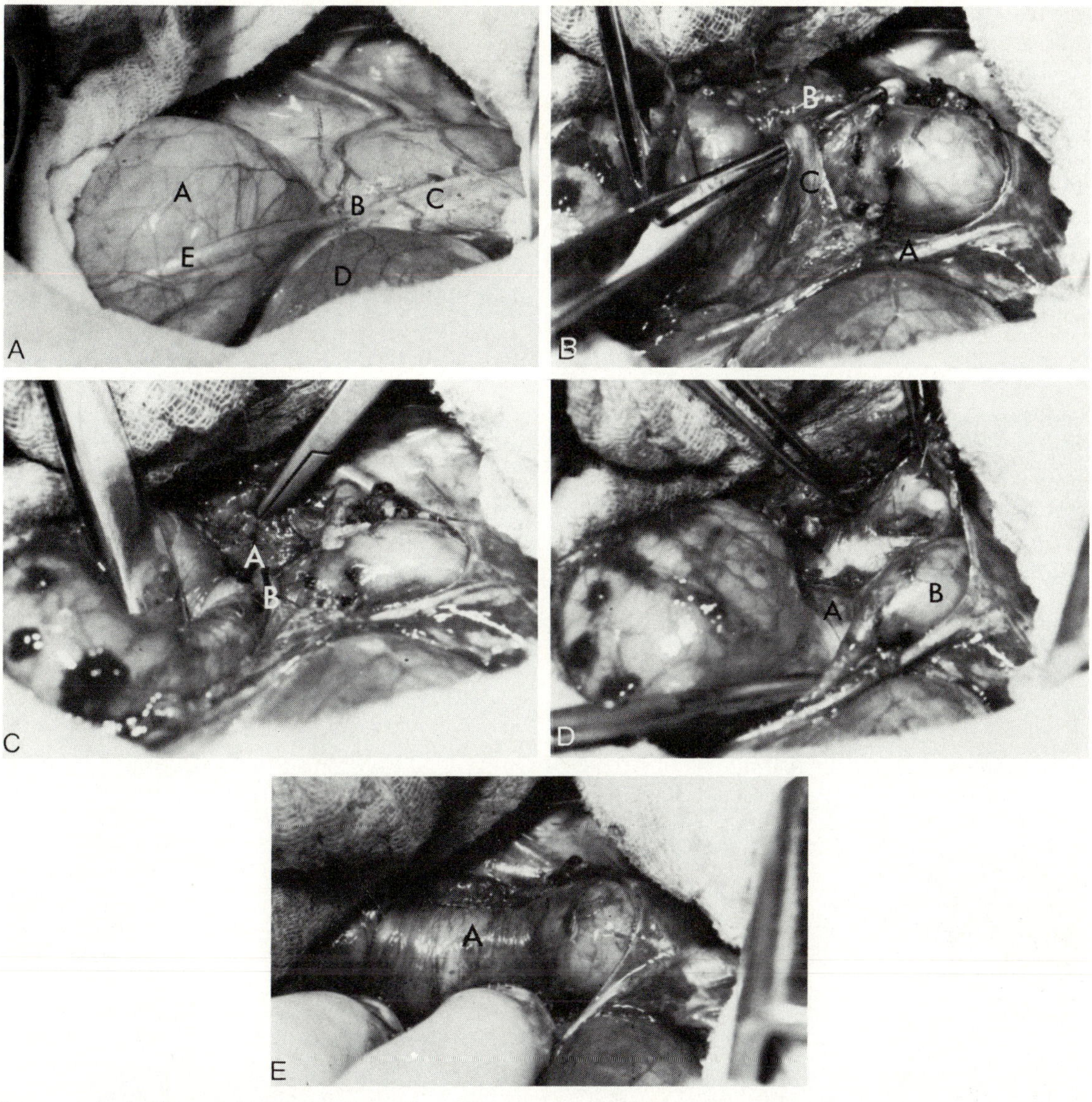

Figure 4–6. *A*, The esophagus has been exposed through a left fourth thoracotomy. The dilated esophagus (A) cranial to the ligamentum arteriosum, the constricted area (B) and the distal esophagus (C) are seen. The heart (D) and the phrenic nerve (E) are seen. The phrenic nerve within the mediastinum must be reflected to expose the ligamentum arteriosum.

B, The portion of the mediastinum with the phrenic nerve (A), has been reflected ventrally, and the other portion dorsally, (B), to expose the constricted area of the esophagus. A right angle forceps has been passed under the ligamentum arteriosum, (C). The bleeding must be controlled so that the operative site may be clearly seen.

C, The ligamentum arteriosum has been double ligated (A & B) and will be divided between the ligatures.

D, The ligamentum arteriosum has been divided. Note that the esophagus still appears constricted (A) when compared with the normal caudal esophagus (B). This constriction is the result of the presence of connective tissue.

E, The connective tissue in the constricted area has been removed. The esophagus (A) has attained the same diameter as the normal caudal esophagus.

PERSISTENT RIGHT AORTIC ARCH REPAIR (Fig. 4–6)

Persistent right aortic arch is the most common of the vascular anomalies producing esophageal stenosis. It is best to perform surgery when the animal is 14 weeks of age. The surgical procedure involves division of the ligamentum arteriosum (LA) and complete mobilization of the esophagus from the connective tissue in the area of the entrapment. The surgeon should treat the ligamentum as if it were patent, as it occasionally is.

The esophagus is approached through a left fourth thoracotomy. The dilated cranial esophagus, the caudal esophagus, the heart, the phrenic nerve, and the area of the constriction are identified. The mediastinum is carefully dissected from the esophagus cranial and caudal to the constricted area, exposing the esophagus.

The area of constriction is dissected until the LA is identified. It is a thick band that crosses over the esophagus. Occasionally, there is an aberrant vessel in the area. If so, it should be either reflected or ligated.

Right-angle forceps are passed between the LA and the esophagus. Two ligatures are passed and tied around the ligament to prevent hemorrhage, if it is patent. The LA is transected. The esophagus usually will not expand because connective tissue is still constricting it. This connective tissue around the esophagus must be dissected to completely free the esophagus. This dissection becomes more difficult in older dogs. When the esophagus is completely denuded

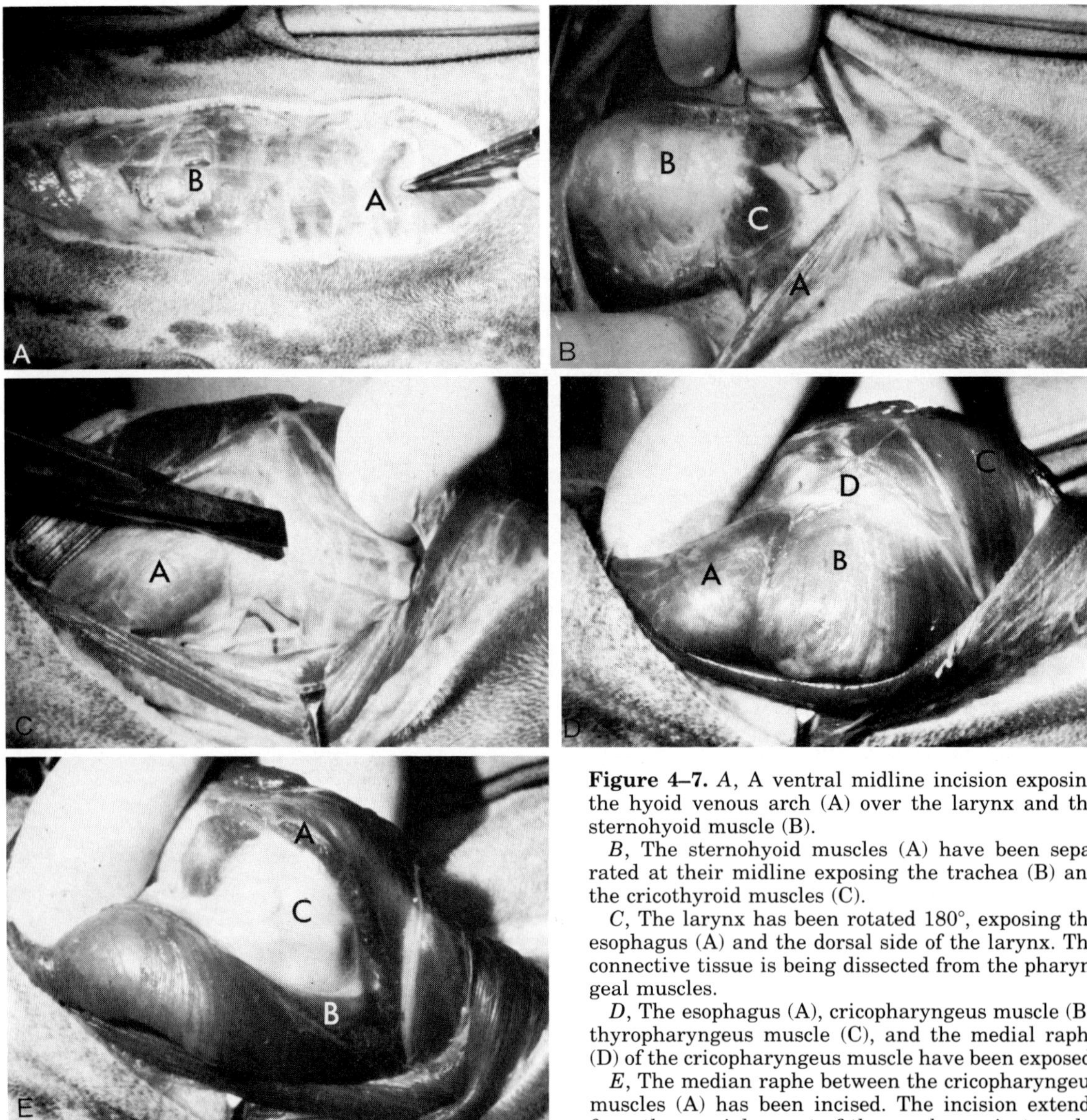

Figure 4–7. *A*, A ventral midline incision exposing the hyoid venous arch (A) over the larynx and the sternohyoid muscle (B).

B, The sternohyoid muscles (A) have been separated at their midline exposing the trachea (B) and the cricothyroid muscles (C).

C, The larynx has been rotated 180°, exposing the esophagus (A) and the dorsal side of the larynx. The connective tissue is being dissected from the pharyngeal muscles.

D, The esophagus (A), cricopharyngeus muscle (B), thyropharyngeus muscle (C), and the medial raphe (D) of the cricopharyngeus muscle have been exposed.

E, The median raphe between the cricopharyngeus muscles (A) has been incised. The incision extends from the cranial aspect of the esophagus just caudal to the cricopharyngeus muscles up to the thyropharyngeus muscle (B). The incision is carried to the pharyngneal submucosa (C). Care must be taken not to penetrate the esophageal or pharyngeal mucosa.

of connective tissue, the constricted area of the esophagus is the same size as the caudal esophagus. The cranial, dilated portion of the esophagus remains unchanged.

Most surgeons do not recommend inversion or excision of the dilated portion of the esophagus. The esophagus caudal to the site of the constricting band is usually normal. Occasionally, a dog has a generalized esophageal dilation in association with a vascular ring. The prognosis, in this case, is poor, unlike the prognosis for a dog with a normal caudal esophagus. If there is a generalized esophageal dilation in association with a vascular ring anomaly, a modified Heller procedure done at the time of vascular ring repair may be beneficial. More study is needed to evaluate this combination of procedures.

CRICOPHARYNGEAL MYOTOMY (Fig. 4–7)

A cricopharyngeal myotomy is performed to allow a dog with cricopharyngeal stage dysphagia to swallow food more easily. It should be remembered, as discussed in Chapter 3, that this procedure may make dogs with pharyngeal stage dysphagia worse.

An 8 cm ventral, cervical skin incision is made from the larynx cranially and caudally. The incision extends past the hyoid venous arch. The sternohyoideus muscles are exposed and separated on the midline to expose the trachea and the cricothyroideus muscles. The larynx is grasped and rotated 180°, exposing the dorsal aspect of the larynx. The connective tissue is dissected free of the esophagus, the cricopharyngeus, and the thyropharyngeus muscles. The cricopharyngeus muscles are incised, beginning on the esophagus caudally and extending to the thyropharyngeus muscles cranially. Care should be taken not to penetrate the esophageal or pharyngeal mucosa. If penetration occurs, the hole should be closed with a simple interrupted absorbable suture, and the surgical site drained.

The larynx is replaced in its normal position, and the strap muscles are apposed with simple interrupted sutures of absorbable material. The subcutaneous tissue and skin are closed routinely.

The dog may be fed and watered the first postoperative day if the mucosa was not penetrated. If the mucosa was penetrated, all oral intake should be avoided for 72 hours. The penrose drains, if placed, should remain in position until the surgeon is sure the mucosal lesion has healed. Healing can be assessed using positive liquid contrast radiography of the cricopharyngeal area.

Postoperative Care

Postoperative care varies with the type of esophageal surgery. It can be divided into three categories.

1. The first category is used after procedures such as esophagoplasty and the modified Heller, in which the esophageal lumen is not penetrated. Animals are kept off food and water for 24 to 48 hours, depending upon the amount of esophageal handling. Oral liquid is started if there is no ileus and no vomiting. Parenteral fluids are administered as needed.

2. After procedures that penetrate the lumen, such as an esophagotomy, diverticulum repair, or after a myotomy incision that inadvertently penetrated, animals are maintained parenterally for 48 to 72 hours. Liquids only are offered for an additional 48 hours. Semi-solid food can be started on the fifth day and solid food on the seventh day postoperatively. When to start oral intake is decided subjectively on the basis of the degree of esophageal damage.

3. After esophageal resection and anastomoses or patch grafting, a feeding gastrostomy tube is installed during surgery and is maintained for 7 days. High-nutrition dietary supplements may be utilized. Fluid intake may be administered by either parenterally or by gastrostomy tube routes. Care is taken to instill less than 100 ml per feeding through the gastrostomy tube so regurgitation will not occur. Feeding through the tube should begin as soon as possible. Oral fluid intake may be started on the seventh day and semi-solid food on the eighth day postoperatively. A positive contrast esophagram using a water-soluble agent may be indicated prior to resumption of oral intake.

Antibiotics are utilized at the discretion of the clinician. One study in cats demonstrated better esophageal healing following resection and anastomosis if antibiotics were started preoperatively.[13]

References

1. Attum AA, Hankins JR, Ngangana J, and McLaughlin JS: Circular myotomy as an aid to resection and end-to-end anastomosis of the esophagus. Ann Thorac Surg 28:126, 1979.
2. Baker GJ, Hoffer RE: Surgical correction of esophageal stenosis in the dog. J Am Vet Med Assoc 15:119, 1965.
3. Bryant LR: Experimental evaluation of intercostal pedicle grafts in esophageal repair. J Thorac Cardiovasc Surg 50:626, 1965.
4. Goldsmith HS, Kiely AA, Randall HT: Protection of intrathoracic esophageal anastomoses by omentum. Surgery 63:464, 1968.
5. Hoffer RE, MacCoy DM, Quick CB, et al.: Management of acquired achalasia. J Am Vet Med Assoc 175:814, 1979.
6. Hoffer RE, Jensen HG: *Stereoscopic Atlas of Small Animal Surgery: Thoracic, Abdominal, and Soft Tissue Techniques*. 2nd ed. C.V. Mosby Co., St. Louis, 1977.
7. Hoffer RE, Barber SM, Kallfelz FA, Petro SP: Esophageal patch grafting as a treatment for esophageal stricture in a horse. J Am Vet Med Assoc 171:1350, 1977.
8. Hopper CL, Berk PD, Howes EL: Strength of esophageal anastomoses repaired with autogenous pericardial grafts. Surg Gynecol Obstet 117:83, 1963.
9. Howard DR, Lammerding JJ, Dewevire PV: Esophageal reinforcement with sternothyroideus muscle in the dog. Can Pract 2:30, 1975.
10. Muangsombut J, Hankins JR, Mason GR, McLaughlin JS: The use of circular myotomy to facilitate resection and end-to-end anastomosis of the esophagus. J Thorac Cardiovasc Surg 68:522, 1974.
11. Nissen R: Bridging of esophageal defect by pedicled flap of lung tissue. Ann Surg 129:142, 1949.
12. Pass MA: Surgical repair of esophageal defects. J Am Vet Med Assoc 154:1453, 1976.
13. Pearlstein L, Azaer IB, Polk HC: An experimental assessment of esophageal anastomotic integrity. Surg Gynec Obstet 146:545, 1978.
14. Pearson H, Gibbs C, Kelly DF: Oesophageal diverticulum formation in the dog. J Small Anim Pract 19:341, 1978.
15. Petrovsky BV: The use of diaphragm grafts for plastic operations in thoracic surgery. J Thorac Cardiovasc Surg 41:348, 1961.
16. Postlethwait RW, Deator, WR, Jr, Bradshaw HH, Williams RW: Esophageal anastomosis: Types and methods of suturing. Surgery 28:537, 1950.
17. Rosin E: Surgery of the canine esophagus. Vet Clin North Am 2:17, 1973.
18. Sumner-Smith G: Oesophagotomy and oesophageal resection. J Small Anim Pract 14:429, 1973.

CHAPTER

5

Medical Diseases of the Stomach

WAYNE E. WINGFIELD
DAVID C. TWEDT

GROSS ANATOMY

The stomach arises as a spindle-shaped dilation of the foregut during embryonic life and is the largest dilation of the alimentary canal. It originally consists of (1) an internal tube of entoderm, the primary tissue that becomes the epithelial lining and glandular ingrowths; and (2) an investing layer of splanchnic mesoderm that specializes into a thick, supporting wall. As development proceeds, the endothelium expands more rapidly than the mesothelium and thus becomes thrown into folds. These folds anticipate future distention by food and provide additional secretory and absorptive surface area.

The fetus grows, and the entire organ increases in length, with the dorsal border growing more rapidly than the ventral wall. This growth produces a convex greater curvature and a passively concave lesser curvature. The fundus arises as a bulge near the cranial end of the stomach and then begins to rotate 90° to the right about its long axis. The greater curvature thus faces caudally, ventrally, and to the left. The lesser curvature faces cranially, dorsally, and to the right. The concave surface of the lesser curvature forms an acute angle, the incisura angularis. This anatomical landmark is important in endoscopy, because it interferes with visualization of the distal stomach unless flexible probes are passed around the angle. The papillary process of the liver lies in this angle.

The topographical anatomy of the stomach is divided into the following regions: cardia, fundus, body, antrum, and pylorus (Fig. 5–1). The cardia is the entrance of the intra-abdominal esophagus into the stomach.

To the left and dorsal to the cardia lies the fundus. When filling with food, the fundus fills first and displaces in a caudodorsal direction. Further filling will then displace the stomach caudoventrally.

The body is the second part of the stomach to fill and expand. It is the largest region of the stomach and is the most capable of dilation. Together with the cardia and fundus, the body is the proximal storage portion of the stomach. This storage capacity occurs with little change in the intragastric pressure and makes this part an important area for secretion of digestive juices.

A line drawn from the incisura angularis to the greater curvature represents the juncture between the body (proximal) and an

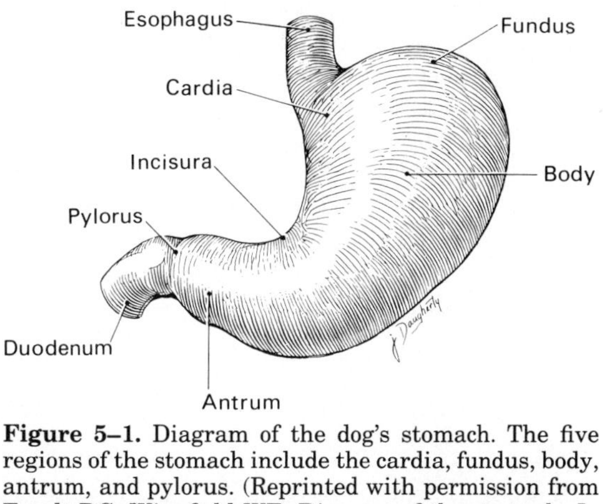

Figure 5–1. Diagram of the dog's stomach. The five regions of the stomach include the cardia, fundus, body, antrum, and pylorus. (Reprinted with permission from Twedt DC, Wingfield WE: Diseases of the stomach. *In* Ettinger SJ (ed): *Textbook of Veterinary Internal Medicine.* 2nd ed. Philadelphia, WB Saunders Co, 1982.)

Table 5–1. ARTERIAL BLOOD SUPPLY TO THE DOG'S STOMACH

Arterial Branch of Celiac Artery	Gastric Segment Supplied	Anastomotic Vessel
Hepatic artery		
Right gastric artery	Pylorus Pyloric antrum (lesser curvature)	Left gastric artery
Right gastroduodenal artery	Pylorus Pyloric antrum (greater curvature)	Right and left gastric artery Left gastroepiploic artery
Left gastric artery	Fundus (lesser curvature) Caudal esophagus	Right gastric artery
Splenic artery		
Left gastroepiploic artery	Cardia Fundus Pyloric antrum (greater curvature)	Right gastroepiploic artery

trum (distal). The antrum forms a region that functions in mechanical digestion and secretion of substances to regulate the release of hydrochloric acid. The antrum is directed cranially and expands with the peristaltic contractions and with the presence of foodstuffs (chyme).

At the junction between antrum and duodenum is an anatomical sphincter, the pylorus. This muscular structure expels chyme into the duodenum and prevents reflux of duodenal contents. A layer of circular smooth muscle several times thicker than the outer longitudinal muscle layer can be seen at the pylorus. There are actually two distinct loops of circular muscle, a right (oral or proximal) loop and a left (aboral or distal) loop. At the lesser curvature, both loops are united in a muscle torus and actually cover 0.5 to 1.5 cm of the gastric wall; they are spread over 2 to 5 cm near the greater curvature. This musculature is thickest as it crosses the greater curvature.

Proximally, the circular muscle fibers form a weak cardioesophageal sphincter. This sphincter is augmented on the greater curvature by transversely directed, inner oblique fibers. Oblique smooth muscle fibers cover the body of the stomach and lie adjacent to the submucosa.

An outer longitudinal coat of smooth muscle covers the circular muscle layer. Longitudinal smooth muscle fibers continue uninterrupted from the esophagus to the duodenum only along the greater curvature. Most longitudinal fibers end before the duodenum.

Ligamentous Supports

Movement of the stomach is restricted. At the gastroesophageal junction movement is inhibited at the passage through the diaphragm. Pyloric movement is restricted by the gastrohepatic ligament and the common bile duct. Additional mesenteric attachments include the greater omentum and the lesser omentum. The gastrosplenic ligament is derived from the greater omentum and attaches the spleen to the greater curvature. The remainder of the double peritoneal sheet constituting the greater omentum attaches along the greater curvature of the stomach.

The lesser omentum loosely spans the lesser curvature of the stomach, the duodenum, and the porta of the liver. The portion of the lesser omentum passing from the liver to the stomach is the gastrohepatic ligament.

Blood Supply

The principal arterial supply to the stomach is derived from the celiac artery. This artery divides into the hepatic, left gastric, and splenic arteries with each branch contributing arterial flow to the stomach (Table 5–1).

Satellite veins to the arteries of the stomach empty into either the gastroduodenal vein on the right or the splenic vein on the left. Both the splenic and gastroduodenal veins join the portal vein just caudal to the hilus of the liver.

Lymphatic drainage from the stomach eventually enters the right or left hepatic lymph nodes. The left hepatic node receives its drainage after the lymph has passed through the splenic and gastric nodes. Lymph drains into the right hepatic node from the stomach after first having passed through the duodenal node.

Nerves

The parasympathetic nerve supply to the stomach comes from the vagus nerves, which stimulate motility of the stomach and the secretion of hydrochloric acid, pepsin, and gastrin. Fibers in the vagi are predominantly afferent.

Ventral vagus branches supply mainly the liver and stomach. Gastric supplies come to the pylorus and the ventral stomach wall. The dorsal vagus supplies the cardia of the stomach and then forms a plexus on the stomach's dorsal surface. Distribution of the dorsal vagus is primarily to the lesser curvature and pylorus. The distribution of the terminal gastric branches of the vagus nerves is segmental.[107, 119]

Sympathetic innervation of the stomach is both efferent and afferent and extends from the celiac plexus. In the dog, autonomic innervation of the cardia differs from that in other parts of the stomach. Sympathetic α-receptors in the cardia act excitatorily and β-receptors inhibitorily, whereas in the stomach both receptors in other parts are inhibitory.[127]

MICROSCOPIC ANATOMY

The surface of the gastric mucosa is composed of mucus-secreting columnar epithelial cells. These lining cells extend into numerous invaginations in the mucosal surface, forming gastric pits. At the base of the gastric pits are mitotic foci, which renew the desquamated surface cells approximately once every one to three days.[8] These cells produce a layer of mucus that lubricates and protects the gastric mucosa. This mucosal cell layer and mucous coat provide the foundation of the gastric mucosal barrier that resists hydrochloric acid and digestive enzymes.

Three types of gastric glands are found in the stomach: cardiac glands, fundic glands (gastric glands), and pyloric glands.[9] These glands open into the base of the gastric pits and extend deep into the mucosa (Fig. 5–2).

Cardiac Gland Region

The cardiac glands, which are found in a narrow zone around the cardia, are composed of mucus-secreting epithelial cells and function in secreting mucus for lubrication.

Fundic Gland Region

The fundic gland region constitutes the largest area of gland distribution and includes the fundus and the body of the stomach. The glands in this region function in digestion by producing hydrochloric acid and pepsinogen. The fundic glands are composed of four cell types: chief cells, parietal cells, mucous cells, and argentaffin cells. The chief cells are in the highest concentra-

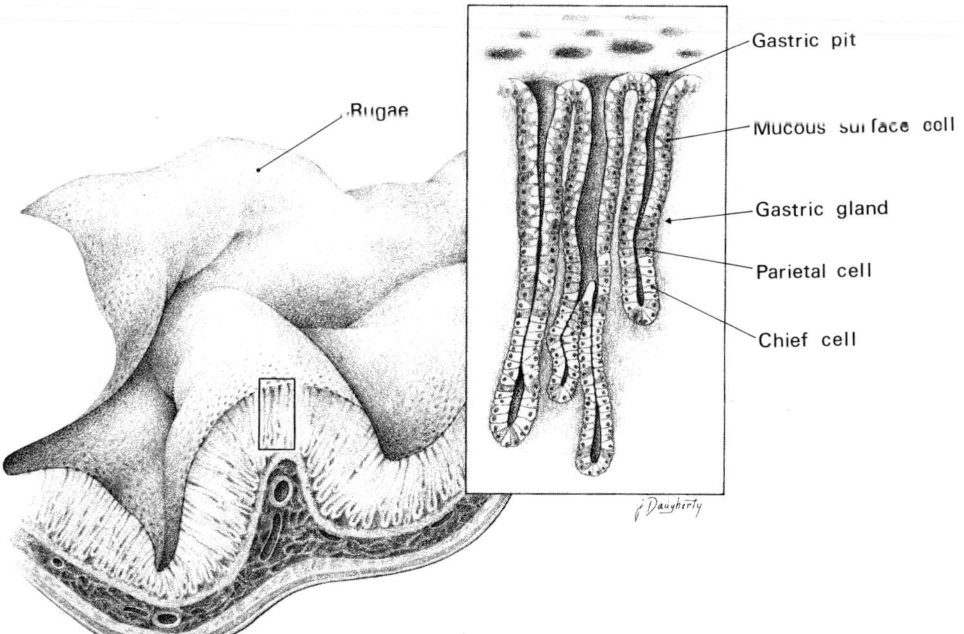

Figure 5–2. Cross-sectional anatomy of the dog's stomach with a microscopic diagram of the fundic glands. (Reprinted with permission from Twedt DC, Wingfield WE: Diseases of the stomach. *In* Ettinger SJ (ed): *Textbook of Veterinary Internal Medicine.* 2nd ed. Philadelphia, WB Saunders Co, 1982.)

tion at the base of the gland and function in the production of pepsinogen. These cells appear basophilic because they have many zymogen granules that contain pepsinogen. The parietal cells (oxyntic cells) are scattered throughout the mid-portion of the gland, stain deeply eosinophilic, and are responsible for hydrochloric acid secretion. The cells are large and contain a complex series of invaginations or secretory canaliculi, which open toward the lumen of the gland. Argentaffin cells are a type of endocrine cell that is scattered throughout the gastric glands. These cells contain granules that hold serotonin, a potent vasoconstrictor. The exact function of these cells is unknown. The mucous cells are relatively few in number and are found in the neck region of the glands.

Pyloric Gland Region

The pyloric glands are found in the antral region of the stomach. The major cell type is the mucous cell. In the mid-gland region are many gastrin-containing cells (G-cells), which are pyramidal and extend long processes into the gastric lumen to detect the nature and pH of the gastric contents. Upon stimulation, the hormone gastrin, a potent stimulator of hydrochloric acid secretion, is released.

Below the glands lies the lamina propria, the connective tissue portion of the gastric mucosal layer. The muscularis mucosa, the deepest layer of the mucosa, consists of a fine smooth muscle layer and is responsible for forming rugal folds or plicae. Between the mucosa and muscular layers is the submucosa, an elastic layer of areolar tissue containing small vessels, nerves, and lymphoid tissue. Scattered throughout both the lamina propria and submucosa are numerous mast cells, which act as mediators of gastric acid secretion.[29] The thick muscular coat is composed of an outer, longitudinal and an inner, circular layer of smooth muscle fibers with an additional oblique layer over the body of the stomach. The serosa, or outer coat, is thin and elastic and is continuous with the omentum.

Normal Physiology

The stomach serves three important functions. First, it provides a rapidly adjustable reservoir for the intake of food. Its volume adjustment occurs without excessive increases in intragastric pressure. Second it serves as a site for mixing gastric contents with gastric secretions. Third, the stomach gradually passes the gastric contents into the intestinal tract for final digestion and absorption.

VOLUME ADJUSTMENT

The filling of the stomach is not an entirely passive process. To a small degree the empty stomach simply unfolds to accommodate a part of the ingested volume.

In order to maintain a rather constant intragastric pressure, the gastric smooth muscle contracts or relaxes with varying stomach volumes. The control over this ability to maintain basal intragastric pressure appears to be partially a centrally mediated reflex. The central reflex (esophagogastric vagovagal relaxatory reflex) is initiated when there is an inhibition of tonic contraction of the proximal stomach in response to swallowing. A local reflex is seen when distention of the stomach by its contents produces reflex activation of the vagal relaxatory fibers. The gastric response to activation of the relaxatory fibers is a markedly prolonged relaxation, primarily affecting the body and fundic regions.

The capacity of the stomach varies from 0.5 to 8.0 liters in the dog. Greater ranges in relative size are noted in puppies than in adult dogs.[50] A capacity of 100 to 250 ml/kg of body weight has been reported by Neumayer and cited by Ellenberger and associates.[49]

GASTRIC SECRETION

The stomach secretes hydrochloric acid, other electrolytes, pepsinogen, gastrin, and mucus into the lumen. Gastrin and pepsinogen are also secreted by the stomach into the blood. These secretions are regulated by the cellular mass of the various mucosal secretory elements and by neural and hormonal stimulants and inhibitors.

Hydrochloric Acid Production

Parietal cells secrete hydrochloric acid into the gastric lumen. The hydrogen ion concentration in the gastric juices is three million times greater than in the blood and tissues. The precise electrical and biochemical events that result in the secretion of hydrochloric acid are not understood. The tremendous increase in hydrogen ion concentration represents a large chemical gradient for the ion to be transported against the concentration gradient and therefore requires considerable energy. Secretion of one liter of hydrochloric acid at a concentration of 160 mEq/L requires 1500 calories of energy.

For each hydrogen ion secreted, a molecule of carbon dioxide (CO_2) derived from arterial blood or mucosal metabolism is converted to bicarbonate and ultimately enters the intestinal fluid. Parietal cells contain a high concentration of the enzyme carbonic anhydrase, which catalyzes this conversion. Active acid secretion produces the alkaline tide, and the amount of bicarbonate entering the blood during secretion is proportional to the amount of acid secreted.

Agonists of gastric acid secretion include acetylcholine, gastrin, histamine, and digested protein. An intestinal hormone called entero-oxyntin has also been suggested as an agonist to gastric acid secretion.[59]

Gastric Acid Secretion

Control of gastric acid secretion is a complex interaction between many neural and humoral factors that dictate secretion at controlled rates and at the proper time. The mechanisms that control secretion have their effect during three different sequential periods of digestion, the cephalic phase, the gastric phase, and the intestinal phase.

Cephalic Phase. The cephalic phase of gastric acid secretion is stimulated by sight, taste, smell, and passage of food through the oropharynx. Higher cortical areas of the brain mediate this phase through efferent vagal fibers. The vagal fibers terminate on gastrin-secreting cells, parietal cells, and chief cells. Thus, the vagus stimulates release of gastrin, hydrochloric acid, and pepsinogen.

Gastric Phase. The gastric phase, the most important determinant of gastric secretion, is initiated by gastric distention and by the presence of digested proteins. Distention of either the fundic gland region or the pyloric gland region results in secretion by the G-cells and parietal cells; the cephalic vagal reflex also causes secretion.[59]

Intestinal Phase. The introduction of protein-containing foods into the small intestine produces a distinct acid secretory response. Three constituents of the intestinal phase can be assessed: direct stimulation of acid secretion, augmentation of maximal response to histamine and gastrin,[42] and release of antral gastrin by food in the intestine.

Role of Histamine. The role of histamine in gastric secretion is not completely understood. Usually, the histamine is not present in the body fluids in any significant quantity. In dogs and cats, histamine is contained in eosinophils and mast cells of the gastric mucosa.[7] Some histamine escapes the gastric mucosa and enters the gastric juice. This observation led to the discovery of H_2 receptors and the correlation between histamine output and the output of gastric juice from the stomach of dogs during psychic and vagal stimulation. Histamine output occurs mainly during the early phases of gastric secretion.[29] The H_2 receptor is postulated to exist on the basement membrane of the parietal cell. When the H_2 receptor is occupied by histamine, and in the presence of acetylcholine, gastrin will act to stimulate maximal acid secretion. If all receptor sites are occupied, and then one site is blocked (i.e., atropine blocking acetylcholine or cimetidine, an H_2 receptor antagonist, blocking histamine), stimulation through the other receptors will result in a response that is less than maximum. Thus, the H_2 receptor on the parietal cell is a major controller of the cell's hydrogen ion production, and use of H_2 receptor antagonists is effective for the control of gastric secretion.

Electrolyte Secretion

Chloride, potassium, and sodium are important electrolytes that are found in significant concentrations in gastric juices. Because of the presence of these electrolytes, the mucosal surface of the stomach is electrically negative compared with the serosal surface. The specific cell responsible for generation of this negative potential has not been identified, but the potential appears to be generated primarily at the cell border of the lumen. The active transport of chloride ions, from the intracellular space into the cell against both concentration and electrical gradients, appears to be the principal source of the potential difference. During secretion of acid, hydrogen ion secretion is coupled with secretion of an equivalent amount of chloride ion; therefore, the potential does not change.

Sodium and hydrogen ion concentrations in gastric juices vary inversely. The basal membrane of the epithelial cell is highly permeable to chloride and less permeable to sodium. As the intracellular concentrations of sodium and chloride are lower than the extracellular concentrations, both ions diffuse into the cell. Sodium is then actively pumped out of the cell.

Potassium concentration in gastric secretions is two to four times greater than plasma potassium concentration. As gastric secretion rates increase, the level of potassium in the juices increases, but after a prolonged period it falls, presumably because the intracellular potassium concentration is depleted. Most potassium in the gastric juices is derived from intracellular stores. Depletion of these stores often is not reflected in a lowering of plasma potassium.

Pepsins

Pepsinogen is the inactive precursor of pepsin, the principal proteolytic enzyme of gastric juices. The chief cell, located in the fundic region of the stomach, stores most of the pepsinogens.

Pepsinogen is secreted into the gastric lumen and its secretion is controlled by the same stimulants as those of acid secretion, with the major exception that secretin inhibits acid secretion and stimulates pepsinogen secretion. In the presence of an acid pH (hydrochloric acid), pepsinogens are autocatalytically converted to pepsins by the cleavage into several small peptides. Pepsin is active at an acid pH and irreversibly inactivated at a neutral or slightly alkaline pH. Thus, the proteolytic activity of pepsin ceases when chyme leaves the stomach and enters the more neutral duodenum.

Mucus

Gastric mucosal cells are coated with a gelatinous material called gastric mucus. This mucus is composed of glycoproteins, proteins, and carbohydrates. Mucus secretion is stimulated in response to local mucosal irritation and cholinergic stimulation. In cats, secretin and pentagastrin also stimulate mucus secretion.[153]

Mucus is assumed to provide lubrication of gastric contents and protection against physical irritants likely to produce surface injury. Mucus provides little impediment to the movement of water and electrolytes. No protection is afforded against either gastric acid or the proteolytic activity of pepsin. Some of the components of mucus provide inhibition of pepsin activity, but they are not effective at the concentrations and pH ranges in the secreting stomach. Mucus has some buffering capacity, which provides neutralization of acid, but this ability is negligible during active acid secretion.

Gastric Hormones

The primary physiological processes of the digestive system are influenced by nervous and hormonal mechanisms. Gastrin, secretin, and cholecystokinin (CCK) have major roles in stimulating gastric acid secretion, pancreatic water and bicarbonate secretion, gallbladder contraction, and pancreatic enzyme secretion, respectively. In addition to the three commonly accepted gastrointestinal hormones, a profusion of peptides has been extracted from gastrointestinal mucosal tissues. There are still events for which physiological evidence suggests hormonal mediation but for which the chemical messenger(s) have not been identified.

Gastrointestinal hormones are produced by amine precursor uptake decarboxylase (APUD) cells that originate in the neural crest of the embryo. All these hormones are polypeptides, have receptor sites in all tissues of the gastrointestinal tract, and affect motility and secretion.[49]

Gastrointestinal hormones are released in response to neural reflexes, the presence of other hormones, and specific stimuli acting on the gastrointestinal mucosa. Both local neural reflexes and neural reflexes of the central nervous system have afferent and efferent fibers in the vagi.

Gastrin. Cells that synthesize gastrin peptides (G-cells) and release the hormones into the circulation when appropriately stimulated are numerous in the antrum of the stomach of the dog. In the canine, gastrin-containing cells are found in the duodenum; none are found distal to the major duodenal papilla.[144] Distribution of feline G-cells is similar to that in the dog.

The regulation of circulating gastrin concentrations follows a basic feedback inhibition loop (Fig. 5–3). When gastrin concentrations rise, the gastric parietal cells are stimulated to secrete acid. When the antral mucosa is bathed in acid, further release of gastrin is inhibited. Feeding is a most important regulator of gastrin release. Partially digested proteins, amino acids (glycine, α- and β-alanine, serine, phenyl-

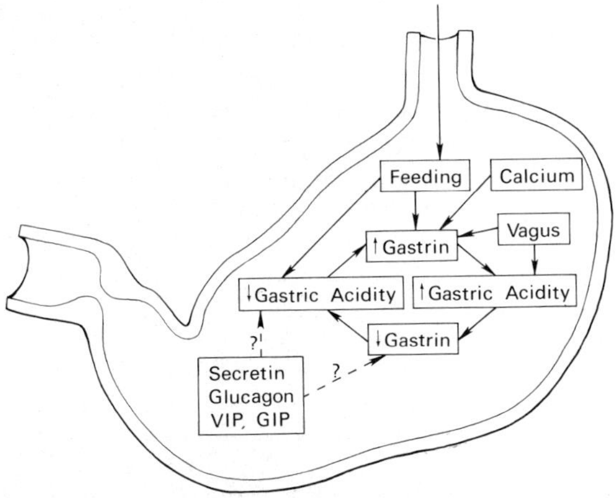

Figure 5–3. Regulation of circulating gastrin concentrations resulting from various feedback inhibition loops. (Reprinted with permission from Twedt DC, Wingfield WE: Diseases of the stomach. *In* Ettinger SJ (ed): *Textbook of Veterinary Internal Medicine. 2nd ed. Philadelphia, WB Saunders Co, 1982.*)

alanine, and lysine),[40] distention of the antrum[41] or fundus,[43] and the presence of calcium are known to cause release of gastrin in the dog.

Gastrin will affect many secretory, absorptive, and smooth muscle activities of the digestive tract (Table 5–2). In the dog, serum gastrin levels increase to a peak of about 160 picogm/ml after eating. The actions of gastrin that will occur at this physiological level are acid secretion, pepsin secretion, increased mucosal blood flow, and the trophic actions. The other actions require much higher levels of serum gastrin. Gastrin is about half as potent as cholecystokinin for stimulation of pancreatic enzyme secretion in the dog.

The kidneys are a major site of removal of gastrin from the circulation and of gastrin metabolism. Other organs, including the small intestine, participate in the metabolism of gastrin. The liver plays a minor role in the inactivation of gastrin.

Secretin. Secretin is released from cells located in the duodenum and jejunum of the dog. The major action of secretin is to stimulate pancreatic secretion of water and bicarbonate. Hydrogen ions are secretogogues for secretin. Acid gastric chyme is rapidly neutralized upon entering the duodenum and requires large volumes of concentrated acid over long segments of the duodenum to stimulate postprandial bicarbonate secretion.[87]

In the stomach, secretin has effects on secretion and motility. Physiological actions of secretin on the pancreas result in elevated water, bicarbonate, trypsin, and insulin secretion. There are increased volume and electrolyte output of bile by the liver, reduced gastric emptying in the stomach, reduced resting and gastrin-stimulated pressure of the lower esophageal sphincter, and decreased motility of the duodenum with secretin release.[123] Removal of secretin from the circulation results from renal excretion.[35]

Cholecystokinin. Fat in the small intestine was noted to release a substance that caused active gallbladder contraction and stimulated pancreatic secretion. The hormone is called cholecystokinin.[123]

Cholecystokinin distribution is limited to the mucosa of the small intestine. In rats, dogs, and baboons, the maximal concentration is in the jejunum, with considerable quantities also located in the ileum and duodenum. Catabolism of cholecystokinin is through the kidney and probably through other tissues.

Newer Gastrointestinal Hormones

In addition to gastrin, secretin, and cholecystokinin, several peptides that function

Table 5–2. ACTIONS OF GASTRIN IN THE DIGESTIVE TRACT*

Action	Organs Affected
Stimulate water and electrolyte secretion	Stomach Pancreas Liver Small intestine Brunner's glands
Stimulate enzyme secretion	Stomach Pancreas Small intestine
Inhibition of water, electrolyte, and glucose absorption	Small intestine
Stimulation of smooth muscle	Lower esophageal sphincter Stomach Small intestine Colon Gallbladder
Inhibition of smooth muscle	Pyloric sphincter Ileocecal sphincter Sphincter of Oddi
Release of hormones insulin and calcitonin	Many sites of action
Increase in blood flow	Small intestine Small intestine Pancreas
Trophic actions	Gastric mucosa Small bowel mucosa Pancreas

*After Walsh JH, and Grossman MI: Gastrin. N Engl J Med *292*:1324, 1975.

as hormones have been identified. Physiological phenomena have been observed that suggest that other substances may be involved with the initiation and modulation of the digestive process. Studies of these peptides, including vasoactive intestinal polypeptide (VIP), gastric inhibitor polypeptide (GIP), glucagon, bombesin, motilin, chymodenin, bulbogastrone, entero-oxyntin, and pancreatic polypeptide, indicate that they may function in digestion.[7] To date, there are many unanswered questions regarding the identity and function of these and other gastrointestinal hormones.[3, 46, 123, 140, 158]

GASTRIC MOTILITY AND EMPTYING

The stomach receives and stores food, mixes it with gastric secretions, and delivers it to the duodenum. It empties liquids faster than solids, and carbohydrates faster than fats. As a motor unit, the stomach has two functional areas: a proximal receptacle (fundus and body) and a distal pump (antrum), which mixes the gastric contents and delivers them to the duodenum. The pylorus, a low-pressure muscular sphincter, has little or no role in regulating gastric emptying of liquids; it is important in preventing the entrance of large food particles into the duodenum and the reflux of duodenal contents.[138]

The fundus is important in gastric motility and emptying. At this site an electrical potential is generated that spreads over the stomach to the pylorus. The electrical control activity is an omnipresent event occurring at a frequency of five cycles per minute in the dog. Whether or not the antrum contracts with each of these cycles depends upon a second electrical event, the electrical response activity, which causes contraction of the antrum. Thus, the number of antral contractions does not always correspond to the number of contractions generated from the electrical control activity of the fundus.

Gastric electrical activity of the muscle and muscle contractions are influenced by a number of factors, including cholinergic, adrenergic, and non-adrenergic inhibitory reflexes. Gastric hormones also affect this activity. Gastrin increases antral electrical activity and muscle contraction frequency, and secretin slows them. Cholecystokinin and gastrin accelerate electrical response activity in the antrum, and secretin slows it. Motilin, a 22–amino acid polypeptide hormone from the upper small intestine, stimulates the motility of the proximal stomach.[44, 142]

Gastric emptying is influenced by the volume and composition of the meal.[31] The nutritive density (Kcal/ml), and not the initial volume, determines the rate of gastric emptying. It has been shown that with isocaloric amounts of fat, protein, and carbohydrates, there will be equal slowing of gastric emptying.[72]

As the fundus and body fill with food they will relax, thus reducing intragastric pressure and decreasing the rate of emptying. If the gastric fundus possesses high motility, the food entering will increase intragastric pressure and accelerate emptying.

The pylorus and antrum are parts of the discriminating mechanism that allows liquids to empty and solids to be retained longer in the stomach. Dietary fats also leave the stomach slowly. This slow release of fats appears to be due to intragastric layering of the oil phase of the aqueous phase and also due to a feedback inhibitory mechanism that is triggered in the intestine by fats.[92]

Digestible and non-digestible solids empty by different gastric mechanisms. Digestible solids are reduced in size to fine particles by the grinding and mixing of the distal antrum. These particles are suspended in fluid, which is then emptied. There are three crucial factors in this process: the grinding pressure waves of the distal antrum, the discriminatory mechanism that allows small suspended particles to leave with liquids and retains longer particles for further grinding in the stomach, and the propulsive forces (mostly fundic) that push the fluids into the duodenum. Non-digestible solids trigger antral grinding contractions, but most of these particles are impervious to this mechanical grinding. The particles are only slightly reduced, to a size that allows emptying. These particles are the last to leave the stomach.

Physical Examination

An animal suspected of having gastric disease should undergo a historical and physical review of all body systems. The animal's hydration is carefully noted, because serious fluid and electrolyte depletion may result from vomiting.

Normally, the stomach cannot be palpated, because it is positioned within the rib cage. Palpation is possible only when the stomach, distended with gas or food, extends past the caudal ribs. It is often easier to palpate the stomachs of small dogs and cats. In some cases, the fingers can be pushed under the rib cage and the stomach palpated. Palpation of the cranial abdomen may be facilitated by elevating the front legs, which allows the abdominal contents to fall caudally.

Pain in the region of the stomach is an inconsistent finding with gastric disease. The gas-distended stomach of the gastric dilatation-volvulus syndrome can be ballotted and percussed as an air-filled density. Auscultation of the abdomen may reveal bowel sounds that occur from gastrointestinal motility caused by the movement of gas over fluid. The strongest and loudest bowel sounds generally originate from the stomach. An empty stomach will usually be silent but becomes vocal with the presence of fluid and gas.[118] Louder sounds may occur in some gastric diseases.

Diagnostic Techniques

LABORATORY TESTS

There are few biochemical and hematological alterations consistently associated with diseases of the stomach. Gastric lesions can occur secondary to other diseases, and laboratory testing is required to rule out these conditions. Acute gastric disease is usually self-limiting and often requires no laboratory evaluation, whereas such conditions as the gastric dilatation-volvulus syndrome result in serious fluid, electrolyte, acid-base, and biochemical abnormalities in which laboratory evaluation, to determine treatment, is essential. The need for laboratory testing is determined on the basis of history, clinical findings, and past clinical experience. The patient that is dehydrated or debilitated or has a history of chronic gastric problems should be assessed by the laboratory.

The hematocrit (PCV) and total serum solids (total serum protein) tests are the minimum laboratory procedures that should be done. These two simple tests give the approximate hydration state of the animal. The fluid loss resulting from vomition and inadequate fluid intake causes dehydration, which is reflected in an increased PCV and higher total serum solids concentration. A normal PCV in a dehydrated animal with an elevated percentage of total solids may suggest a pre-existing anemia (e.g., gastric ulceration).

A complete blood count (CBC) will provide useful information in the animal with gastric disease. Most animals whose vomiting is caused by gastric disease have a stress leukogram (mature neutrophilia, lymphopenia, and eosinopenia). The presence of lymphocytosis and eosinophilia in a vomiting animal that does not have a stress leukogram should suggest the possibility of adrenocortical insufficiency (Addison's disease). An increase in the total eosinophil count may also occur with gastrointestinal parasites, eosinophilic gastritis, or in food allergies. Anemia from blood loss in gastric disease is characterized by regeneration of blood with reticulocytosis, nucleated red blood cells, anisocytosis, and polychromasia. Chronic gastrointestinal blood loss eventually results in an iron deficiency anemia with microcytic hypochromic red blood cell indices.

Biochemical profiles and urinalysis should be done to exclude systemic causes of gastric disease. Common conditions such as liver disease, uremia, and pancreatitis are easily ruled out by most biochemical profile screens.

Vomiting caused by gastric disease may result in electrolyte and acid-base abnormalities. Substantial losses of water, chloride, and sodium and, to a lesser degree, losses of hydrogen and potassium result from vomiting. Traditionally, vomiting has been associated with a metabolic alkalosis resulting from the loss of gastric acid. Clinically, the majority of cases of vomiting in small animals with acid-base abnormalities have a metabolic acidosis.[32] Acidosis occurs because of the loss of fluid and electrolytes and results in contraction of the extracellular fluid volume with a minimal loss of acid. The normal empty stomach of a dog has a negligible amount of basal acid secretion, and when hydrogen ions are actively secreted, there is a transient extracellular alkalosis. This alkalosis is normally corrected by an equivalent loss of bicarbonate through bile and pancreatic juices. Because of the simultaneous loss of refluxed alkaline-rich duodenal fluid and the reabsorption of hydrogen and chloride ions that may pass from the stomach into the intestine, an acid deficit does not occur with vomiting. Hypokalemia frequently occurs in conjunction with vomiting, predominately through urinary losses and, to a lesser extent, through losses in gastric juices.

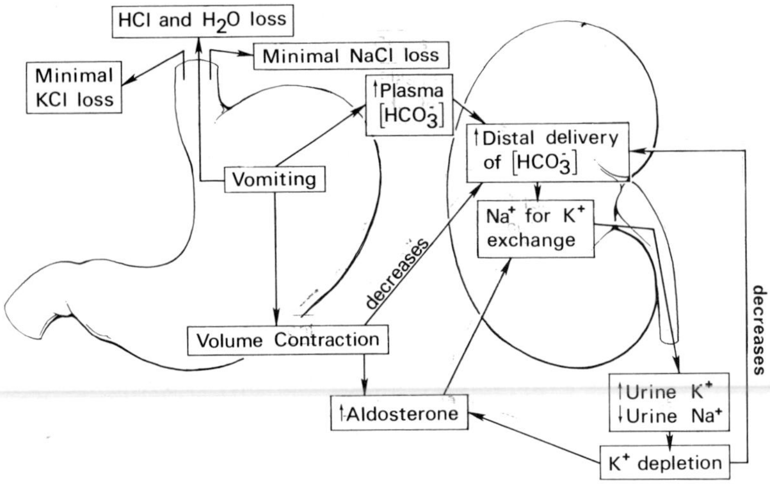

Figure 5–4. Pathophysiological events present perpetuating metabolic alkalosis and renal potassium depletion. (Reprinted with permission from Twedt DC, Wingfield WE: Diseases of the stomach. *In* Ettinger SJ (ed): *Textbook of Veterinary Internal Medicine.* 2nd ed. Philadelphia, WB Saunders Co, 1982.)

Metabolic alkalosis can be precipitated by a net loss in hydrogen ions occurring from frequent and profuse vomiting or because of a pyloric outflow obstruction. Gastric alkalosis is also perpetuated through chloride depletion and contraction of extracellular volume or through hypokalemia.[48]

In normal animals, most of the sodium and bicarbonate entering the kidney is reabsorbed. When the plasma concentration of bicarbonate rises and the capacity for renal absorption is exceeded, excess bicarbonate escapes in the urine, resulting in an increase in urine pH. Urinary bicarbonate excretion continues until homeostasis is again achieved. Metabolic alkalosis may, however, be perpetuated when renal bicarbonate absorption occurs concurrently with elevated plasma bicarbonate levels. This situation can be caused by a contracted extracellular volume and chloride depletion. With losses of salt and water, the effective arterial blood volume contracts, which leads to increased stimulation for proximal nephron reabsorption of sodium. Sodium is reabsorbed with chloride anions; if chloride levels are reduced, then another anion, bicarbonate, must be reabsorbed to maintain electrical neutrality. Thus, extracellular fluid depletion, especially when associated with hypochloremia caused by vomiting, results in inadequate bicarbonate excretion leading to or maintaining a state of metabolic alkalosis.

Potassium deficiency often occurs with metabolic alkalosis. The development of this deficiency may result from etiologic factors that caused hydrogen and chloride losses (i.e., vomiting), renal wasting of potassium, and increased aldosterone secretion with volume depletion. Loss of cellular potassium will also cause a shift of extracellular hydrogen ions (derived from carbonic acid) into cells, and thereby produce an increase in extracellular bicarbonate, thus perpetuating peripheral metabolic alkalosis.

Renal wasting of potassium occurs when there is a disparity between the availability of reabsorbable anion (chloride) in the glomerular filtrate and the simultaneous need to conserve body sodium (Fig. 5–4).[126] With these conditions, sodium-hydrogen exchange, as well as sodium-potassium exchange, in the distal tubule of the kidney is accelerated. With a severe hypokalemia, sodium will exchange only with hydrogen ions. When a metabolic alkalosis occurs in conjunction with renal bicarbonate reabsorption and a sodium-hydrogen exchange, a paradoxical aciduria will exist.[56]

The stool should be examined for evidence of gastrointestinal parasites and upper gastrointestinal bleeding. Obvious melena may be the consequence of severe gastric bleeding, whereas mild hemorrhage is not evident grossly. The stool can be evaluated for occult blood by using Hematest tablets.* Animals eating a meat protein diet will often show a false-positive occult test. The animal should be on a meat-free diet for several days prior to the test.

Gastric Fluid Analysis

In addition to the gross examination of the vomitus, certain laboratory tests can be performed to analyze gastric contents. Samples collected from the vomitus, by aspira-

*Hematest tablets, Ames Company, Elkhart, IN.

tion during endoscopy or from a gastric tube that was placed during pharyngostomy,[19] are analyzed.

Normal gastric contents of a fasted animal should be clear and should contain small amounts of mucus and saliva. The pH of the gastric fluid will approach neutrality. With gastric acid stimulation the pH of the gastric contents may fall to a level of 2 or less. The pH of vomitus indicates its origin. With regurgitation caused by esophageal disease, the pH will most often be alkaline. The presence of bile-stained gastric juice, which is caused by duodenal reflux, will also elevate the pH of the fluid.

Microscopic examination of the sediment of a centrifuged sample may reveal red blood cells, white blood cells, epithelial cells, bacteria, parasites, foreign material, or food particles. Owing to the acidity of the gastric juice, only nuclear remnants of cellular elements may remain. In cases of suspected neoplasia, a gastric lavage may retrieve neoplastic cells. Normal saline is instilled into the stomach of an animal that has fasted by means of a stomach tube and a syringe. The stomach is flushed by vigorously swishing the solution back and forth prior to retrieval. The fluid is collected and centrifuged, and the sediments examined.

RADIOLOGY

Gastric position, shape, intraluminal radiopaque foreign bodies, gastric wall abnormalities, and gastric emptying can be demonstrated radiographically.

When possible, animals should be fasted for at least 12 hours before abdominal films are to be taken. A radiograph taken in right lateral recumbency usually shows fluid in the pyloric antrum and gas within the gastric body, whereas a left lateral radiograph usually demonstrates gas in the pyloric antrum.

Gastric size, shape, and location can usually be evaluated on routine abdominal radiographs. Changes in gastric position and shape are usually due to extragastric causes or gastric wall lesions. The condition of the rugal folds is difficult to assess on routine films. Complete evaluation of the luminal surface usually requires contrast studies and distention of the stomach. Radiopaque gastric foreign bodies are easily observed, whereas radiolucent foreign bodies are more difficult to discern. Contrast studies are performed in animals with chronic signs of gastric disease and normal routine films.

Negative-Contrast Study

A negative-contrast study of the stomach is performed using either air or carbon dioxide. A stomach tube is passed into the stomach, and gas is introduced until the stomach is moderately distended. This contrast method is an inexpensive and easy means of outlining many intraluminal gastric foreign bodies or for evaluating gastric wall thickness.

Positive-Contrast Study

A positive-contrast study is one employing a radiopaque contrast material. In most cases, barium sulfate is used. Commercially prepared micropulverized contrast agents (30 per cent weight per volume) give consistent homogeneous gastric filling. The suggested dosage, administered by stomach tube, is 8 to 12 ml/kg body weight in small dogs and cats and 5 to 7 ml/kg body weight for large dogs,[125] given by stomach tube.

Contrast studies provide a crude method of evaluating gastric wall motility and emptying. Being a dynamic process, fluoroscopy is the best means of evaluating gastric wall motility. Without fluoroscopy, multiple radiographs must be taken to observe the changes in the gastric wall caused by peristaltic contractions. A fixed, rigid, or nondistensible region of the stomach suggests a gastric wall lesion. Delayed gastric emptying results from gastric motility disorders or from gastric outflow obstruction. Normally, the duodenum begins to fill in 5 to 15 minutes and the stomach empties in approximately 1 to 4 hours.[53] Total retention of the contrast material in the stomach for longer than 30 minutes generally indicates some degree of pyloric occlusion.[57] The rate of gastric emptying can be altered by excitement, nervous inhibition, or various anticholinergic drugs or tranquilizers. If tranquilization is required, acepromazine maleate* is reported not to affect gastric transit time.[169]

Double-Contrast Study

Double-contrast studies of the stomach involve using both negative and positive

*Acepromazine, Ayerst Laboratories, New York, NY.

contrast agents. This technique is useful in outlining gastric foreign bodies, gastric wall contour, and the mucosal surface. It is most beneficial when gastric foreign bodies absorb or are coated by the positive contrast agent. The technique involves giving approximately 1 ml/kg body weight of micropulverized barium sulfate (30 per cent weight per volume, W/V).[108] The animal is rolled to coat the mucosal surface with contrast material, a stomach tube is reintroduced, and the stomach is distended with gas.

ENDOSCOPY

Endoscopy enables the clinician to visually examine the luminal surface of the stomach. Older rigid endoscopes, either hollow tubes or solid optics, had only limited value in the examination of the small animal stomach. They have been useful in aiding in the removal of various gastric foreign bodies.

With the development of flexible fiberoptics, examination of the gastrointestinal system has improved.[77, 168] The entire stomach can now be adequately visualized. The distal tip of the endoscope is directed through either a two- or a four-way control knob in the handpiece. In addition to the optical fiber bundles, two channels are present. One allows a variety of endoscopic tools (biopsy forceps, cytology brushes, aspirating tubes, snares, and grasping forceps) to be passed into the stomach and stomach fluids to be suctioned. The other channel carries air for insufflation of the stomach or for passing water to wash mucus and other material from the viewing window of the endoscope. A separate light source with pump for instillation of fluid and air and a separate suction apparatus are required.

GASTRIC BIOPSY

Peroral biopsy capsules are available.[12] These instruments are relatively simple, non-invasive, and can be passed into the stomach to obtain a small mucosal biopsy specimen. All the capsules are attached to long, flexible tubes. Suction is created by the operator, who uses a syringe and a vacuum gauge to draw a piece of mucosa into a small hole in the capsule. A knife, attached to a cable, is pulled and removes the piece of tissue. The mucosal biopsy specimen is retained inside the capsule.

One type of capsule found suitable for gastric biopsy in small animals is a Sielaff's gastric biopsy probe.* Other instruments that are useful include the multi-purpose suction biopsy tube† and the Carrie gastrointestinal biopsy capsule‡ (see Chapter 2).

Surgical Biopsy

An exploratory celiotomy provides the best means of establishing a definitive diagnosis of gastric disease. Surgery provides the opportunity to palpate the stomach, examine the luminal surface, obtain a full-thickness biopsy specimen of the gastric wall, and remove gastric foreign bodies. Surgery is often required for the removal of gastric ulcers, polyps, and tumors and to correct gastric outflow obstructions. At surgery, the animal should be carefully evaluated for other intra-abdominal problems such as pancreatitis, enlarged regional lymph nodes, and small gastrin-secreting tumors of the pancreas.

GASTRIC SECRETORY TESTING

The collection of gastric secretions and the analysis of the acid content will help the clinician recognize hyperacidic secretory states. Clinical gastric acid collection in the dog is best achieved by temporarily placing a gastric tube via pharyngostomy into the antral region of the stomach.[1] Basal gastric acid output (BAO) secretions are collected from the fasted dog every 15 minutes. The sample is titrated by means of a pH meter to a neutral pH and the acidity is expressed in milliequivalents of hydrogen ion per 15-minute period.[74] Basal gastric acid output in the normal, fasted dog is usually negligible. The potential acid-secreting ability of the stomach is directly proportional to the parietal cell mass.[93] The maximal acid output (MAO) can be stimulated by various secretogogues such as histamine, betazole, and pentagastrin.§

Pentagastrin contains the C-terminal active site of natural gastrins and therefore acts as a physiological gastric acid stimula-

---

*Sielaff's gastric biopsy probe, Richard Wolf Medical Instruments Corp., Rosemont, IL.

†Multi-purpose suction biopsy tube, Quinton Instrument Co., Seattle, WA.

‡Gastrointestinal biopsy capsule, Precision Instruments.

§Peptaulon, Ayerst Laboratories, New York, NY.

tor and is preferred for evaluating gastric secretory function. Pentagastrin given at the rate of 6 μg/kg body weight, subcutaneously or intravenously, will cause a maximal acid secretion within 1 hour.[13] In the normal dog, a wide range of MAO values are reported, depending on the method of measurement used. Ranges of 3 to 12 mEq of hydrogen ion per 15 minutes are reported.[17, 58, 67]

Gastric Diseases

ACUTE GASTRITIS

Acute gastritis is a common disease that occurs in small animals. By strict definition, acute gastritis is a description of the inflammation and mucosal damage that has occurred in response to an insult to the gastric mucosa. Rarely do conditions of acute gastritis warrant biopsy and histological confirmation; therefore the diagnosis of acute gastritis is given when signs of gastric disease are acute and self-limiting.

History and Physical Examination

Vomiting is the principal clinical sign of acute gastritis. Observation of vomiting enables the clinician to differentiate gastric disease from regurgitation associated with esophageal disease or from coughing and expulsion of phlegm associated with respiratory or cardiovascular disease. Vomiting is preceded by a period of nausea with licking, salivation, or multiple attempts at swallowing. This period is followed by retching or several forceful, simultaneous diaphragmatic and abdominal contractions and, with the head lowered, expulsion of gastric contents.

Observation of the amount, color, and consistency of vomitus is useful. If the vomitus consists of food, the degree of digestion suggests the length of time it has remained in the stomach. Vomitus may contain mucus and fluid from gastric and swallowed salivary secretions. Yellow or green stained vomitus indicates intestinal reflux of bile into the stomach. Fresh blood from gastric bleeding may be present as small, red flecks or as large blood clots. Blood that has remained in the stomach soon becomes partially digested and has as a brown "coffee grounds" appearance. The presence of blood in vomitus generally signifies a more serious gastric disease.

Other physical signs associated with gastric disease include nausea, belching, polydipsia, and pica. Melena, or black tarry stools, is seen with upper gastrointestinal bleeding and may imply gastric disease. Coughing may occur because of an aspiration pneumonitis. Animals with gastric pain may exhibit a position of relief, or "praying position," with the rear legs elevated.[143]

Etiology

In most cases of acute gastritis, the etiology is never determined. There is a paucity of published cases of spontaneously occurring acute gastritis in contrast to the number of reports of experimentally induced lesions. Acute gastritis has been associated with a multitude of factors, mainly resulting from dietary indiscretions of dogs and cats. It is most often associated with ingestion of rancid or spoiled foodstuffs that leads to a "garbage-can" intoxication. The agent incriminated in cases of acute gastritis is usually the fermentation or putrefaction of food products, various bacterial enterotoxins, and various mycotoxins.[62]

Ingestion of foreign material such as food wrappings, bones, plastic, rocks, and small toys mechanically damages the gastric mucosa. The incidence of ingested foreign bodies is higher in young animals, possibly because of their chewing habits and curious natures. Trichobezoars (hairballs) are frequently encountered in the stomachs of some long-haired cats and dogs. Certain drugs (e.g., aspirin, indomethacin, phenylbutazone, and corticosteroids) and chemicals (e.g., heavy metals, cleaning agents, fertilizers, and herbicides) are reported to cause gastritis in the dog and cat.

Many types of plants and plant toxins cause an acute gastritis, possibly the most common being associated with the ingestion of grass. The ingestion of grass and plants is probably a normal instinctual behavior; however, animals with gastric disease, for some unknown reason, seem to ingest and commonly vomit plant material. Ingestion of many common household plants will also cause acute gastritis.[6]

Infectious agents are associated with acute gastritis. The incidence of bacterially induced gastritis is low because the gastric lumen, which is very acidic, generally contains few bacteria.[160] Viruses such as canine distemper, canine hepatitis, coronavirus, and parvovirus may cause gastric lesions as a part of a more extensive disease condition. Mycotic infections of the stomach have been reported in the dog.[11, 70, 112] Parasites generally do not produce gastric lesions or clinical signs; *Physaloptera* spp., and infrequently ascarids and tapeworms, are the most common parasitic agents of gastritis and vomiting. Spirochetes have been observed in the mucous layer and the parietal cells of the stomachs of some dogs and cats, and may be a factor in the cause of gastritis.[162]

Acute gastritis may result from an allergic reaction to an antigen to which the animal was previously sensitized. It is often suggested that clinical conditions are simple food allergies. Other disease conditions including uremia,[27] liver disease, neurological disease, shock, sepsis, and even stress may play a role in the etiology of acute gastritis.

Pathophysiology

Acute lesions may be localized or diffuse. Necrosis of surface cells with extravasation of blood and plasma from the damaged vessels in the lamina propria produces superficial erosions, edema, and hemorrhage. There are variable amounts of polymorphonuclear (PMN) leukocyte and lymphocyte infiltration of the lamina propria. Occasionally, inflammation may become a purulent gastritis with necrosis and extensive PMN leukocyte infiltration.

The parietal cells of the gastric mucosa produce hydrochloric acid, generating a luminal secretion with a low pH. The unique ability of the stomach to withstand concentrated acid without cellular damage is referred to as the gastric mucosal barrier.[75] This barrier resists the "back-diffusion" of hydrogen ions from the gastric lumen into the mucosa and prevents sodium loss into the lumen. The anatomical makeup of the barrier consists of two parts—the mucous layer, lining the surface of the epithelial cells, and the mucosal cells, which compose the epithelial membrane. The true function of the mucous layer is believed to be predominately in lubrication. Mucus has only a weak neutralizing and buffering capacity, and acid will readily diffuse through the mucous layer. The gastric epithelial cells are the most important anatomical barrier.[133]

The back-diffusion of luminal acid into the mucosa is essential in the pathogenesis of gastric mucosal damage. Normally, there is minimal leakage of secreted acid back into the mucosa. Such leakage occurs at a very slow rate, and the acid is rapidly removed by the vascular system.[26] The topical action of many endogenous and exogenous agents can alter this barrier, thereby increasing mucosal permeability to acid. With increased entry of acid, the direct damage to the mucosa is followed by destruction of the subepithelium. Mast cells present in the submucosa and lamina propria degranulate and release histamine upon contact with acid. The release of histamine stimulates parietal cell secretion of hydrochloric acid as well as local inflammation and edema. Acid may also damage blood vessels and stimulate nerves of the gastric wall, leading to increased muscular contractions.

Diagnosis

A diagnosis of acute gastritis is made on the basis of history, clinical signs, and physical findings. Since acute gastritis is more common than other causes of gastric disease, symptomatic therapy is usually initiated without extensive diagnostic procedures. A rapid and complete response to therapy confirms the diagnosis. Cases involving severely ill animals or patients that fail to respond to symptomatic therapy require further diagnostic testing.

Treatment

Most patients with acute gastritis show improvement within 24 hours following little or no therapy. Such animals are usually treated on an outpatient basis. Those animals displaying frequent vomiting, evidence of dehydration, or failing to respond to previous conservative measures require further medical and laboratory evaluation. The basic principles in the therapy of gastric disease include removing the initiating agent, providing proper conditions to promote mucosal repair, correcting secondary complications of gastritis (vomiting, abdominal pain, and infection), and correcting fluid, electrolyte, and acid-base abnormalities.

Dietary restriction is the initial therapy for acute gastritis. Ingestion of food or liquids results in gastric distention, increased gastric motility, and further vomiting. Food will increase gastric acid production by stimulating both the cephalic and gastric phases of secretion, resulting in further back-diffusion of hydrogen ions and further mucosal injury. Food also serves as an exogenous source of bacteria that could potentially invade the damaged gastric mucosa.

An animal with acute gastritis should be fasted for a minimum of 12 hours. If no vomiting has occurred during that time, the animal is frequently offered small amounts of water or ice cubes, enough to keep the mouth moist and to supply a modest fluid replacement. After a minimum of 24 hours from the onset of signs, food is reintroduced. Small amounts of a bland, carbohydrate diet are fed—cooked rice or cooked cereals supplemented with cottage cheese; lean, boiled ground beef; or baby foods. Commercial diets formulated for gastrointestinal disease (e.g., Prescription Diet I/D)* may also be prescribed. If a favorable response is obtained with dietary management, the regular diet is gradually reintroduced over several days.

Parenteral fluids are initiated when electrolyte or acid-base imbalances or dehydration occur. The quantity of fluids given should be enough to supply daily maintenance needs (approximately 40 to 60 ml/kg/day), to correct existing dehydration, and to replace fluid losses that may occur with continued vomiting. Vomiting in acute gastritis generally results in volume depletion and losses of sodium, chloride, and potassium with a *metabolic acidosis*. An isotonic, balanced electrolyte solution such as Ringer's lactate solution is usually given.[151] Infrequently, in profuse vomiting or a gastric outflow obstruction, a severe hypochloremia, hypokalemia, or metabolic alkalosis may exist. Normal (0.9 percent) saline is the fluid of choice for correcting metabolic alkalosis resulting from vomiting. Therapy with chlorides rectifies the deficit and allows renal excretion of bicarbonate.[51] In either acidosis or alkalosis, potassium levels are depleted, and often additional potassium chloride must be added to the fluids.[130] The amount of potassium chloride added is based on the existing serum potassium levels.[149]

Antiemetic drugs are given to control refractory vomiting when the presence of a pyloric obstruction or a gastric foreign body has been ruled out. These drugs inhibit vomiting but do little for primary treatment of gastritis. Antiemetic drugs act centrally by suppressing either the chemoreceptor trigger zone (CTZ), the emetic center, or the vestibular apparatus. Drugs that depress only the CTZ are generally not useful unless the gastritis is the result of toxins that may directly stimulate the trigger zone. The phenothiazine tranquilizers (e.g., chlorpromazine)* have a broad-spectrum pharmacological effect in blocking the chemoreceptor trigger zone and the emetic center, in addition to some anticholinergic action.[38] These drugs are effective in blocking viscerally stimulated vomiting caused by gastritis and should be used in patients with repeated vomiting. The phenothiazines should not be used in a dehydrated or a hypotensive animal because of their alpha-adrenergic blocking action, which causes arteriolar vasodilatation and, thus, a secondary hypotension.

Anticholinergic drugs reduce gastric motility and spasms. In addition to blocking the parasympathetic stimulation of smooth muscles of the gastric wall, these drugs block the cephalic and gastric phases of gastric acid secretion, but they do not block histamine or gastrin-stimulated acid secretion. These drugs have the undesirable effect of reducing gastric emptying, which results in gastric distention and further gastric acid secretion. Overuse of these drugs may cause gastric hypotonia and a pharmacologic gastric outflow obstruction and, thus, continued vomiting. Anticholinergic drugs used in the therapy of gastric disease include atropine, methylscopolamine, isopropamide,† and propantheline.‡ These drugs often are combined with an antiemetic for veterinary use. Opiates (e.g., camphorated tincture of opium and diphenoxylate) have a similar action in decreasing gastric motility and emptying.

Oral protectants such as kaolin and pectin and antibiotics are generally not indicated in the treatment of acute gastritis. Protectants may bind certain bacteria or toxins, but they do not coat or protect the injured gastric mucosa. Any potential benefit is frequently outweighed by difficulty in owner administration and vomiting that may occur

*Prescription Diet I/D Hill's Pet Products, Inc., Topeka, KS.

*Thorazine, Smith, Kline & French Laboratories, Philadelphia, Pa. Dosage: 0.5 mg/kg.

†Darbazine, Norden Laboratories, Lincoln, NB. Dosage: 4 lbs to 15 lbs No. 1 capsule BID
15 lbs to 30 lbs No. 1 capsule 2 BID
30 lbs No. 3 capsule 1 BID

‡Pro-banthine, Searle & Co., San Juan, PR. Dosage:
Small 5 to 7.5 mg q8h PO
Medium 15 mg q8h PO
Large 30 mg q8h PO

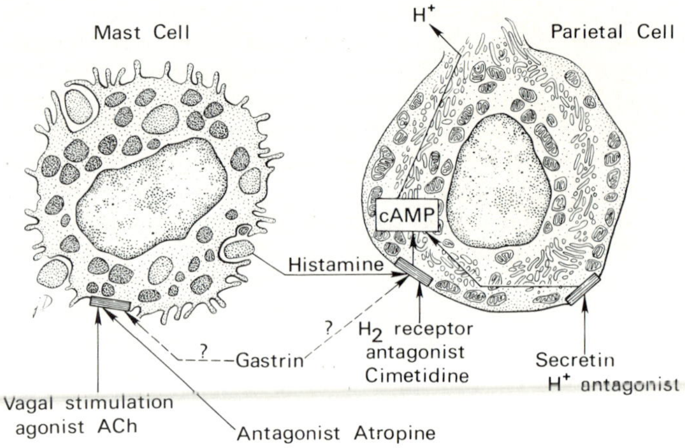

Figure 5–5. Relationship betwen H_2 receptors, histamine, and secretion of hydrochloric acid from the parietal cell. It is postulated that histamine may be the final mediator in parietal cell stimulation. Blockade of receptor sites will result in less than maximal acid secretion. (Reprinted with permission from Twedt DC, Wingfield WE: Diseases of the stomach. *In* Ettinger SJ (ed): *Textbook of Veterinary Internal Medicine.* 2nd ed. Philadelphia, WB Saunders Co, 1982.)

because of gastric distention. For the same reasons, antibiotics are not required unless a bacterial infection is suspected.

Antacid therapy is not usually prescribed for simple cases of acute gastritis (see "Gastric Ulcers").

H_2 receptor antagonists (e.g., cimetidine)* are effective in reducing gastric acid production in the dog and cat by blocking the histamine receptor of the parietal cells (Fig. 5–5). Use of these drugs has been advocated in the treatment of duodenal and gastric ulcers, in esophagitis from gastroesophageal reflux, in the prevention and treatment of acute gastric hemorrhage, and in syndromes resulting in gastric acid hypersecretion.[92] They may be useful in the treatment of some types of gastritis, Zollinger-Ellison syndrome, and gastric ulcers caused by mast cell tumors. On the basis of studies in the dog, a dosage of 4 mg/kg QID has been suggested. No toxic effects have yet been noted at this dosage.

Severe gastric hemorrhage should be treated as an emergency. Whole blood and fluids should be given to replace losses. Attempts are directed at controlling bleeding through gastric lavage and local vasoconstriction (see "Gastric Ulcer").

All gastric foreign bodies should be removed. The most accepted procedure is gastrotomy. Surgery also offers the chance to examine the other sections of the gastrointestinal tract for foreign bodies or other abnormalities. A less invasive measure, endoscopy, can be used, since some gastric foreign bodies can be successfully removed using grasping forceps or snares under endoscopic visualization. Alternative methods of removal include retrieving metallic foreign bodies with magnets and passing grasping forceps under fluoroscopic direction.

With ingestion of small objects such as needles or pins and no signs of gastric disease, one may elect to allow natural passage of the foreign object. A high-fiber diet and lubricants are given, and the animal is kept under strict observation. Failure to pass the object in 48 hours requires surgical removal of the foreign body. Emetics to initiate vomiting should be used with extreme caution. Their use should be attempted only when the foreign body is small and has smooth surfaces that will not cause laceration, perforation, or esophageal obstruction. The animal should be fed cotton balls to coat the foreign object before initiation of vomiting. Vaseline or other petroleum products are used to lubricate passage of small trichobezoars through the gastrointestinal tract. Owners should not be advised to administer mineral oil for fear it may cause an aspiration pneumonitis. Large indurated trichobezoars require surgical removal.

CHRONIC GASTRITIS

Chronic gastritis is an uncommon clinical diagnosis. Because gastric biopsy specimens that correlate the clinical with the histological finding are rarely obtained, little is known regarding chronic gastric disease in dogs and cats.

Etiology

The etiology of chronic gastritis is seldom determined. Most lesions probably occur as a result of repeated exposure to a variety of

*Tagamet, Smith Kline & French Lab Co., Carolina, P.R.

extrinsic influences that results in damage to the gastric mucosa. In addition, certain immune mechanisms or allergic conditions have been suggested as causes of chronic gastritis in the dog.

Many chemicals, drugs, and physical agents will cause lesions of chronic gastritis. Most of these agents have also been incriminated as causes of acute gastritis, but repeated exposure to them may result in chronic lesions. The long-term ingestion of aspirin, for example, causes chronic gastritis. Gastric foreign bodies, if left in the stomach, will cause chronic gastric mucosal irritation and lesions of chronic gastritis. Atrophic gastritis has experimentally been produced in the dog by repeated immunization with gastric juices,[83] but naturally occurring immune-mediated gastric disease has not been documented. Hypertrophic gastritis may result from chronic mucosal inflammation or possibly from the trophic actions of histamine or gastrin on the gastric mucosa.

Pathophysiology

The most common form of chronic gastritis is generally characterized by an excessive inflammatory cell infiltration and fibrosis of the mucosa and submucosa.[155] The inflammatory component consists of lymphocytes, plasma cells, and neutrophils. Superficial mucosal erosions, edema, and hemorrhage may be present. With most chronic gastritis there is no obvious change in mucosal thickness, but long-standing irritation to the gastric mucosa may cause a thickened mucosa from metaplasia, hyperplasia, or cyst formation (hypertrophic gastritis)[80] or a thinned mucosa from atrophy of the gastric glands (atrophic gastritis).

Chronic Atrophic Gastritis. *Chronic atrophic gastritis* is a diffuse lesion that involves the body and fundus of the stomach. Atrophy is evidenced by a thinner than normal mucosa with a reduction in size and depth of the gastric glands. The number of chief and parietal cells is reduced and these cells are replaced by mucus-secreting cells. An inflammatory component is almost always present.

Chronic atrophic gastritis associated with achlorhydria is reported in the dog.[45] Though not convincingly documented, a reasonable assumption is that a hypochlorhydria would exist because of the reduction in the parietal cell mass. A further assumption is that an animal is predisposed to the development of gastric ulcers when the negative feedback inhibition of gastrin by acid secretion is lost, and an abnormally high serum gastrin level occurs.[136]

Chronic Hypertrophic Gastritis. *Chronic hypertrophic gastritis* is characterized by macroscopic thickening of the gastric mucosa and large rugal convolutions. These features result from mucosal hypertrophy and hyperplasia of gastric glands, an inflammatory cell response, and cystic dilation of mucous glands. Lesions may occur as either focal polypoid areas that clinically resemble neoplasms,[80] or as a diffuse hypertrophy of the rugae involving the majority of the stomach.[154] Giant hypertrophic gastritis, reported in basenjis,[156] occurs as a gastropathy in which protein is lost through the hypertrophic gastric mucosa.

Eosinophilic Gastritis. *Eosinophilic gastritis* is a rare condition characterized by a diffuse eosinophilic and granulation tissue infiltration involving many or all layers of the stomach wall or, less frequently, by discrete single or multiple granulomatous nodules.[63, 141] Eosinophilic lymphadenitis and vasculitis also are stated to occur in this condition. Hayden and Fleischman[63] describe the gross lesions of diffuse eosinophilic gastritis as scirrhous thickenings of the gastric wall resembling gastric neoplasia.

The cause of the eosinophilic infiltration in the stomach is unknown but likely is immunologically mediated and possibly allergic or parasitic in nature. In a study of diffuse eosinophilic gastritis in a dog, micro filaria were observed in some histological sections.[18] Dogs experimentally infected with *Toxocara canis* had focal eosinophilic gastritis, but the lesions rarely contained larvae, and vasculitis was not found.[64] Eosinophilic gastritis may be similar to the syndrome eosinophilic gastroenteritis, in which there is either a segmental or a diffuse infiltration of eosinophils into the mucosa and submucosa of the stomach and intestine. Though the clinical manifestations of the two conditions may be similar, they differ significantly in pathological features.

History and Physical Examination

The signs of chronic gastritis are ill-defined, often obscure, and exacerbated periodically. Many dogs show symptoms for several months before they are presented, while some are asymptomatic. Vomiting is reported to be the most common sign observed in chronic gastritis, although it does not occur in every case.[155] Vomiting is usually infrequent and may or may not be associated with eating. Owners may describe periodic, early morning vomiting of a bile-tinged fluid. Frequent and severe vomiting occurs with gastric outflow obstruction or in advanced gastritis. With gastric mucosal ulceration, the vomitus may contain either digested or undigested blood. Other signs of chronic gastritis may include a poor appetite, weight loss, abdominal pain, depression, and polydipsia. With gastric bleeding, anemia and melena may occur. The physical examination is usually unrevealing.

Diagnosis

Routine laboratory evaluations generally do not contribute to the diagnosis but help to exclude gastritis secondary to some other disease. Anemia, electrolyte imbalance, and dehydration may occur with chronic gastritis and will be reflected in laboratory values. Plasma proteins, both albumin and globulin, will be depressed in conditions resulting from a protein-losing gastropathy. A leukocytosis with an absolute eosinophilia occurs in most cases of eosinophilic gastritis. A presumptive diagnosis of eosinophilic gastritis can be made in animals with signs of chronic gastric disease, a peripheral eosinophilia, and a positive response to a trial dose of corticosteroids. At present, gastric acid analysis has little use except to confirm suspected states of hypochlorhydria or hyperchlorhydria.

Very few, if any, radiological signs are pathognomonic for chronic gastritis. Contrast studies may demonstrate a paucity of rugal folds in atrophic gastritis, large rugal folds in hypertrophic gastritis, granulomatous nodules or a thickened gastric wall in eosinophilic gastritis, gastric ulcers, or delayed gastric emptying.

Gastroscopy is a useful tool in the diagnosis of chronic gastritis.[52] Mucosal erosions, hemorrhage, and large gastric ulcers are readily observed. Atrophic gastritis is easily visualized because the submucosal vessels can be seen through the thinner than normal mucosa. Large prominent mucosal folds, especially in the antral region, may occur with hypertrophic gastritis, gastric edema, or neoplasia. Gastric biopsies are required for a definitive diagnosis of chronic gastritis.

Treatment

The primary aim of therapy in chronic gastritis should be the removal of the etiological agent. With this removal, prognosis is good. The etiology of most cases is never determined, and the therapy must be directed in a logical but often trial-and-error approach. The prognosis in such cases is variable. No clinical studies evaluating the effectiveness of therapies for chronic gastritis in the dog and cat have been reported.

Dietary control should be attempted in the treatment of chronic gastritis in which it is suspected that the etiological agent has been ingested. A positive response to dietary elimination confirms the suspicion. Strombeck reports that dogs with eosinophilic gastritis placed on controlled diets showed clinical improvement and resolution of previous peripheral eosinophilia.[141] Diets high in antigenic proteins (meat diets) and those with many supplements should be avoided. Multiple small feedings of a bland, predominately carbohydrate diet may be beneficial. Prescription diets developed for (allergic) gastrointestinal disease (e.g., Prescription diet D/D)* may also be useful.

Corticosteroids are indicated to control chronic gastritis that results from an immune mechanism or those conditions suggestive of an immune response. Corticosteroids will stimulate regeneration of gastric parietal cells and may be beneficial in treating some cases of atrophic gastritis.[76] Corticosteroids enhance the ulcerogenic potential of mucosal lesions.

Cimetidine, used to inhibit gastric acid secretion, may play an important role in the therapy of chronic gastritis with hyperchlorhydria. Some dogs with chronic simple gastritis and mild mucosal atrophy have shown a positive response to this drug. Frequent administration of antacids may be equally beneficial in these cases. Long-term anticholinergic therapy should be avoided, for it may result in a hypotonic stomach and continued vomiting.

Surgical resection is required for the removal of areas of focal hypertrophic gastritis, granulomas, or large gastric ulcers. A

*Prescription Diet D/D, Hill's Pet Products, Inc., Topeka, KS.

partial gastrectomy is indicated when a protein-losing gastropathy occurs with chronic hypertrophic gastritis. If gastric lesions result in delayed gastric outflow, either pyloromyotomy, pyloroplasty, or gastric bypass surgery is indicated.

GASTRIC ULCERS

Ulcers of the gastric mucosa are more frequently diagnosed in the dog and cat than in previous years, probably because of increased professional awareness, improved drug and surgical therapy, and the pursuit of clinical diagnosis through necropsy.

Gastric ulcers are usually peptic. The presence of gastric acid and pepsin is, by definition, a prerequisite for the development of peptic ulcers. Peptic ulcers are usually benign, acute or chronic, circumscribed mucosal defects that extend through the muscularis mucosa and have a firm, raised margin. They occur in adult dogs ranging from 2½ to 12 years of age. Females have a higher incidence than males and there is no breed predilection.[105]

Etiology

Gastric ulceration in the dog may result from any of the agents causing acute or chronic gastritis. In addition to these agents, stress and mastocytosis are important etiological factors.

Stress Ulceration. Stress ulceration results in the development of multiple erosions in the gastric, duodenal, or colonic mucosa of acutely ill patients. The lesions are usually superficial to the muscularis mucosa and are thus usually only erosions, but occasionally a penetrating ulcer is seen. Stress ulceration is reported in the dog infrequently, but when present it may have a significant mortality rate.[2, 68, 100, 146]

Systemic Mastocytosis. With systemic mastocytosis, histamine produced by mast cells is released in large quantities and is associated with gastric lesions. Gastric ulcers secondary to mast cell neoplasms in dogs[24, 69] and cats[132] have been reported. In the dog, the concentration of histamine in mast cell tumors varies considerably, with up to 3000 μg of histamine base per gram of wet tissue.[71] Lesions in the dog's stomach are most common with mastocytomas.[69]

The mechanism of induction of the gastroduodenal lesions with mastocytomas is not completely understood. Interestingly, heparin has been shown to prevent mucosal ulceration in the stomachs of guinea pigs[161] and dogs.[69] Thus, in dogs there may be a pronounced histamine intoxication without a concomitant heparinemia. The mast cell contains an abundance of both compounds. Therefore, it follows that in mastocytomas either the heparin is not released in significant amounts, or it is bound or rapidly metabolized following liberation. In canine mastocytoma the neoplastic cells are anaplastic and contain little cytoplasmic metachromasia, indicating the lack of heparin.[69]

Mucosal lesions in mastocytoma are associated with mucosal ischemia and intravascular thrombosis. Small vascular thrombi were observed in eight of 24 stomachs of dogs with mastocytoma.[69]

Pathophysiology

Most peptic ulcers occur in the zone between the body and fundus (where acid is secreted) and the proximal duodenum. Between these two sites lies the pylorus, separating the stomach (with a mucosa highly adapted to withstand acid) from the duodenum (with a mucosa adapted to withstand bile and pancreatic juice).

Luminal acid is generally accepted as essential for the pathogenesis of gastric ulceration. Other factors that affect the resistance of the gastric mucosa to injury include mucosal permeability and blood flow, secretory state, acid-base balance, and the presence of pepsin.[81] Nutritional status is also important.[134]

Stress ulceration most frequently involves the body of the stomach. The mechanism of this ulceration is not entirely known, but it is most frequently thought to be mucosal ischemia, which in most clinical circumstances is due to an episode of hypotension. Focal mucosal necrosis may also result from an energy deficit that is particularly severe in the body of the stomach because of its primarily aerobic energy metabolism.[96] Gastric acid secretion will fall during acute stress and then recover as the patient improves. The foci of ischemic necrosis then undergo acid peptic digestion with bleeding.

As mentioned previously, hydrogen ions are a requisite for the genesis of erosive gastritis. Interestingly, in all species except the rabbit, stress does not lead to a break in the mucosal cation barrier.[99]

The precise role of stress in the genesis of acute erosions remains obscure. The effect of stress on central or autonomic neural pathways,[39, 124] neurohumoral factors, and the release of histamine from mast cells have been suggested as possible influences.

History and Physical Examination

Vomiting is the most common clinical sign of gastric ulcers. The vomitus may be tinged with partially digested blood ("coffee grounds" appearance) or fresh blood and clots in severe ulcers. Melena, a variable appetite, and weight loss are often reported. With severe blood loss the patient may show anemia. With vomiting, dehydration and a secondary polydipsia may be noted. Some dogs may be asymptomatic with gastric ulcers, while others have perforation which rapidly results in death.

Abdominal pain is the most frequently encountered physical finding. The stomach's location prevents actual palpation, but abdominal splinting should include gastric ulceration as a possible diagnosis. If present, anemia, hematemesis, and melena are all indications of ulceration. The presence of cutaneous mastocytomas may result in significant gastric disease.

Diagnosis

A regenerative anemia is one indication of peptic ulcer. In 16 of 22 cases of peptic ulceration in dogs, liver disease was also noted. Pathological changes in the liver range from severe disease to fatty and degenerative changes.[105] Lead poisoning may also result in gastric ulcers.[128]

The presence of gastric ulcers, mucosal niches, craters, or fissures of varying sizes is demonstrated by contrast radiography. Superficial stress erosions cannot usually be seen on a barium contrast examination.

Endoscopy affords the best objective evidence of gastric ulcers. With acute ulcers, the mucosal lesions may be bleeding, have an inflammatory appearance around their periphery, and usually have no evidence of fibrin in the ulcer crater. Chronic ulcers may show little inflammatory response and have a fibrin-filled crater and a wrinkled mucosa peripheral to the ulcer. With stress ulceration, early in the post-stress period, focal areas of pallor and cyanosis are seen. Later, discrete areas of extravasation of red blood cells may be observed. Numerous small, well-delineated punctate lesions can be identified along the crests of the rugae within the proximal stomach. These lesions are usually only a few millimeters in diameter. Biopsy of the ulcer periphery is indicated in all patients.

Exploratory gastrotomy can be a useful diagnostic tool in gastric ulceration. This condition can occur in association with benign and malignant neoplasms of the stomach. Cytological and histopathological studies should be included in the work-up of cases of gastric ulceration.

Treatment

Secretion of gastric acid perpetuates mucosal lesions and is required for new lesions to occur. Treatment is intended either to decrease hydrogen ion and peptic activity or to increase the ability of the gut to deal with and resist the effects of these agents. Two pharmacological agents are practical and useful in the management of gastric ulceration—antacids and the newer histamine analogues like cimetidine.

Antacids function to reduce the total amount of available hydrogen ions. They also irreversibly inactivate pepsin if the gastric contents can be brought above pH 6. A third effect of antacids on gastric juice is to diminish peptic activity, because the pH is raised above the range for optimal proteolysis.

Antacids must be given as frequently as once every 2 hours. Infrequent antacid administration may result in a rebound hypersecretion of acid, because acid pH in the antrum inhibits the release of gastrin. Antacid neutralization of gastric contents removes this inhibition and gastrin release continues and, thus, leads to a greater quantity of acid secretion. The rebound effect is most frequently noted when antacids are given 2 to 3 times a day. The rate of gastric emptying is a major determinant of antacid effectiveness. Thus, with the exponential emptying characteristic of the stomach, the administration of a given quantity of antacid in large, infrequent doses is less likely to provide sustained buffering. Aluminum-containing antacids will delay gastric emptying in some species.[73]

Various preparations are available (Table 5–3), but no antacid is free of hazard. So-

Table 5–3. COMMONLY USED LIQUID ANTACIDS

Antacid	Manufacturer	Ingredients (per 5 ml)	Acid Neutralizing Capacity* (mEq)	Usual Dose† (ml)
Amphojel	Wyeth Laboratories	320 mg aluminum hydroxide	13	10
Di-Gel	Plough, Inc.	282 mg aluminum hydroxide	18	10
		87 mg aluminum hydroxide 20 mg simethicone		
Gelusil	Parke-Davis	200 mg aluminum hydroxide 200 mg magnesium hydroxide 25 mg simethicone	24	10
Maalox	William H. Rorer, Inc.	225 mg aluminum hydroxide 200 mg magnesium hydroxide	27	10–20
Mylanta	Stuart Pharmaceuticals	200 mg aluminum hydroxide 200 mg magnesium hydroxide 20 mg simethicone	12.7	5–10
Riopan	Ayerst Laboratories	480 mg magaldrate	13.5	5–10

*The mEq of acid neutralized in a 15 minute standardized test by the lowest used dose recommended by the manufacturer.
†Recommended by the manufacturer for human use.

dium bicarbonate may produce sodium overload and systemic alkalosis. Magnesium preparations may lead to severe diarrhea and are hazardous to renal failure patients. Calcium carbonate may cause hypercalcemia, renal impairment, and stimulation of gastric secretion. Aluminum hydroxide may lead to phosphate depletion, with consequent muscle weakness, bone resorption, and hypercalciuria.[101] Milk is not considered an antacid.

In the veterinary patient clinical assessment of histamine analogue drugs like cimetidine is lacking, although it has been reported to be effective in one dog with gastric ulceration.[131] Cimetidine dosage for the dog is 4 mg/kg QID and is given intravenously or orally. In dogs, research showed that this drug had different effects on experimentally induced ulcers; duodenal ulcers evidenced an enhancement of healing, whereas gastric ulcers showed no significant improvement.[109]

With acute gastrointestinal bleeding (i.e., stress ulceration), an H_2 receptor antagonist like cimetidine is less effective than antacids in providing adequate prophylaxis. Its relative ineffectiveness results from the impairment of the secretory state of the mucosa, decreases intracellular buffering capacity, and inadequately reduces intraluminal acidity.[120] Antacids may be more beneficial because they do not affect the secretory state of the mucosa and, thus, do not affect its buffering capacity and also because they reduce intraluminal acid in a more reliable fashion.

Not infrequently, antacids and cimetidine are simultaneously prescribed. No reports are available in the veterinary literature concerning the bioavailability of cimetidine when given with an antacid. In humans, antacids containing aluminum hydroxide, magnesium hydroxide, or both inhibit absorption of oral cimetidine.[137] Thus, by reducing absorption of cimetidine, antacids may diminish its acid-suppressive effects should the two be taken simultaneously.

With severe gastric blood loss, intragastric lavage with iced water is indicated. Norepinephrine* can be added to the iced water at a rate of 8 mg/500 ml. This potent β-adrenergic vasoconstrictive agent is almost completely destroyed in one passage through the normal liver. The fluid is instilled into the stomach and left for 30 minutes and removed; the lavage is repeated to determine whether or not gastric bleeding has ceased. Caution should be exercised to avoid mucosal ischemia and necrosis with norepinephrine lavage.

Occasionally, surgical therapy is required for gastric ulceration. A partial gastrectomy is generally used to remove the ulcer. This technique, along with pyloromyotomy and vagotomy, has been successfully used in the

*Levophed, Breon Laboratories, New York, NY.

dog.[37] With peritonitis secondary to perforation of a gastric ulcer, immediate surgery is indicated.

GASTRIC RETENTION AND PARESIS

Retention of gastric contents is often associated with pyloric dysfunction, motility disorders of the stomach, or both. The pylorus is an anatomical scapegoat because of its location at the distal end of the stomach and because it acts to impede emptying and to prevent duodenal reflux.

Etiology

Pyloric dysfunction may result from intrinsic, extrinsic, or obturative lesions. Intrinsic lesions of the pylorus result either from hypertrophy of the circular muscle fibers or from intrinsic pyloric neoplasia. Extrinsic pyloric lesions include hepatic and pancreatic abscesses, neoplasms, and inflammatory lesions. Histoplasmosis may lead to intrinsic or extrinsic lesions. Foreign bodies, gastric and duodenal ulcers, antral mucosal hypertrophy, and antral polyps cause obturative pyloric lesions.

Acute stress, trauma, psychogenic factors, and inflammatory disease reduce motility in the digestive tract, resulting in the retention of gastric contents. Inhibition of gastric motility is generally associated with stimulation of the sympathetic nervous system. Drugs, hypokalemia, recurring gastric dilation, and chronic obstruction of the pylorus also contribute to gastric hypomotility and retention.

Pylorospasm has been described as an abnormal contraction of the pyloric musculature that closes the sphincter. Although the pyloric sphincter in the dog does have a high pressure zone,[21] its effect on gastric emptying is minor.[138, 139] In fact, because of the anatomical continuity of the antrum and pylorus, these two segments function as a single muscle unit.[139] As noted previously, the grinding and emptying of solids are primarily functions of the gastric antrum, whereas emptying of liquids depends on tonic activity in the fundus. The retardation of gastric evacuation is due to decreased antral peristalsis.[121]

Pathophysiology

Pyloric stenosis may result from the excessive secretion of gastrointestinal hormones. With antral distention, the G-cells are stimulated to release gastrin, ultimately leading to a decrease in gastric pH. Gastrin has a potent trophic effect on gastric smooth muscle.

Pyloric stenosis may also be associated with neurogenic dysfunction. The overall number of myenteric ganglion cells and nerve fiber tracts is reduced in the pyloric region, and the circular muscle of the pylorus is hypertrophied.[14] A non-organic stenosis accompanied by antral dilation and muscular hypertrophy can be produced by selective destruction of the intramural ganglia of the pylorus.[110]

Partial obstruction of gastric outflow results in gastric hypersecretion in the dog. An obvious consequence of this outflow obstruction is gastric distention. With chronic distention gastric mucosal hyperplasia arises as a consequence of increased secretory cell mitosis.[34]

Gastric retention either is present at birth or develops with age. With gastric retention comes the worsening of outflow obstruction from gastrin's trophic actions on smooth muscle and mucosa. Gastric dilation results from chronic outflow destruction leading to a loss of motility of the antrum. No loss of motor function is noted, nor is there always constriction of the pylorus, suggesting that there is poor filling of the antrum with each contraction and, thus, greater gastric retention and less rapid gastric emptying.

History and Physical Examination

Vomiting at regular intervals following ingestion of solid foods, with accompanying gastric distention, is the primary sign of gastric retention. The vomitus is usually undigested food and is rarely bile-stained. Chronic vomiting generally is associated with some weight loss and dehydration.

Patients with gastric retention exhibit projectile vomiting; the vomitus occurs abruptly and without the warning of increased salivation and retching. In most instances, the vomitus is thrown for a considerable distance and readily empties the stomach.

Brachycephalic breeds of dogs have a high incidence of gastric retention, as do Siamese cats.[116] No specific sex incidence is reported for the dog or the cat. The existence of two female kittens with pyloric stenosis has been reported, suggesting the possible inheritable nature of the disease.[147]

There are no specific findings on physical

examination of an animal with gastric retention. Observation of emesis may be useful. Vomiting of undigested or only partially digested food when the stomach should be empty is diagnostic of gastric retention. Normally, the stomach should be completely empty within 6 to 8 hours after eating. After vomiting, the animal will usually resume feeding, only to vomit again at variable intervals.

Diagnosis

Laboratory assessment usually shows the hematological changes caused by dehydration. With severe gastric outflow obstruction and vomiting, there may be a metabolic alkalosis.

Because of enhanced proximal bicarbonate reabsorption, smaller concentrations of bicarbonate are delivered to the distal nephron, and urinary sodium and bicarbonate levels decrease. Paradoxical aciduria in the presence of a metabolic alkalosis is the result.[56]

Radiography affords the most definitive method of diagnosing gastric retention. The presence of gastric distention with food or air long after the ingesta should be in the intestine is diagnostic of gastric retention.[57] In the cat with gastric retention, although the fundus and body become elongated craniocaudally because of an increase in gastric volume, they remain on the left side of the midline. Also in this condition, the mucosal folds are stretched and have a smooth appearance.[116] The pyloric antrum is often enlarged, and the pyloric canal narrow and elongated.

Contrast radiography is helpful in assessing the rate of gastric emptying. Less than 30 minutes is reported to be normal gastric emptying time. Normally, barium is retained for 5 to 15 minutes. The presence of barium in the stomach for longer than 12 to 24 hours is abnormal and should be considered a sign of gastric retention. The stress of chemical[169] or manual restraint may delay gastric emptying.

Fluoroscopy with contrast material is useful for assessing gastric motility. Many times the peristaltic waves are of normal rate and intensity but result only in a dilation of the antrum, with little barium passing through the pyloric canal. Filling defects of the antrum or pylorus may be identified.

The usefulness of gastroscopy in the canine patient with hypertrophy of the pyloric musculature is not well documented. One report suggests the pyloric orifice is fixed or narrowed and that peristaltic waves result in the incomplete closure of the orifice.[168] One should remember that the pyloric orifice of the dog is usually partially open. With the presence of foreign bodies, ulcers, neoplasms, inflammation, or granulomatous changes, biopsy specimens may be obtained to determine diagnosis and prognosis.

Treatment

Obstruction of gastric outflow is generally managed surgically. Intrinsic hypertrophy of the pylorus is successfully treated with pyloromyotomy or pyloroplasty (see Chapter 6).[4, 5, 86, 147, 148] With either technique, the surgeon must extend the incision well on to the antrum and the duodenum in order to free the area from hypertrophied muscle.

Obturative lesions must be carefully assessed. With severe mucosal damage and ulceration, surgical excision of the affected area may be required. Occasionally, the severity of the lesion necessitates the elaborate surgical dismemberment of the pylorus with such procedures as gastroduodenostomy[23] and gastrojejunostomy.

Surgery on the pylorus in normal dogs has little effect on the emptying of solids and causes a slight acceleration of emptying of liquids.[66]

Motility disorders of the stomach have received no attention in veterinary literature. Therapy has been directed toward the control of symptoms, mainly by use of centrally acting antiemetics. Gastric stimulation with a cholinergic agent such as bethanechol* or metoclopramide† has been tried.[135]

Surgery for gastroparesis has not been objectively studied in veterinary patients. Guidelines similar to those used in humans may be useful in assessing veterinary patients with gastric emptying disorders involving decreased motility. Only patients with objective abnormalities in gastric motor function and stasis whose symptoms cannot be controlled by medical therapy should

---

*Urecholine, Merck Sharp & Dohme, West Point, PA. Dosage: 5-25 mg Q8H PO

†Reglan, A. H. Robins Co., Pharmaceutical Division, Richmond, Va. Dosage: 0.2–0.4 mg/kg Q8H

be considered for surgery, and some attempt should be made to verify that other motor disturbances of the digestive tract are absent.[91]

GASTRIC NEOPLASIA

The rate of occurrence of benign and malignant gastric neoplasia in the dog and cat is low. Adenocarcinoma is the most common neoplasm reported in the canine stomach; it accounts for 1 per cent of all malignant neoplasms and constitutes from 42 to 72 per cent of all gastric malignancies.[115] The incidence of feline gastric neoplasia is unknown but is lower than that of canine gastric neoplasia. In reports of gastrointestinal neoplasms in the cat, the stomach was the least affected organ[22] and lymphosarcomas were the most common neoplasms.[152]

The signs of gastric neoplasia, regardless of cell type, are usually the result of either altered motility of the gastric wall or gastric outflow blockage. The most common signs include persistent vomiting and weight loss.

Benign Tumors. Benign adenomatous polyps occur as pedunculated or polypoid nodules of mucosal proliferation that protrude above the gastric surface. Although there are a few reported cases of adenomatous polyps in the dog and the cat,[65, 106] the incidence of clinically silent polyps may actually be higher. Most occur as either single or multiple solitary nodules ranging from a few millimeters to a few centimeters in diameter; however, diffuse, multiple polyps invading the entire gastric mucosa have been reported.[30, 61] Gastric adenomatous polyps are often incidental findings during endoscopy or necropsy. They generally cause no clinical signs unless they are diffuse or occlude the pyloric antrum. Although the etiology of adenomatous polyps is unknown, many feel that they occur secondary to chronic gastric mucosal damage. It has been suggested, although not proven in the dog, that adenomatous polyps have a premalignant tendency.

Leiomyomas. Leiomyomas are the second most common gastric tumor found in older dogs (average age 15 years).[115] These tumors vary in size and arise from the muscle layers of the gastric wall. Most are found incidentally at necropsy, distributed randomly and involving different segments of the muscular layer. Ulceration is infrequent, and the tumor exerts its effect by mass involvement, altering either motility or pyloric outflow.

Malignant Tumors. Adenocarcinoma is the most common malignant tumor in the stomach of the dog; however, it is exceedingly rare in the cat. The average age of dogs diagnosed with gastric adenocarcinoma is 8 years,[89] and males are more commonly affected than females. Grossly, these gastric tumors appear either as a raised plaque with a central ulcer, as a polypoid lesion projecting into the lumen, or as a very firm, diffusely infiltrating mass invading the stomach wall. Most tumors have superficial mucosal ulcerations, and more than half originate in the pyloric antral area.

Patnaik and associates[115] describe two main histological types of adenocarcinoma, diffuse and intestinal, each with several subtypes. The most common and most malignant is the diffuse type, which lacks a distinct glandular structure. The neoplastic cells of this type, in some unknown way, stimulate mesenchymal elements and produce a tremendous fibrous connective tissue component of the tumor.[85] The other histological type, the intestinal adenocarcinoma, has a glandular structure. This type often manifests as a raised mass in the gastric wall. Regardless of the histological type, metastasis is frequent, extending into regional lymph nodes, liver, lungs, and adrenals.

Primary sarcomas of the stomach occur most commonly as lymphomas, which are the most common gastric tumors in the cat. The majority of cats with these tumors are FeLV negative. The lesions occur either as raised masses or as a diffuse infiltration of the gastric wall with various-sized ulcers in the gastric mucosa. Other, less common malignant tumors of the stomach include leiomyosarcomas and fibrosarcomas. Rarely, metastatic tumors result from adenocarcinomas (of mammary glands, GI tract, liver, or pancreas), lymphosarcomas, or hemangiosarcomas.

History and Physical Examination

The most consistent sign of gastric neoplasia is vomiting. The vomiting may vary in both frequency and time of onset after eating, with the severity of signs often being related to the amount of gastric wall involvement of pyloric outflow obstruction. With a complete pyloric obstruction, the vomiting may become projectile. Hematemesis and melena occur with mucosal ulceration and bleeding. Malignant gastric neoplasia often results in anorexia, chronic debilitation, and weight loss. The duration of clinical signs for dogs, in one report, ranged from 2 weeks to 3 months.[129]

Gastric neoplasia should always be suspected in the older animal displaying chronic vomiting. Abdominal palpation is generally unrevealing; however, occasionally a gastric mass may be palpated. Gastric pain is inconsistent, unless perforation of the tumor, which is rare, has resulted in peritonitis. Anemia with melena is a common finding with chronic bleeding lesions. Ascites, jaundice, or respiratory distress may result from metastasis to other areas.

Diagnosis

In addition to routine laboratory evaluation, radiology should be an early step in the diagnosis of gastric neoplasia. Plain films are usually non-diagnostic but with extensive involvement may demonstrate a mass or a thickened gastric wall. When a neoplasm is suspected, a constrast study is required to definitively demonstrate the gastric lesion. In many cases, a double-contrast study best outlines lesions of the gastric wall. Certain characteristic radiographic findings are suggestive of gastric neoplasia. These include thickening and rigidity of the gastric wall, which can be seen on multiple radiographs, distortion of the gastric lumen and derangement of the rugal folds, filling defects, ulcers, and a delay in gastric emptying. Because gastric neoplasia often alters motility and pyloric emptying, fluoroscopy is beneficial in evaluating some lesions. Lesions invading the gastric wall without a mass involvement may not be apparent without the use of fluoroscopy.

Endoscopy is used to confirm suspected gastric lesions that were observed with radiology. A skilled endoscopist often can detect lesions not demonstrated on gastric contrast studies.[84] Polyps, ulcerations, or raised masses protruding into the luminal surface are easily observed. Gastric neoplasia without mass or mucosal involvement is more difficult to perceive. The endoscopist must be aware of areas that have lost distensibility or normal rugal fold patterns. Gastric adenocarcinomas of the linitis plastica type with predominantly submucosal involvement are often missed on endoscopic examination. When lesions are observed, biopsy forceps or cytology brushes can be directed, under endoscopic control, to obtain samples, with good results.

Gastric lavage and cytologic analysis may retrieve diagnostic cells of gastric neoplasia, but there have been no reports using this technique in dogs.

Surgery is the best diagnostic method for evaluating gastric neoplasia. The surgeon is able to palpate the stomach wall for inconsistencies, perform a gastrotomy, evaluate the mucosal surface and pyloric canal diameter, and obtain a full-thickness biopsy specimen of the gastric wall. Surgery also allows evaluation of the regional lymph nodes, liver, and adjacent organs for evidence of metastasis.

Treatment

The current treatment of choice for most gastric neoplasia is surgical removal. Partial gastrectomy or segmental resection is usually indicated. Since the majority of the gastric neoplasms involve the pyloric antral area, resection of the pylorus may be required. In such cases, surgical anastomosis of the remaining stomach to the intestines (gastroduodenostomy or gastrojejunostomy) is required; however, this procedure is not without complications. Palliative surgery in malignant gastric neoplasia may be justified, because it may increase survival times by several months.[47, 95] Chemotherapy, which has been suggested for lymphosarcomas following surgical removal of single or multiple solitary masses, has resulted in good responses in some cases.[90] Therapy for sarcomas involves using vincristine,* cyclophosphamide,† and prednisone combinations. Patients with sarcomas in which there is diffuse infiltration of the gastric wall and who are not surgical candidates show a poor response to chemotherapy. Chemotherapy may also be used as an adjunct to surgical removal of other malignant gastric tumor types.[98]

The prognosis for patients with malignant gastric neoplasia is generally poor because

*Oncovin, Eli Lilly & Company, Indianapolis, IN.

†Cytoxan, Mead Johnson & Company, Evansville, IN.

of the advanced nature of the disease at the time of diagnosis, surgical complications of gastric resection, and frequent metastasis.

ACUTE GASTRIC DILATATION-VOLVULUS

Overeating by immature animals, and occasionally adults, results in gastric distention. This gluttony is often relieved by vomiting. Acute gastric dilatation in mature, large breed dogs may result in rotation of the stomach. The greater curvature of the stomach moves ventrally with gastric distention, and in a dog with a deep chest conformation, an eventual laxity of the gastrohepatic ligament results. With this laxity the pylorus is free to move dorsally, cranially, and to the left, resulting in a volvulus of the stomach.

Gastric dilatation-volvulus (GDV) is a serious, life-threatening syndrome. Gastric gas and fluid accumulate and cannot pass via the esophagus or the duodenum. This distention of the stomach results in additional fluid generation and complicates fluid and electrolyte losses. If the stomach distention is not promptly relieved, death may rapidly ensue.

Incidence

Large breed, deep-chested dogs are most frequently affected by GDV. To date 28 breeds have been reported to be affected by this syndrome.[145] Among them are breeds that do not conform to the typical characteristics, such as dachshunds and Pekingese. Domestic cats have also been reported to have GDV.[79] Other species that are affected by GDV are reviewed by Van Kruiningen.[157] Most dogs with GDV are mature, middle-aged, or older.[145] Males are affected more often than females in a ratio of 2:1.[16]

Etiology

Gastric dilatation precedes volvulus. In order for GDV to occur, there must be a source of gas and an obstruction to the relief of the distention. Gastric distention with gas occurs in both postprandial and fasting stomachs. Aerophagia appears to be the source of gas in dogs.[25] In two studies, gastric gas analysis revealed gas concentrations consistent with atmospheric air and an absence of significant concentrations of either hydrogen or methane.[25, 157]

Bacterial fermentation is not important in the formation of gas in the normal empty stomach. Only after feeding do bacterial numbers increase. The sources of these bacteria are the oral cavity and the diet. *Clostridium perfringens* has been found in the stomach of dead dogs and was thought to be a source of gas in GDV.[157] More recently, it was reported there was no difference in clostridial incidence between the stomachs of healthy dogs and of dogs with gastric dilatation-volvulus.[160] Because of the acuteness of GDV and the inconsistent ability to isolate gas-forming bacteria, it is unlikely that bacteria are responsible for the gas.

The role of diet in gastric dilatation-volvulus is unclear. GDV develops in animals whether they are being fed (1) free-choice or selective diets, (2) meat or cereal, (3) soybean-containing or soybean-free foods, or (4) small or large quantities.[33] Attempts at reproducing GDV by dietary manipulation have been unsuccessful. If there is a relationship between diet and gastric dilatation-volvulus, it is likely to be associated with anatomic changes and resultant development of laxity of the gastrohepatic ligament and of gastric paresis of the body and fundus, which would thus allow eventual rotation of the stomach.

History and Physical Examination

Young animals presented with gastric dilation rarely have tympany upon percussion of the abdomen. The animals often will be lethargic and reluctant to move, and will make grunting sounds with respiratory effort. Attempts to palpate the abdomen encounter abdominal splinting and increased respiratory grunting. In most instances, the animals make no effort to retch or vomit.

Dogs with acute gastric dilation have cranial abdominal distention with tympany. The abdomen is tensed upon palpation. Increased respiratory efforts, hyperpnea, and open-mouthed panting are frequently noted.

Abdominal palpation may provide evidence of splenomegaly. The spleen may be oriented cranially to caudally along the ventral midline of the abdomen.

Retching with an inability to vomit is an important clinical finding in GDV. The retching may become quite violent without producing vomitus. With increasing efforts to retch, the abdomen further distends with gas via aerophagia.

As gastric distention progresses, the clinical signs of shock are manifested. A weak femoral pulse, tachycardia, and prolonged capillary refill time in the mucous membranes are commonly noted. Increased venous pressures can be observed by placing the dog in lateral recumbency and observing the saphenous vein. As the leg of a normal animal is slowly raised to the level of the right atrium, this vein disappears. In dogs with GDV, the leg may be extended well above the level of the right atrium before the vein collapses, suggesting increased venous congestion.

The ability to pass an orogastric tube was once believed to rule out the diagnosis of volvulus of the stomach. This technique is *not a diagnostic test* for GDV. Passage of a gastric tube does *not* eliminate the possibility of volvulus.

As the duration of gastric distention increases, the shock state of the animal progresses. Pathological changes proceed and death may rapidly ensue.[166] Animals may be presented to the hospital unable to rise, in severe shock, and moribund.

Pathophysiology

Following gaseous distention, the stomach is unable to relieve itself. This may be due to an abnormal gastroesophageal angulation that interferes with belching or vomiting, a compression of the duodenum by the dilated stomach that prevents passage of gas into the small bowel, or a disturbance of extrinsic innervation of the stomach.

As the stomach dilates, the gastrosplenic ligament causes passive movement of the spleen. Thus, any movement of the greater curvature also moves the spleen. Eventually, the splenic vessels come to lie ventrally across the esophagus and become partially obstructed, leading to venous congestion and a secondary splenomegaly. Rotation of the spleen also is important in the development of an area of gastric necrosis.[10] The site is almost always on the greater curvature of the fundus where the short gastric arteries anastomose with the left epigastric artery. Torsion of the splenic pedicle may occur independently or in association with gastric volvulus.

The dilating stomach exerts pressure upon the caudal vena cava.[165] The vessel is partially occluded, and blood is shunted via the ventral vertebral sinuses and azygos vein to the cranial vena cava. Rotation of the stomach actively occludes the portal vein, leading to venous congestion of abdominal splanchna. This occlusion promotes the onset of severe shock.

As intragastric pressures increase, the peristaltic activity decreases, creating ischemic hypoxia. Severe damage to the ganglion cells of Auerbach's plexus may result and may contribute to the large, atonic stomach frequently noted at surgery. If the hypoxia is corrected within 3½ to 4 hours, the neurological insult is reversible.

Arterial pressure to the stomach is maintained even with gastric dilation, whereas venous drainage is compromised and intravascular venous stasis arises. Gastric mucosal injury results and may lead to subepithelial hemorrhage and edema. Erosions and ulcers may arise in the gastric mucosa.

With continued gastric distention, the systemic arterial pressure falls and the caudal vena caval pressure rises. Blood becomes sequestered in organs draining to the caudal vena cava. With the blood sequestration, oxyhemoglobin desaturation occurs in the caudal vena cava and right atrium.[97]

The decreased venous return to the right atrium results in a decreased cardiac output. Neurogenic stimulation of the splanchnic sympathetics by the distended stomach may also result in hypotension. The consequences of this hypotension and decreased circulating blood volume are manifested by a low velocity of flow. At low velocity, blood tends to increase in viscosity, and the ability to perfuse tissues decreases.[94] This sludging also promotes disseminated intravascular coagulation in gastric volvulus.[88]

Portal venous occlusion may initiate septic shock in dogs with GDV. When the portal vein is experimentally occluded, a high mortality rate is noted.[20, 78] Death is caused by hypovolemia, a neurogenic enhancement of the shock state, or a failure of the reticuloendothelial system's capacity to neutralize endotoxins. Gram-negative bacteria within the gut release their endotoxins with portal vein occlusion.[111] These endotoxins enter the circulatory system either via the peritoneal surface[36] or via the lymphatic channels.[55, 111]

The encroachment of the dilated stomach on the thoracic space initially decreases tidal volume and increases respiratory rate, in order to maintain minute volume. The decrease in lung compliance that occurs in gastric dilation may result in a compromised ventilation-perfusion ratio.[117]

Diagnosis

Definitive diagnosis of gastric volvulus is by means of abdominal radiography. Because enforced manipulation for positioning increases stress and risk to the patient, radiography is performed after the initial shock therapy and gastric decompression. A lateral projection as well as dorsal recumbency is necessary for assessment of gastric position. Barium is occasionally administered.

The radiographic course of events after successful gastric decompression shows great variation among cases. Sometimes, the stomach returns to a normal position immediately or within hours. In other cases, the stomach remains malpositioned for days or weeks without functional disturbance.[53]

As the stomach dilates, the pylorus moves caudodorsally, and the greater curvature lies along the ventral abdominal wall. Gradually, the pylorus moves dorsally, cranially, and toward the left. The spleen follows the greater curvature as it moves toward the right. A large gas- and fluid-filled stomach is generally seen. A soft-tissue density often separates the fundus from the pylorus.[82]

Treatment

Gastric decompression is achieved most quickly by passing a stomach tube or by gastrocentesis (trocarization). A colt-sized (9.5 mm), moderately stiff stomach tube can frequently be passed, and the gastric contents removed by lavage. In the event a stomach tube cannot be passed, the stomach may be trocarized with a 12 to 16 gauge needle to achieve decompression. Partial relief of gastric gas will often allow passage of the orogastric tube.

Gastrostomy. Gastrostomy may be employed as a decompressive procedure (see Chapter 6). Use of this technique at one institution reduced the mortality rate of GDV from 68 per cent[114] to 33 per cent.[159] An assessment of tissue viability is possible with gastrostomy. A definitive surgical procedure is required to realign the stomach and spleen. The gastrostomy must be closed first.

Improved cardiovascular function follows gastric decompression. Cardiovascular function is further enhanced by rapid volume replacement using intravenous, isotonic fluids. Surprisingly, clinical patients with GDV have not been in the severe acidosis state of experimental dogs.[103, 167] At present, bicarbonate therapy is no longer condoned in routine treatment of this disease.[167]

A transient hyperkalemia results from gastric decompression.[164] Of greater consequence is the total body hypokalemia that occurs. Intravenous replacement of potassium is found to decrease the incidence of postoperative cardiac dysrhythmias and muscle weakness.

It is important to gather baseline laboratory parameters prior to large-volume fluid replacement. A simple packed cell volume (PCV) and a total serum solids value (total serum protein) will provide information useful in assessing the need for fluid replacement. Determining a complete blood count (CBC) and blood glucose level is useful in assessing the presence of septic shock. Leukopenia (<3000 leukocytes/mm^3), a significant left shift, and hypoglycemia (<60 mg glucose/dl) suggest septicemia.

Corticosteroids are routinely used in the management of shock.[122] Their beneficial effects are attributed to competitive inhibition of endotoxin, stabilization of lysosomal membranes, improved cell metabolism, antagonism of vasoactive substances released in shock, and improved cardiac performance. Fluid therapy *always* precedes corticosteroid therapy.

Broad-spectrum antibiotics are useful in controlling bacterial numbers preoperatively and postoperatively. Currently, bacteriocidal drugs are favored for lessening the severity of endotoxemia.

Surgical Therapy. Numerous surgical techniques have been attempted to prevent recurrence of GDV. These include gastropexy,[162] gastrocolopexy,[28] "permanent" gastropexy,[15] and tube gastrostomy.[113] Recently a circumcostal gastropexy has been employed in dogs for prophylaxis.[60] Experience to date has shown the superiority of this technique over previous prophylactic procedures. Advantages of this procedure include the use of the pyloric antrum (the area least damaged in GDV), the physiological positioning of the stomach, and the firm adhesion between the stomach and peritoneum that develops.

Complications. Postoperative difficulties are associated with shock, hypokalemia, cardiac dysrhythmia,[102] and gastrostomy complications. Fluid therapy and patient monitoring are important in the recognition and treatment of possible complications. Because of the gastritis, the animal receives no oral nourishment for 24 to 48 hours. During this interval, it is important to maintain electrolyte balance and fluid needs.

The cardiac dysrhythmias include supraventricular dysrhythmias, such as atrial premature contractions and atrial fibrillation. Ventricular premature contractions, paroxysmal ventricular tachycardia, ventricular tachycardia, and multifocal ventricular tachycardia are also noted postoperatively.[102, 104] These dysrhythmias are often resistant to therapy with intravenous lidocaine hydrochloride or intravenous or oral procainamide hydrochloride* to re-establish sinus rhythm. With potassium replacement these dysrhythmias are less frequently encountered.

Gastrostomy complications result from premature removal of the Foley catheter or leakage. Peritonitis results when the tube is in place for less than 5 days. This complication usually requires an immediate laparotomy and medical management.

Prognosis. Because the cause of gastric dilatation-volvulus is unknown, it is difficult to advocate preventive measures. As mentioned previously, no specific foodstuff, homemade or commercial, can prevent GDV.

Application of various principles of gastric emptying may be useful. It is important to feed the animal small quantities frequently to decrease gastric distention. Moistening dry foods and preventing postprandial exercise and excitement may help. Most large breed dogs are fed dry foodstuffs because they provide more calories on a weight to volume basis. Dry foodstuffs generally provide about 1500 kcal per pound, whereas semimoist and canned foods only yield about 500 kcal per pound. The presence of soybeans as a protein source does not result in a high incidence of GDV.

The presence of fat in the diet will generally delay emptying of the stomach. Alternatively, by increasing the fat content it is possible to decrease the volume of food needed to satisfy the caloric demands of the dog.

Antifoaming antacids are of no use in GDV because a frothy bloat does not exist in the dog.

*Pronestyl, E. R. Squibb & Sons, Inc., Princeton, NJ.

Gastric dilatation-volvulus is a life-threatening disease that requires prompt recognition and aggressive medical and surgical therapy. Newer surgical procedures have decreased recurrence of gastric volvulus. Unless the etiology is specifically identified in future research, one can only rely upon principles of gastric physiology to lessen the incidence and the mortality rate of GDV in the dog.

References

1. Aagaard P, Fischerman K, Funding J: Augmented histamine test in dogs. Methods of aspiration technique. Scand J Gastroenterol 7:279, 1972.
2. Ader P: Penetrating gastric ulceration in a dog. J Am Vet Med Assoc 175:710, 1979.
3. Ambinder RF, Schuster MM: Endorphins: New gut peptides with a familiar face. Gastroenterology 77:1132, 1979.
4. Archibald RM, Milton AR: Surgical relief of pyloric stenosis in the dog. Can J Comp Med 18:394, 1954.
5. Archibald JA, Cawley AJ, Reed JH: Surgical technic for correcting pyloric stenosis. Mod Vet Pract 41:28, 1960.
6. Atkins CE, Johnson RK: Clinical toxicities of cats. Vet Clin North Am 5:623, 1975.
7. Aures D, Hakanson R, Owman C, et al: Cellular stores of histamine and monoamines in the dog stomach. Life Sci 7:1147, 1968.
8. Baker BL: Cell replacement in the stomach. Gastroenterology 46:202, 1964.
9. Banks WJ: Digestive System. *In* Banks WJ (ed): *Applied Veterinary Histology.* Baltimore, Williams & Wilkins Company, 373, 1981.
10. Baronofsky I, Wangensteen OH: Obstruction of splenic vein increases weight of the stomach and predisposes to erosion and ulcer. Proc Soc Exp Biol Med 59:234, 1945.
11. Barsanti JA, Attleberger MN, Henderson RA: Phycomycosis in a dog. J Am Vet Med Assoc 167:293, 1975.
12. Batt RM: Technique for single and multiple peroral jejunal biopsy in the dog. J Small Anim Pract 20:259, 1979.
13. Baron JH: Maximal stimuli. *In* Baron JH (ed): *Clinical Tests of Gastric Secretion.* New York, Oxford University Press, 25, 1979.
14. Belding HH III, Kernohan JW: A morphologic study of the myenteric plexus and musculature of the pylorus with special reference to the changes in hypertrophic pyloric stenosis. Surg Gynecol Obstet 97:322, 1953.
15. Betts CW, Wingfield WE, Rosin E: "Permanent" gastropexy—as a prophylactic measure against gastric volvulus. J Am Anim Hosp Assoc 12:177, 1976.
16. Betts CW, Wingfield WE, Green RW: A retrospective study of gastric dilatation-torsion in the dog. J Small Anim Pract 15:727, 1974.
17. Bilski R, Kowalewski K, Secord DC: The effect of L–amino acids given intravenously on gastric secretion stimulated by pentagastrin in dogs. Digestion 18:240, 1978.
18. Bishop L, Sheffield WD, Strandberg JD: Eosino-

philic gastritis in a dog associated with microfilaria. Manuscript in preparation, 1985.
19. Bohning RJ Jr, DeHoff WE, McElkinney A, Hofstra PC: Pharyngostomy for maintenance of the anorectic animal. J Am Vet Med Assoc 156:611, 1970.
20. Boyce FF, Lambert R, McFetridge EM: Occlusion of the portal vein. J Lab Clin Med 20:935, 1935.
21. Brink BM, Schlegel JF, Code CF: The pressure profile of the gastroduodenal junctional zone in dogs. Gut 6:163, 1965.
22. Brody RS: Alimentary tract neoplasms in the cat: A clinicopathologic survey of 46 cases. Am J Vet Res 27:74, 1966.
23. Butler HC: Gastroduodenostomy in the dog. J Am Vet Med Assoc 155:1347, 1969.
24. Carrig CB, Seawright AA: Mastocytosis with gastrointestinal ulceration in a dog. Aust Vet J 44:503, 1968.
25. Caywood DH, Teagne D, Jackson DA, et al: Gastric gas analysis in the canine gastric dilatation-volvulus syndrome. J Am Anim Hosp Assoc 13:459, 1977.
26. Cheung LH, Chang N: The role of gastric mucosal blood flow and H^+ back-diffusion in the pathogenesis of acute gastric erosions. J Surg Res 22:357, 1977.
27. Cheville NF: Uremic gastropathy in the dog. Vet Pathol 16:292, 1979.
28. Christie LR, Smith CW: Gastrocolopexy for prevention of recurrent gastric volvulus. J Am Anim Hosp Assoc 12:173, 1976.
29. Code CF: Reflections of histamine, gastric secretion, and the H_2 receptor. N Engl J Med 296:1459, 1975.
30. Conroy JD: Multiple gastric adenomatous polyps in a dog. J Comp Pathol 79:465, 1969.
31. Cooke AR: Control of gastric emptying and motility. Gastroenterology 68:804, 1975.
32. Cornelius LM, Rawlings CA: Arterial blood gas and acid-base values in dogs with various diseases and signs of disease. J Am Vet Med Assoc 178:992, 1981.
33. Cott B, Shelton M, DeYoung DW: Preliminary report on AGD/V questionnaire. Pure-Bred Dogs Am Kennel Gazette April:76, 1976.
34. Crean GP, Hogg DF, Rumsey RDE: Hyperplasia of the gastric mucosa produced by duodenal obstruction. Gastroenterology 56:193, 1969.
35. Curtis PJ, Rayford PL, Thompson JC: Renal extraction of circulating secretin in dogs. Physiologist 18:181, 1975.
36. Cyevas P, Fine J: Route of absorption of endotoxin from the intestine in nonseptic shock. J Reticuloendothel Soc 11:535, 1972.
37. Damiano S: Chronic follicular hypertrophic gastritis in a dog. Acta Med Vet 13:363, 1967.
38. Davis LE: Pharmacologic control of vomiting. J Am Vet Med Assoc 176:241, 1980.
39. Davis RA, Brooks FP: Experimental peptic ulcer associated with lesions on stimulation of the central nervous system. Surg Gynecol Obstet 116:307, 1963.
40. Debas HT, Yamagishi T, Dryburgh JR: Motilin enhances gastric emptying of liquids in dogs. Gastroenterology 73:777, 1977.
41. Debas HT, Slaff GF, Grossman MI: Intestinal phase of gastric acid secretion: Augmentation of maximal response of Heidenhain pouch to gastrin and histamine. Gastroenterology 68:691, 1975.
42. Debas HT, Walsh JH, Grossman MI: Evidence for oxynto-pyloric reflex for release of antral gastrin. Gastroenterology 68:687, 1975.
43. Debas HT, Crendes A, Walsh JH, et al: Release of antral gastrin. *In* Chey WP, Brooks SP (eds): *Endocrinology of the Gut.* Thorofare, NJ, Charles B. Slack, Inc., 222, 1974.
44. Debas HT, Konturek SJ, Walsh JH, et al: Proof of a pyloro-oxyntic reflex for stimulation of acid secretion. Gastroenterology 66:526, 1974.
45. Ditchfield J, Phillipson MH: Achlorhydria in dogs, with report of a case complicated by avitaminosis C. Can Vet J I:396, 1960.
46. Dockray GJ: Molecular evaluation of gut hormones: Application of comparative studies on the regulation of digestion. Gastroenterology 72:344, 1977.
47. Douglas SW, Hall LW, Walker RG: The surgical relief of gastric lesions in the dog: Report of seven cases. Vet Rec 86:743, 1970.
48. Dumler F: Primary metabolic alkalosis. Am Fam Physician 23:193, 1981.
49. Ellenberger W, Baum H: *Handbuch der Vergleichender Anatomie der Haustiere.* Berlin, Springer-Verlag, 1943.
50. Evans HE, Christensen GC: *Anatomy of the Dog.* Philadelphia, WB Saunders Company, 476, 1979.
51. Finco DR: Fluid therapy for profuse vomiting. J Am Anim Hosp Assoc 8:200, 1972.
52. Fung WP, Papadimitriou JM, Matz LR: Endoscopic, histological, and ultrastructural correlations in chronic gastritis. Am J Gastroenterol 71:269, 1979.
53. Funkquist B: Gastric torsion in the dog. I. Radiological picture during nonsurgical treatment related to the pathological anatomy and to the further clinical course. J Small Anim Pract 20:73, 1979.
54. Funkquist B, Garmer L: Pathogenetic and therapeutic aspects of torsion of the canine stomach. J Small Anim Pract 8:523, 1967.
55. Gans H: The escape of endotoxin from the intestine. Surg Gynecol Obstet 139:395, 1974.
56. Gardham JRC: Pyloric stenosis: An experimental study of alkalosis and the paradox of acid urine in dogs (abst). Br J Surg 56:628, 1969.
57. Gibbs C, Pearson H: The radiological diagnosis of gastrointestinal obstruction in the dog. J Small Anim Pract 14:61, 1973.
58. Grossman MI, Konturek SJ: Inhibition of acid secretion in dog by metiamide, a histamine antagonist acting on H_2 receptors. Gastroenterology 66:517, 1974.
59. Grossman MI: The chemicals that activate the "on" switches of the oxyntic cell. Mayo Clin Proc 50:515, 1975.
60. Fallah AM, Lumb WV, Nelson AW, et al: Circumcostal gastropexy in the dog. A preliminary study. Vet Surg 11:9, 1982.
61. Happe RP, Van Der Gaag I, Wolvekamp W, Van Toorenburg J: Multiple polyps of the gastric mucosa in two dogs. J Small Anim Pract 18:179, 1977.
62. Harris WF: Clinical toxicities in dogs. Vet Clin North Am 5:605, 1975.
63. Hayden DW, Fleischman RW: Scirrhous eosinophilic gastritis in dogs with gastric arteritis. Vet Pathol 14:441, 1977.
64. Hayden DW, Van Kruiningen HI: Experimentally induced canine toxocariasis: Laboratory exami-

nations and pathologic changes, with emphasis on the gastrointestinal tract. Am J Vet Res 36:1605, 1975.
65. Hayden DW, Nielsen SW: Canine alimentary neoplasia. Zentralbl Veterinaermed 20:1, 1973.
66. Hinder RA, Bremmer CG: Relative role of pyloroplasty size, truncal vagotomy, and milk meal volume in canine gastric emptying. Am J Dig Dis 23:210, 1978.
67. Hirschowitz BI, Gibson RG: The effect of cimetidine on stimulated gastric secretion and serum gastrin in the dog. Am J Gastroenterol 70:437, 1978.
68. Hoerlein BF, Spano JS: Non-neurological complications following decompressive spinal cord surgery. Arch Am Coll Vet Surg IV:11, 1975.
69. Howard EB, Sawa TR, Nielsen SW, Kenyon AJ: Mastocytoma and gastroduodenal ulceration. Path Vet 6:146, 1969.
70. Howard EB: Acute mycotic gastritis in a dog. Vet Med Small Anim Clin 61:549, 1966.
71. Howard EB, Kenyon AJ: Canine mastocytoma: Altered α-globulin distribution. Am J Vet Res 26:1132, 1965.
72. Hunt JN, Stubbs DF: The volume and energy content of meals as determinants of gastric emptying. J Physiol (Lond) 245:209, 1975.
73. Hurwitz A, Robinson RG, Vats TS, et al: Effects of antacids on gastric emptying. Gastroenterology 71:268, 1976.
74. Isenberg JI: Gastric secretory testing. *In* Sleisenger MH, Fordtran JS (eds): *Gastrointestinal Disease,* 2nd ed. Philadelphia, WB Saunders Company, 714, 1978.
75. Ivey KJ: Gastritis. Med Clin North Am 58:1289, 1974.
76. Jeffries GH: Gastritis. *In* Sleisenger MH, Fordtran JS (eds), *Gastrointestinal Disease,* 2nd ed. Philadelphia, WB Saunders Company, 733, 1978.
77. Johnson GF, Twedt DC: Endoscopy and laparoscopy in the diagnosis and management of neoplasia in small animals. Vet Clin North Am 7:77, 1977.
78. Johnstone FRC: Acute ligation of the portal vein. Surgery 41:958, 1957.
79. Key DM: Dilatation and torsion of the stomach in a cat. Fel Pract 7:38, 1977.
80. Kipnis RM: Focal cystic hypertrophic gastropathy in a dog. J Am Vet Med Assoc 173:182, 1978.
81. Kivilbakso E, Silen W: Pathogenesis of experimental gastric-mucosal injury. N Engl J Med 301:364, 1979.
82. Kneller SK: Radiographic interpretation of the gastric dilatation-volvulus complex in the dog. J Am Anim Hosp Assoc 12:154, 1976.
83. Krohn KJE, Finlayson DC: Interrelations of humoral and cellular immune responses in experimental canine gastritis. Clin Exp Immunol 14:237, 1973.
84. Laufer MD, Mullers JE, Hamilton J: The diagnostic accuracy of barium studies of the stomach and duodenum—correlation with endoscopy. Radiology 115:569, 1972.
85. Laurén P: The two histological main types of gastric carcinoma: diffuse and so-called intestinal-type carcinoma. An attempt at histo-clinical classification. Acta Pathol Microbiol Scand 64:31, 1965.
86. Lawther WA: Pyloric stenosis in a puppy. Aust Vet J 37:317, 1961.
87. Lee KY, Tai HH, Chey WY: Plasma secretin and gastrin responses to a meat meal and duodenal acidification in dogs. Am J Physiol 230:784, 1976.
88. Lees GE, Leighton RL, Hart R: Management of gastric dilatation-volvulus and disseminated intravascular coagulation in a dog: A case report. J Am Anim Hosp Assoc 13:463, 1977.
89. Lingeman CH, Garner FM, Taylor DON: Spontaneous gastric adenocarcinomas of dogs: A review. J Natl Cancer Inst 47:137, 1977.
90. MacEwen EG: Canine lymphosarcoma. *In* Kirk RW (ed): *Current Veterinary Therapy VII.* Philadelphia, WB Saunders Company, 419, 1980.
91. Malagelada JR: Physiologic basis and clinical significance of gastric emptying disorders. Dig Dis Sci 24:657, 1979.
92. Malagelada JR, Cortot A: H_2-receptor antagonist in perspective. Mayo Clin Proc 53:184, 1978.
93. Marks IN, Kemarov SA, Shay H: Maximal secretory response to histamine and its relation to parietal cell mass in the dog. Am J Physiol 199:579, 1960.
94. Matheson NA: Factors in tissue perfusion. The microcirculation in shock. Postgrad Med 45:530, 1969.
95. McDonald AE: Primary gastric carcinoma of the dog: Review and case report. Vet Surg 7:70, 1978.
96. Menguy R, Masters YF: Gastric mucosal energy metabolism and "stress" ulceration. Am Surg 180:538, 1974.
97. Merkely DF, Howard DR, Eyster GE, et al: Experimentally induced acute gastric dilatation in the dog: Cardiopulmonary effects. J Am Anim Hosp Assoc 12:143, 1976.
98. Moertel CG: Current concepts in cancer: Chemotherapy of gastrointestinal cancer. N Engl J Med 299:1049, 1978.
99. Moody FG, Cheung LY, Simons MA, Zalewsky C: Stress and the acute gastric mucosal lesion. Am J Dig Dis 21:148, 1976.
100. Moore RW, Withrow SJ: Gastrointestinal hemorrhage and pancreatitis associated with intervertebral disk disease in the dog. J Am Vet Med Assoc 180:1443, 1982.
101. Morrissey JF, Barreras RF: Antacid therapy. N Engl J Med 290:550, 1974.
102. Muir WW: Gastric dilatation-volvulus in the dog, with emphasis on cardiac arrhythmias. J Am Vet Med Assoc 180:739, 1982.
103. Muir WW: Acid-base and electrolyte disturbances in dogs with gastric dilatation-volvulus. J Am Vet Med Assoc 181:229, 1982.
104. Muir WW, Weisbrode SE: Myocardial ischemia in dogs with gastric dilatation-volvulus. J Am Vet Med Assoc 181:353, 1982.
105. Murray M, Robinson PB, McKeating FJ, Lauder IM: Peptic ulceration in the dog: A clinico-pathological study. Vet Rec 91:441, 1972.
106. Murray M, McKeating FJ, Baker GJ, Lauder IM: Primary gastric neoplasia in the dog: a clinico-pathological study. Vet Rec 91:474, 1972.
107. Nogoaka K: Electromyography study on the mechanism of delayed gastric emptying after vagotomy in dogs. Tokaku J Exp Med 95:1, 1968.
108. O'Brien TR: Stomach. *In* O'Brien TR (ed): *Radiographic Diagnosis of Abdominal Disorders in the Dog and Cat.* Philadelphia, WB Saunders Company, 204, 1978.
109. Okabe S, Takeuchi K, Murata T, Urushidni T: Effects of cimetidine on healing of chronic gastric and duodenal ulcers in dogs. Dig Dis 23:166, 1978.
110. Okamoto E, Iwasaki T, Kakutani T, Uera T:

Selective destruction of the myenteric plexus: Its relation to Hirschsprung's disease, achalasia of the esophagus and hypertrophic pyloric stenosis. J Pediatr Surg 2:444, 1967.

111. Olkay I, Kitaham A, Miller RH, et al: Reticuloendothelial dysfunction and endotoxemia following portal vein occlusion. Surgery 75:64, 1974.
112. Osborne AD, Wilson MR: Mycotic gastritis in a dog. Vet Rec 85:487, 1969.
113. Parks JL, Greene RW: Tube gastrostomy for the treatment of gastric volvulus. J Am Anim Hosp Assoc 12:168, 1976.
114. Pass MA, Johnston DE: Treatment of gastric dilation and torsion in the dog. Gastric decompression by gastrostomy under local analgesia. J Small Anim Pract 14:131, 1973.
115. Patnaik AK, Hurvitz AI, Johnson GE: Canine gastric adenocarcinoma. Vet Pathol 15:600, 1978.
116. Pearson H, Gaskell CI, Gibbs C, Waterman A: Pyloric and oesophageal dysfunction in the cat. J Small Anim Pract 15:487, 1974.
117. Peters RM: Physiologic review—coordination of ventilation and perfusion. Ann Thorac Surg 6:570, 1968.
118. Politzer JP, Devroede G, Vasseur C, et al: The genesis of bowel sounds. Influence of viscus and gastrointestinal content. Gastroenterology 71: 282, 1976.
119. Polyak RI, Gresew VV, Fisher AA: Parasympathetic innervation of the stomach. Bull Exp Biol Med 71:373, 1971.
120. Priebe HJ, Skillman JJ, Bushnell LS, et al: Antacid versus cimetidine in preventing acute gastrointestinal bleeding. N Engl J Med 302:426, 1980.
121. Quigley JP, Bauor HJ, Read MR, Brofman BL: Evidence that body irritations or emotions retard gastric evacuation, not by producing pylorospasm but by depressing gastric motility. J Clin Invest 22:839, 1943.
122. Rawlings CA, Wingfield WE, Betts CW: Shock therapy and anesthetic management of gastric dilatation-volvulus. J Am Anim Hosp Assoc 12:158, 1976.
123. Rayford PL, Miller TA, Thompson JC: Secretin, cholecystokinin and newer gastrointestinal hormones. N Engl J Med 294:1093, 1976.
124. Reed JD, Saunders DJ, Thorpe V: The effect of splanchnic nerve stimulation on gastric acid secretion and mucosal blood flow in the anesthetized cat. J Physiol (Lond), 214:1, 1971.
125. Root CR, Morgan JP: Contrast radiography of the upper gastrointestinal tract in the dog. J Sm Anim Pract 10:279, 1969.
126. Sabatini S, Arruda JA, Kurtzman NA: Disorders of acid-base balance. Med Clin North Am 62:1223, 1978.
127. Sakamoto H: A pharmacological study on the autonomic innervation of cardia, corpus and pylorus in the dog stomach. Fukuoka Acta Med 60:561, 1969.
128. Sass B: Perforating gastric ulcer associated with lead poisoning in a dog. J Am Vet Med Assoc 157:76, 1970.
129. Sautler JH, Hanlon GF: Gastric neoplasms in the dog: A report of 20 cases. J Am Vet Med Assoc 166:691, 1975.
130. Schaer, M.: Disorders of potassium metabolism. Vet Clin North Am 12:399, 1982.
131. Schulman J: Control of gastric ulcers in a dog using cimetidine. Can Pract 6:42, 1979.
132. Seawright AA, Grono LR: Malignant mast cell tumor in a cat with perforating duodenal ulcer. J Pathol Bacteriol 87:107, 1964.
133. Skillman JJ, Silen W: Gastric mucosal barrier. Surg Ann 4:213, 1972.
134. Smale BF, Mullen JL, Rosato EF: Experimental gastric mucosal injury. N Engl J Med 302:61, 1980.
135. Snape WJ Jr, Battle WM, Schwartz SS, et al: Metoclopramide to treat gastroparesis due to diabetes mellitus: A double-blind, controlled trial. Ann Intern Med 96:444, 1982.
136. Sorour VE: The relationship between atrophic gastritis and gastric ulcer. S Afr J Surg 14:47, 1976.
137. Steinberg WM, Lewis JH, Katz DM: Antacids inhibit absorption of cimetidine. N Engl J Med 307:400, 1982.
138. Stemper TJ, Cooke AR: Effect of a fixed pyloric opening on gastric emptying in the cat and dog. Am J Physiol 230:813, 1976.
139. Stemper TJ, Cooke AR: Gastric emptying and its relationship to antral contractile activity. Gastroenterology 69:649, 1975.
140. Straus E: The explosion of gastrointestinal hormones. Med Clin North Am 62:21, 1978.
141. Strombeck DR: Chronic gastritis, gastric retention and gastric neoplasms. *In: Small Animal Gastroenterology*. Davis, CA, Stonegate Publishing, 110, 1979.
142. Thomas PA, Kelly KA, Go VLW: Does motilin regulate canine interdigestive gastric motility? Dig Dis Sci 24:577, 1979.
143. Thrall DE, Bovee KC, Biery DN: Demonstration of a position of relief in dogs with lesions of the stomach or small bowel. J Am Anim Hosp Assoc 14:343, 1978.
144. Tobe T, Chen ST, Henmi K, Fukuchi K: Distribution of gastrin in canine, cat, and human digestive organs. Am J Surg 132:581, 1976.
145. Todorff RJ: Gastric dilatation-volvulus. Comp Cont Ed I:142, 1979.
146. Toombs JP, Caywood DD, Lipowitz AJ, Stevens JB: Colonic perforation following neurosurgical procedures and corticosteroid therapy in four dogs. J Am Vet Med Assoc 177:68, 1980.
147. Twaddle AA: Congenital pyloric stenosis in two kittens corrected by pyloroplasty. NZ Vet J 19:26, 1971.
148. Twaddle AA: Pyloric stenosis in three cats and its correction by pyloroplasty. NZ Vet J 18:15, 1970.
149. Twedt DC: Jaundice, hepatic trauma, and hepatic encephalopathy. Vet Clin North Am 11:121, 1981.
150. Twedt DC, Wingfield WE: The stomach. *In* Ettinger SJ (ed): *Textbook of Veterinary Internal Medicine,* 2nd ed. Philadelphia, WB Saunders Company, 1982.
151. Twedt DG, Grauer GF: Fluid therapy for gastrointestinal pancreatic and hepatic disorders. Vet Clin North Am 12:463, 1982.
152. Tyler DE: Gastric neoplasia in the dog and cat. (Abst) Arch Am Coll Vet Surg 6:47, 1977.
153. Vagne M, Fargier MC: Effect of pentagastrin and secretin on gastric mucus secretion in conscious cats. Gastroenterology 65:757, 1973.
154. Van Der Gaag I, Happe RP, Wolvekamp W: A boxer dog with chronic hypertrophic gastritis resembling Menetrier's disease in man. Vet Pathol 13:172, 1976.
155. Van Der Gaag I, Happe RP, Wolvekamp W: In-

the stomach while the work is being performed and will prevent unnecessary spillage of stomach contents into the abdominal cavity once the incision has been made (Fig. 6–10*A*). The remaining and avulsed attachments of the greater omentum and the associated vascular supply along the area to be resected should be ligated and divided. All severely devitalized tissue should be resected, but the decision of how much to resect should be based upon the appearance of the serosal and muscular walls, not on the appearance of the mucosal surface. In most cases of gastric volvulus that require gastric resection, the major portion of the mucosal surface looks severely damaged but will recover if the gastric musculature is viable.

Before resection, the stomach is packed off with warm, moistened laparotomy sponges to help prevent contamination of the abdominal cavity. After the stomach is opened, the gastric contents should be aspirated to prevent contamination and to improve visualization of the tissue (Fig. 6–10*B*).

After resection of damaged tissue is complete, the incision should be inspected for adequate hemostasis.

Closure is made with two layers of sutures in continuous inverting patterns. A Connell suture pattern is used for the first layer and a Lembert pattern for the second. If the closure is long, it is advisable to tie the continuous suture once or twice along the incision line while performing the closure. Recommended suture materials are 2/0 to 0 chromic gut, but the use of synthetic absorbable material throughout, or of non-absorbable material in the second layer of sutures, is acceptable (Fig. 6–10*C* and *D*).[17, 31]

Partial Gastrectomy—Area of the Lesser Curvature, Pyloric Antrum, and Pylorus

Gastric ulcers and neoplasia are most commonly located in the area of the lesser curvature, pyloric antrum, and pylorus. A complicating factor in this region is the possibility that the duodenal tissue, into which the pancreatic ducts and the common bile duct drain, may also require resection. A Billroth I type of anastomosis is employed for closure if, after resection of the diseased tissue, the duodenum can be anastomosed with the stomach without interfering with the pancreatic ducts and the bile duct. A Billroth II type of anastomosis is recommended if the diseased segment of duodenum extends beyond the entrance of the biliary and pancreatic duct systems. Closures that most nearly restore the original anatomical orientation of the duodenum with the stomach are usually physiologically superior.[15, 27, 31]

Resection of this area of the stomach is begun by ligating and dividing the vessels that supply the region and the lesser omentum close to their attachments to the lesser curvature, working from the animal's left to its right. The line of dissection continues, freeing the pylorus on its cranial border by ligation and division of the hepatogastric and hepatoduodenal ligaments. The common bile duct and its entrance into the duodenal wall are identified. Care must be exercised because the stretched common bile duct can appear similar to a hepatogastric ligament. After cranial borders of the gastric and pyloric tissues are freed, the dissection is started at the tissue along the greater curvature, once again proceeding from the animal's left to its right. The dissection should be close to the gastric and pyloric walls avoiding the pancreas and its blood supply. Duodenal lymph nodes are commonly encountered near the junction of the pylorus and pancreas. The nodes should be removed with the resected tissue if cancer is suspected.

Once the region to be resected is freed of its vascular attachments, the area should be isolated with warm, moistened laparotomy pads. Traction sutures are placed in the gastric and duodenal tissues that are to remain. An incision is made through the ventral gastric wall first, and the stomach is emptied. The incision is continued, transecting the stomach. This procedure is continued in the same manner, transecting the duodenum at the intended location. All diseased tissue is removed. The transected lumens that remain should be held in a way that will prevent spillage of their contents and will aid inspection for additional disease. The gall bladder should be expressed to identify its orifice into the duodenum. The common bile duct must be functional. If gastric cancer is present, the tissue deep to the resected area is closely inspected for any enlarged lymph nodes around the portal vein. Nodes that are accessible and enlarged should be removed.

Billroth I Anastomosis. Billroth I type of gastroduodenal anastomosis is performed for those cases in which the pancreatic and bile ducts are not involved. It is started by closing the gastric opening from the lesser curvature towards the greater curvature (Fig. 6–11*A*). A double-layer continuous inverting suture pattern is used. The large gastric opening is closed except for an area near the greater curvature, which should have an opening of the same diameter as the duodenal opening to facilitate anastomosis with the duodenum (Fig. 6–11*B*). A single-layer, simple interrupted approximating suture pattern is used to anastomose the duodenum to the stomach (Fig. 6–11*C* and *D*). To ensure good apposition, the junction of the duodenal-gastric anastomosis with the gastric closure should be closely inspected.[15, 27, 31]

Suture materials recommended for the closure are sizes 2/0 to 0 chromic gut or synthetic absorbable material. Single-layer, simple interrupted anastomotic techniques work well for anastomosis of the duodenum to the stomach. Double-layer techniques may narrow the lumen too much. The simple interrupted "crushing" technique of intestinal anastomosis should be employed if non-absorbable sutures are used to anastomose the duodenum to the stomach.

Billroth II Anastomosis. Billroth II type of closure can be utilized if the resection of the stomach and pylorus also requires resection of the duodenum beyond the entrance of the common bile duct and the pancreatic ducts.

The procedure that was previously described for resection of the involved segment of the gastrointestinal tract should be employed; added care must be taken in handling the common bile duct and the pancreas. The common bile duct should be ligated and transected near its junction with the duodenum. The pancreas should be gently dissected free from the duodenum, with the fact kept in mind that the right lobe of the pancreas shares its blood supply with the duodenum through the cranial and caudal pancreaticoduodenal arteries and veins. Minimal amounts of pancreas should be dissected from the duodenum to allow for proper resection. The right lobe of the pancreas should be amputated if extensive duodenal resection is required. The pancreatic ducts should be ligated when encountered.

Surgical closure must maintain patency of the anastomosis for gastric contents and bile to pass into the small intestine. It is also physiologically desirable to salvage the

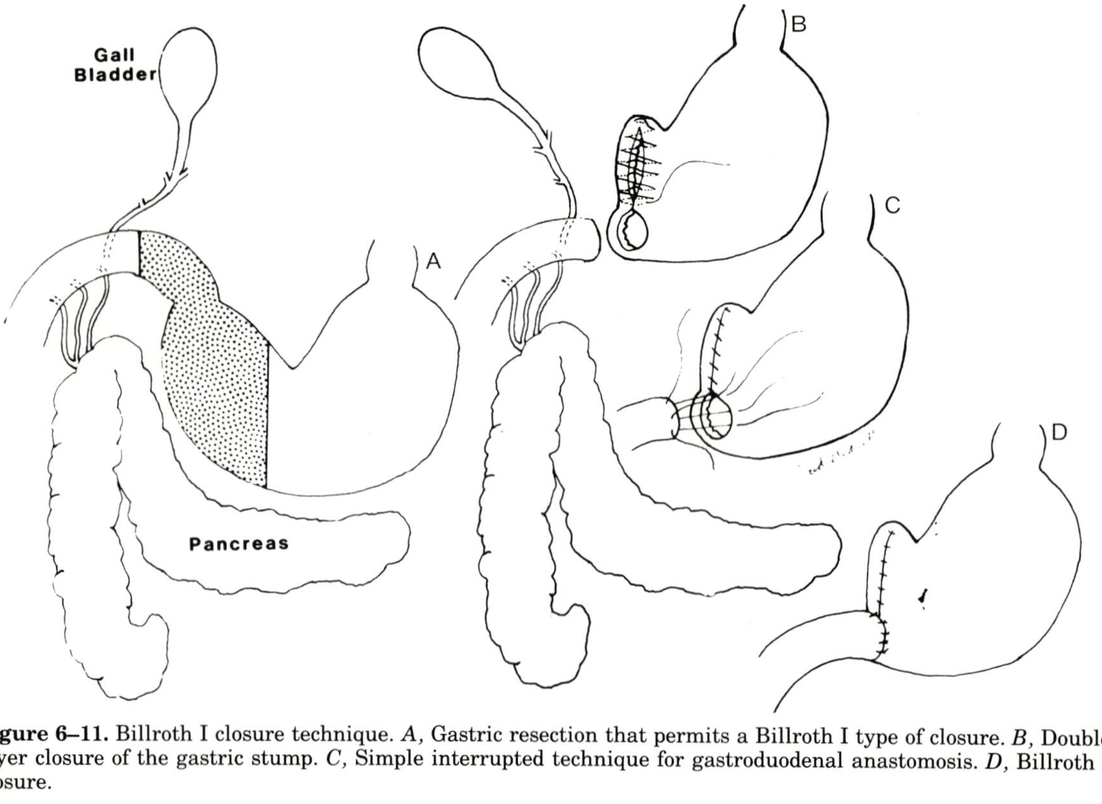

Figure 6–11. Billroth I closure technique. *A*, Gastric resection that permits a Billroth I type of closure. *B*, Double layer closure of the gastric stump. *C*, Simple interrupted technique for gastroduodenal anastomosis. *D*, Billroth I closure.

exocrine pancreatic ducts, but the technical and postoperative complications associated with pancreatic ductal anastomosis into the intestine discourage the performance of such a procedure. Ligation of the exocrine ducts of the pancreas will lead to atrophy of the exocrine portion of the pancreas, requiring permanent supplementation of the diet with pancreatic enzymes. Endocrine activity is not altered (Fig. 6–12*A*).

As a general rule, the closer the reconstruction of anatomical relationships be-

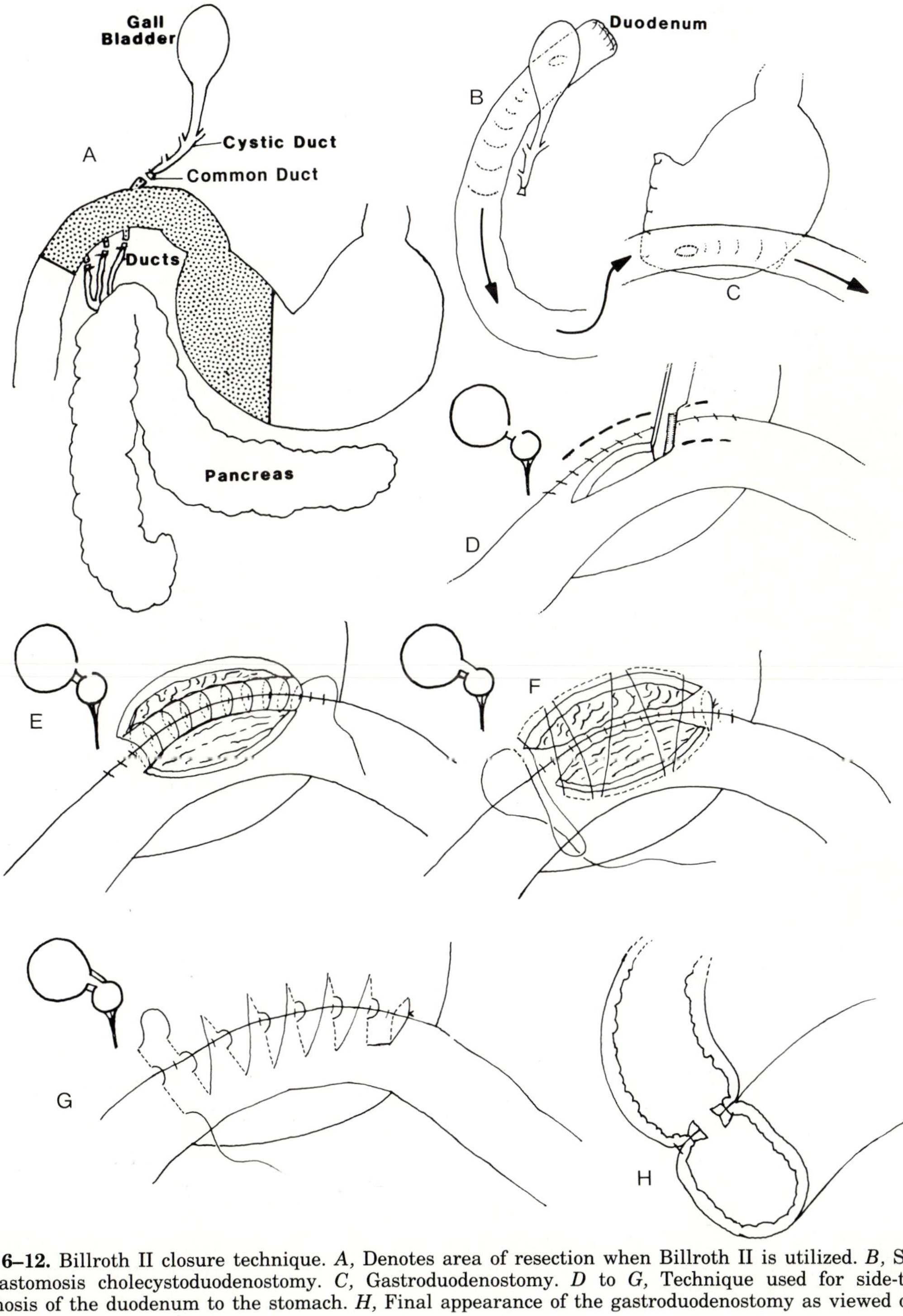

Figure 6–12. Billroth II closure technique. *A,* Denotes area of resection when Billroth II is utilized. *B,* Side to side anastomosis cholecystoduodenostomy. *C,* Gastroduodenostomy. *D* to *G,* Technique used for side-to-side anastomosis of the duodenum to the stomach. *H,* Final appearance of the gastroduodenostomy as viewed on the cut section.

tween the stomach and biliary system is to the original orientation, the better the prognosis. After a major resection of this nature, closure is begun by completely closing the stump of the stomach, utilizing a two-layer, continuous inverting suture pattern. The duodenum is closed with an inverting pattern using a continuous or interrupted suture pattern in one or two layers. Next, a cholecystoduodenostomy (an opening between the gall bladder and the duodenum) and a gastroduodenostomy or gastrojejunostomy (an opening between the stomach and duodenum or jejunum) are performed. It is important that both anastomoses are positioned so that tension on the suture lines is prevented. A gastroduodenostomy is preferred over a gastrojejunostomy because it approximates the normal flow of gastric contents. If the duodenum will not lie against the stomach without tension, then a gastrojejunostomy should be performed, uniting the proximal jejunum to the stomach.[17, 18, 19]

Cholecystoduodenostomies and gastroduodenostomies are performed similarly to a side-to-side anastomosis (Fig. 6–12*B* and *C*).

Cholecystoduodenostomy. Cholecystoduodenostomy is usually performed as a side-to-side anastomosis between the fundic portion of the gall bladder and an area close to the blind-ended stump of the duodenum. The opening into the duodenum should be along the antimesenteric border. The size of the opening of the anastomosis should be about ¼ to ½ inch long. Small openings, resembling the normal diameter of the common bile duct, have a tendency to close or to become obstructed.

To begin the anastomosis, a stay suture is placed, with the needle attached, at each corner of the planned opening in the gall bladder, to help mark the length of the opening and aid traction on the tissues being sutured. Before the incision is made, the first row of continuous sutures should be placed from the duodenum to the gall bladder between the two stay sutures. Next, the incisions into the gall bladder and the duodenum are made, with care taken to avoid cutting the first row of sutures (Fig. 6–12*D*). The cut edges of the gall bladder and the duodenum are sutured in a continuous pattern to form the new circular opening. When the circular opening is sutured, it should be tied at the half-way point before completing the top half of the circle (Fig. 6–12*E* and *F*). The last layer of sutures is then placed on top, using the same continuous pattern between the two corner sutures as was used in the first row that was placed on the bottom; this completes the anastomosis (Fig. 6–12*G* and *H*).[27, 31]

The recommended suture material is 3/0 to 2/0 chromic gut, which should be placed by swaged needles. Because the gall bladder is often very thin-walled, the needles should be intestinal types, and care must be taken to avoid tearing the wall during suturing.

Gastroduodenostomy or Gastrojejunostomy. The tissues to be anastomosed must be gently manipulated to minimize the inflammatory response, which can be excessive. The opening in the stomach should be on the ventral surface near the blind-ended stump. The opening into the intestine should be at the antimesenteric border. The size of the opening when the anastomosis is complete should be about the same as the diameter of the relaxed pylorus. To avoid tension between the stomach and small intestine once the anastomosis is complete, the most proximal portion possible of the small intestine is used.

Stay sutures are placed apposing the stomach and the intestine. The first row of sutures is a continuous pattern placed between the two stay sutures before the incisions are made. Since the incision into the small intestine is along the antimesenteric border, the first row of sutures in the intestine should be placed midway between the mesenteric and antimesenteric borders. Incisions into the stomach and small intestine are made next (Fig. 6–12*D*). The second row of sutures is placed in a continuous pattern joining the closest edges of the intestine and the stomach incisions, again in a line between the two stay sutures (Fig. 6–12*E*). The third row of sutures joins the far edges of the stomach and the intestinal incisions, thereby closing the opening (Fig. 6–12*F*). A fourth row of sutures is placed in a similar pattern over the third row (Fig. 6–12*G*). Each line of sutures is a half circle, so the completed anastomosis is a two-layer closure (Fig. 6–12*H*).[15, 27, 31]

The recommended suture material is 3/0 or 2/0 chromic gut or a synthetic absorbable material. If the outer row of sutures does not penetrate the lumen, a non-absorbable suture material may be used.

PYLOROPLASTY

. The following two techniques enlarge the lumen of the pylorus. The procedure credited to Fredet and Ramstedt does not enter the lumen of the pylorus but expands the pylorus' diameter by cutting the longitudinal and circular muscles surrounding it.[4] It is referred to as a pyloromyotomy. Heineke and Mikulicz's procedure opens the area of the pylorus more than the myotomy technique and is more reliable in keeping the pylorus open once the tissues are healed. It is a more aggressive procedure than the myotomy because the lumen is opened. A number of different pyloroplasties designed for use in humans can be utilized in the canine and feline.[4, 9, 10, 15, 27, 31]

Fredet-Ramstedt Pyloromyotomy

To perform the Fredet-Ramstedt pyloromyotomy, the pylorus should be mobilized toward the abdominal incision with the use of traction sutures in the stomach and finger traction from beneath the pylorus. The pylorus should be freed from the gastrohepatic ligaments that run from the liver toward its cranial border. The common bile duct lies lateral and very close to the ligaments in some animals and should be identified before mobilizing the pylorus.

A short incision is made on the ventral surface of the pylorus, midway between cranial and caudal borders of the pylorus, starting on the duodenal side and crossing the pylorus to the wall of the stomach. The incision should be deepened over the stomach wall through the longitudinal and circular muscle fibers, permitting the submucosa to bulge outward. It is on the gastric side of the pylorus that the submucosa is more easily freed from the muscle portion of the wall, enabling the desired plane of tissue to be well visualized. The incision should then be deepened back across the pylorus until the submucosa is bulging along the entire incision. Close inspection should be made to see if any circular muscle fibers remain. If so, they should be incised so that the submucosa bulges free of any restriction. When attempting to cut the remaining circular muscle fibers, the surgeon should cut along a different longitudinal path to avoid entering the lumen. If the lumen is entered, it is safer to perform a Heineke-Mikulicz pyloroplasty than to attempt closure of the small opening. If hemorrhage occurs, which it often does near the submucosa, a sponge applied with light pressure to the area for a few minutes will control most of the bleeding. Those vessels that continue to bleed should be ligated. If

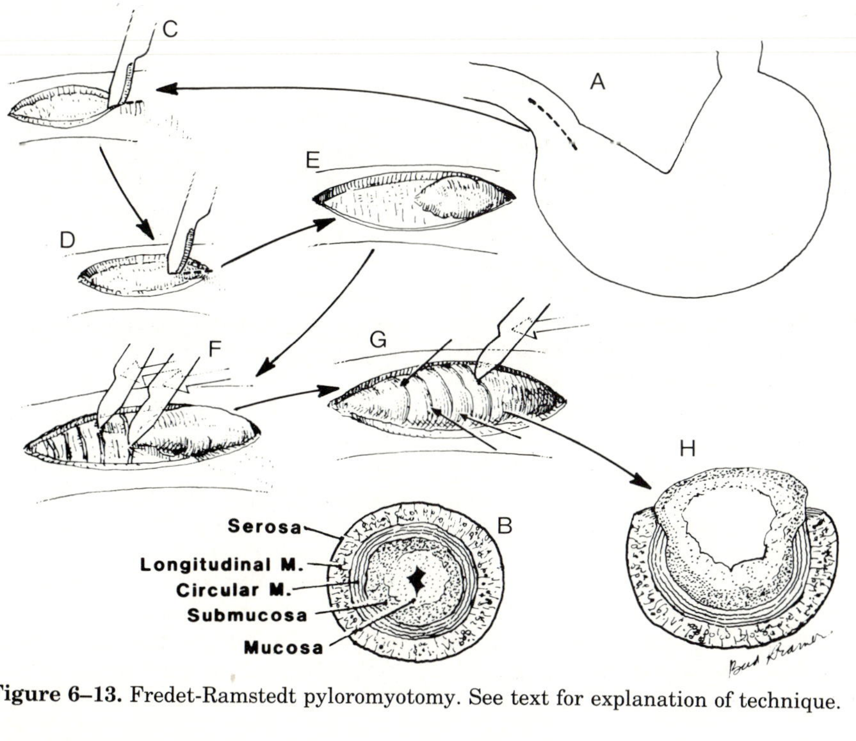

Figure 6–13. Fredet-Ramstedt pyloromyotomy. See text for explanation of technique.

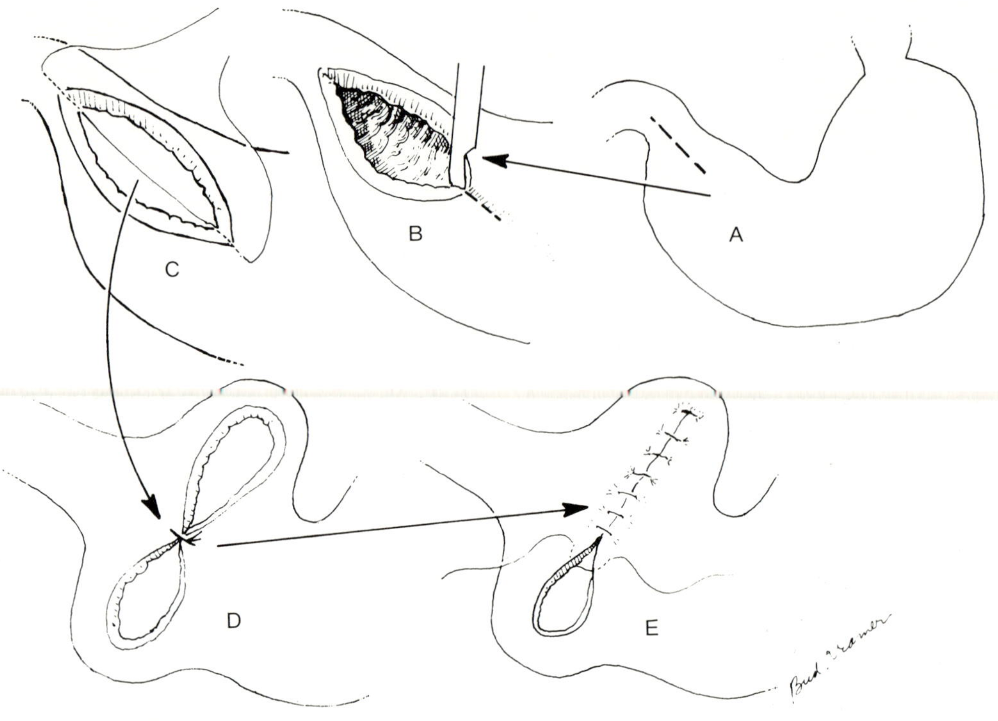

Figure 6–14. Heineke-Mikulicz pyloroplasty. See text for explanation of techinque.

electrosurgical means are used to control bleeding, care should be taken not to burn the submucosa because, with burning, the submucosa can slough 2 to 3 days later (Fig. 6–13).[4, 9, 15, 27, 31]

Heineke-Mikulicz Pyloroplasty

To perform the Heineke-Mikulicz pyloroplasty, the pylorus should be mobilized toward the abdominal incision as in the Fredet-Ramstedt pyloromyotomy. The surgical area should be isolated with warm, moistened laparotomy sponges to prevent contamination of the abdominal cavity, since in this technique the intestinal and gastric lumens are opened. An incision, which enters the lumen and crosses longitudinally from the pyloroduodenal junction to the pylorogastric junction, should be made on the ventral surface of the pylorus. This longitudinal incision is to be sutured, forming a transverse suture line that shortens and widens the pyloric canal. This procedure removes the ability of the pylorus to contract effectively. A single row of simple interrupted approximating sutures is recommended for closure. The first suture should be placed through all layers of the bowel, entering the serosa and exiting through the mucosa at the angle of the incision on the duodenal side, and then it should be carried to the angle of the incision on the gastric side, going through all layers of tissue from mucosa to serosa. When this suture is tied, the longitudinal incision is transformed into a transverse incision. Closure is completed with a simple, interrupted suture pattern that is similar to the first suture.[4, 15, 27, 31] Recommended suture material is 3/0 to 0 chromic gut, depending upon the size of the animal. Care should be taken to ensure that the corners or angles are adequately approximated when closure is complete (Fig. 6–14).

PHARYNGOSTOMY-GASTROSTOMY TUBE PLACEMENT

The animal should be placed in lateral recumbency with its head and neck in a neutral position. To determine the length of tubing needed to extend from the pharyngostomy site into the stomach, the distance from the posterior border of the mandible to the eleventh rib is measured. An oral speculum should be used to hold the mouth wide open. A finger is inserted into the pharynx near the base of the tongue and the posterior border of the mandible and the hyoid appa-

ratus are palpated. The tongue should not be held extended forward as this moves the hyoid apparatus forward out of position. The space between the epihyoid cartilage of the hyoid apparatus and the posterior border of the body of the mandible is called the piriform fossa. The skin will bulge outward if a finger is flexed laterally in this pouch. Large curved forceps are substituted for the finger to maintain the outward bulge. An incision wide enough to permit passage of the tube is made through all layers of skin, with care taken not to cut into the muscle. The tip of the forceps is pushed out through the hole in the skin with a short, sharp jab. Blunt dissection with the forceps through the pharyngeal tissue produces minimal hemorrhage (Fig. 6–15).

The end of the tubing is grasped firmly and pulled into the mouth. The tubing is then threaded down the esophagus. A radiograph of the stomach is beneficial to ensure that the tube has entered the stomach but is not too long, since excessive length would put pressure on the gastric mucosa.

The tube should be secured to the skin with one or two sutures. A purse-string suture should not be placed around the orifice. Petroleum jelly should be used on the skin under the pharyngostomy to serve as a "drainboard" to prevent exudate from building up and causing a dermatitis.

Feeding can begin as soon as the animal awakens from the anesthesia. The first few feedings should be small until the animal's ability to tolerate food has been determined. Animals can eat, drink, and vomit around the pharyngostomy-gastrostomy tube.

A cap should be placed on the tube, provided that it is not being used to relieve stomach gas, in order to prevent fluids from draining out of the tube when the animal is recumbent.

To remove the pharyngostomy-gastrostomy tube (1) the tube is flushed with water; (2) the skin sutures are removed; and (3) the tube is extracted from the pharyngostomy site with a steady, gentle pull. When this procedure is performed, the animal should be awake and should have a normal swallowing reflex. The wound should be cleaned. It will seal itself in 3 to 5 days. No sutures are required.

The tubing diameter varies with the size of the animal and the consistency of food to be fed. With the production of good, complete liquid diets, it is not necessary to use a large-bore catheter as has been recommended in the past. A 14 gauge or smaller intravenous catheter can be used success-

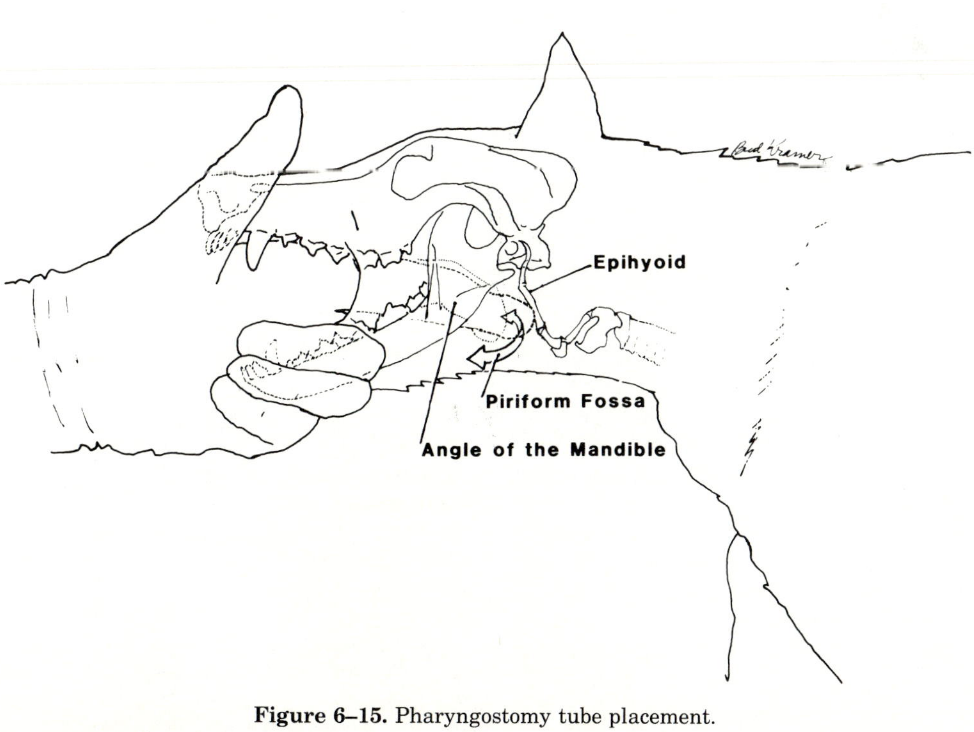

Figure 6–15. Pharyngostomy tube placement.

fully. It is important to understand that tubing passing through the lower esophageal sphincter will decrease its competency. If the food need only be presented to the esophagus, the tubing should not be placed into the stomach.[7]

ESOPHAGEAL HIATUS PLICATION AND CARDIOESOPHAGEAL GASTROPEXY

Esophageal hiatus plication and cardioesophageal gastropexy are two techniques that are recommended specifically for the correction of chronic recurrent gastroesophageal intussusceptive hiatal hernias in the cat and dog.[28] Anatomically, the esophageal hiatus is formed by the separation of the medial portion of the lumbar crus into left and right segments. The thickened fascia that is a continuation of this muscle attaches to the esophagus, forming a seal. The thickened fascia is referred to as the phrenicoesophageal ligament.[12, 30]

In this type of hiatal hernia, the fundus of the stomach herniates or intussuscepts into the esophagus only when the animal vomits or regurgitates. Following vomition, the stomach returns to its original position in the abdomen.[28, 30]

Surgical exploration of the area permits confirmation of the diagnosis. Diagnosis can be made by invaginating the gastric wall into the gastroesophageal junction with a finger. An elliptical, sphincter-like muscle wall should be palpable in the area where the diaphragm joins the cardia. If absence of a sphincter-like muscle is found by palpation and clinical signs of the disease are present, with or without radiographic confirmation, the diagnosis is made. Often, the ventral fundic surface will show increased vascularity where it has been invaginating into the esophagus (Fig. 6–16*A* and *B*).

For repair of a chronic recurrent gastroesophageal intussusceptive hiatal hernia, the left half of the liver must be mobilized, with the lobes reflected to the right of the cardia, and packed off with warm moistened laparotomy sponges. The liver's two left triangular ligaments, which run from the cranial surface of the liver to the diaphragm near the cardia, are incised to mobilize the organ. These ligaments are usually avascular and should be divided in the middle. This maneuver permits good visualization of the diaphragm, cardia, and fundus.

The defect is not a hole in the diaphragm but either a lack of musculature in the diaphragm around the hiatus or a stretching of the phrenicoesophageal ligament. The

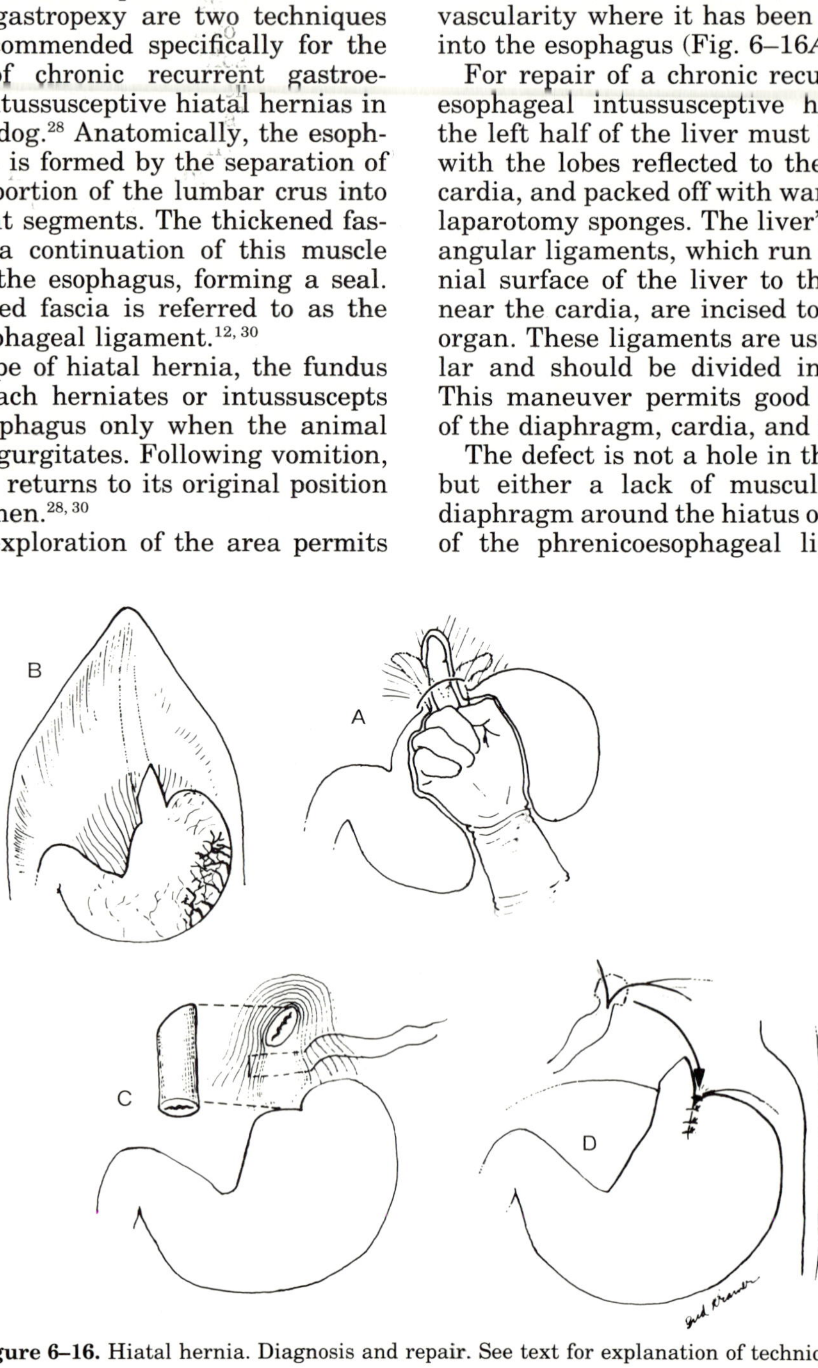

Figure 6–16. Hiatal hernia. Diagnosis and repair. See text for explanation of technique.

most common area for the defect is the supraesophageal region of the diaphragm, beneath the cardia as viewed on the surgery table. This is the location of the medial lumbar crus (Fig. 6–16*C*).

The repair technique, esophageal hiatus plication, consists of placing one or two mattress sutures in the edges of the normal diaphragm musculature of the supraesophageal area. The sutures are pulled tight enough to re-establish a palpable muscular sphincter around the cardia but not tight enough to excessively narrow the internal diameter of the gastroesophageal junction. This task is accomplished by placing the sutures and then reinvaginating the stomach wall into the esophagus with a finger. The stomach wall should enter the esophagus, the diaphragm should act as a continuous sphincter-like muscle around the cardia, and the lumen should be expandable. If the sphincter is too tight, the sutures should be removed and placed closer to the hiatus, and the stomach once again reinvaginated. If the sphincter is too loose, another suture should be placed and the cardia checked once again.

The next step, cardioesophageal gastropexy, is performed by suturing the fundus of the stomach to the cardia and the diaphragm. A line of interrupted sutures starts at the angle made by the fundus and the cardia, and ends at the junction of the cardia and the diaphragm. The last suture goes through the fundus, cardia, and diaphragm. Depending on the size of the animal, 2/0 or 1/0 chromic gut is usually used for all sutures (Fig. 6–16*D*).[28] The liver is replaced in its original position and the abdomen is closed.

Surgical Diseases

GASTRIC FOREIGN BODIES

Clinicians should be aware of the possibility of being presented with specific types of gastric foreign bodies at different times of the year: the Christmas and New Year holiday times, when a variety of materials such as tinsel, small tree ornaments, and toothpicks from hors d'oeuvres are present; the spring, when many puppies and kittens are at the inquisitive age; fishing season, when fish hooks and line are available; and early fall, when peach seeds and corn cobs can be found.

Taking a good history from the owner will often lead the clinician to place gastrointestinal foreign bodies high on the list of differential diagnoses. Ask the owner questions such as: Is the pet's favorite toy missing? Is chewing on objects a problem? Is raiding the garbage a common or recent occurrence? The owner should be queried about changes in the animal's environment, with such questions as, Is there a new baby in the house? Are any of the children's toys missing? Is there an opportunity for the animal to get into sewing materials? Has the animal been confined to a different part of the yard for any reason?

Some foreign bodies are found accidentally while the animal is being radiographed for other problems. Usually such a foreign body has been in the stomach for some time without causing signs of gastric disease, but it can eventually cause problems. If repeat films, taken in 2 or 3 days, show that the material is not moving, surgical removal should be considered. This type of material is either too big to pass through the pylorus or has become attached to the stomach wall by eroding the mucosa or by penetrating the stomach wall. Bottle caps and rough stones can become embedded in the mucosa, and needles can penetrate the gastric wall. Bezoars of hair and plant material can become quite large before creating clinically recognizable problems. Animals that eat grass or have very fine, long hair and are always grooming themselves are good candidates for developing these large stomach masses. The bezoar is found when a barium series is peformed or if metallic materials become entrapped in the mass.

Large gastric foreign bodies, such as sticks, glass, and sharp metal objects, can become lodged in the stomach and create an emergency surgical problem when they rupture the wall. With this type of problem, the prognosis is guarded without early diagnosis and surgical intervention. It is difficult for the omentum and surrounding tissue to seal off severe contamination in the cranial abdominal cavity. Pyothorax can be a sequela of peritonitis in the cranial abdominal cavity. The pathophysiology of pyothorax is believed to be related to the carrying of material from the area of contamination, across the diaphragm, and into the thoracic cavity by the lymphatics in the omentum.[12]

Another emergency surgical situation due to the presence of large foreign bodies within the stomach is complete pyloric obstruction. The seriousness of this problem is due to the severe electrolyte and fluid disturbances it creates and the associated projectile vomition, which is difficult to control. The history of an animal with complete pyloric obstruction might include the eating of a large object, such as a rock, or the fact that a favorite ball is missing.

The presence of a type of gastric foreign body that causes partial pyloric obstruction or periodic complete obstruction is similar to the presence of a body that causes complete pyloric obstruction. This type of obstruction is more difficult to diagnose because the foreign body, for example a ball, rolls in and out of the pylorus. The animal may exhibit signs that vary from those of complete obstruction to no signs at all. Partial obstructions caused by non-radiopaque materials, such as wooden toys and baby nipples, markedly reduce the rate of pyloric outflow and mimic severe pyloric hypertrophy, except in the acute onset of signs. The animal is able to ingest liquids, but not bulk food. Because of the acute onset of signs, many diseases are included in the differential diagnosis. Radiographic contrast studies usually are required to interpret the often puzzling signs of partial or periodic complete obstruction.

A radiograph should be taken just prior to surgical intervention to ensure that the foreign body has not left the stomach through the gastrointestinal tract, in vomit, or by digestion.

A long incision into the body of the stomach is recommended to permit a thorough examination of the gastric pockets. This examination should be continued after the foreign material believed to have caused the problem has been located. It is not uncommon for an animal to have eaten a number of different objects, some of which are not radiopaque. The stomach mucosal wall should be inspected for erosions and hemorrhage. Internal palpation of the cardia and pylorus will often reveal unsuspected foreign material. Linear foreign bodies traversing the stomach cavity are commonly found along the surface of the lesser curvature. Secondary gastritis and pyloric dysfunction may be a postoperative problem.

The oral cavity and the intestines should always be closely inspected for additional foreign bodies, especially in cases of linear gastric foreign bodies. For instance, there may be more than one piece of string. Although string-like foreign materials are commonly found around the base of the tongue, they can be found caught on dental calculi and around the epiglottis. If the material has been present around the tongue for an extended period, it may cut through the frenulum and may be visualized only as it enters the esophagus. Similar circumstances exist when the material is attached to a needle that is buried in tissues of the oral cavity.[4, 5]

Although the stomach heals rapidly following an operation, the animal should be returned to its regular feeding schedule gradually. Bland soft foods divided into small quantities are recommended. The caloric requirements are greater for any animal following surgery and a good quality protein diet will enhance healing. Postoperative gastritis and associated vomition must be treated. Firm stomach contractions during vomition cause pain, which may lead to anorexia. The contractions may also disrupt healing. Vomition is also a sign of other diseases that can follow gastric surgery, such as pancreatitis and peritonitis. If vomition occurs after gastric foreign body removal, treatment should include proper nutrition and the administration of antiemetics, gastric coating agents, and parenteral fluids.

GASTRIC DILATATION-TORSION-VOLVULUS

Gastric dilatation-torsion-volvulus ranks among the most challenging surgical gastrointestinal problems encountered in clinical practice today. Much has been written regarding the clinical course of the disease, the investigative findings, and the variety of surgical techniques that are employed in its treatment, but to date, no one etiology has been agreed upon. The disease is believed by many workers to be the final stage in a variety of initiating problems. Investigators have made some progress toward understanding this disease, and an increased survival rate and decreased rate of recurrence have resulted.[5, 6, 9, 10, 14, 16, 18, 20, 22, 23, 24, 26, 29, 32, 33]

The clinical work of the past 10 years has produced valuable findings. Early decompression, with multiple trocarizations, if necessary to quickly relieve the severe gastric distention, provides time to stabilize the animal prior to surgery and helps to decrease some of the more serious postoperative problems.[21,24] The technique of creating a permanent gastropexy has been responsible for the tremendous decrease in recurrence rates. This procedure is probably the most important contribution to the treatment of the disease made in the past 10 years.[6,13,16,18,20,25,29,34] Awareness of the ventricular arrhythmias associated with this condition and their treatment has added new complexity to the management of gastric dilatation-torsion-volvulus and has also increased survival rates.[22,23,32] Recent reevaluation has led to cases that had previously been diagnosed only as gastric dilatation now being diagnosed as partial twisting of the stomach. In these cases, radiographic contrast studies are indicated once the animal is stable. If the stomach is found to be malpositioned, surgery is recommended on an elective basis. There is at present an increased awareness on the part of clinicians of the gastric dilatation-torsion-volvulus syndrome in animals of susceptible breeds that have recurring gastrointestinal problems. Gastric radiographic studies are used to demonstrate a malpositioned stomach before gastric dilatation torsion-volvulus develops. Surgery is recommended for these animals.

A major problem for the clinician is the continuing inability to prognose the outcome of individual cases. All prognoses must be somewhat guarded until a few days after surgery.

The pathophysiology of the gastric dilatation-torsion-volvulus complex is believed to be initiated by the gaseous distention of the stomach. This distention has devastating effects on systemic circulation. It decreases caudal vena caval blood flow and portal venous return, leading to a reduction in cardiac output. The continuation of these events results in a lower arterial blood pressure, thereby decreasing tissue perfusion. The stomach, besides being affected by poor perfusion, has a disorder of its own. The distention collapses the venous system and encourages twisting of the stomach. The pylorus moves cranially as the body of the stomach enlarges. As the distention of the stomach continues, the pylorus moves from the right side to the left, passing ventral to the stomach (Fig. 6–17*A* and *B*). The stomach's arteries are stretched and twisted as the organ distends. The arterial branches most severely damaged are the left gastro-

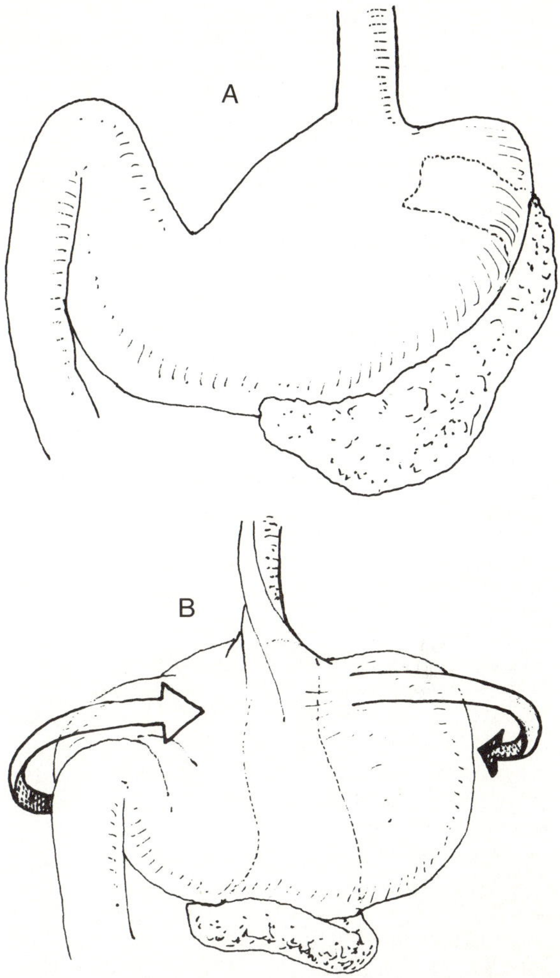

Figure 6–17. *A*, Normal position of the stomach as viewed at the surgical table. *B*, Direction of rotation of most gastric torsion as viewed at the surgical table.

epiploic arteries and the short gastric arteries, which are the major suppliers to the left half of the stomach in the area of the greater curvature.

The spleen is usually engorged with blood because its venous drainage is obstructed. As the stomach twists, the gastrosplenic ligaments are stretched. The spleen is pulled cranial and dorsal to the stomach. In some cases the spleen continues to twist on its pedicle, creating a splenic torsion. The vessels thrombose, further complicating the pathophysiological events.[21,22,23,24,26,32,33]

Treatment

Successful treatments, to date, have most often been associated with early diagnosis, vigorous therapeutic regimens, and close monitoring during the postoperative period. Accomplishing these goals with the desired level of consistency requires pre-planned, organized treatment.

The first goal of therapy is to relieve the gastric distention. It is desirable to attempt non-invasive techniques if the animal will permit them. If invasive techniques are employed to decompress the stomach, abdominal exploration is recommended as soon as the animal is stable. Radiographs for initial diagnostic work are not recommended until some decompression has been accomplished. The animal is often quiet, holds its neck slightly extended, and breathes through its open mouth. Its cranial abdomen bulges on both sides. Palpation reveals a large, firm, balloon-like mass filling the cranial abdomen.

Stomach Tube. A large-bore, firm, flexible stomach tube should be used to relieve gas pressure. To avoid rupturing the stomach, the tube should be pre-measured, so that its length equals the distance from the nose to the eleventh rib, and marked. An oral speculum or mouth gag will aid in starting the tube through the esophagus. Lubricants should be used on the stomach tube.

If the tube passes into the stomach, gas pressure should be relieved and the tube left in place until the stomach can be lavaged. The stomach is severely stretched; it will not regain tone or ability of eructation for hours or days.

The animal's vital signs should be closely monitored and the abdomen should be palpated to ensure that the spleen is also decreasing in size. If the animal is responding well, no further emergency treatment is required. If the tissue perfusion does not decrease, or the animal is oliguric, the implementation of shock therapy is indicated. Such therapy consists of the placement of a large-bore intravenous catheter for administration of lactated Ringer's solution, broad-spectrum intravenous antibiotics, sodium bicarbonate, and cortisone. An electrocardiogram should be done if the animal's condition does not improve, since a number of animals with this disease develop ventricular arrhythmias. If an arrhythmia is found, lidocaine is effective. It is also beneficial to obtain baseline data on the animal, including a complete hematological profile, a laboratory evaluation of electrolyte and blood gas concentrations, and a set of abdominal radiographs.[22]

After gastric distention has been relieved via stomach tube and the animal has stabilized, it should be evaluated with gastric contrast radiographs. If the stomach is in the proper position, the animal can be gradually put back onto an acceptable feeding program. If the stomach or pylorus is displaced, abdominal exploration as an elective procedure is recommended to correct the problem and to prevent recurrence of the disease.

Needle Trocarizations. If a stomach tube cannot be passed, needle trocarization should be tried to relieve the distention. A large-bore needle is used to tap the stomach through the abdominal wall. The needle should be removed and replaced when the gas flow slows or stops. Once the stomach size has been reduced, the stomach tube should once again be used to more completely decompress the stomach and flush out its contents, if possible.

The question of when to explore the abdomen continues to be highly debated. Decisions are based upon the facilities and personnel available, the treatment plans developed at the different hospitals, and the condition of the animal. The animals, whose physiological state quickly stabilizes after decompression and whose radiographs show a slight displacement of the stomach or the pylorus, are recommended for elective abdominal exploration as soon as possible.

Abdominal Surgery. Animals in which a stomach tube still cannot be passed following needle trocarization are recommended for emergency surgery as soon as they are physiologically stable. Emergency surgery is also suggested for those animals that do not adequately respond to therapy.

If the definition of elective surgery is surgery performed at the earliest convenient opportunity, i.e., during the hospital's or the surgeon's regular working hours, and emergency surgery is dictated by the patient's state, then the major points to be considered are that the animal should be stable before surgery and the length of time the procedure can be delayed.

Most animals can be adequately stabilized for surgery in 1 to 2 hours following decompression; many could be more completely stabilized if additional time were available.[25, 29] However, most cases are not benefited by delays extended beyond the time required for adequate stabilization.

1. Those in which the stomach is developing a necrotic area where it is supplied

by the left gastroepiploic and short gastric arteries.

2. Those in which varying degrees of splenic torsion have been sustained.

3. Those in which the arterial blood supply has been avulsed.

4. Those in which the stomach is maximally twisted.

Because it is difficult to predetermine the extent of injury that has occurred or that is occurring, surgical intervention as soon as stabilization is adequate is recommended for all these animals.

Anesthesia level should be monitored closely, and assisted respiration should be continued throughout the procedure. Fluids should be administered through large-diameter intravenous catheters at a rapid rate until tissue perfusion is good. Monitoring urine production, heart rate, mucous membrane refill time, and lung sounds for the development of pulmonary edema are all beneficial for determining fluid requirements. Acid-base balance and determination of electrolyte concentration improve the quality of patient assessment. The use of broad-spectrum intravenous antibiotics and intravenous corticosteroids has been shown to directly benefit treatment of shock.[26]

Sodium bicarbonate is given if the acid-base status of the animal requires it. Acid-base determinations are commonly not available, but past cases have shown that animals that are in extreme shock and that are not responding to treatment require about 0.5 mEq/lb intravenously every 30 minutes during the surgical procedure. Animals with gastric dilatation-torsion-volvulus that stabilized quickly have not needed the addition of bicarbonate to their treatment regimens.

The surgery should be well organized and accomplished in an efficient manner (see "Surgical Techniques"). Before the stomach can be repositioned more gases may have to be evacuated. This maneuver is easily accomplished by tapping the stomach with a needle attached to the suction apparatus. The stomach should then be replaced into proper position by grasping the gastric or pyloric tissue located along the left abdominal wall and pulling outward and toward the right abdominal wall.

Once the stomach has been repositioned, it and the spleen should be examined closely for thrombosis and necrosis. If the splenic vessels have been severely thrombosed or if the spleen is severely infarcted and has not diminished in size, a splenectomy is recommended. The splenectomy should not be performed unless the spleen is damaged beyond repair.

The stomach should be closely examined for necrotic areas. The area that most commonly becomes necrotic in cases of gastric volvulus is at or near the left side of the greater curvature in the region of the body and fundus. If necrotic tissue is present, a partial gastrectomy must be performed. (See "Partial Gastrectomy: Area of the body and fundus of the stomach along the greater curvature".)

Pyloroplasty has been recommended for a number of years. The Heineke-Mikulicz technique is acceptable, but the Fredet-Ramstedt technique is preferred if time is critical because it can be performed more quickly. (See "Pyloroplasty.")

The last step before closure of the abdominal incision is to create a permanent gastropexy between the ventral surface of the pyloric antrum and the right abdominal wall. The use of this procedure has nearly ended recurrence of the disease.

The right-side tube gastrostomy technique is currently recommended, because it has been a consistently successful means of promoting a permanent gastropexy that prevents disease recurrence. The short-term benefits of this procedure are that it prevents gaseous distention of the stomach postoperatively because the tube is left open. The degree of hemorrhage into the stomach can be monitored. If the animal is intractable and reluctant to eat postoperatively, fluids, nutrients, and medications can be administered via the tube. (See "Right-Side Tube Gastrostomy-Gastropexy.")

Immediate postoperative monitoring is critical. Body temperature, which commonly drifts below 94° F, must be raised. Assisted respiration should continue until the animal will no longer tolerate intubation. Intravenous fluid to replace fluid deficits and meet maintenance requirements should continue. Efforts to improve and maintain renal function should be intensified. Knowledge of the animal's blood gas and electrolyte status will greatly enhance the quality of therapy in the immediate postoperative period.[22]

The heart should be monitored electrocardiographically. Ventricular arrhythmias are prevalent and, if untreated, can be fatal. A general rule to follow is that if the heart rate remains above 150 beats per minute and pulse deficits are present, or electrocardiograms document regular runs of ventricular arrhythmias, treatment should be initiated. The initial drug of choice is intravenous lidocaine administered in bolus form at a dose of 2 to 4 mg/kg. This can be repeated once, if needed. If there is no response or if the arrhythmias return, a continuous infusion is begun. The recommended dosage for lidocaine infusion is 30 to 70 μg/kg/minute. This dosage is administered in intravenous fluids. As a rule of thumb, an animal receiving maintenance fluids of 30 ml/lb/day intravenously needs about 20 to 30 ml of 2% lidocaine* in each 500 ml bottle of its maintenance fluids. Lidocaine is neurotoxic. If toxic signs such as seizure activity occur, Valium† is the drug of choice. The lidocaine is discontinued and restarted at a lower dose, after the animal is stable. If a constant infusion is started, it should be maintained for a minimum of 12 hours after the arrhythmias have ceased. Not all arrhythmias respond to this therapy. If they do not, underlying heart disease may be present, and an alternative therapy must be instituted.

Postoperatively, no food or water should be offered for 24 to 48 hours, depending upon the severity of the animal's condition. Monitoring electrolyte concentration is important, since severe imbalances do arise. Oral feeding is resumed gradually, starting with small amounts of water every few hours and gradually including a good quality protein broth. If the animal is stable and tolerates the food, it should receive its total caloric requirement in small quantities offered four to eight times a day by the third or fourth day. Once the animal starts to eat and drink, intravenous fluid should be discontinued. Antibiotics should be continued 7 to 14 days after surgery, depending on the animal's condition. The gastrostomy tube, if used to create the permanent gastropexy, can be removed 5 to 7 days postoperatively.

It is recommended that when the animal goes home the owner continue to feed it good quality, easily digested foods three to four times per day. It is recommended that the animal never return to a once-a-day feeding schedule, and that the owner stay with one brand of food and regulate the animal's exercise to avoid heavy feeding and watering just before or just after vigorous activity.

Some animals are presented with a history and physical appearance that are similar to those of gastric dilatation-torsion-volvulus complex, but passage of the stomach tube does not relieve the distention. Severe intestinal obstruction, such as that caused by intestinal volvulus or herniation of the intestine through a rent in the mesentery, is a possibility. Confirmation of the disease is made on the basis of the clinical signs of acute shock, radiographic indication of intestinal blockage, palpable fluid and gas-filled loops of bowel, and a rising packed cell volume with severe acidosis. Immediate surgical intervention and aggressive endotoxic shock therapy are required.

PYLORIC MUSCLE DYSFUNCTION

Clinically, pyloric muscle dysfunction is most commonly evidenced by delayed emptying of the stomach and projectile vomiting.

The surgical procedures designed to alleviate the problem are called pyloroplasties. The two most commonly used pyloroplasty techniques in veterinary medicine today are the Fredet-Ramstedt procedure and the Heineke-Mikulicz procedure. Both pyloroplasty techniques enlarge the diameter of the lumen of the pylorus and significantly decrease function of the sphincter-like muscle. The loss of function of the pyloric sphincter from these pyloroplasties appears to cause little, if any, problem for the animal.[4, 17]

Pyloric dysfunction, for which surgery should be considered, is divided into three general categories, none of which is well documented in the veterinary literature.

The first and most frequently discussed type of pyloric dysfunction is congenital pyloric hypertrophy. Whether the condition is congenital, inherited, or developmental remains to be discovered. This type of pyloric dysfunction is manifested as animals are being weaned and placed on solid food. The usual history is a ravenous appetite with projectile vomiting at a regular interval within 1 hour following feeding. These animals may be weakened because of the significant electrolyte disturbances from the chronic vomition and nutritional deficits. Initial treatment should be aimed at stabilizing the animal and supporting its electrolyte and nutritional needs. This is best ac-

*Lidocaine 2%, Abbott Laboratories, North Chicago, IL.

†Valium, Roche Laboratories, Nutley, NJ.

complished by separating the animal from its litter-mates and feeding it small amounts of liquid slowly and frequently in order to re-establish nutritional and electrolyte needs. Most of these animals can retain liquid but not solid foods. Solid foods should again be started once the animal has regained its strength; this process usually takes a few days. The animal should frequently be offered small amounts of food, and it should remain separated from its litter-mates. Surgery is not necessary if solid food is tolerated. Radiographs of the stomach using contrast material mixed with food should be taken if food is not tolerated. Delayed gastric emptying and an abnormally large stomach cavity will be present in pyloric stenosis. A pyloroplasty is indicated if this diagnosis is confirmed. At surgery, the pylorus will be firm and thickened. A Fredet-Ramstedt pyloromyotomy is recommended. Postoperatively, the animal should be returned to small, multiple feedings. The animal usually has no problem retaining solid foods immediately after surgery.

The second category of pyloric dysfunction is similar to the first in that it is manifested by projectile vomiting, usually within 1 hour of eating, ravenous appetite, and chronic weight loss. The vomiting after eating develops gradually. The affected animals range in age from young adults to the very old. They are in good general health, and laboratory data are usually normal. The history of vomiting after eating can be reproduced in the hospital setting. Radiographs of the stomach utilizing contrast material mixed with food show a greatly enlarged stomach with prolonged and often incomplete gastric emptying.

A Fredet-Ramstedt pyloromyotomy or a Heineke-Mikulicz pyloroplasty is recommended. The pylorus is usually large and firm. The circular muscle layer is the location of the problem. When cut, the layer will be many times its normal thickness. A biopsy of the cut muscle should be done to confirm the diagnosis and rule out the possibility of neoplasia.

The stomach, and particularly the pyloric outflow tract, should be palpated for increased thickness and polyp-like masses. It is possible that the circular muscle of the pylorus has thickened secondary to a luminal obstruction arising from the gastric mucosa. This development is more likely to be seen in animals that have confirmed cases of chronic gastritis and in older animals that may have gastric cancer. It is for these reasons, and because it permits visualization of the pyloric and gastric mucosae, that the Heineke-Mikulicz technique is preferred. If the Fredet-Ramstedt technique is employed, a small gastrotomy near the pyloric antrum will permit palpation of the gastric and pyloric mucosae. If the gastric mucosa is obstructing the pylorus, it should be resected. Resection is easily accomplished by excising redundant mucosa. Closure is with an absorbable suture material in a continuous pattern.

The postoperative recovery from pyloric stenosis is dramatic. The animal usually stops vomiting immediately, and weight gain is rapid. The animal should be kept on multiple, small feedings to permit reduction of stomach size and regulation of gastric secretion. There have been no reports of restenosis following the operation.

The third category of pyloric dysfunction is believed to be a problem in animals that have gastric dilatation-torsion-volvulus. The existence of this type of pyloric dysfunction has not been unquestionably confirmed. These animals usually do not show muscular hypertrophy as do the animals in the first two categories. It has been shown that a gastric dilation can cause gastric volvulus.[21] Therefore, if the pylorus did not function properly, gastric distention could occur. Other studies have shown that animals with gastric volvulus treated by pyloroplasties had a better prognosis.[34] It is hoped that as additional research is performed, the role the pylorus plays in the gastric dilatation-torsion-volvulus complex will become more evident. At present, a pyloroplasty is performed because it is believed to help and because it is not known to cause harm. Another reason for performing the technique in gastric dilatation-torsion-volvulus cases is that right-side permanent gastropexy techniques may inhibit normal gastric emptying into the duodenum.

CHRONIC RECURRENT GASTROESOPHAGEAL INTUSSUSCEPTIVE HIATAL HERNIA

Hiatal hernia is not a common clinical diagnosis in veterinary medicine, but it does

occur in dogs and cats. This condition is well described in veterinary pathology texts as an agonal entity. It is a common clinical diagnosis in humans, in whom it is well documented.[5, 27, 31]

The term hiatal hernia refers to any tissues that herniate through the esophageal hiatus of the diaphragm. In the canine and feline this condition is seen as an intraesophageal herniation of the stomach.[11] It is usually diagnosed because of its progressive chronicity of recurrence. This hernia is not associated with trauma; it is believed to be a developmental disease.

The defect is the loss or the stretching of a segment of mucle tissue in the diaphragm that surrounds the esophageal hiatus as a muscle sling. The diaphragm should be in contact with the esophagus and cardia of the stomach. When the muscle segment is missing, the fascial tissue continues uninterruptedly as a replacement. The most common site for a loss of muscle tissue is in the supraesophageal region, where the muscle separates as it encircles the esophagus.[28]

The most common sign is recurrent vomition with increasing frequency that is associated with feeding. Animals vomit daily for days or weeks. Their conditions may improve and then worsen again. There is no breed or sex predilection reported, but hiatal hernias do appear to be more common in cats. The short-haired cats with chronic vomition should be suspected of being af-

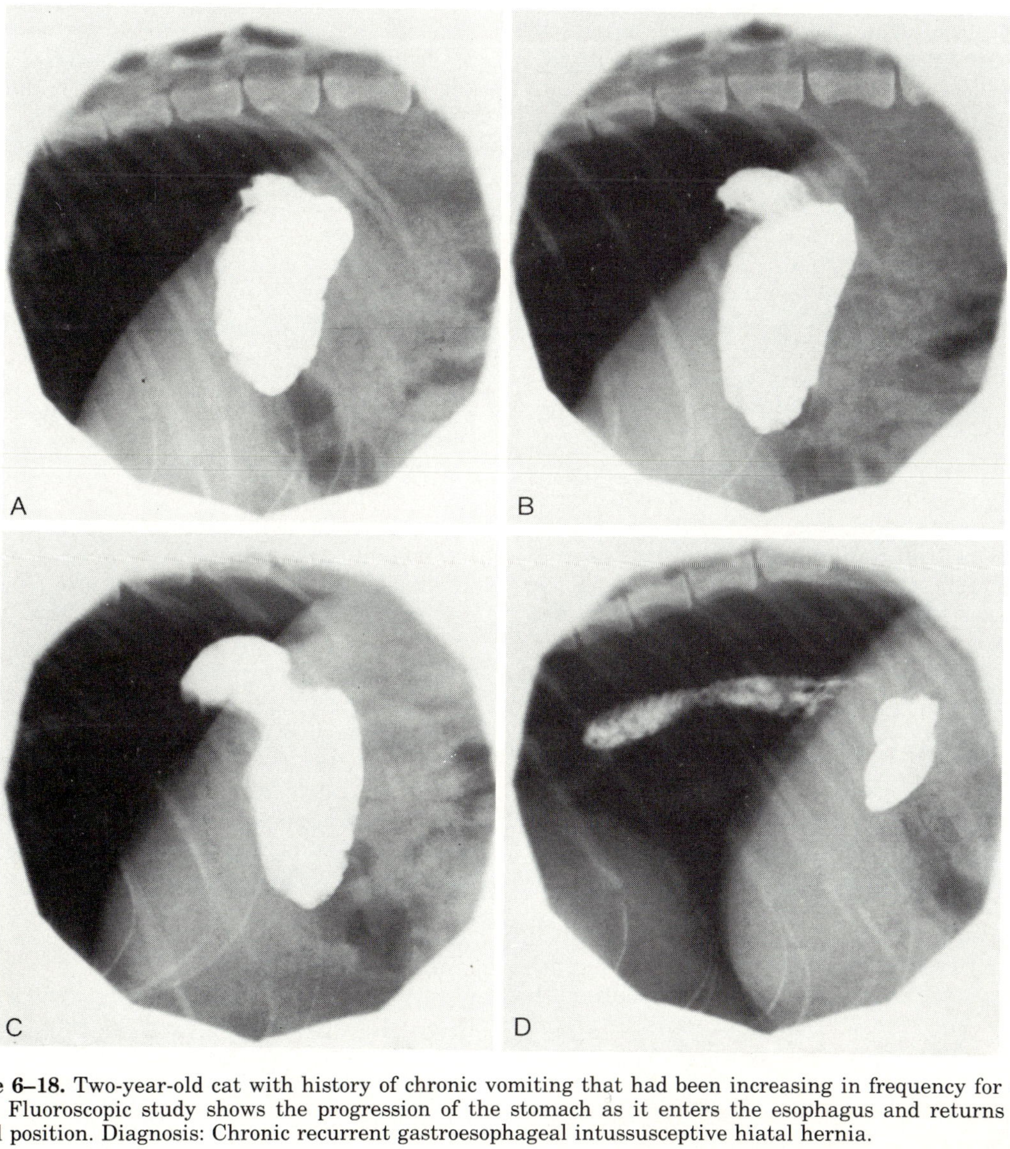

Figure 6–18. Two-year-old cat with history of chronic vomiting that had been increasing in frequency for 4 to 6 weeks. Fluoroscopic study shows the progression of the stomach as it enters the esophagus and returns to its normal position. Diagnosis: Chronic recurrent gastroesophageal intussusceptive hiatal hernia.

fected. Mixed breeds of both species have been diagnosed with the disease. In the dog, it has also been diagnosed in a wide variety of purebreds of all sizes, ranging from collies to Chihuahuas.[1, 2, 28]

The diagnosis of chronic recurrent gastroesophageal intussusceptive hiatal hernia is difficult to make without abdominal exploration. The history is fairly consistent in all cases. The diagnostic work-up does no more than to rule out other conditions that are more easily observed, such as gastritis. Radiographic contrast studies can demonstrate the disease if the rugal folds of the stomach protrude into the esophagus during the study and then seconds later drop back into a normal position (Fig. 6–18). Visualization of the stomach herniating into the esophagus can be improved by filling the stomach with contrast material and then inducing vomition (Fig. 6–19). Suspending the animal head down on an acutely angled radiographic table, as is done in humans in the search for the herniating tissue, is also helpful.

Non-surgical means of treatment are based upon methods that are useful in humans. They include changing the animal's diet to more easily digested foods, limiting roughage, having the animal feed and drink in an upright position, and feeding it small meals.

The animal is usually in good health because it is able to maintain its nutritional needs. If non-surgical methods can control or reduce the frequency or severity of the problem, many owners are pleased to choose that route.

Surgery is recommended if the diagnosis has been confirmed radiographically and if the repeated vomition cannot be adequately controlled by non-surgical means. Surgery is often performed as an abdominal exploration for diagnostic purposes, since all diagnostic tests may demonstrate a normal animal that continues to have repeated episodes of vomition. Abdominal exploration performed on an animal in good health should be a low-risk procedure that could be of significant diagnostic and therapeutic value.

When an abdominal exploration for chronic recurrent vomition is performed, the liver, biliary system, pancreas, pylorus, stomach, spleen, and esophageal hiatus should be closely examined.

In cases of chronic recurrent gastroesophageal intussusceptive hiatal hernia, the stomach's ventral serosal surface, near the junction between the fundus and body, will have an area of increased serosal vascularity. The diagnosis is confirmed by invaginating or herniating the site of increased vascularity into the esophagus with the index and middle fingers. With the stomach held inside the esophagus, the sphincter-like pressure of the wall of the diaphragm against its junction with the esophagus can be felt. This muscular wall should be palpated as a continuous encirclement around the esophagus and should permit the esophagus to dilate when the fingers are spread apart. If a muscular defect in the diaphragm exists around its junction with the esophagus, a gap will be felt in the area of muscular encirclement.[28]

If the defect is found, plication of the esophageal hiatus's area of weakness and cardia gastropexy are recommended (see "Surgical Techniques").

Postoperatively, the animal should be started on small, multiple feedings and

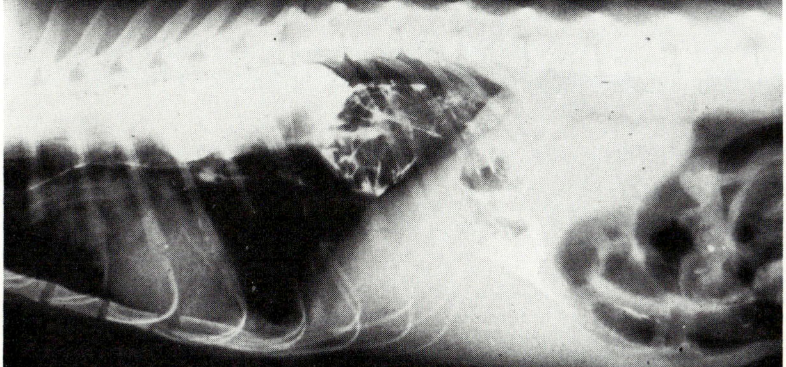

Figure 6–19. Mature cat with a chronic history of increasingly frequent vomiting. Lateral radiograph taken as the cat vomited. Diagnosis: Chronic recurrent gastroesophageal intussusceptive hiatal hernia.

gradually returned to its regular feeding habits. Vomition in the immediate postoperative period is to be avoided to prevent tearing and breakdown of the plicating sutures. In some animals, the use of antiemetic drugs and topical treatment for secondary esophagitis, if present, may be required.

References

1. Ackerman N, Millman T: Esophageal hiatal hernia in the dog. Vet Radiol 23:107, 1982.
2. Alexander JW, Hoffer RE, MacDonald JM et al: Hiatal hernia in the dog: A case report and review of the literature. J Am Anim Hosp Assoc 11:793, 1975.
3. Andersen PH, Woodward ER: Gastrostomy, an evaluation of the Dragstedt method. Am J Surg 124:581, 1972.
4. Arnoczky SP, Ryan WW: Gastrotomy and pyloroplasty. Symposium on surgical techniques in small animal practice. Vet Clin North Am 5:343, 1975.
5. Bellenger CR, Archibald J: Stomach. *In* Archibald J, Catcott ES (eds): *Canine and Feline Surgery,* Vol I. American Veterinary Publications, Inc., Santa Barbara, 105, 1984.
6. Betts CW, Wingfield WI, Rosin E: Permanent gastropexy—as a prophylactic measure against gastric volvulus. J Am Anim Hosp Assoc 12:77, 1976.
7. Bohning RH, DeHoff WD, McElhinney A, Hofstra PC: Pharyngostomy for maintenance of the anorectic animal. J Am Vet Med Assoc 156:611, 1970.
8. Crowe DT: Closure of abdominal incisions using a continuous polypropylene suture: Clinical experience in 550 dogs and cats. Vet Surg 7:24, 1978.
9. DeHoff WD, Greene RW: Gastric dilatation-complex. *In* Kirk RW (ed): *Current Veterinary Therapy V*. Philadelphia, W. B. Saunders Company, p. 733, 1974.
10. DeHoff WD, Greene RW: Gastric dilatation and the gastric torsion complex. Vet Clin North Am 2:141–152, 1972.
11. Dorland's Illustrated Medical Dictionary, 26th ed. Philadelphia, W. B. Saunders Company, 1981.
12. Evans HE, Christensen GC (eds): *Miller's Anatomy of the Dog,* 2nd ed. Philadelphia, W. B. Saunders Company, p. 467, 1979.
13. Fallah AM, Lumb WV, Nelson AW, et al: Circumcostal gastropexy in the dog. A preliminary study. Vet Surg 11:1, 1982.
14. Gupta CD, Gupta SC, Agarwal VK: Area distribution of gastric arteries in dog's stomach. Anat Anz 443:490, 1978.
15. Harkins HN, Nyhus LM: *Surgery of the Stomach and Duodenum,* 2nd ed. Boston, Little, Brown & Company, pp. 555–590, 1969.
16. Johnson RG, Barrus J, Greene RW: Gastric dilatation-volvulus: Recurrence rate following tube gastrostomy. J Am Anim Hosp Assoc 20:1, 1984.
17. Larsen LH, Bellenger CR: Stomach and small intestines. *In* Archibald JA (ed): *Canine Surgery*. American Veterinary Publications, Inc., Santa Barbara, 1974.
18. Levine SH, Caywood DD: Biomechanical evaluation of gastropexy techniques in the dog. Vet Surg 12:166, 1983.
19. Markowitz J, Archibald J, Downe HG: *Experimental Surgery*. Baltimore, Williams & Wilkins, p. 123, 1964.
20. Mattiesen DT: The gastric dilatation-volvulus complex: Medical and surgical considerations. J Am Anim Hosp Assoc 19:925, 1983.
21. Merkley DR, Howard DR, Eyster GE: Experimentally induced acute gastric dilatation in the dog: Cardiopulmonary effects. J Am Anim Hosp Assoc 12:143–148, 1976.
22. Muir WW: Acid-base and electrolyte disturbances in dogs with gastric dilatation-volvulus. J Am Vet Med Assoc 181:229, 1982.
23. Muir WW, Lipowitz AJ: Cardiac dysrhythmias associated with gastric dilatation-volvulus in the dog. J Am Vet Med Assoc 172:683, 1978.
24. Orton EC, Muir WW: Hemodynamics during experimental gastric dilatation-volvulus in dogs. Am J Vet Res 44:1512, 1983.
25. Parks JL, Greene RW: Tube gastrostomy for the treatment of gastric volvulus. J Am Anim Hosp Assoc 12:168, 1976.
26. Rawlings CA, Wingfield WE, Betts CW: Shock therapy and anesthetic management in gastric dilation-volvulus. J Am Anim Hosp Assoc 12:158, 1976.
27. Sabiston DC (ed): *Textbook of Surgery,* 10th ed. Philadelphia, W. B. Saunders Company, p. 817, 1972.
28. Schmidt DH, DeHoff WD: Diagnosis and surgical technique for repair of chronic recurrent gastroesophageal intussusceptive hiatal hernia in the dog and cat. Kleint Prax 28:399, 1984.
29. Walshaw R, Johnston DE: Treatment of gastric dilatation-volvulus by gastric decompression and patient stabilization before major surgery. J Am Anim Hosp Assoc 12:162, 1976.
30. Watrous B: Esophageal disease. *In* Ettinger SJ (ed): *Textbook of Veterinary Internal Medicine,* 2nd ed. Philadelphia, W. B. Saunders Company, p. 1220, 1983.
31. Welch CE: *Surgery of the Stomach and Duodenum,* 4th ed. Chicago, Year Book Medical Publishers Inc., 1966.
32. Wingfield WE, Twedt DC, Moore RW et al: Acid-base and electrolyte values in dogs with acute gastric dilatation-volvulus. J Am Vet Med Assoc 180:1070, 1982.
33. Wingfield WE, Betts CW, Rawlings CA: Pathophysiology associated with gastric dilatation-volvulus in the dog. J Am Anim Hosp Assoc 12:136, 1976.
34. Wingfield WE, Betts CW, Greene RW: Operative techniques and recurrence rates associated with gastric volvulus in the dog. J Small Anim Pract 16:427, 1976.

CHAPTER

7

Medical Diseases of the Small Intestine

ROBERT T. FRANKLIN
BRENT D. JONES
BERNARD F. FELDMAN

Anatomy of the Small Intestine

The small intestine is the longest part of the gastrointestinal system. The average length of the small intestine is five times the length of the body.[92] It is divided into three portions: (1) the duodenum, (2) the jejunum, and (3) the ileum. The duodenum begins at the pylorus and is approximately 10 per cent of the small bowel. It receives the contents from the stomach, common bile duct, and pancreatic ducts. The *descending* part lies to the right of the median plane where it is usually in direct contact with the parietal peritoneum. Caudally the duodenum turns on itself, forming the caudal duodenal flexure. It continues toward the stomach as the *ascending* part. Endoscopic examinations can be made to the caudal duodenal flexure. The middle portion is the jejunum, which is the longest part of the small intestine and fills the mid-abdomen. The terminal portion of the small intestine is the ileum, which terminates at the ileocolic orifice.

The cranial mesenteric artery is the major source of blood for the small intestine. The cranial aspect of the duodenum receives its blood supply from the gastroduodenal artery, which originates from the common hepatic branch of the celiac artery. Venous drainage is by the cranial and caudal mesenteric vein and the gastroduodenal vein into the portal vein and is filtered by the liver. Intestinal lymphatic vessels are usually found with the intestinal arteries and veins. They drain into the mesenteric lymph nodes, which are drained by the intestinal lymphatic trunks. These trunks form the cisterna chyli, the dilated caudal portion of the thoracic duct, which finally empties into the venous circulation.

Innervation of the small intestine is by the autonomic nervous system, which is divided into extrinsic and intrinsic systems. The vagus (parasympathetic) and the splanchnic nerves (sympathetic) supply the extrinsic innervation. The myenteric and submucosal plexuses are involved in intrinsic innervation of the small intestines. The myenteric plexuses are located between the circular and longitudinal muscle layers, whereas the submucosal plexuses are located throughout the submucosa.

The intestinal wall is divided into seven layers: (1) mucosal columnar epithelium, (2) basement membrane, (3) lamina propria, (4) muscularis mucosae, (5) submucosa, (6) circular and longitudinal muscle layer, and (7) serosa (Fig. 7–1). The mucosa is folded and has villi projecting into the lumen (Fig. 7–2). The villi are lined with a single layer of specialized cells that have microvilli on their luminal surface. This microvillous border is coated with a glycoprotein, called glycocalyx (Fig. 7–3). The glycocalyx is continuously synthesized by the Golgi apparatus of the epithelial cells, transported to the microvillous surface, and eventually shed into the lumen. The microvillous plasma membrane and its glycocalyx constitute the digestive-absorptive unit. Several enzymes such as disaccharidases, aminopeptidases,

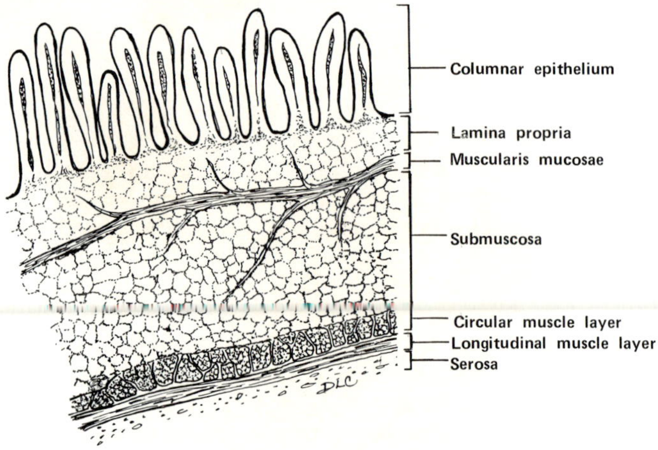

Figure 7–1. Cross-section of the small intestine demonstrating the various layers.

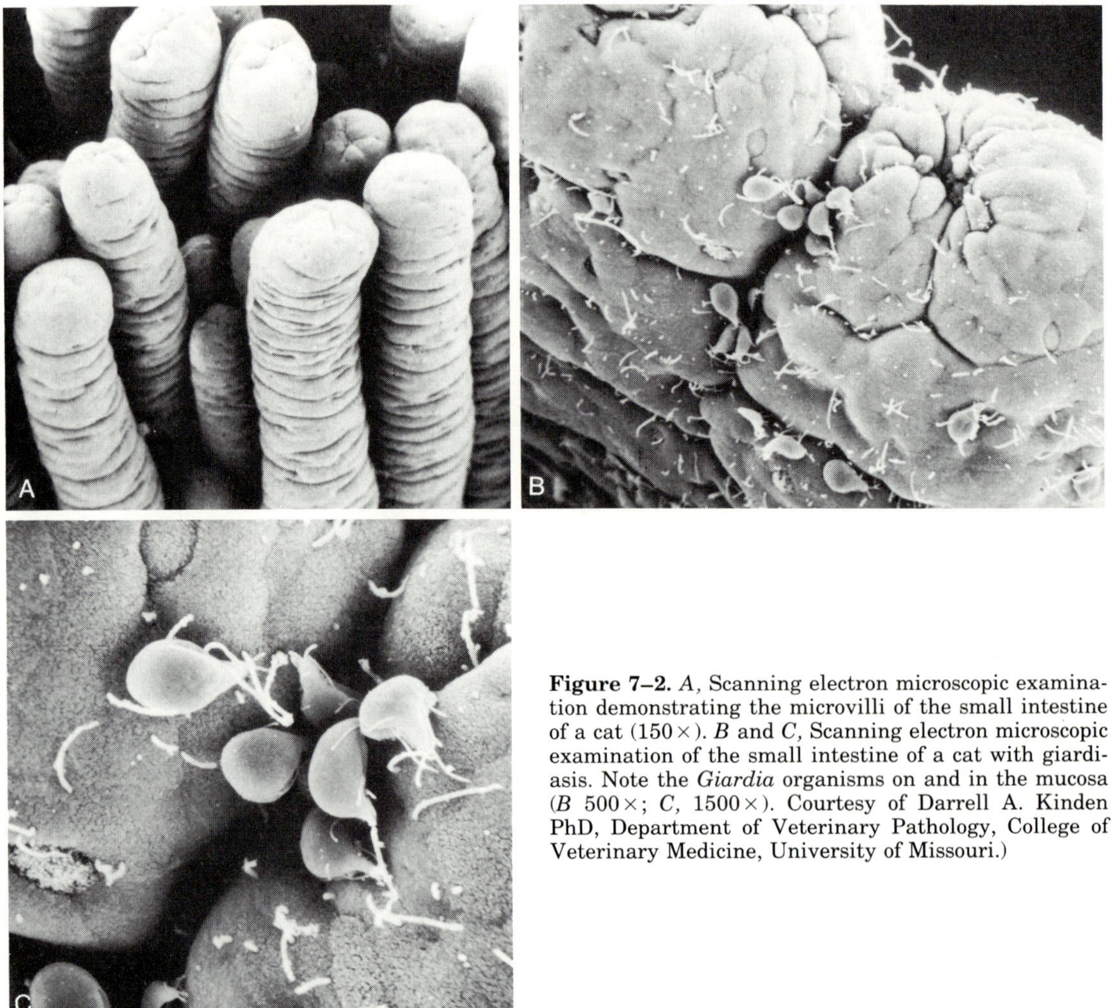

Figure 7–2. *A,* Scanning electron microscopic examination demonstrating the microvilli of the small intestine of a cat (150×). *B* and *C,* Scanning electron microscopic examination of the small intestine of a cat with giardiasis. Note the *Giardia* organisms on and in the mucosa (*B* 500×; *C,* 1500×). Courtesy of Darrell A. Kinden PhD, Department of Veterinary Pathology, College of Veterinary Medicine, University of Missouri.)

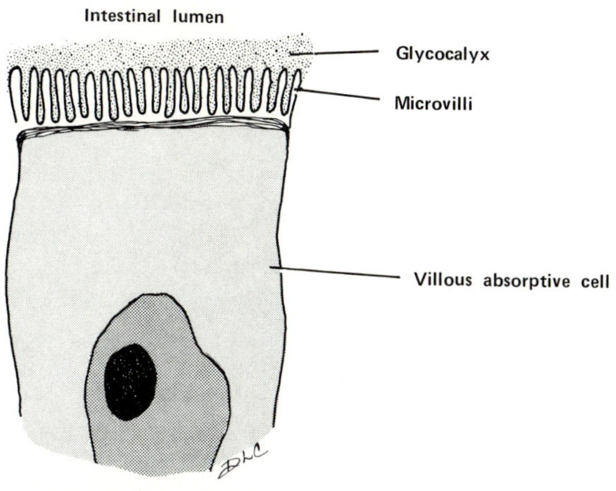

Figure 7–3. The microvillous border is coated with a glycoprotein called glycocalyx. The microvillous plasma membrane and its glycocalyx constitute the digestive-absorptive unit.

and dipeptidases are located within this unit. The active transport of glucose, galactose, and amino acids is mediated by receptors and carriers that are localized to this region. Surface of the villi and linings of the crypts are covered primarily with five types of cells: (1) the enterocyte (columnar cell), whose functions are digestion and absorption and which is the most populous cell; (2) the goblet cell, which secretes mucus; (3) Paneth's cell, whose function is suspected to be secretory; (4) the enteroendocrine cell, whose function is to secrete hormones after chemical stimuli; and (5) the undifferentiated crypt cell.

There is a constant turnover of intestinal epithelial cells. Normally the undifferentiated cells of the crypts replicate, and the cells produced migrate up the villi (Fig. 7–4). These cells are eventually extruded at the tips of the villi. As these cells migrate up the villi they undergo morphologic and biochemical functional maturation to become villous absorptive cells, goblet cells, or Paneth's cells. This process takes from two to six days,[120] depending on the species and villous length. Epithelial cell turnover time can be accelerated or prolonged by various factors. Intestinal disease and surgical resection can increase cellular turnover. Uremia, radiation, chemotherapeutic agents that inhibit DNA synthesis, and food withdrawal decrease cellular turnover times. Cellular turnover is faster in animals with a normal flora than in gnotobiotic animals.[120]

Intestinal Immunology

Considerable attention has been centered on the immunological system of the small bowel. Experimental studies of the structure and function of lymphoid tissue in the intestine of animals and of immunodeficiency disorders in animals have emphasized the importance of the gut as a lymphoid organ.[136]

Before birth, T cells predominate in the aggregated lymphoid tissues such as Peyer's patches, but after birth, following antigenic stimulation by ingested viral, bacterial, and dietary antigens, B cells proliferate in germinal centers. Antigen and immunologically competent cells come into apposition, probably through specialized cells overlying the Peyer's patches. From here, IgA precursor cells migrate to mesenteric lymph nodes, enter the thoracic duct, and via the blood circulation, home selectively to the gut mucosa. During migration, they develop the capacity to produce IgA. In the lamina propria over 90 per cent of lymphoid cells are IgA-secreting plasma cells. Two units of monomeric IgA produced by plasma cells are linked to a glycoprotein, the secretory component, by the J-chain to form secretory IgA. The secretory component facilitates the transport of secretory IgA into the lumen and protects it from proteolysis. Secretory IgA is involved in local immunity, particularly with respect to viruses and bacteria, and may help to regulate antigen absorp-

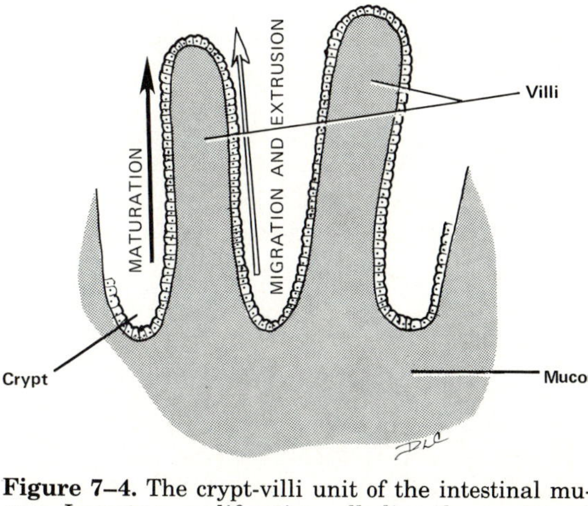

Figure 7–4. The crypt-villi unit of the intestinal mucosa. Immature proliferative cells line the crypts and mature digestive-absorptive cells line the villi. The crypt cells proliferate to supply new cells that migrate onto the villi.

tion. The precise mechanisms are not clear but probably include a non-specific effect as well as specific local antibody production. IgM can combine with the secretory component and has the capacity to compensate for IgA in selective IgA deficiency. IgA in secretions may be important in the control of parasitic infections. A cell-mediated immune response, as well as IgG and IgM circulating antibody, operates once antigen has crossed the mucosal surface.[3, 136, 146]

Although an understanding of these basic immune mechanisms in the gut may provide insight into the pathogenesis of some of the disorders to be discussed, there is little evidence that qualitative or quantitative immunological defects are operative.[146]

The gastrointestinal tract is often affected in the severe immunodeficiency disorders (for example, combined immunodeficiency of Arab foals), but these are rare in small animals. Gastritis and small intestinal abnormalities may occur in humans with spontaneous variable hypogammaglobulinemia or selective IgA deficiency. The cause of malabsorption in these patients is complex, but bacterial overgrowth and infection with *Giardia lamblia* are often implicated. Selective IgA deficiency may be associated with a true gluten-sensitive enteropathy but not with bacterial overgrowth, presumably because of compensation by IgM.[146]

Alpha-chain disease in man, a neoplastic disorder in which there is lymphoid proliferation involving the IgA secretory system, may provide interesting information regarding the role of antigenic stimulation from the gut in the development of neoplasia.[3]

Physiology of the Small Intestine

The primary function of the small intestine is the assimilation of food. This process involves digestion and absorption and is accomplished by the secretion of enzymes into the gut lumen, mucosal brush border breakdown of ingesta, and absorption into the blood and lymph circulation. These processes are enhanced by several properties of the small intestine: (1) the looped and folded, hollow tubular structure; (2) the folds and villi of the mucosal lining; and (3) the specialized cells that have microvillous borders. In general the assimilation process involves three phases: luminal, mucosal, and delivery. The luminal phase includes the digestive activity within the lumen of the gastrointestinal tract. The mucosal phase involves the digestive activities of the mucosal cell surface, absorption of the nutrient into the mucosal cell, and any processing of the nutrient within the mucosal cell. The delivery phase includes the transfer of nutrients from the mucosal cell to the blood.

Of the three classes of nutrients—carbohydrates, protein, and fats—digestion and absorption of fats is the most complex. This process is also very efficient. Approximately 95 per cent of ingested fat is absorbed from the intestinal lumen.[120] This is true even for patients that are on a high-fat diet. Most of the remaining fat in feces is due to desquamated colonic cells, colonic secretions, and bacterial synthesis.

Fatty acids are composed of three chains of triglycerides on a glycerol backbone. The normal diet contains mostly long-chain triglycerides, 16 to 18 carbons in length. A small amount contains medium-chain triglycerides (6 to 12 carbons). The mechanisms of assimilation of long- and medium-chain triglycerides differ; both will be discussed.

Fat digestion takes place entirely in the small intestine. The stomach's only role is in regulation of the gastric emptying of fat into the duodenum, which is prolonged compared to other food stuffs. This action is influenced by neurohormones. Once fats reach the duodenum, cholecystokinin (CCK) is released. CCK stimulates pancreatic enzyme secretion and causes contraction of the gallbladder allowing both lipase and bile to enter the duodenum. The luminal phase of fat assimilation involves emulsification, hydrolysis, and micellarization. Emulsification occurs due to the normal motility patterns of the stomach and intestinal tract. Fat hydrolysis is aided by bile salts, which emulsify the intraluminal fats, thus aiding in hydrolyzation of triglycerides by lipase, as lipase activity is best at a water-oil interface. However, lipolysis can take place without the presence of bile salts. Lipase splits off the two alpha fatty acids, leaving only the beta fatty acid attached to the glycerol backbone, a betamonoglyceride (Fig. 7–5).

After hydrolysis takes place, micellarization occurs. This happens also with the aid of bile salts. Bile salts are amphipathic, having hydrophobic and hydrophilic portions. Once a significant concentration of bile salts is reached, they form spheres. In these spheres the hydrophilic region faces toward the luminal water and the hydrophobic region faces toward the center of the sphere. In the center of the sphere, fatty acids, monoglycerides, and the fat-soluble vitamins (A, D, E, and K) are found in a solubilized state. These spheres are called micelles. Their purpose is to present the fatty acids, monoglycerides, and fat-soluble vitamins to the intestinal epithelium for absorption. When the micelles reach the epithelial cells, disaggregation occurs. The fatty acids and monoglycerides are passively diffused across the cell membrane, while the bile salts remain in the lumen. In the cell the fatty acids and monoglycerides are re-esterified back into triglycerides. The bile acids are eventually reabsorbed in the terminal ileum. Approximately 95 per cent of the bile salts are reabsorbed during each cycle of the enterohepatic circulation.

After the triglycerides are re-formed, they are aggregated with lipoproteins, cholesterol, and phospholipid to form chylomicrons. The chylomicrons exit the cell into the lamina propria and are transported by the central lacteals of the villi to the draining lymphatics. This is aided by the pumping action of the smooth muscle found in the villi. After the chylomicrons reach the draining lymphatics, they are transported to the thoracic duct and eventually to the venous circulation, where they may cause postprandial lipemia.

The events just discussed occur in the assimilation of long-chain triglycerides, the predominant fat in the diet. As mentioned earlier, digestion and absorption of medium-chain triglycerides differs from that of long-chain triglycerides. Pancreatic lipase cleaves off all three fatty acids, leaving a minimal monoglyceride. Medium-chain fatty acids form micelles more readily, although micellarization may not be necessary, since they are more water soluble than long-chain fatty acids. Approximately 30 per cent of all medium-chain triglycerides can be absorbed without lipolysis.[121] Once absorbed by the epithelial cell, the medium-chain fatty acids leave the cell "as is," enter the venous capillary system of the villi, and are then transported to the liver via the portal system.

The process of digestion and absorption of fat is so complex that its assimilation is easily affected by other factors. Further, the cells at the tip of the villus are highly specialized for fat assimilation and are also extremely susceptible to mucosal injury. These are possible reasons why fecal fat excretion is a good indicator of malassimilation.

Carbohydrates are absorbed as monosaccharides. Dietary forms of carbohydrates include disaccharides (sucrose, lactose) and polysaccharides (starch, glycogen).

When ingesta enter the duodenum, CCK is released, stimulating secretion of pancreatic enzymes. One of the pancreatic enzymes is amylase, which cleaves starch into several oligosaccharides (maltose, maltotriose, and two dextrins). The resulting oligosaccharidases and the dietary disaccharides are further digested to monosaccharides (glucose, fructose, and galactose) by oligosaccharidases (for example, maltase, isomaltase, sucrase, lactase, amyloglucosides), found at the brush border. The monosaccharides are then absorbed by active transport mechanisms.

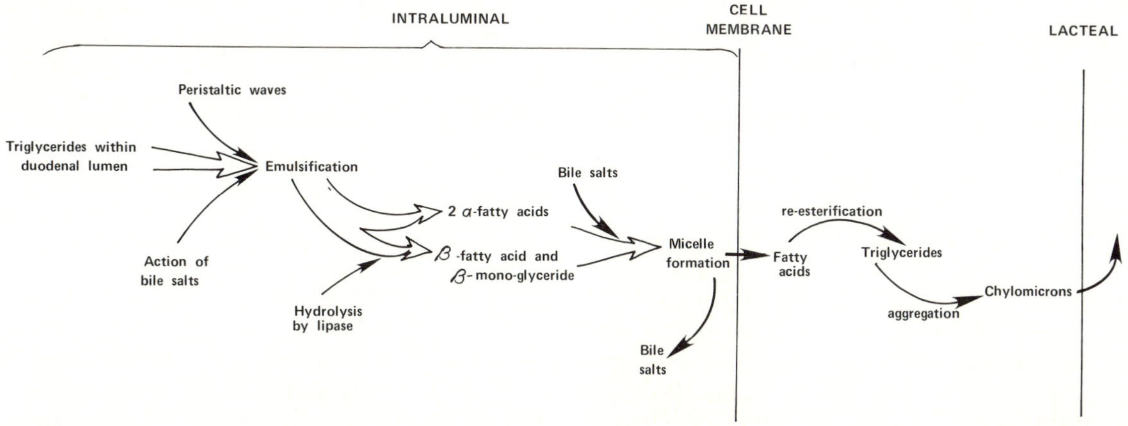

Figure 7–5. Diagrammatic representation of the major steps in the digestion and absorption of dietary fat.

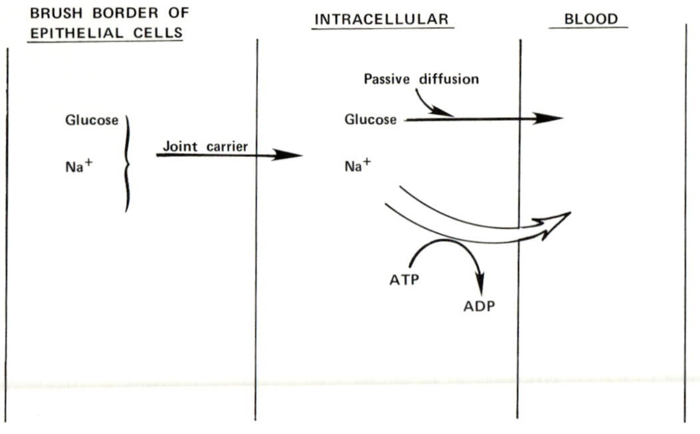

Figure 7–6. Carrier-mediated Na^+-coupled transport of glucose. The glucose molecule and Na^+ are bound to the joint mobile carrier at the luminal border of the microvilli. The carrier transports both to the other surface of the membrane where glucose and Na^+ are released.

The active transport mechanisms are the rate-limiting step in carbohydrate absorption. The action of lactase may be an exception; in this case hydrolysis by lactase may be the rate-limiting step.[120] Glucose and galactose are absorbed into the intestinal epithelial cells by a protein-carrier mediated process. This process is coupled with sodium entry into the intestinal epithelial cell and requires energy (Fig. 7–6). Fructose is absorbed by facilitated diffusion that requires a carrier mechanism, but not sodium entry. After being absorbed into the cell, they are released from their carrier proteins and exit the cell via a concentration gradient through the lamina propria, into the capillaries of the portal venous system.

Malassimilation of carbohydrates can occur for of several reasons: (1) deficiency of amylase (maldigestion); (2) impaired hydrolysis of oligosaccharides (maldigestion); (3) impaired monosaccharide absorption, secondary to diffuse mucosal disease (malabsorption); and (4) impaired monosaccharide absorption due to infiltrative diseases of the lamina propria (malabsorption). In humans congenital deficiencies of brush border enzymes and monosaccharide carrier proteins have been described but are rare. These deficiencies cause carbohydrate malassimilation and they have not been described in the dog and cat.[6]

Protein is primarily digested in the duodenum and jejunum, although some protein digestion occurs in the stomach by the action of pepsin. The digestion of protein is aided by pancreatic proteases. CCK stimulates the excretion of proteolytic enzymes in an inactive state, called proenzymes. The secretion of these enzymes can also occur secondary to vagal activity. Trypsinogen, the inactive form of trypsin, is converted to trypsin in the lumen by enterokinase, a duodenal brush border enzyme. Activated trypsin activates the other proteases and further activates trypsinogen. A pH of 7 is needed for optimal pancreatic protease activity. This is accomplished by the secretion of bicarbonate-rich pancreatic juice. This secretion is stimulated by the hormone secretin.

Proteases are divided into exo- and endopeptidases, depending on their site of action. Endopeptidases cleave internal peptide bonds, resulting in small peptides. Exopeptidases cleave terminal peptide bonds, resulting in small peptides and some amino acids. Trypsin, elastase, and chymotrypsin are classified as endopeptidases; carboxypeptidases A and B are exopeptidases.

The resulting small peptides are cleaved further to amino acids at the intestinal brush border. Peptidases needed for this are found within the brush border membrane. Some peptides are absorbed into the cell and broken down there. The enzymes found in the cell and the brush border membrane appear to be distinctly different. The amino acids are then absorbed across the cell membrane by protein carrier-mediated mechanisms. Four mechanisms are known; they are for a specific group of amino acids, require active transport, and are sodium dependent. After entry into the cell, the amino acids exit into the capillaries and are delivered to the portal venous system.

Maldigestion of proteins can occur secondary to exocrine pancreatic insufficiency. Also, severe mucosal disease can lead to impaired absorption and impaired mucosal digestion.

The small intestine and colon are capable of absorbing a tremendous amount of water. Diet normally contributes approximately 25 per cent, whereas secretions from the mouth, stomach, biliary tract, pancreas, and intestinal wall contribute approximately 75 per cent of the total intestinal water content. About one-half of this total amount is absorbed by the jejunum and a majority of the remaining water is absorbed by the ileum. The colon is capable of handling most of the remaining fluid, so that small amounts (1 to 4 per cent of total intestinal water) are excreted in the stools per day. A delicate balance exists between secretion and absorption, with a net positive absorption. This results in a formed instead of a liquid stool.[49, 80]

Water transport involves both passive and active processes, with passive diffusion accounting for most of the water movement.[95] Movement of water and solutes occurs intercellularly through pores and transcellularly. In transcellular transport, water primarily follows the movement of solutes. The movement of solutes is usually by active transport. Intercellular movement of water accounts for the bulk of water movement. This occurs through pores in the junctions between epithelial cells and is influenced by electrochemical, osmotic, and hydrostatic pressure gradients.[95, 120, 134]

The enterosystemic cycles of protein, water, fat, and bile salts are important in the conservation of these substances. In an enterosystemic cycle, a substance is secreted or lost in a location proximally and reabsorbed distally for reutilization. Bile salts are secreted into the duodenum and are reabsorbed by the terminal ileum. Water and ions are secreted and absorbed by the small intestine, with absorption exceeding secretion. Also, large amounts of protein and fat enter the lumen by secretion and from extruded cells. If this protein and fat were not absorbed, the body would have a net deficiency, since more protein enters the gastrointestinal lumen from endogenous sources than is eaten daily.[120]

The intestine has two types of motility: rhythmic segmentation and peristalsis. These aid in mixing of the chyme with intestinal secretions, and digestive juices. In addition, motility aids in increased contact with absorptive surfaces.

Peristaltic activity starts in the proximal duodenum and progresses down the length of the gut to the ileum. It transports bowel contents in an aboral direction. In addition to propulsive peristaltic waves, there are circular contractions of the intestinal muscle that do not progress. These segmentation contractions occur rhythmically and at recurrent sites along the gut. They have a mixing effect that gives ingesta greater contact with digestive enzymes and with the intestinal mucosa. This effect also slows down passage of nutrients so that digestion and absorption can take place.

In dogs fasted over 12 hours, interdigestive motility occurs. Contractions start at the stomach and move distally. It is thought that the purpose of these contractions may be to cleanse the gastrointestinal tract of undigested materials and bacteria before the next meal.

Intestinal motility is primarily determined by the electrical control activity of smooth muscle. This basal electrical rhythm is influenced by hormones, neural activity, feeding, and disease states. Neural effects on gastrointestinal motility are regulated by the autonomic nervous system. Parasympathetics increase motility, whereas sympathetics decrease motility. Chemoreceptors and mechanoreceptors give sensory input into intestinal motility. Chemoreceptors are stimulated by osmolarity, pH, and digestive products, while mechanoreceptors are stimulated by pressure, movement, and volume.

The intestine produces a variety of polypeptide hormone products. These include cholecystokinin (CCK), secretin, gastrin, enteroglucagon, vasoactive intestinal polypeptide (VIP), somatostatin, motilin, and gastric inhibitory peptide. These polypeptides are produced by APUD (Amine Precursor Uptake and Decarboxylation) cells, which are found scattered among the mucosal cells. APUD cells are also found in the pancreatic islets. These polypeptides are released and act locally, performing a paracrine function. Some of these peptides are also close to neural structures within the gut wall, suggesting a possible neurocrine function.

There are other factors besides the immune system, which has been discussed previously, that help decrease the possibility of disease. These include normal microflora, gut motility, primary peristalsis, and alimentary secretions.

Diarrhea

PATHOPHYSIOLOGY

Diarrhea is defined as an increase in the frequency of bowel evacuation and water content of the stool. The mechanisms of diarrhea are broken down into four categories: (1) osmotic, (2) secretory, (3) increased permeability, and (4) motility disorders. Classifying diarrhea in one of the four categories can aid in treatment. Most diarrheal problems involve one or a combination of the above mechanisms.[95]

Osmotic Diarrhea

Osmotic diarrhea is the result of poorly absorbed materials that retain water in the gut lumen. Causes of osmotic diarrhea include maldigestion, malabsorption, failure to transport a dietary non-electrolyte, and some laxatives.

Non-absorbable solutes in the intestine retard water absorption and by their osmotic effect tend to cause a net water movement from plasma to the gut lumen. This is because the effective osmotic pressure of luminal contents containing non-absorbable solutes is higher than that of plasma. Unabsorbed carbohydrates have a greater effect as a cause of osmotic diarrheas than do fats, because carbohydrates are very water soluble whereas fats are not. Carbohydrates are hydrolyzed to small organic acids by colonic bacteria, which further increases their osmotic activity.[120]

A characteristic of osmotic diarrhea is that it often resolves when the patient is fasted. Osmotic diarrheas have an osmol gap. Patients with an osmotic diarrhea have a fecal osmolality greater than two times the sum of the fecal sodium and potassium levels, e.g., 2 (fecal Na^+ + fecal K^+). (The total of 2 (Na^+ + K^+) is less than the measured osmolality of the fecal fluid.) Also, fecal pH is usually low because of the breakdown of carbohydrates to organic acids.[120]

Secretory Diarrhea

Secretory diarrhea results when fluids and electrolytes are secreted by mucosal cells at an exaggerated rate. This occurs independent of changes in permeability, absorptive capacity, or exogenously generated osmotic gradients.[95] Most of the secretion takes place in the crypts, whereas absorption occurs at the villus. Usually absorption exceeds secretion and a normal stool results. When secretion exceeds absorption, diarrhea can occur. Intestinal secretion is thought to be controlled by cyclic adenosine monophosphate (cAMP), and mucosal cell cAMP levels are thought to be regulated by hormones.[95]

E. coli entertoxin, cholera in humans, and *Salmonella* toxin are felt to produce secretory diarrheas. Extensive studies done on the cholera toxin have increased our knowledge in this area.

It is thought that the cholera toxin stimulates adenyl cyclase which in turn appears to elevate the levels of cAMP intracellularly. As a result of this increase in cAMP, there is hypersecretion. These secretions are usually isotonic, and the fecal osmolality is equal to 2 (Na^+ and K^+). The consequences of increased secretion include electrolyte loss, acidosis due to bicarbonate loss, and isotonic dehydration.[95, 120]

Prostaglandins, serotonin, gastrointestinal hormones, parasympathetic stimulation, dihydroxy bile acids, hydroxylated fatty acids, and certain laxatives are also known to stimulate intestinal secretions.[120]

In humans, secretory diarrheas have been identified secondary to neoplasias, both pancreatic and non-pancreatic. Thyroid medullary carcinoma and hypergastrinemia secondary to a pancreatic tumor have been described in the dog as causing secretory diarrhea.[120]

Increased Permeability

There are continuous fluxes of water and electrolytes across the intestinal border. In the normal animal, absorptive fluxes exceed secretory fluxes, resulting in net absorption.[96] These fluxes are primarily accomplished by passive diffusion, which occurs through pores in the junction between epithelial cells. These pores are too small to be seen even with the aid of microscopy.[95] Changes in surface area or specific abnormalities in mucosal cell membranes may increase "pore size" in the mucous membranes, resulting in increased flow from the blood to the intestinal lumen. If the amount exuded exceeds the absorptive capacity of the intestines, diarrhea results.[95]

The size of the particles that leak through the mucosa depends on the magnitude of the increase in pore size. Small increases permit increased diffusion of small molecules such as fructose, creatine, mannitol, erythritol, and inulin. Transudation of large amounts of these molecules can result in diarrhea. Large increases in pore size permits exudation of plasma proteins into the lumen. Such disorders are characterized as "protein-losing enteropathies." The increase in size of existing pores can be due to (1) an increase in hydraulic pressure in the mucosa because of obstructed lymph flow; or (2) the action of chemical mediators of an inflammatory process, acting directly to increase pore size. The channels that appear in protein-losing enteropathies, allowing protein movement from plasma to the intestinal lumen, are ultrastructurally recognizable separations of the junctional complexes between epithelial and endothelial cells.[95]

For hemorrhagic diarrheas to occur, a greater than 10,000-fold increase in the pore size must occur. This allows the leakage of red blood cells, leading to hemorrhagic diarrhea.[95]

Motility Disorders

In theory, increased peristalsis, by either increased frequency or intensity, could cause diarrhea by accelerating transit of ingesta and secretion. In actuality, there is no evidence that this occurs as a primary problem or even as a major contributing problem.[95] What has been shown is that in some diarrheal diseases *decreased* motility occurs, which can allow intestinal bacterial overgrowth to occur, thus causing diarrhea.[95] Stagnant loop syndrome is an example of this phenomenon.

Diagnosis

In the diagnosis of diarrheal problems it is helpful to classify the problem as acute or chronic. Also, the separation of diarrheal problems into small and large bowel disease is helpful in setting up a diagnostic plan; in most cases, the above can be determined by history and physical examination.

Acute diarrheas are more common than chronic and are usually self-limiting. They usually respond to symptomatic therapy. In animals that do not respond to the initial symptomatic treatment, the problem often becomes chronic. In man, chronic diarrhea is defined as lasting longer than 10 days. Although no definition has been determined in veterinary medicine, the authors feel that this 10-day period is a valid time interval for differentiating between acute and chronic diarrheas. In chronic cases an accurate diagnosis is needed to initiate specific therapy and to give an accurate prognosis.[22]

History and Physical Examination in Disorders of Small Intestine

As mentioned, the history is very important when trying to distinguish acute versus chronic, and small bowel versus large bowel disease. Significant factors include duration of the diarrhea, presence of vomiting, diet, appearance of the feces, frequency of defecation, appetite, tenesmus, and weight loss.[22]

Duration of diarrhea is important in assessing the problem. If the diarrhea has been evident longer than 10 days, it is seldom self-limiting and usually requires a thorough examination of the patient. Diarrheas that are continuous tend to be associated with organic disease, while intermittent diarrheas tend to be functional disorders.[22]

The appearance of the feces can aid in localizing lesions. Bulky stools usually indicate small bowel disease; the stool may be light in color, watery, frothy, free of blood and mucus, and foul-smelling. In large bowel problems, the feces are usually scant and contain fresh blood or mucus.[22]

Tenesmus is usually associated with distal large bowel disease. Excess mucus suggests an inflammatory condition of the colon. Vomiting is more commonly associated with proximal gastrointestinal disease; however, as many as 30 per cent of dogs with colitis will also have a history of vomiting.[22] The vomiting tends to be intermittent and not associated with eating, and bile and blood are not present.[22]

In summary, small bowel disease is associated with vomiting, weight loss, melena, excessive borborygmus, flatulence, and voluminous and malodorous stools. Large bowel disease is associated with tenesmus and urgency and scant stool containing fresh blood and mucus.[22, 120, 139]

Physical examination is important in diagnosis. Palpation of the abdomen can identify neoplasia, thickened bowel loops, foreign bodies, plication of intestine (linear foreign body), and painful abdomen (pancreatitis, peritonitis, etc.). When performing the physical examination it is also important to look at the general condition of the patient, examining for emaciation. The color of the mucous membranes should be noted; if pale, enteric blood loss must be considered. A perineal region that is greasy or oily is suggestive of steatorrhea. Ascites, pleural effusion, or edema may be indicative of hypoalbuminemia secondary to a protein-losing enteropathy.[22, 120]

MINIMUM DATA BASE

The initial work-up should consist of fecal analysis (direct and flotation), a complete blood count (CBC), serum biochemical profile, and urinalysis.

Three fecal tests, both direct and flotation, should be done to eliminate endoparasitism as a cause. Zinc sulfate, ($ZnSO_4$) and saturated sucrose are two media that may be used for flotation analysis.

The hemogram should include examination of the erythron, leukon, and platelets. Relative polycythemia may be associated with dehydration in many gastrointestinal diseases. A prime example is hemorrhagic gastroenteritis. Normocytic and normochromic anemia is associated with either chronic gastrointestinal inflammatory disease or chronic malnutrition. Microcytic hypochromic anemia may be found in chronic gastrointestinal hemorrhage (e.g., hookworms and neoplasia) and iron depletion. Increased numbers of nucleated red blood cells and basophilic stippling of these cells as well as of adult red cells may be found in lead poisoning. On rare occasions distemper inclusion bodies may be found in red blood cells as well as leukocytes. Leukocytosis, especially a regenerative neutrophilia, can be indicative of infectious or inflammatory problems. Leukopenia is associated with feline parvovirus enteritis, FeLV-associated panleukopenia-like syndrome, canine parvoviral enteritis, and early canine distemper, as well as *Salmonella* and *Escherichia coli* enteric infections. Lymphopenia may be noted in intestinal lymphangiectasia. Eosinophilia can suggest eosinophilic gastroenteritis, although endoparasitism and hypoadrenocorticism cannot be excluded. *Histoplasma* may be discovered in the monocytes of patients in which gastrointestinal infections are suspected. Thrombocytosis is associated with chronic blood loss.

A serum biochemical profile can help rule out metabolic disorders such as renal failure, pancreatitis, liver disease, and hypoadrenocorticism. Hypercalcemia has been noted with intestinal lymphoma, whereas hypocalcemia may occur in association with protein-losing enteropathies secondary to hypoalbuminemia. Hypercholesterolemia has been associated with renal and gastrointestinal albumin loss.

Although the half-life of serum alkaline phosphatase is quite short, the serum level of intestinal isoenzyme may be mildly elevated due to inflammation of the small intestine. Serum urea nitrogen may be elevated due to dehydration in gastrointestinal fluid loss. Gastrointestinal bleeding will also cause a marked elevation in serum urea nitrogen. This is most identifiable in patients with apparent normal hydration and normal urinalysis.

Although the urinalysis does not lend itself to specific diagnoses of gastrointestinal disease, it should be recalled that specific gravity will elevate during dehydration in all patients free of renal disease. Negative or minimal amounts of protein in the urine will rule out proteinuria as a cause of hypoalbuminemia. Alkaline urine may be due to diet or metabolic alkalosis associated with vomition. Metabolic acidosis, most commonly associated with diarrhea, intestinal volvulus, or ischemia, may cause production of acid urine.

SCREENING TESTS

When malassimilation of chronic diarrhea is suspected there are several tests that can be done to further classify the problem. These tests include fecal trypsin activity, Sudan III or IV staining with or without acetic acid for fats, Lugol's iodine stain for fecal starch, plasma turbidity tests, and fecal occult blood and fecal cytology stains.

New Methylene blue or Wright's stain can be used to identify inflammatory cells in the feces. Inflammatory exudate is primarily seen in large bowel problems.[140] Also, colonic mucosal scrapings can diagnose inflammatory disease; the best example is enteric histoplasmosis, in which the organism can be observed in macrophages obtained from colonic scrapings.

Lugol's iodine stain can be used for the detection of undigested starch. A small aliquot of stool suspension is mixed with 1 to 2 drops of 2 per cent Lugol's iodine and a coverslip placed over it. The slide is examined microscopically for bluish-black stained particles. If large numbers are seen, this indicates that undigested starch is present in the feces (amylorrhea). This is suggestive of exocrine pancreatic insufficiency. Talcum powder may mimic dietary starch if the sample is contaminated with surgical glove powder.

The Sudan stain is a qualitative test for fecal fats. It is simple to perform and it has been shown to correlate very well with quantitative methods.[13] Direct and indirect tests can help differentiate malabsorption from maldigestion. In the direct test a small aliquot of stool is mixed with Sudan stain III or IV and examined microscopically.

Fatty acids are present as lightly staining flakes or as needle-like crystals that do not stain. Soaps also do not stain and appear as well-defined amorphous flakes or as rounded masses or as coarse crystals. Neutral fats appear as large red or orange droplets (Fig. 7–7). In the normal dog there should not be more than two to three fat droplets per low-power field; if there are more, this is indicative of maldigestion.

The indirect test is performed by taking a small aliquot of feces mixed with two drops of 36 per cent acetic acid and two drops of Sudan III or IV. The suspension is then heated to boiling. This converts the neutral fats and soaps to fatty acids and then melts the fatty acids, causing them to form droplets that stain strongly with Sudan stain. The slide should be examined while still warm. If positive on the indirect test and negative on the direct test, this is indicative of malabsorption. If there is an equal amount of droplets in *both* preparations, the patient most likely has maldigestion of fats. It has been our experience that due to the low fat content of some commercial dog foods, a patient with malassimilation that is being fed commercial food may not have any fat drops per low-power field. We suggest putting the patient on a food with a moderate fat content* for 24 hours before the test is done.

Fecal trypsin activity can be crudely measured by x-ray film digestion and gelatin tube tests. The x-ray film digestion test is performed by adding 1 ml of feces to 9 ml of 5 per cent sodium bicarbonate to make a

*c/d, Hill's Pet Products, Inc., Topeka, KS.

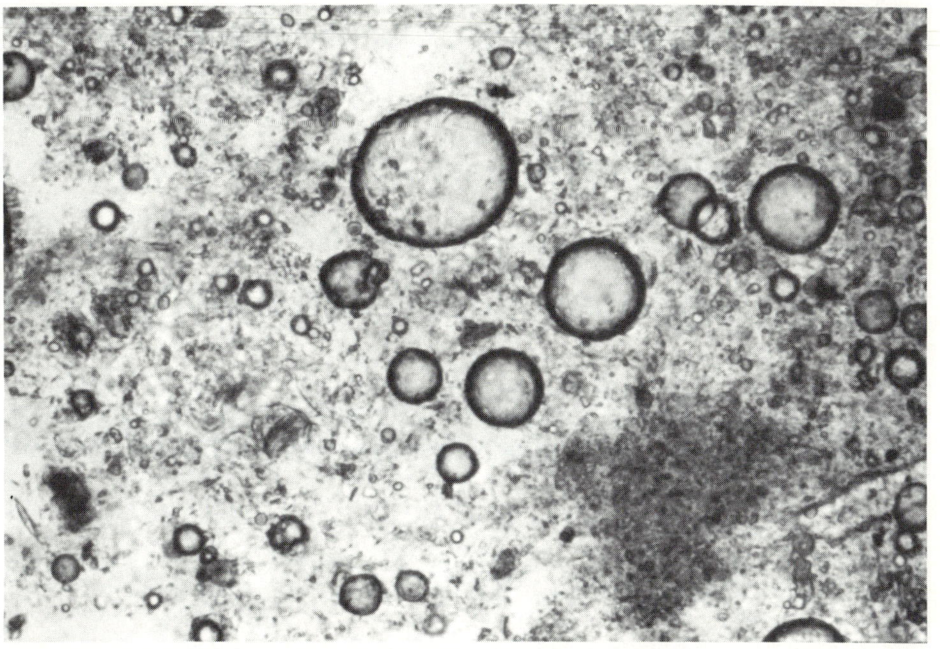

Figure 7–7. Fecal smear stained with Sudan stain demonstrating excess amount of fecal fat. The fat droplets stain a tannish orange color. (Courtesy of Donald Schmidt, DVM, PhD, Department of Veterinary Pathology, University of Missouri.)

total of 10 ml. A strip of x-ray film is then placed in the solution and allowed to stand for 2½ hours at room temperature or 1 hour at 37°C. The film is then rinsed with tap water. If the film is cleared, then trypsin is present.

For the gelatin tube test, dilute feces with water to a 1:10 dilution. Heat two gelatin tubes to 37°C; add 1 ml of 5 per cent sodium bicarbonate and 1 ml of feces to one tube. To the other tube add 1 ml of 5 per cent sodium bicarbonate (the second tube is negative control). Agitate both tubes and heat to 37°C for 1 hour or let stand at room temperature for 2½ hours. Then refrigerate at 5°C for 20 minutes. If the gelatin solidifies, digestion did not occur, indicating that trypsin is not present. The negative control should solidify.

Both tests are crude measurements of trypsin activity and exocrine pancreatic insufficiency. False negative results can occur because of bacterial degradation of trypsin, dilution of trypsin by the increased fecal water, or by indigestible x-ray film coatings. False positive results can occur because of bacterial proteases. In one study 57 per cent of dogs with pancreatic exocine insufficiency had positive fecal gelatin digestive tests.[23] The film digestion tests and gelatin digestion test are simple to run but one should be aware that their diagnostic accuracy is quite low.

The plasma turbidity test, or fat absorption test, is another screening test for malabsorption-maldigestion problems. The patient should be fasted overnight. A presample is taken to ensure that the plasma is clear. Then Lipomal* or corn oil (6 ml/kg) is given orally. Post-samples are taken 2 and 3 hours later, and plasma is checked for turbidity. If the plasma is clear, the patient has malassimilation of fats. To rule out exocrine pancreatic insufficiency the test is repeated on a different day with pancreatic enzymes† at a dose of 1 teaspoon per 10 kg of body weight. If the plasma then becomes lipemic, this is indicative of maldigestion (Fig. 7–8). If the plasma remains clear, diagnosis of malabsorption is supported.

When examining the feces, blood can often be seen grossly. If the bleeding is from the upper gastrointestinal tract, the stool is often "tarry black," whereas lower gastrointestinal bleeding may show unchanged blood, coloring the stool red. If occult blood is present in the stool, it can be measured by simple chemical tests or orthotoluidine tests. These tests, however, are extremely sensitive and yield a great many false positives. The guaiac test is less sensitive and when coupled with a meat-free diet, such as cottage cheese and rice, for 48 to 72 hours prior to testing may be more consistent and revealing. Prior to doing an occult blood test on the feces, the patient's diet should be checked for occult blood. Since many commercial diets contain meat or meat-by-products they will test positive; therefore, the fecal occult blood tests will be falsely positive in patients on these diets.

*The Upjohn Co., Kalamazoo, MI.
†Viokase, Viobin Corp., Monticello, IL.

TESTS TO DIFFERENTIATE MALABSORPTION FROM MALDIGESTION

There are several tests to differentiate malabsorption from maldigestion. None of the tests alone are diagnostic, and often several different tests are required to make a diagnosis. Probably the most useful tests are the D-xylose absorption test, the BT-PABA (*N*-benzoyl-L-tryosyl-*p*-aminobenzoic acid) digestion test, and quantitation of fecal fats. The quantitation of fecal trypsin levels has been used in conjunction with quantitation of fats for the diagnosis of malabsorption or maldigestion.[23]

The quantitation of fecal fat, if elevated, is diagnostic of malassimilation, but it does not differentiate malabsorption from maldigestion. There are three ways to determine fecal fat: (1) amount of fat in feces (gm/day), (2) per cent assimilation of ingested fat, and (3) amount of fat in feces per weight of the patient in kg per day (gm/kg/day).

When quantitating fecal fats, it is advised to feed a known quanity of fat for 3 days prior to collecting feces. Canned c/d* is frequently used as it contains 8.4 per cent fat on a dry weight basis. After the diet has been standardized, the feces should be collected for 48 to 72 hours and weighed. The feces are then sent to a lab for fat analysis.

Reported normal values in the dog vary: less than 7 gm/day[140]; 0.24 ± 0.01 gm/kg of body weight; 90 per cent assimilation on a cereal-based diet or 96.9 per cent assimilation on a meat-based diet.[23, 89] Fecal fat values of 2.08 gm/kg of body weight per day

*Hill's Pet Products, Inc., Topeka, KS.

have been associated with exocrine pancreatic insufficiency, whereas values of 1.14 gm/kg of body weight per day have been associated with malabsorption.[23] In the cat, excretion of greater than 3.59 gm of fat per day is diagnostic for malassimilation.[83]

Fecal trypsin activity has also been measured with fecal fats. Dogs fed a meat-based diet had a fecal trypsin activity of 4.96 mg/kg of body weight per day. Dogs with exocrine pancreatic insufficiency had significantly lower fecal trypsin activity (0.49 mg/kg of body weight per day), whereas dogs with malabsorption had significantly higher fecal trypsin activity (15.2 mg/kg of body weight per day).[23, 89]

The D-xylose absorption test helps to rule out malabsorption. D-Xylose is a five-carbon sugar that is absorbed passively. Assimilation of D-xylose does not require intraluminal digestion. An abnormal D-xylose test usually indicates small bowel mural disease or bacterial overgrowth.

Before running the test, the patient is fasted for 12 to 24 hours. The D-xylose is given as a 5 per cent solution, at a dose of 0.5 g/kg orally. Samples are collected at 0, 30, 60, 90, 120, and 180 minutes. In normal dogs a net plasma xylose of at least 45 mg/dl is seen by 60 to 90 minutes. Values less than 45 mg/dl are indicative of malabsorption.[59] It is our opinion that normal dogs have a net plasma xylose level of at least 60 mg/dl by 60 to 90 minutes. Values that are falsely decreased can be obtained secondary to delayed gastric emptying or bacterial degradation of xylose in the intestinal lumen because of bacterial overgrowth.[9] It has been stated that sequestration of D-xylose in ascitic fluid can falsely lower plasma D-xylose levels.[120] Since D-xylose is excreted in the urine, renal failure could potentially give falsely elevated values.[59, 120]

The BT-PABA absorption test is specific for the activity of chymotrypsin.[133] Chymotrypsin hydrolyzes the BT-PABA peptide bond, releasing PABA, which is absorbed by the intestine and excreted in the urine within 6 hours. Blood levels or urinary levels can be used in this test.[118, 133] The patient is fasted for 12 hours and either 50 mg/kg or 150 mg/kg of a 3 per cent BT-PABA solution is administered orally. The urine is then collected for 6 hours, or blood samples are taken at 0, 30, 60, 90, 120, and 150 minutes. Normally, by 60 to 90 minutes, blood levels greater than 10 μm/ml are detected with a dosage of 50 mg/kg, and greater than 30 μg/ml with a dosage of 150 mg/kg.[131] If measuring urinary excretion after 6 hours, 60 per cent of the PABA should be excreted. If a chymotrypsin deficiency exists, less than 15 per cent will be excreted. Values less than 46 per cent may be indicative of partial exocrine pancreatic insufficiency.[133] Because the D-xylose absorption test evaluates for malabsorption and the BT-PABA test evaluates for maldigestion, these tests have been run together for the diagnosis of malassimilation.[9, 118, 131]

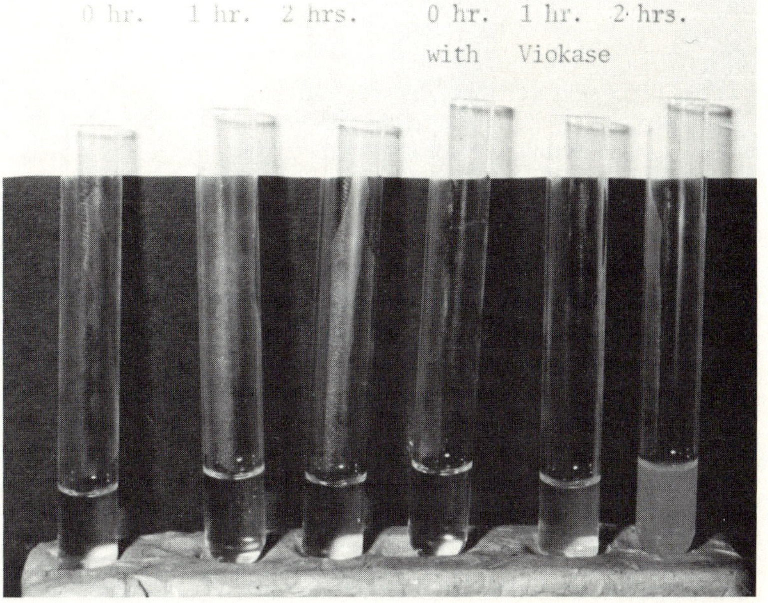

Figure 7–8. Plasma tubes from a patient after a fat absorption test. The patient had pancreatic exocrine insufficiency. Note that the plasma from the initial test (without enzymes) is clear in all three tubes on the left; after adding enzymes it becomes turbid by two hours (three tubes on the right).

The use of the BT-PABA and D-xylose tests in cats may not be as reliable as it is in dogs. In one study on cats there was great variation in normal values. Also, the values were less in the cat than in the dog. Mean peak PABA concentration was 7.5 ± 3.2 μg/ml and mean peak D-xylose levels were 42.8 ± 17.8 mg/dl. Further studies need to be done to determine the reliability of BT-PABA and D-xylose tests in the cat.[121]

The tests that have been described are the more common ones used in the diagnosis of malassimilation. Two other tests that can aid in the diagnosis of fat malassimilation are vitamin A absorption tests and oleic acid^{125}I and triolein^{131}I absorption tests.

In the vitamin A absorption test, 200,000 units of vitamin A, given as cod liver oil concentrate, is administered orally. Blood samples are taken at 0, 2, 4, 6, 8, and 24 hours. The blood is kept away from light to minimize vitamin A deterioration. In normal dogs, the vitamin A value increases three- to fivefold over normal resting levels in 6 to 8 hours. A drawback of the test is that the results tend to be inconsistent.[54]

The principle of the oleic acid^{125}I and triolein^{131}I test is based on the fact that triolein needs lipase to be absorbed and oleic acid does not. In normal dogs, 13 per cent of the oleic acid and 11 per cent of the triolein is absorbed. In dogs with a lipase deficiency (exocrine pancreatic insufficiency), the oleic acid^{125}I will be absorbed normally and the triolein^{131}I will have decreased absorption. If there is malabsorption, both will be decreased. A disadvantage of this test is the requirement for radioactive isotopes and special analysis, which limits its availability.[71]

The glucose tolerance, lactose tolerance, and starch digestion tests also have been used for measuring carbohydrate absorption. The oral glucose tolerance test is not as accurate as the D-xylose test, but it is useful in the diagnosis of malabsorption. In this test, the patient is fasted for 12 to 24 hours and then given 2 gm/kg of a 25 per cent dextrose solution orally. Blood samples are collected at 0, 15, 30, 60, 120, and 180 minutes. Normal dogs will have a glucose peak greater than 140 mg/dl between 60 and 90 minutes. The peak should return to normal in 2 hours. This test is useful in the diagnosis of malabsorption. Several factors can affect the test, including individual variation, amount of glucose given, period of starvation before the test, carbohydrate content of dyes, gastric motility, stress, cardiovascular lesions, insulin, and obesity.[126]

The starch digestion test is similar to the oral glucose tolerance test, in that both look for a rise in blood glucose. The difference is that starch needs to be digested first by amylase. The patient is fasted overnight and then given starch orally at a dose of 3 gm/kg (1.5 ml of hot water is mixed with each 3 gm). Blood samples are then taken every 30 minutes for 2½ hours. Normally the blood glucose reaches a level of 125 mg to 130 mg/dl in 1 hour. This test has the same limitations as the glucose tolerance test.[88]

The lactose tolerance test is used to evaluate brush border disaccharidase activity (lactase). For this test to be of value the absorption of glucose must be normal. The patient is given 2 gm/kg of a 12½ per cent solution of lactose orally. By 90 minutes the blood glucose should be approximately 127 mg/dl.[88]

The measurement of serum folate and vitamin B_{12} levels may be an aid in the diagnosis of malassimilation. Folate is absorbed from the jejunum and vitamin B_{12} is absorbed from the ileum. This fact makes it possible to localize lesions in the small intestine. If both serum folate and vitamin B_{12} are decreased, this indicates severe changes in the jejunum and ileum. If serum folate is decreased and vitamin B_{12} is normal, this suggests damage to the proximal small intestine. If serum folate levels are increased and vitamin B_{12} is decreased, bacterial overgrowth is suspected. This occurred in dogs with severe exocrine pancreatic insufficiency and may be due to secondary bacterial overgrowth or defective degradation of a vitamin B_{12}–binding protein, which has been observed in humans.[7]

The vitamin B_{12} absorption (Schilling) test, which is used in human medicine, may have an application in veterinary medicine. In human medicine it is used when achlorhydria, intrinsic factor deficiency, or small intestinal disease is suspected. This test has been applied experimentally in veterinary medicine, but not clinically.[88]

A test using ^{51}Cr-labeled albumin has been developed to aid in the diagnosis of protein-losing enteropathies. In this test, ^{51}Cr-labeled albumin (1.47 μC/kg) is injected intravenously. The feces are then collected and analyzed. The dog normally secretes less than 2 per cent over a period of 3 days; in protein-losing enteropathies, greater amounts are detected in the feces.[37]

Radioimmunoassays (RIA) of gastrointestinal hormones are used in human medicine.[101] Normal values are known in the dog, but these assays are not routinely available.[121] The diagnosis of canine gastrinoma (Zollinger-Ellison syndrome) has been aided by RIA of plasma gastrin levels.[132]

Assays of specific mucosal border enzymes have been determined for canine jejunal mucosa. These assays may have clinical application in the future.[8, 10, 120]

MISCELLANEOUS PROCEDURES

Fiberoptic endoscopy is useful in the diagnosis of small intestinal disease. It is possible to pass the fiberoptic endoscope through the pylorus and examine the descending duodenum.[66] If passing the endoscope through the pylorus meets with resistance, glucagon can be given intravenously at a dose of 0.05 mg/kg, not to exceed 1 mg. This will relax the pylorus and help passage of the endoscope.[66] Metoclopramide hydrochloride* is another drug that may be of value in relaxing the pylorus. After passage, biopsy and aspirations can be taken. The diagnosis of giardiasis can be aided by the use of endoscopy.[140]

An upper gastrointestinal radiographic series may aid in the diagnosis of obstruction, infiltrative disease, chronic inflammatory disease, and neoplasia. All other testing should be completed before a barium series is carried out, since it can interfere with other tests.

When the diagnosis cannot be made by any other method, intestinal biopsies by exploratory celiotomy should be considered. Biopsies should be taken even if the organs and intestines look normal.

Selected Diseases

NON-SPECIFIC ACUTE DIARRHEA

Non-specific acute diarrhea is one of the most common problems for small animal veterinarians. Often the etiology is never determined. These cases usually have an acute onset, with a duration of 24 to 48 hours prior to presentation. The diarrhea is often watery and may contain blood. It is important to differentiate self-limiting acute diarrhea from fulminating diarrheas, which are often infectious. The latter, which can be life-threatening and often need vigorous treatment, will be discussed later.

Physical examination findings vary, depending on severity. Dehydration is the most common finding. The patient should be examined carefully to rule out multisystemic diseases.

Clinical pathology work-up should include at least a fecal smear and flotation analysis for parasites. At least three fecal examinations are needed to rule out parasites. Often, if the problem is mild, this may be all that is necessary and the patient is treated symptomatically. If the diarrhea is severe, further investigation is needed, including initially a CBC, serum biochemical profile, and urinalysis.

Often the diagnosis can be made from the history and physical examination and treatment instituted. The treatment will vary with the severity of the problem.

Initially the patient should have food and water withheld (nothing per os, NPO) for 12 to 24 hours and without food for at least 24 to 48 hours. The reasons for not feeding the patient are multiple:

1. When inflammation is present in the gastrointestinal tract, the loss of mucosal cells is accelerated. Food acts as an abrasive and increases mucosal cell loss.
2. Bacteria are present in food and, due to the fact that the normal flora in the intestinal tract can be upset in the diarrheic state, transient bacteria may colonize the intestinal tract. Fasting the patient helps decrease the number of transient bacteria entering the intestine.
3. The small intestinal mucosa can lose brush border enzymes during diarrhea, thereby losing the ability to digest disaccharides. The inability to digest food, especially carbohydrates, can lead to an osmotic diarrhea and compound the existing diarrhea.

Once the patient has been fasted, food intake should be reinstituted slowly. The diet should be bland, consisting mainly of carbohydrates and protein. Since fat assimilation is complex, fats should be severely limited. Initially the patient should be given a small amount of food to make sure it will be tolerated.

There are several other measures that may be used to treat acute diarrheas. These include fluid replacement, intestinal protectants and salicylates, antimotility drugs, and antibiotics.

*Reglan, A. H. Robins Co., Richmond, VA.

In severe cases of diarrhea, fluid therapy is extremely important. Proper fluid therapy is based on the state of hydration and serum electrolyte and acid-base studies. If serum electrolytes and blood gas studies are unavailable, it is best to use a balanced electrolyte solution (e.g., lactated Ringer's solution). Oral fluid therapy may be of value in the rehydration of patients with diarrhea. The basis of oral rehydration is the fact that active intestinal absorption of glucose or amino acids is associated with sodium and potassium absorption.[24] The use of oral fluid therapy has greater application in diarrheas in which the absorptive ability of the mucosa is intact. The net result should be an increase in absorption that offsets the net secretion. Oral rehydration has been used effectively in the treatment of human cholera and diarrhea in calves, pigs, and small animals.[24] To be effective, these solutions must contain the necessary amounts of glucose, amino acids, sodium, potassium, and chloride and must be isotonic.[24] Commerical preparations for oral rehydration are available.*

Protectants and salicylates have been used in veterinary medicine in the treatment of diarrheas. It appears that they are neither beneficial nor detrimental, as they have not been shown to alter fluid and electrolyte losses. However, there is some evidence that pectin plus salicylates† can adsorb and inactivate enterotoxins, such as those produced by *E. coli*. One of the actions of salicylates is inhibition of prostaglandins, which may decrease enterotoxin-induced intestinal secretion.

The use of antimotility drugs is warranted in the treatment of some diarrheas. The rationale behind their use is a decrease in peristalsis and increase in segmentation contraction. Anticholinergics are not beneficial. With their use, motility can be stopped, which allows bacterial overgrowth (stagnant loop syndrome), thus compounding the problem. Narcotic analgesics (paregoric, loperamide hydrochloride,‡ and diphenoxylate hydrochloride§ are of benefit in the treatment of diarrhea. These drugs increase segmental contraction while decreasing peristalsis.[120] If the diarrhea is caused by an infectious agent such as *Salmonella,* narcotic analgesics may be detrimental because they may trap organisms and toxins within the intestine.[24] Loperamide has been shown to have anti-secretory properties; this may make loperamide beneficial in entertoxin-induced diarrheas.[24]

The use of antibiotics in the treatment of diarrhea is controversial. If antibiotics only succeed in inhibiting the normal flora, they are detrimental. In patients with acute diarrhea, antibiotic therapy is warranted when there is evidence of an inflammatory reaction in the gastrointestinal tract (numerous bacterial and inflammatory cells in the feces), invaded intestinal mucosa (blood in the stool), a generalized inflammatory reaction (pyrexia, leukocytosis), or abnormal fecal culture results. Ideally, controlled studies need to be done to determine when antibiotic therapy is needed in dogs and cats with diarrhea. The use of protectants with antibiotics has some contraindications. Protectants will absorb some antibiotics and therefore neutralize them. Ampicillin is less susceptible to this action than cationic antibiotics such as lincomycin.[24]

BACTERIAL DISEASES CAUSING ACUTE DIARRHEA

The small intestine has a resident population of bacteria known as the microflora. The microflora is established shortly after birth. Anaerobic bacteria are the principal components of the normal flora and outnumber aerobes 1000 to 1. There are approximately 10^6 to 10^7 organisms per gram of feces in the small intestine.[134] The bacterial organisms found in the small intestine are predominantly *Clostridium perfringens, Lactobacillus, E. coli,* and enterococci.

Normally the microflora lives in a symbiotic relationship with the host. Under normal conditions the microflora presents no problem and actually acts as a defense mechanism. By colonizing the mucosa, the microflora takes up space and prevents other organisms from colonizing. The metabolic products produced by these bacteria are inhibitory to the growth of other bacteria. This helps to prevent overgrowth by any one particular organism. There are also other factors that help regulate the normal flora. These include intestinal motility, pH, bile

---

*Pedialyte, Ross Laboratories, Columbus, OH; Infalyte, Pennwalt Corp., Rochester, NY.

†Pepto-Bismol, Ross Laboratories, Columbus, OH.

‡Imodium, Janssen Phamaceutica, Piscataway, NJ.

§Lomotil, Searle & Co., San Juan, Puerto Rico.

acids, diet, mucosal surface, and oxygen availability.[133]

Bacteria that cause disease of the gastrointestinal tract are classified as enteropathogenic. Enteropathogenic bacteria can be further grouped depending on their action. Bacteria that attach to the mucosa and cause diarrhea by releasing an enterotoxin are classified as enterotoxigenic. Enterotoxigenic organisms include *E. coli, Clostridium perfringens, Salmonella* spp., *Yersinia enterocolitica, Klebsiella pneumoniae,* staphylococci, and *Vibrio cholerae.* Other bacteria cause diarrhea by invading the mucosa and submucosa. Invasive organisms include invasive strains of *E. coli, Salmonella, Campylobacter,* and *Shigella.*

Salmonella

Clinical salmonellosis in the dog and cat is uncommon. *Salmonella* has been cultured from the feces of 28 per cent of the dog population.[25] In the United States the carrier rate in the dog for *Salmonella* is thought to be 10 per cent.[76a] In the cat the carrier rate has been reported to range from 0.5 to 13.6 per cent.[40] Several different serotypes have been isolated from the dog and cat.[98]

The most common *Salmonella* species isolated from the dog are *S. typhimurium* and *S. anatum.*[93, 134] In the cat *S. typhimurium* is the most common isolate.[40]

Salmonella infections are important because of their zoonotic potential. There have been several reports of these types of cases.[97] The transmission of the *Salmonella* organisms is by the fecal/oral route, usually through contaminated food and water. Fecal shedding of the organism in naturally occurring infections has been reported to persist for at least six weeks.[98] Salmonellosis affects primarily young, debilitated, and pregnant animals. Clinical signs of salmonellosis include malaise, depression, incoordination, pyrexia (40 to 41.2°C), anorexia, diarrhea, bloody feces, dehydration, stillbirth, abortion, and metritis. Partial posterior paralysis, cough, nasal hemorrhage, hyperirritability, and "running-barking fits" have been seen in more severe cases.[97] Most dogs infected with *Salmonella* are asymptomatic and tend to become occult fecal shedders. If the *Salmonella* invasion is limited to the mucosa, usually a self-limiting gastroenteritis occurs. The acute phase usually runs a four- to ten-day course, but a chronic intermittent diarrhea lasting three to four weeks has been observed in some patients.[97, 98] The CBC may show neutropenia and lymphopenia. This leukopenia is suspected to be the result of microvascular leukocyte sequestration and may be an effect of enterotoxin released by *Salmonella* organisms. As the patient improves, the lymphocyte count is elevated first, followed by a rise in the neutrophils.[138]

Salmonella can cause an acute septicemia, and in these instances thrombocytopenia and a non-regenerative anemia may be observed. The septicemia may be severe enough to initiate disseminated intravascular coagulation (DIC).[79] Pathological lesions include congestion or petechial hemorrhages of the mucosa; blood and mucus may be present in the intestinal lumen; and mesenteric lymph nodes may be enlarged. Other lesions often seen include areas of necrosis that appear as yellow-white foci in the liver, spleen, and mesenteric lymph nodes.[40] If septicemia occurs, petechiation and ecchymosis can be seen in mucous membranes and hairless areas. If DIC occurs, thromboembolism may be seen in all tissues.[79] The diagnosis of salmonellosis is confirmed by fecal culture. Diagnosis of salmonella septicemia is by blood culture.

Treatment is primarily concerned with keeping the patient well hydrated. Oral fluid therapy can be effective if the intestine is not too severely damaged. Balanced electrolyte solutions (e.g., lactated Ringer's) should be used. The use of antibiotics is controversial. If the animal has only mucosal invasion and no evidence of septicemia, antibiotics are contraindicated. They appear to have no beneficial effects and animals tend to shed *Salmonella* organisms longer if they have received antibiotics.[88, 134] However, if signs of septicemia are present, systemic antibiotics are warranted. The choice of antibiotic should be based on culture and sensitivity. Chloramphenicol, gentamicin, and trimethoprim/sulfa have been reported to be effective.[120, 134] A strong reason not to use antibiotics indiscriminately is because *Salmonella* organisms can pass on antibiotic resistance to *E. coli* by plasmids.[40] If endotoxic shock is present, treatment with glucocorticoids may be indicated. Other agents that may have value are acepromazine (1.1 mg/kg) to counteract endotoxin-mediated intestinal vasoconstriction and 5 per cent dextrose in water if hypoglycemia is present.[138]

Escherichia coli

E. coli is a normal inhabitant of the intestines. Because of this, its role in enteric disease is controversial. *E. coli* is considered by some to be the most common cause of bacterial enteritis in the dog.[19]

There are two classifications of enteropathogenic *E. coli:* enterotoxigenic and invasive. Enterotoxigenic *E. coli* attaches to the mucosa and releases an enterotoxin that activates the secretory mechanism of the mucosa. This stimulation of the secretory mechanism results in diarrhea.[134] The increase in secretion is manifested by an increase in adenyl cyclase, which in turn increases intracellular cAMP. The end result is loss of isotonic fluid into the intestinal lumen. This mechanism is partially supported by the observation that *E. coli* enterotoxins, isolated from humans with secretory diarrhea, stimulated adenyl cyclase and isotonic fluid secretion in canine jejunum.[51]

Invasive *E. coli* organisms invade the epithelial cells and release a cytotoxic enterotoxin, which results in disruption of the mucosal surface and acute enterocolitis.[134] *E. coli* can cause a septicemia that is manifested by shock, collapse, and death within 24 hours.[88] Clinical signs include diarrhea (possibly hemorrhagic), dehydration, and acidosis. This problem occurs primarily in young animals.[19]

Laboratory test results are consistent with dehydration and acidosis. The hematocrit and total serum protein may be elevated secondary to dehydration.

Since *E. coli* is part of the normal flora, it is difficult to interpret positive fecal cultures and to make a definitive diagnosis of *E. coli* infection. Serotyping has been done, but is not totally reliable.[88, 120] The most reliable way to diagnose enterotoxigenic *E. coli* is by fecal inoculation of intestinal loops of young mice or by adrenocortical tissue cultures.[88] Invasive *E. coli* is diagnosed by the organism's ability to induce a conjunctivitis within 24 hours after application in the eye of a guinea pig (Sereny test).[39, 88] Radioimmunoassay (RIA) and enzyme-linked immunosorbent assay (ELISA) have been used to determine enterotoxins.[52]

Therapy is primarily aimed at rehydration and correction of acidosis. Oral fluid therapy can be of value in these cases. Parenteral fluids are indicated if the disease is severe and should consist of balanced electrolyte solutions (e.g. lactated Ringer's). Antibiotic use in these cases is controversial. With no evidence of sepsis, antibiotics should not be used. Antibiotics that are effective are gentamicin (2 mg/kg/TID) and kanamycin (5 mg/kg/BID).[135] Bismuth subsalicylate* has clinical application in *E. coli* diarrheas. Bismuth subsalicylate can absorb unbound toxin and the salicylate component probably has local anti-prostaglandin activity that counteracts the effects of the enterotoxin.[88]

Campylobacter

Campylobacter jejuni is a gram-negative, motile, microaerophilic curved rod. Within the past few years *C. jejuni* has been recognized as a major human enteric pathogen.[41] The exact role that *C. jejuni* plays in disease of small animals is unknown, but the fact that *C. jejuni* has been cultured from the feces of dogs and cats makes this organism of public health significance. *C. jejuni* has been cultured from both normal dogs and dogs with diarrhea.[33, 62, 114] Experimentally, *C. jejuni* of human and canine origin given orally to gnotobiotic dogs produced signs of disease, including lethargy, anorexia, mild diarrhea, and tenesmus. A mild, superficial colitis was noted.[114] Studies performed on normal puppies induced a seven- to ten-day course of semiformed-to-watery stools with mucus and occasional blood, tenesmus and occasional vomiting. In these cases involvement of the jejunum and ileum was seen.[33]

There have been several reports of transmission from dogs and cats to man.[12, 62] In Great Britain it is estimated that 5 per cent of human cases of *C. jejuni* are associated with canine and feline infections.[62] The route of infection is thought to be fecal/oral primarily in contaminated food and water.

The prevalence of *Campylobacter* organisms in normal dogs and cats varies, depending on the study. It has been reported to be highest (49 per cent of dogs and 45 per cent of cats) in immature animals (< 6 months of age), especially animals housed in crowded conditions (e.g., kennel, pound). A 1.6 per cent incidence has been reported in adult cats and dogs raised in households.[125]

The significance of *Campylobacter* in dogs and cats is unknown, although the organism

*Pepto-Bismol, Ross Laboratories, Columbus, OH.

may be the cause of diarrhea in these animals. In humans, the organisms are thought to be invasive, which may also be the case in dogs and cats.[41]

In a study done at one hospital, eight cases of *Campylobacter jejuni* were diagnosed over a nine-month period. The dogs' clinical signs were mucus-laden and watery diarrhea from one to several days' duration, with blood apparent in some cases, as well as decreased appetite, vomiting, and slight fever.[41] Not enough is known about *Campylobacter* in dogs to be able to assess CBC and biochemical profile changes.

The diagnosis of *Campylobacter* diarrhea is made by fecal culture on special media. The organism is microaerophilic and has an optimal growth temperature of 37°C to 42°C. The organism will not grow at 25°C. When sending fecal swabs to the laboratory they should be kept at 4°C in anaerobic transport medium.[33] A presumptive diagnosis can be made by dark-field or phase-contrast microscopy. Motile curved rods are visualized.[33] Recommendations for treatment with antibiotics vary. In human medicine, erythromycin is the drug most often used. In dogs and cats with *Campylobacter,* erythromycin (40 mg/kg/day) has been recommended.[42, 62] If vomiting is a problem secondary to erythromycin administration, tylosin (45 mg/kg/day) may be substituted.[62] Other antimicrobials reported to be successful by in vitro sensitivity include aminoglycosides, chloramphenicol, tetracycline, furazolidone, and clindamycin.[42] Some *C. jejuni* produce β-lactamase, making them resistant to penicillins.[42]

Yersinia enterocolitica

Yersinia enterocolitica, a gram-negative rod, has been recognized as a pathogen in man.[120] The most frequent signs of infection in people are fever, abdominal pain, and diarrhea. Meningitis, septicemia, polyarthritis, and abscesses associated with *Y. enterocolitica* have been reported.[105]

Because *Y. enterocolitica* has been isolated from dogs,[36, 105] public health consideration may be warranted. The carrier incidence in the United States (0.4 per cent) and Canada (0.6 per cent) is low, but in Japan and the Scandinavian countries the carrier incidence is reported as 6 per cent.[105]

In the dog there have been only two reported cases of *Y. enterocolitica* enteritis.[105] There is one previous report of a dog with chronic enteritis in which *Y. enterocolitica* was isolated after necropsy.[36] In both clinical cases the dogs presented with diarrhea of two weeks' duration. The stools ranged from semi-liquid to normal, and the feces were covered with mucus and blood. Tenesmus was noted and appetite was normal. On fecal culture *Y. enterocolitica* was isolated, and the dogs were treated. Subsequent attempts to culture *Y. enterocolitica* were negative.[105]

Chloramphenicol, tetracycline, and gentamicin are usually effective as treatment. The significance of *Y. enterocolitica* as an enteric pathogen is not known and cannot be assessed until more cases are diagnosed.

Bacillus piliformis

Bacillus piliformis is a spore-forming, gram-negative, pleomorphic bacillus that is the etiologic agent of Tyzzer's disease. Rodents are the primary reservoirs for *B. piliformis*. Tyzzer's disease has been reported in dogs and cats, but this is rare.[111, 116, 120] It was reported as a complication of canine distemper and mycotic infection in one dog.[111] The disease is seen primarily in puppies and kittens but does occur in adults. Animals treated with radiation or cortisone that are immunosuppressed may be susceptible to the disease.[111]

The diagnosis is made by the use of special stains (Warthin-Starry, Gomori's methenamine silver, Giemsa, and periodic acid–Schiff) on sections taken from the margins of hepatic and intestinal abscesses.[111, 120] Numerous filamentous organisms are seen intracellularly.

Tyzzer's disease is characterized by a hemorrhagic enterocolitis and multifocal hepatic necrosis and is fatal.[111, 120]

Other Bacterial Diseases

Clostridium perfringens has been associated with two cases of peracute hemorrhagic gastroenteritis.[112] The association was made because large numbers of *C. perfringens* organisms were found adhering to the necrotic epithelial surfaces in parts of the gastrointestinal tract and large numbers of *C. perfringens* organisms were recovered from the intestine.[112]

Enterotoxin produced by *Staphylococcus aureus* has been shown to cause food poisoning in people. In Japan, enterotoxigenic staphylococci were isolated in 26 of 451 dogs.[73] This may have public health significance. Food poisoning by staphylococci may be of canine origin via persons who have had contact with a carrier dog.[73]

Shigella spp. have been isolated from dogs but have not been shown to cause disease.[98] This is significant because the dog may be a source of human infections.[98]

SALMON POISONING DISEASE AND ELOKOMIN FLUKE FEVER

Salmon poisoning disease and Elokomin fluke fever are rickettsial diseases of dogs. They are primarily seen in the Pacific Northwest. Dogs acquire the diseases by digestion of raw salmon or trout that is infected with the metacercaria of the fluke *Nanophyteus salmincola*. The fluke harbors the rickettsia *Neorickettsia helminthoeca* and the rickettsial-like agent called Elokomin fluke fever agent. Together they are responsible for the signs of salmon poisoning.[35] The disease has been shown to be transmitted by aerosols and rectal contact, demonstrating that the disease is communicable but not highly contagious.[15]

Salmon Poisoning Disease

The incubation period for salmon poisoning disease is five to seven days after ingestion of the raw fish. Clinical signs are pyrexia (39.7° to 41.7°C) that then decreases for six to eight days, followed by hypothermia and death. Severe depression, anorexia, extreme thirst, emesis, lymphadenopathy, and progressive and often bloody diarrhea are seen after the temperature peak. Mucopurulent nasal and conjunctival exudate are common findings. If untreated, 50 to 90 per cent of the dogs die.[35]

The disease is diagnosed by fecal examination using the washing-sedimentation technique to demonstrate the fluke egg. Properly stained aspirates from the mandibular lymph nodes may demonstrate rickettsia-like bodies (morulae).

Treatment consists of symptomatic therapy and correction of the dehydration with fluid therapy using a balanced electrolyte solution. The antibiotic of choice is oxytetracycline, given intravenously at a dosage of 11 mg/kg of body weight, followed by a subsequent dosage of 6.6 mg/kg.[35] If the dog recovers, strong immunity develops.

Elokomin Fluke Fever

The Elokomin fluke fever agent has been shown to cause disease by itself. The incubation period is 5 to 12 days.[35] Clinical signs include pyrexia that reaches a plateau for 4 to 7 days and gradually returns to normal in dogs that survive. Subnormal temperatures are seen in dogs before death. Other symptoms include mucopurulent ocular discharge, vomition, diarrhea, and dehydration. Severe depression and ataxia may occur in some dogs. Lymphadenopathy is seen in all infected dogs. It can persist for weeks and the infectious agent can be recovered for months in normal dogs.[35]

The diagnosis of Elokomin fluke fever is made by clinical signs and the presence of fluke eggs in the feces. Treatment is the same as for salmon poisoning disease.

Prevention

To prevent both diseases, raw fish should not be fed to dogs. Cooking or freezing inactivates the fluke and prevents the diseases.

VIRAL DISEASES

Many viruses have been isolated from the feces of dogs and cats. The significance of all of them is not known. In the dog, parvovirus and coronavirus are recognized causes of disease. Rotavirus and astrovirus may have clinical importance, but to what extent is unknown. Other viruses that have been identified in dogs are minute virus (parvovirus distinct from enteritis-producing parvovirus), adenovirus, paramyxovirus-like virus, picornavirus, human echovirus, and coxsackievirus.[43, 120, 143]

Parvovirus is the most important virus in the cat, but other viruses have been identified, including coronavirus, rotavirus, astrovirus, calcivirus, reovirus type III, and non-culturable enteric picornaviridae-like virus.[4, 120] In cats with diarrhea problems, feline leukemia virus (FeLV) and feline infectious peritonitis (FIP) virus must be considered in the diagnosis, especially in cats refractory to treatment.

Canine Parvovirus (CPV)

Canine parvovirus is an extremely small (22 nm) single-stranded DNA virus. It was recognized as a clinical entity in 1978. Serological investigations of dog sera prior to 1978 have failed to recognize any parvovirus antibodies.[86, 110] CPV is an epitheliotropic virus that can replicate only in rapidly dividing cells. Because of this, the virus attacks crypts, bone marrow, and lymphoid cells. CPV is transmitted primarily by direct fecal/oral contact. However, it can exist outside the host for at least six months[67]; thus, indirect transmission does occur. The exact incidence of CPV enteritis is unknown but is significantly less at the present time than during the first three years after the disease was recognized.[110] The virus is ingested in most cases, and invasion occurs at the oropharyngeal ring, producing the initial viremia. Localization and multiplication of the virus occurs in the marrow and lymphoid tissue. There are two syndromes seen in dogs: myocarditis and enteritis. Myocarditis usually occurs in dogs 4 to 6 weeks of age.[145] The puppies are usually infected postnatally. With the vaccination of bitches, CPV myocarditis has become extremely rare.[67, 110] The incubation period for CPV is usually five to seven days.

CPV can infect dogs of any age but frequently infects dogs between 6 to 16 weeks. Often the puppy has just been acquired by the owners. Initial clinical signs are lethargy and anorexia. This is often followed by diarrhea (watery to hemorrhagic) and vomiting. On physical examination, the dog will be depressed and dehydrated. The patient is sometimes febrile and occasionally there is pain on abdominal palpation. Some of the patients show only depression, or they may collapse and die within 24 hours after presentation.

In puppies presenting with myocarditis, there is acute heart failure. Signs include crying, depression, and respiratory diseases. Acute death is common between 3 and 6 weeks of age. A subacute form is seen in dogs 6 to 12 weeks of age; these animals may succumb to heart failure several months later.[67] The myocardial form is usually not seen with the enteric form, and vice versa. Mild and inapparent infections are fairly common.

The hemogram consistently shows a leukopenia, especially in the granulocytes. The total white blood cell count often ranges between 500 and 2000 per $mm.^3$ Frequently the leukopenia does not occur for 24 to 72 hours after initial signs. Serial complete blood counts are often needed for diagnosis and for monitoring recovery. In our opinion, fecal cultures for bacteria are warranted. There is one report of isolation of *Campylobacter* organisms from 23 of 49 dogs with CPV, and one report of isolation of toxigenic *C. perfringens,* type A.[119, 137] It has been the experience at our institution (University of Missouri–Columbia, UMC) that abnormal numbers of *C. perfringens* are cultured from the stool in approximately 80 per cent of animals with CPV infection.

The diagnosis of CPV infection can be made utilizing several methods. Usually the diagnosis is accomplished from clinical signs and evidence of a leukopenia. Electron microscopy of feces during the acute phase can identify the virus particles. Cell culture of the feces is available for viral isolation. Hemagglutination (HA) of the feces is available to detect the virus in the feces, although the value of this test has not been determined. High CPV titers have been seen in healthy dogs and negative titers have been found in dogs that met all other criteria for parvovirus infection. A hemagglutination inhibition test is available for serodiagnostic evaluation.[28] Since the titer can remain high for longer than one year, a high titer is not diagnostic. A high IgM titer to CPV is indicative of recent infection. Immunofluorescent antibody studies of infected tissue can be used to diagnose CPV infection, and an ELISA test has been recently described for diagnosis.[93, 110]

Treatment of CPV enteritis is mainly symptomatic. Fluid therapy is required for dogs that are dehydrated or vomiting and have diarrhea. The use of a balanced electrolyte solution, such as lactated Ringer's, is recommended. If hypoglycemia is a finding, a bolus of 50 per cent dextrose IV followed by fluids supplemented with dextrose is needed. Antibiotics are strongly recommended in these cases. Since there is a severe leukopenia, a bactericidal antibiotic is recommended. At UMC Ampicillin (22 mg/kg TID) is used. This is effective against *C. perfringens,* which frequently shows heavy growth on fecal cultures, as previously described.

The use of motility modifiers is controversial. Narcotic analgesics will help decrease the diarrhea by increased segmental contraction, but increased enterotoxin absorption may occur. If there are signs of shock, glucocorticoid therapy is warranted.

Prognosis is extremely variable. Mortality

seems to be higher among younger animals. If fluid and electrolyte balance can be successfully restored, the prognosis is good.[87] Some authors have proposed that the lower the leukocyte count, the worse the prognosis.[110, 120] It has been the experience at UMC that the leukocyte count has no relationship to prognosis.

Postmortem findings reveal mild to severe intestinal congestion. The intestines feel thickened and the serosal surface has a roughened, granulated appearance.[67] The mucosa may appear hyperemic with ulceration. Intestinal contents may be watery with a fetid odor or there may be frank hemorrhage and mucosal sloughing.[14] Lymphadenopathy is also seen. Histologically, there is a severe degenerative necrotic enteritis. Sloughing of intestinal crypt cells leads to crypt aplasia and mucosal collapse.[86] In young animals, thymus atrophy is seen. Bone marrow changes reflect an extreme marrow toxicity and reactivity with increased turnover and destruction of normal elements.[14] In puppies with myocarditis, large, dense intranuclear inclusion bodies can be seen.[145]

Prevention of CPV infection is best accomplished by vaccination. Since feline panleukopenia virus (FPV) and CPV are antigenically similar, the following types of vaccines have been used: killed FPV and CPV vaccines and modified live CPV and FPV vaccines. The modified live CPV vaccines seem to give the best results.[110] When vaccinating puppies it is best to start at 6 to 8 weeks, vaccinate every 2 to 4 weeks until 16 weeks of age, and then give yearly boosters. Most puppies that have received maternal antibodies will become susceptible to CPV between 6 and 16 weeks of age. During this time there is a 1-to 3-week period when puppies may not respond to vaccination and yet are susceptible to infection.[47, 110]

Vaccination of puppies infected with parvovirus is contraindicated. In one study, five gnotobiotic dogs were vaccinated with canine distemper, adenovirus type 2, and parainfluenza viruses, and *Leptospira canicola–L. icterohaemorrhagiae* bacterin; they were then infected orally with CPV. Two of the dogs developed canine distemper virus encephalomyelitis secondary to the vaccine.[78]

Control of the spread of CPV in infected environments is aided by disinfection with 1:30 chlorine bleach in runs and housing areas, although complete elimination of the virus from the premise is extremely difficult.[121]

Feline Panleukopenia Virus (FPV)

FPV is a highly contagious parvovirus infection of cats. Like CPV, the virus replicates in rapidly dividing cells , such as the crypt cells of the intestine, bone marrow, and lymphoid tissue.[120, 122] The end result is enteritis, leukopenia, and lymphoid depletion. Young kittens (parturition to 10 days) that become infected with FPV can show signs of cerebellar hypoplasia. The cerebellar cells replicate until about 10 to 14 days after parturition.

In utero infection can occur and results in resorption of fetuses, mummification, abortion, stillbirth, and birth of weak or fading kittens.[111] Cerebellar hypoplasia, thymic atrophy, and blindness due to retinal dysplasia can occur up to 10 days postnatally.

FPV can be viable for longer than one year outside the host. Infection occurs by ingestion or inhalation of the virus. Initial replication occurs in the oropharynx, followed by a viremic phase. The virus then locates in a secondary lymphoid replication site.[70]

Clinical signs of FPV infection include anorexia, depression, vomiting, dehydration, fever, and abdominal pain. The cat may present with peracute signs, collapsed or dead. If the cerebellum has been affected, ataxia and hypermetria may be seen. Neurologic and enteric signs are rarely seen together.

The severity of signs seems to be dependent on the microflora. Gnotobiotic cats infected with the virus showed no signs of illness, whereas specific pathogen-free cats had only slight changes and anorexia for five to six days.[27] Clinical pathology reveals a leukopenia of varying severity. Often the WBC count is less than 1000 cells per mm^3.

Histopathologically, mucosal collapse is seen. The virus replicates in the crypt cells, resulting eventually in villous atrophy and collapse. These lesions are primarily seen in the small intestine, but similar less severe and more focal lesions are seen in the colon.[122]

The diagnosis is primarily based on the CBC and on clinical signs. For a definitive diagnosis, electron microscopic viral identification from the feces and immunofluorescent studies of infected tissue may be utilized.

Treatment is basically the same as for CPV enteritis (fluids, broad-spectrum bactericidal antibiotics, and so forth). The prognosis is generally considered guarded.

Prevention is best achieved by vaccination. The recommended procedure is vaccination of kittens at the time of the first office visit and every four weeks until 14 weeks of age, followed by yearly boosters.[110]

Canine Corona Virus (CCV)

Canine corona virus has been recognized as a pathogen since 1971 when it was recovered from military dogs.[75] CCV affects the epithelial cells of the villi. The virus is contagious and transmission is usually by the fecal/oral route. Once ingested, the virus penetrates into the enterocytes between microvilli, possibly by pinocytosis.[135] The infected cells are sloughed from the villi, resulting in shortening, blunting, and fusion of the villi and lengthening of the crypts.[13, 75] CCV affects the small intestine, particularly the ileum.[135] Histologically, in addition to shortening of the microvilli and blunting of the villi, intracellular vacuolization, infiltration of the lamina propria with inflammatory cells and intercellular edema are seen.[74] The end result is malabsorption and diarrhea.

The patient may develop signs of disease one to three days following exposure. The clinical signs can vary from inapparent infection to rapid death.[110] Diarrhea is the main presenting sign and is usually foul-smelling, loose to mucoid, and orange in color and may contain blood. Vomiting may also occur.

Physical examination findings include lethargy, depression, anorexia, and slight dehydration. The temperature is usually normal to subnormal.[110] Clinical pathology is usually within normal limits. The disease in most cases is self-limiting and symptoms resolve in five to ten days. Occasionally diarrhea will persist for two to three weeks.

A definitive diagnosis is usually not made. The presumptive diagnosis is made on history, clinical signs, and absence of leukopenia. For a definitive diagnosis electron microscopic identification of virus in feces, isolation of virus from feces, and immunofluorescence studies of the affected tissues can be performed. Serum neutralizing antibody titers are available but only indicate possible infection.

Treatment depends on the severity of disease and is symptomatic. The prognosis is usually good and most dogs will recover uneventfully.

Feline Coronaviruses

Three coronaviruses may infect the cat: feline infectious peritonitis (FIP), feline enteric corona-1 (FEC-1), and feline enteric corona-2 (FEC-2). FEC-1 is morphologically distinct from FIP and is found in approximately 10 per cent of cats. Studies are being done on the clinical and serological differentiation of FIP and FEC-1.[4]

FEC-2 is antigenically closely related to FIP virus.[108] FEC-2 has been shown to produce an inapparent to mildly severe enteritis in kittens 4 to 12 weeks of age. These cats can show positive titers to FIP virus. FEC-2 is thought to be ubiquitous in nature and prevalent in all catteries.[4] There are several differences betwen FIP virus and FEC-2. FIP virus is not highly infective per os and does not cause clinically apparent enteritis in kittens; it does cause peritonitis, pleuritis, and disseminated granulomatous disease. FEC-2 is highly infective orally, causes enteritis in kittens, and does not cause feline infectious peritonitis.[108]

Clinical signs of FEC-2 infection include inapparent to mild diarrhea. FEC-2 has an affinity for the mature apical columnar epithelium of the villi. If the infection is severe enough, sloughing of the tips of the villi occurs and villous atrophy results.[108] The lesions are seen from the duodenum to the cecum. Treatment is usually not necessary, although supportive care is recommended in more severe cases.

Rotavirus—Dogs and Cats

Rotavirus has been associated with neonatal diarrhea in people, cattle, foals, swine, sheep, mice, antelope, and deer.[34] Rotavirus is the most common cause of non-bacterial enteritis in human neonates in most countries.[43] In human neonates the infection is often asymptomatic but can be severe enough to cause death.[90]

Two reported cases of neonatal diarrhea in dogs have been reported. One case involved a 3-day-old puppy that subsequently died, and the other was a 12-week-old puppy that survived infection.[34, 43] In both cases rotavirus was isolated.

In humans the virus replicates primarily in the enterocytes of the small intestine. In severe cases the villi are shortened and somewhat edematous.[90] The villus then becomes populated by immature cells that have migrated from the crypts at an accelerated rate. This leads to a net secretory flux and the loss of sodium and chloride, causing a secretory diarrhea. In the dog these same changes appear to occur, as demonstrated in gnotobiotic dogs infected with rotavirus.[66] Rotavirus has been isolated from cats but has not been associated with disease.[4] The exact importance of rotavirus in dogs and cats still needs to be determined.

Other Viruses

Astroviruses have been known to produce diarrhea in humans, turkeys, and sheep.[4] Astrovirus-like particles have been found in beagle puppies and in one cat.[4, 143] The significance of astrovirus infections in dogs and cats is unknown. Feline leukemia virus (FeLV) has been shown to infect the crypt epithelial cells of cats. Mucosal collapse can occur, resulting in diarrhea. FeLV infection may result in a panleukopenia-like syndrome. If the patient has diarrhea lasting longer than one week, FeLV should be considered in the diagnosis. Diagnosis is made via a positive FeLV test.[4]

Feline calicivirus (FCV) has been isolated from the feces of cats with diarrhea. FCV that causes upper respiratory signs may have a variant form that causes diarrhea and possibly malabsorption.

MYCOTIC INFECTION

Mycotic infection of the small intestine is rare. Due to the opportunistic nature of fungal infections, they are usually seen secondary to prolonged use of antibiotics or corticosteroids, immunosuppressive therapy, malnutrition, or debilitating diseases.[88, 120] The most common causes of mycotic intestinal disease are *Histoplasma capsulatum, Candida albicans,* Phycomycetes, and *Aspergillus* spp. Mycotic infections can present as acute fulminating disease or chronic diarrhea with weight loss.

Candida albicans can infect the mucosal surface. The diagnosis is made from fecal culture or the presence of large numbers of yeast bodies in a fecal smear stained with Wright stain.[89] The treatment of candidiasis is oral ketoconazole* (30 mg/kg/day/divided TID). Other treatments that are effective are nystatin per os and IV amphotericin B.†

Phycomycosis is an infection caused by a broad group of fungi. These fungi are characterized by non-septate branching hyphae and are ubiquitous in nature.[44] Patients with Phycomycetes infections of the small intestine will usually present for vomiting. On physical examination dogs with phycomycosis usually have a palpable abdominal mass.[44] Gastrointestinal phycomycosis has been reported in dogs and cats by several authors.[2, 44, 94] It is a fairly common canine fungal disease in states bordering the Gulf of Mexico.[94] Medical treatment tends to be difficult and surgical removal of the mass is probably warranted.[44]

Aspergillosis has been diagnosed in mycotic intestinal disease.[130] Aspergillosis is characterized by diffuse infiltration of the intestinal submucosa with branching septate hyphae. The diagnosis can be made with fecal cultures.

Aspergillosis responds poorly to medical treatment. A combination of 5-fluorocytosine (100 mg/kg/day) and amphotericin B IV (0.1 mg/1b given on Monday, Wednesday, Friday) can be effective in the treatment of aspergillosis. When amphotericin B is used alone, it should be started at 0.15 mg/kg IV in 25 to 30 ml of 5 percent dextrose in water and given over a 30-minute period. Therapy should be every other day. During the second week of therapy, the dosage may be gradually increased to 0.20 mg/kg. Blood urea nitrogen should be monitored before each treatment during therapy because of the nephrotoxicity of amphotericin B.

Histoplasmosis

Histoplasmosis is caused by the pleomorphic fungus *Histoplasma capsulatum.* Histoplasma is found endemically in 31 states.[32] *H. capsulatum* can be found in the soil in the mycelial form as a saprophyte and is often found in areas enriched with fecal material of avian species and bats.[139]

*Nizoral, Jessen Pharmaceutical, New Brunswick, NJ.

†Fungizone, E. R. Squibb & Sons, Inc., Princeton, NJ.

It is believed that *Histoplasma* organisms gain entry via inhalation. The organism then localizes in the lung where most of the time it causes focal lung necrosis and later is encapsulated and calcified. These lesions are the benign form. In some cases hematogenous spread occurs during early pulmonary infections, but this is usually self-limiting. Occasionally the disease progresses to the disseminated form with involvement of the reticuloendothelial system.[32, 129] Some investigators think that the disseminated form occurs with invasion of the intestinal wall and then spreads via lymphatics and the portal blood supply to the regional lymph nodes and the hepatic reticuloendothelial cells.[32, 127]

Animals that present with disseminated histoplasmosis generally have a history of a chronic problem. This can include weight loss, diarrhea that may be bloody, depression, and anorexia. Physical examination findings depend on the organs involved. The animal will often appear emaciated, with pale mucous membranes. On abdominal palpation the liver, spleen, and lymph nodes may be enlarged and the intestine may feel thickened. Respiratory signs may also be evident.

Clinical pathology depends on which organs are affected. Often the animal presents with a non-regenerative anemia. Malabsorption and protein-losing enteropathies may be seen in animals with histoplasmosis.

Diagnosis can be made by identification of the organism in neutrophils or monocytes from a buffy coat smear of the peripheral blood or in colonic scrapings. Other available tests are complement fixation, immunodiffusion, fluorescent antibody technique, and antiglobulin hemagglutination.[77]

Treatment of histoplasmosis traditionally has been with amphotericin B. Ketoconazole, an imidazole, has also been reported to be successful against histoplasmosis.[100] At UMC ketoconazole (30 mg/kg/day TID) has been used successfully in the treatment of one case of gastrointestinal histoplasmosis. The prognosis for animals with histoplasmosis is always guarded.

ACUTE HEMORRHAGIC GASTROENTERITIS (HGE)

Acute hemorrhagic gastroenteritis is a disease of dogs that is characterized by peracute onset of vomiting and severe bloody diarrhea. The etiology and exact mechanisms are unknown. The rapid onset of clinical signs and the similarity to experimental endotoxic shock suggest that HGE may result from an allergic or anaphylactic response to bacterial endotoxins.[21] Another mechanism that has been suggested is an immune-mediated pathogenesis.[134]

The clinical history often reveals that the dog was fine four to five hours prior to presentation and then abruptly started vomiting or having bouts of diarrhea, or both. In a short time, the vomiting or diarrhea becomes hemorrhagic and the patient is depressed. HGE affects a wide variety of breeds but miniature schnauzers, miniature and toy poodles, and miniature and toy breeds as a group seem to be more susceptible.[21] There seems to be an age range of 2 to 4 years.[21]

Physical examination reveals depression and hemorrhagic diarrhea or "raspberry-jam" stool. Rectal temperature is usually normal. Judged by skin turgor, the patient does not appear to be dehydrated; some patients, however, will present in hypovolemic shock. Disseminated intravascular coagulopathy may also be a finding in patients with HGE.

Clinical pathology varies, depending on severity. Most of the abnormalities are secondary to fluid loss due to diarrhea. The white blood cell counts are usually normal throughout the course of the disease. The most consistent finding is an elevated packed cell volume (PCV) secondary to fluid loss. In a review of 107 dogs with HGE, the median PCV was 69.0 per cent. A mean PCV of 73 per cent was seen in dogs that died.[21] Prerenal azotemia is often a finding in dogs with HGE.

Loops of darkened congested small bowel were found at necropsy in dogs with HGE. Also, frank hemorrhage was seen in the gut lumen and the mucosal surface was dark reddish-black in color.[21]

Treatment is primarily concerned with fluid replacement. Patients may not exhibit dehydration clinically, but they have extracellular dehydration, evidenced by increased PCV and total protein. Fluids should be given intravenously and started immediately after hospitalization. Often the patient is acidotic; therefore, a balanced fluid such as lactated Ringer's solution is recommended. Fluids with bicarbonate added may be warranted but blood gas measurements should be obtained first. Often, fluid therapy is needed only for a short time. In these cases, a jugular catheter should be used. The initial dosage of fluids should be 30 to 60 ml/kg of body weight in the first 15 to 30 minutes. Once the animal is stabilized, the amount of fluids can be reduced to maintenance levels. Glucocorticoids may be necessary in patients in hypovolemic shock.

The use of antibiotics is controversial. At UMC 90 per cent of the patients have a heavy growth of *Clostridia* spp. on fecal cultures. For this reason we believe that antibiotics are warranted. Penicillin antibiotics appear to be the antibiotic of choice because of their effectiveness against anaerobic bacteria and their minimal effect on normal flora. Intestinal protectants are not needed, but bismuth salicylate (Pepto-Bismol) may be of benefit because of the salicylate component. Motility modifiers are usually not needed because of the short duration of the diarrhea; however, they may be necessary if the diarrhea is severe or long-lasting.

With proper therapy, the prognosis of most patients is excellent; however, some will die even with prompt treatment. Usually the patient responds in 24 to 48 hours and is released in 48 to 72 hours.

Endocrine Diarrheas

Many metabolic and endocrine disorders affect the small intestine indirectly and cause diarrhea. Diseases such as hypoadrenocorticism (Addison's disease) and diabetes mellitus are well documented as causes of intestinal upsets. Several others have been determined to be part of a diarrhea syndrome.

Thyroid Disorders

In the canine, medullary carcinoma has been associated with a watery diarrhea. In one report a patient presented with a diarrhea of three months' duration.[81a] A mass was palpated in the right cervical region and was removed surgically. The diarrhea resolved the second day postoperatively.

A syndrome in humans exists in which a secretory diarrhea is associated with medullary thyroid carcinoma. The mechanism of the diarrhea is poorly understood but it is felt to be due to a humoral agent secreted by the tumor that stimulates adenyl cyclase.[119a, 120] Calcitonin has been shown to stimulate jejunal secretion of water and electrolytes and is a likely choice.[119a] Medullary carcinoma of the thyroid also secretes prostaglandins that stimulate intestinal motility and may be the cause of the diarrhea.[119a]

Feline hyperthyroidism is a multisystem problem arising from elevated circulating T_3 and T_4 levels.[109] Functional thyroid adenomas are the most common cause of feline hyperthyroidism, although thyroid carcinoma may also rarely be a cause. These adenomas primarily occur in cats ten years and older.[63]

Clinical signs are weight loss, increased appetite, and hyperactivity. Gastrointestinal signs include vomiting, increased frequency of defecation, and increased volume of feces. Malabsorption is seen in some cats with hyperthyroidism. This can be detected by increased fecal fat excretion. Polyuria and polydipsia are also frequent findings.[109] On physical examination, the cat will often be emaciated and hyperactive. Tachycardia with systolic murmur or gallop rhythm may be auscultated. These cats may sometimes present with congestive heart failure. Palpation of the cervical area often reveals one or more masses.

Clinical pathological findings vary. Leukocytosis with eosinopenia is often present, secondary to stress. There may be an increase in the PCV, which is induced by the effects of thyroid hormones on erythroid elements, with the subsequent production of erythropoietin.[109] Often there are increased levels of serum alanine aminotransferase, serum aspartate aminotransferase, and serum alkaline phosphatase. Most important, T_3 and T_4 levels are elevated, although in some cases the T_3 value may be normal.[109]

A conclusive diagnosis can be made and the extent of the tumor can be determined using a thyroid scan. Bilateral enlargement is found in 70 per cent of cats with hyperthyroidism.[109] Thyroid scans can also detect regional and distant metastases of functional thyroid carcinomas.[63]

There are three possible treatments for feline hyperthyroidism: surgical removal, antithyroid drug therapy, and radioactive iodine therapy. Surgical removal is considered the most effective treatment. Preoperatively, in order to lower T_3 and T_4 levels, the cat should receive propylthiouracil* (PTU) (50 mg/kg/TID). T_3 and T_4 values

*Eli Lilly & Co., Indianapolis, IN.

should be monitored at 7 to 14 day intervals. Usually the values return to normal in two to three weeks; if not, the dosage may need to be increased to 200 to 300 mg/kg/day. Once thyroid levels are normal, surgery should be performed. It is important that at least one functional parathyroid gland is left intact. The patient will probably require supplementary thyroid medication after surgery.

PTU has many side effects; if the drug cannot be used safely, propranolol (2.5 to 5.0 mg TID) can be substituted. Propranolol is a beta-adrenergic blocker that negates many of the cardiovascular and neuromuscular effects of thyrotoxicosis.[109] If the cat is in congestive heart failure, propranolol is contraindicated. If the owners elect not to have surgery performed, PTU can be used for long-term therapy. Its disadvantage is that PTU does not alter the underlying problem. Also, the dosage may have to be altered eventually, and potential side effects of the drug may occur.[109]

The third possible treatment for hyperthyroidism, radioactive iodine (^{131}I), selectively destroys functional thyroid tissue.[109]

Prognosis is variable depending upon the type of tumor, size, duration, ease of removal, and the compliance of the owner in medicating the cat regularly.

Zollinger-Ellison–Like Syndrome

Zollinger-Ellison syndrome in humans was described in 1955. This syndrome consists of recurrent peptic ulcers, hypersecretion of gastric acid, and a non–beta-islet cell tumor of the pancreas. The tumor produces gastrin which stimulates hypersecretion of gastric acid and causes peptic ulcers and diarrhea.[53] The resulting low intestinal pH causes mucosal ulceration, inactivation of lipase, and precipitation of bile salts, leading to fat malassimilation and protein loss in the gut. This syndrome has been reported in the dog.[53, 68] The condition is rare in both humans and dogs.

Clinical signs include vomiting, diarrhea, poor appetite, and weight loss. Previous treatments usually have been unsuccessful. Physical examination findings are non-specific, with generalized lethargy and weight loss.

Clinical pathology also is usually nonspecific, although hypoalbuminemia is common and steatorrhea may be present.

Diagnosis is confirmed by evidence of ulceration, high serum gastrin levels, and histopathology of the pancreatic islet cell tumor. Barium upper gastrointestinal series may show duodenal or jejunal ulcers. Laparoscopy or exploratory celiotomy may reveal multiple small nodules in the pancreas, and there may be metastases to regional lymph nodes and the liver. Serum gastrin levels determined by radioimmunoassay (RIA) are elevated. Fasting serum gastrin levels in the normal dogs range from 23 to 104 pg/ml.

The pathological lesion consists of non–beta-islet cell pancreatic tumors with or without metastases to the regional lymph nodes and liver. The entire gastrointestinal tract may show ulcerations due to gastrin secretion and elevated gastric acid production. C-cell hyperplasia of the thyroid glands can occur secondary to gastrin's effect on calcitonin release.

Treatment consists of surgical excision of the pancreatic tumors.

There has been one reported case of a gastrin-secreting tumor in a 12-year-old cat.[92]

CHRONIC DIARRHEA

Chronic diarrheas are generally more challenging to diagnose and to treat than are acute diarrheas. In small animals chronic diarrheas are seen with much less frequency than are acute forms. Chronic diarrheas can be divided into four groups: protein-losing enteropathies, inflammatory bowel disease, maldigestion, and malabsorption. Often the disease causing the chronic diarrhea will overlap into more than one of these broad categories.

Protein-Losing Enteropathies (PLE)

Protein-losing enteropathies are characterized by the loss of excess protein into the intestinal lumen. This often leads to panhypoproteinemia. If the decrease in albumin is great enough, edema, ascites, and pleural effusion can occur. Causes of PLE include lymphangiectasia, restrictive pericarditis, congestive heart failure, and inflammatory and ulcerative diseases. Definitive diagnosis of PLE can be made using ^{51}Cr-labeled albumin. In one report 30 μc were administered to dogs with suspected PLE. The feces were collected for three days and measured for radioactivity. Control dogs excreted less than 6 per cent of the labeled albumin, whereas dogs with PLE excreted a great deal more.[5]

Inflammatory Small Bowel Disease

Chronic inflammatory small bowel disease is characterized by distention of the lamina propria and occasionally the deeper layers of the bowel wall with inflammatory cells. Examples are eosinophilic gastroenteritis and lymphocytic-plasmacytic gastroenteritis. These conditions are often steroid responsive.[100]

Maldigestion

Maldigestion problems are due primarily to exocrine pancreatic insufficiency. These are treated by dietary supplementation with pancreatic enzymes. (See Chapter 12.)

Malabsorption

Malabsorption can be the result of several diseases, including infiltrative diseases such as intestinal lymphosarcoma. Malabsorption may occur secondary to parasitism and bacterial overgrowth. Inflammatory small bowel disease and massive intestinal resection can lead to malabsorption. Tests for identification of a malabsorption problem have been discussed previously.

Non-Specific Treatment of Malabsorption.

There are several possible non-specific treatments for malabsorption. Dietary management is one important aspect of treatment. A high-protein and high-carbohydrate diet that contains low amounts of fats is recommended. This can be supplemented with medium-chain triglycerides* (MCT) (a mixture of triglycerides synthesized from cocoanut oil) to add calories.[117] In animals with possible lactase deficiency, milk products should be avoided. It does not appear that restriction of protein and carbohydrates, except for lactose, is needed in malabsorption conditions. There is some indication that the use of high quantities of high-quality protein facilitates intestinal adaptation and recovery from the disease.[120] The restriction of long-chain triglycerides (LCT) is advised in the treatment of malabsorption. This can be accomplished by the use of low-fat commercial diets such as r/d.†

*MCT Oil, Mead-Johnson and Co., Evansville, IN.
†Hill's Pet Products, Inc., Topeka, KS.

These diets can be supplemented with MCT, which are assimilated differently than LCT.

The diet should be supplemented with vitamins and minerals, because deficiencies often occur. The fat-soluble vitamins (A, D, E, and K) are most important, along with folic acid and vitamin B_{12}. Deficiencies of the water-soluble vitamins rarely occur.[117]

The use of antibiotics is warranted, especially if bacterial overgrowth is the cause of the malabsorption. Stasis of the intestines can allow colonic bacteria to migrate into the small intestine, and this can cause malabsorption secondary to bile deconjugation by bacteria.[117] Since most of the bacteria in the colon are anaerobic, penicillin antibiotics are usually effective.[117]

Parasites have also been shown to cause malabsorption. In these cases, treatment with appropriate anthelmintics is indicated.

In humans, parenteral hyperalimentation and liquid elemental diets have been used to prevent malnutrition in malabsorptive states. Parenteral hyperalimentation is used when there is almost a complete inability to use the gastrointestinal tract.[120] This is done primarily in the hospital, but home hyperalimentation can be performed.[96] These solutions are tailored to the individual patient's needs.

Elemental diets are of the most value during the "adaptation" phase of recovery, when mucosal growth in the remaining small intestine occurs.[118] Elemental diets also aid in the conversion from intravenous to oral nutrition. Elemental diets are made up of amino acids, dextrins, trace elements, and vitamins.[117] The main consideration in using these methods in veterinary medicine is the high cost.

Chronic Small Intestinal Disease

EOSINOPHILIC GASTROENTERITIS

Eosinophilic gastroenteritis was first described in 1937 as a clinical entity in humans. It has been well described in the veterinary literature, but the etiology is still not known. Dietary allergens are thought to be the most likely cause,[115, 134] although there is a report of eosinophilic gastroenteritis secondary to parasitic infiltration (visceral larval migrans).[55]

It is believed that dietary antigens are absorbed from the intestine. This causes increased permeability, which allows for protein loss (PLE). Once the antigens are absorbed, an immune response occurs that results in accumulation of eosinophils in the lamina propria. Several mechanisms have been proposed as to what then occurs.[134]

Eosinophils are attracted by a chemotactic factor released by mast cells and basophils; therefore, an immediate hypersensitivity-type reaction has been theorized as a mechanism. Since chemotactic factors are also released by sensitized T lymphocytes and some components of complement,[134] it is possible that an Arthus or delayed cell-mediated hypersensitivity is involved. Eosinophils prevent basophilic granular release and phagocytize granules released from mast cells. Slow-reacting substances of anaphylaxis are also inhibited by eosinophils. The main action of eosinophils in these cases is to modify an allergic reaction.[134]

The immediate type of hypersensitivity may result from an antigen entering the gastrointestinal tract repeatedly. In this proposed mechanism, IgE is produced in response to the antigen. The IgE binds to mast cells and on re-exposure the mast cells degranulate. Eosinophils are brought into the area and attenuate the hypersensitivity response, thus making the signs milder and of a chronic nature.[135] In the case of visceral larval migrans, migrating larvae are perceived as foreign antigens by immunologic defense mechanisms, resulting in eosinophilia and formation of granulomatous lesions.[55] A similar syndrome has been reported in cats; in one report they did not respond to treatment as successfully as dogs.[58]

Clinical signs include vomiting, diarrhea that may be bloody, abdominal pain, anorexia, and weight loss. It is common for these patients to have borborygmus followed by vomiting or diarrhea. The gastrointestinal signs usually last two to three days and resolve until the next cyclic episode. The cycles are usually very regular but may vary from six days to two months, depending on the individual case.

Physical examination is usually unremarkable but the patient may appear thin. Other findings may include thickened bowel loops, enlarged mesenteric lymph nodes, and bloody diarrhea.

Clinical pathology varies. An eosinophilia may be seen on the hemogram; however, this is not a consistent finding. Fecal examination may reveal large numbers of parasite ova. The feces may be positive for fecal fat on the indirect Sudan test. Absorption studies (D-xylose, glucose, fat) are usually normal but may be abnormal, depending on the severity of the problem. Serum biochemistries may show a hypoproteinemia; with normal liver screening tests and urinalysis, a diagnosis of protein-losing enteropathy can be supported. This can be confirmed by doing a ^{51}Cr-labeled albumin fecal loss study, but in most cases it is unnecessary.[37]

The diagnosis of eosinophilic gastroenteritis is confirmed by biopsy. Histopathology reveals that all layers of the affected small intestine are thickened. The lamina propria of the mucosa shows an eosinophilic infiltrate, which is seen even in the villi. Increased numbers of lymphocytes and plasma cells are also seen. If visceral larval migrans is the underlying cause, cross-sections of the larva surrounded by an eosinophilic granuloma may be observed.[55] Biopsies can be obtained from the colon and stomach by endoscopy. Since the disease is often diffuse, the stomach and colon may also be involved. Biopsies of the stomach mucosa will often provide the diagnosis and spare the patient an abdominal celiotomy. Sometimes the diagnosis can be made from a colon biopsy; however, this is less common than by stomach biopsy.[134] If neither stomach nor colon biopsies confirm the diagnosis, an abdominal celiotomy with biopsies of the small intestine is warranted.

If the owners are unwilling to have surgery performed, a tentative diagnosis can be made by the findings of an eosinophilia in peripheral blood and of thickened bowel loops with irregularity of the mucosa on barium series. If treatment resolves the clinical signs, this would be further evidence to support the clinical impression of eosinophilic gastroenteritis.

The treatment of eosinophilic gastroenteritis is a controlled diet and corticosteroid therapy. A bland diet, such as i/d,* is recommended for these patients. One author recommends a formulated diet of just a single source of carbohydrates initially; when clinical response is noted, a single source of protein is then added. So long as the stools are normal, a new nutrient is added to the diet. In this way the foods that are not tolerated can eventually be determined.[134]

Most authors recommend oral prednisolone therapy at a dosage of 2.2 mg/kg/day, which is gradually tapered over a two- to

*Hill's Pet Products, Inc., Topeka, KS.

three-week period.[88] Occasionally long-term steroid therapy is needed. In these cases the lowest possible dosage is recommended to control the problem, and it is advisable to attempt alternate-day therapy.

If visceral larval migrans is suspected, anthelmintic therapy, in conjunction with steroids, may be considered. No currently approved anthelmintic for use in the dog is effective against visceral larval migrans.[120] Fenbendazole,* which has recently been marketed for the dog, may be efficacious (25 to 30 mg/kg.). Although not approved for use in the dog, thiabendazole† and levamisole‡ may also be efficacious.[121]

The prognosis in dogs is good, so long as visceral larval migrans is not the cause. Dogs with eosinophilic gastroenteritis usually respond well to steroid therapy. This is not the case in cats. Cats respond poorly to therapy and most die or have to be euthanized.[58]

LYMPHOCYTIC-PLASMACYTIC ENTERITIS

Lymphocytic-plasmacytic enteritis is characterized by infiltrates of lymphocytes and plasma cells in the mucosa of the small intestine.[56] The lymphocytes and plasma cells are found diffusely in the affected mucosa or concentrated in the villi or the lamina propria.[56] This disease is one of the two most common causes of protein-losing enteropathy in dogs.[88]

Clinical signs include frequent defecation (six to seven times a day), stools that are soft to liquid in consistency, and mucus in the stools. Other signs may be a dull hair coat and modest weight loss.[56] Physical examination is generally unremarkable, except that the dog looks thin.

Clinical pathology may reveal hypoproteinemia; blood test results are otherwise unremarkable. Steatorrhea is a finding in dogs with lymphocytic-plasmacytic enteritis. In a study performed on five German shepherds, 24-hour fecal fat levels ranged from 4.98 to 12.9 gm (2.37 gm is normal in dogs).[56] In this study fecal nitrogen was elevated in the two dogs checked—8.38 and 11.7 gm, respectively, per 24 hours (3.54 gm per 24 hours is normal in dogs).[56] Barium studies can show flocculation and segmentation in the small intestines, indicating small bowel disease.[56] Absorption studies appear to be within normal limits, but may be altered in severe cases.[56]

*Panacur, American Hoechst, Somerville, NJ.
†Thiabendazole, Merck & Co., Westpoint, PA.
‡Levasole, Pitman-Moore, Washington Crossing, NJ.

The diagnosis is made by intestinal biopsy. Because the colon and stomach may be involved, endoscopy with biopsy of the colon and stomach is warranted. If the biopsies are normal or inconclusive, abdominal celiotomy is necessary to confirm the diagnosis. It is important to advise the owner that celiotomy can be risky, because these patients have an impaired healing capacity.[88]

Necropsy findings are generally unremarkable. The small bowel mucosa may be congested and covered with mucus and bile. Lymphoid tissue may be prominent in the intestine.[56]

The actual mechanism of the disease is unknown, but the increased number of immunocytes suggest an immune-mediated pathogenesis.[140]

Treatment consists of antibiotics, steroids, and diet control. Since immune-complexing disease is suspected, prednisolone is given at a dosage of 2.2 mg/kg/day slowly tapered over two to three weeks. Tylosin has been reported to be effective in some cases.[88] Because lymphangiectasia may be associated with lymphocytic-plasmacytic enteritis, diet management is warranted. Long chained triglycerides should be excluded from the diet and replaced with medium-chain triglycerides.* Vitamin supplementation is recommended, especially of the fat-soluble and B-complex vitamins. Two homemade diets are listed in Table 7–1.

*MCT Oil, Mead-Johnson Co., Evansville, IN.

Table 7–1. TWO RECOMMENDED DIETS FOR TREATMENT OF LYMPHOCYTIC-PLASMACYTIC ENTERITIS*

Diet 1 (550 k-calories)
1 Cup boiled rice (dry)
1 Pound uncreamed cottage cheese
2 Teaspoons dicalcium phosphate
Balanced vitamin and mineral supplementation
300 ml MCT Oil†
Diet 2 (1980 k-calories)
2 Cups of Portagen†
12 Ounces uncreamed cottage cheese
4 Medium-size baked potatoes
2 Cups rice (dry)
2 Ounces MCT Oil†
Balanced vitamin and mineral supplementation

*Courtesy of Gerald Johnson, DVM., New York, NY.
†Mead-Johnson Co., Evansville, IN.

The prognosis for patients with lymphocytic-plasmacytic enteritis is poor, especially in long-standing cases in which the animals are hypoproteinemic and debilitated.[88]

GRANULOMATOUS ENTERITIS

Granulomatous enteritis is a chronic inflammatory bowel disease of unknown etiology. Regional enteritis in humans closely resembles granulomatous enteritis in dogs. The lesions can be found anywhere in the gastrointestinal tract. Nine cases of granulomatous enteritis have been reported in dogs.[31] Trichuriasis was suspected as the etiology in one dog. All of the affected dogs were under four years of age, and all but one were males. Clinical signs were predominantly chronic diarrhea and weight loss.

Other findings are ventral edema and ascites.[88] History may reveal that although the dog is polyphagic, it is losing weight.[88]

On physical examination, the dog is thin, and abdominal pain may be elicited on palpation. Thickened bowel loops and enlarged mesenteric lymph nodes may also be noted on abdominal palpation. Perianal fistulas associated with regional enteritis were seen in one dog.[31] Fistula formation is common in humans.[31]

Hypoproteinemia is the most common clinical pathological finding. CBC and serum biochemical profiles are usually within normal limits. Barium series may show a scalloped mucosal surface or thickened intestinal wall.[88] Fat absorption and D-xylose tests may be altered, depending on the severity of the problem. The diagnosis is made by full-thickness biopsies of the affected bowel segments. This requires an abdominal celiotomy.

The intestines can be affected in one or multiple sites. In cases in which multiple sites are affected, the intestine between lesions appears normal.[31] Also, the mesenteric lymph nodes may appear enlarged. On biopsy a granulomatous inflammation is seen. All four layers of the intestine are affected. Histopathology reveals macrophages, multinucleated giant cells, lymphocytes, plasma cells, eosinophils, and neutrophils.[31]

The treatment of granulomatous enteritis has not been very rewarding. Medical treatment in humans consists of glucocorticoids and salicylazosulfapyridine (sulfasalazine).[88] Sulfasalazine* is cleaved by intestinal bacteria to sulfapyridine, which is an antibacterial, and 5-aminosalicylic acid, which has anti-inflammatory and anti-prostaglandin synthetase activity.[88] Azathioprine† and metronidazole‡ have also been used successfully for the treatment of regional enteritis in people.[88] Surgical resection can be performed if the enteritis is localized. In humans there is a high recurrence at the anastomosis site.[31]

The prognosis for dogs with granulomatous enteritis is poor. Long-term response to therapy has been unsatisfactory.

LYMPHANGIECTASIA

Lymphangiectasia was first described in people in 1961.[20, 85] In 1968, Campbell and colleagues[26] reported the first case in dogs. Since that time several cases have been reported.[20, 50, 57, 85, 87, 103] Intestinal lymphangiectasia is characterized by cystic dilatation of the lymphatics within the mucosa and submucosa of the villus.[20] Lymphangiectasia can be a primary (congenital) insufficiency of the lymph vessels or secondary to obstruction.[20] Congestive heart failure, restrictive pericarditis, lymphosarcoma, histoplasmosis, and inflammatory bowel disease, such as granulomatous enteritis and lymphocytic-plasmacytic enteritis, have been implicated as causes of lymphangiectasia.[20, 57]

Dogs with lymphangiectasia can present with various clinical signs. Diarrhea and weight loss are the most common. Edema, ascites, hydrothorax, vomiting, anorexia, and weakness may be other presenting signs.

Physical examination findings depend on the extent of the disease. Often the dogs are thin, with diarrhea. Respiratory difficulty is present if hydrothorax has developed. If ascites is present, the abdomen may be distended.

Clinical pathology is variable; hyproproteinemia is the most common finding. Lymphangiectasia is considered the most common cause of protein-losing enteropathies.[20] There are several proposed mechanisms of how this occurs. Obstruction of the intes-

---

*Azulfidine, Pharmacia Laboratories, Piscataway, NJ.

†Imuran, Burroughs Wellcome Co., Research Triangle Park, NC.

‡Flagyl, Searle & Co., San Juan, Puerto Rico.

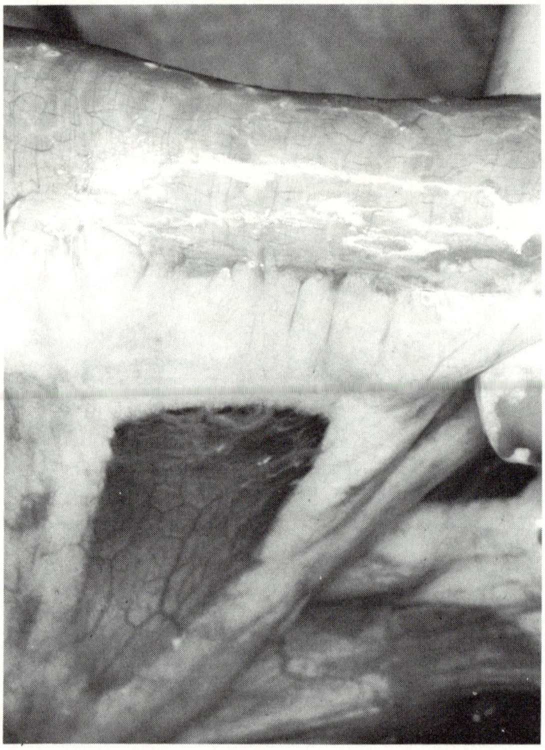

Figure 7–9. Serosal surface of the small intestine of a dog with lymphangiectasia. Note the dilated lymphatics on the serosal surface. This is commonly seen in patients with lymphangiectasia.

tinal lymphatics increase lymph leakage, causing protein loss into the intestinal lumen. Transudation through ulcerated mucosa and alterations in mucosal cell metabolism can lead to excessive intestinal protein loss. Rupture of dilated lymphatic vessels results in discharge of their contents, causing large amounts of protein loss in some cases. It is also theorized that diffusion of protein from intestinal capillaries occurs through an intact epithelium.[103] All of the above can eventually lead to hypoproteinemia, which can result in edema, ascites, and hydrothorax. Protein-losing enteropathy can be diagnosed using ^{51}Cr-labeled albumin.

Another clinical pathology finding is steatorrhea on Sudan fecal stain or 24-hour fecal fat tests. Lymphopenia is often seen on the hemogram. Cholesterol values are commonly decreased, secondary to fat malabsorption and loss of body stores of fat in chyle.[20] Hypocalcemia may be a finding, primarily due to the low albumin level. Vitamin D malabsorption and formation of calcium–fatty acid complexes within the intestine can also play a role in low calcium values.[20]

Results of malabsorption studies are variable. Fat absorption tests are usually abnormal with and without pancreatic enzymes. D-Xylose absorption tests are usually normal but have been reported to be abnormal.[20, 103]

Radiography usually is not helpful in the diagnosis of lymphangiectasia. Delayed emptying, hypermotility, prominent mucosal folds, and patchy uneven filling of intestinal loops have been seen on barium studies.[20]

The definitive diagnosis can be made only by abdominal celiotomy and biopsy of the small intestine. Abdominal exploratory surgery can be risky, especially when the patient's albumin level is decreased, because healing is often delayed or impaired.

The lymphatics of the small intestinal serosal surface may be dilated and irregular. Numerous smooth, cream-colored nodules, primarily on the mesenteric border, can be observed (Fig. 7–9). These intestinal nodules are granulomas composed of actively phagocytic macrophages and occasional fibroblasts.[20] Histopathology reveals dilatation of lymphatic vessels in the villous submucosa (Fig. 7–10).

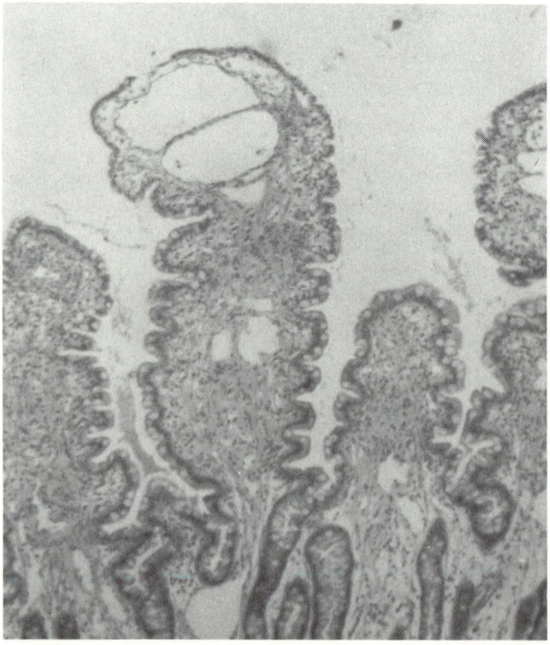

Figure 7–10. Photomicrograph of the intestinal villi of a dog with lymphangiectasia. Note the dilated lymphatics. They frequently rupture, leaking their contents into the intestinal lumen.

Treatment consists of correcting the primary cause, if it can be identified, and dietary management with vitamin and mineral supplements. The main objective in treating lymphangiectasia is the use of low-fat diets and, in particular, avoidance of long-chain triglycerides.

One recommendation is the use of r/d,* which contains 1.1% fat but has only 330 kCal per can, supplemented with medium-chain triglycerides (MCT Oil†). There are 115 kCal per tablespoon of MCT Oil.[57] Recommended dosage for MCT Oil is 30 ml/10 kg.[87]

The two diets shown in Table 7–1 that are recommended for treatment of lymphocytic-plasmacytic enteritis can be used in the treatment of lymphangiectasia.

It is most important that the patient receives adequate calories. The weight used as the basis for determining caloric intake should be the animal's optimal weight. Therefore, in planning the diet, maintenance energy needs must be considered and the diet should be adjusted for weight gain if necessary. One recommendation is 28 kCal/lb/day[57]; a more accurate determination is 150 × kg body weight in kg.[87] In some cases the patient can be slowly weaned from the special diet and return to a regular diet.[57]

The prognosis is considered guarded for patients with lymphangiectasia. Not all patients will respond to dietary control.

DIARRHEAL SYNDROME IN BASENJIS

A chronic diarrheal syndrome that seems to be worsened by stress has been reported in basenjis.[17, 18] It is believed that this syndrome has an autosomal recessive hereditary component.[17]

These dogs present with a history of chronic intractable diarrhea, chronic weight loss, intermittent anorexia, and occasional vomiting.[17, 18] In pups, swelling of buccal lymph nodes, adverse reactions to vaccinations, and transient neurological signs are features of this syndrome.[18] Neurological signs include incoordination, paresis, seizures, and contracture of the facial musculature.[17] Stressful situations appear to cause exacerbation of anorexia and diarrhea in dogs with the diarrheal syndrome.[18]

*Hill's Pet Products, Inc., Topeka, KS.
†Mead-Johnson Company, Evansville, IN.

Clinical pathology shows a consistent hypoalbuminemia and a hypergammaglobulinemia. There is some indication that the albumin level decreases and gammaglobulins increase as the disease progresses.[16] Plasma turbidity tests with and without pancreatic enzymes are abnormal, along with the D-xylose absorption test, which supports malabsorption as a component of this syndrome.

Protein-losing enteropathy is suspected to occur, but in the two cases in which a ^{51}Cr-labeled albumin test was done the results were abnormal in one and normal in the other.[16] Further studies are needed to clarify whether PLE actually exists in this syndrome.

The diagnosis is made by intestinal biopsy, but the survival rate of dogs subjected to surgery is extremely poor.[17, 18] When the above findings are present, surgery in these dogs must be carefully considered, and the owners must be well informed as to the potential dangers involved.

Necropsy reveals uniformly thickened small intestines. Histological examination findings include lymphocytic-plasmacytic infiltration with loss of villous epithelium and shortening and fusion of the villi.[17, 18] Lymphangiectasia has been seen in some basenjis with this syndrome.[17, 18] Owing to the fact that infiltration by immunologically active cells occurs, chronic antigen stimulation has been suggested as playing a role in this disease.[17] Diet appears to be involved in the pathogenesis of some cases.[18] Two diets that have lessened the severity of the diarrhea in some cases or eliminated it completely in others are IAMS* and Advanced Nutritional Formula.* Both these diets lack soybean protein, which may be the reason for the apparent improvement.[18]

Treatment has not been well worked out, although several recommendations have been made. Dietary manipulation and minimizing stress have been advocated. Tylosin appears to be beneficial in treatment of the disease. Prednisolone has been advocated at a dosage of 2 mg/kg/day divided BID for five days, after which alternate-day low-dose therapy is utilized for maintenance.[18]

Additional studies need to be done to further characterize the problem and develop better control measures.

*IAMS Co., Lewisberg, OH.

PROTEIN-LOSING ENTEROPATHY IN LUDENHUNDS

A protein-losing enteropathy (PLE) in Ludenhunds has been reported by one investigator[38] and is suspected of having a hereditary component. The disease is characterized by intermittent diarrhea, vomiting, weight loss, ascites, and edema.

Clinical signs include a history of intermittent bouts of vomiting and diarrhea. A distended abdomen and edematous swelling may also be seen. Weight loss and anorexia are other symptoms reported in these dogs.

On physical examination, the dog is thin, often with pale mucous membranes. Ascites may be noted on abdominal palpation. Ventral edema or edematous swelling of the legs may be present. The animal also may be dehydrated.

Laboratory investigation findings include hypoproteinemia, particularly hypoalbuminemia. Serum calcium levels are often decreased secondary to the decrease in albumin. The remainder of the serum biochemical profile is normal. In the one report of this disease no absorption studies were done.[38]

Necropsy showed emaciation of varying degrees; the small intestinal mucosa was thickened and enlarged, and roughened villi were seen in clumps or spread diffusely. Histopathology revealed thickened mucosa of both the duodenum and jejenum. Villi were blunt and usually shorter than normal. Edema and infiltration of mononuclear cells, primarily plasma cells, were seen in the lamina propria. The lymph vessels in the submucosa were distended. The mucosal changes lessened gradually toward the ileum.

Treatment recommendations are similar to those discussed for other PLE problems. More studies are needed to determine a specific treatment for this syndrome.

The etiology of this problem is unknown, although hereditary factors have been suggested.[38] One suggested possible mechanism is a combined immunological deficiency and partial hypoplasia of the lymphatics.[38]

Prognosis has to be considered very guarded for dogs with this condition.

IDIOPATHIC VILLOUS ATROPHY

In humans a primary malabsorption disorder has been described that results from atrophic changes of the mucosa of the small intestine. Two forms of primary intestinal malabsorption are recognized: non-tropical sprue (synonyms: celiac disease, gluten enteropathy) and tropical sprue.[76] There have been several reports of a non-tropical sprue–like condition in the dog.[72, 88, 134, 141] Villous atrophy that resembles tropical sprue has also been reported in the dog.[8a]

Non-tropical sprue in people is the result of hypersensitivity to the protein gliadin.[88] Gliadin is a gluten found in many grains, such as wheat, barley, rye, buckwheat, and oats.[88, 134] In this condition malabsorption occurs, resulting in weight loss, steatorrhea, and anemia. The anemia can be secondary to vitamin B_{12} and folate malabsorption or associated with malabsorption of iron.[76]

Histopathological changes seen in human non-tropical sprue include severe blunting and distortion of the villi. The enterocytes become cuboidal and the microvilli are reduced in size. Within the lamina propria a chronic inflammatory cell reaction is seen, the predominant cell types affected being lymphocytes and plasma cells.

In dogs malabsorption has been reported in cases that resemble non-tropical sprue. The dogs presented with weight loss, vomiting, diarrhea, and anorexia. Laboratory evaluation revealed hypoproteinemia and anemia.[72] Results of absorption studies were abnormal for both lipids and carbohydrates.[72, 76]

Histopathologically, the small intestinal villi were irregular in length and width and the surfaces were slightly blunted. The epithelium at the tips of the villi was cuboidal. No microvilli could be detected, but there were many irregular projections and invaginations. Other pathology findings included mucosal cysts that contained mucin and neutrophils, and excessive numbers of plasma cells and lymphocytes in the lamina propria.[72]

Tropical sprue is characterized by similar changes, but they are usually less severe.[76] The disease is believed to be secondary to infection by an unidentified agent.[121]

The diagnosis of idiopathic villous atrophy is made by biopsy. This can be accomplished by laparotomy or by a biopsy capsule passed orally.[8]

The treatment for idiopathic villous atrophy varies depending on the cause. Dietary management is necessary if the problem is truly a gluten-induced enteropathy; this can only be determined by a positive response to removal of gluten from the diet and return of signs when gluten is reintroduced. Gluten-free diets are d/d and i/d Prescription Diets,* Science Maximum Stress* and Canine Growth Diets,* and IAMS Chunks,† or Eukanuba.†[120, 134] Homemade diets consisting of lean meat, rice, and corn can be used. Vitamin B_{12}, folic acid, and fat-soluble vitamin supplementation should also be considered.[88]

Long-term antibiotic therapy has proved successful in some cases, especially with tetracycline and tylosin.[88] The use of corticosteroids—for example, prednisolone, 2 mg/kg/day divided BID initially—has been shown to help alleviate signs in some cases.[88, 134] Combination therapy of antibiotics and prednisolone has been reported effective by some authors.[88]

The prognosis in these cases should always be considered very guarded to unfavorable. Although some patients respond to therapy, many do not.

BACTERIAL OVERGROWTH

Bacterial overgrowth has been reported as a cause of malabsorption in the dog.[60, 123] In humans, bacterial overgrowth (synonyms: stagnant and blind loop syndromes) is a major cause of malabsorption.[48, 64] The potential causes of bacterial overgrowth include decreased gastric acid secretions, decreased motility, and partial obstructions such as gastrointestinal strictures.

Deconjugated bile acids have been proposed as a major factor in this malabsorption syndrome.[48, 64] According to one theory, bacteria deconjugate bile acids, which decreases the effective luminal concentration of conjugated bile salts to a level below the critical micellar concentration.[64] This then leads to steatorrhea. Another possible mechanism is the role of deconjugated bile acids as a cause of mucosal dysfunction, leading to steatorrhea.[64]

Carbohydrate absorption can also be interfered with by bacterial overgrowth. The suspected mechanism is an abnormally low level of brush border enzymes, which is due to an abnormally rapid turnover of glycoproteins. It has been shown experimentally in rats that the luminal bacteria produce an elastase-like enzyme that degrades glycoproteins, leading to malabsorption of carbohydrates.[64]

*Hill's Pet Products, Inc., Topeka, KS.
†IAMS Co., Lewisberg, OH.

In people, hypoalbuminemia is commonly seen with bacterial overgrowth.[64] Some of the proteins may be deaminated. It is believed that hepatic protein synthesis is impaired by absorption of some toxic bacterial metabolites from the portal circulation.[64] The impairment of albumin synthesis has been reported in blind loop rats and is probably a non-specific effect of hepatic damage.[64]

Vitamin B_{12} malabsorption may occur with bacterial overgrowth. Several mechanisms are suspected. Several types of bacteria have the ability to bind vitamin B_{12}. Anaerobic bacteria, especially *Bacteriodes,* have a high affinity to bind both vitamin B_{12} and intrinsic factor–cobalamin complex.[64] Other bacteria, including *Clostridium* spp., *E. coli,* and *Propionibacteria,* have the ability to metabolize cobalamin to inactive substances known as cobamides.[64] Both these mechanisms can lead to malabsorption of vitamin B_{12}.

Mucosal damage seems to be minimal in bacterial overgrowth and does not appear to play a large role in the development of malabsorption.[64]

Malabsorption in the dog secondary to bacterial overgrowth has been reported in a few cases, but probably occurs more commonly than reported.[60, 123] In two cases reported, the dogs presented with chronic diarrhea that had been unresponsive to treatments. Weight loss was evident in both dogs.

Clinical pathology revealed an abnormal D-xylose absorption test. Results of a BT-PABA test in one of the dogs were normal.[60] Results of fat absorption studies in the other dog were abnormal.[123] Fecal trypsin activity in both dogs was normal. In one animal, a heavy growth of *Pseudomonas aeruginosa* was cultured from the feces. Both dogs recovered when treated with antibiotics. Results of absorption studies after treatment were within normal limits. The diagnosis of bacterial overgrowth is confirmed by quantitative bacterial cultures for both anaerobes and aerobes. Samples of small intestinal fluid can be obtained by intestinal intubation or laparotomy.[120] However, this is many times impractical to do. Correction of abnormalities secondary to treatment is often sufficient to make the diagnosis. Barium radiography may be of assistance, especially if a stricture is present.

Treatment is therapy with broad-spectrum antibiotics that are effective against anaerobes, such as tetracycline (25 mg/kg TID) and metronidazole.* Other antibiotics that may be effective are ampicillin, chloramphenicol, clindamycin, erythromycin, lincomycin, and tylosin. Vitamin supplementation is recommended, especially vitamin B_{12}. If a stricture is present, surgical correction is warranted.

SHORT BOWEL SYNDROME

The short bowel syndrome is the result of surgical removal of a large part of the small intestine. Clinical signs include diarrhea, weight loss, and various nutritional deficiencies.[144] This syndrome is well documented in humans and has been reported in the dog.[69, 144]

The diagnosis is confirmed by history of intestinal resection. Subsequent to surgery, the patient develops a chronic diarrhea and weight loss.

In one of the cases reported in the literature, dilated bowel loops were visible radiographically and a barium series demonstrated decreased transit time[144]; 24-hour fecal fats were elevated and Sudan stain for split and unsplit fats showed a large portion of digested fats; D-xylose absorption and BT-PABA tests were abnormal.[144]

The pathogenesis of short bowel syndrome probably involves several mechanisms: maldigestion, malabsorption, bacterial overgrowth, bile salt– and fatty acid–mediated diarrhea, and gastric hypersecretion.[144] The mechanism of bile salt– and fatty acid–mediated diarrhea has been discussed previously. Maldigestion may occur because secretin and cholecystokinin, which are normally released from the wall of the duodenum and upper jejunum, will be reduced if portions of these intestinal segments are resected. Rapid transit time may also contribute to maldigestion. Activity of mucosal-cell border digestive enzymes is decreased in dogs in which 75 per cent of the proximal small bowel has been resected, causing further maldigestion.[144] The effects of bacterial overgrowth have been discussed. The resection of the ileocolic valve removes one of the barriers that prevents colonic bacteria from invading the small intestine. Malabsorption may result from a combination of rapid transit time and reduced small intestinal surface area.[144] In addition to the malabsorption of fats, carbohydrates and protein that has been noted in the short bowel syndrome, deficiencies of calcium, magnesium, iron, zinc, vitamin D, vitamin B_{12}, and folate have also been reported in man.[144] Gastric hypersecretion has been documented in both man and dogs with the short bowel syndrome. In humans, fasting and postprandial serum gastrin levels are elevated, whereas in the dog only postprandial levels are increased.[144]

Resection of part of the ileum can also induce diarrhea. In this case it is caused by an excess of bile acids, which are normally resorbed by the ileum. Steatorrhea does not occur unless large amounts of the ileum are removed.[61]

After bowel resection, the remaining intestine undergoes compensatory changes.[144] The bowel increases in diameter, the small intestinal villi and crypts enlarge, and the number of mucosal cells per unit length of gut increases. Oral feeding seems to play a major role in stimulating adaptive hyperplasia.

Treatment has not been well worked out in the dog. General guidelines include a low-fat diet* supplemented with medium-chain triglycerides. Vitamin and mineral supplements are warranted. Other products that may be of value are readily absorbable diet supplements containing free amino acids, simple sugars, vitamins and minerals, pancreatic enzymes, and oral antibiotics. Frequent, small meals are recommended.[144] Cimetidine† to decrease gastric acid hypersecretion may be of some benefit. In treating bile diarrhea, cholestyramine‡, a binding agent of bile acids, has been used successfully in people.[61]

The use of an intestinal pacer to cause peristalsis has been effective in treatment of experimentally induced short bowel syndrome in dogs.[45, 46, 81] The value of this in veterinary medicine remains to be seen. The studies were performed on dogs only to evaluate the pacer's possible use in humans. The prognosis for short bowel syndrome has to be considered guarded.

DUODENAL ULCERS

Spontaneous duodenal ulcers in dogs and cats are fairly rare, although there have

---

*Flagyl, Searle & Co., San Juan, Puerto Rico.

*r/d, Hill's Pet Products, Inc., Topeka, KS.

†Tagamet, Smith, Kline & French Laboratories, Philadelphia, PA.

‡Questran, Mead Johnson Pharmaceutical Co., Evansville, IN.

been reported cases of spontaneous duodenal ulcers in the dog.[1, 65] Ulceration of both the stomach and duodenum has been reported in dogs and cats with disseminated mastocytosis.[29] The ulcerations appear to be secondary to histamine release by mast cells, which causes increased gastric acid secretion.

Gastrointestinal ulcers are also seen in association with renal disease. Gastrin is normally removed from the blood by renal excretion. In patients with renal disease gastrin blood levels become increased, which causes hypersecretion of gastric acid.[134] High gastric ammonia may also play a role. Urea diffuses from the intestinal fluid into the lumen of the stomach. The urea is converted by urease to ammonia by bacteria and gastric mucosal cells. Ammonia levels in the stomach are believed to increase to levels that are toxic to the mucosal cells, resulting in mucosal ulcerations.[134]

Liver disease has also been related to ulcerations, although the exact mechanism is unknown. One proposed mechanism in chronic liver disease, particularly hepatic cirrhosis, is that ulceration occurs secondary to increases in blood gastrin and histamine levels.[134]

Drugs have been shown to induce ulcers: these include aspirin, corticosteroids, indomethacin, and cinchophen.[128, 134]

As has been discussed, gastrinomas can cause ulcerations in dogs. Dogs with gastric or duodenal ulcers present with vomiting, melena, weight loss, and abdominal pain. Blood is often present in the vomitus. Perforations and blood loss are potential complications of ulceration.

Barium series may be of benefit in the diagnosis of gastric and duodenal ulcers. The definitive diagnosis is made by endoscopic examination of the stomach and duodenum.

Treatment involves both the correction of the primary problem and the administration of symptomatic therapy. The most important consideration is resting the gastrointestinal tract. Food is abrasive to the mucosa and can aggravate the problem when feeding is resumed.

Only small amounts of food should be fed at frequent intervals. The meal should consist of easily digested foods. Initially carbohydrates should be fed (primarily starch—for example, rice), and proteins should be gradually introduced. Generally the diet should consist of carbohydrates and small amounts of protein and have a low fat content.[134]

Cimetidine* has beneficial effects in cases of gastroduodenal ulcerations. Cimetidine is an H_2 blocker that decreases gastric acid secretion. It also has been found to accelerate the healing of duodenal ulcers, but this effect is not seen with gastric ulceration.[102]

Antacids are effective in neutralizing gastric acid but, unless given frequently, they may make the problem worse. Normally, an acid pH on the antral mucosa inhibits gastrin release. Neutralization of the acids removes the inhibitory effect, resulting in increased acid secretion.[134] For this reason the administration of antacids only two to three times a day results in greater acid secretion.[134]

Non-specific protectants are of minimal benefit in the treatment of ulcers. Specific protectants are carbenoxolone, lauryl glycyrrhizinic acid, and cholestyramine.† These prevent the adverse effects of bile acids. Carbenoxolone has aldosterone-like properties that lead to sodium retention and potassium wasting, making its use less desirable.[134]

Because of their antipepsin activity, sulfated mucopolysaccharides and glycoproteins may be useful in treating acute lesions. These agents bind to the mucosal surface, preventing the digestion of the membrane by pepsin.

Oral cimetidine should not be used at the same time as protectants, as these decrease the absorption of cimetidine.

The prognosis depends on the cause and the extent of the ulcerations.

Neoplasia

Several types of neoplasia have been reported involving the intestine; these include lymphosarcoma, adenocarcinoma, adenoma, leiomyoma, leiomyosarcoma, fibrosarcoma, mast cell tumor, and polyps.[99, 104, 106, 120] Lymphosarcoma and adenocarcinoma are the most common types.

Intestinal lymphosarcoma is divided into two morphologic classifications: diffuse and nodular.[120] In the diffuse type villous atro-

---

*Tagamet, Smith, Kline & French Laboratories, Philadelphia, PA.

†Questran, Mead-Johnson Pharmaceutical Co., Evansville, In.

phy occurs secondary to infiltration of all layers of the small intestine. This can result in malabsorption, chronic diarrhea, and weight loss.[88] On physical examination the bowel may feel thickened. Palpation may also reveal splenomegaly, hepatomegaly, enlarged mesenteric lymph nodes, or peripheral lymphadenopathy. In the nodular form, a segmental thickening of the small intestine occurs. This is most often seen in the ileocecocolic region and may cause partial obstruction.[120] The diagnosis is made by intestinal biopsy. The FeLV test in cats is unreliable because in the majority of cases it will be negative.[88] Several chemotherapeutic protocols can be used in treatment of lymphosarcoma; however, the prognosis is generally poor.

Adenocarcinoma is seen predominantly in older animals, eight to nine years of age in dogs and greater than 11 years in cats.[84] In cats, males and the Siamese breed may be predisposed.[107] Adenocarcinomas of the intestines in dogs are most often seen in the rectum, colon, and duodenum, whereas in cats they are found most often in the ileum and jejenum.[84, 106] Adenocarcinoma may cause segmental thickening within the bowel wall and act like an expanding mass. It can also grow inward, producing an annular constriction and a partial obstruction (Fig. 7–11).[120] Clinical signs are varied depending on where the tumor is located and the relative size of the tumor. Projectile vomiting is common in cats. Melena can also be evident secondary to mucosal ulceration. Other clinical signs include depression, weight loss, and ascites.[107] The definitive diagnosis is made by intestinal biopsy. Barium series may detect a partial obstruction. Treatment is surgical resection of the affected intestines. Prognosis is generally poor. There is one report of 28-month survival time after intestinal resection.[107]

Metastasis has usually occurred by the time clinical diagnosis is made, either by route of the lymphatics and veins or through implantation.[30] Metastasis in the dog frequently involves the liver, lungs, regional and mesenteric lymph nodes, and peritoneum. There has been one report of metastasis to the vertebrae.[30, 99] In cats infiltration of neoplastic cells into the mesentery and omentum is common, and metastasis to regional lymph nodes, spleen, lungs, and kidneys also occurs.[107]

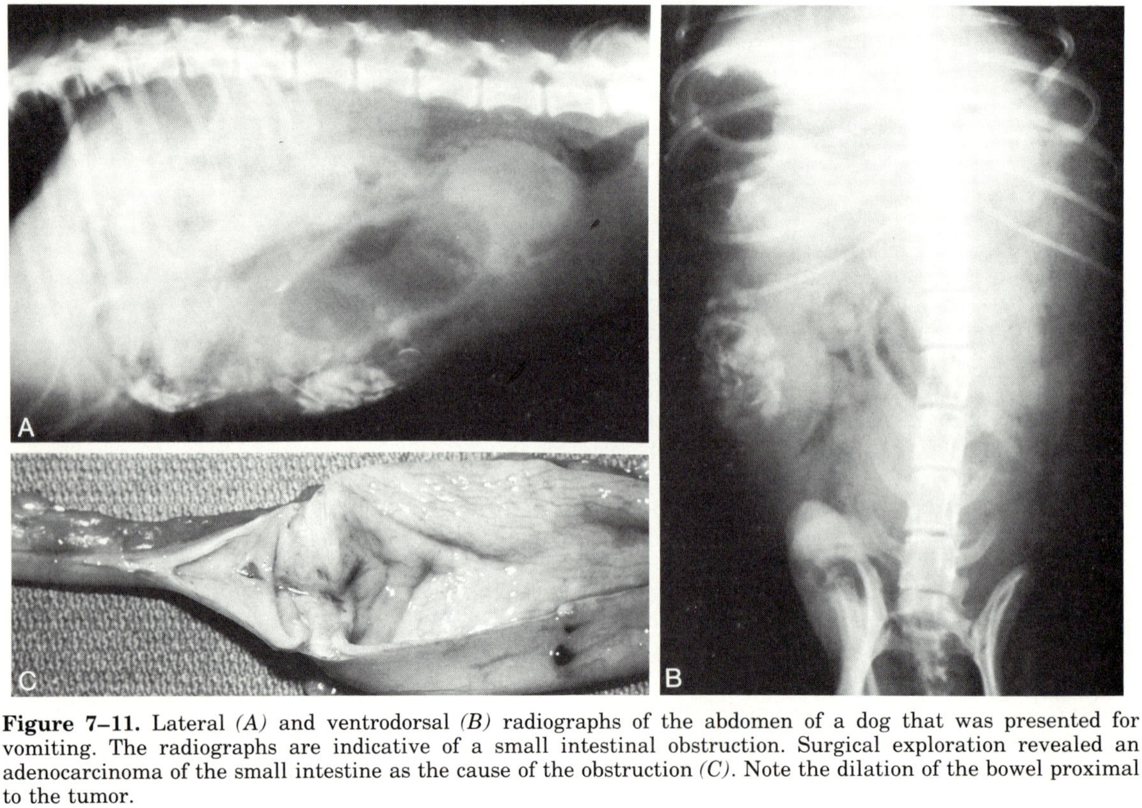

Figure 7–11. Lateral *(A)* and ventrodorsal *(B)* radiographs of the abdomen of a dog that was presented for vomiting. The radiographs are indicative of a small intestinal obstruction. Surgical exploration revealed an adenocarcinoma of the small intestine as the cause of the obstruction *(C)*. Note the dilation of the bowel proximal to the tumor.

References

1. Ackerman N, Root C. Benign duodenal ulceration and perforation in a dog. Vet Radiology 22:19–21, 1981.
2. Ader PL: Phycomycosis in fifteen dogs and two cats. J Am Vet Med Assoc 174:1216–1223, 1979.
3. Amos HE: Allergic Drug Reactions, Edward Arnold, London, 211, 1978.
4. Baldwin S: Feline enteric diseases. *In* Kirk, RW (ed), *Current Veterinary Therapy VIII*, W. B. Saunders Company, Philadelphia, 1168–1171, 1983.
5. Barton CL, Smith C, Troy G, et al: The diagnosis and clinicopathological features of canine protein-losing enteropathy. J Am Anim Hosp Assoc 14:85–91, 1978.
6. Batt RM: The molecular basis of malabsorption. J Small Anim Pract 20:555–569, 1980.
7. Batt RM: Role of serum folate and vitamin B_{12} concentrations in the differentiation of small intestinal abnormalities in the dog. Res Vet Sci 32:17–22, 1982.
8. Batt RM, Bush BM, Peters TJ: Biochemical changes in jejunal mucosa of dogs with naturally occurring exocrine pancreatic insufficiency. Gut 20:709–715, 1979.

8a. Batt RM, Bush BM, Peters TJ: Morphologic and biochemical studies of naturally occurring enteropathy in the dog resembling chronic tropical sprue in man (Abstract). Gastroenterology 76:1096, 1979.

9. Batt RM, Mann LC: Specificity of BT-PABA test for the diagnosis of exocrine pancreatic insufficiency in the dog. Vet Rec 108:303–307, 1981.
10. Batt RM, Peters TJ: Subcellular fractionation studies on peroral jejunal biopsies from the dog. Res Vet Sci 25:94–100, 1978.
11. Blaser J, Cravens J, Powers BW, et al: Campylobacter enteritis associated with canine infection. Lancet 2:979–981, 1978.
12. Blaser MJ, Weiss SH, Barrett TJ: Campylobacter enteritis associated with a healthy cat. JAMA 247:816, 1982.
13. Bohl EH: Coronaviruses: diagnosis of infections. *In* Kurstak E, Kurstak C (eds), *Comparative Diagnosis of Viral Diseases,* Vol. 4: Vertebrate Animal and Related Viruses, Part B, Academic Press, New York, 301–323, 1981.
14. Boosinger TR, Rebar AH, DeNicola DB, et al: Bone marrow alterations associated with canine parvoviral enteritis. Vet Path 19:558–561, 1982.
15. Bosman DD, Farrell RK, Gorham JR: Non-endoparasite transmission of salmon poisoning disease of dogs. J Am Vet Med Assoc 156:1907–1910, 1970.
16. Breitschwerdt EB, Barta O, Waltman C: Serum proteins in healthy Basenjis and Basenjis with chronic diarrhea. Am J Vet Res 44:326–328, 1983.
17. Breitschwerdt EB, Halliwell WH, Foley CW: A hereditary diarrhetic syndrome in the Basenji characterized by malabsorption, protein-losing enteropathy and hypergammaglobulinemia. J Am Anim Hosp Assoc 16:551–560, 1980.
18. Breitschwerdt EB, Waltman C, Hagstad HV, et al: Clinical and epidemiologic characterization of a diarrheal syndrome in Basenji dogs. J Am Vet Med Assoc 180:914–920, 1982.
19. Buckner RG: The small intestine. *In* Catcott EJ, (ed), *Canine Medicine,* Vol. I. American Veterinary Publications, Santa Barbara, CA, 336–351, 1979.
20. Burns MG: Intestinal lymphangiectasia in the dog. A case report and review. J Am Anim Hosp Assoc 18:97–105, 1982.
21. Burrows CF: Canine hemorrhagic gastroenteritis. J Am Anim Hosp Assoc 13:451–458, 1977.
22. Burrows CF: Chronic diarrhea in the dog. Vet Clin North Am (Gastroenterology) 13:521–540, 1983.
23. Burrows CR, Merritt AM, Chiapella AM: Determination of fecal fat and trypsin output in the evaluation of chronic canine diarrhea. J Am Vet Med Assoc 174:62–66, 1979.
24. Bywater RJ, Newsone PM: Diarrhea. J Am Vet Med Assoc 181:718–720, 1982.
25. Calvert CA, Leifer CE: Salmonellosis in dogs with lymphosarcoma. J Am Vet Med Assoc 180:56–58, 1982.
26. Campbell RSF, Brobst D, Bisgard G: Intestinal lymphangiectasis in a dog. J Am Vet Med Assoc 153:1050–1054, 1968.
27. Carlson JH, Scott FW, Duncan JR: Feline panleukopenia. I: Pathogenesis in germfree and specific pathogen-free cats. Vet Pathol 14:79–88, 1977.
28. Carmichael LE, Joubert JC, Pollock RVH: Hemagglutination by canine parovirus: serologic studies and diagnostic applications. Am J Vet Res 41:784–791, 1980.
29. Carrig CB, Seawright AA: Mastocytosis with gastrointestinal ulceration in a dog. Aust Vet J 44:503–506, 1968.
30. Cho DY, Friedman LS, Strafuss AC: Adenocarcinoma in the duodenum and vertebrae in a dog. J Am Vet Med Assoc 169:317–319, 1971.
31. DiBartola SP, Rogers WA, Boyce JT, et al: Regional enteritis in two dogs. J Am Vet Med Assoc 181:904–908, 1982.
32. Dillon AR, Teer PA, Powers RD, et al: Canine abdominal histoplasmosis: A report of four cases. J Am Anim Hosp Assoc 18:498–502, 1982.
33. Dillon AR, Wilt GR: The role of campylobacter species in the dog and cat. A cause for concern? Vet Clin North Am 13:647–652, 1983.
34. England JJ, Poston RP: Electron microscopic identification and subsequent isolation of a rotavirus from a dog with fatal neonatal diarrhea. Am J Vet Res 41:782–783, 1980.
35. Farrell KR: Canine rickettsiosis. *In* Kirk RW (ed), *Current Veterinary Therapy V,* W. B. Saunders Company, Philadelphia, 985–987, 1974.
36. Farstad L, Landsverk T, Lassen J: Isolation of *Yersinia enterocolitica* from a dog with chronic enteritis. Acta Vet Scand 17:261–263, 1976.
37. Finco DR, Duncan JR, Schall WP, et al: Chronic enteric disease and hypoproteinemia in nine dogs. J Am Vet Med Assoc 163:262–271, 1973.
38. Flesjå K, Yri T: Protein-losing enteropathy in the Lundehund. J Small Anim Pract 18:11–23, 1977.
39. Formal SB, O'Brien A, Gemski P, et al: Invasive *Escherichia coli.* J Am Vet Med Assoc 173:596–598, 1978.
40. Fox JG: Feline salmonellosis. *In* Kirk RW (ed), *Current Veterinary Therapy VIII,* W. B. Saunders Company, Philadelphia, 1305–1307, 1980.
41. Fox JG, Moore R, Ackerman JI: *Campylobacter jejuni*–associated diarrhea in dogs. J Am Vet Med Assoc 183:1430–1433, 1983.
42. Fox JG, Moore R, Ackerman JI: Canine and feline campylobacteriosis: Epizootiology and clinical and

public health features. J Am Vet Med Assoc 183:1420–1424, 1983.
43. Fulton RW, Johnson CA, Pearson NJ, et al: Isolation of a rotavirus from a newborn dog with diarrhea. Am J Vet Res 42:841–843, 1981.
44. Gaunt PS: Intestinal phycomycosis in a dog: A case report. Southwest Vet 35:51–53, 1982.
45. Gladen HE, Kelly KA: Enhancing absorption in the canine short bowel syndrome by intestinal pacing. Surgery 88:281–286, 1980.
46. Gladen HE, Kelly KA: Electrical pacing for short bowel syndrome. Surg Gynecol Obstet 153:697–700, 1981.
47. Gooding GE, Robinson WF: Maternal antibody, vaccination and reproductive failure in dogs with parvovirus infection. Aust Vet J 59:170–174, 1982.
48. Gracey M: Intestinal absorption in the contaminated small-bowel syndrome. Gut 12:403–410, 1971.
49. Greenberger NJ, Winship DH: *Gastrointestinal Disorders: A Pathophysiologic Approach.* Yearbook Medical Publishers, Chicago, 104, 1976.
50. Griffiths GL, Clark WT, Mills JW: Lymphangiectasia in a dog. Aust Vet J 59:187–188, 1982.
51. Guerrant RL, Ganguly V, Casper AGT, et al: Effect of *Escherichia coli* on fluid transport across canine small bowel. J Clin Invest 52:1707–1714, 1973.
52. Gyles CL: Comments on detection and importance of enteropathogenic *Escherichia coli* in diarrheal disease of human beings. J Am Vet Med Assoc 173:598–600, 1978.
53. Happe RP, VanderGaag I, Lamers CBHW: Zollinger-Ellison syndrome in three dogs. Vet Pathol 17:177–186, 1980.
54. Hayden DW, VanKruiningen HJ: Control values for evaluating gastrointestinal function in the dog. J Am Anim Hosp Assoc 12:31–36, 1976.
55. Hayden DW, VanKruiningen HJ: Eosinophilic gastroenteritis in German shepherd dogs and its relationship to visceral larva migrans. J Am Vet Med Assoc 162:379–384, 1973.
56. Hayden DW, VanKruiningen HJ: Lymphocytic-plasmacytic enteritis in German shepherd dogs. J Am Anim Hosp Assoc 18:89–96, 1982.
57. Heise KM: Lymphangiectasia and protein-losing enteropathy in a German shepherd dog. VM/SAC 78(1):67–71, 1983.
58. Hendrick M: A spectrum of hypereosinophilic syndromes exemplified by six cats with eosinophilic enteritis. Vet Pathol 18:188–200, 1981.
59. Hill FWG, Kidder DE, Frew J: A xylose absorption test for the dog. Vet Rec 87:250–255, 1970.
60. Hoenig M: Intestinal malabsorption attributed to bacterial overgrowth in a dog. J Am Vet Med Assoc 176:533–535, 1980.
61. Hofmann AF: Bile acid malabsorption caused by ileal resection. Arch Intern Med 130:597–605, 1972.
62. Holt PE: The role of dogs and cats in the epidemiology of human campylobacter enterocolitis. J Small Anim Pract 22:681–685, 1981.
63. Holzworth J, Theran P, Carpenter JL, et al: Hyperthyroidism in the cat: ten cases. J Am Vet Med Assoc 176:345–353, 1980.
64. Isaacs PET, Kim YS: Blind loop syndrome and small bowel bacterial contamination. Clin Gastroenterol 12:395–414, 1983.
65. Jackson RF, Simpson CF, Wallace LJ: Spontaneous duodenal ulcers in a dog. J Am Vet Med Assoc 148:892–893, 1966.
66. Johnson GF: Endoscopic examinations. *In* Anderson NV (ed), *Veterinary Gastroenterology,* Lea & Febiger, Philadelphia, 1980.
67. Johnson RH, McCandlish IAD, Wilson JHG: The present status of canine parovirus Vet Q 5:86–88, 1983.
68. Jones BR, Nicholls MR, Badman R: Peptic ulceration in a dog associated with an islet cell carcinoma of the pancreas and an elevated plasma gastrin level. J Small Anim Pract 17:593–598, 1976.
69. Joy CL, Patterson JM: Short bowel syndrome following surgical correction of a double intussusception in a dog. Can Vet J 19:254–259, 1978.
70. Kahn DE: Pathogenesis of feline panleukopenia. J Am Vet Med Assoc 173:628–630, 1978.
71. Kallfelz FA, Norrdin RW, Neal TM: Intestinal absorption of oleic acid ^{131}I and triolein ^{131}I in the differential diagnosis of malabsorption syndrome and pancreatic dysfunction in the dog. J Am Vet Med Assoc 153:43–46, 1968.
72. Kaneko JJ, Moulton JE, Brodey RS, et al: Malabsorption syndrome resembling non-tropical sprue in dogs. J Am Vet Med Assoc 146:463–573, 1965.
73. Kato E, Kaji Y, Kaneko K: Enterotoxigenic staphylococci of canine origin. Am J Vet Res 39:1771–1773, 1978.
74. Keenan KP, Binn LN, Takevchi A: Animal model of human disease—acute nonbacterial gastroenteritis. Am Assoc Path 94(2):439–442, 1979.
75. Keenan KP, Jervis HR, Marchwicki RH: Intestinal infection of neonatal dogs with canine coronavirus 1–71: Studies by virologic, histologic, histochemical and immunofluorescent techniques. Am J Vet Res 37:247–256, 1976.
76. Kelly DF: Idiopathic villous atrophy of the small intestine. *In* Andrews EJ (ed), *Spontaneous Animal Models of Human Disease,* Vol. I, Academic Press, New York, 22–25, 1979.
76a. Ketaren K, Brown J, Shotts EB, et al: Canine salmonellosis in a small animal hospital. J Am Vet Med Assoc 179:1017–1018, 1981.
77. Khansari N, Segre D, Segre M: Diagnosis of histoplasmosis and blastomycosis by an antiglobulin hemagglutination test. Am J Vet Res 43:2279–2283, 1982.
78. Krakowka S, Olsen RG, Axthelm MK, et al: Canine parvovirus infection potentiates canine distemper encephalitis attributable to modified live-virus vaccine. J Am Vet Med Assoc 180:137–139, 1982.
79. Krum SH, Stevens DR, Hirsh DC: *Salmonella arizonae* bacteremia in a cat. J Am Vet Med Assoc 170:42–44, 1977.
80. Lawry JV: *Essential Concepts of Clinical Physiology.* Sinauer Associates, Sunderland, MA, 188, 1977.
81. Layzell T, Collin J: Retrograde electrical pacing of the small intestine—a new treatment for the short bowel syndrome? Br. J. Surg 68:711–713, 1981.
82. Letaren K, Brown J, Shotts EB, et al: Canine salmonellosis in a small animal hospital. J Am Vet Med Assoc 179:1017–1018, 1981.
83. Lewis LD, Bolulay JP, Chow FHC: Fat excretion

and assimilation by the cat. Feline Pract 9:46–49, 1979.
84. Lingeman CH, Garner FM: Comparative study of intestinal adenocarcinomas of animals and man. J Natl Cancer Inst 48:325–346, 1972.
85. Mattheeuws D, DeRick A, Thoonen H, et al: Intestinal lymphangiectasia in a dog. J Small Anim Pract 15:757–761, 1974.
86. McCandlish IAP, Thompson H, Fisher EW, et al: Canine parvovirus infection. In Practice 3:5–14, 1981.
87. McDonald J: Protein-losing enteropathy due to lymphangiectasia. Canine Pract 9:22–27, 1982.
88. Merritt AM: Small Intestinal Diseases in Veterinary Gastroenterology. *In* Anderson NV (ed), *Veterinary Gastroenterology* Lea & Febiger, Philadelphia, 463–522, 1980.
89. Merritt AM, Burrows CF, Cowgill L, Streett W: Fecal fat and trypsin in dogs fed a meat-base or cereal-base diet. J Am Vet Med Assoc 174:59–61, 1979.
90. Middleton PJ: Pathogenesis of rotaviral infection. J Am Vet Med Assoc 173:544–545, 1978.
91. Middleton DJ, Watson ADJ, Vasak E, et al: Duodenal ulceration associated with gastrin-secreting pancreatic tumor in a cat. J Am Vet Med Assoc 183:461–462, 1983.
92. Miller ME: The abdomen, pelvis and pelvic limb. *In Guide to the Dissection of the Dog*. Edwards Brothers, Ann Arbor, MI, 1962.
93. Miller J, Evermann J, Ott R: Immunofluorescence test for canine cornavirus and parvovirus. Western Veterinarian. 17–18:14–19, 1980.
94. Miller RI, Qualls CW, Turnwald GH: Gastrointestinal phycomycosis in a dog. J Am Vet Med Assoc 182:1245–1246, 1983.
95. Moon HW: Mechanisms in pathogenesis of diarrhea: A review. J Vet Med Assoc 172:443–447, 1978.
96. Morris JA, Selivanor V, Sheldon GF: Nutritional management of patients with malabsorption syndrome. Clin Gastroenterol 12:463–474, 1983.
97. Morse EV, Duncan MA: Canine salmonellosis: Prevalence, epizootiology, signs, and public health significance. J Am Vet Med Assoc 167:817–820, 1975.
98. Morse EV, Duncan MA, Estep DA, et al: Canine salmonellosis: A review and report of dog to child transmission of *Salmonella enteritidis*. Am J Public Health 66:82–84, 1976.
99. Nielsen SW: Classification of tumors in dogs and cats. J Am Anim Hosp Assoc 19:13–60, 1983.
100. Noxon JO, Digilio K, Schmidt DA: Disseminated histoplamosis in a cat: successful treatment with ketoconazole. J Am Vet Med Assoc 181:817–820, 1982.
101. O'Dorisio TM, O'Dorisio MS, Cataland S: Overview: Endocrinology of the gastrointestinal tract. Proceedings of 6th Kal Kan Symposium, Columbus, October 16–11, 1982.
102. Okabe S, Takeuchi K, Murata T, et al: Effects of cimetidine on healing of chronic gastric and duodenal ulcers in dogs. Dig Dis 23:166–168, 1978.
103. Olson NC, Zimmer JF: Protein-losing enteropathy secondary to intestinal lymphangiectasia in a dog. J Am Vet Med Assoc 173:271–274, 1978.
104. Orr CM, Groffydd-Jones TJ, Kelly DF: Ileal polyps in Siamese cats. J Small Anim Pract 21:669–674, 1980.
105. Papageorges M, Higgins R, Gosselin Y: *Yersinia enterocolitica* enteritis in two dogs. J Am Vet Med Assoc 182:618–619, 1983.
106. Patnaik AK, Hurvitz AI, Johnson GF: Canine intestinal adenocarcinoma and carcinoid. Vet Pathol 17:149–163, 1982.
107. Patnaik AK, Johnson GF, Greene RW, et al: Surgical resection of intestinal adenocarcinoma in a cat with survival of 28 months. J Am Vet Med Assoc 178:479–481, 1981.
108. Pedersen NC, Boyle JF, Floyd K: An enteric coronavirus infection of cats and its relationship to feline infectious peritonitis. Am J Vet Res 42:368–377, 1981.
109. Peterson MF: Diagnosis and treatment of feline hyperthyroidism. Proceedings of 6th Kal Kan Symposium, Columbus, October 16–17, 1982.
110. Pollock RVH: Canine viral enteritis. *In* Kirk RW (ed), *Current Veterinary Therapy VIII*, W. B. Saunders Company, Philadelphia 1164–1168, 1983.
111. Poonacha KB, Smith HL: Naturally occurring Tyzzer's disease as a complication of distemper and mycotic pneumonia in a dog. J Am Vet Med Assoc 169:419–420, 1976.
112. Prescott JF, Johnson JA, Patterson JM, et al: Haemorrhagic gastroenteritis in the dog associated with *Clostridium welchii*. Vet Rec 103: 116–117, 1978.
113. Prescott JF, Manninen KI, Barker IK: Experimental pathogenesis of *Campylobacter jejuni* enteritis—Studies in gnotobiotic dogs, pigs, and chickens. *In Campylobacter: Epidemiology, Pathogenesis and Biochemistry,* MIP Press Ltd., Lancaster, UK, 170–171, 1982.
114. Prescott JF, Munroe DL: *Campylobacter jejuni* enteritis in man and domestic animals. J Am Vet Med Assoc 181:1524–1530, 1982.
115. Quigley PJ, Henry K: Eosinophilic enteritis in the dog: A case report with brief review of the literature. J Comp Path 91:387–392, 1981.
116. Qureshi SR, Carlton WW, Olander HJ: Tyzzer's disease in a dog. J Am Vet Med Assoc 168: 602–604, 1976.
117. Regan PT, Dimagno EP: The medical management of malabsorption. Mayo Clin Proc 54:267–274, 1979.
118. Rogers WA, Stradley RP, Sherding RG, et al: Simultaneous evaluation of pancreatic exocrine function and intestinal absorptive function in dogs with chronic diarrhea. J Am Vet Med Assoc 117:1128–1131, 1980.
118a. Saad MF, Ordonez G, Rashed RK, et al.: Medullary carcinoma of the thyroid. A study of the clinical features and prognostic factors in 161 patients. Medicine 63:314–342, 1984.
119. Sandstedt K, Wierup M: Concomitant occurrence of *Campylobacter* and parvoviruses in dogs with gastroenteritis. Vet Res Comm 4:271–273, 1981.
120. Sherding RG: Diseases of the Small Bowel. *In* Ettinger, SJ (ed), *Textbook of Veterinary Internal Medicine,* 2nd ed, W. B. Saunders Company, Philadelphia, 1983.
121. Sherding RG, Stradley RP, Rogers WA, Johnson SE: Bentiromide:xylose test in healthy cats. Am J Vet Res 43:2272–2273, 1982.
122. Shindel NM, VanKruiningen HJ, Scott FW: The colitis of feline panleukopenia. J Am Anim Hosp Assoc 14:738–747, 1978.
123. Simpson JW: Bacterial overgrowth causing intes-

tinal malabsorption in a dog. Vet Rec 110: 335–336, 1982.

124. Skirrow MB: Campylobacter enteritis in dogs and cats: A "new" zoonosis. Vet Res Comm 5:13–19, 1981.
125. Skirrow MB: Campylobacter enteritis—the first five years. J Hyg (Cambridge) 89:175–184, 1982.
126. Smyth GB: Factors that affect the response of the oral glucose tolerance test. (Abstract) Aust Vet 13:26, 1983.
127. Stark DR: Primary gastrointestinal histoplasmosis in a cat. J Am Anim Hosp Assoc 18:154–156, 1982.
128. Stewart THM, Hetenyi C, Rowell H, et al: Ulcerative enterocolitis in dogs induced by drugs. J Path 131:363–378, 1980.
129. Stickle JE, Hribernik TW: Clinicopathological observation in disseminated histoplasmois in dogs. J Am Anim Hosp Assoc 14:105–110, 1978.
130. Stokes K: Intestinal mycosis in a cat. Aust Vet J 49:499–500, 1973.
131. Stradley RP, Stern RJ, Heinhold N: A method for the simultaneous evaluation of exocrine pancreatic function and intestinal absorptive function in dogs. Am J Vet Res 40:1201–1205, 1979.
132. Straus E, Johnson GF, Yalow RS: Canine Zollinger-Ellison syndrome. Gastroenterology 73:380–381, 1977.
133. Strombeck DR: New method for evaluation of chymotrypsin deficiency in dogs. J Am Vet Med Assoc 173:1319–1323, 1978.
134. Strombeck DR: *Small Animal Gastroenterology,* Stonegate, Davis, CA, 1979.
135. Takouchi A, Binn LN, Jervis HR, et al: Electron microscope study of experimental enteric infection in neonatal dogs with a canine coronavirus. Lab Invest 34:539–549, 1976.
136. Thompson RA: *The Practice of Clinical Immunology,* Edward Arnold, London, 105, 1978.
137. Tilton RC, VanKruiningen HJ, Kvasnik I, et al: Toxigenic *Clostridium perfringens* from a parvovirus infected dog. J Clin Microbiol 14:697–698, 1981.
138. Timoney JF: Feline *salmonellosis.* Vet Clin North Am 6:395–398, 1976.
139. Twedt DC, Pitts RP, Mallie KA: Comparison of duodenal aspiration with fecal flotation for diagnosis of giardiasis in dogs. J Am Vet Med Assoc 182:1210–1211, 1983.
140. VanKruiningen HJ, Hayden DW: Interpreting problem diarrheas of dogs. Vet Clin North Am 2:29–47, 1972.
141. Vernon DF Jr: Idiopathic sprue in a dog. J Am Vet Med Assoc 140:1062–1067, 1962.
142. Watson DW, Sodeman WA Jr: The small intestine. *In* Sodeman WA Jr, Sodeman TM, *Pathologic Physiology: Mechanisms of Disease,* 6th ed, W. B. Saunders Company, Philadelphia, 824–859, 1979.
143. Williams FP: Astrovirus-like, corona-virus–like and parvovirus-like particles detected in the diarrheal stools of Beagle pups. Arch Virol 66:215–226, 1980.
144. Williams DA, Burrows CF: Short-bowel syndrome—A case report in a dog and discussion of the pathophysiology of bowel resection. J Small Anim Pract 22:263–275, 1981.
145. Wood GL: Canine myocardial diseases. *In* Kirk RW (ed), *Current Veterinary Therapy VIII,* W. B. Saunders Company, Philadelphia, 321–329, 1983.
146. Wright R: *Immunology of Gastrointestinal and Liver Diseases,* Edward Arnold, London, 27, 1977.

CHAPTER

8

Surgery of the Small Intestine

M. JOSEPH BOJRAB

The small intestine is that portion of the alimentary tract that extends from the pylorus to the cecum. Procedures involving the small intestine play an important role in small animal surgery. The surgeon should have a thorough knowledge of the anatomy, physiology, and pathology of the small intestine. This knowledge becomes particularly important when a small intestinal disorder leads to an acute abdomen, a condition in which quick decisions must be made.

Surgical Anatomy

GROSS ANATOMY

The length of the small intestine is approximately three and one-half times the length of the body, making it the longest portion of the alimentary tract.[29] The duodenum is the first and most fixed part of the small intestine.[12] It begins at the pylorus to the right of the median plane of the body. After a short dorsocranial course, the duodenum turns, creating the cranial duodenal flexure, and continues caudally on the right as the descending duodenum. At approximately the level of the sixth lumbar vertebra, the duodenum turns, forming the caudal duodenal flexure, and then continues cranially as the ascending portion.[12, 29] The ascending portion lies to the left of the root of the mesentery; cranially it forms the duodenojejunal flexure.

The jejunum and ileum compose 91 per cent of the small intestine.[29] They form the coils that occupy the ventrocaudal part of the abdominal cavity. The jejunum is the longest portion of the small intestine.[12] The ileum ends by opening into the proximal part of the ascending colon at the ileocolic orifice. The ileocolic orifice generally lies to the right of the median plane between the descending and ascending portions of the duodenum. Unlike the relatively fixed duodenum, the jejunum and ileum are freely moveable within the abdominal cavity.[29] They are suspended by the mesentery from the cranial part of the sublumbar region in the area of the first lumbar vertebra.[25, 29]

The blood supply to the small intestine is composed of the cranial mesenteric and the celiac arteries. The duodenum receives branches from both the cranial (celiac) and caudal (cranial mesenteric) pancreaticoduodenal arteries. The most proximal jejunal artery anastomoses with the most distal duodenal branch of the caudal pancreaticoduodenal artery. The jejunum is supplied by 12 to 15 jejunal arteries from the cranial mesenteric artery.[29] These arteries form a series of anastomotic arches in the mesentery near the intestine (Fig. 8–1). The ileum is supplied on its mesenteric side by a branch of the accessory cecal artery, and on its antimesenteric side by the ileal branches of the ileocecal artery; all of these vessels are branches of the cranial mesenteric artery. Those branches coursing along the antimesenteric border of the ileum serve as excellent landmarks for the distal ileum.

The short, irregular vasa recta that arise from the terminal arcades lie closely adjacent to the intestine; they run variable distances on the mesenteric half of the intestinal musculature before perforating it to supply the submucosa and the mucosa.[29]

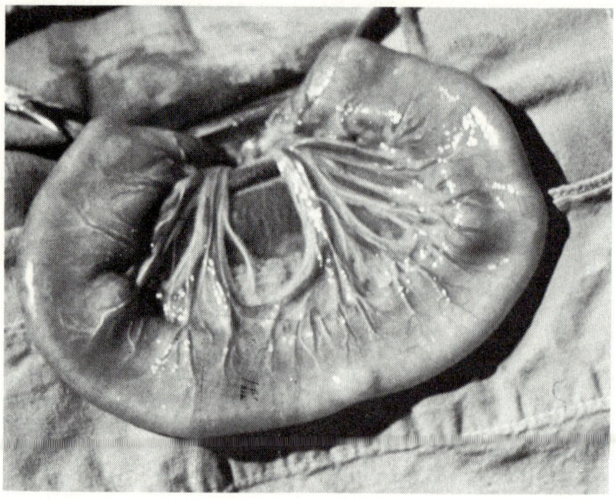

Figure 8–1. The normal appearance of small intestine. Note the arcadial vessel in the mesentery and the communication of the vasa recta with the mesenteric border of the intestine.

Lymph from the duodenum is carried to the hepatic lymph nodes and to the duodenal lymph node when it is present.[29] The mesenteric lymph nodes lie along the vessels in the root of the mesentery. Lymphatic vessels from the jejunum and ileum drain primarily into the right and left mesenteric lymph nodes. Lymphatics from the ileum also drain into the colic lymph nodes.

MICROSCOPIC AND ULTRASTRUCTURAL ANATOMY

An important anatomical characteristic of the small intestine is the large surface area it provides for absorption. The gross, microscopic, and ultrastructural features of the small intestine that account for this characteristic are: the length of the intestine and the presence of mucosal folds, villi, and microvilli.[40] The small intestine is made up of four layers, which from the lumen outward are the mucosa, the submucosa, the muscularis, and the adventitia or serosa.

The mucosa of the small intestine is composed of three layers: the epithelium, the lamina propria, and the muscularis mucosa. The mucosal surface has two important structural features, the villi and intestinal crypts. Because of the presence of highly developed microvilli, the absorptive surface of the small intestine is approximately 15 to 25 times greater than that of the mucosal surface.[25]

The lamina propria lies between the intestinal epithelium and the muscularis mucosa. It contains blood and lymphatic vessels, nerve fibers, smooth muscle fibers, fibroblasts, macrophages, plasma cells, lymphocytes, eosinophils, mast cells, and connective tissue elements.

The second layer of the small intestine is the submucosa. This is a strong fibroelastic and areolar connective tissue layer containing blood vessels, nerves, and lymphoid tissue. The fibroelastic and connective tissue components of the submucosa account for the holding power when the small intestine is sutured. Therefore, any method of intestinal suturing should include sutures through the submucosa.

The tunica muscularis, the muscular portion of the small intestine, is formed by two distinct layers of smooth muscle, an outer longitudinal coat and an inner circular coat.

Preoperative Considerations

PATIENT STABILITY

In elective situations the patient should be fasted for 12 to 24 hours prior to surgery. Attempts should be made to submit appropriate blood samples to a lab for determination of a CBC, the biochemical profile, and serum electrolyte levels. If the animal is dehydrated, intravenous fluids should be started prior to surgery in an attempt to correct the hydration status and the electrolyte and acid-base imbalances. Following the correction of these imbalances, maintenance fluid therapy should be initiated with lactated Ringer's solution with 5% dextrose at a rate of 20 ml/kg TID via a slow continuous intravenous drip. When the solution is given slowly, the renal threshold will not be exceeded and there will be no glucosuria.

Oral and systemic antibiotics should be started 24 hours prior to surgery, if possible. Oral neomycin sulfate at a dose of 20 mg/kg every 6 hours is effective in suppressing the bacterial flora of the small intestine. While gross contamination of the abdomen is to be avoided, it is often an inevitability, and may lead to serious complications.

It is best to start broad-spectrum systemic antibiotics or a combination of antibiotics before surgery. A combination of procaine penicillin G (40,000 IU/kg SID) and kanamycin (5 mg/kg BID) provides excellent protection and is relatively safe. Problems encountered with this combination of antibiotics are due to the ototoxicity and nephrotoxicity of kanamycin.

ACUTE ABDOMEN

The acute abdomen has been loosely defined as "medical slang for any acute condition within the abdomen demanding immediate operation."[8a] A more elegant and more succinct definition is, "The acute abdomen is one that requires an acute decision."[4] Lesions of the small intestine that may be involved in this clinical syndrome include those caused by: foreign bodies, intussusceptions, volvulus, strangulations, trauma caused by a blunt object, hemorrhage, trauma caused by a sharp object, gunshot wounds, and neoplasia. Patient stability in these cases is of primary concern to the practitioner.[2]

It must be emphasized that regardless of the type of lesion, patient stability is required prior to surgical intervention. Surgery must often be delayed until after shock therapy has been initiated. A large-bore catheter should be placed in any easily accessible vein. If the animal is in shock or is extremely hypotensive, a cutdown may be necessary. Lactated Ringer's solution is infused at a rate of up to one blood volume (80 ml/kg) during the first hour. The patient is then re-evaluated and the appropriate adjustment is made in fluid delivery rate.

Adjustment of acid-base status is best done after the measurement of arterial pH and PCO_2 and the calculation of bicarbonate concentrations and base deficits. If blood gas and pH analyses are not available, sodium bicarbonate solution should be administered at a dosage of 1 to 4 mEq/kg, according to the apparent severity of the animal's condition. Half the amount should be given slowly intravenously, and the remainder should be added to the intravenous fluid and given over the next 4 to 6 hours.[22] Corticosteroids are believed to be beneficial especially for the management of endotoxic shock.[22] Both dexamethasone at 2 mg/kg and prednisone sodium succinate at 10 to 20 mg/kg given intravenously early in the course of therapy are helpful. Intravenous antibiotics given during the initial stabilization period aid in controlling bacterial infection in septic shock and in preventing bacteria invasion in other forms of shock. Choices of antibiotics include chloramphenicol sodium succinate at 50 mg/kg q6h IV, penicillin G sodium at 50,000 to 100,000 IU/kg q4h IV, and ampicillin sodium at 10 to 20 mg/kg q6h IV.

The initial period of patient stabilization with intense fluid and corticosteroid therapy generally lasts 30 to 60 minutes. The patient should be carefully evaluated through this period; pulse, capillary refill time, and the presence of tachycardia should be noted. If the patient is cooperative, the abdomen is clipped and prepared for surgery during this time.

Surgical Principles

GENERAL PRINCIPLES

A standard mid-line approach to the abdomen is utilized. The length of the incision depends on the individual patient. Technique should not be compromised by inadequate exposure.[43] A Balfour retractor* is helpful in providing good surgical exposure. The entire small intestine from the pylorus to the cecum should be examined. Often, more than one lesion will be present. A thorough exploratory laparotomy will lessen the chances of having to repeat an operation.

Meticulous atraumatic surgical techniques must be practiced when intestinal surgery is performed. Poor surgical technique may result in a disrupted blood supply, contamination, leakage, ileus, peritonitis, and a breakdown in the mucosal barriers to the ever-present intestinal bacteria and toxins. If surgical trauma occurs, the result is tissue death and subsequent lysosomal membrane rupture with enzyme release. The enzymes, in turn, digest and kill other cells, leading to a perpetuation of the "vicious circle." This sequence of events, in small intestinal surgery, results in mucosal lining destruction and, thus, permeability to bacterial toxins, which leads to endotoxic shock and death. This process occurs from several hours to several days postoperatively and accounts for a number of the unexplained deaths surgeons see after intestinal surgery.

The principles of atraumatic technique dictate the following recommendations concerning intestinal surgery: (1) a "clampless" technique (i.e., utilizing an assistant's fingers instead of intestinal clamps) for intestinal resection and anastomosis (Fig. 8–2*A*); (2) careful and gentle handling of the intes-

*Balfour Self-Retaining Abdominal Retractor, American V. Mueller, Chicago, IL.

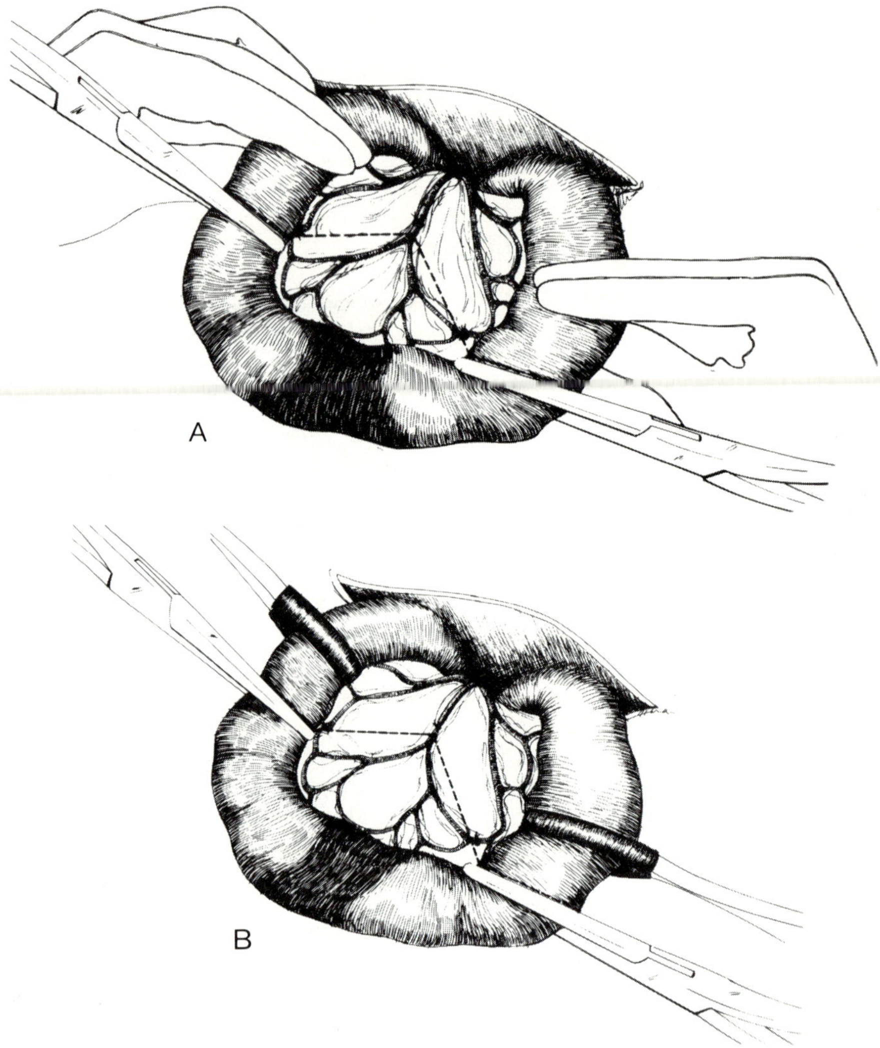

Figure 8–2. *A,* The preferred method of occluding the bowel is by the use of an assistant's fingers. This should prevent the spillage of intestinal contents into the peritoneal cavity. *Broken lines* indicate the angle of resection. *B,* non-crushing clamps (Doyen or Vascular clamps) are placed across the point of excision *(broken line).* Non-crushing clamps are used to prevent spillage of ingesta if an assistant is not available to do it with his fingers. (Reprinted with permission from Krahwinkel DJ Jr, Richardson DC: Surgery of small intestine. *In* Bojrab MJ (ed): *Current Techniques in Small Animal Surgery.* 2nd ed. Philadelphia, Lea and Febiger, 1983.)

tine; (3) prevention of tissue dehydration; and (4) the use of a scalpel rather than scissors as the cutting instrument.

Atraumatic intestinal forceps may be used to handle the intestine (Fig. 8–2*B*); however, the least traumatic way to hold a piece of intestine involves the use of an assistant's fingers. During a surgical procedure, the ends of intestine should be padded with moistened gauze sponges and held gently between two fingers. It is extremely difficult to hold and suture the intestine at the same time; therefore, it is necessary to have an assistant. This makes the procedure less traumatic and decreases the incidence of contamination.

BIOPSY

A biopsy of the small intestine is indicated whenever the lesion or disease syndrome is uncertain and is related to the small intestine. A complete systematic exploratory laparotomy should be performed to carefully examine the small intestine from the pylorus to the cecum. Blood supply and lymphatic drainage should always be evaluated.

In general, a biopsy should be done only

to tissues that are abnormal, as determined by visualization, palpation, radiograph, or laboratory test. All regional lymph nodes should be examined by inspection, palpation, and biopsy. When possible, the lesion and its margins should be submitted for histological examination and bacterial and fungal culture.

Small biopsy specimens may be taken by simple, full-thickness excision through the intestinal wall. These biopsy specimens may be in the form of a wedge, a longitudinal, or a transverse resection. Small biopsy incisions are easily closed by several simple interrupted sutures using 2/0 or 3/0 synthetic absorbable suture material. More extensive biopsies may involve complete resection of a segment of the small intestine. When small excisional biopsy specimens are taken, they should be secured on something flat. This can be either a piece of cardboard, foam,* or a tongue depressor. If these specimens are put on something flat, and then put in a formalin solution, the tisses are fixed and stay in one plane. This makes it easier for the pathologist to section the tissues at a 90° angle and to visualize the full length of the villi.

GUIDELINES FOR INTESTINAL RESECTION

It is often difficult to determine whether a segment of small intestine is viable. The guidelines generally used in determining bowel viability are: (1) color, which is pink to blue-black; (2) motility, which is demonstrated by peristaltic waves and segmented contractions; (3) a glistening serosal coat; and (4) a visible arterial pulsation.[2] If the viability of the intestine is questionable, the bowel segment should be released, placed on a warm, saline-moistened sponge for a few minutes, and then re-examined. If normal color has returned, peristalsis is evident, and an arterial pulse is visible, it is probably safe to retain the segment. If there is a reasonable doubt as to the viability of the bowel, it should be resected.

Resection of 80 per cent of the small intestine is reasonably safe, if the ileocolic valve is intact. When the valve itself is resected, not more than 50 per cent of the small intestine may be resected.[19] It should be noted, however, that when massive resection of the bowel is performed, and especially when the ileocolic valve is involved, more adjunctive surgical procedures are helpful. Common to all of these adjunctive procedures is the construction of a nonrefluxing valve. In dogs with the valve, mortality that is associated with a decrease in weight and with bacterial overgrowth is significantly decreased when compared to dogs without a valve.[9, 44, 46]

*Gelfoam, The Upjohn Company, Kalamazoo, MI.

Surgical Techniques

INTESTINAL ANASTOMOSIS TECHNIQUES

There are four broad classifications of end-to-end anastomoses in the dog: inverting, everting, approximating, and invaginating.

Inverting Technique

Inversion of a large, internal cuff of tissue accounts for the pathophysiology that is often seen with a double-layer closure. The submucosal blood vessels are bent at a 90° angle; and thus, the blood flow to the inverted portion of the intestine is greatly inhibited, resulting in hemodynamic compromise.

With the single-layer inverting technique there is less distortion of the submucosal blood vessels, allowing more adequate blood supply with a decrease in necrosis and edema. There is less reduction of lumen diameter with the single-layer closure.[1]

The inverting technique offers the advantage of serosa-to-serosa contact, forming an excellent seal. This contact is desirable in the septic abdomen or colon, where serosal apposition is important.[17, 25]

Everting Technique

The everting technique produces an external cuff of tissue without reducing the internal luminal diameter. Some mucosa is trapped between sutures and becomes necrotic; however, a fibrin seal cements the remainder of the mucosal layer within 3 hours of the anastomosis. Early regeneration of the mucosa and aggregation of fibrin provide a water-tight seal within 3 days. There is conflicting evidence as to when arterial anastomosis occurs across the suture line in the everting technique. Ravitch reported that it occurs early.[14, 41] Abramowitz found that vessels crossed the incision at 1 week with the inverting technique and showed minimal crossing at 3 weeks when the everting suture pattern was used.[1, 14]

In terms of absence of inflammation and closer apposition of the anastomotic surfaces, the everting anastomosis is superior to the inverting anastomosis. However, the healing process seems to be delayed in the everting technique, because of the degeneration of the trapped mucosa. Also, because the everted mucosa causes more inflammation outside the lumen, peritoneal response is enhanced and adhesions are more pronounced than in the inverting technique. If the inflammatory response and fibrous adhesion formation are excessive, stricture of the anastomotic site may occur.[14, 33]

Approximating Technique

Approximation of the bowel wall with the crushing technique provides rapid regeneration of the mucosa over the incision, and causes less collagen and fibrous connective tissue deposition and less inflammatory cell infiltration than with either the everting or the inverting techniques. The everting, inverting, and crushing techniques have been compared in dogs, and the greatest amount of fibrosis has been found with the everting technique and the least with the crushing technique.[3, 10, 12, 14, 30]

Histological evaluation of the simple, interrupted non-crushing approximating technique is not available, but one would expect the healing resulting from it to be similar to that occurring in the crushing technique.[14] Technically, both the crushing and non-crushing appositional patterns are difficult to perform without some eversion of the mucosa occurring; and therefore, some modification of healing, similar to that described for everting patterns, may take place.[14]

Invaginating Technique

As described by Frier, the invaginating technique involves pulling the distal segment of a resected bowel into the proximal segment with mattress sutures and allowing the invaginated portion of the distal segment to slough off.[13] Grier performed an extensive evaluation of the invaginating technique in the dog. He dissected mucosa from the distal segment in one group of six dogs, resected the muscularis externa of the proximal segment and removed mucosa from the distal segment in 12 dogs, and resected the muscularis externa of the proximal segment only in four dogs. The invagination anastomoses were held in place with mattress sutures. Grier concluded that until a rapid and efficient method for total dissection of mucosa of the distal segment is achieved, the invaginating technique is not recommended over a conventional anastomosis.[15]

RESECTION AND ANASTOMOSIS TECHNIQUE

The arcadial vessels and the communicating branches of the vasa recta vessels along the mesenteric border that supply the diseased segment of the intestine are identified and ligated with absorbable suture material. When ligating these communicating vessels, the serosa should be incorporated into each ligature (Fig. 8–3). Fingers should be used to hold the intestine, while it is transected with the vasa recta ligatures remaining with the healthy tissue. The intestine should be transected at an angle of approximately 30° from transverse, leaving more tissue on the mesenteric border. This will help to insure an adequate blood supply to the antimesenteric border.

One of the approximation techniques involves use of the "crushing suture technique."[3, 14, 30] This suture pattern is a simple interrupted through-and-through one-layer closure. Absorbable sutures (2/0 or 3/0) are most commonly employed; those made of

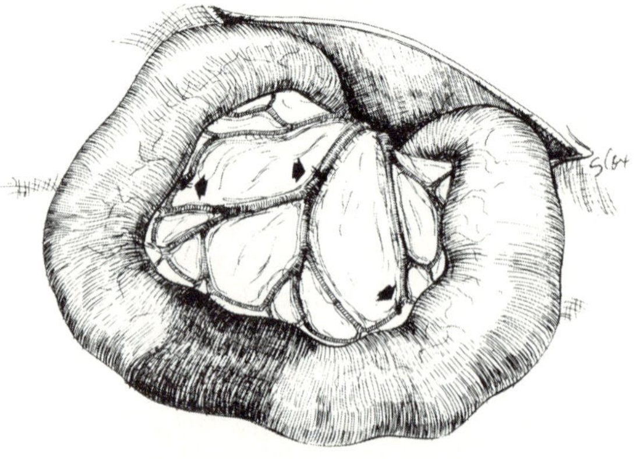

Figure 8–3. The segment of bowel to be resected along with a short section of normal bowel on either side is isolated from the remaining viscera. The mesenteric and arcadial vessels are ligated *(arrows)*. (Reprinted with permission from Krahwinkel DJ Jr, Richardson DC: Surgery of small intestine. *In* Bojrab MJ (ed): *Current Techniques in Small Animal Surgery*. 2nd ed. Philadelphia, Lea & Febiger, 1983.)

polyglycolic acid,* polyglactin 910,† and polydioxanone‡ have some theoretical advantages over surgical gut. Gut is susceptible to rapid proteolytic digestion in the entire gastrointestinal tract and causes significantly more inflammation than the synthetic absorbable suture material.[8] In a very debilitated patient, for example, one with hypoproteinemia, when slow healing is anticipated, the use of non-absorbable suture material such as 2/0 or 3/0 monofilament nylon§ or Ethibond|| is advisable. Regardless of the suture material used, a swaged-on taper or taper-cut needle¶ is desirable because it is less traumatic.[8]

*Dexon, American Cyanamid Co., Princeton, NJ.

†Vicryl, Pitman-Moore, Inc., Washington Crossing, NJ.

‡P. D. S., Pitman-Moore, Inc., Washington Crossing, NJ.

§Ethilon, Ethicon, Inc., Somerville, NJ.

||Ethibond, Ethicon, Inc., Somerville, NJ.

¶Tapercut needles, Ethicon, Inc., Somerville, NJ.

The "crushing suture technique" is begun by placement of two initial sutures, one mesenteric and one antimesenteric, approximately 3 mm from the cut serosal edge (Fig. 8–4*A*). The needle passes through the tissue from serosa to mucosa and then crosses the incision line. On the opposite side, it starts at the mucosal surface and exits through the serosa, again 3 mm from the cut surface (Fig. 8–4*B*). The suture is then tied slowly, cutting through the serosa and mucosa down to the strong fibroelastic submucosal layer, thus only incarcerating this one layer (Fig. 8–4*C*). The simple interrupted pattern apposes the submucosa of the two edges, thereby producing an accurate apposition of the mucosal and serosal layers of each side.[3, 28] Sutures are placed approximately 2 to 3 mm apart. After the suture line is complete, it should be tested for leaks by occluding each side and injecting sterile saline into the lumen. If there are any leaks, an additional simple interrupted suture may be needed.

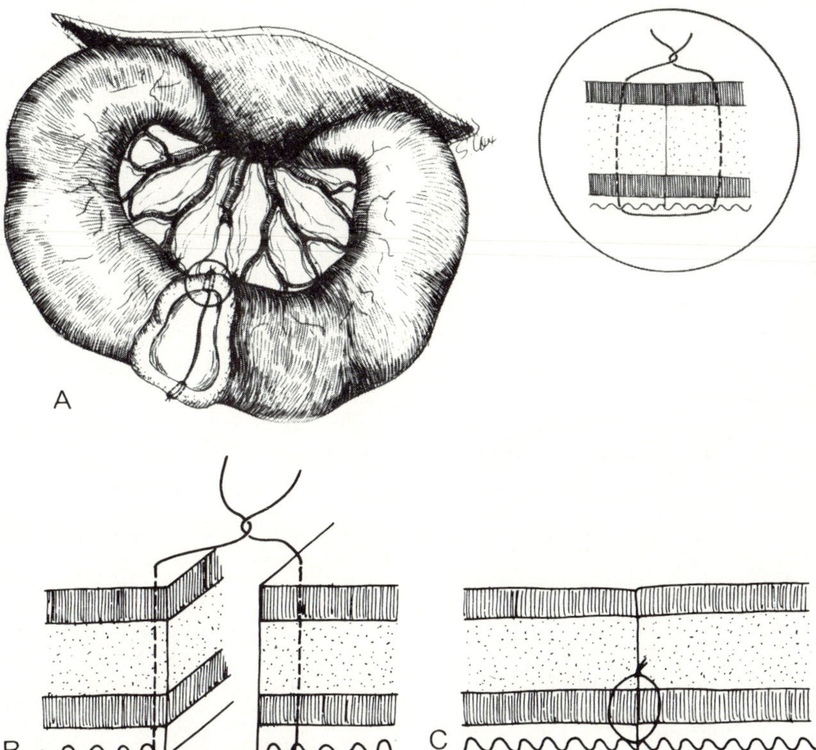

Figure 8–4. Crushing suture technique. *A,* The first suture is placed at the mesenteric border and the second at the antimesenteric border. *Inset,* the placement of a crushing suture before it is tightened to include only submucosa. It includes 2–3 mm of the cut end of the bowel. *B,* Untied crushing suture placed through the serosa to mucosa and then, crossing the transection line, passing from mucosa to serosa. Both passages are placed 3 mm from the cut edge. *C,* Crushing suture pulled tight to include only the submucosa. (*A* Reprinted with permission from Krahwinkel DJ Jr, Richardson DC: Surgery of small intestine. *In* Bojrab MJ (ed): *Current Techniques in Small Animal Surgery.* 2nd ed. Philadelphia, Lea & Febiger, 1983.)

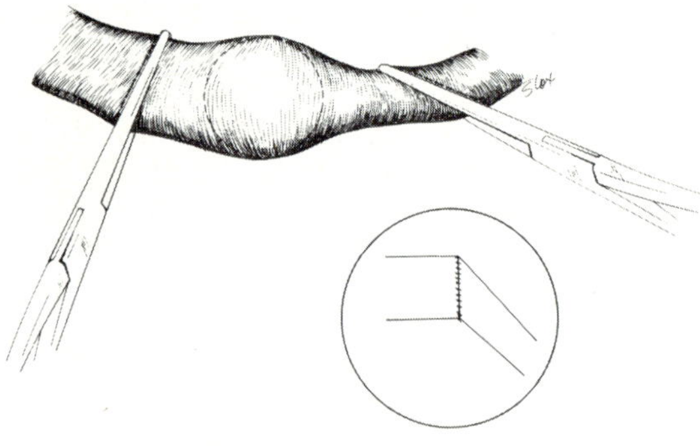

Figure 8–5. To accommodate unequal lumen sizes, the small end is cut at an acute angle and the large end at nearly 90° *(broken lines)*. *Inset,* the resulting anastomosis is at an angle. (Reprinted with permission from Krahwinkel DJ Jr, Richardson DC: Surgery of small intestine. *In* Bojrab MJ (ed): *Current Techniques in Small Animal Surgery*. 2nd ed. Philadelphia, Lea & Febiger, 1983.)

When confronted with anastomosing ends of different diameters (i.e., the proximally dilated portion and the normal distal segment of obstructed bowel) the practitioner should incise the smaller segment at a more oblique angle in order to enlarge its lumen (Fig. 8–5). If the size differential can not be compensated for in this way, a longitudinal incision into the antimesenteric border of the smaller piece should be made to enlarge its lumen.

Rents in the mesentery should be sutured with a simple, continuous pattern, using an

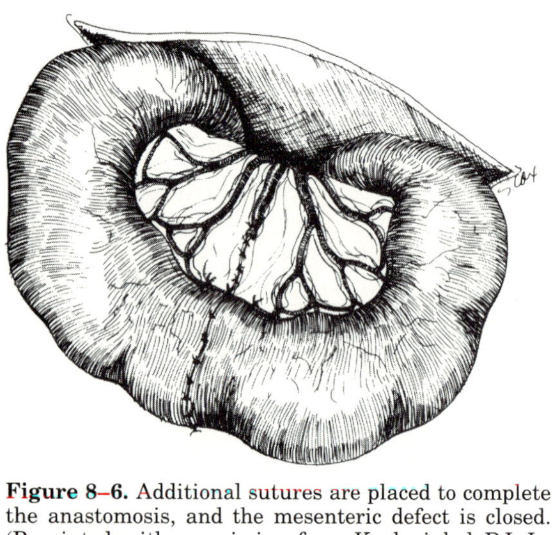

Figure 8–6. Additional sutures are placed to complete the anastomosis, and the mesenteric defect is closed. (Reprinted with permission from Krahwinkel DJ Jr, Richardson DC: Surgery of small intestine. *In* Bojrab MJ (ed): *Current Techniques in Small Animal Surgery*. 2nd ed. Philadelphia, Lea & Febiger, 1983.)

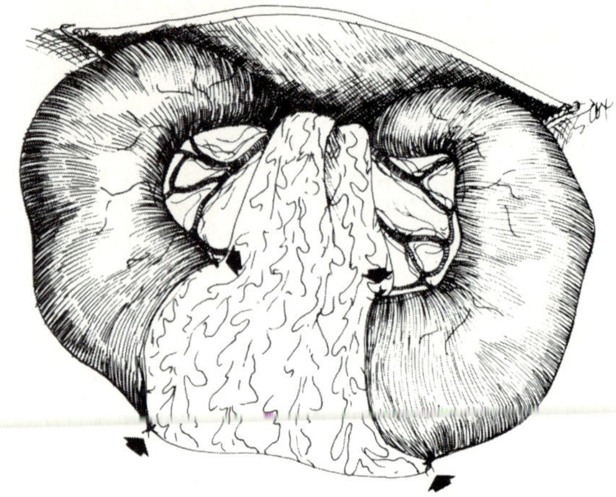

Figure 8–7. A pedicle of omentum can be used to reinforce the anastomosis. Sutures are used to hold the omentum in place *(arrows)*. (Reprinted with permission from Krahwinkel DJ Jr, Richardson DC: Surgery of small intestine. *In* Bojrab MJ (ed): *Current Techniques in Small Animal Surgery*. 2nd ed. Philadelphia, Lea & Febiger, 1983.)

absorbable suture material. This additional step is done to eliminate any possibility of postoperative strangulation of intestine or omentum (Fig. 8–6). Care should be taken not to trap the arcadial vessels in the closure.

When the health and viability of the ends of the intestine to be anastomosed are precarious, the anastomotic site should be covered with a pedicle of omentum. The omentum should be wrapped around the intestine and sutured to the serosa with absorbable suture material (Fig. 8–7). This step will help prevent leakage and subsequent peritonitis. However, this technique should never be used as a substitute for proper anastomosis.

Peritonitis

Before the abdomen is closed, the peritoneal cavity should be thoroughly irrigated with warm, sterile saline or lactated Ringer's solution. If gross contamination of the peritoneal cavity occurs either because of the lesion (e.g., ruptured bowel, penetrating trauma) or because of faulty technique, an antibacterial agent should be added to the final flush. Probably the best lavage solution consists of 10 ml of 1 per cent Betadine

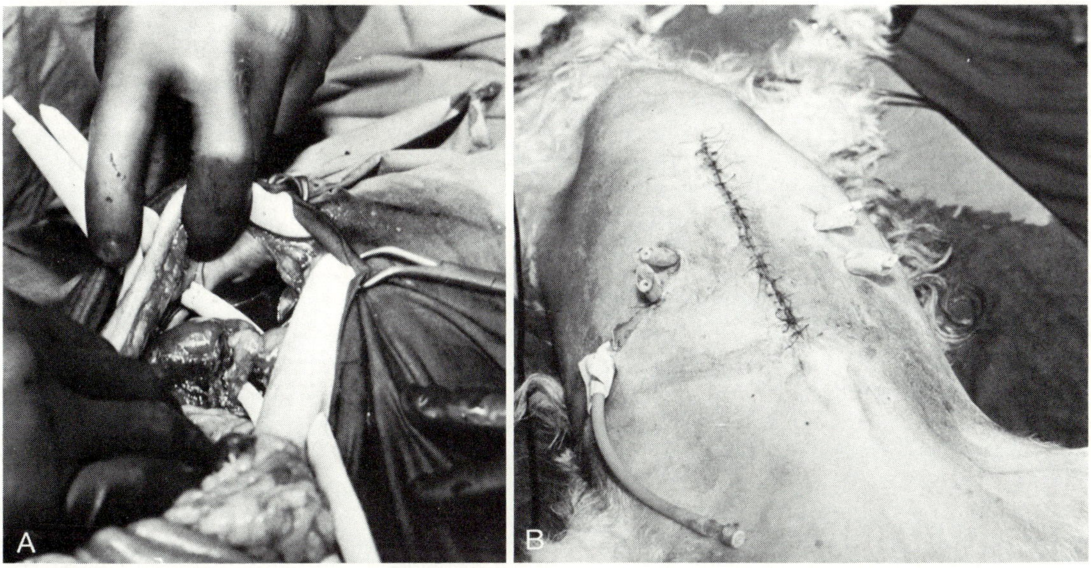

Figure 8–8. *A,* If the peritoneal cavity is contaminated, a sump-Penrose drain needs to be applied. Drains are applied two centimeters from middle incision prior to closure. *B,* Sump-Penrose drain applied.

solution* in 1 liter of sterile saline or lactated Ringer's solution. This lavage solution has excellent antibacterial properties and is non-irritating.[28] If material from the peritoneal cavity is to be cultured, it should be removed prior to lavage. Antibiotics that are efficacious for the final peritoneal lavage are penicillin G soduim, aqueous chloramphenicol, ampicillin, kanamycin, and cephalothin added at a dose of 1 g/l of warmed, sterile lactated Ringer's or saline solution. Heparin is also added to the lavage solution at a ratio of 2,500 units per liter. Dogs weighing less than 13.50 kg receive 500 ml of the lavage solution, while dogs weighing more than 13.50 kg receive 1 liter of solution.[35]

If the peritoneal cavity is grossly contaminated, it is wise to place peritoneal drains prior to closure. Sump-Penrose drains work well for peritoneal drainage and are constructed by placing a fenestrated piece of a tube made of polymeric silicone† within a perforated Penrose drain. This particular type of drain is utilized because adjacent tissues frequently seal off the openings of a single-bore drain. The sump-Penrose drain allows air or lavage fluid to enter the drained area through the central drain, thus displacing fluid into the Penrose drain. Fluid flow, dependent upon gravity, is through the Penrose drain and around the central sump drain.[42] Placement of the peritoneal sump-Penrose drain is accomplished by making an incision in the skin 2 cm from the mid-line incision. Carmalt forceps are used to tunnel 4 to 6 cm subcutaneously. The forceps are pushed through the abdominal muscle, grasp the sump-Penrose drain, and pull it through the skin. The tube is fixed to the skin with a non-absorbable mattress suture. The tip of the tube should be placed close to the point of insult (Fig. 8–8*A* and *B*). In one controlled study, the percentage volume recovered from the abdomens of mongrel dogs after the lavage solution was instilled, was 72 per cent with the sump-Penrose drain and only 40 per cent with the simple Penrose drain.[16]

Peritoneal lavage is performed two to three times daily, if necessary. The exterior of the drain is cleaned with antiseptic, and the warm solution is allowed to run into the abdomen by gravity flow. If the animal experiences any discomfort or dyspnea, the flow is discontinued. When the abdomen has been filled, the drain is clamped and the solution is left in place for 10 to 20 minutes. The clamp is then removed, and the lavage solution allowed to drain. A disposable diaper is taped over the drain to prevent retro-

*1% Betadine Solution, Purdue Frederick Co., Norwalk, CT.

†Silastic, Dow-Corning Corporation, Medical Products Division, Midland, MI.

grade contamination and to lift and store any continual drainage. Lavage is continued until the signs of peritonitis have resolved and the lavage fluid has remained clear on two successive lavages.[47, 48]

Side effects and complications arising from the use of peritoneal lavage include: peritoneal irritation, adhesion formation, respiratory depression by neuromuscular blockade caused by aminoglycoside antibiotics used in the lavage solution, ascending peritonitis, hypoproteinemia, hypokalemia, and chewing out of drains by the patient.

Closure of the abdomen depends upon whether there was contamination during the operation. If no gross contamination occurred, the abdomen is closed in a routine manner. The peritoneum is apposed with absorbable suture material in a simple continuous pattern, and the rectus fascia is sutured with similar suture material in a simple interrupted pattern. The subcutaneous tissue is closed with a simple continuous or running suture pattern using absorbable material. The skin is apposed with a non-absorbable suture material in a simple interrupted pattern.[40] If contamination of the abdomen occurred during surgery or if the patient is very large and has a long incision, the use of larger non-absorbable suture material in the rectus fascia is indicated. Appropriate materials would be 2/0 Ethibond or 3/0 monofilament stainless steel.

Postoperative Care

Postoperative care following any surgical procedure involving the small intestine is dictated by several factors. The two factors that will most influence postoperative care are patient stability and the type of lesion treated.

Relatively minor procedures such as biopsies and small enterotomies require minimal postoperative care. Oral and systemic antibiotics, as discussed along with preoperative care, should be continued for 3 to 5 days following surgery. Intravenous fluids should be continued for 24 hours following surgery. At this time, oral intake can be allowed. Small amounts of an I/D* (intestinal diet) gruel or baby food should be offered 3 or 4 times for the first day following operation. Oral intake should be increased daily so that in 2 or 3 days the patient is back on a regular diet and can be discharged from the hospital.

*Prescription Diet I/D, Hill's Pet Products, Inc., Topeka, KS.

Postoperative care in a very debilitated patient is much more extensive. Oral and systemic antibiotics, along with maintenance fluid therapy (lactated Ringer's Solution), should be continued until the patient is able to take oral fluid and food. Electrolyte, blood gas, and CBC evaluations should be encouraged and are often essential. Hydration should be carefully monitored, clinically by assessing skin elasticity, enophthalmia, and urine formation, as well as by PCV and total serum protein values.

Anemia, hypoproteinemia (hypoalbuminemia), and electrolyte disturbances occur as a consequence of both lavage therapy and peritonitis. Protein losses of from 40 to 247.9 gm/24 hours have been reported in humans as a result of repeated peritoneal dialysis. In experimental dogs with peritonitis, protein was removed at a mean rate of 35.5 gm/24 hours. It was shown that the frequency of dialysis, rather than the fluid volumes used, was the most important factor in protein loss.[28, 35] The increased removal of protein in the presence of peritonitis constitutes an additional drain on body stores.

Electrolyte disturbances are associated with clinical signs of weakness and depression. Serum sodium and potassium levels are decreased. Proper intravenous therapy with potassium and sodium supplementation counters these complications.

In the very debilitated patient, total serum protein values often are good indicators not only of dehydration but also of prognosis. A patient with a falling total serum protein value that is in a normal state of hydration is a more severe postoperative risk than a patient with a normal total serum protein level. Plasma transfusions should be encouraged whenever the albumin value drops below 1 gm/dl. Transfusions are often essential in a patient with severe peritonitis or in a patient undergoing peritoneal lavage.[35]

Surgical Diseases

FOREIGN BODIES

Linear Foreign Bodies

Cats are notorious for ingesting string and other linear foreign objects such as fishing line and pieces of electrical cord. Physical

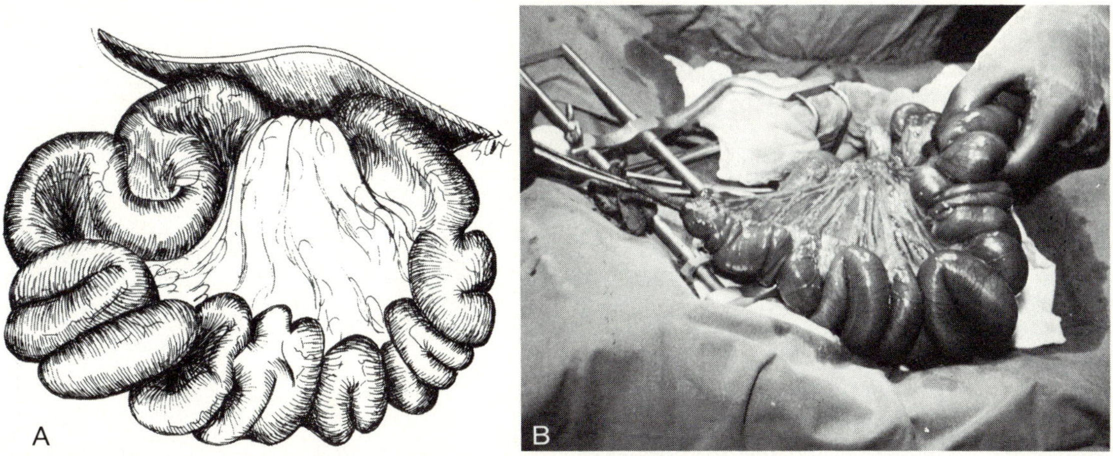

Figure 8–9. *A,* The accordion pleating of the intestine is diagnostic of a linear foreign body. *B,* Actual case of linear foreign body before removal through several enterotomy incisions along antimesenteric border. (*A* Reprinted with permission from Krahwinkel DJ Jr, Richardson DC: Surgery of small intestine. *In* Bojrab MJ (ed): *Current Techniques in Small Animal Surgery.* 2nd ed. Philadelphia, Lea & Febiger, 1983.)

examination will often reveal a moderately painful abdomen. On palpation of the abdomen the intestines will be bunched together in a compact mass. The possibility that a string may be looped around the base of the tongue should always be investigated. Radiographs help confirm the diagnosis of a linear foreign body and will reveal a plicated, irregular, compact mass of intestine with a characteristic gas pattern. A positive-contrast series of radiographs is seldom needed to confirm the diagnosis. A barium series may be harmful to the patient if the small intestine is perforated. The contrast material of choice when a perforated bowel is suspected is a water-soluble compound such as Renografin.*

Surgery is always indicated in patients in which a perforated bowel is suspected and should be considered an emergency. Although it rarely occurs, a dog or cat may pass the string. An exploratory laparotomy should be performed with the involved loops of intestine identified and packed off from the rest of the intestine with saline-moistened sponges (Fig. 8–9*A* and *B*). Sometimes the foreign body is short and may easily be removed through a small enterotomy. If the foreign body is long it should be removed through numerous small enterotomies along the antimesenteric border. It is dangerous to remove a long, linear foreign body through one incision. While the foreign body is being pulled out, it may saw through the mesenteric border of the intestinal wall. Each enterotomy incision should be closed with two or three interrupted, crushing sutures.

Before closing the abdomen, the mesenteric border of the entire small intestine should be checked for perforations. Small rents must be carefully debrided, checked to ensure they have an adequate vascular supply, and then closed with several simple interrupted sutures using the crushing technique.

It is important to check the stomach in cases of linear foreign bodies, since many extend from the stomach. A gastrotomy should be performed if part of the foreign body is in the stomach. Closure of the abdomen is routine, with drains being utilized if contamination is present.

Non-Linear Foreign Bodies

A variety of foreign objects can become lodged in the small intestine. The clinical signs will vary, depending on whether a complete or partial obstruction is present. Partial obstructions may occur because of trauma to the small intestine, which results in adhesions and stenosis, neoplasia, and intussusception, or because of the presence of soft foreign bodies. The more complete the obstruction and the more proximal in the intestinal tract the foreign body is located, the more serious and urgent is the need for surgery. Some animals may be presented with a one-day history of anorexia and vomiting, while others may have a his-

*Renografin–76, E. R. Squibb & Sons, Inc., Princeton, NJ.

tory of illness extending over several weeks.

Many foreign bodies can be diagnosed during the physical examination by carefully and thoroughly palpating the abdomen. The diagnosis is usually confirmed by plain abdominal radiographs, which may suggest a radiolucent foreign body with varying degrees of ileus. At times, especially with a partial obstruction, a positive-contrast series may be required. Care should be exercised with positive-contrast material; if perforation is suspected, a water-soluble contrast agent should be used instead of barium. After the diagnosis of a foreign body has been made, the state of the patient and the nature of the obstruction dictate how soon the surgery should be performed. A complete obstruction high in the intestinal tract warrants surgery as soon as the patient is stable (Fig. 8–10).

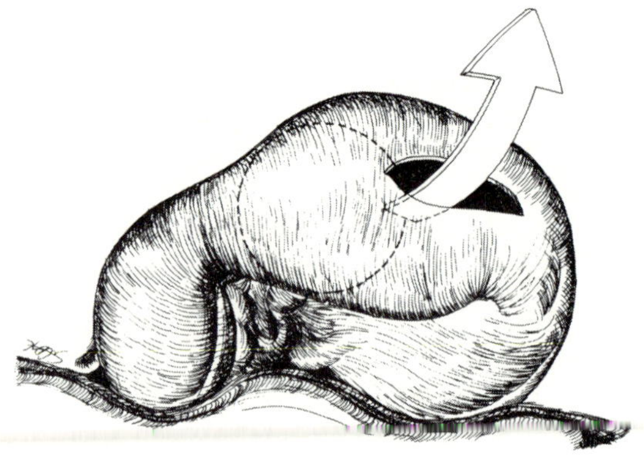

Figure 8–11. A longitudinal enterotomy is performed in the intestine distal to the obstruction. *Arrow* indicates direction in which the foreign body is "milked" through the incision. (Reprinted with permission from Krahwinkel DJ Jr, Richardson DC: Surgery of small intestine. *In* Bojrab MJ (ed): *Current Techniques in Small Animal Surgery.* 2nd ed. Philadelphia, Lea & Febiger, 1983.)

The surgical procedure chosen depends upon many factors. A thorough laparotomy should always be performed. Small foreign bodies can be removed through a single enterotomy. This enterotomy should be aboral to the foreign body in healthy tissue to decrease the possibility of postoperative complications due to a dehiscence at the enterotomy site (Fig. 8–11).[43] As previously described, this enterotomy is sutured with 2/0 or 3/0 synthetic absorbable material in a simple crushing pattern (Fig. 8–12).

Large foreign bodies may require resection and anastomosis, especially if the tissues are becoming dark and friable. When possible, the foreign body should first be removed through an aboral enterotomy, which should then be sutured. The involved segment of intestine should be wrapped in a warm, saline-moistened sponge for approximately 5 minutes. Often the vascularization will improve in this segment, and a complete resection will not be required. If the color and motility do not return, the involved segment should be resected back to normal tissue, as previously discussed.

Postoperative care should include both oral and systemic antibiotics. Maintenance fluid therapy should continue until the patient is eating again. With a very debilitated patient, serial postoperative blood counts and blood gas and electrolyte determinations should be done. The heart should be carefully monitored for the first 24 to 48 hours following surgery, as cardiac arrhythmias are not uncommon, especially in the giant breeds, following severe obstruction. These arrhythmias are generally ventricu-

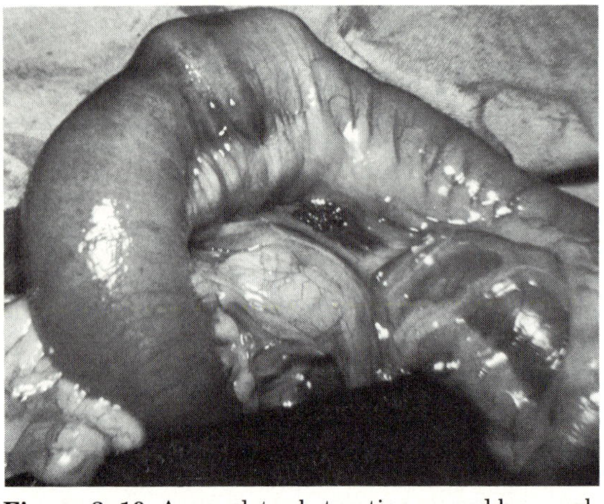

Figure 8–10. A complete obstruction caused by a cork.

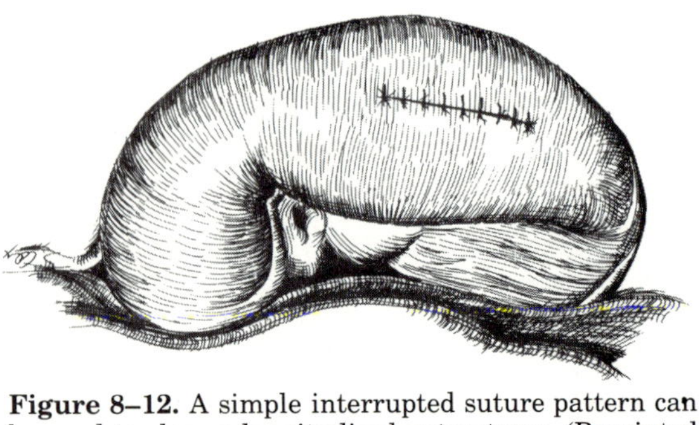

Figure 8–12. A simple interrupted suture pattern can be used to close a longitudinal enterotomy. (Reprinted with permission from Krahwinkel DJ Jr, Richardson DC: Surgery of small intestine. *In* Bojrab MJ (ed): *Current Techniques in Small Animal Surgery.* 2nd ed. Philadelphia, Lea & Febiger, 1983.)

lar in origin and, thus, are classified as either serious or potentially lethal. The most probable cause of ventricular arrhythmias is myocardial ischemia and hypoxia, as a consequence of shock from the electrolyte loss due to the location of the obstruction.[22]

TRAUMA

Signs of intra-abdominal injuries are largely non-specific and often subtle. Since such injuries are usually the result of violent trauma in which multiple system injury is common, it is important to search for intra-abdominal injury when signs compatible with their pathophysiological effects are seen.

The most common signs of abdominal injury are those related to hemorrhage. Depression, shock, diffuse abdominal tenderness, and accumulation of fluid in the abdomen are seen. In the case of intestinal rupture, septic peritonitis develops within 6 to 24 hours, resulting in pyrexia, anorexia, depression, emesis, abdominal tenderness, ileus, intraperitoneal fluid accumulation, and hypotension.[20] The small intestine may be involved in the initial trauma, e.g., rupture at the time of injury, or it may begin to fail several days following injury.[39]

Diagnostic aids to be used include careful physical examination, which should consist of careful, gentle palpation of all regions of the abdomen. Rectal palpation should be done to detect lacerations of the rectum and blood in feces. The abdomen should be ausculated at intervals, because the persistent absence of normal intestinal sounds is considered a reliable sign of intraperitoneal injury.[20]

Radiography of the abdomen is useful in establishing a diagnosis. Both plain films and positive-contrast gastrointestinal studies will provide evidence of rupture of the bowel. If perforation of the small or large bowel is suspected, a suitable water-soluble contrast material should be used.

Exploratory celiotomy is the most direct and expeditious means of confirming the presence of an intra-abdominal injury. In cases in which signs of intra-abdominal injury are present but such injury cannot be confirmed by other means, exploration is warranted.

Abdominocentesis is an extremely accurate means of diagnosing intra-abdominal injury such as rupture of a bowel or any hollow viscus.[7,21] Two techniques of paracentesis are the four-quadrant method, which uses an 18 gauge, 1½ inch needle on a syringe,[32] and paracentesis utilizing a polyethylene peritoneal dialysis catheter*.

The technique of diagnostic paracentesis and lavage in dogs, using a peritoneal dialysis catheter, is similar to the technique used in humans.[31,45] The dog is placed in lateral recumbency, the urinary bladder is emptied, and the area around the umbilicus is prepared as for surgery. Aseptic technique is used throughout the procedure. The skin is draped, and local anesthetic is infiltrated into the skin 1 cm caudal to the umbilicus. Additional anesthetic is infiltrated down to the peritoneum. A small stab incision is made through the skin to the fascia of the transverse abdominal muscle. The catheter and stylet unit is grasped near its tip so that the stylet will not be thrust too deeply into the abdominal cavity. After the peritoneum is penetrated, the stylet is withdrawn and the catheter is carefully advanced in a dorsocaudal direction so that the spleen, pancreas, and liver are not likely to be injured. If fluid flows from the catheter, a sample is obtained and the catheter is withdrawn. If fluid is not obtained, the dog is carefully rolled to its other side or the catheter is repositioned. If fluid again is not obtained, lavage is performed by introducing physiological saline solution into the abdominal cavity at a rate of 20 ml/kg of body weight. At the end of the infusion, the dog's abdomen is massaged to mix the fluid. It is not necessary to collect all the lavage fluid infused; only a representative sample is needed. The catheter is withdrawn, and a suture is used to close the stab incision. Aliquots of the collected fluid are analyzed cytologically and biochemically.[21]

A comparison of the catheter technique with that of the needle shows that there is greater accuracy in diagnosing abdominal trauma when the catheter is used. The catheter has also proved to be more efficient in recovering fluid when paracentesis is used with abdominal lavage. The catheter can recover a volume of fluid (1.0 to 4.0 ml of fluid/kg of body weight) sufficient for a number of cytological and biochemical tests, whereas the needle has been shown, at times, to be ineffective in recovering fluid, even when large volumes are present.[21]

---

*Trocath, McGraw Laboratories, Division of American Hospital Supply Company, Glendale, CA.

In evaluating the results of lavage, a syringe with dark printing on its barrel is placed under the connective tubing that has been filled with returning fluid. Results are interpreted on the basis of the degree of turbidity of the fluid. If the printing on the syringe barrel can be read through the tubing, regardless of the fluid color, results are considered negative, indicating the lack of serious injury. If the fluid is opaque, so that the printing on the syringe cannot be read, results are considered positive, indicating serious hemorrhage, peritonitis, or soilage from visceral contents.[7]

The catheter technique is very safe; however, serious complications may arise if the catheter and trocar are used improperly, causing laceration of the small bowel. The only inadequacy of the procedure reported is its inability to detect isolated retroperitoneal injuries.[32, 45]

Injuries to the intestine include: contusions, intramural and mesenteric hematomas, mucosal and serosal tears, avulsions of the mesentery, ruptures, and punctures. The most important consequence of intestinal injuries is leakage of contents into the peritoneal space with resulting peritonitis.[20] A wound to the intestine is debrided and sutured as an enterotomy or an anastomosis. The peritoneal cavity is then lavaged.

Laceration or avulsion of the mesentery is seen with blunt or penetrating trauma. Avulsion of the mesentery is most likely to occur at points of attachment, e.g., at the root mesentery or distally where the mesentery attaches to the bowel.[20] Consequences of mesenteric trauma include: ischemia of a segment of bowel, and strangulation of a loop of bowel that is incarcerated through a rent in the mesentery. Treatment of mesenteric injuries involves resection of the affected portion of bowel and anastomosis.

INTUSSUSCEPTION

Intussusception is most commonly seen in the dog but does occur in the cat. It primarily occurs in young animals.

The cause of intussusception is intestinal irritation. This irritation may be from several causes, such as canine distemper virus and intestinal parasites. In general, it occurs most often in the area of the ileocecal valve (Fig. 8–13*A* to *C*).[6]

The cardinal signs of intussusception are pain, vomiting, passage of mucus and blood in the stool, and the presence of a palpable, cylindrical mass, usually in the right sublumbar region. During palpation of the abdomen, it is advisable to raise the animal's forequarters, in order to slide the ileocecal area caudally from behind the ribs. Diagnosis is confirmed with abdominal radiographs. Results of plain film radiography depend on whether the intussusception is causing a complete or an incomplete obstruction. If the obstruction is complete, dilated gas and fluid-filled loops of bowel are seen proximal to the intussusception. The colon will be empty. If the obstruction is incomplete there is little, if any, distention of the bowel and feces are usually present in the colon. Occasionally, the mass of the intussusception is dense enough to be visible radiographically.[18]

Probably the most satisfactory method of demonstrating an intussusception is the barium enema. The reasons the barium enema is favored over the barium swallow are that the time taken to demonstrate the intussusception is much shorter with an enema, and the oral administration of barium may cause emesis.[18]

When an intussusception is diagnosed, surgery is indicated. Being able to manually reduce an intussusception depends on its duration. One hand is used to hold the ensheathing layer (intussuscipiens) while the other hand pushes the apex of the invaginating layer (intussusceptum) proximally and exerts gentle traction on the intestine proximal to the intussusception. After manual reduction of the intussusception, the intestine and mesentery should be carefully checked for viability. If the involved segment is non-viable, then that segment should be resected, and the remaining ends anastomosed.

In intussusceptions of longer duration, manual reduction may be impossible. Adhesions often develop as a result of congestion and production of a fibrinous exudate from the serosal surfaces.[25] With time, the circulatory embarrassment causes an ischemic necrosis, often with a localized peritonitis. In chronic cases, in which manual reduction is impossible because of adhesions and congestion, or if the segment of intestine is no longer viable, resection and anastomosis are necessary.

The greatest postoperative surgical complication, barring peritonitis, is the recurrence of the intussusception because of a localized irritation. This may occur whether

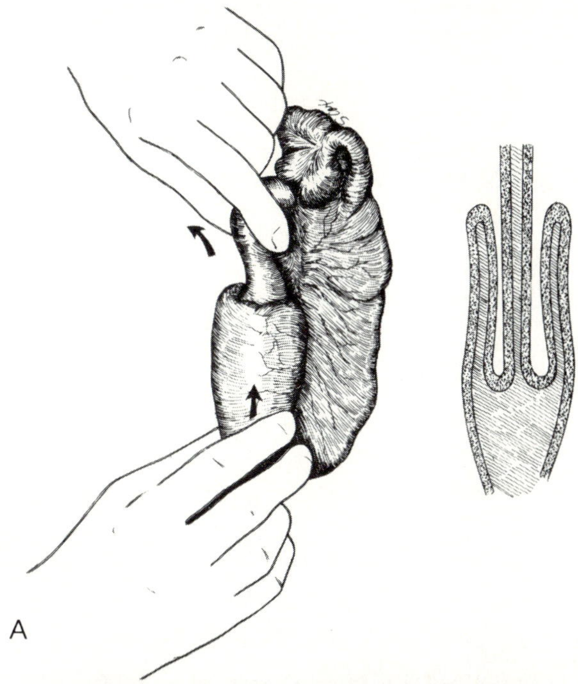

Figure 8–13. *A,* An intussusception is reduced by applying gentle pressure on the invaginated end while simultaneously "milking" the opposite end. *B,* Actual intussusception found on celiotomy. *C,* Reduction of intussusception by technique shown in *A*. (*A* Reprinted with permission from Krahwinkel DJ Jr, Richardson DC: Surgery of small intestine. *In* Bojrab MJ (ed): *Current Techniques in Small Animal Surgery*. 2d ed. Philadelphia, Lea & Febiger, 1983.)

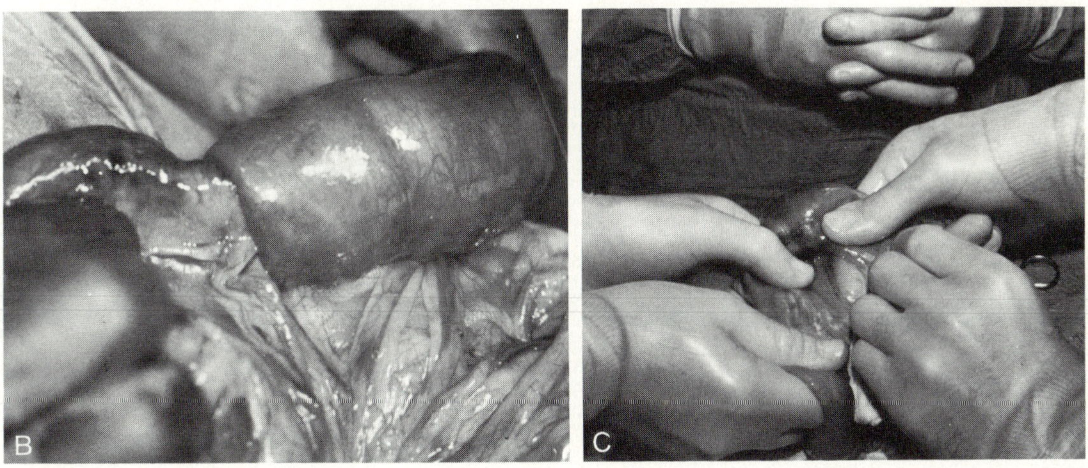

manual reduction or resection was performed.

If the intussusception recurs, it may be helpful to double the intestine upon itself so that the portion causing the problem lies at the turn of a U-shaped segment. The serosa of the segments proximal and distal to the site of the intussusception is sutured together at the antimesenteric border with absorbable suture material. Three loops of plicated bowel should be used proximal and distal to the intussusception (Fig. 8–14).[11] This procedure will help decrease the chances of recurrence.

It is important to determine the cause of the intussusception. If it is due to hypermotility secondary to parasite-induced enteritis, the appropriate anthelmintic should be administered.

VOLVULUS

Volvulus is the rotation of the intestine about its mesenteric axis, with the degree of rotation dictating the amount of circulatory embarrassment. The duodenum is seldom involved in this problem, as its position is relatively fixed. The jejunum and ileum, however, because of their long mesenteric attachments, are more likely to rotate.

This condition is rare in the dog and cat. The signs, those of an acute obstruction,

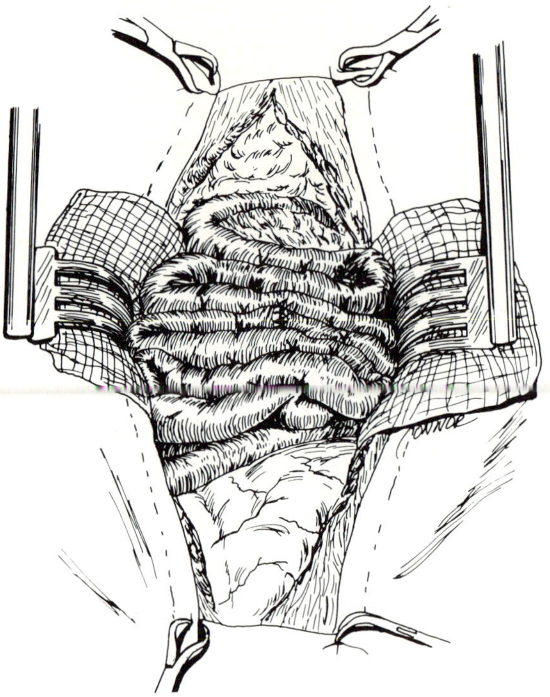

Figure 8–14. Bowel plication after resection of anastomosis to prevent recurrent intussusception. (Reprinted with permission from Engen MH: Bowel plication for preventing recurrent intussusception. *In* Bojrab MJ (ed): *Current Techniques in Small Animal Surgery*. 2nd ed. Philadelphia, Lea & Febiger, 1983.)

include anorexia, vomiting, and passing of bloody, mucoid stools. The problem demands early surgical intervention. The affected portion of gut shows signs of circulatory embarrassment; the severity of the lesion is directly related to the amount of intestinal rotation and the subsequent ischemia. Surgical treatment of this problem involves derotation of the affected portion of gut and ascertaining the viability of the intestine. If the intestine appears necrotic or devitalized, resection and anastomosis should be performed.

Prognosis depends on the length of time the volvulus is present, the amount of bowel involved, and the physical status of the patient. If diagnosis and surgical intervention are prompt and a small percentage of the small intestine is involved, the prognosis is favorable.

STRANGULATION

Strangulation refers to the constriction of a portion of bowel when it slips through an opening in the mesentery, omentum, or abdominal wall and subsequent obstruction. As with any acute obstruction, early surgical intervention is advisable. The rent, whether in the abdominal wall, omentum, or mesentery, should be repaired. If the small intestine is obviously non-viable, the involved section should be resected and the ends anastomosed.

NEOPLASIA

Lymphosarcomas and adenocarcinomas are the most common gastrointestinal tumors of dogs and cats.[5,26,36,37] Less commonly encountered neoplasms include leiomyoma, mastocytoma, leiomyosarcoma, fibrosarcoma, and carcinoid tumors.[38] Gastrointestinal neoplasia usually develops in a slow, insidious manner with only vague clinical signs. Anorexia and weight loss may be the only early signs, but often diarrhea, vomiting, dehydration, and anemia may result.

Intestinal lymphosarcoma (LSA) occurs as two different morphological forms, diffuse and nodular, to which any age animal is susceptible. In diffuse LSA, extensive infiltration of the lamina propria and submucosa with neoplastic lymphocytes may cause malabsorption, steatorrhea, diarrhea, and weight loss. In nodular LSA, a segmental thickening of the bowel, most often in the ileocecocolic area, may cause lumen narrowing and partial obstruction. Metastasis to regional lymph nodes is common with both forms of intestinal lymphosarcoma.

Adenocarcinomas affect older animals and may cause bowel obstruction in either of two ways. There may be a segmental thickening within the bowel wall with the effect of an expanding mass, or the tumor may grow inward toward the lumen, producing an annular, fibrous constricting band with little outward enlargement (Fig. 8–15).

The tentative diagnosis of intestinal neoplasia can be made from the history, clinical signs, plain films and contrast radiography, and abdominal palpation. Nodular LSA, outwardly expanding adenocarcinomas, and most of the less common tumors can be palpated as firm, irregular abdominal masses. Diffuse LSA palpates as a thickened gut loop, whereas the stricture type of adenocarcinoma may not be palpable. Definitive diagnosis can be made by obtaining a biopsy specimen during surgery. The prognoses for LSA and adenocarcinoma are poor because

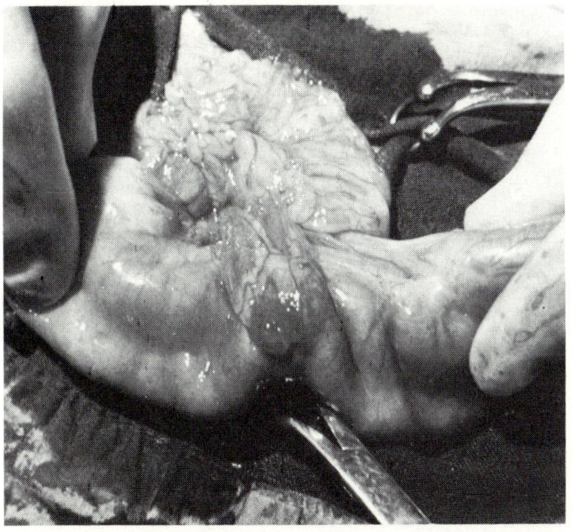

Figure 8–15. Adenocarcinoma as it appeared on the intestine.

the surgical margins and the regional lymph nodes are usually invaded. Chemotherapy is available for some cases of lymphosarcoma.[34] Whenever neoplasia is suspected, the chest should also be radiographed for evidence of metastasis.

Surgery involving the small intestine is used in treating several lesions, including trauma, obstruction, and neoplasia. Regardless of the type of lesion, careful, thorough, aseptic, and atraumatic surgery should always be performed. When a few rigid guidelines are followed, few complications should be encountered in the preoperative, operative, or postoperative periods. Knowing the pathophysiology of this dynamic organ will enable the surgeon to anticipate complications before they become life-threatening and to compensate for or correct them either preoperatively or when they are encountered.

References

1. Abramowitz HB, McAlister WH: A comparative study of small bowel anastomoses by angiography and microangiography. Surgery 66:654, 1969.
2. Anderson NV: Disorders of the small intestine. *In* Ettinger SJ (ed): *Textbook of Veterinary Internal Medicine.* W. B. Saunders Company, Philadelphia, 1150, 1975.
3. Bennett RR, Zydeck FA: A comparison of single layer suture patterns for intestinal anastomosis. J Am Vet Med Assoc 157:2075, 1970.
4. Botsford TW, Wilson RE: *The Acute Abdomen: An Approach to Diagnosis and Management.* W. B. Saunders Company, Philadelphia, 1977.
5. Brodey RS: Alimentary tract neoplasms of the cat. A clinicopathological survey of 46 cases. Am J Vet Res 27:74, 1966.
6. Butler HC: Survey of the small intestine and colon. Vet Clin of North Am 1:60, 1972.
7. Crowe DT, and Crane SW: Diagnostic abdominal paracentesis and lavage in the evaluation of abdominal injuries in dogs and cats: Clinical and experimental investigations. J Am Vet Med Assoc 168:700–705, 1976.
8. Deveney KE, Way LW: Effect of different absorbable sutures on healing of gastrointestinal anastomoses. Am J Surg 73:86, 1977.

8a. Dorland's Illustrated Medical Dictionary, 25th ed. W. B. Saunders Company, Philadelphia, 1974.

9. Diego MD, deMiguel E, Lucea CM et al: Short gut syndrome: A new surgical technique and ultrastructural study of the liver and pancreas. Arch Surg 117:789, 1982.
10. Ellison GW: End to end anastomosis in the dog: A comparison of techniques. Comp Cont Ed 3:486, 1981.
11. Engen MH: Bowel plication for preventing recurrent intussusception. *In* Bojrab MJ (ed): *Current Techniques in Small Animal Surgery,* 2nd ed. Lea & Febiger, Philadelphia, 183, 1983.
12. Evans HE, deLahunta A: *Miller's Guide to the Dissection of the Dog,* 2nd ed. W. B. Saunders Company, Philadelphia, 1971.
13. Frier PA: A simplified method of intestinal anastomosis. Mod Vet Pract 47:71, 1966.
14. Grier RL: Techniques for intestinal anastomosis. *In* Bojrab MJ (ed): *Current Techniques in Small Animal Surgery,* 2nd ed. Lea & Febiger, Philadelphia, 119, 1975.
15. Grier RL: Evaluation of invagination techniques in small bowel anastomosis in the dog. J Am Vet Med Assoc 153:528, 1968.
16. Hanna EA: Efficiency of peritoneal drainage. Surg Gynecol Obstet 131:983, 1970.
17. Hoffer RE: The peritoneum. *In* Bojrab MJ (ed): *Current Techniques in Small Animal Surgery,* 2nd ed. Lea & Febiger, Philadelphia, 165, 1975.
18. Kealy JK: Gastrointestinal tract. In: *Diagnostic Radiology of the Dog and Cat.* W. B. Saunders Company, Philadelphia, 1979.
19. Knecht CD, Allen AR, Williams DJ, Johnson JH: *Fundamental Techniques in Veterinary Surgery,* 2nd ed. W. B. Saunders Company, Philadelphia, 1981.
20. Kolata RJ: Diagnostic abdominal paracentesis and lavage: Experimental and clinical evaluation in the dog. J Am Vet Med Assoc 168:697, 1976.
21. Kolata RJ: Burrows CF, Soma LR: Shock: Pathophysiology and management. *In* Kirk RW (ed): *Current Veterinary Therapy VII.* 32, 1980.
22. Kolata RJ: Abdominal trauma. Comp Cont Ed 1:445, 1979.
23. Krahwinkel DJ Jr, Richardson DC: Surgery of small intestine. *In* Bojrab MJ (ed): *Current Techniques in Small Animal Surgery,* 2nd ed. Lea & Febiger, Philadelphia, 162, 1983.
24. Larsen LH, Bellenger CR: End to end intestinal anastomosis. *In* Archibald J (ed): *Canine Surgery,* 2nd ed. American Veterinary Publications, Inc., Santa Barbara, p. 555, 1974.
25. Larsen LH, Bellenger CR: Stomach and small intestines. *In* Archibald J (ed): *Canine Surgery,* 2nd ed. American Veterinary Publications, Inc., Santa Barbara, p. 555, 1974.

26. Lineniann CH, Garner FM: Comparative study of intestinal adenocarcinomas of animals and man. J Nat Cancer Inst 48:325, 1972.
27. MacCoy DM: *In* Kirk RW (ed): *Current Veterinary Therapy VI*. W. B. Saunders Company, Philadelphia, p. 52, 1977.
28. Meenes W, Green JA, Weller JM: Peritoneal clearance of urea and potassium and protein removal during acute peritonitis in dogs. J Lab Clin Med 76:903, 1970.
29. Miller ME, Christensen GC, Evans HE: *Anatomy of the Dog*. W. B. Saunders Company, Philadelphia, 1964.
30. Neal TM: Crushing technique for closure of incisions and resections in the small intestine. *In* Bojrab MJ (ed): *Current Techniques in Small Animal Surgery*, 2nd ed. Lea & Febiger, Philadelphia, 125, 1975.
31. Olsen WR, Heldreth DH: Abdominal paracentesis and peritoneal lavage in blunt abdominal trauma. J Trauma 11:824, 1971.
32. Osborne CA, Perman V, Low DG: Clinical and laboratory evaluation of abdominal body fluid accumulation. Part I. Techniques of paracentesis. Proc 40th Ann Meet, Anim Hosp Assoc 610, 1973.
33. Ott BS, Doyle MD, Greenawald KA: Single layer everted intestinal anastomosis. J Am Vet Med Assoc 153:142, 1968.
34. Owen LN: Cancer chemotherapy and immunotherapy. *In* Ettinger SJ (ed): *Textbook of Veterinary Internal Medicine,* 2nd ed. W. B. Saunders Company, Philadelphia, 368, 1981.
35. Parks J, Gahring D, Greene RW: Peritoneal lavage for peritonitis and pancreatitis in twenty-two dogs. J Am Anim Hosp Assoc 9:442, 1973.
36. Patnaik AK, Hurvitz AI, Johnson GF: Canine intestinal adenocarcinoma and carcinoid. Vet Pathol 17:149, 1980.
37. Patnaik AK, Hurvitz AI, Johnson GF: Canine gastrointestinal neoplasms. Vet Pathol 14:547, 1977.
38. Patnaik AK, Liu SK, Johnson GF: Feline intestinal adenocarcinoma. A clinicopathologic study of twenty-two cases. Vet Pathol 13:1, 1976.
39. Perry JF Jr: Blunt and penetrating abdominal injuries. Curr Probl Surg 8:1, 1970.
40. Postlethwait RW: Principles of operative surgery: Antisepsis, technique, sutures, and drains. *In* Sabiston DC Jr (ed): W. B. Saunders Company, Philadelphia, 300, 1972.
41. Ravitch MM, Canalis F, Weinshelbaum A et al.: Study in intestinal healing. 3. Observations on everting intestinal anastomoses. Ann Surg 166: 670, 1967.
42. Renegar WR: The use of sump-Penrose drains for intraperitoneal drainage. Review and case report. Missouri Vet 29:6, 1979.
43. Richardson DC: Intestinal surgery: A review. Comp Cont Ed 3:259, 1981.
44. Ricotta J, Zuidema GD, Gadacz TR, Sadri D: Construction of an ileocecal valve and its role in massive resection of the small intestine. Surg Gynecol Obstet 152:310, 1981.
45. Root HE, Hausen DW, McKinley GR et al: Diagnostic peritoneal lavage. Surgery 57:633, 1965.
46. Stacchini A, DiDio LJ, Primo ML et al: Artificial sphincters as surgical treatment for experimental massive resection of small intestine. Am J Surg 143:721, 1982.
47. Thal ER, Shires GT: Peritoneal lavage in blunt abdominal trauma. Am J Surg 126:64, 1973.
48. Waterman NG, Watsky R, Kasdon ML, Abrams BL: The treatment of acute hemorrhagic pancreatitis by sump drainage. Surg Gynecol Obstet 126:963, 1968.
49. Wingfield WE: The stomach. *In* Bojrab MJ (ed): *Pathophysiology in Small Animal Surgery*. Lea & Febiger, Philadelphia, 1981.

CHAPTER

9

Medical Diseases of the Colon

COLIN F. BURROWS

The large intestine of higher mammals is an extremely versatile organ, functioning in the maintenance of fluid and electrolyte balance, as a potential site of nutrient absorption, as a temporary store for excreta, and as a major reservoir for billions of microorganisms. Disease can disrupt these complex and interrelated functions in a variety of ways, but in all species disruption is usually manifested as either diarrhea or constipation.

Anatomy of the Colon

Compared with the proximal portion of the mammalian gastrointestinal tract, the colon exhibits large interspecies variations in anatomy; these variations are believed to be at least partly related to diet.[28, 69, 88] Herbivores have a very large colon and cecum, omnivores a somewhat smaller colon and cecum, and carnivores a relatively small colon and a virtually vestigial cecum. The carnivore colon is occasionally referred to as a "simple" organ. This term is misleading, since the colon carries out a number of disparate and complex functions, which contribute to both fluid and electrolyte homeostasis and to the storage and regular elimination of excreta.[28]

As in all species, the large intestine of the dog or cat is divided into the cecum, colon, rectum, and anal canal, with the colon and anorectum forming a continuous tube (Fig. 9–1). However, unlike herbivores and omnivores, these two species have small cecums with no known specific functions. The cecum forms a diverticulum from the proximal portion of the colon, with distinct cecocolic and ileocolic junctions or sphincters. The colon has traditionally been divided into ascending, transverse, and descending segments. Although anatomically appropriate, these terms fail to correlate with the regionalized functions of the organ, and division into proximal, intermediate, and distal segments has been proposed as more logical, since the terms are applicable to different species.[37] However, in both the dog and cat the proximal colon correlates neither anatomically nor functionally with the ascending colon of other species, and in this context these two species can be considered to have little or no proximal colon.[28] From an anatomical and clinical viewpoint, therefore, the traditional classification is perhaps more appropriate, inasmuch as it provides readily identifiable landmarks, which facilitate the localization of disease processes.

The ascending colon is short, about 3 to 8 cm in the dog and 1 to 2 cm in the cat. It begins at the ileocolic sphincter and runs cranially, adjacent to the right limb of the pancreas, and terminates at the right-angled right colic or hepatic flexure. The transverse colon is longer, about 5 to 8 cm in the dog and 2 to 4 cm in the cat. It runs across the dorsal, cranial abdomen, in contact with the left limb of the pancreas, and terminates at the left colic or splenic flexure. The descending colon is the longest segment, varying in length with the size of the animal. It begins at the left colic flexure and runs caudally, usually following the curvature of the left abdominal wall and terminates at the rectum. The organ forms the shape of a question mark, with some dogs having a

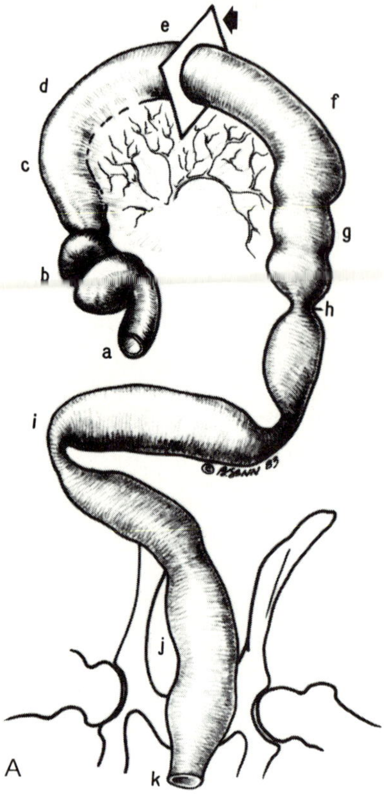

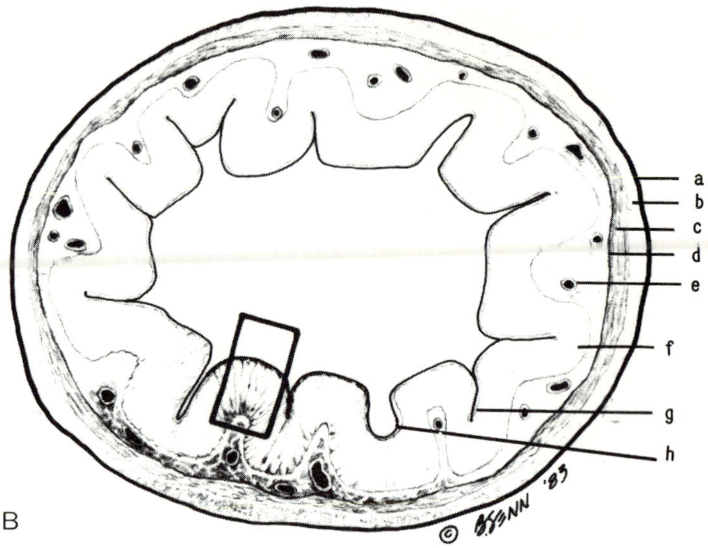

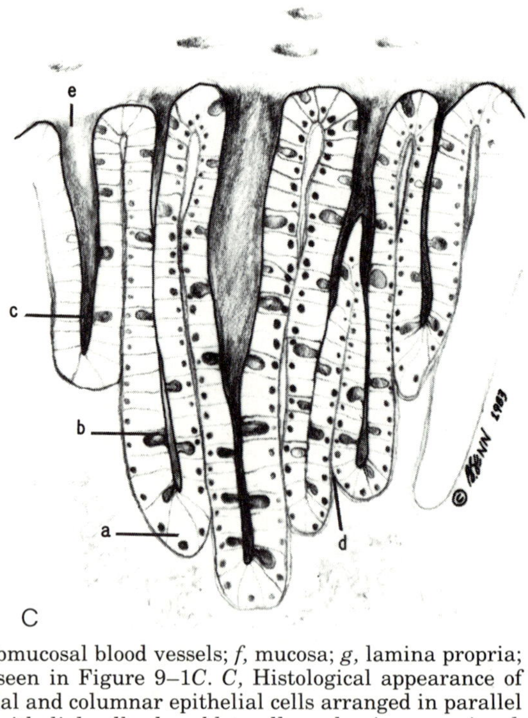

Figure 9–1. *A,* Anatomy of the canine colon. The colon is divided into three parts: ascending, transverse, and descending. The ascending colon is short; beginning at the ileocolic sphincter and running cranially to terminate at the right-angled right colic flexure. (The cecum is a small, distinct diverticulum distal to the ileocolic sphincter.) The transverse colon runs across the dorsal cranial abdomen and terminates at the left colic or splenic flexure. The descending colon, which is the longest segment, begins at the left colic flexure and runs caudally to terminate at the rectum. Some dogs, as depicted here, have a distinct flexure of the distal colon, which is analogous to the sigmoid flexure of the human colon. *a,* terminal ileum; *b,* cecum; *c,* ascending colon; *d,* hepatic flexure; *e,* transverse colon; *f,* splenic flexure; *g,* descending colon; *h,* segmental contraction; *i,* sigmoid (distal) flexure; *j,* rectum; *k,* anal canal; Plane (arrow). *B,* Cross-section of the transverse colon. *a,* serosa; *b,* longitudinal muscle; *c,* circular muscle; *d,* submucosa; *e,* submucosal blood vessels; *f,* mucosa; *g,* lamina propria; *h,* longitudinal folds of mucosa; box: histological structures seen in Figure 9–1*C*. *C,* Histological appearance of colonic mucosa. The colon lacks villi and is composed of cuboidal and columnar epithelial cells arranged in parallel crypts. The crypts are richly supplied with goblet cells. *a,* epithelial cells; *b,* goblet cells; *c,* lamina propria; *d,* crypts; *e,* crypt opening.

distinct flexure of the distal part, rather like the sigmoid flexure of the human colon. The descending colon is continuous with the rectum which is generally considered to begin at the pelvic inlet.[66] The rectum runs through the pelvic canal and terminates in the anus and anal sphincter.

Histologically the colon and rectum are composed of four layers: the mucosa, submucosa, muscle layer, and serosa (Fig. 9–1*C*). The mucosa usually appears to be folded longitudinally when the organ is viewed in the contracted state, but circular folds are apparent if it is actively contracting. However, unlike those of the small intestine, most mucosal folds in the colon can be readily eliminated by stretching or distention. Colonic mucosa also has a more compact microstructure than the small-intestinal mucosa. It lacks villi and is composed of cuboidal and columnar epithelial cells arranged in perpendicular and parallel crypts; the organ is also richly supplied with goblet cells (Fig. 9–2). The submucosa is abundantly provided with nerves, blood vessels, and lymphoid nodules. Some submucosal nerves terminate in the mucosa. When viewed through an endoscope, the submucosal blood vessels appear as an interlacing network, and the ability to see them is an important criterion of normality. The muscle coat is composed of inner circular and outer longitudinal layers, and the colon is covered by a serosal coat, which is a reflection of the peritoneum; no part of the colon is retroperitoneal.

Physiology of the Colon

The colon has two major physiological functions: the absorption of electrolytes and water from the luminal contents and the storage and periodic expulsion of the resulting fecal material.[69, 82] Absorption of electrolytes and water occurs primarily in the ascending colon, transverse colon, and the proximal parts of the descending colon,[7, 72] whereas storage takes place in the distal part of the organ.[69]

ABSORPTION AND SECRETION

The colon is an important site of electrolyte and water absorption, but it is also capable of secretion. Absorption is important for fluid homeostasis in both normal animals and those with small intestinal diarrheal disease, in which the colon increases salt and water absorption to com-

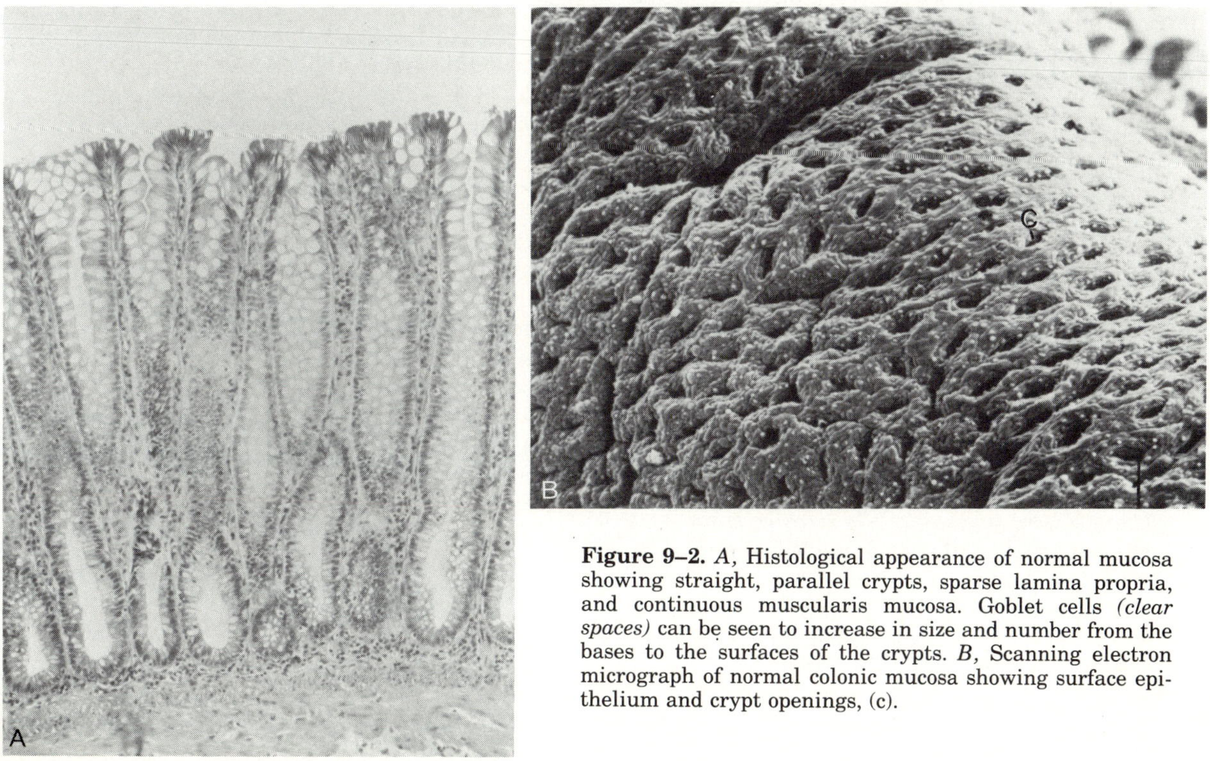

Figure 9–2. *A,* Histological appearance of normal mucosa showing straight, parallel crypts, sparse lamina propria, and continuous muscularis mucosa. Goblet cells *(clear spaces)* can be seen to increase in size and number from the bases to the surfaces of the crypts. *B,* Scanning electron micrograph of normal colonic mucosa showing surface epithelium and crypt openings, (c).

pensate for extra fluid delivered from the small intestine.[77] This ability to increase fluid absorption, termed "colonic absorptive reserve capacity," is an important concept in the pathophysiology of diarrheal disease.[17, 71]

Most salt and water absorption occurs in the proximal colon, since the distal colonic and rectal mucosae have much less efficient absorptive processes. No evidence exists to suggest that colonic water transport is other than a passive accompaniment to solute transfer.[69]

Colonic sodium absorption is primarily an active process, as evidenced by the high concentration of sodium-potassium ATPase in colonic mucosal tissue.[69] The colonic mucosal sodium pump is very effective and is capable of generating a transmucosal potential difference of about 40mV.[45] Absorption of sodium coupled with volatile fatty acids (primarily acetic acid) also occurs in the colon and accounts for some osmotic water absorption.[54] Both exogenous and endogenous glucocorticoids and mineralocorticoids have been shown to enhance colonic sodium absorption, particularly in states of water depletion or dehydration.[69] The colonic mucosa has tight epithelial junctions that prevent back-diffusion of sodium against a concentration gradient. This tight epithelial barrier is disrupted in inflammatory disease, with subsequent decreases in the transmucosal potential difference and absorptive capacity.[36, 74]

Colonic potassium absorption is believed to be passive, with partition along electrochemical gradients.[46] There is some evidence, however, that the colon regulates potassium transport by both absorptive and secretory mechanisms and that a carrier-mediated process probably regulates both methods of transport.[53] Chronic diarrhea frequently leads to hypokalemia, with the colon being the major source of potassium loss. Under these circumstances, potassium may be secreted into the lumen under the influence of aldosterone; desquamation of epithelial cells that contain high concentrations of potassium is probably also important. Colonic mucus is another important source of potassium loss, particularly in colitis.[69]

Colonic chloride absorption is an active process. In most species absorption is electrically neutral, chloride being exchanged one-for-one with bicarbonate, but there is evidence that the canine colon absorbs, rather than secretes, bicarbonate.[62] Bicarbonate may also be important in maintaining the pH at approximately 6.5 in the canine colon; however, other factors such as dietary composition and the bacterial flora also are important.[54, 69]

There is little evidence to suggest that secretion of electrolytes and water plays a major physiological role in the normal carnivore colon, but secretion does become important in a variety of diarrheal diseases. A diverse group of both exogenous and endogenous chemical and physical factors are now recognized as evoking colonic secretion.[70] In the dog and cat, dihydroxy bile acids and long-chain dietary fatty acids that pass into the colon in malabsorptive steatorrheal disease are the major secretogogues, but bacterial enterotoxins may also be important. Substances that cause colonic secretion can also increase colonic permeability, and bacteria as well as inert molecules may gain access to the mucosa when permeability is increased. There has been speculation that this increased permeability may be the cause of some of the as yet unexplained chronic inflammatory diseases of the colon.

VOLATILE FATTY ACIDS

In contrast to the situation in herbivore and omnivore colons, there is no evidence to suggest that microbial digestion of luminal contents in the dog and cat colon serves any nutritional function. However, the concentration of volatile fatty acids (i.e., acetic, propionic, butyric, and valeric acids) is high in the canine colon regardless of the nature of the diet,[9, 18, 54] and these compounds all facilitate the absorption of sodium.[54] Although the colon can absorb large quantities of volatile fatty acids, not all organic anions are absorbed, and those that are not form the major osmotic component of fecal water. Organic anions are particularly important in osmotic diarrhea, in which degradation by colonic bacteria of unabsorbed carbohydrate to osmotically active volatile fatty acids is thought to be the major reason for the increase in fecal water output.

THE BACTERIAL FLORA

The large intestine normally contains billions of organisms. Quantitative fecal analysis has revealed concentrations as high as 10^{14} bacteria per gram.[69] The majority of these bacteria are anaerobes, the importance of which was unrecognized until quite recently, when their precise cultural requirements were defined. There is such a nosological complexity of colonic flora that a biochemical classification of organisms based on their enzymic effects on luminal substrate may be more realistic than a classic microbiological taxonomy.[69] Diet appears to play a major role in defining the colonic flora of each individual, but the complex relationships between dietary composition and bacterial population remain to be elucidated.

Bacterial enzymes are important in both health and disease through their metabolism of both endogenous and dietary substrates and because of their ability to metabolize certain drugs. Long-chain, unsaturated fatty acids, for example, can be hydrated by fecal flora to form hydroxyfatty acids, which are more potent secretogogues than the parent unsaturated compounds.[5] Ricinoleic acid, the active ingredient of castor oil, is a potent colonic secretogogue that differs chemically from oleic acid (olive oil) by only a single hydroxyl group. Hydroxylation of unabsorbed fatty acids and their subsequent stimulation of colonic secretion to increase fecal water output is important in steatorrheal disease.[11] Similarly, cholic acid, a primary bile acid, is inert, but its bacterial dehydroxylation yields the potent secretogogue deoxycholic acid.[69] Bacterial enzymes also deconjugate bile acids, a process that increases their lipophilic properties and facilitates their reabsorption from the gut. Bacteria are also important in nitrogen metabolism. Generation of ammonia from urea by bacterial ureases and the colonic absorption of ammonia are normally of no clinical importance; however, ammonia is implicated in the clinical syndrome of hepatic encephalopathy. Bacterial enzymes also play a role in the metabolism of a number of drugs, most important of which is probably sulfasalazine,* a drug used in the treatment of colitis. The azo bond in this drug can be split by a variety of colonic bacteria to form 5-amino-salicylate and sulfapyridine.[47]

There have been no studies of colonic bacterial flora in diarrheal disease in either the dog or cat, but it is probable that changes in the bacterial population could play an important role in the clinical manifestations of diarrhea.

*Azulfidine, Pharmacia Laboratories, Piscataway, NJ.

COLONIC MOTILITY AND THE MOVEMENT OF INTRALUMINAL CONTENTS

The second major function of the colon is the regulation of the orderly distal movement of luminal contents in order to maximize the absorptive process, store the resulting fecal residue, and ensure its regular elimination. Distal movement and regular elimination of luminal contents are achieved by organized and complex patterns of colonic smooth muscle contractile activity.

All segments of the intestinal tract can store or at least delay the passage of luminal contents so as to maximize nutrient digestion and absorption. Whereas passage through the proximal gastrointestinal tract is measured in hours, transit through the canine colon can take as long as 1 to 3 days. In the normal dog the first portion of a meal reaches the proximal colon within 5 hours of ingestion, but it can be 48 hours more before the residue is excreted.[8, 19, 20] This delay in excretion is one of the major functions of colonic smooth muscle, and is aimed at facilitating salt and water absorption, particularly in the proximal part of the organ. Therefore, although initially considered a paradox, it is perhaps not surprising that colonic smooth muscle is much more active in constipation than in diarrhea.[30]

Unlike the stomach and small intestine, which share a similar structure and function in all mammals, the colon exhibits remarkable interspecies differences, which have so far precluded the development of any overall concept of colonic motor function. While the contractile processes of the canine and feline colon are now beginning to receive more attention, it has become apparent that although basic functions are similar, there are a number of distinct species differences in contractile activity. Retrograde peristalsis (ring contractions moving cephalad), for example, acts to impair the distal movement of luminal contents and appears to be the dominant motor activity of the proximal colon of the cat, but it does not occur in the dog.[18, 37] In contrast, segmentation (co-ordinated circular contractions that may be either stationary or progress over short distances in either direction) appears to be the dominant motor activity of the intermediate colon in both species. Segmental contractions are generally thought to mix luminal contents and facilitate absorption. The distal colon functions as a fecal reservoir, and in both species the dominant motor activity appears to be caudad moving, strong rings of contraction or "mass movements."

Most information about colonic motility in the conscious animal has been obtained from the concurrent monitoring of electrical and contractile activities of colonic smooth muscle.[15, 18, 44, 106] The electrical activity of gastrointestinal smooth muscle is characterized by a continuous oscillation of the resting membrane potential of individual muscle cells, a process called a slow wave or a basic electrical rhythm. The slow wave of a number of smooth muscle cells in a localized area of the gut wall can be measured by the application of an electrode to the serosal surface.[13] When the membrane oscillation becomes great enough or the voltage of the resting membrane potential is stimulated to reach threshold through a variety of nervous, hormonal, or other factors, the cell depolarizes completely. Depolarization is signaled electrically by action, or spike potentials, which are associated with muscular contraction.[13] The organization of slow waves and their associated spike potentials provides orientation for the direction of contractile activity and the subsequent movement of luminal contents. In both the feline and canine colon, spike potentials occur in two distinct forms. In the first form, spike potentials are phase-locked to individual slow waves, which occur at a frequency of about 5 cycles per minute (cpm). The function of associated contractile activity seems to be antiperistalsis or segmentation. The second form is unique to the colon and is composed of bursts of spike potentials that are completely unrelated to slow waves and that last from 30 seconds to more than 1 minute.[18] Individual bursts appear in groups, which in turn last from 5 minutes to more than 30 minutes. Since the bursts are propagated distally with a corresponding movement of luminal contents, they have been called migrating spike bursts.[18, 27] Migrating spike bursts appear to be composed of phasic contractions that arise from the circular muscle at a frequency of about 5 cpm. These contractions are superimposed on tonic contractions of the longitudinal muscle, which occur at a frequency of about 0.5 to 1 cpm (Fig. 9–3). This activity is cholinergically mediated, since it is inhibited by atropine,[26, 38] and is virtually abolished in colonic inflammatory disease, an observation that supports the concept of an overall decrease in motility in some diarrheal diseases.

Colonic motility is under extensive autonomic neural control, with innervation from both the parasympathetic and sympathetic nervous systems. Preganglionic parasympathetic fibers synapse in the myenteric plexus, and stimulation of colonic smooth

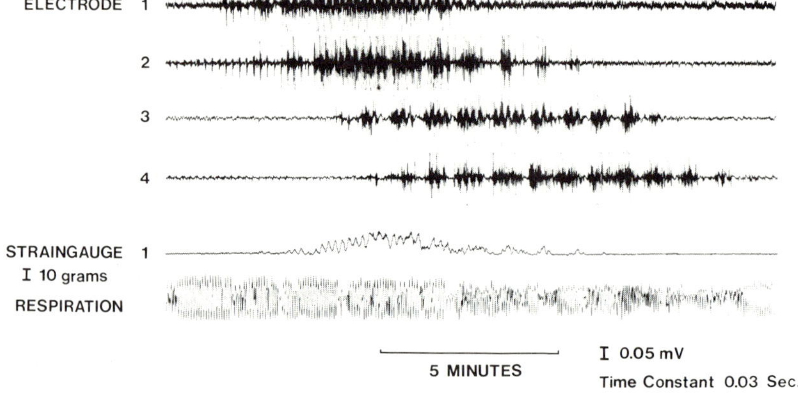

Figure 9–3. Myoelectrical and contractile activity of the canine colon recorded from four bipolar electrodes attached to the serosal surface of the transverse colon at 3-cm intervals. Contractile activity is recorded by means of a straingauge attached in the circular plane adjacent to electrode #2. The distally-moving pattern of electrical spiking on all four electrodes is called a migrating spike burst (MSB) and is associated with the aboral movement of luminal contents. Contractile activity measured by the straingauge correlates well with the intensity of spike activity. (Adapted from Burrows CF, Merritt AM: Influence of alpha-cellulose on myoelectrical activity of the proximal canine colon. Am J Physiol *245*:9301, 1983.)

muscle cells is caused by the release of acetylcholine from postganglionic parasympathetic nerves. The sympathetic nervous system innervates the colon through the thoracic, splanchnic, and lumbar colonic nerves. Adrenergic nerves inhibit colonic motility predominantly through beta-receptors. When the colonic nervous system is intact, the dominant neural response is inhibition. Neural modulation of colonic motility is important in modifying overall activity of the colon, but other factors such as gastrointestinal hormones and the nature of the luminal contents also play a role.

In humans, a marked increase in colonic motility occurs after a meal, a process that results mainly through the effect of the hormones cholecystokinin and gastrin on colonic smooth muscle.[84] Feline colonic smooth muscle is also sensitive to these hormones but no immediate postprandial increase in colonic motility can be detected in the dog.[26] Luminal factors also influence colonic motility, particularly the increase in fecal bulk, which follows ingestion of a relatively undigestible substance such as dietary fiber.[18] Fiber decreases overall colonic motility in the dog, especially the duration of migrating spike bursts, and fiber intake is correlated with an increase in speed of colonic transit (decreased transit time).[18, 20] The effect of fiber to decrease colonic motility supports the use of bulking agents in the treatment of both constipation and diseases associated with an increase in colonic contractile activity, such as the irritable colon syndrome. (See "Irritable Colon Syndrome.")

Colonic Disease: General Considerations

We know little of normal colonic function in the dog and cat and even less about colonic function in naturally occurring colonic disease of these two species. Much of what we know, or perhaps more correctly assume, is extrapolated from studies in humans, and may not be relevant to dogs and cats. It is known, however, that the absorption of water and electrolytes from the colon is markedly reduced when the organ is inflamed[7, 36, 74] and that colitis reduces aspects of colonic motility.[29, 30, 35, 60, 84]

The incidence of colonic disease in the dog is probably much higher than is generally appreciated. In the author's practice, approximately 50 per cent of dogs with chronic diarrhea have some form of colonic dysfunction, with idiopathic and whipworm-induced colitis being the most frequently diagnosed diseases.[21] Even though the author practices in a referral center and treats more dogs with chronic diarrhea than the typical small animal practitioner, the high percentage gives an indication of the incidence of colonic diarrheal disease, which is similar to that in humans.[73] The incidence of diseases that lead to constipation is unknown.

In the cat, colonic disease is uncommon and colitis is extremely rare. The reasons for this marked species difference are unclear, but there are several possible explanations. Whipworm infection, a major cause of colitis in the dog, is very rare in the cat; the absence of this infection could go a long way toward explaining the difference. The cat is also more fastidious in its selection of food and is less likely to suffer the toxic and traumatic sequelae of dietary indiscretion that occur so often in the dog. The character, use, housing, and temperament of cats also probably play roles. Cats generally lead a quieter, more independent, and less stressful life than dogs; moreover, cats are neither subjected to obedience training nor used for a variety of potentially stressful functions such as guard or police work. Exposure to stressful situations could be significant, since stress in its varied forms has been implicated as a major etiological factor in colonic disease in humans[3, 82] and to a lesser extent in the dog.[59]

PHYSICAL EXAMINATION

Like most of the gastrointestinal tract, the colon does not readily lend itself to physical examination, but it is more accessible than the more proximal regions of the gut. Abdominal palpation and rectal examination are the best methods of detecting deviations from normal. Abdominal palpation should be routine in any animal with signs of colonic disease, since it may suggest for example, the presence of an intraluminal foreign object, an ileocolic intussusception, colonic impaction, or abnormal thickening of the colonic wall. Most animals with colonic disease appear normal at physical examination; therefore, the clinician must rely primarily on the history and a variety of ancillary aids to make a specific diagnosis.

Rectal examination is extremely important in any animal in which signs suggest some type of large bowel disease, but examination of the perineum for inflammatory or neoplastic lesions should precede rectal examination. Tail carriage in some animals may suggest the nature of the underlying process. For example, a dog that carries its tail away from the perineum may have a painful perineal inflammatory or neoplastic disease.

After examination of the perineum, a lubricated, gloved finger should be gently inserted into the anal canal, and the anal sphincter should be examined for tone, strictures, and irregularities. The finger is then inserted further, and the rectum is examined for strictures, foreign material, rectal masses, any abnormality of the rectal wall, or any extraluminal lesion in the pelvic canal that may be related to the patient's signs. Fecal material obtained by rectal examination should be examined for color and appearance as well as for the presence of bones, foreign material, blood, or mucus. A sample of feces should be examined microscopically for parasites and stained for inflammatory cells using new methylene blue.

SIGNS OF COLONIC DISEASE

The several colonic diseases of the dog and cat have only a relatively small number of presenting signs. Although none are pathognomonic, two signs predominate, namely diarrhea and constipation (Table 9–1). These are frequently accompanied by other signs suggesting large bowel disease, such as tenesmus, dyschezia, and hematochezia.

Diarrhea

Diarrhea is one of the most frequent complaints in veterinary medicine and from a historical and diagnostic viewpoint is usually considered to originate in either the small or large bowel.[17] The location of the disease can usually be determined from the history.[17,19] The major differences between small and large bowel diarrhea are summarized in Table 9–2.

Diarrhea in colonic disease results from a decreased ability of the colon to absorb water and electrolytes from the bowel lumen coupled perhaps with some secretion of electrolytes and water.[10] In severe disease these two factors are also accompanied by exudation of blood and tissue fluid into the bowel lumen. The role that deranged motility plays in the pathogenesis of colonic diarrhea is unknown. Except for special cases such as hypermotility induced by the presence of hydroxyfatty acids or bile salts,[83,89] it is

Table 9–1. SIGNS OF COLONIC DISEASE AND ANORECTAL DISEASE IN THE DOG AND CAT

Sign	Comments
Diarrhea	Frequently but not invariably mucoid, less often bloody. The frequency of defecation is usually increased, and tenesmus may be present. The dog or cat may have "accidents" in the house, and defecation is often associated with a sense of urgency.
Constipation	Caused by a number of disorders that interfere with or prevent normal colonic function and defecation. If untreated, constipation may become intractable (obstipation). Secondary degenerative changes in colonic muscle are common.
Tenesmus	Tenesmus of alimentary tract origin must be differentiated from that associated with the urogenital tract. The relationship of tenesmus to defecation can be useful in diagnosis.
Vomiting	Occurs in about 30% of dogs with colitis. Vomiting does *not* necessarily indicate gastric or small intestinal involvement in the dog with chronic vomiting and diarrhea.
Dyschezia	Crying or whimpering during defecation is usually associated with a lesion or foreign body in the rectum or anus. The animal may not defecate if pain is severe. Lack of defecation can result in constipation.
Hematochezia	Fresh blood in the feces is a reliable sign of colonic or rectal disease.
Fecal incontinence	The inability to retain feces and defecate normally. It occurs most often after surgical trauma to the rectum or anus but may also occur as a complication of neurogenic disease.
Biting the perineal area	Biting the skin around the anus, tail chasing, or rubbing the perineum along the ground are reliable signs of anal irritation and are most frequently associated with anal sac disease.
Weight loss	A slowly progressive loss of weight may be seen in severe colonic disease. It results from either increased inflammatory protein loss in the feces or a decreased food intake.

Table 9–2. DIFFERENTIATION OF SMALL INTESTINAL DIARRHEA FROM LARGE INTESTINAL DIARRHEA IN THE DOG

Parameter	Small Intestinal Diarrhea	Large Intestinal Diarrhea
Feces		
Volume	Markedly increased	Normal or decreased
Mucus	Rarely present	Common
Melena	May be present	Absent
Hematochezia	Absent except in acute hemorrhagic diarrhea	Fairly common
Steatorrhea	Present with maldigestive or malabsorptive disease	Absent
Undigested food	May be present with maldigestion	Absent
Color	Color variations occur, e.g., creamy brown, green, orange, or clay-colored	Color variations rare; may be bloody
Defecation		
Urgency	Absent except in acute or very severe disease	Usually but not invariably present
Tenesmus	Absent	Frequent, but not invariably present
Frequency	2 to 3 times normal for the patient	Usually greater than 3 times normal
Dyschezia	Absent	Present with distal colonic or rectal disease.
Ancillary Signs		
Weight loss	May occur in maldigestive or malabsorptive disease	Rare except in severe colitis, diffuse tumors, or histoplasmosis
Vomiting	May be present in inflammatory diseases	Uncommon, but occurs in up to 25–30% of dogs with colitis
Flatulence and borborygmus	May be reported with maldigestion and malabsorption	Absent
Halitosis in the absence of oral disease	Present with maldigestion or malabsorption	Absent

generally agreed that colonic motility is decreased or absent in colitis.

The character of colonic diarrhea and the patterns of defecation vary, depending on the underlying disease, the location of the lesion, and its severity (Table 9–3). The classic description of colonic diarrhea is that it is of small volume, frequently mucoid, and bloody.[21, 79] Defecation is frequent and often associated with tenesmus and a sense of urgency; even a well-trained dog may defecate in the house or suddenly beg to be

Table 9–3. CHARACTERIZATION OF COLONIC DIARRHEA

Parameter	Comments
Frequency of defecation	Is usually increased to at least 2 or 3 times normal; some dogs may defecate as frequently as every 2 hours. Defecation is frequently associated with a sense of urgency; the animal may have accidents in the house.
Act of defecation	Is usually prolonged and associated with tenesmus. Many afflicted dogs will remain squatting for a considerable time period and will move around in this position, intermittently producing small quantities of fecal material.
Appearance of the feces	Varies from semi-formed to liquid. Mucus is frequently present and may be passed as such flecked with blood, or mixed with the feces. Fresh blood is a helpful diagnostic sign but is present in little more than half the afflicted animals. Frank dysentery is rare.
Microscopic examination	May reveal whipworm or hookworm eggs. New methylene blue–stained mucosal smears reveal inflammatory cells. Steatorrhea is absent.

let outside to defecate. While these signs are helpful in the diagnosis of colonic diarrhea it is important to realize that they are not present in all dogs with colitis, and that their absence by no means excludes colonic disease. Diarrhea does not even have to be continuous; in diseases associated with a primary disorder of colonic motility, for example, diarrhea may alternate with periods of normal defecation.

Constipation

Constipation is another prominent sign of colonic disease. Most clinicians interpret constipation as infrequent defecation, excessively hard or dry feces, increased straining to defecate, or a reduced fecal volume.[73] Many clients, however, equate constipation with tenesmus, a comparison that is not necessarily correct, since tenesmus may also be associated with disease of other systems.[105] Constipation must also be differentiated from obstipation—intractable constipation, which results when feces are retained in the bowel for a prolonged period and become excessively hard and dry. Under these circumstances defecation becomes progressively more difficult until it is virtually impossible. Obstipation is invariably associated with a guarded prognosis, since degenerative changes in the bowel wall may be irreversible.

Constipation is often confused with megacolon, a condition of extreme dilatation of the colon.[87] The two terms are not synonymous, however, since animals with megacolon are always constipated, but constipated animals do not necessarily have megacolon. Constipation, moreover, is a sign, whereas megacolon is a disorder primarily of function and secondarily of structure.

Megacolon may be either primary or secondary. The cause of primary megacolon in the dog and cat is still unknown but may be due to a defect in colonic smooth muscle innervation. Secondary megacolon may follow any lesion or disease that prevents normal defecation for a prolonged period.

A large number of factors may predispose to constipation (Table 9–4). Dietary and environmental constipation is most common; when mixed with feces, substances such as bone, foreign material, or hair can form hard masses or concretions, which the animal is unable to eliminate. Changes in environment, such as occur when an animal is hospitalized or deprived of the opportunity for defecation (e.g., removal of the litter box or failure to exercise), can also result in constipation. Painful lesions of the anorectum, such as anal sacculitis, anal abscesses, perianal fistulae, and rectal strictures are other well-recognized causes. Defecation is often painful in anorectal disease, and after a few initial attempts, the animal may suppress the urge to defecate. Inability to adopt the position for defecation, such as may occur in an animal with a fractured femur or pelvis or in animals with a variety of neurological diseases, may also result in constipation. Intraluminal or extraluminal lesions that obstruct normal fecal transit are other causes and occur, for example, in perineal hernia, in pelvic fractures that have healed leaving a narrowed pelvic canal, and in association with rectal, colonic, or pelvic tumors. Some metabolic and endocrine diseases may also result in constipation either as a consequence of severe dehydration that causes enhanced colonic water absorption or as an impairment of gastrointestinal smooth muscle function due to muscle weakness or electrolyte imbalances.

Tenesmus

Tenesmus is defined as an ineffectual effort to defecate.[87] In veterinary medicine the term has been expanded to encompass severe straining due to abnormalities in or around the lower alimentary or urogenital systems, including straining during parturition.[105] Tenesmus is *not* synonymous with painful defecation. Tenesmus caused by disease of the gastrointestinal tract must always be differentiated from that caused by disease of other organ systems. Tenesmus of alimentary tract origin is usually associated with inflammatory diseases of the rectum and anus and may be associated with either diarrhea or constipation. Tenesmus preceding defecation usually suggests constipation, whereas tenesmus occurring after defecation is usually associated with diarrheal disease—indicating the colonic or rectal mucosa may be inflamed. Continuous tenesmus is rare, but is most often associated with either a rectal foreign body or a tumor. The position the animal adopts to defecate can be useful in differentiating the cause of tenesmus. Tenesmus with the animal squatting is usually associated with colitis (Fig. 9–4*A*), whereas a half-squatting, restless

Table 9–4. A CLASSIFICATION OF THE CAUSES OF CONSTIPATION

Dietary and Environmental	
Dietary	Bones, hair, or foreign material mixed with feces and impacted in the colon
Environmental	Lack of exercise
	Change of habit or environment (e.g., hospitalization or lack of a litter box)
Painful Defecation	
Anorectal disease	Anal sac disease
	Perianal fistula
	Anal stricture
	Anal spasm
	Anal foreign body
	Ulcerating tumor
	Pseudocoprostasis
Trauma	Fractured pelvis
	Fractured limb
	Dislocated hip
	Bite wounds
	Abscess in the perineum
Obstructive	
Extraluminal obstruction	Healed pelvic fracture with narrowed pelvic canal
	Prostatic hypertrophy
	Pelvic tumor
	Anal tumor
	Pseudocoprostasis
Intraluminal obstruction	Colonic tumor
	Rectal tumor
	Perianal hernia
Neurogenic	
Central nervous system dysfunction	Spinal cord disease
	Disc disease
	Paraplegia
Intrinsic colonic nerve dysfunction	Idiopathic megacolon
Metabolic and Endocrine	
Disruption of colonic smooth muscle function	Hyperthyroidism
	Hypothyroidism
	Hyperparathyroidism
Debility	Generalized muscle weakness and dehydration

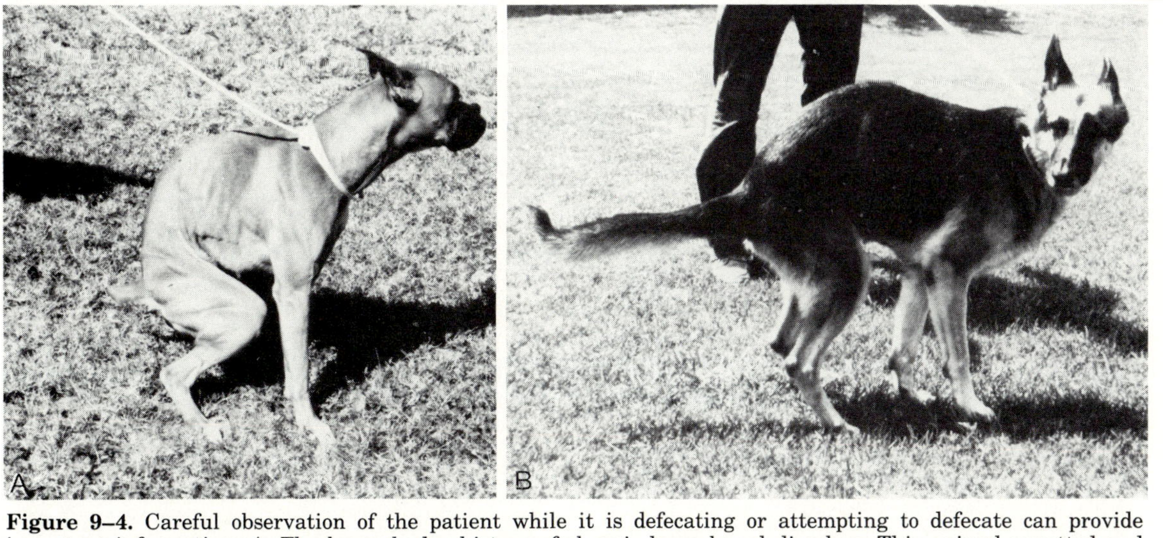

Figure 9–4. Careful observation of the patient while it is defecating or attempting to defecate can provide important information. *A,* The boxer had a history of chronic large bowel diarrhea. This animal squatted and strained for more than 4 minutes to produce a small quantity of feces. Colonoscopy and biopsy confirmed the clinical impression of colitis. *B,* This German shepherd was presented with a diagnosis of colitis that had failed to respond to treatment. When outdoors, the dog would assume the stance shown and would not attempt to squat normally or to defecate; such continuous tenesmus suggests a severe lesion of the distal colon. At examination, the dog was found to have a rectal stricture with secondary colonic impaction. Colonoscopy confirmed the presence of a ring-like lesion in the rectum, and biopsy disclosed a rectal adenocarcinoma. In both patients, a careful history combined with *direct observation* provided a great deal of useful information.

walk can be associated with an obstructive lesion (Fig. 9–4*B*).

Vomiting

Vomiting can occur in association with any inflammatory disease of the intestinal tract and is relatively common in both severe colitis and prolonged constipation. In one study, 29 per cent of dogs with colitis had vomiting as one of the presenting signs, and it was suggested that vomiting resulted from stimulation of the chemoreceptor trigger zone by absorbed toxins.[40]

Dyschezia

Painful or difficult defecation is usually associated with lesions in or near the anus. The animal may cry out as it attempts to defecate or may not defecate at all. Diseases associated with dyschezia include pseudocoprostasis, perianal fistula, anal spasm, and perineal hernia.

Hematochezia

Fresh blood in the feces is a reliable sign of colonic, rectal, or anal disease. Dysentery is uncommon and is associated with severe colonic inflammatory disease. Streaks of blood in normal feces suggest a solitary bleeding lesion such as an ulcerating tumor.

DIAGNOSTIC TECHNIQUES

A variety of diagnostic studies are used in the evaluation of colonic disease. The results of the hemogram, blood chemistry studies, and urinalysis are often more important for the diseases that they rule out than for those that they implicate.[19] A complete fecal examination is mandatory in every animal with colonic disease, and should include both macroscopic and microscopic examination of the feces; bulk, color, consistency and the presence of blood and mucus should always be ascertained. Microscopic examination by both direct (smear), and indirect (flotation) techniques for evidence of parasitic infection is essential. Staining a fresh fecal or colonic smear with new methylene blue for leukocytes is useful in the diagnosis of inflammatory bowel disease.[51, 63]

Other more direct means of diagnosing colonic disease include colonoscopy, colonic biopsy, and contrast radiographic studies. Specific diagnosis of most types of colonic disease, and certainly all those associated with diarrhea, is made by colonoscopy in conjunction with mucosal biopsy. Biopsy is important for differentiation of the various types of colitis from non-inflammatory colonic disease, and a biopsy specimen should be obtained even if the colonic mucosa appears normal on gross examination.[6, 21, 25, 50] Colonoscopy and biopsy are simple diagnostic steps that should be routine in any veterinary practice; the necessary equipment is inexpensive, and the diagnostic yield so high that it is difficult to understand why the use of these techniques is not more widespread. In terms of time and skill, colonoscopy and biopsy cost less than ovariohysterectomy, and in an average practice the initial expenditure for equipment is usually recouped in about 6 to 12 months.

Two types of colonoscope are available, the rigid colonoscope (human sigmoidoscope) and the flexible fiberoptic endoscope; both can be used to examine the colon, and each has advantages and disadvantages. Rigid colonoscopes allow examination of only the descending colon and rectum; this is not a major handicap however, since most colonic disease in the dog and cat involves the distal colon. Flexible colonoscopes are much more expensive but permit examination, biopsy, and photography of the whole organ.

Two sizes of rigid colonoscope* allow examination of virtually all patients. A 15 cm × 15 mm colonoscope is suitable for colonoscopy in cats and small dogs, and a 25 cm × 15 mm instrument can be used in medium and large breeds of dogs. Most rigid colonoscopes are provided with a light source, air insufflation equipment, suction tube, and biopsy forceps (Fig. 9–5). Disposable human colonoscopes are inexpensive and can be reused in animals.

The technique for colonoscopy is simple.[23, 79] Food should be withheld for 24 to 36 hours before the procedure, and a cleansing warm-water enema should be given the night before, followed by a warm physiological saline enema given 1 to 2 hours before the examination. On both occasions the enema should be repeated until the effluent is clear. In order to avoid overdistention of the colon the volume infused should never exceed 10 to 20 ml/kg. A more thorough

*Rigid colonoscope, Welch Allen Inc., Skaneateles Falls, NY.

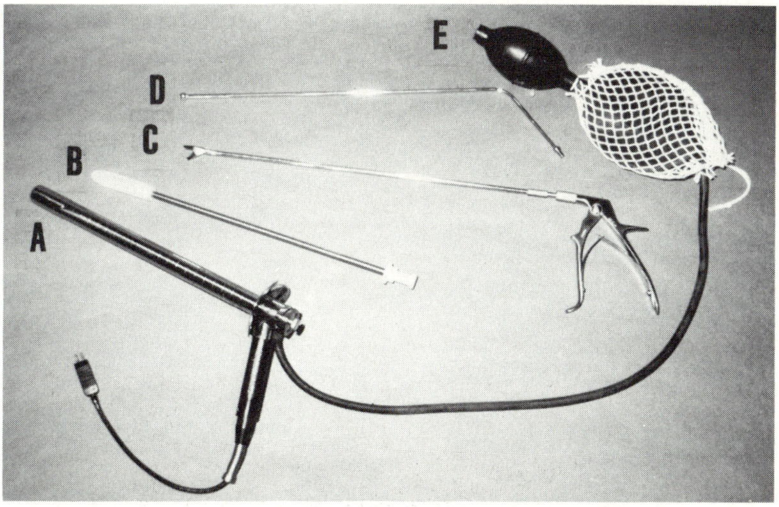

Figure 9–5. Welch-Allen rigid sigmoidoscope with ancillary equipment. *A,* 20 cm × 1.8 cm rigid sigmoidoscope with light source; *B,* Obturator, which is placed inside the colonoscope during insertion; *C,* Biopsy forceps, which provide a good sample of tissue, and are invaluable for biopsy of specific lesions; *D,* suction tube for removal of liquid feces and mucus from the colonic lumen; *E,* rubber bulb for insufflation of air into the colon. Air insufflation dilates the colon and facilitates examination.

preparation is necessary for fiberoptic endoscopy. A typical regimen includes a 48-hour fast and 150 to 300 ml of magnesium trisilicate solution in conjunction with 2 to 4 bisacodyl tablets,* (5 mg/tablet) depending on body size, administered the evening before the procedure. An enema (saline or tap water) should be given the morning of the procedure and should be repeated until the effluent is clear.

In human patients, it has been emphasized that proctoscopy should be done without preparatory cleansing enemas in order to avoid mucosal distortion and washing away of mucosal exudate.[57] Since the canine or feline colon frequently contains large amounts of feces, cleansing enemas are essential for thorough mucosal examination. The only contraindication to routine enemas is in patients with severe anorectal disease in which passage of the enema tube might either be excessively painful or cause mucosal damage. It is sometimes necessary to perform colonoscopy without an enema in dogs with both severe colitis and watery diarrhea. In these patients liquid feces can be removed by suction.

In most animals, rigid colonoscopy can be performed without sedation or anesthesia, with the patient either standing or in *right* lateral recumbency. The latter position reduces gravitational flow of feces to the distal colon. Tilting the table so that the animal's head is slightly lowered also facilitates examination. General anesthesia is required only in animals with severe inflammation, excessive scarring, or strictures in which examination would otherwise be too painful. Narcotic analgesics are best avoided, since they stimulate intestinal motility and increase the rate of fluid delivery to the large bowel. Fiberoptic endoscopy should be done with the patient heavily tranquilized or anesthetized and in *left* lateral recumbency.

For rigid colonoscopy, the lubricated colonoscope is gently inserted through the anus with the obturator in place (Fig. 9–6). After insertion, the obturator is removed, the glass window is inserted or closed (depending upon the type of colonoscope), and a small quantity of air is insufflated. Air insufflation distends the colon and facilitates insertion and passage of the colonoscope. The instrument is then passed up the descending colon as far as it will go without the use of force (Fig. 9–6*B*). During insertion the mucosa is carefully examined for color, texture, ulcerations, parasites, and other lesions. After full insertion, the instrument is slowly withdrawn and appropriate biopsy specimens are taken.

The normal colonic mucosa is smooth and glistening and uniformly reflects the endoscopic light from a broad area. Normal colonic mucosa is pink, but the shade depends on such factors as the type of light in the colonoscope and the type of preparation the patient has undergone (Fig. 9–7). Superficial submucosal blood vessels are usually visible through the mucosa. Normal colonic mucosa does not bleed when gently rubbed with the tip of the colonoscope, and the colon readily distends when air is insufflated.[23]

Biopsy of focal lesions can be carried out under direct observation using uterine biopsy (alligator) forceps passed through the

*Dulcolax, Boehringer Ingelheim, Ridgefield, CT.

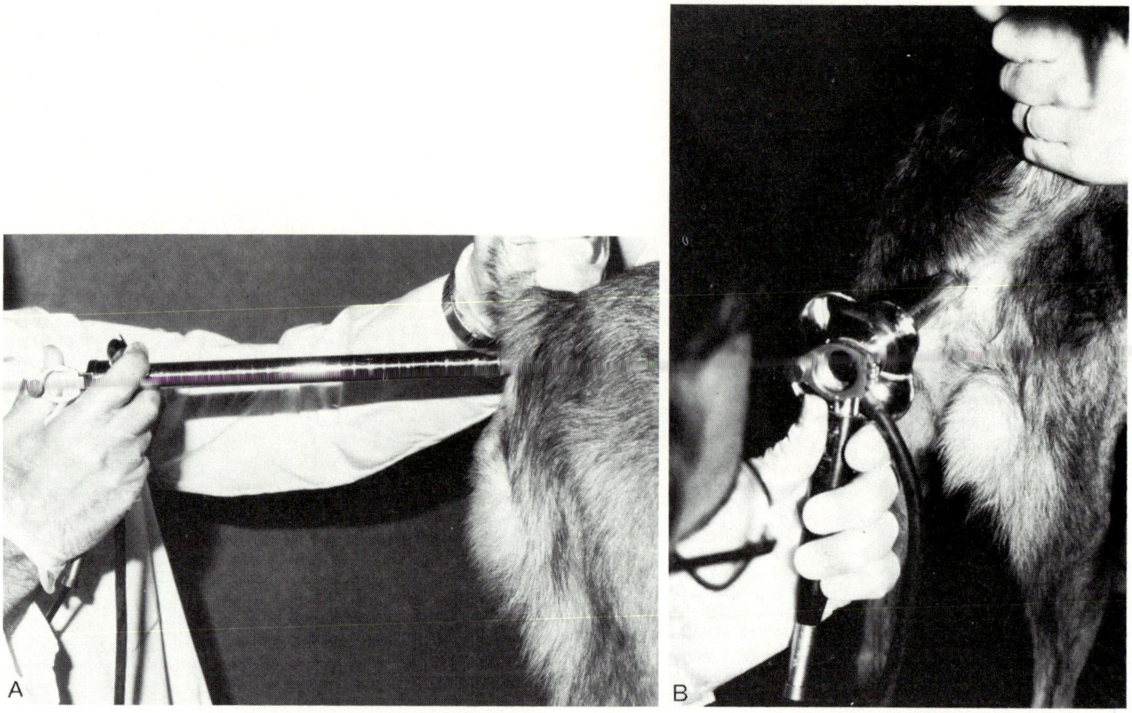

Figure 9–6. *A,* Insertion of the colonoscope. The lubricated colonoscope is gently inserted through the anus with the obturator in place. In this case, the dog was standing and had been given no tranquilizers. Examination was uneventful. *B,* Examination of the colon. After insertion of the colonoscope, the obturator is removed, the magnifying glass window is closed, and a small quantity of air is insufflated. The instrument is then passed up the colon as far as it will go under *direct observation and without the use of force.* The mucosa is examined *during insertion.*

colonoscope (Fig. 9–8).[6, 56] For this technique the mucosa is lightly grasped with the forceps, gentle backward pressure is exerted to "tent" the mucosa and pull it away from the submucosa, and the mucosa is then cut as the forceps are firmly closed—this technique minimizes the chance of colonic perforation (Fig. 9–9). The forceps are then withdrawn, the specimen is gently removed, is placed flat on a piece of filter or blotting paper, and is put into an appropriate fixative (Bouin's or formalin). Impression smears made from the mucosal surface of the biopsy specimen may be helpful in the diagnosis of some

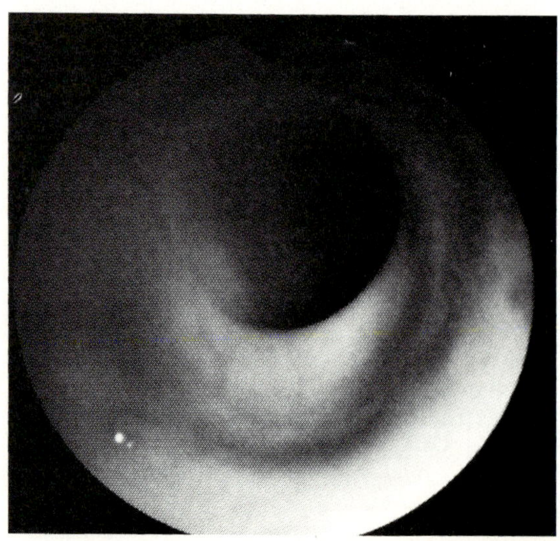

Figure 9–7. Normal colonic mucosa is viewed through a flexible fiberoptic colonoscope. The mucosa is creamy pink or pink and reflects light uniformly. Blood vessels are usually apparent in the submucosa; failure to see these vessels is a reliable sign of colonic disease and suggests the presence of inflammation, congestion, or edema. See Color Plate.

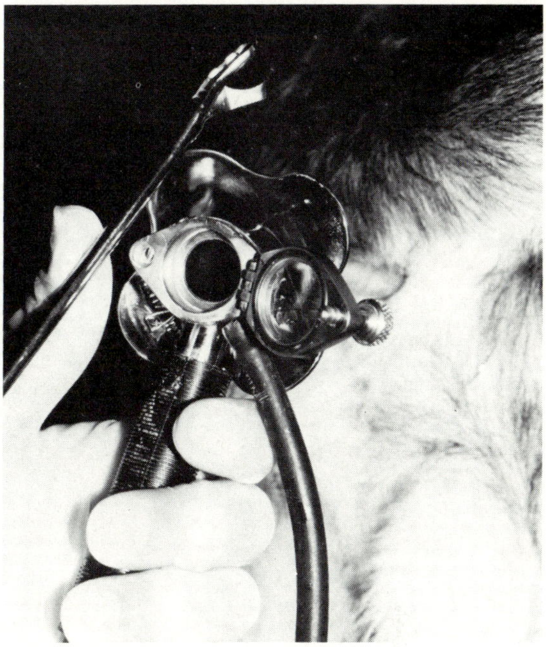

Figure 9–8. Preparation for colonic biopsy. When a lesion or site for biopsy has been identified, the glass window is opened, and the biopsy forceps are inserted.

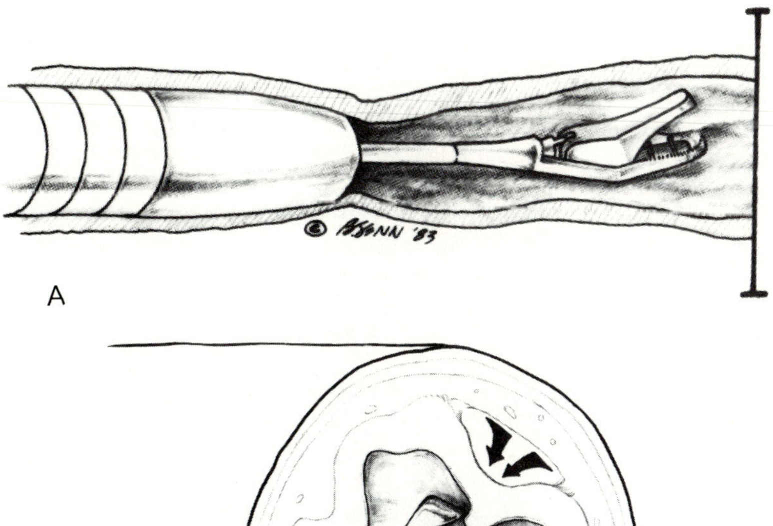

A

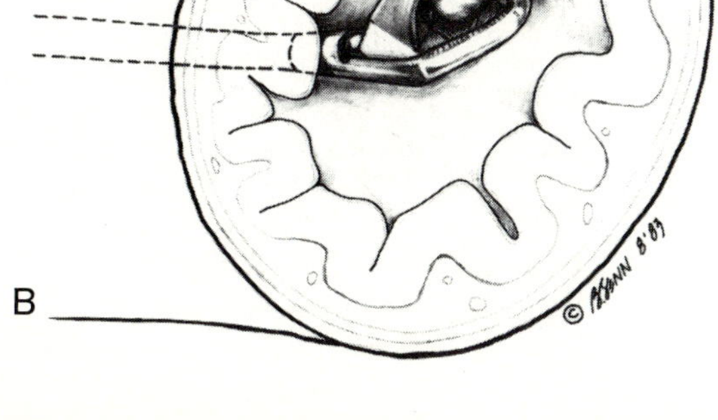

B

Figure 9–9. Technique for colonic biopsy. *A*, The biopsy forceps are passed through the colonoscope and a fold of mucosa is lightly grasped. *B*, To complete the biopsy, gentle backward pressure is applied to "tent" the mucosa and to pull it away from the underlying muscles *(arrows)*. The forceps are then firmly closed, the biopsy specimen is taken, and the forceps are withdrawn.

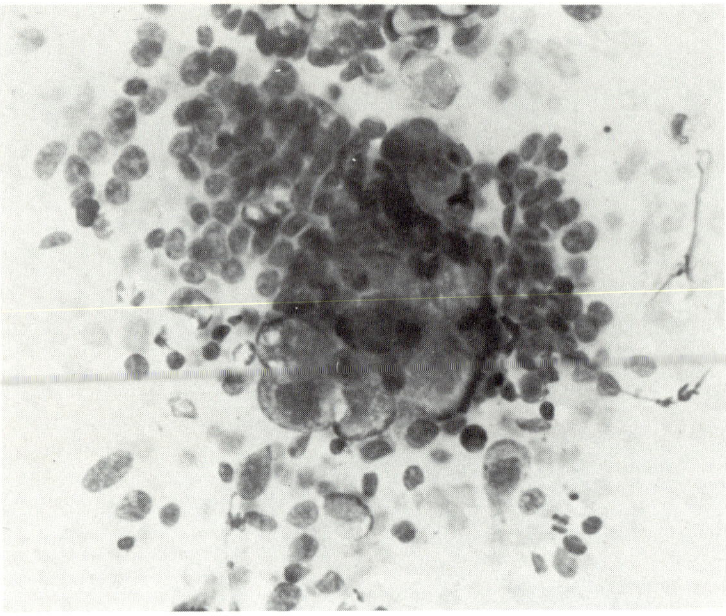

Figure 9–10. Cytological examination of a touch preparation made from a biopsy specimen can be diagnostic. In this example, the diagnosis is a carcinoma *in situ*. The biopsy specimen taken from an obviously abnormal, friable, proliferative mass seen in the distal colon of a dog with a history of hematochezia. A clump of large neoplastic cells surrounded by normal colonic epithelial cells is seen (× 200). (Courtesy of Dr. D. J. Meyer.)

diseases such as histoplasmosis and certain tumors. A safer and more efficient biopsy instrument for diagnosis of diffuse colonic disease is the Quinton multiple purpose suction biopsy instrument.[56]* (See Chapter 2.)

Cytological examination of direct fecal smears, or preferably of a rectal or colonic smear, stained with new methylene blue or Loeffler's methylene blue is useful in the diagnosis of colonic disease (Fig. 9–10).[51] Erythrocytes and inflammatory cells are frequently present in smears made from animals with colitis, and the diagnostic importance of these smears is enhanced because in mild colitis the smear may be abnormal, even when the mucosa appears normal and is not friable. Smears allow more rapid diagnosis than biopsy, can be taken from multiple sites, never cause serious bleeding, and will not delay barium enema examination. Large cotton swabs† can be used to test for mucosal friability and to obtain mucosal smears for cytological and parasitological examination.

Evaluation of the large bowel by barium contrast radiography is useful in the diagnosis of certain colonic diseases, particularly those localized to the proximal colon, which cannot be examined with a rigid colonoscope. Contrast radiography is also useful in the evaluation of the colon above an area of stricture. However, the technique is not routinely used in the diagnosis of colonic disease, since it is time-consuming, messy, expensive, and is no substitute for a thorough colonoscopic examination. To avoid any risk of colonic perforation or rupture, a barium enema should not be done for at least 3 to 4 days after a colonic biopsy specimen has been taken. The techniques and procedures for contrast radiography are outlined in chapter 14 and in standard radiology texts.[48, 68]

*Multi-purpose Suction Biopsy Instrument, Quinton Instrument Company, Seattle, WA.

†Scopettes, Parke-Davis, Morris Plains, NJ.

Colonic Diseases with Diarrhea as the Principal Sign

Diarrhea is the principal sign in the majority of the colonic diseases. Diarrhea can result from either inflammatory diseases or disorders of colonic motility.

The group of diseases that share the common factor of colonic inflammation (Tab. 9–5) are an important cause of chronic diarrhea in the dog. In the past, there has been an unfortunate tendency to treat canine colitis as a single disease entity,[40] rather than as a group of separate, albeit as yet poorly defined diseases that often need specific, individualized treatment.[21, 99] Uncommon colonic diseases, such as histiocytic ulcerative colitis in the boxer, have also been overemphasized at the expense of more common disorders such as idiopathic chronic colitis.

ACUTE NON-SPECIFIC COLITIS

Acute non-specific colitis is an uncommon, poorly defined group of diseases with multiple causes that occur almost exclusively in the dog. The specific cause is seldom identified, but occasionally the history may incriminate ingestion of garbage or foreign material. In other instances parasites are found on fecal examination, or the history and laboratory studies may suggest a food-induced allergic colitis. In the case of garbage ingestion, it has been postulated that abrasive foreign material damages the colonic mucosa and allows secondary bacterial invasion and development of bacterial colitis. Since many of the causes of acute colitis also cause gastric and small intestinal disease, signs of colonic involvement usually accompany non-specific acute gastroenteritis. A small number of such cases progress to chronic colitis.

History. The syndrome is characterized by the sudden onset of severe, watery, and occasionally bloody, mucoid diarrhea. Vomiting may be present in dogs with acute non-specific gastroenteritis or a history of scavenging or garbage ingestion. Animals are usually presented for veterinary examination within 48 hours of the onset of signs. There are no reports of age, breed, or sex predisposition.

Physical Findings. The physical findings depend on the severity and nature of the initial insult as well as on the amount of body fluid lost from vomiting and diarrhea. Fever may be present and abdominal palpation may elicit pain. Rectal examination may reveal foreign material such as pieces of bone, plastic, wood, or aluminum foil in dogs with a history of garbage ingestion.

Diagnosis. The hemogram is compatible with the severity of dehydration; a leukocytosis may also be present but neither the hemogram nor results of blood chemical analysis is diagnostic. A fecal examination

Table 9–5. A CLASSIFICATION OF COLONIC DISEASE IN THE DOG AND CAT

Diseases with Diarrhea as the Principal Sign	
Inflammatory diseases	Acute non-specific colitis
	Chronic colitis
	Parasitic colitis
	Whipworm-induced colitis
	Hookworm-induced colitis
	Amebic colitis*
	Giardiasis*
	Balantidiasis*
	Infectious colitis
	Histoplasmosis
	Salmonellosis*
	Protothecosis*
	Granulomatous colitis*
	Uremic colitis
	Histiocytic ulcerative colitis*
	Eosinophilic colitis
	Segmental colitis (secondary to chronic pancreatitis)
	Inflammation caused by trauma
	Antibiotic associated—pseudomembranous*
	Colitis cystica profunda*
Tumors	Lymphosarcoma
	Adenocarcinoma
Non-inflammatory colonic diarrheal disease	Irritable colon (spastic colitis, functional diarrhea, irritable bowel syndrome)
	Cecal inversion*
Diseases with Constipation and Dyschezia as the Principal Signs	Colonic impaction
	Idiopathic megacolon
	Rectal and anal stricture
	Rectal and anal foreign bodies
	Anal spasm*
	Anal trauma
	Perineal hernia
	Perianal fistula
	Anal sac disease
	Pseudocoprostasis
	Tumors of the colon, rectum, and anus

*Uncommon or rare diseases

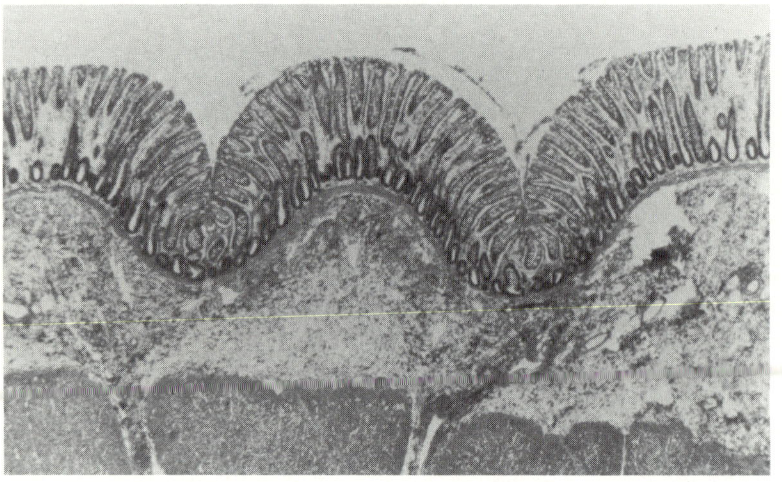

Figure 9–11. Acute canine colitis. Histological appearance of a biopsy specimen taken from a dog with a 4-day history of progressively more severe diarrhea. Diarrhea began after the dog had ingested garbage containing chicken bones. The feces became increasingly mucoid and bloody. Colonoscopy revealed a diffusely inflamed colon that bled readily when touched with the tip of the colonoscope. In this specimen the mucosa appears to be of normal thickness. There is some dilatation of the crypts and accumulation of mucus. The submucosa was infiltrated with neutrophils, plasma cells, and erythrocytes.

is mandatory and should include both direct smear and flotation studies for gastrointestinal parasites. Colonic biopsy reveals changes typical of acute colitis (Fig. 9–11).

Treatment. The extent and vigor of treatment must be tailored to the severity of the clinical signs. Intravenous administration of balanced electrolyte replacement solutions is indicated if dehydration is evident; broad-spectrum antibiotics are indicated if the dog is febrile. (Chloramphenicol, ampicillin, and tetracyclines have been used effectively by the author.) Non-absorbable oral antibiotics such as neomycin* are contraindicated, since they disrupt enteric flora and frequently prolong morbidity. Liquid antidiarrheal drugs, such as bismuth subsalicylate† and antispasmodics such as diphenoxylate‡ and propantheline bromide§ may also be beneficial. Anthelmintics should be administered if infection with gastrointestinal parasites is diagnosed.

Dietary manipulation is important; the principle of resting the gastrointestinal tract is well established in acute disturbances.[92, 93] Dogs with acute colitis appear to do better if fasted for a minimum of 24 hours after the onset of signs, even if they show a desire to eat. Water, however, is not contraindicated and should always be freely available. Feeding can be resumed on the second or third day after onset of signs. Food should initially be bland and bulky; examples of suitable foods are cottage cheese, chicken, hamburger, and rice. One to two tablespoons of bran or psyllium mucilloid* should be added to each feeding.

*Biosol, The Upjohn Company, Kalamazoo, MI.
†Pepto-Bismol, Procter and Gamble, Cincinnati, OH.
‡Lomotil, Searle & Co., San Juan, PR.
§Pro-Banthine, Searle & Co., San Juan, PR.

Prognosis. The prognosis for complete recovery is usually good. With appropriate treatment, feces appear normal or near normal by the third day. There are, however, a few dogs that fail to recover from the initial acute episode and develop chronic colitis. More extensive diagnostic studies and a different therapeutic regimen are indicated in these patients. Management is discussed in the next section.

CHRONIC COLITIS

There is some overlap between the designations acute colitis and chronic colitis. However, the diseases described in this section will be discussed as chronic diseases, even if they sometimes have an acute onset, since it is their persistence that is of greatest concern to the client. This group includes chronic (idiopathic), parasitic, eosinophilic, infectious, granulomatous, traumatic, and iatrogenic colitis and the specific but very rare entity canine histiocytic ulcerative colitis. (See Table 9–5.)

Chronic Idiopathic Colitis

Chronic colitis, the single most common form of canine colitis, may well be a group of as yet poorly identified, distinct disease entities that await specific pathological classification.[21] There is no known cause; clinical signs are typical of any form of chronic canine colitis and there is no single specific

*Metamucil, Searle Laboratories, Chicago, IL.

diagnostic feature. The disease has been called idiopathic ulcerative colitis,[59] and a comparison has been made with human ulcerative colitis.[96] Ulcerative colitis is probably not a good term for the canine disease, since there is currently little evidence to justify comparison with human ulcerative colitis, and colonic ulceration is not a reliable diagnostic feature.

Etiology. The precise etiology and pathogenesis of chronic idiopathic canine colitis have yet to be defined. It is possible that there are several causes, all resulting in a common, predictable, and typical colonic response that may be self-perpetuating long after the inciting cause is removed. The disease, for example, may follow a bout of non-specific gastroenteritis or may be the cause of chronic diarrhea, originally attributed to whipworm or hookworm infection, that persists long after the parasites have been eliminated. The histological appearance of the colonic mucosa is the same no matter what the cause; therefore, specific differentiation of the etiological agent is impossible. It is possible that as in humans, psychogenic, genetic, or immunological factors may be involved in the development of the disease.[24]

History. The disease affects dogs of all ages and breeds, but animals between 6 months and 4 years seem particularly susceptible. The history is typically one of chronic large bowel diarrhea that, in most cases, has failed to respond, or has responded only temporarily, to conventional antidiarrheal therapy.

The feces vary in consistency from semiformed to liquid; hematochezia may be present in more severely afflicted animals, especially if they have been previously treated with corticosteroids. Mucus is usually, but not invariably present, and the feces may be flecked with fresh blood; dysentery is rare. The frequency of defecation is increased from two or three times normal to as much as 10 to 12 times per day. Unlike that of small intestinal diarrhea, which animals seem better able to control, defecation is frequently associated with a sense of urgency. However, the individual fecal volume at each defecation is frequently less than normal and the total daily fecal weight is increased only slightly over normal.[22] Tenesmus after passage of liquid or semiformed feces may also be reported. The presence of tenesmus and a history of mucus in the feces are two of the most important facts to be elicited when obtaining the history from the client. These signs suggest some type of colitis, although it should be emphasized that their absence does not eliminate the diagnosis.

Some dogs are presented with a history of both chronic vomiting and diarrhea,[40] and if it is not recognized that vomiting can be a feature of canine colitis, the wrong diagnostic study might be chosen at the expense of the veterinarian's time and the client's money and patience.

Physical Findings. Physical findings are normal in most dogs with chronic idiopathic colitis. However, some dogs may appear underweight or dehydrated in long-standing or severe disease. Long-haired breeds may have fecal contamination of the perianal hair and an associated painful, moist perineal dermatitis. Fever is rare; abdominal palpation is usually normal but signs of pain are occasionally elicited on deep palpation of the caudal abdomen. Rectal examination may sometimes initiate tenesmus if the distal part of the bowel is involved.

Diagnosis. Diagnosis of chronic idiopathic colitis is based on a combination of clinical and pathological criteria, the appearance of the colonic lesions, and the exclusion of other forms of colitis.

There are no characteristic hematological changes; a neutrophilia with a left shift may be present in some patients, and a mild microcytic hypochromic anemia may be observed if chronic gastrointestinal blood loss has occurred. Repeated fecal examination for gastrointestial parasites is necessary in order to differentiate chronic idiopathic colitis from parasite-induced colonic inflammatory disease.

Endoscopic features of chronic colitis are variable; one of the most prominent changes is the disappearance of submucosal blood vessels as the mucosa becomes edematous and inflamed. Irregular mucosal thickening with a change in the patterns of reflected light from smooth and glistening to granular results from the inflammation of the mucosa. As inflammation intensifies, the fine granularity appears coarser and the mucosa appears dry. Increased vascularity may be appreciated as hyperemia. Excessive amounts of thick, tenacious mucus may be observed to adhere to the mucosa or to accumulate within the lumen; unlike that of the normal colon, the mucosa may bleed readily when touched with the tip of the colonoscope (Fig. 9–12). Ulceration is vari-

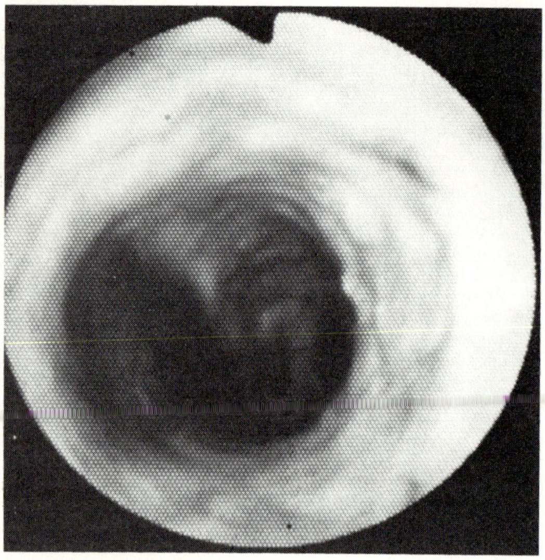

Figure 9–12. Colon of a dog with chronic idiopathic colitis viewed through a colonoscope. No submucosal blood vessels are visible; the mucosa reflects light abnormally, and several large erythematous areas can be seen. These areas bled readily when rubbed with the tip of the colonoscope. See Color Plate.

able and is present in less than half of the dogs with colitis. Small ulcers are most common and appear as areas of pinpoint hemorrhage; large, deep, bleeding ulcers with tags of epithelial tissue around the edges are rare. Although the extent of mucosal change at colonoscopy reflects the overall severity of disease, the true extent of the lesion is revealed only by histological examination of a biopsy specimen.

The typical histological appearance is one of either acute or chonic inflammation that is focal, invariably limited to the colonic mucosa, and rarely ulcerated. Both acute and chronic reactions may be present in a single biopsy specimen suggesting a progressive disease process (Fig. 9–13). The acute reaction is represented by edema of the lamina propria and infiltration by acute inflammatory cells. Colonic glands are dilated and lined by predominantly columnar epithelial cells. The lamina propria is fibrosed and the colonic glands appear to be more separated. Reactive hyperplasia, characterized by an increase in length and tortuosity of the glands, is present in some patients (Fig. 9–14). As in the acute form, the numbers of goblet cells are usually depleted, a finding that in human patients suggests active disease.

Contrast radiographic studies of the colon may reveal fine mucosal irregularities. Filling defects indicative of ulcers, or changes in colonic length and pliability suggestive of more than mucosal involvement, are seen in more severely afflicted patients or in those with long-standing disease. The value of contrast radiography must be weighed against the likely benefit. The procedure is time-consuming and expensive and reveals diagnostic changes in only half the patients studied.[68]

Differential Diagnosis. The initial diagnostic evaluation should consider all causes of chronic diarrhea; however, small intestinal disease can usually be eliminated by a complete history.[17] The signs of colonic diarrhea are presented in Table 9–3. Dogs with chronic idiopathic colitis are usually presented with a history of mucoid, small volume, high-frequency diarrhea; variable quantities of blood may also be noted in the feces. Chronic idiopathic colitis is differentiated from non-inflammatory colonic diarrheal disease (see p 248) by colonoscopy and biopsy, and from parasitic colitis by the

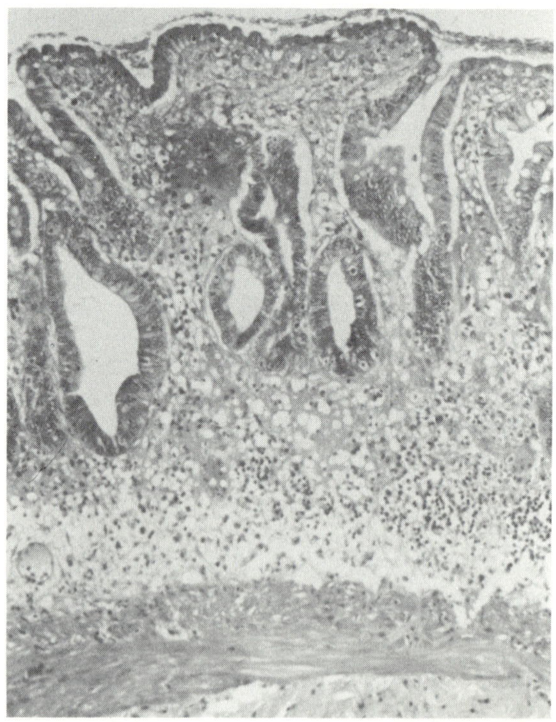

Figure 9–13. Histological section of the colon of a dog with chronic idiopathic colitis. There is dramatic disruption of the normal architecture of the crypts (compare with Figure 9–2). The crypts are fused, truncated, and shortened, and the surface is covered by intact, slightly flattened epithelium, which shows lack of differentiation to goblet cells. The underlying lamina propria is infiltrated with lymphocytes and plasma cells.

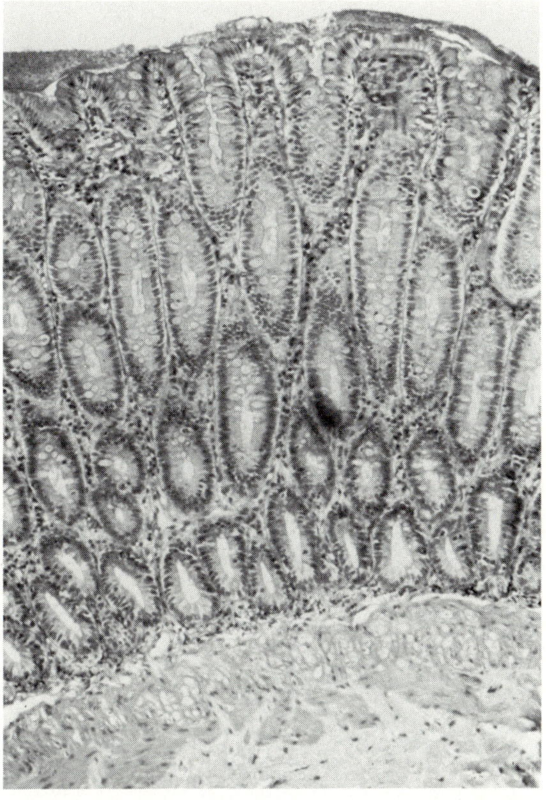

Figure 9–14. Colonic mucosal hyperplasia. The mucosa is increased in thickness (compare with Figure 9–2) and the glands are increased in length and are more tortuous than normal. Intact glands are seldom seen in such specimens no matter how carefully the section is cut. There is an increase in the number of goblet cells with dilatation of the crypts and glands. A few inflammatory cells are present in the lamina propria, but the submucosa is normal. This is a common finding in dogs with either chronic small intestinal disease and malabsorption (in which the colon reacts to unabsorbed materials from above) or non-inflammatory colonic diarrhea.

absence of parasitic infection and characteristic histopathological findings. Colonoscopy and biopsy also differentiate chronic idiopathic colitis from other less common types of canine colitis.

Treatment. The fact that there is no universally effective therapeutic regimen for chronic idiopathic colitis indicates the complexity of the disease process and its several causes. Treatment falls into three categories: (1) antibacterial, (2) antispasmodic, and (3) dietary. In severely afflicted patients treatment with parenteral fluids and perhaps blood or plasma may also be indicated.

The drug of choice in the treatment of canine colitis is sulfasalazine.* This drug, a combination of sulfapyridine and 5-aminosalicylate, has been shown to be useful in the treatment and prophylaxis of ulcerative colitis in humans[31, 47] and chronic colitis in the dog.[21, 40] Sulfasalazine is supplied only in 500-mg tablets; an effective canine dose is 25 to 40 mg/kg body weight administered 3 times daily. Most dogs respond well to sulfasalazine and need only a short (3 to 4 week) course of treatment. This is in contrast to the treatment of human ulcerative colitis, in which the drug must usually be administered for prolonged periods. A few dogs also require a long period of maintenance therapy, and in these, the minimum dose needed to suppress signs of colitis must be found by trial and error. Side effects of sulfasalazine in the dog are rare. Keratoconjunctivitis sicca has been observed in dogs treated with the maximum dose for a long period,[2] but may also occur as an acute reaction if there has been prior exposure to sulfonamides. Allergic dermatitis, nausea and vomiting, and cholestatic jaundice have also been reported as rare occurrences.[40]

Efficacy and dosage have not been determined in the cat. It is likely, however, that lower doses are indicated in this species because of its sensitivity to salicylates. The few cats that the author has treated with this drug have shown signs of salicylate toxicity at the recommended dose.

Metronidazole† has also been used in the treatment of colitis. It is an effective antibacterial drug, but is much less effective than sulfasalazine in the treatment of colonic inflammatory disease.

There is no place for the routine use of anticholinergics in the treatment of colitis. Inflammation depresses colonic motility, and there is no therapeutic benefit in further inhibition. Narcotic analgesics are of potential benefit, since these drugs apparently act directly on colonic smooth muscle to inhibit propulsive movement and reduce diarrhea. They are useful in the initial symptomatic treatment of severe colitis.[81] Compounds that act in this way are a mixture of diphenoxylate and atropine,‡ codeine, and loperamide.§

There is no specific nutritional treatment for canine colitis, but diets should always be nutritionally balanced and palatable. Canned all-meat or meat-based dog foods

---

*Azulfidine, Pharmacia, Laboratories, Piscataway, NJ.

†Flagyl, Searle Laboratories, Chicago, IL.

‡Lomotil, Searle & Co., San Juan, PR.

§Imodium, Janssen Pharmaceutica, Piscataway, NJ.

help to control diarrhea in colitis, whereas dry, cereal-based foods, although of comparable nutritional value, produce bulkier, heavier feces in normal dogs[64] and much more voluminous feces in virtually every type of diarrheal disease, especially colitis.

Low-residue diets have been recommended in colitis on the incorrect premise that they decrease colonic motility.[59, 93] In fact, high-residue foods cause a reduction in overall colonic motility,[18] and the addition of bran to the food of some dogs with colitis can bring about a reduction of diarrhea.[21] For these reasons, dogs with colitis should receive frequent (at least TID) feedings of a meat-based or all-meat food or its home-prepared equivalent, to which has been added 2 to 4 tablespoons of coarse bran for each 2 cans (approximately 400 gm) of food.

The indications for corticosteroid therapy in chronic colitis remain to be clarified; some dogs with colitis reportedly deteriorate when treated with steroids.[40] Since chronic canine colitis is an inflammatory disease of unknown etiology, a trial of steroids may be warranted in those patients that are unresponsive to conventional treatment. Oral prednisolone at a dose of 1 to 2 mg/kg/day is occasionally effective when sulfasalazine fails to bring about a remission of signs.

Prognosis. There have been no long-term studies of either the recovery rate or recurrence of idiopathic canine colitis. In the author's experience, about 70 to 80 per cent of afflicted dogs recover completely and show no recurrence when treated with sulfasalazine. Some dogs, however, require long-term treatment, and clients should always be advised of the possibility of long-term drug treatment and its potential cost. Colonic fibrosis may develop in long-standing cases and result in a decrease in colonic surface area and permanent impairment of absorptive function; the prognosis in these animals is very poor.

Parasitic Colitis

A variety of parasites affect the canine colon, causing diseases of varying severity that are usually manifested as colitis. Most important from a clinical viewpoint are whipworm and hookworm infections; much less important are entamoebiasis, giardiasis, and balantidiasis.

The prevalence of parasitic infection in the dog mandates one or more fecal examinations in any dog presented with a history of chronic diarrhea. The failure to rule out gastrointestinal parasitism before progressing to more complex diagnostic studies is a very serious and potentially costly omission.

Whipworm-induced Colitis. The incidence of whipworm-induced colitis is as high as that of chronic colitis. Although trichuriasis is very common, it does not cause overt colitis in all infected dogs. Signs of infection, primarily diarrhea, depend on the number of parasites and the individual response of the host. Signs of whipworm-induced colitis are similar to those of idiopathic chronic colitis, except that the parasite stimulates mucosal goblet cell hyperplasia, causing increased mucus in the feces.

History. Dogs with whipworm-induced colitis are presented with a history of diarrhea, which is more often mucoid than bloody. Tenesmus is rare but the history is otherwise similar to that of chronic colitis. Signs of typhlitis such as biting at the flank and irritability are occasionally observed.

It must be emphasized that not all dogs with trichuriasis have colitis or diarrhea; light infections may cause no signs or be presented with unexplained weight loss in the face of a normal appetite. Infection is acquired by ingestion of material infected with eggs and in some dogs seems to recur with surprising frequency. The history in these patients often reveals exposure to a contaminated environment such as a dirt run or a park frequented by a large number of dogs.

Physical Findings. As in chronic idiopathic colitis, the results of a physical examination are seldom helpful. Body weight and the state of hydration vary in proportion to the duration and severity of the infection. Dogs may appear thin and slightly dehydrated if diarrhea has been severe. The rectum feels normal on digital examination and tenesmus is rare, since the disease process seldom extends that far distally.

Diagnosis. The most important aspect of diagnosis is detection of *Trichuris* eggs on microscopic examination of the feces. Dogs with whipworm-induced colitis usually have eggs in their feces. However, shedding of eggs by the adult parasite is not continuous, and at least three examinations made over a 3 to 6 day period must reveal no eggs for infection to be ruled out. Adult whipworms have been reported in the descending colon of dogs whose fecal examinations repeatedly revealed no evidence of infection.[21, 58]

Colonoscopy typically reveals the colon to be hyperemic with excessive amounts of mucus, both free in the lumen and adhering to the mucosa. Ulceration is very rare, but areas of focal hemorrhage may occur (Fig. 9–15*A*). In severe infections, large numbers of creamy-white adult worms, each about 5 to 10 mm long, may be seen attached to the mucosa. Histological examination of a biopsy specimen reveals extensive mucosal hyperplasia, with the parasites surrounded by an intense cellular reaction and a proliferation in the number of goblet cells. There are also plasma cell and lymphocyte accumulations in the mucosa and submucosa, and an increase in mononuclear cellularity of the lamina propria. Sections of adult worms may also be present (Fig. 9–15*B*).

Hematological and blood chemical changes in whipworm infection are nondiagnostic. Radiographic examination is seldom helpful. Plain films of the abdomen occasionally reveal an enlarged, gas-filled cecum. Contrast radiography is a waste of time and money, except in those very few dogs in which diagnosis is difficult and which may have severe lesions confined to the proximal colon and cecum.

Differential Diagnosis. Whipworm-induced colitis and typhlitis are differentiated from other causes of colonic diarrhea by detection of eggs in the feces or by finding adult parasites at colonoscopy or biopsy.

Treatment. Successful treatment is predicated upon adequate and repeated anthelmintic therapy. This is not always easy, because whipworms are one of the most difficult parasites to eliminate, and reinfection is common if good husbandry is not simultaneously practiced.

Anthelmintics that are effective against whipworms include dichlorvos,* butamisole,† fenbendazole, and mebendazole.‡ Follow-up fecal examinations are essential to confirm that the parasites have been eliminated, and more than one course of treatment is frequently necessary for success. Concurrent therapy with sulfasalazine may also be indicated in severe cases.

Hookworm-induced Colitis. Hookworms are generally thought of as parasites of the small intestine, but they may be found in fairly large numbers in the colon, where they cause colitis.[65] The disease is usually chronic and characterized by mucoid, occasionally bloody diarrhea. Hookworm-induced colitis should be suspected if a dog

*Task, Shell Chemical Co., Animal Health Division, Houston, TX.

†Styquin, American Cyanamid Co., Princeton, NJ.

‡Telmintic Powder, Pitman-Moore Inc., Washington Crossing, NJ.

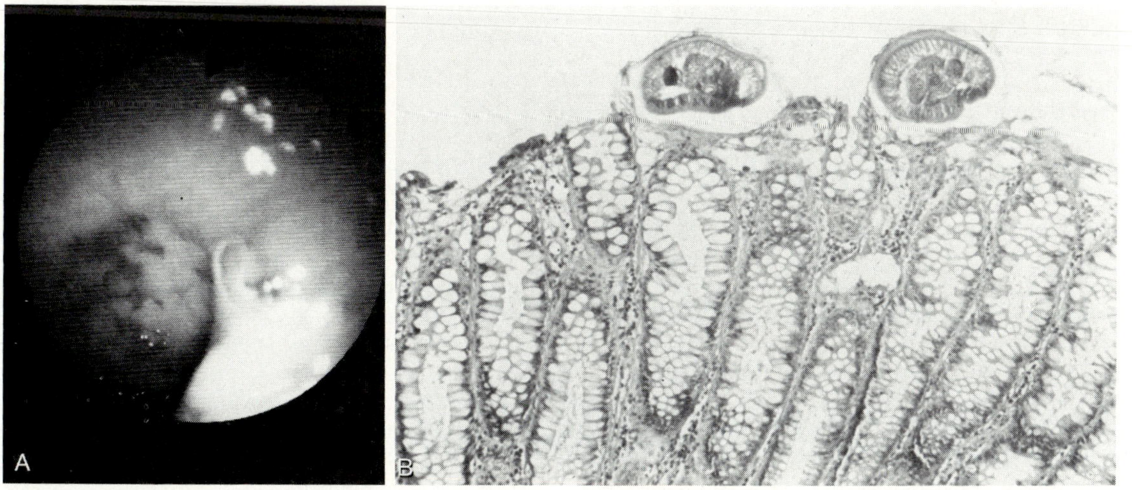

Figure 9–15. *A,* endoscopic appearance of whipworm-induced colitis. The mucosa reflects light unevenly *(bright areas),* indicating excessive mucus secretion. There are several areas of obvious mucosal hemorrhage, and a whipworm can be seen attached to the mucosa. Numerous other whipworms were found throughout the proximal colon. The patient, an 11-year-old mixed-breed dog, had a 6-month history of intermittent bloody diarrhea. Repeated fecal examinations had failed to reveal parasitic ova. Appropriate anthelmintic treatment in conjunction with sulfasalazine brought about an almost immediate cessation of signs. Whipworm infection would not have been confirmed without endoscopy. See Color Plate. *B,* Histological appearance of a biopsy specimen taken from a dog with chronic whipworm infection. Two whipworms can be seen in cross-section on the surface of the mucosa. There is a marked increase in the number of goblet cells with dilatation of the crypts. Inflammatory reaction is minimal.

with chronic weight loss, diarrhea, and hookworm eggs in its feces has signs of colonic involvement (mucoid feces, increased frequency of defecation, and occasional fresh blood in the feces). The colonic mucosa of these dogs appears hyperemic, and small ulcers are occasionally seen at colonoscopy. Many dogs have an eosinophilia.

Several drugs are effective in the treatment of hookworms, including: dichlorvos, butamisole, mebendazole, disophenol,* fenbendazole† and pyrantel pamoate.‡ At least two doses administered 2 to 3 weeks apart are necessary to eliminate the parasite. Husbandry should be improved concurrently with anthelmintic therapy in order to decrease the possibility of reinfection. Treatment for hookworms is usually sufficient to control colitis but in some dogs, the signs of colonic involvement persist long after elimination of the parasite. Treatment for these patients should be the same as for colonic idiopathic colitis.

Other Parasite-induced Colonic Inflammatory Disease. There are occasional reports of canine colitis due to infection with *Entamoeba histolytica, Giardia canis,* and *Balantidium coli.*[39, 52, 55]

Infection with *Entamoeba histolytica* is rare; it has been reported sporadically in the southern part of the United States as well as in India, China, Indochina, Egypt, and Panama. Signs of infection vary, depending on the number of parasites involved and host susceptibility. Signs range from mild, gelatinous, occasionally mucoid diarrhea to acute fulminating dysentery.[55] Infection may be diagnosed by the identification of trophozoites in fresh feces that are mixed with an equal volume of physiological saline, by staining with iodine or iron hematoxylin, or by colonic mucosal biopsy. Colonoscopy may reveal focal ulceration or diffuse mucosal friability and bleeding. The disease must be differentiated from chronic colitis as well as from other cases of dysentery such as hemorrhagic gastroenteritis and parvovirus infection. The optimal treatment is unclear, but metronidazole (30 mg/kg once a day for 7 to 10 days) appears to be the drug of choice and should be combined with appropriate supportive therapy.

Giardia canis infection is generally thought to be a disease of the small intestine. However, canine giardiasis can purportedly present as chronic ulcerative colitis.[41]

The history and clinical signs of giardia-induced colitis are similar to those of chronic colitis, and diagnosis is by detection of *Giardia canis* cysts in the feces. Giardiasis is uncommon in the cat and seems to be primarily a disease of the small intestine. However, rectal prolapse associated with severe diarrhea has been reported in one animal.[14] Treatment with quinacrine hydrochloride or metronidazole is effective. Specific therapy for chronic colitis can be given if indicated.

Balantidium coli is a protozoan that normally resides in the mucus lining the colonic mucosa. The organism produces disease in humans, pigs, and horses, and there are sporadic reports of infection in dogs.[8, 39, 52] All instances of canine infection have been associated with a concomitant severe *Trichuris* infection, with the implication that mucosal damage caused by whipworms may allow the *B. coli* to penetrate the mucosa. After penetration, proteolytic secretions of the organism cause further ulceration and extensive necrosis of the colonic mucosa.[59] Diagnosis is by identification of the organism in a fresh fecal smear. Treatment with metronidazole is reportedly effective, but elimination of *Trichuris* alone may be sufficient.

Infectious Colitis

Infectious colitis is an uncommon entity in the dog; colitis associated with infection by *Salmonella,* algae of the genus *Prototheca,* and *Histoplasma capsulatum* are the only currently recognized causes.

Salmonellosis generally presents as a generalized enterocolitis and, at least in the author's practice, is uncommon. The clinical signs, diagnosis, and treatment of salmonellosis are discussed in Chapter 8.

Protothecal infection is an extremely uncommon cause of colitis in the dog.[18, 102, 103, 105] The disease is caused by pathogenic algae of the genus *Prototheca.* The algae colonize the lamina propria and submucosa of the intestinal tract, with a predilection for the colon. The inflammatory response results in a severe transmural colitis with secondary lymphadenitis and occasional lymphangiectasia. Colonoscopy reveals thickened, corrugated, friable mucosal folds and variable ulceration.[101] Diagnosis is made either by

---

*DNP, American Cyanamid Co., Princeton, NJ.
†Panacur, American Hoechst Corp., Somerville, NJ.
‡Nemex, Pfizer, Inc., New York, NY.

detection of the organism in the feces or by biopsy. There is no reported treatment. Systemic infection with central nervous system involvement may also occur.[96]

Histoplasmosis is a chronic, systemic fungal infection that invades the body via the respiratory tract, although direct infection of the gastrointestinal tract also reportedly occurs.[32] *Histoplasma capsulatum* colonizes the intestinal lamina propria and submucosa and elicits a prominent macrophage response. Macrophages filled with the organism distend the mucosa and submucosa, causing distortion and corrugation. The affected segment of intestine becomes thickened, and the lumen is narrowed. Infiltration of the colonic wall results in a decreased ability to absorb water and electrolytes and a change in motility, both of which can result in diarrhea. The history of the dog with histoplasma-induced colitis is one of severe, chronic diarrhea and weight loss. Cough, abdominal distention, and depression also occur in disseminated disease with secondary colonic involvment; these signs are important diagnostic features in dogs with chronic diarrhea.[33, 90] Restriction of the disease to the colon is rare. The diarrhea is typical of colonic disease but is frequently profuse and watery when the small intestine is involved. Signs associated with malabsorption may also be present. Physical findings are compatible with a chronic, debilitating fungal disease; rectal examination reveals a thickened mucosa with a narrowed lumen, and the iliac lymph nodes are frequently enlarged.

Infection is best documented by colonoscopy and biopsy. The mucosa appears corrugated and ulcerated, and it has been reported that the colon does not distend readily following air insufflation.[101] Organisms may be demonstrated in the biopsy specimen or in smears made from the colonic mucosa (Fig. 9–16). Other causes of a transmural colitis, such as histiocytic ulcerative colitis, protothecal enterocolitis, granulomatous colitis, regional enteritis of the colon, and colonic lymphosarcoma,[101] should be considered and ruled out by biopsy when the lesions are restricted to the colon.

Other Chronic Inflammatory Diseases of the Colon

Granulomatous Colitis. Granulomatous colitis, or regional enteritis of the colon, which is reportedly analogous to regional enteritis of humans (Crohn's disease),[98, 101] was first described in cocker spaniels in 1954.[91] It is an uncommon disease of unknown etiology, characterized by severe patchy inflammation with extensive intestinal scar tissue formation. There is no apparent breed predilection; the disease has been described in the cocker spaniel, Weimeraner, Labrador retriever, dachshund, German shepherd, and bassett hound.[32, 75, 101] The disease has also been described in a foxhound in association with an aberrant *Trichuris* infection.[107] Most afflicted dogs are under 4 years old and there is no apparent sex predilection.

History. The dog with granulomatous co-

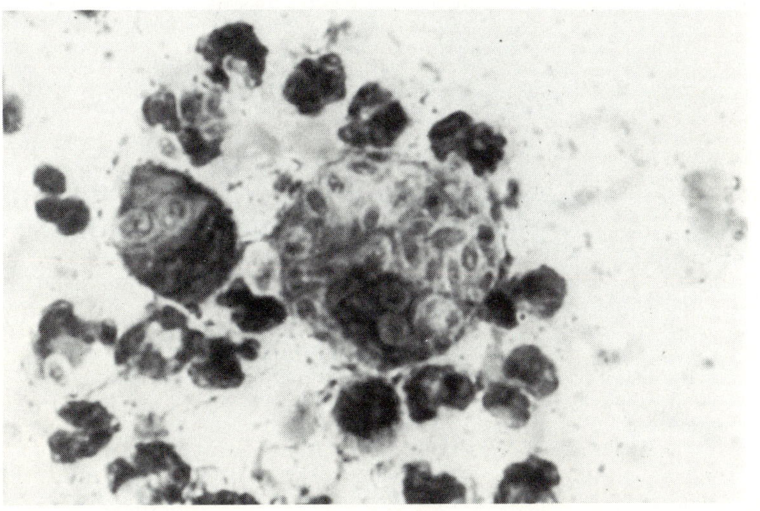

Figure 9–16. Cytological appearance of a touch preparation made from a biopsy specimen from a dog with histoplasmosis of the colon. The macrophages containing numerous *Histoplasma capsulatum* organisms are surrounded by neutrophils. (Wright's Giemsa, × 400) (Courtesy of Dr. D. J. Meyer.)

litis is usually presented with chronic, bloody, occasionally mucoid diarrhea, in conjunction with listlessness, inappetence or anorexia, and progressive weight loss. Tenesmus is also present if the distal colon and rectum are involved, and constipation rather than diarrhea may be the presenting complaint if the lesions cause a stricture of the distal rectum and anus (Fig. 9–17). Vomiting may also occur in some patients.

Physical Findings. The nature of the physical findings depends on the duration, location, and severity of the disease process. The general appearance is that of a severely sick and malnourished animal. Dehydration is common and some dogs may be febrile. Abdominal palpation may reveal thickened loops of intestine if concurrent granulomatous enteritis is present. Rectal examination may reveal strictures, a thickened mucosa, and enlarged iliac lymph nodes.

Diagnosis. The hemogram characteristically shows a mild anemia and leukocytosis with a shift to the left; an eosinophilia or monocytosis may also be present. Hypoalbuminemia and concurrent hypocalcemia are common. Colonoscopy reveals extensive granulomatous mucosal proliferation with a narrowed lumen and failure to dilate following air insufflation. The colonic mucosa appears corrugated and hyperemic, and bleeding ulcers are frequently observed. However, unlike most types of canine colitis, the whole length of the colon is not necessarily involved, and lesions are usually interspersed between relatively normal areas of colonic mucosa.

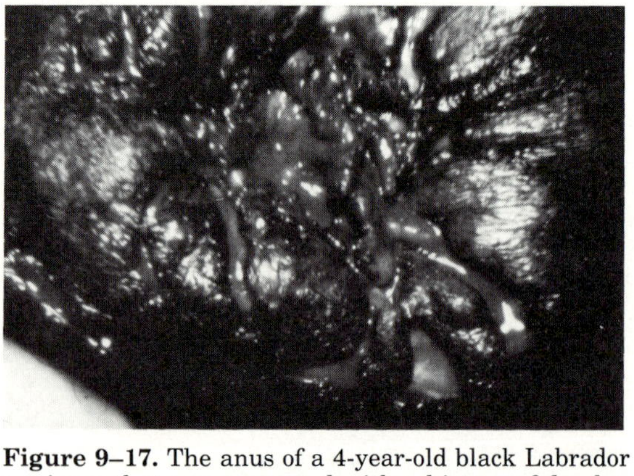

Figure 9–17. The anus of a 4-year-old black Labrador retriever that was presented with a history of dyschezia. Abdominal radiographs revealed an impacted, dilated colon, but rectal examination showed the lesion to involve only the anal sphincter. The nature and severity of the lesion were such that resection of the anus was considered the only possible choice of treatment. After surgery, the dog made an uneventful recovery and continued to work as a gundog. Histological examination of the resected material revealed changes compatible with a diagnosis of granulomatous colitis.

Contrast radiographs should be made if colonoscopy reveals a normal colon, since the lesions may involve only the terminal ileum, the ileocolic junction, or the ascending colon and may not be visible through the rigid colonoscope. Radiographs are likely to reveal a segmental constriction of the lumen with mucosal serration and ulceration. Only biopsy is diagnostic. Published reports of the histopathology describe the lesion to be characterized by ulceration of the mucosa and submucosa.[32, 75, 91, 107] These structures are edematous, with substantial infiltration of mononuclear cells, eosinophils, and polymorphonuclear leukocytes. Lymphoid nodules, granulomatous aggregates of epithelial cells, transmural fissures, and microabscesses may also be observed in the submucosa.

Treatment. Surgical excision is indicated if the lesions are sparse and localized. In other cases, corticosteroids (1 to 2 mg/kg/day) and tylosin (20 mg/kg/day), or corticosteroids and sulfasalazine (25 to 40 mg/kg TID), administered for weeks or months are reported to occasionally halt or at least to retard the progression of the disease process.[100] The prognosis is grave; complete recovery is rare and, the disease may occur even after surgical excision.

Histiocytic Ulcerative Colitis. Canine histiocytic ulcerative colitis is an extremely rare chronic inflammatory disease of the mucosa and submucosa of the intestine; it is confined almost exclusively to the boxer. It is characterized by infiltrates of large periodic acid–Schiff–positive (PAS) macrophages and progressive superficial ulceration.[49] Until recent reports of isolated cases in a French bulldog[97] and a cat,[98] the disorder had been reported only in pure-bred boxers.

Histiocytic ulcerative colitis has probably received far more attention in the literature than its incidence deserves. The disease is now much less common than it used to be and in the author's practice accounts for less than 2 per cent of all cases of colitis. The cause is unknown, but possible causes and pathogenic mechanisms have been reviewed.[59] It is probable that a genetic predisposition underlies the disease process.[78]

History. The disease affects young boxers

of either sex, with most dogs showing signs before 2 years of age. The presenting complaint is often one of bloody, mucoid diarrhea with the maintenance of overall good body condition. The appetite is usually good, and only in severe or long-standing cases do animals appear debilitated. Diarrhea is similar to that of other forms of colitis, with tenesmus becoming increasingly more frequent and severe (see Fig. 9–4A). Bloody diarrhea is more frequent in histiocytic ulcerative colitis than in most other types of colitis.

Physical Findings. Physical examination is usually unrewarding, with the dog initially appearing in good condition; weight loss and cachexia occur late in the disease. Dehydration and fever are rare but digital rectal examination may reveal a thickened and corrugated rectal mucosa.

Diagnosis. The hemogram is usually unremarkable, although some dogs may exhibit a leukocytosis and mild anemia. Examination of a fecal smear or rectal mucosal smear stained with new methylene blue reveals numerous erythrocytes and neutrophils. Colonoscopy reveals thickened mucosal folds with variable ulceration (Fig. 9–18). The findings range from mucosal hyperemia and edema to isolated or multiple strictures and deep, bleeding ulcers. Biopsy is diagnostic. Microscopically, there is thickening of the lamina propria and submucosa caused by histiocytes, plasma cells, and lymphocytes, and in some cases there is ulceration and neutrophil infiltration. The majority of the histiocytes are periodic acid–Schiff–positive; detailed histological appearances of all stages of the disease have been described.[49, 97]

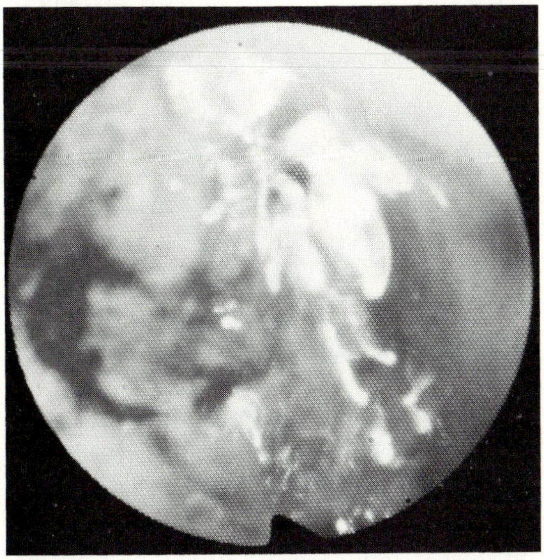

Figure 9–18. Endoscopic picture of the colon of a 2-year-old female boxer with histiocytic ulcerative colitis. Changes in the colon wall are more extensive than those seen in chronic idiopathic colitis. Areas of extensive hemorrhage and desquamated epithelium (*yellow material*) are obvious. No submucosal blood vessels are visible, and the mucosa reflects light unevenly, indicating excessive mucus secretion. See Color Plate.

Treatment. Treatment is symptomatic and never curative. It has been reported that some dogs respond to a combination of chloramphenicol and tylosin,[99] but all need life-long treatment. Sulfasalazine has also been used with moderate success, but corticosteroids, with or without antibacterial agents, seem to have little beneficial effect. The prognosis is guarded, and most patients are euthanized after an unsuccessful course of therapy.

Eosinophilic Colitis. Eosinophilic colitis is uncommon as a specific disease entity, being more commonly seen in association with eosinophilic gastroenteritis. The cause is unknown; allergy is frequently blamed but trials of elimination diets are unsuccessful and other causes or manifestations of allergic reactions are rare. The clinical signs are similar to those of chronic colitis; characteristic findings include infiltration of the colonic mucosa with eosinophils and peripheral eosinophilia. Diagnosis is made by identification of eosinophils in the rectal smear or by finding eosinophilic infiltration of the colonic mucosa in a biopsy specimen. Corticosteroids are the treatment of choice, since it is seldom possible to identify and eliminate the underlying or predisposing cause. High doses (1 to 2 mg/kg/day) of prednisolone should be given initially, and the dose gradually tapered to a maintenance level over 3 to 4 weeks. The lowest dose required to eliminate clinical signs should be identified by trial and error and should in turn be slowly tapered over 6 to 8 weeks. Relapse is uncommon when this regimen is used, but long-term steroid therapy is required in a few animals. Oral cromolyn sodium* has been used for the treatment of food allergy in humans[104] and is an approach that may merit trial in dogs that require long-term therapy. Other symptomatic and supportive treatment as described for

*Intal, Fisons Corporation, Bedford, MA.

chronic idiopathic colitis may be indicated as concurrent therapy.

Colitis Secondary To Chronic Pancreatitis. Hematochezia, diarrhea, and mucoid feces are occasional complaints in dogs suffering from subacute, recurrent, or chronic pancreatitis. The transverse colon is adjacent to the pancreas in the dog, and if pancreatitis is sufficiently severe and prolonged this portion of the colon can become involved secondarily. Colonic stenosis may occur in humans but has not been reported in the dog. Diagnosis is made from the clinical and laboratory signs and is confirmed by fiberoptic endoscopy and biopsy of the transverse colon.[1, 67] Contrast radiographs may show disease localized to the transverse colon. Treatment is based on the addition of sulfasalazine at the normal dose (25 to 40 mg/kg TID) to the treatment regimen for pancreatitis; corticosteroids are contraindicated.

Lymphocytic-Plasmacytic Colitis in the Cat. Colitis characterized by infiltration of the lamina propria with lymphocytes and plasma cells has been described in the cat.[109] These animals have typical large bowel diarrhea; small intestinal involvement is variable. It is believed that the condition is due to exposure of the immune system to dietary antigens, since diarrhea resolves when patients are fed lamb and rice, a diet to which they have not been previously exposed. Some cats are able to be maintained free from diarrhea on a commercial prescription diet.* Sulfasalazine† may be useful as adjunctive therapy.

LESS COMMON FORMS OF COLITIS

The colon is subjected to many different types of insult. The most common causes and their accompanying clinical syndromes have been described in the preceding sections. There are, however, many other causes of colonic inflammation that may result in an animal being presented with signs of colitis. Most are represented by single case reports and include: mycotic colitis, traumatic colitis, antibiotic-associated pseudomembranous colitis, self-limited proctitis, colitis of feline panleukopenia, lymphocytic mucosal colitis, and colitis cystica profunda.[12, 21, 100] In all cases, treatment is predicated on removal of any known inciting cause in conjunction with specific drug therapy, which usually includes sulfasalazine.

NON-INFLAMMATORY COLONIC DIARRHEAL DISEASE

Not all diarrhea of colonic origin is associated with inflammatory disease. About 10 to 15 per cent of dogs with chronic diarrhea in which the history apparently suggests a colonic origin have no evidence of colitis on colonoscopy or biopsy and are assumed to have a primary defect in colonic motility. The precise nature of this defect has not yet been defined; indeed, no definitive evidence for colonic motor dysfunction yet exists in the dog, but clinical experience strongly suggests that it does. The syndrome has been called irritable colon or spastic colon[59] and may be similar to human irritable bowel syndrome. This latter disease is a very common clinical disorder characterized by either diarrhea or constipation in the absence of any organic bowel disease.[86] There is evidence that abnormal myoelectrical activity produces colonic dysfunction[85] but there is still very little objective information concerning either the cause or pathophysiology of irritable bowel syndrome. It may be stress-related, since the irritable bowel syndrome is frequently associated with life-stress and emotional tension.[3]

History. Dogs with non-inflammatory colonic diarrhea are usually presented with a history similar to that of dogs with chronic colitis. Diarrhea is typically mucoid, frequently intermittent, and of long duration. Defecation, however, is seldom associated with quite the same urgency as in dogs with colitis, and defecation in the house at night is uncommon; hematochezia, tenesmus, and vomiting are rare. Many afflicted dogs also have a long history of failure to respond to various dietary changes or to conventional antidiarrheal preparations, including sulfasalazine.

The disorder appears to have a predilection for the larger breeds and may have an unusually high incidence in working dogs such as Seeing Eye, guard, and police dogs. It is helpful if an association can be made between the onset of diarrhea and changes in environment or behavior. It has been

---

*Prescription Diet C/D, Hill's Pet Products, Inc., Topeka KS.

†Azulfidine, Pharmacia Laboratories, Piscataway, NJ.

reported that signs of disease may be evident only during periods of separation from the owner or following the birth of a child in the family.[59] Afflicted dogs are not necessarily hyperexcitable or unmanageable.

Diagnosis. Afflicted dogs appear clinically normal. Until the establishment of objective diagnostic criteria, diagnosis must be made by the exclusion of organic colonic disease and other functional diarrheas. There are no hematological or blood chemical changes; microscopic examination of a fecal or colonic smear reveals an absence of the inflammatory cells and erythrocytes, and when present, parasite eggs are only an incidental finding.

A carefully taken history, including that of regular medications, is essential, since an idiosyncratic sensitivity to such drugs as styquin given on a daily basis for control of heartworms and hookworms can cause diarrhea that mimics the irritable colon syndrome.

Colonoscopic examination and biopsy are essential for diagnosis in that they rule out organic colonic disease. At colonoscopy the mucosa may appear normal but there is more often a generalized hyperemia of varying severity, together with large amounts of mucus, both adhering to the mucosa and free in the lumen. In some dogs the colonic mucosa may look extremely congested, with a purple or plum-colored appearance. Ulcers are absent, areas of petechial hemorrhage are rare, and the mucosa does not bleed when gently rubbed with the tip of the colonoscope. The colon occasionally appears hypermotile even in the heavily sedated dog, and insertion of the colonoscope and distention of the mucosa by air insufflation may be difficult, presumably because of active contraction of the smooth muscle in the colon wall.

Histological examination of colonic biopsy specimens reveals no characteristic abnormalities; the lamina propria may occasionally be reported as thickened, or the mucosa engorged with erythrocytes. The extremely congested colonic mucosa may bleed excessively after biopsy. If hemorrhage occurs it may be controlled by packing the colon with sponges soaked in epinephrine diluted 1:10,000 with saline; tranquilization with a hypotensive drug such as promazine may help reduce blood loss.

Treatment. Treatment consists of a combination of anticholinergics, sedatives, and dietary modification. An attempt should also be made to alleviate any contributing environmental factors. At this time no available treatment is curative, and the client must be advised of the probable necessity for long-term drug therapy. Anticholinergic drugs such as propantheline bromide* or clidinium bromide may be effective but may need to be combined with sedation in some patients. Darbazine† or chlordiazepoxide in combination with clidinium bromide‡ appears to be effective for long-term regulation of the syndrome, but no controlled studies of the efficacy of these drugs have been carried out. Phenobarbital or chlorpromazine is also useful in excessively nervous dogs, especially before periods of anticipated stress.

The addition of fiber in the form of coarse bran (2 to 5 tablespoons per can of food) or a commercial cellulose preparation§‖ (1–2 tablespoons per can of food) to the diet of dogs suffering from irritable colon helps to alleviate diarrhea. Fiber is currently of considerable public and scientific interest because inadequate intake has been associated with a number of common human diseases,[16] some of which are associated with abnormal colonic motor activity,[76] including the irritable bowel syndrome.[61]

Dietary fiber decreases colonic motility in the dog.[18] A low-fiber diet has been recommended for the treatment of gastrointestinal disturbances,[4] and increasing fecal bulk has been advocated as a treatment for both diarrhea and constipation in the dog.[92] Sterculia gum, a bulking agent with the capacity to absorb large amounts of water, reportedly has the same effect.

Prognosis. The prognosis is guarded, inasmuch as treatment is symptomatic and may be needed for the remainder of the patient's life. Clients are much more likely to accept this situation if the nature of the disease is adequately explained and will stop moving from one veterinarian to another in the hope of obtaining a more successful treatment and favorable prognosis. Some clients find it difficult to accept that their pet's problem may be attributable, either directly or indirectly, to their relationship with the animal.

---

*Quarzan, Roche Laboratories, Nutley, NJ.
†Darbazine, Norden Laboratories, Lincoln, NB.
‡Librax, Roche Laboratories, Nutley, NJ.
§Metamucil, Searle Laboratories, Chicago, IL.
‖Siblin, Parke-Davis, Morris Plains, NJ.

Colonic Diseases with Constipation and Dyschezia as the Principal Signs

There are a large number of colonic and rectal diseases that may, either directly or indirectly, cause constipation and dyschezia, including colonic impaction, idiopathic megacolon, anal stricture and spasm, perineal hernia, perianal fistula, anal sac disease, and pseudocoprostasis (See Table 9–4).

COLONIC IMPACTION

When mixed with feces, many undigested materials form hard masses, which the animal finds difficult to eliminate, and impaction of the colon with a mixture of feces and ingested hair is probably the most common cause of constipation in the dog and cat. The incidence of colonic impaction increases with age, with the feeding of highly digestible (low-residue) diets, and with co-existing, painful anorectal disease.

Impaction is more common in the cat, presumably because this species is observed to defecate less frequently and because of its tendency to ingest hair during the grooming process. It is a recurrent problem in some apparently susceptible animals, especially the long-haired breeds, and may lead to the development of secondary megacolon.

Any lesion that obstructs the normal passage of feces or that causes pain on defecation can cause secondary colonic impaction. Such lesions include rectal stricture, colonic tumor, rectal tumor, perineal hernia, rectal foreign bodies, perianal fistula, anal sac disease, prostatic hypertrophy, and a narrowed pelvic canal following a fractured pelvis.

History. The animal with colonic impaction is usually presented with a history of failure to defecate for days to weeks. The client may have observed the animal making frequent unsuccessful attempts to defecate and, in some cases, to have passed small amounts of liquid feces, often containing blood or mucus, with a great deal of straining. Such animals may be presented with a spurious complaint of diarrhea. If defecation has not been observed, the patient may be presented only because it is dull, listless, inappetent or anorexic, or vomiting intermittently.

Diagnosis. Animals with colonic impaction may appear depressed and are often dehydrated. Mucous membranes may be hyperemic and the coat may have a dull unkempt appearance. Cats may adopt a crouching, hunched attitude indicative of abdominal discomfort. Obvious abdominal distention is occasionally observed, and abdominal palpation usually reveals a hard fecal mass that may fill the whole length of the colon. Digital rectal examination usually reveals an empty rectum with an accumulation of very hard feces at the pelvic rim. Rectal examination combined with abdominal palpation is useful in localizing the fecal mass and in identifying any underlying lesion such as a rectal foreign body, prostatic hypertrophy or a narrowed pelvic canal. Rectal sacculation or dilation may also be identified by digital examination, even if obvious signs of perineal hernia are

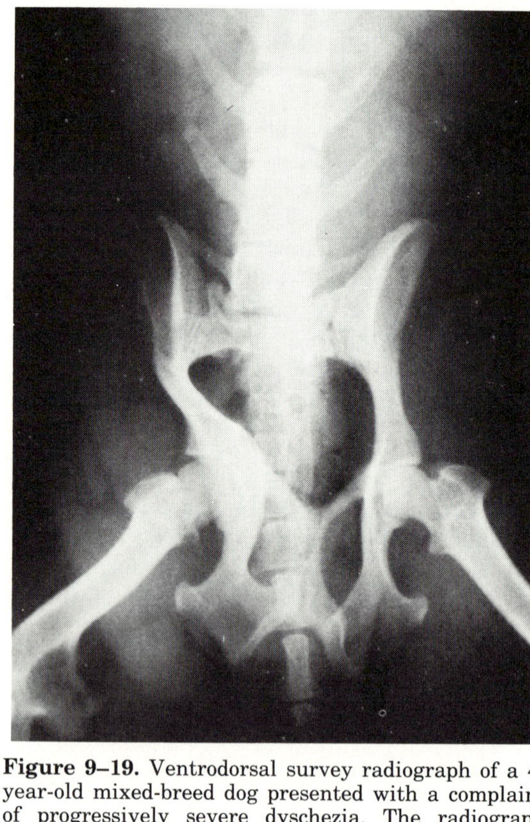

Figure 9–19. Ventrodorsal survey radiograph of a 4-year-old mixed-breed dog presented with a complaint of progressively severe dyschezia. The radiograph showed an old pelvic fracture that had healed with displacement. The dog had suffered a pelvic fracture when hit by a car 13 months previously. Rectal examination revealed a hard bony mass in the right ventral pelvis, which caused rectal deviation and extraluminal obstruction to the passage of feces. Surgical realignment of the pelvis was considered impractical, and fecal softeners (bran) methylcellulose and bisacodyl were prescribed. These resulted in decreased dyschezia, but signs recurred when therapy was withdrawn; such clients are now resigned to long-term medical therapy.

absent. Abdominal survey radiographs confirm the presence of colonic dilation and impaction in some instances and may reveal its cause (Figs. 9–19 and 9–20).

Treatment. Treatment of colonic impaction consists of gentle removal of fecal concretions and, if possible, of identification and removal of any underlying cause. Breakdown and removal of fecal masses impacted in the colon should be accomplished as slowly and gently as possible. It is less traumatic for the patient if the feces are softened and removed over 2 to 4 days than if removal of all feces is attempted at one time. The severely constipated animal is often cachexic and dehydrated and may need corrective fluid and electrolyte therapy before any attempt can be made to remove the impaction.

Impaction can be treated with oral laxatives, with enemas, or by manual removal of fecal material with the patient under general anesthesia following administration of enemas and laxatives. Simple impaction of relatively short duration is best treated by oral administration of lubricants such as mineral oil. This can be given either alone or in combination with dioctyl sodium sulfosuccinate (DSS)* at a total dose of 10 to 50 mg per patient. DSS, which is both a wetting agent and a colonic irritant, acts to stimulate colonic secretion;[34] therefore, the patient must be well hydrated before compounds containing this substance are administered.

Another useful irritant laxative is bisacodyl; this compound exerts its action on colonic mucosal nerve plexuses. Stimulation is reportedly segmental and axonal, producing contraction of the entire colon independent of resting tone. The compound is supplied in 5-mg tablets—1 tablet is usually sufficient for a cat or small dog and 2 to 4 tablets for larger dogs.

In severely constipated patients it may be necessary to manually remove fecal concretions piece by piece with the aid of a small pair of whelping forceps or sponge forceps.

After initial relief, attention must be directed to the prevention of recurrence. If appropriate, bones should be eliminated from the diet, regular grooming should be instituted, and the opportunity should be provided for regular defecation. Prevention of recurrence may be difficult in patients with long-standing impaction that have developed secondary megacolon. In all instances the therapeutic goal should be to have the patient form soft feces and defecate regularly. To this end, fecal bulking and

*Colace, Mead Johnson & Company, Evansville, IN.

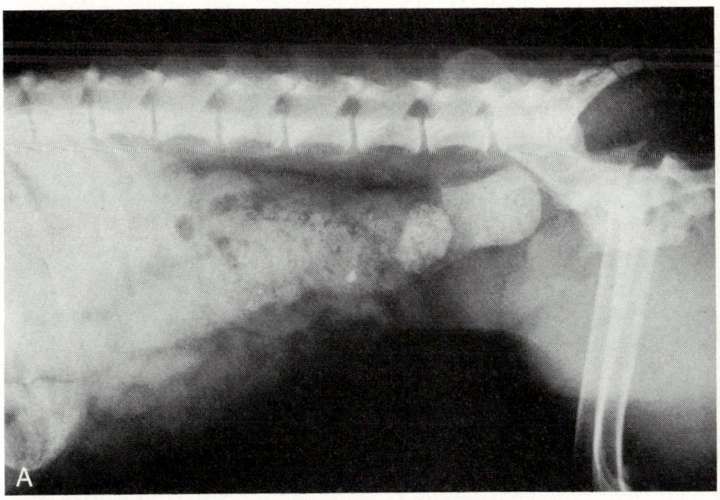

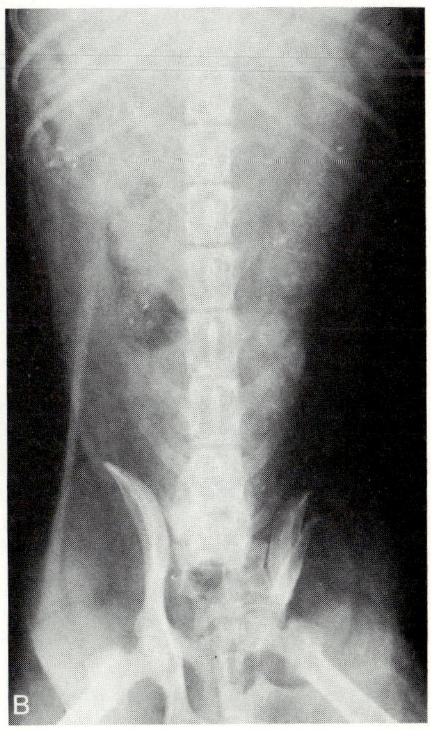

Figure 9–20. *A* and *B*, lateral and ventrodorsal radiographs of colonic impaction secondary to a fractured pelvis. A pelvic fracture in a 3-year-old golden retriever 7 days after being hit by a car. Pelvic displacement was minimal, and cage rest was the recommended treatment. Even though no neurological defects were found, the dog had neither stood nor defecated since the accident. Enemas relieved the colonic impaction; fecal softeners were prescribed, and support of the caudal abdomen with a sling during urination and defecation was recommended. This treatment resulted in the passage of soft feces, and an uneventful recovery.

softening agents containing methylcellulose, psyllium hydrophilic mucilloid, bisacodyl, or DSS can be added to the diet; fiber supplements in the form of bran (2 to 4 tablespoons per 14 oz can of food) are also useful, but low-residue diets are contraindicated. Commercial veterinary laxatives containing petrolatum as the active ingredient are useful for preventing hair impaction in cats.

IDIOPATHIC MEGACOLON

Primary or idiopathic megacolon is more common in the cat than in the dog but is an unusual cause of constipation in either species. The cause is unknown but is perhaps related to a degeneration or relative absence of myenteric ganglion cells in the colonic wall. The disorder has erroneously been called Hirschsprung's disease, a human disorder that is diagnosed in childhood and is caused by the absence of ganglion cells in a constricted but otherwise normal distal rectal segment. In idiopathic megacolon, fecal material is unable to pass through the aganglionic segment, and feces gradually distend the proximal colon, causing severe constipation. Also, the internal anal sphincter functions abnormally in Hirschsprung's disease.[94] The absence of ganglion cells in the colon and abnormal anal sphincter function have not yet been documented to occur concurrently in either the dog or cat.

History. Idiopathic megacolon may occur in the cat at any time after approximately 5 years of age. Afflicted cats are usually presented with a history similar to that described for colonic impaction. Depression, loss of appetite, and occasional vomiting are the common complaints. The disease is insidious in onset and seemingly progressive in nature, since recurrent episodes of constipation of increasing severity and frequency may occur before their significance is realized.

The disease is extremely rare in the dog but the presenting history is similar to that in the cat.

Diagnosis. Most afflicted cats are depressed and have an unkempt appearance. The rectum is usually found to be empty and dilated on digital examination, but a mass of hard feces is usually felt at the pelvic inlet. Abdominal palpation usually confirms the presence of a large colonic fecal mass, although survey abdominal radiographs help to differentiate it from alimentary lymphosarcoma (Fig. 9–21).

Treatment. Treatment is the same as for colonic impaction. Preventive measures are needed for the duration of the animal's life and include dietary modification and the regular administration of laxatives such as bisacodyl. The diet should include laxative foods such as raw liver, and bulking agents such as methylcellulose or bran.

Idiopathic megacolon is a very difficult disease to manage, and most clients eventually tire of the continued need for laxatives and enemas and request euthanasia. Surgical resection of the atonic colon has been described and is now the treatment of choice when colonic dilatation appears irreversible.[42, 108] Cats appear to do extremely well after colectomy; most cats pass normal feces after anastomosis of the distal ileum colon to the rectum. The disease, however, is always associated with a guarded prognosis, and the client must be warned of the necessity for persistence with preventive and long-term therapeutic measures.

COLONIC PERFORATION

Resulting as it so frequently does in acute peritonitis, septic shock, and death, colonic perforation is, fortunately, a rare event. Perforation has a variety of causes, including trauma, biopsy procedures, erosion by tumors, and the administration of high doses of corticosteroids to animals that have undergone a neurosurgical procedure.[95] Perforation commonly follows colonic biopsy or neurosurgery with corticosteroid therapy.

Perforation of the colon releases fecal contents containing large numbers of bacteria into the abdominal cavity. Bacterial proliferation and the subsequent release and uptake of bacterial toxins cause acute peritonitis and the rapid deterioration of the patient. Death results from a combination of septic and hypovolemic shock.

Signs of perforation are associated with acute peritonitis and include abdominal pain, fever, vomiting, and diarrhea that is often bloody; in rare instances perforation may result in constipation. Signs of septic and hypovolemic shock may be the first evidence of perforation in dogs receiving high doses of corticosteroids. Bleeding may be an indication of perforation in dogs that have undergone a colonic neurosurgical procedure, and all patients so far reported in

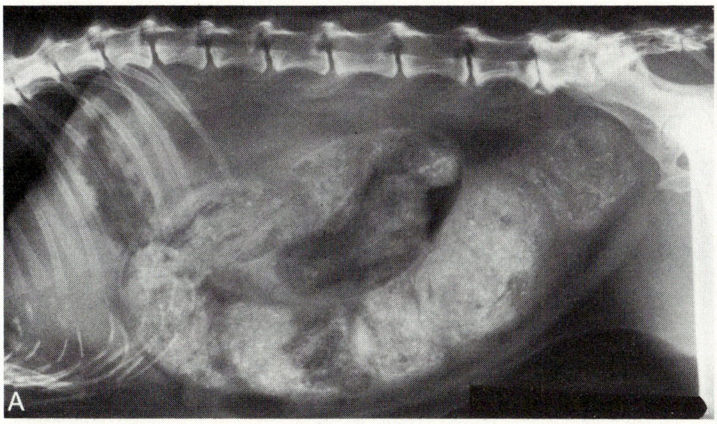

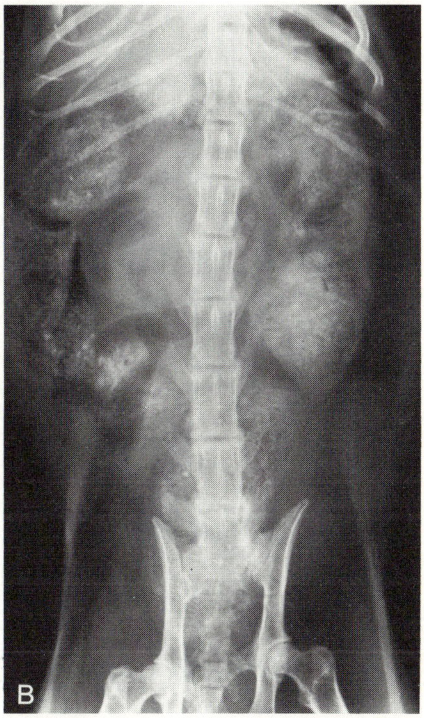

Figure 9–21. Lateral *(A)* and ventrodorsal *(B)* radiographs of a 6-year-old cat with a 2-year history of constipation. Radiographs show colonic impaction with secondary megacolon. The ventrodorsal radiograph reveals evidence of previous pelvic damage. Enemas and stool softeners prescribed on an intermittent basis over the previous two years had failed to permanently resolve the problem. The colonic impaction shown in the radiographs was relieved by means of multiple saline enemas administered during a three-day period. A more vigorous regimen of dietary modification and fecal softeners was then prescribed. This treatment resulted only in temporary improvement, and the cat underwent colonic resection. After surgery the cat passed four to six soft bowel movements per day, but the frequency of defecation decreased to two per day over a four-week period. The owner now describes defecation as normal and the problem appears to have been resolved. This reveals the practical value of colectomy in the treatment of megacolon.

this category have died.[95] In all these animals perforation occurred in the proximal descending colon at the site where the vagal and lumbosacral parasympathetic innervations overlap. The possible etiological implications of this observation, however, remain to be elucidated.

Laboratory studies in afflicted dogs reveal a leukocytosis and a left shift that may be degenerative; serum lipase and amylase activities may be elevated owing to the escape of fecal contents and reabsorption of luminal enzymes into the circulation. Survey abdominal radiographs reveal free air in the abdominal cavity together with other signs of peritonitis. Peritoneal lavage is diagnostic in animals whose signs may be depressed or altered by high doses of corticosteroids.

The major differential diagnosis is acute pancreatitis, but other causes of acute peritonitis must also be considered.

Treatment is surgical; in most instances the patient is stabilized and treated for shock before laparotomy, surgical repair of the colon, and extensive abdominal lavage.

The prognosis depends on the underlying cause. It ranges from good in perforation associated with biopsy procedures to grave in dogs in the corticosteroid-neurosurgical group.

References

1. Abcarian H, Eftaiha M, Kraft AK, Nyhus LM: Colonic complications of acute pancreatitis. Arch Surg 114:995, 1979.
2. Aguirre G: Letter to the editor. J Am Vet Med Assoc 162:8, 1973.
3. Almy TP: Wrestling with the irritable colon. Med Clin North Am 62:203, 1978.
4. Amand WB: Diet and gastrointestinal problems. *In* Kronfeld DS (ed): *Canine Nutrition*. University of Pennsylvania, Philadelphia, 48, 1972.
5. Ammon HV, Phillips SF: Inhibition of colonic water and electrolyte absorption by fatty acids in man. Gastroenterology 65:744, 1973.
6. Anderson NV: Biopsy of the gastrointestinal system. Vet Clin North Am 4:317, 1974.
7. Argenzio RA: Physiology of diarrhea—large intestine. J Am Vet Med Assoc 173:667, 1978.
8. Bailey S, Williams AG: Balantidium infection in the dog. J Am Vet Med Assoc 115:238, 1949.
9. Banta CA, Clemens ET, Krinsky MM, Sheffy BE:

Sites of organic acid production and patterns of digesta movement in the gastrointestinal tract of dogs. J Nutr 109:1592, 1979.
10. Binder HJ: Net fluid and electrolyte secretion: The pathophysiologic basis for diarrhea. *In: Mechanisms of Intestinal Secretion.* Alan R. Liss, Inc., New York, 1, 1979.
11. Binder HJ: Fecal fatty acids—mediators of diarrhea? Gastroenterology 65:847, 1973.
12. Bolton GR, Brown TT: Mycotic colitis in a cat. Vet Med (Small Anim Clin) 67:978, 1972.
13. Bortoff A: Myogenic control of intestinal motility. Physiol Rev 56:418, 1976.
14. Brightman AH, Slonka GF: A review of five clinical cases of giardiasis in cats. J Am Anim Hosp Assoc 12:492, 1976.
15. Bueno L, Garcia-Villar R, Ruckebusch Y: Electrical colonic activity in the conscious dog. Seances Acad Sci [III] 285:1463, 1977.
16. Burkitt DP: Epidemiology of large bowel disease: The role of fibre. Proc Nutr Soc 32:145, 1973.
17. Burrows CF: Chronic diarrhea in the dog. Vet Clin North Am Small Anim Pract 13:521, 1983.
18. Burrows CF, Merritt AM: Influence of alpha-cellulose on myoelectrical activity of the proximal canine colon. Am J Physiol 245:9301, 1983.
19. Burrows CF: Diarrhea and constipation. *In* Ettinger SJ (ed): *Textbook of Veterinary Internal Medicine,* 2nd ed. W. B. Saunders Company, Philadelphia, 56, 1982.
20. Burrows CF, Kronfeld DS, Banta CA, Merritt AM: Effects of fiber on digestibility and transit time in dogs. J Nutr 112:1726, 1982.
21. Burrows CF: Diseases of the colon and anorectum in the dog and cat. *In* Anderson NV (ed): *Veterinary Gastroenterology.* Lea & Febiger, Philadelphia, 553, 1980.
22. Burrows CF, Merritt AM, Chiapella AM: Determination of fecal fat and trypsin output in the evaluation of chronic canine diarrhea. J Am Vet Med Assoc 174:62, 1979.
23. Canfield PJ, Bennett AM, Watson ADJ: Large intestinal biopsies from normal dogs. Res Vet Sci 28:6, 1980.
24. Cello JP, Meyer JH: Ulcerative colitis. *In* Sleisenger MH, Fordtran JS (eds): *Gastrointestinal Disease,* 2nd ed. W. B. Saunders Company, Philadelphia, 1597, 1978.
25. Chambers TJ, Morson BC: Large bowel biopsy in the differential diagnosis of inflammatory bowel disease. Invest Cell Pathol 3:159, 1980.
26. Chiapella AM, Burrows CF: The effect of feeding on the myoelectrical activity of the canine colon. (abst.) Gastroenterology 78:1150, 1980.
27. Christensen J: Myoelectric control of the colon. Gastroenterology 68:601, 1975.
28. Christensen J: Colonic motility. *In* Duthie HJ (ed): *Gastrointestinal Motility in Health and Disease.* University Park Press, Baltimore, 367, 1972.
29. Christensen J, Weisbrodt NW, Hauser RL: Electrical slow wave of the proximal colon of the cat in diarrhea. Gastroenterology 62:1167, 1972.
30. Connell AM: Motility of the pelvic colon. II. Paradoxical motility in diarrhea and constipation. Gut 3:342, 1962.
31. Das KM, Sternlieb I: Salicylazosulfapyridine in inflammatory bowel disease. Am J Dig Dis 20:971, 1975.
32. Dibartola SP, Rogers WA, Boyce JT, Grimm JP. Regional enteritis in two dogs. J Am Vet Med Assoc 181:904, 1982.
33. Ditchfield WJB: Mycotic disease. *In* Catcott EJ (ed): *Canine Medicine.* American Veterinary Publications, Inc, Santa Barbara, 172, 1968.
34. Donowitz M, Binder HJ: Effect of dioctylsodium sulfosuccinate on colonic fluid and electrolyte movements. Gastroenterology 60:941, 1975.
35. Duff WM: Intracellular recordings of slow waves from inflamed smooth muscle of the colon. (Abstr) Gastroenterology 72:1052, 1977.
36. Edmunds CJ, Pilcher D: Electrical potential difference and sodium and potassium fluxes across rectal mucosa in ulcerative colitis. Gut 14:784, 1973.
37. Elliot TR, Barclay-Smith E: Antiperistalsis and other muscular activities of the colon. J Physiol 31:272, 1904.
38. El-Sharkaway TY, Bardakjian BL, MacDonald WM, Diamont N: Origins of the multiple patterns of electrical control activity in the colon. *In* Wienbeck WM (ed): *Motility of the Digestive Tract.* Raven Press, New York, 491, 1982.
39. Ewing GO, Aldrete AV: Canine giardiasis presenting as chronic ulcerative colitis: A case report. J Am Anim Hosp Assoc 9:52, 1973.
40. Ewing GO, Gomez JA: Canine ulcerative colitis. J Am Anim Hosp Assoc 9:395, 1973.
41. Ewing SA, Bull RW: Severe chronic canine diarrhea associated with Balantidium–trichuris infection. J Am Vet Med Assoc 149:519, 1966.
42. Fellenbaum S: Partial colectomy in the treatment of recurrent obstipation/megacolon in the cat. Vet Med/Small Anim Clin 73:737, 1978.
43. Fennell C: The use of sterculia gum for controlling intestinal tone in the dog and cat. J Sm Anim Pract 17:543, 1976.
44. Fioramonti J, Garcia-Villar R, Bueno L, Ruckebusch Y: Colonic Myoelectrical activity and propulsion in the dog. Dig Dis Sci 25:641, 1980.
45. Frizzell RA, Schultz SG: Models of electrolyte absorption and secretion by gastrointestinal epithelia. *In* Crane RK (ed): *Gastrointestinal Physiology III.* University Park Press, Baltimore, 205, 1978.
46. Giller J, Phillips SF: Electrolyte absorption and secretion in the human colon. Am J Dig Dis 17:1003, 1972.
47. Goldman P, Peppercorn MA: Sulfasalazine. New Engl J Med 293:20, 1975.
48. Gomez JA: The gastrointestinal contrast study. Vet Clin North Am 4:805, 1978.
49. Gomez JA, Russell SW, Trowbridge JO, Lee J: Canine histiocytic ulcerative colitis. Am J Dig Dis 22:485, 1977.
50. Goodman MJ, Kirsner JB, Riddell RH: Usefulness of rectal biopsy in inflammatory bowel disease. Gastroenterology 72:952, 1972.
51. Harris JC, Dupont HL, Hornick RB: Fecal leukocytes in diarrheal illness. Ann Intern Med 76:697, 1972.
52. Hayes FA, Jordan HE: Canine helminthiasis complicated with Balantidium species. J Am Vet Med Assoc 129:161, 1956.
53. Hayslett JP, Halevy J, Pace PE, Binder HJ: Demonstration of net potassium absorption in mammalian colon. Am J Physiol 242:G209, 1982.

54. Herschel DA, Argenzio RA, Southworth M, Stevens CE: Absorption of volatile fatty acid, Na, and H_2O by the colon of the dog. Am J Vet Res 42:1118, 1981.
55. Jordan HW: Amebiasis *(Entamoeba histolytica)* in the dog. Vet Med/Small Anim Clin 67:61, 1967.
56. Kasper J, Chiapella AM: Gastrointestinal biopsy. *In* Kirk RW (ed): *Current Veterinary Therapy VIII*. W. B. Saunders Company, Philadelphia, 962, 1980.
57. Krejs GL, Fordtran JS: Physiology and pathophysiology of ion and water movement in the human small intestine. *In* Sleisenger MH, Fordtran JS (eds): *Gastrointestinal Disease,* 2nd ed. W. B. Saunders Company, Philadelphia, 297, 1978.
58. Krook A, Danielsson D, Kjellander J, Jarnerot G: The effect of metronidazole and sulfasalazine on the fecal flora in patients with Crohn's Disease, Scand J Gastroenterol 16:183, 1981.
59. Lorenz MD: Diseases of the large bowel. *In* Ettinger SJ (ed): *Textbook of Veterinary Internal Medicine,* 2nd ed. W. B. Saunders Company, Philadelphia, 1346, 1983.
60. MacPherson BR, Shearin NL, Pfeiffer CJ: Experimental diffuse colitis in cats: Observations on motor changes. J Surg Res 25:42, 1976.
61. Manning AP, Heaton KW, Harvey RF, Uglow P: Wheat fibre and the irritable bowel syndrome. A controlled trial. Lancet 2:417, 1977.
62. Mekhjian HS, Phillips SF: Perfusion of the canine colon with unconjugated bile acids: Effects of water and electrolyte transport, morphology and bile acid absorption. Gastroenterology 59:120, 1970.
63. Merritt AM: Gastrointestinal function testing. *In* Anderson NV (ed): *Veterinary Gastroenterology*. Lea & Febiger, Philadelphia, 247, 1980.
64. Merritt AM, Burrows CF, Cowgill LD, Street W: Quantitation of canine fecal fat and trypsin output from normal dogs on a meat-base or cereal-base diet. J Am Vet Med Assoc 174:59, 1979.
65. Migasena S, Gilles HM, Maegraith BG: Studies in *Ancylostoma caninum* infection in dogs II. anatomical changes in the gastrointestinal tract. Ann Trop Med Parasitol 66:203, 1972.
66. Miller WE, Christensen GC, Evans HE: *Anatomy of the Dog*. W. B. Saunders Company, Philadelphia, 1964.
67. Negro P, De Bernardinis G, Tuscano D et al: Stenosis of the colon following pancreatitis. Ital J Gastroenterol 10:241, 1978.
68. O'Brien TR: Large intestine. *In: Radiographic diagnosis of Abdominal Disorders in the Dog and Cat*. W. B. Saunders Company, Philadelphia, 352, 1978.
69. Phillips SF, Devroede GJ: Function of the large intestine. *In* Crane RK (ed): *Gastrointestinal Physiology III*. University Park Press, Baltimore, 263, 1979.
70. Phillips SF, Gaginella TS: Intestinal secretion as a mechanism in diarrheal disease. *In* Glass GBT (ed): *Progress in Gastroenterology III*. Grune and Stratton, New York, 481–504, 1977.
71. Phillips SF, Giller J: The contribution of the colon to electrolyte and water conservation in man. J Lab Clin Med 81:733, 1973.
72. Phillips SF: Absorption and secretion by the colon. Gastroenterology 56:966, 1969.
73. Polish EO: The pathophysiology of common gastrointestinal symptoms. *In* Brooks FP (ed): *Gastrointestinal Pathophysiology*. Oxford University Press, New York, 7, 1974.
74. Rask-Madsen J, Jensen B: Electrolyte transport capacity and electrical potentials of the normal and the inflamed human rectum in vivo. Scand J Gastroenterol 8:169, 1973.
75. Rechenberg VR: Enteritis regionalis beim Hund. Monats Vet Med 29:352, 1974.
76. Reilly RW, Kirsner JB (eds): *Fiber Deficiency & Colonic Disorders*. Plenum Publishing, New York, 1975.
77. Rubens RD, Lambert HP: The homeostatic function of the colon in acute gastroenteritis. Gut 13:915, 1972.
78. Russell SW, Gomez JA, Trowbridge JO: Canine histiocytic ulcerative colitis. Lab Invest 25:509, 1971.
79. Sherding RG: Canine large bowel diarrhea. Comp Contin Ed 2:279, 1980.
80. Shindel NM, Van Kruiningen HJ, Scott FW: The colitis of feline panleukopenia. J Am Anim Hosp Assoc 14:738, 1978.
81. Sleisenger MH: Clinical pharmacology. *In* Sleisenger MH, Fordtran JS (eds): *Gastrointestinal Disease*. W. B. Saunders, Philadelphia, 418, 1973.
82. Smith FW, Sleisenger MH: Physiology of the colon. *In* Sleisenger MH, Fordtran JS (ed.): *Gastrointestinal Disease,* 2nd ed. W. B. Saunders Company, Philadelphia, 1523, 1979.
83. Snape WJ, Shiff S, Cohen S: Effect of deoxycholic acid on colonic motility in the rabbit. Am J Physiol 238:G321, 1980.
84. Snape WJ, Matarazzo SA, Cohen S: Abnormal colonic myoelectrical and motor responses to eating in ulcerative colitis (Abstr). Gastroenterology 74:1978.
85. Snape WJ, Carlson GM, Matarazzo SA, Cohen S: Evidence that abnormal myoelectrical activity produces colonic motor dysfunction in the irritable bowel syndrome. Gastroenterology 72:383, 1977.
86. Snape WJ, Carlson GM, Cohen S: Colonic myoelectric activity in the irritable bowel syndrome. Gastroenterology 70:326, 1976.
87. *Stedman's Medical Dictionary,* 24th Ed. Williams & Wilkins Company. Baltimore, 1982.
88. Stevens CE: Comparative physiology of the digestive system. *In* Swenson MJ (ed): *Physiology of domestic animals*. Cornell University Press, Ithaca, NY, 1977.
89. Stewart JJ, Bass P: Effects of ricinoleic and oleic acids on the digestive contractile activity of the canine small and large bowel. Gastroenterology 70:371, 1976.
90. Stickle JE, Hribernik TN: Clinicopathological observations in disseminated histoplasmosis in dogs. J Am Anim Hosp Assoc 14:105, 1978.
91. Strande A, Sommers SC, Petrak M: Regional enterocolitis in cocker spaniel dogs. Arch Path 57:357, 1964.
92. Strombeck DR: Dietary management of gastrointestinal problems. *In* Kronfeld DS, Low DA (eds): *Diet and Disease in Dogs*. University of California, 1975.
93. Strombeck DR: *Small Animal Gastroenterology*. Stonegate Publishing, Davis, CA, 1979.
94. Tobin F, Reid NCRW, Talbert JL, Schuster MM: Non-surgical test for the diagnosis of Hirschsprung's disease. N Engl J Med 278:188, 1968.
95. Toombs JP, Caywood DD, Lipowitz AD, Stevens

JB: Colonic perforation following neurosurgical procedures and corticosteroid therapy in four dogs. J Am Vet Med Assoc 177:68, 1980.
96. Tyler DE, Lorenz MD, Blue JL, et al: Disseminated protothecosis with central nervous system involvement in a dog. J Am Vet Med Assoc 176:987, 1980.
97. Van der Gaag I, Van Toorenburg J, Voorhart G, et al: Histiocytic ulcerative colitis in a French bulldog. J Small Anim Pract 19:283, 1978.
98. Van Kruiningen HJ, Dobbins WO: Feline histiocytic colitis. Vet Pathol 16:215, 1979.
99. Van Kruiningen HJ: Letter to the editor. J Am Anim Hosp Assoc 10:210, 1974.
100. Van Kruiningen HJ: Canine colitis comparable to regional enteritis and mucosal colitis of man. Gastroenterology 62:1128, 1972.
101. Van Kruiningen HJ, Hayden DW: Interpreting problem diarrheas in dogs. Vet Clin North Am 2:29, 1972.
102. Van Kruiningen HJ: Protothecal enterocolitis in a dog. J Am Vet Med Assoc 157:56, 1970.
103. Van Kruiningen HJ, Garner FM, Schiefer B: Protothecosis in a dog. Path Vet 6:348, 1969.
104. Vaz GA, Ton LKT, Gerard JW: Oral cromoglycate in treatment of adverse reaction to foods. Lancet 1:1066, 1978.
105. Weaver AD: Differential diagnosis of tenesmus in the dog. J Small Anim Pract 15:609, 1974.
106. Wienbeck M, Christensen J, Weisbrodt NW: Electromyography of the colon in the unanesthetized cat. Am J Dig Dis 17:356, 1972.
107. Widmer WR, Van Kruiningen HJ: Trichuris-induced transmural ileo-colitis in a dog, an entity mimicking regional enteritis. J Am Anim Hosp Assoc 10:581, 1974.
108. Yoder JT, Dragstedt LR, Starch CJ: Partial colectomy for correction of megacolon in a cat. Vet Med/Small Anim Clin 63:1049, 1968.
109. Nelson RW, Dimperio ME, Long GG: Lymphocytic-plasmacytic colitis in the cat. J Am Med Assoc *184*:1133, 1984.

CHAPTER

10

Surgery of the Large Bowel

C. W. BETTS

Surgery of the large bowel has been performed more frequently and with greater success as our diagnostic acumen and surgical prowess have improved. Because of this increasing sophistication and greater client awareness, the veterinarian should be familiar with available techniques. Complications arising during surgery on the large bowel are often serious, thus there is the need for strict attention to the techniques of aseptic surgery and preservation of the blood supply.

Preoperative Considerations

Ongoing investigation in human surgery has documented the value of antibiotic prophylaxis.[16, 17, 40, 51, 84] However, controversy exists as to the ideal agent or combination of agents, the duration of therapy, and the route of administration. A preparation of neomycin and erythromycin* given orally the day before surgery provides adequate intestinal antisepsis without the hazards of prolonged preoperative administration.[52, 84] A combination of oral preoperative and parenteral perioperative antibiotics is more effective than oral antibiotics alone.[51] Using a cephalosporin or gentamicin† parenterally provides protection against any gram-negative organisms that may develop resistance to the oral antibiotic.[51] For select, uncomplicated procedures, such as simple biopsy, preoperative antibiotics are not necessary.[61] Vigorous mechanical cleansing of the bowel reduces the total number of microorganisms and should be combined with antibiotic prophylaxis.[16] Several warm-water or Fleet enemas* may be necessary.

When feasible, the animal should be fed an easily digested, low-residue diet that contains minimal fat[77] for 3 to 4 days prior to bowel preparation. In humans, cleansing enemas are recommended approximately 36 hours prior to surgery, and they should be continued until no solid feces are returned. A 10 per cent Betadine solution is easily prepared, well tolerated, and quite effective as an enema preparation.[6] A liquid diet with supplemental intravenous fluid should be considered for the day prior to surgery. Potassium levels should be evaluated before anesthesia is given, especially in animals that have had chronic mucinous diarrhea or several cleansing enemas. The sodium-potassium-ATPase system is stressed by malabsorption and diarrhea, and a 5 to 10 per cent decrease in total body potassium occurs postoperatively.[53] Preoperative antibiotics, if used, should be started approximately 12 to 16 hours before surgery. On the day of surgery the animal should be taken outside to defecate prior to administration of medication for anesthesia.

Along with the change in emphasis on antibiotics, new suture materials are avail-

*Neomycin Sulfate Tablets, 20 mg/kg QID/OS. Eli Lilly and Company, Indianapolis, IN.

Erythromycin (Erythrocin), 10 mg/kg TID. Abbott Pharmaceuticals, North Chicago, IL.

†Cephalexin (Keflex), 20 to 22 mg/kg TID or 30 to 33 mg/kg BID. Eli Lilly and Company, Indianapolis, IN.

Gentamicin (Gentocin), 4 mg/kg IM or SQ BID × 1 day, then 2.2 mg/kg IM, SQ, or IV TID. Schering Corporation, Kenilworth, NJ.

*Fleet enema, C.B. Fleet Co., Inc., Lynchburg, VA.

able that are superior to chromic gut. Several factors determine the desirability of a suture material: (1) its initial tensile strength, (2) the rate of gain of tissue strength, and (3) the interaction between the suture and the tissue. The tensile strengths of 3/0 polyglactin 910* (4.8 lb) and polyglycolic acid suture† (3.9 lb) are slightly greater than those of chromic gut (3.8 lb) of the same size.[19] Gut approximates the new absorbable synthetic sutures in rate of strength loss, although synthetic polymer sutures may perform better because of higher initial tensile strength. A polydioxanone suture‡ has superior long-term tissue breaking strength and the advantage of being a monofilament, synthetic absorbable suture. The mechanism of absorption contributes to the duration of suture strength. Gut, an animal protein, is subject to dissolution by proteolytic enzymes liberated by the inflammatory process around the suture. The synthetic polymers are hydrolyzed, a slower process that occurs at the same rate in all tissues. Gastrointestinal secretions dissolve gut in 1 week, whereas a polyglycolic acid suture and polyglactin 910 remain invulnerable for at least 3 weeks. In the stomach and duodenum, absorption of gut occurs within 1 day when it is exposed to intraluminal contents.[19]

The strength of the suture material holding the intestinal ends in apposition and the strength of the normal tissue on either side determine the integrity of the anastomosis in the first 3 to 5 days. A comparison of colonic anastomoses done with different suture materials showed that chromic gut, polyglycolic acid suture, and braided silk cause considerable damage to the submucosa when passed through the tissue. Polypropylene suture§ and Teflon-coated braided Dacron‖ caused minimal damage; however, the Teflon coat flaked off in places, providing access to the interstices of the Dacron for bacteria. Hairline cracks were shown on the knot with Prolene, possibly reducing its tensile strength. Numerous small blood vessels course through the collagen network of the submucosa, and distortion of the tissue may damage or compress these vessels, with secondary damage to the submucosa and mucosa through ischemia. Suture material causing less tissue damage is more conductive to wound healing.[56] Polyglactin 910 was not evaluated.

WOUND HEALING

Fortunately, the colon has a very rapid system of wound healing. Postinjury bursting strength returns to normal in 5 to 7 days.[78] There is some controversy about the role of new and old collagen in the healing process.[78] Collagen lysis takes precedence over synthesis during the first postoperative days owing to rapid breakdown and turnover of insoluble collagen. The breaking strength of the anastomosis is lowest on the 3rd to 4th postoperative day, but by the 7th day synthesis exceeds lysis and strength returns rapidly.[44, 45] Total colonic collagen mass does not seem to decrease because of the injury, but edema and extravasated proteins may decrease the collagen concentration. It has been established that new collagen, represented by acute, labeled ^{3}H-hydroxyproline, is formed close to the site of injury and is limited to that area.[78]

The submucosa of the colon consists of long, thin plates of collagen. When viewed under a scanning electron microscope, these plates may appear moth-eaten owing to the disappearance of the submucosal collagen after incision of the colon, hypoxia, and repeated anesthesia. In this instance, lysis of collagen occurs without synthesis of new collagen, and the anastomosis may fail. In contrast, when healing occurs normally, a new network of disorderly collagen fibers covers and adheres to the existing orderly submucosal fibers. The new fibers intersperse between the plates and span the tissue gap. A battle then ensues between lysis, which causes reduced tensile strength, and new collagen synthesis, which increases strength. The final determinant of these cellular activities is circulation.[71]

Preserving the blood supply and avoiding tension on the suture line are tenets for successful wound healing. The cardinal rule is not to suture ischemic tissue.[71] In large bowel surgery, particularly anastomoses, consequences of wound dehiscence are disastrous. A recent study showed a significant incidence of anastomotic leakage in rectal resections when the middle hemorrhoidal vessels were sacrificed and no leakage when the vessels remained intact. These results

---

*Vicryl Sutures, Ethicon, Inc., Somerville, NJ.
†Dexon, Davis and Geck, American Cyanamid Co., Pearl River, NY.
‡PDS, Ethicon, Inc., Somerville, NJ.
§Prolene, Ethicon, Inc., Somerville, NJ.
‖"Silky" II Polydek Deknatel, Queens Village, NY.

were somewhat influenced by the increased technical difficulty of handling a distal anastomosis in which the vessels must be sacrificed rather than the more proximal resection in which the blood supply can be preserved. A supplemental measure of documented benefit is to protect the incision by securing the omentum to the surgery site. Free omental grafts provide no significant mechanical protection, however, because revascularization is delayed.[28] Marlex mesh* is highly effective in sealing the suture line but it is imperative that minimal contamination occurs.[37] Peritonitis and death are potential complications of significant leakage and contamination.

In recent years, a one-layer technique for small bowel anastomosis has gained popularity in human and veterinary surgery. The one-layer technique is now being advocated for large bowel anastomosis.[33, 46, 50, 67] This technique causes less tissue trauma and disturbance of circulation, and improves anatomical precision and speed.[46] Also, experimental evidence favors the one-layer method because it causes a small reduction in luminal diameter, decreases tissue strangulation, and increases anastomotic strength after the 5th postoperative day.[50] Histologically, mucosal continuity and muscle realignment occur more rapidly.

A comparison of an end-to-end simple interrupted crushing suture pattern and an end-to-end, interrupted, inverting suture pattern using 3/0 polyglycolic acid suture material yielded similar clinical results.[67] The inverting pattern produced a 63 per cent loss of lumen diameter compared with 30 per cent loss from the crushing pattern, but no clinical significance was noted. Normal bursting pressures were present 28 days after surgery with the inverting pattern, but anastomoses using the crushing technique were significantly weaker. However, histologically, the end-to-end, crushing pattern had less inflammatory response, the mucosa had bridged the anastomotic site, the remaining layers were becoming aligned, and minimal fibrous tissue proliferation was noted. The anastomotic site where the inverting pattern was used did not have a mucosal bridge, a bud of granulation tissue was present, and a marked inflammatory cell response and fibrous tissue proliferation were seen.

*Marlex Mesh, Bard Implants Division, C. R. Bard Inc., Billerica, MA 01821.

Mechanical stapling devices are available for colorectal surgery.[23, 49, 52, 86] A comparative study of the GIA stapler* and an end-to-end two-layer technique in 242 human patients using 3/0 chromic and 3/0 silk or cotton suture materials for colonic anastomoses by experienced surgeons established that operating time, return of intestinal activity, and length of the postoperative hospital stay were not significantly affected by the anastomotic technique.[70] For low colorectal anastomoses, the EEA stapling device† is considered superior to hand sewing because of the inherent technical advantage.[52] A potential advantage of the use of the EEA stapler for low anastomoses in animals with suitable lesions is that there is no need for a protective colostomy.[86]

Whether a suture or stapling technique is used, clean bowel ends are important, especially with low anastomosis. The integrity of the anastomosis can be checked by instilling fluid into the rectum or by insufflating air into the rectum with lavage fluid covering the anastomotic site.[52]

Postoperative wound dehiscence is always a major concern. Traumatized animals undergoing large bowel surgery are at higher risk for anastomotic leakage because of depressed circulation and less collagen synthesis. They need antibiotic coverage. The nutritional status of the postoperative patient, especially one with chronic disease and inanition, may contribute to poor wound healing. The importance of vitamins and minerals for wound healing should not be ignored.[71]

Failure of the anastomosis, in most cases, can be avoided by adherence to sound surgical principles. Guidelines for large bowel surgery are as follows:

1. Preoperative mechanical cleansing of the bowel.
2. Preoperative and intraoperative antibiotics followed by only 1 or 2 days of postoperative antibiotic therapy if the recovery is routine.
3. Preserve adequate blood supply to involved tissue.
4. Minimize fecal spillage and contamination by using fluid-resistant drapes, and discard soiled instruments, gowns, and gloves after the bowel is closed.
5. When signs of peritoneal or systemic

*GIA, United States Surgical Corporation, New York, NY.

†EEA Stapler, United States Surgical Corporation, New York, NY.

infection appear, diligently search for the source using abdominal paracentesis and lavage and survey and contrast radiography. Surgical exploration should be performed early; antibiotics are not a substitute for drainage.

6. Promptly discontinue ineffective antibiotics; avoid nephrotoxic antibiotics in critically ill patients.

7. Use the most conservative surgical steps in high-risk patients.[18]

HISTORY

An accurate history and knowledge of breed predilections will aid in establishing a diagnosis of large bowel disease. Although the age, breed, and disposition of the dog should be considered, certain symptoms are significant in any animal. It is important to first establish whether a small or large bowel problem is present. The absence of vomiting and the retention of appetite associated with diarrhea, tenesmus, and dyschezia are indicative of large bowel problems. Melena usually indicates gastric or small bowel hemorrhage; frank blood clots, and hemorrhage are more characteristic of large bowel disease. The presence of large amounts of mucus in or coating the stool reflects irritation and inflammation of the large bowel.

The onset, duration, and severity of the signs should be well defined. Tenesmus of several weeks' duration with increasing severity would be suggestive of intussusception in a young dog, whereas the same history in an old dog could be associated with a perineal hernia or a colonic or rectal tumor. Breed predilection would support the suspicion of perianal fistulas in an adult German Shepherd. The cardinal signs of colonic disease are tenesmus, high-frequency, low-volume defecation, and the presence of mucus and blood in the stool.[48]

PHYSICAL EXAMINATION

All dogs should be given a thorough general physical examination prior to examination of the large bowel. In old dogs, careful scrutiny for primary tumors or metastatic lesions that are causing the large bowel signs is important. In young dogs, a second congenital lesion may be found, which could influence the overall prognosis or the client's desire to maintain the animal.

Careful palpation of the abdomen is essential. One should take note of any abnormal masses, unusually large amounts of fluid or gas in the intestines, or colonic impaction. Sensitivity to or resentment of abdominal palpation must be interpreted in terms of the dog's personality.

Rectal palpation should always be done as part of the physical examination and is usually well tolerated if done properly. The client should stand at the animal's head to provide assurance and a well-trained assistant should restrain the dog. It is preferable for the dog to be standing while a gloved, well-lubricated index finger is gently inserted into the rectum. The perineum and anus should be inspected immediately prior to rectal examination to minimize the dog's discomfort. The tail should be gently elevated no higher then necessary for visual inspection and finger insertion. During rectal examination, the tail should be released and the free hand used simultaneously to palpate the caudal abdomen. Palpation of the abdomen is often revealing, particularly when the prostate gland is being examined. One should also assess the degree of discomfort exhibited and check carefully for dyssymmetry in bony or soft tissue architecture. Fecal flotation is done if a sufficient amount of stool is extracted, and the fecal material on the glove is examined for blood, mucus, or foreign material. If further diagnostic studies are necessary or if in-patient therapy is required, the animal should be hospitalized and samples should be collected for a data base.

Data Base

For any animal admitted to the hospital a minimum data base appropriate to its age, condition, and possible mode of therapy should be established. The data base includes a determination of packed cell volume and plasma total solids, a check for microfilaria, a urinalysis and a fecal flotation for young healthy animals. A complete blood count and serum chemistry profile are added for serious cases and older patients.

The data base can be expanded as necessary. Lesions palpable through the rectum can be directly examined with the aid of an anoscope or proctoscope. Such a procedure may require sedation or general anesthesia. The latter should not be performed without prior assessment of the laboratory profile and physical findings to determine anesthetic risk. In the interim, the animal can be prepared for survey radiographs. Warm-

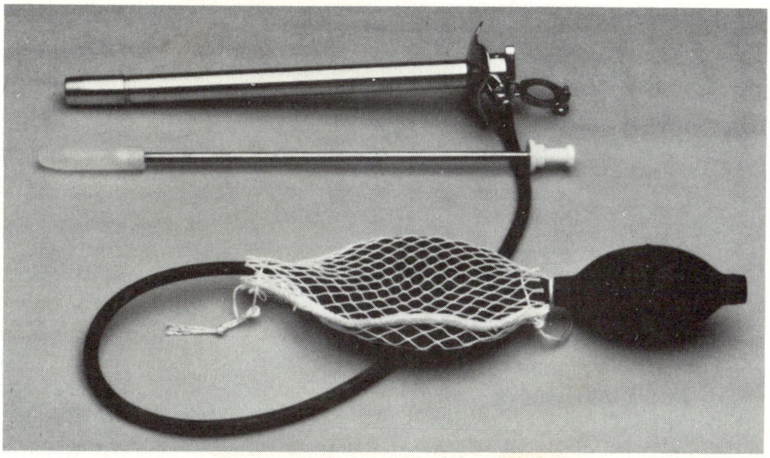

Figure 10–1. Colonoscopy can be performed using an 11 mm to 23 mm by 25 cm rigid proctoscope. This proctoscope has a magnifying lens, an obturator that is removed once the scope is inserted, and an inflation bulb.

water enemas are usually sufficient to stimulate evacuation of the fecal mass. Animals with an electrolyte imbalance or dehydration should not be given enemas, satisfactory cleansing may be achieved by administration of 1 tablet given orally (do not dissolve or crush) of bisacodyl* for dogs up to 22 or 23 kg, or two tablets if the animals are larger. The medication is given in the afternoon or evening and the radiographs are taken the following morning. Food (but not water) should be withheld that evening. Correction of fluid and electrolyte imbalance should be initiated concurrently.

If an intramural or intraluminal lesion is suspected after survey radiography, proctoscopic or endoscopic examination should be done prior to contrast studies. If the contrast studies are done first, the lesion may become coated with barium, which may cause misinterpretation of the results. For lesions in the anorectum, an anoscope or vaginal speculum with a suitable light source is sufficient for the examination. An otoscope may be more appropriate for very small animals. Lesions of the descending colon are best seen through a rigid proctoscope. The rigid proctoscope has been very satisfactory for lesion evaluation and biopsy procedures (Fig. 10–1). The flexible endoscope (Fig. 10–2) is used to evaluate and biopsy more proximal lesions, but the quantity of biopsy tissue that can be obtained is limited. The flexible fiberoptic sigmoidoscope has proved to be vastly superior to the rigid sigmoidoscope (proctoscope) in human patients, in that its accuracy is two or three times greater in diagnosis and removal of polyps and surveillance of the colon for cancer.[59] Because of the instrument's flexibility and length,

*Dulcolax, Boehringer Ingelheim, Ridgefield, CT.

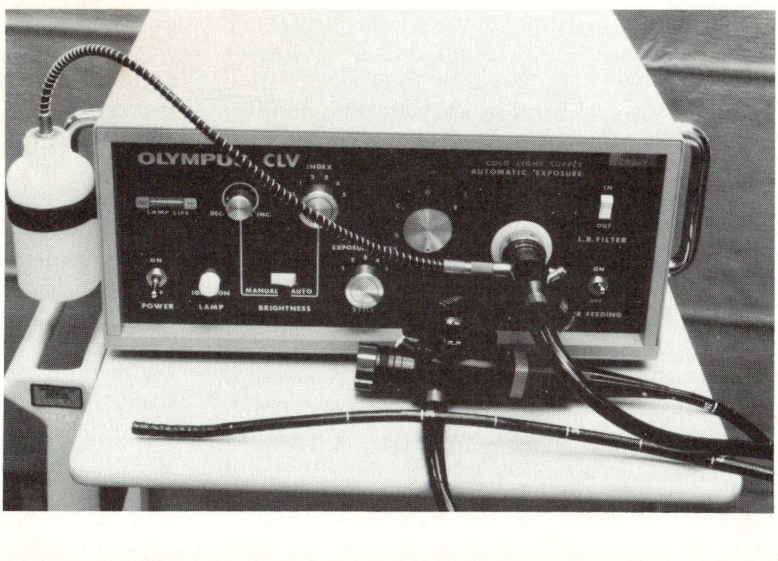

Figure 10–2. A flexible fiberoptic endoscope with a light source is an excellent instrument for colonoscopy and colonic biopsy.

total colonic surveillance is possible, markedly increasing the detection of synchronous (occurring at the same time) and metachronous (occurring at different times) lesions.[48, 66] In a study of 157 human cancer patients who underwent 175 colonoscopic procedures, 13.6 per cent of the cancers were missed on double-contrast barium enema examination.[66] Flexible fiberoptic colonoscopy is indicated for diagnosis, surveillance, and therapy. Use of the rigid scope is indicated for delineation and localization of lesions of the rectum and descending colon. Because the rigid sigmoidoscope is marked in centimeter increments the examiner is able to make critical rectal measurements. The flexible sigmoidoscope has 5-cm increments. Both can be used for surveillance of disease states or anastomoses, for rectal biopsy, and for rectal or descending colon polypectomy in animals.[59] A representative biopsy specimen may enable one to render a diagnosis and prognosis of sufficient accuracy to preclude surgical intervention in poor-risk patients.

To reiterate, a thorough history and physical examination in conjunction with laboratory and radiographic evaluation provide the subjective and objective data bases. Having sufficient data to generate an accurate assessment, one can formulate an appropriate plan for the problem.

Surgical Diseases of the Large Bowel

DISEASES OF THE CECUM

Cecal disease occurs infrequently but warrants consideration because surgery may be the definitive treatment. Clinical conditions affecting the cecum are typhlitis, inversion (invagination), impaction, dilation, and neoplasia.[14, 20, 34, 36, 55] The client may report that the dog has exhibited any of the following signs: depression, anorexia, vomiting, weight loss, tenesmus, and diarrhea with or without melena.[20, 41]

Abdominal tenderness may be present with inflammatory lesions. A mass palpated to the right of and cranial to the umbilicus may be suggestive of cecal involvement. The ileocecocolic region is a common site for intussusception. This is primarily a problem in young dogs with characteristic palpable definition. Whipworms reside in the cecum and large bowel, and a fecal examination should always be part of the data base. Although whipworm infestation responds well to modern anthelmintics, a severe or unresponsive case might warrant typhlectomy.

Survey radiographs may confirm the presence of a mass or intussusception involving this region of the bowel. Dilation of the cecum may be present with inflammatory disease along with radiographic evidence of ileus.[41] A barium enema may be necessary to define the cecum, and a double-contrast study may provide additional detail.[34] The cecocolic area can be examined endoscopically. Foreign body impaction rarely occurs but will usually be evident on palpation and on radiography.

The clinical interpretation of the disease should always be based on evaluation of all established parameters. Disease is indicated by the presence of a palpable lesion in the region of the cecum. This diagnosis is reinforced by radiographic evidence and a correlative history. The animal's general condition also should be assessed by physical examination and laboratory evaluation.

With the exception of whipworm infection, medical therapy seldom cures cecal disease. Surgical intervention is indicated for most problems and may be necessary for diagnosis as well as therapy in some cases.

Treatment

Typhlotomy. Typhlotomy for cecal impaction and cecal biopsy can be done with the same ease and confidence of success as the more familiar enterotomy of the small bowel. With the dog under general anesthesia, a caudal, ventral midline incision is made starting at the umbilicus. Incision length should be sufficient to allow easy placement of moistened laparotomy pads and a Balfour self-retaining retractor. After the cecum, which should be in the right caudal quadrant, is located, it should be isolated; the mesentery of the descending colon should be draped over the small intestine and the cecum should packed off with laparotomy pads moistened with warm saline or lactated Ringer's solution. The addition of Betadine solution to a warm lavage solution at a dilution of 1:20 is recommended for application to the exposed bowel and the laparotomy pads to prevent drying of the tissue and to minimize the effect of minor contamination. Stay sutures help provide stability and should be placed a sufficient distance apart on the antimesenteric border to allow an adequate incision into the cecum. A linear incision is made parallel to the long axis of the cecum. A stab incision is used to enter the lumen and the incision is lengthened with Metzenbaum scissors. Any contaminated debris is gently removed with a moistened sponge. Foreign material is removed with a forceps, and the interior surface of the cecum is inspected. If a biopsy is needed, a suture should be placed in a through-and-through fashion between the stay sutures. Then an elliptical piece of tissue that extends through all layers is removed by sharp dissection around the suture (Fig. 10–3). This technique eliminates distortion of the tissue by thumb forceps. The excised tissue, with the suture, is placed in formalin. Wound closure is identical to that for the typhlotomy and biopsy incisions.

The wound can be closed with the conventional two-layer, inverting suture pattern. However, no problems have been encountered with the use of a one-layer, simple interrupted, full-thickness pattern with 3/0 to 4/0 polypropylene or nylon* sutures on a tapered needle placed 3 to 6 mm apart. Additional sutures should be placed if leakage results from the movement of bowel contents into the cecum. The tissue is gently irrigated with antiseptic solution since contamination should be minimal. The laparotomy pads are removed and counted, and the cecum is replaced within the abdominal cavity. Omentum should be draped over the cecum before the abdomen is closed. A routine closure of the abdominal wall is done with polyglycolic acid suture material, polyglactin 910, or polydioxanone suture material. If contamination was excessive, monofilament stainless-steel wire (3/0 to 2/0) or polypropylene (2/0 to 0) might be used for average-sized to large dogs.

*Ethilon, Ethicon, Inc., Somerville, NJ.

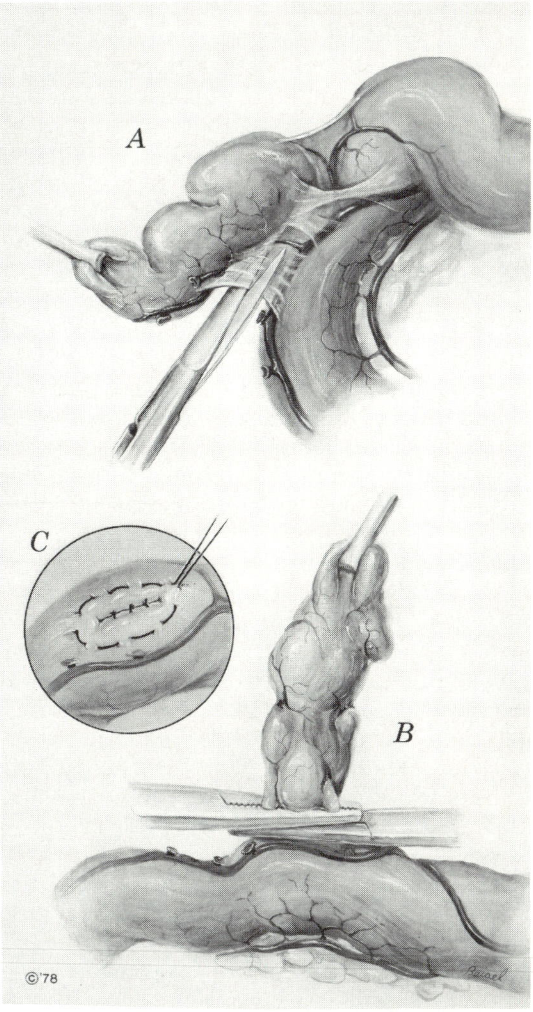

Figure 10–4. Typhlectomy procedure.

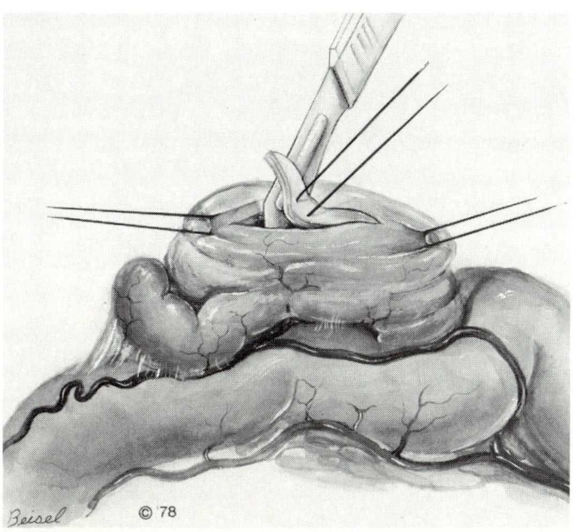

Figure 10–3. The location and technique for typhlotomy or cecal biopsy.

Typhlectomy. Typhlectomy may be the definitive treatment for typhlitis, cecal inversion, and neoplasia. The precautionary measures used for isolation of tissue, control of contamination, and prevention of tissue drying apply to removal of the cecum the same as for typhlotomy. The cecum is freed from its colonic attachment by gentle soft-tissue dissection of the peritoneal reflection. The vascular supply, which arises from the ileocecal artery, is double-ligated and divided between ligatures as close as possible to the cecum (Fig. 10–4*A*). Once the cecum is completely mobilized, the base is double-clamped, the cecum is excised between the clamps, and the cecocolic valve area is inverted with a Parker-Kerr closure over the remaining clamp (closest to the colon) using 3/0 to 2/0 polyglycolic acid or polyglactin 910 suture (Fig. 10–4*B*). Chromic gut or polydioxanone suture materials may be preferred for this suture pattern because they cause less suture drag. An alternative method that has simplistic appeal involves: (1) isolation of the cecum as described, (2) placement of simple, interrupted sutures at the oral and aboral edges of the cecocolic orifice, and (3) excision of the cecum. The wound in the colon is then closed with through-and-through, simple, interrupted sutures of gut, polyglycolic acid or polyglactin 910. If inadequacy of tissue closure is suspected, an additional suture line is placed, using a continuous Lembert or a purse-string pattern (Fig. 10–4*C*).

Postoperative Management. The animal should be checked carefully for fever, peritonitis, overt abdominal pain, depression, and anorexia. These complications may warn of possible wound dehiscence. Small amounts of food should be offered several times a day, starting 12 to 24 hours after surgery. A normal feeding routine can be resumed 2 to 3 days after surgery. Free access to water is allowed after recovery from anesthesia. Small amounts of water should be given frequently to prevent overindulgence and regurgitation.

Recent evidence supports the use of short-term preoperative oral antibiotics only.[16, 84] A combination of neomycin and erythromycin is recommended.

DISEASES OF THE COLON AND RECTUM

Intussusception

The ileocolic region is the most common site of intussusception.[87] For a complete discussion of this problem see Chapter 8.

Torsion of the Colon

Colonic torsion results in rapid deterioration of the affected animal and requires immediate surgical intervention. Torsion occurs when the bowel twists on its long axis. Torsion is not possible without a tear in the mesocolon. The subjective signs are consistent with an "acute abdomen." The finding of a painful mass in the caudal abdomen and the radiographic evidence of enlargement of the colon from gas or fluid that ends abruptly at the pelvic inlet provide evidence of colonic torsion.[21] A complete data base should be obtained as quickly as possible because it is informative; however, its absence does not justify a delay in therapy.

An aggressive plan that directs full attention to combating shock and toxemia is essential. There are many anesthetic and surgical parameters to consider in devising this plan, but a minimum of shock-level fluid therapy and a high dose of broad-spectrum antibiotics are mandatory. Surgical correction usually involves a colectomy because of tissue ischemia secondary to the torsion. The procedure is described later in this chapter. If the bowel appears viable, reduction of the torsion and colopexy are sufficient.

Megacolon

Megacolon was originally described in 1691 as a postmortem finding. The pathological changes and clinical picture were not delineated until Hirschsprung, in 1886, defined the problem as an agangliogenesis in the dilated area of colon. In 1948, it had become apparent that the aboral undilated segment was the problem, and Swenson and Bill pioneered a successful surgical technique for correction of the disease with experimental work on dogs.[58] This technique has become known as a "pull-through" and has been successfully adopted for use in human and veterinary surgery.

History. Cases resembling congenital megacolon or Hirschsprung's disease in animals are seen occasionally, but actual Hirschsprung's disease has not been documented. The majority of animals have acquired the disease secondary to pelvic fracture, obstructive disease, or pica. The history is consistent with that of any cause of constipation or terminal bowel blockage; a variety of signs can be noticed by the clients. Tenesmus is reported most commonly, in addition to diarrhea, which is often accompanied by abdominal distention and vomiting. As the disease progresses, the animal becomes unthrifty and inappetent. Animals with congenital megacolon manifest these symptoms at a very early age.

Physical Examination. The distinguishing feature found on physical examination is a large, dilated colon that is full of feces and often palpable in its entirety. Other physical parameters may be normal, depending on the duration of the disease. Documentation of the diagnosis is provided by cleansing enemas, proctoscopy, barium enema, and rectal biopsy. Theoretically, the histological findings should distinguish acquired from true or congenital megacolon in that there should be an absence of ganglia from Meissner's and Auerbach's plexuses in the involved segment.

Pathophysiology. If there is no evidence for acquired megacolon (narrowed pelvic canal from trauma, a stricture of the colon or rectum by scar tissue, or an obstructive lesion such as a tumor or congenital anorectal lesions), the diagnosis is congenital megacolon, although the disease entity seen in humans is not well documented in animals.

The pathophysiology of congenital megacolon in humans (Hirschsprung's disease) results from abnormal innervation of the distal bowel beginning at the internal anal sphincter and extending proximally for varying distances. The basic histological finding is the absence of ganglia from Meissner's and Auerbach's plexuses in the involved segment. When ganglia are absent, there are large nerve trunks lying between the circular and longitudinal muscles.[58] Staining for acetylcholinesterase to identify cholinergic nerves and the use of the catecholamine fluorescent techniques to recognize adrenergic nerves have provided new insight into the pathophysiology of Hirschsprung's disease.[42]

Surgery. In acquired megacolon, the underlying cause must be dealt with. The innervation of the bowel should be normal unless atonicity from chronic dilation develops. In one study, after the cause (e.g., scar tissue, narrowed pelvic canal) was removed or corrected, linear excision of redundant colon to construct a smaller lumen was recommended,[54] but partial colectomy is a more effective procedure.[54]

A variety of procedures have been used in children. The original pull-through procedure is recommended, but it is technically demanding and requires a team effort. The procedure is also applicable for low colonic or rectal neoplasms.

Pull-through Procedure. Preoperative preparation with cleansing enemas, diet restriction, and antibiotics is essential. The dog is positoned in dorsal recumbency with the hind legs slightly flexed and abducted. Well-monitored and assisted inhalation anesthesia with adequate fluid therapy is advised. The abdomen and perineum are clipped and prepared, then draped separately. A ventral, midline incision is made from the midabdomen to the pubic brim by the abdominal team. Balfour retractors are used to enhance exposure, and the small bowel and omentum are packed-off cranially with warm, saline-moistened laparotomy pads. The descending colon is mobilized and the funnel-shaped transition zone from proximal, normal to dilated bowel is identified (Fig. 10–5*A*). The bowel is divided in the transitional zone between intestinal clamps and is oversewn with a Parker-Kerr pattern using 2/0 to 3/0 chromic gut (Fig. 10–5*B*). The multifilament, synthetic, absorbable sutures are less satisfactory for this pattern because of tissue drag.

Traction is applied to the dilated bowel to facilitate dissection. The rectum should be freed by blunt dissection as far into the pelvic canal as possible. Electrocautery can be used judiciously to control hemorrhage. The major part of the dilated bowel is removed by incising between the clamps, and the stumps are then oversewn. Every attempt must be made to preserve the blood supply by ligating the branches of the left colic artery as close to the colon as possible. The two ends of the bowel are tied together with silk sutures (Fig. 10–5*C*). In congenital megacolon, the surgeon must examine a frozen section to confirm that the aganglionic bowel has been removed and that the ends to be anastomosed have normal-appearing innervation, or the problem will recur.

A member of the team working from the anus passes a long Allis tissue clamp into the rectal pouch, clamps the inverted tissue of the stump, and everts the distal segment, simulating a prolapse. Simultaneously, the surgeon working in the abdomen guides the attached proximal segment into the prolapsed distal segment, creating an intussusception (Fig. 10–5*D*). Any mesenteric or peritoneal attachments that create tension must be released to avoid compromising the blood supply. If the rectal segment has been sufficiently freed, the mucocutaneous junction is easily prolapsed and grasped through the dilated anal orifice. The everted rectal mucosa is cleansed with sterile saline, and an incision is made into the rectum parallel to the anal ring approximately 1 to 2 cm from the mucocutaneous junction. The silk sutures are grasped and the proximal segment of the bowel is exteriorized through

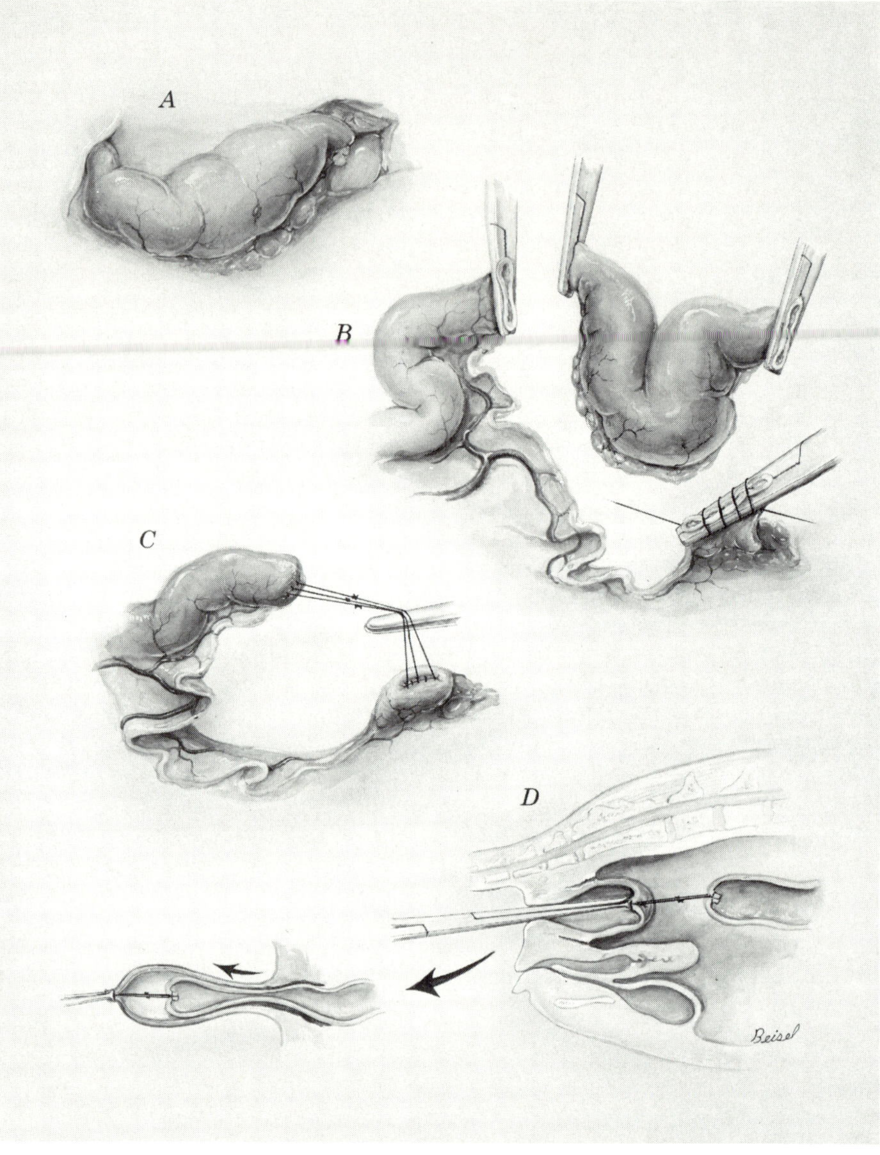

Figure 10–5 ABCD. Pull-through procedure.

the rectal cuff. The proximal segment should descend 2 to 3 cm beyond the rectal cuff without tension. Additional release of the bowel and its mesentery is necessary if tension is required to maintain the proximal segment in this position.

The outer wall of the colon is now sutured to the adjacent seromuscular layer of the anorectum with simple, interrupted sutures of 4/0 to 6/0 polyglycolic acid or polyglactin 910 (Fig. 10–5*E*). The stitches are placed 3 to 5 mm apart. As the suture line progresses, the initial anorectal incision is extended. At the conclusion of the seromuscular suture line, the intussuscepted end of the proximal bowel is excised and the mucosal layers, separated by the intervening seromuscular layers, are closed with simple, interrupted, 3/0 to 4/0 polyglycolic acid or polyglactin 910 sutures. These sutures should be placed in order to include some submucosa (Fig. 10–5*F*). The everted anastomosis is gently reduced (Fig. 10–5*G*). The abdominal closure is routine.

Postoperative Management. Antibiotics should be continued for 3 to 5 days, and the animal should be carefully monitored for wound dehiscence. Leakage at the an-

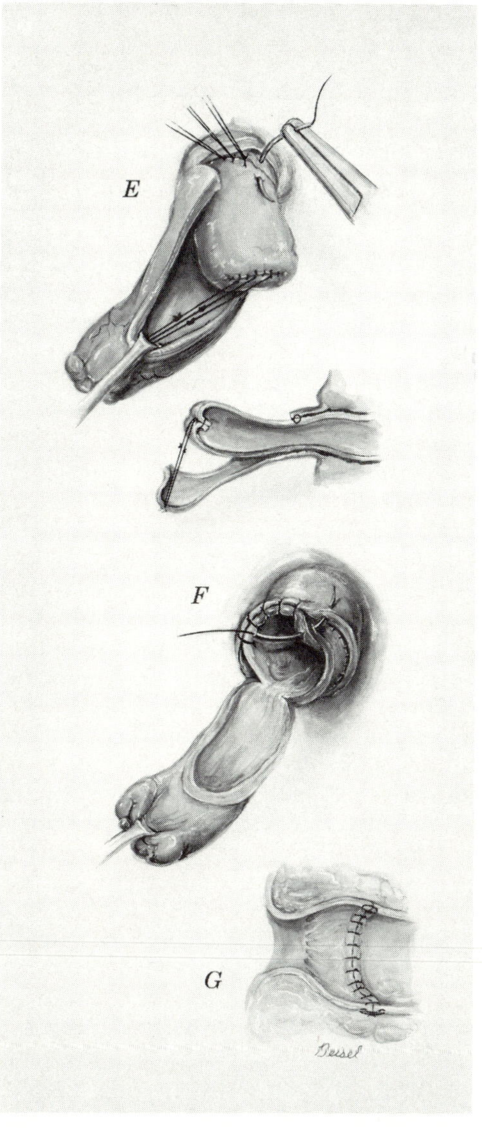

Figure 10–5 EFG. Pull-through procedure continued.

astomotic line may result in a perirectal abscess that can be drained either through the perineum, or abdominally if it is located cranial to the perirectal fossa. If major complications arise, the need for reoperation must be determined. Peritonitis must be treated vigorously to prevent septic shock. Failure to preserve the blood supply and failure to eliminate tension on the anastomotic line are the most common causes of wound disruption.

Water consumption is encouraged 4 to 6 hours after surgery, with supplemental parenteral fluid therapy provided as needed. Feeding should resume with the return of intestinal peristalsis in 48 to 72 hours. A highly digestible low-residue diet* (i/d) that assures an easily eliminated stool is needed. Stool softeners† should be used if tenesmus occurs.[63]

A modification of the classic Swenson's technique has been used successfully in cats for very low rectal lesions.[26] The colon is

*Hill's Prescription Diet, Hill's Pet Products, Inc., Topeka, KS.

†Docusate sodium, 100 to 300 mg BID PO (dogs), Upsher-Smith Laboratories, Inc., Minneapolis MN.

clamped and divided in an area of normal tissue on the oral side of the lesion, and the normal colonic stump is oversewn. The tumor-containing bowel is exteriorized as much as possible on the abdominal side. It is transected on the anal side of the mass close to the anal sphincter from the abdominal approach. The oversewn normal colon is then exteriorized through the anal orifice and anastomosed to the remaining rectal cuff. For isolated lesions involving only the rminal rectum, a rectal pull-through involves less surgery.[0,02]

Subtotal colectomy has been advocated for chronic incapacitating constipation in humans[7] and in cats with chronic constipation/obstipation[24,88] that have developed idiopathic megacolon. If this procedure is unsuccessful, a pull-through can still be performed. Additional intra-abdominal procedures, such as ovariohysterectomy, can be done safely in conjunction with the colectomy.[9]

The social problem of anorectal incontinence after extensive lower bowel surgery and pull-through procedures is a major postoperative concern with human patients[60] and house pets. In patients with mucosal disease, e.g., chronic ulcerative colitis and familial polyposis, an initial transanal mucosal stripping is advantageous to ensure elimination of diseased tissue on the anorectal side of the anastomosis[80] and less interference with sphincter mechanisms. A terminal ileal—pelvic reservoir, which has been created for humans after total colectomy, has resulted in continence, absence of postoperative perineal excoriation, and an acceptable frequency of stool passage.[60] This procedure would be feasible for selected veterinary patients.

Colorectal Stricture

This condition may manifest as a problem with constipation characterized by tenesmus and passage of thin, soft, ribbon-like stools.

History. The history reflects a chronic progressive problem with unsatisfactory relief from medical management. The age, diet, and personality of the dog may be relevant factors. Some dogs exhibit a fondness for eating sticks and other debris and often have a history of fecal impactions. In other dogs, particularly older animals, these signs are suggestive of a tumor or an idiopathic problem.

Physical Examination. An impacted large bowel may be palpated, depending on the degree of obstruction and the location of the stricture. Rectal palpation may be unrevealing unless the strictured area is within the pelvic canal. Survey abdominal radiographs seldom define the problem. Cleansing enemas should be given and a proctoscopic examination should be performed. A biopsy may be indicated. Additional information can be gained by performing a barium enema if the proctoscope fails to pass the area of stricture. If possible, an endoscopic examination with a flexible fiberoptic instrument should be attempted prior to the barium enema.

An assessment of the objective data is essential to formulating a plan. If the stricture appears to be secondary to scar tissue, e.g., bone impaction, the prognosis, plan, and postoperative management may be straightforward. However, a stricture secondary to an intraluminal or intramural neoplasm may necessitate a pull-through procedure and a more guarded prognosis. On rare occasions, an intrapelvic mass or a prostatic tumor may compress the colorectal junction, but alleviation of the compression is a secondary consideration.

Table 10–1. SURGICAL PLAN FOR COLORECTAL STRICTURES

Stricture secondary to cicatrix	Resection and anastomosis—colectomy Narrow band—longitudinal incision and transverse closure
Stricture secondary to neoplasm	Colectomy Pull-through procedure Transanal mucosal resection

Colorectal Trauma

Trauma to the large bowel is uncommon and infrequently diagnosed in veterinary patients. Traumatic injuries that result from gunshot wounds or automobile accidents and cause damage to a normal colon that is full of feces are usually fatal unless treated promptly and correctly.

Animals with abdominal gunshot wounds should undergo an immediate exploratory laparotomy. Stab wounds that manifest no evidence of visceral injury must be monitored for signs of peritonitis, but emergency surgery may not be necessary. Blunt trauma to the abdomen should also be monitored. Administration of broad-spectrum antibiotics is imperative in all instances. Copious abdominal lavage at the end of operation to remove all particulate matter is important;

the subcutaneous tissue and skin can be left open to heal by secondary intention in the event of gross contamination.[1] The entire abdominal wall may be left open for drainage, if necessary. A loose continuous pattern of 0 or 2/0 prolene suture is placed in the rectus sheath, and the wound is bandaged appropriately with a sterile, absorptive dressing. When the animal has stabilized and the wound environment is acceptable, a secondary closure is done.

The method of repair will vary from resection and anastomosis to simple suture repair for isolated tears. Criteria to be considered for primary repair include: (1) the interval between injury and surgery, (2) the size of the wounds, (3) the magnitude of the fecal spill, (4) the location of the wound on the antimesenteric or mesenteric surface, (5) the presence of associated injuries, and (6) the manifestation of shock.[1] It is important to remember that death due to a colorectal injury is largely preventable with early diagnosis and proper treatment. Barium enema is contraindicated as a diagnostic tool because a colorectal injury with barium peritonitis is generally fatal.[1]

Neoplasms of the Colon and Rectum

The frequency of neoplasia of the terminal bowel in dogs is low,[47, 57, 64] but approximately half of gastrointestinal neoplasms involve the colon and rectum,[38] and adenocarcinoma occurs most commonly.[11, 38] Descriptions of the different tumor types are available in other texts.[33, 57, 64] Benign tumors of this region include adenomatous polyps, leiomyomas, and papillary adenomas.[57]

History. The clinical signs, to some degree, reflect the type of tumor. Tenesmus is common. Bloody-streaked, solid stools or bloody, mucoid diarrhea is typically seen with colonic and rectal polyps. The infiltrative and obstructive tendencies of colonic and rectal carcinomas cause constipation with intermittent, bloody, mucoid diarrhea. Ulcerative lesions result in a bloody stool.[57] In addition to those signs attributable to the lesion, there may be others that involve the major organ systems because the majority of affected animals are middle-aged or older and because malignant tumors of the colon and rectum frequently metastasize. Large bowel signs predominate early, and the animals are usually seen before systemic involvement occurs.

Physical Examination. A thorough physical examination that includes a careful digital investigation of the rectum must be done. The colon can be palpated simultaneously with the rectum, enabling one to detect low colonic lesions. Polyps are frequently numerous, bleed easily, and are friable. Hemorrhage may also result from palpation of ulcerative lesions, but other characteristics allow them to be distinguished. It is critical to determine the lesion's size, location, and degree of fixation or extension into adjacent tissue prior to surgery. A preoperative intravenous pyelogram is recommended in humans in order to document that both kidneys are functional in case extensive resection is necessary. A barium enema or colonoscopic examination is advised to determine the presence of a second primary tumor.[15, 66, 75] In addition to careful palpation of the abdomen and the regional lymph nodes (medial iliac, lumbar, middle colic),[62] thoracic and abdominal radiogaphs are indicated. In the absence of palpable or radiographic evidence of metastatic lesions, a biopsy is necessary to establish malignancy.

In humans, suspicion is aroused by finding occult blood in a stool sample from a patient that eats a high-bulk, meat-free diet.[65, 75] Biochemical factors, known as tumor markers, have received a lot of attention because they aid in diagnosis and preoperative disease staging. Carcinoembryonic antigen (CEA), an oncofetal glycoprotein, is considered of prognostic value by some researchers.[10, 82] A preoperative CEA level that is less than 5.0 ng/ml indicates a more favorable prognosis and a higher longevity than higher values. A level above 20 ng/mg strongly suggests metastasis to the liver or disseminated disease.[82] For a tumor marker to have value (1) it must have sufficient sensitivity to detect the presence of malignancy in a significant proportion of cancer patients, (2) elevations in marker level should not occur in non-malignant states, (3) the absolute level of the marker should be indicative of tumor bulk, and (4) the tumor marker should be readily available at a reasonable cost.[31] Tennessee antigen is a tumor-associated antigen that is believed to have high sensitivity for colorectal cancer; however, serum values were variable, difficult to interpret, and clinically unreliable when compared with values obtained with CEA in one study.[30, 31] No comparative values are available for animals, and the difficulty in gathering significant numbers for evaluation precludes use of these tumor markers in animals.

Because of the potentially poor prognosis with colorectal tumors, careful assessment of data is essential. In advanced disease, surgery is palliative at best. Radiation and immunostimulants are not well-established alternatives or supplemental measures. Location, size and biological behavior of the tumor directly influence the feasibility of surgery or radiation.[39] The effect of low dose preoperative irradiation and high dose/low dose preoperative irradiation on subsequent distal colorectal anastomosis has been studied in dogs.[12, 69] It is recommended that surgery take place 3 weeks after irradiation.

A uniform treatment plan for all cases is not practical. In humans, treatment of adenocarcinoma of the colon and rectum by surgery presents the best hope of cure.[75] Surgery is a reasonable approach to the treatment of many of veterinary patients; however, a realistic attitude toward the outcome must be maintained.

Biopsy. Prior to definitive operation, a biopsy is indicated. Determination of an accurate prognosis and treatment feasibility may be possible after histopathological evaluation of a biopsy specimen. There is usually a single lesion with adenocarcinoma. If diffuse disease is seen (e.g., inflammatory disease, multiple polyps, or lymphosarcoma) multiple biopsies are not necessary because the histological features of the large bowel are similar throughout the colon.[13] Preoperative bowel preparation is essential to minimize technical difficulty and to decrease contamination. Antibiotics should be started 12 to 24 hours prior to biopsy. Preparation for colonic inspection includes a 12 to 24 hour fast and several warm-water enemas. One enema should be given the evening before the examination and one or two enemas on the day of the procedure, but the latter should not be given within one or two hours of biopsy. Residual fluid, tissue congestion, and hyperemia are avoided when this regimen is followed. Although productive, irritant enemas induce transient inflammatory change in the bowel wall that can be confused with colitis. Alligator-jaw biopsy forceps are recommended for this procedure because they cut more sharply and require less tugging and tissue shredding than clamshell biopsy forceps.[3] These instruments are easily passed through the rigid colonoscope. The normal mucosa will appear glistening and smooth and will be easily distensible.[48] As the colonoscope is withdrawn, the mucosa is examined for color (e.g., pink, reddened, grayish), appearance (e.g., velvety, granular, pebbled, thickened, eroded, ulcerated, glistening, dull), the amount of mucus, the presence of intraluminal masses, and changes in luminal diameter.[3] Lymphoid follicles that appear as small, glistening plaques are normal. Lesion location should be recorded. For further detail on biopsy of the large bowel, see Chapter 9.

Surgery. The objective of surgical treatment of large bowel cancer is to remove the primary tumor and any regional spread without causing further dissemination of the tumor while leaving the patient with a reasonable quality of life.[79] A preliminary discussion of surgical principles relative to cancer surgery of the bowel is relevant.[76] A wide resection of the tumor-bearing segment of bowel along with wide removal of the lymphatic drainage of that segment should be done. Wide removal of large portions of the colonic mesentery that contain the lymphatic drainage enhances removal of the bowel segment containing the tumor.

The same techniques that minimize bacterial contamination are used to minimize cancer cell contamination. The abdomen should be thoroughly explored for metastatic lesions before the tumor is handled. Further isolation of the tumor by packing away the adjacent viscera with laparotomy pads is recommended. Manipulation of the tumor should be kept to a minimum; contaminated gloves should be washed frequently. After tumor excision, the field should be gently irrigated. Contaminated packs and gloves should be changed. Any crushed tissue should be excised, and the contents of the two bowel segments should be aspirated before an anastomosis is performed. Swabbing the mucosa and the open ends of the bowel with a skin preparation agent* is recommended. Finally, all contaminated drapes and gloves should be replaced before the abdominal wall is closed.[75]

Prior to 1967, the conventional method of operation in humans involved a limited, segmental resection of the colon with little inclusion of mesentery. Turnbull published data on a series of cases in which he used a "no-touch" technique that emphasizes isolation and division of the lymphovascular pedicle, division of the colon at selected sites

---

*Betadine solution, Purdue Frederick Co., Norwalk, CT.

of resection, and excision of the associated mesentery and peritoneum. The tumor is not touched or handled by the surgeon or the assistants before or during the operation.[83] Using Duke's classification (Fig. 10–6),[25] survival for patients with A, B, and C lesions following no-touch resections were 68 per cent versus 52 per cent with conventional resection. The most significant results were in class C lesions, with 5-year survival rates of 57.8 per cent compared with 28 per cent with conventional surgery.

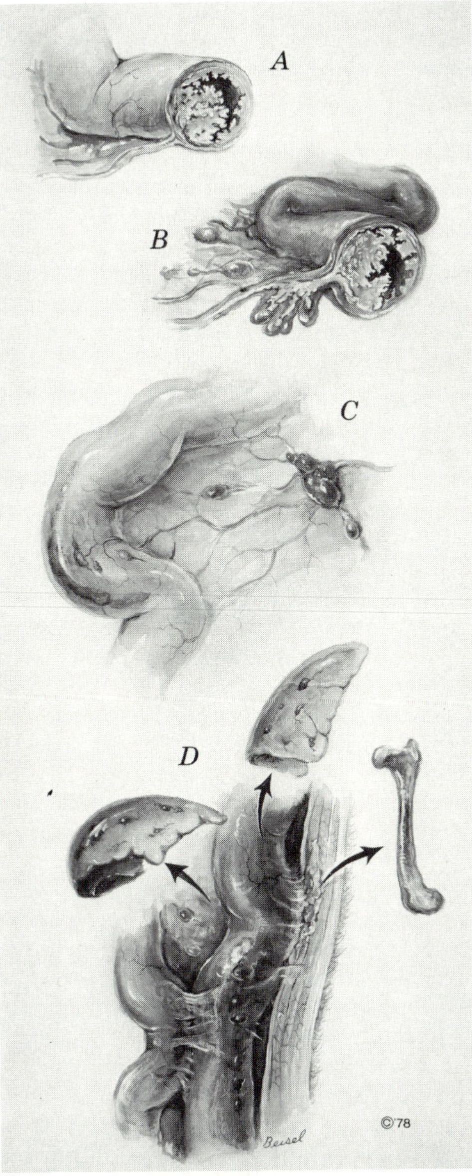

Figure 10–6. Duke's clinicopathological classification of cancers of the colon: Class A, tumor limited to all coats of the bowel but not beyond; Class B, extension into fat; Class C, metastasis of tumor to lymph nodes only; and Class D, extension into adjacent organs, metastasis to liver, lungs, bone, and extension into parietes.

In both humans and dogs, the lymphatics of the colon drain centrally in the mesentery, paralleling the vascular supply.[62, 75] Similar results to Turnbull's have been achieved by wide resection of the mesentery to the vascular origin of the respective mesenteric vessel. Comparison of the two techniques leads one to conclude that the adequacy of cancer resection is the key to increased survival rates.[22, 79] Justification for the no-touch technique lies in the demonstration of an increased number of tumor cells in the iliac veins after handling of carcinomas of the colon.[68] Also, lymph flow has been shown to increase markedly after manipulation and massage of the intestine.[2] More recently, it has been shown that high arterial ligation of the appropriate major arteries, followed by ligation of the marginal vessels running close to the colon in the area of clamp application, results in negligible lymphatic and venous flow. The remainder of the mesocolon including the lymphatic channels and veins is clamped, cut, and tied. The standard no-touch technique is then employed.[2] This approach apparently combines the best qualities of both techniques. One has to be quite careful to preserve the common colic artery when excising portions of the descending colon, in the dog.[34]

The extent of local resection of an isolated lesion that is necessary to establish an adequate soft tissue margin has been evaluated extensively in humans.[29] The same guidelines are appropriate for use in animals. Several studies comparing survival rates with the extent of the margin of resection suggest that a margin of less than 5 cm is associated with diminished survival. Margins greater than 5 cm are not worthwhile for extensive disease owing to the existence of disseminated lymphatic metastases. After a study of 1500 consecutive cancer specimens of the rectum and rectosigmoid, a distal margin of 2.5 cm was considered adequate for carcinoma of average or low-grade frequency in humans.[29] Because of the correspondingly smaller size of the veterinary patient, 2.5 cm should provide an adequate soft tissue margin, but the margins of the biopsy should be carefully checked for microscopically visible spread.

Adhesion of adjacent structures or organs is a poor prognostic sign. Tumor cells are found at the interface of the primary tumor and the adjacent structure, resulting in residual malignant cells that can be left behind if the tissues are separated. Survival may result after *en bloc* resection of involved organs or structures, but this extensive degree of surgery is seldom worthwhile in animals because of the poor prognosis and the management problems.

The extent of lymphatic resection that is considered adequate is controversial. The lymphatic drainage of the colorectal area in humans is well documented and correlates with the structure and function in dogs and cats. The nodes closest to a large bowel cancer are the epicolic nodes, which are located in direct apposition to the bowel wall. The paracolic nodes are in the mesentery directly adjacent to the bowel wall. The major lymph flow from these nodes follows the arterial blood supply rather than the portal venous system. The intermediate nodes are in the mesentery along the course of the major arteries. The principal nodes lie at the origins of the larger arteries; the para-aortic nodes drain into the cisterna chyli or other lymphatic channels and then into the thorax. The colon and upper one-third of the rectum drain along the lymphatic channels following the portal vein. The lower two thirds of the rectum drains upward along the superior hemorrhoidal vessels to the retroperitoneal and portal lymphatics. A second drainage system flows laterally into the internal iliac nodes, along the middle hemorrhoidal vessels and the levator ani muscle to the common iliac nodes and then to the retroperitoneal lymph nodes. Another drainage area for low rectal cancers is through the inferior hemorrhoidal system to the superficial inguinal lymph nodes. On postmortem examination of 11 human patients who died after large bowel resection, it was concluded that four patients with residual metastasis in the resected specimen potentially could have been cured by more radical lymphatic resection.[27] Tumor metastases progress in an orderly fashion from the primary tumor along a lymph node chain. Survival rates are better if lymphatic metastases are a distance from the highest ligature on the resected specimen; these rates support the previous observations.[79] A retrograde lymphatic metastasis may occur a distance from the relevant lymphatic arcade when lymph nodes become plugged by metastatic tumor cells.[35] None of the patients in whose specimens this type of spread was seen were salvaged. Owing to the number of factors involved, one group suggests that radical resection of the colon should be advised only for young patients with an excellent surgical risk and when no added morbidity or mortality from the radical procedure is expected.[79] This advice seems appropriate for the veterinary patient.

The management of exfoliated intraluminal tumor cells deserves mention. These cells will implant on the surfaces of the anastomotic site and are implicated in the high recurrence rate (10 to 35 per cent) after resection of the large bowel for cancer. The increased incidence of left-side and colocolic anastomotic recurrences may be related to closeness of the tumor to the anastomosis, increased manipulation of the primary tumor with resection of a low-lying lesion, more than adequate bacterial cleansing by enemas of the left colon prior to surgery, failure of exfoliated tumor cells to survive or implant within the intestinal lumen in the presence of small bowel digestive enzymes, and the additional opportunity for tumor cells to survive or implant because of delayed peristalsis with colocolic anastomoses. Precautionary techniques are recommended to reduce the number of exfoliated cells that are available to implant in the bowel lumen. Water or a cytotoxic chemical is maintained within the lumen with constricting tapes. This technique allows a thorough lavage to be performed and the exfoliated cells to be combined with the segment that is to be removed. Iodized suture materials are recommended for the anastomosis.[79]

Colectomy. General anesthesia with careful monitoring of vital signs and fluid replacement adequate to maintain intravascular fluid volume and blood pressure are essential prerequisites for successful surgery in any seriously ill patient, particularly animals with malignant disease of the bowel, since most are older, often are debilitated, and may have pre-existing electrolyte and acid-base disturbances. Clipping and preparation of the abdomen adequate for an exploratory laparotomy is often possible before induction of anesthesia.

A ventral midline incision is made caudally from the cranial abdomen. Sufficient exposure for visual inspection and palpation of cranial abdominal organs is essential, and the incision should be adjusted accordingly. Sterile laparotomy pads are used to line the incision, and Balfour retractors are placed for maximum exposure of the caudal abdomen. The abdomen should be thoroughly and systematically examined for metastatic lesions. The entire course of the gastrointestinal tract, including each adjacent organ, should be carefully checked to avoid mistakes. The temptation to immediately work on the colonic lesion should be resisted. Manipulation of the lesion during this exploration should be avoided. Any metastatic lesions found must be evaluated for resectability and influence on the prognosis. Disseminated disease will usually preclude excision of the colonic lesion. The colonic biopsy procedure is the same as that for cecal biopsy.

The colonic lesion is isolated with laparotomy pads, and the small bowel and omentum are sequestered in the cranial abdomen. Careful attention must be paid to the blood supply in the area to be resected. Most of the transverse and descending colon is supplied by the middle colic branch of the common colic artery, which arises from the cranial mesenteric artery. The descending colon is also supplied by the left colic artery; a branch of the caudal mesenteric artery descends along the distal colon to supply numerous branches to the proximal rectum. There is no arterial arcade in this region; the marginal vessels are the short vasa recti. The arterial supply is ligated as close as possible to its origin without jeopardizing the blood supply to the remaining bowel (Fig. 10–7*A*). Any marginal vessels in the areas to be resected are then ligated. If possible, the intervening mesentery is excised, with concurrent ligation of the lymphovascular channels. Intestinal clamps, preferably rubber-shod, or umbilical tapes are applied to the segment of bowel containing the lesion (Fig. 10–7*B*). This segment is then excised between clamps, with as much mesentery as possible. The lesion should not be handled. The blood supply of the dog is not suitable for primary arterial and marginal vessel ligation followed by wide excision of intervening mesentery and lymphovascular channels; therefore, the no-touch technique may be more important in dogs than in humans. If primary arterial ligation does not appear feasible, a segmental colectomy,[34] which preserves the major blood supply, is recommended. However, this method closely resembles the conventional technique of limited resection, which in humans was statistically inferior to Turnbull's no-touch technique.[83] Crushed tissue is excised, the bowel ends are gently lavaged, and an anastomosis is performed. A simple, interrupted suture pattern is preferred, using 3/0 to 4/0 polyglycolic acid sutures or polyglactin 910 with a through-and-through stitch (Fig. 10–7*C*). The mesenteric border is approximated first, then the antimesenteric border, followed by closure of each respective side. A single-layer closure is sufficient if the sutures are placed 3 to 5 mm apart. Tension on the anastomotic line must be avoided. The Balfour retractor is removed, the laparotomy pads are counted and discarded, and the abdomen is thoroughly lavaged with warm lactated Ringer's solutions. Omentum is secured over the anastomosis and the abdomen is closed with polypropylene suture or monofilament stainless steel wire. If drainage is necessary because of excessive contamination, sump-type drains are placed adjacent to the anastomosis and exited through the body wall lateral to the abdominal incision. Two drains are usually sufficient, and they should be removed in 36 to 48 hours if there is no significant drainage.

Postoperative Management. Antibiotics should be continued for 3 to 5 days after surgery. Feeding is resumed 12 to 24 hours after surgery. A low-residue diet is recommended for the first 10 to 14 days to minimize fecal bulk and straining. Stool softeners may be used, but enemas are discouraged. Any suggestion of wound dehiscence merits immediate attention, since death will be the sequela to septic peritonitis. Gentle exercise by leash walking should be encouraged.

Pull-through Procedure. Lesions of the distal colon or the colorectal junction are more amenable to a pull-through procedure than to a segmental colectomy. Unless a clamp can easily be placed a sufficient distance distal to the lesion to ensure healthy tissue for the anastomosis and to provide adequate tissue for technical proficiency, the intra-abdominal colectomy will fail.

Polyps

In humans, polyps are considered precancerous lesions. Some precancerous polyps have been reported in the dog,[74] but canine polyps are generally considered benign. Polyps may be located in the colon or rectum,

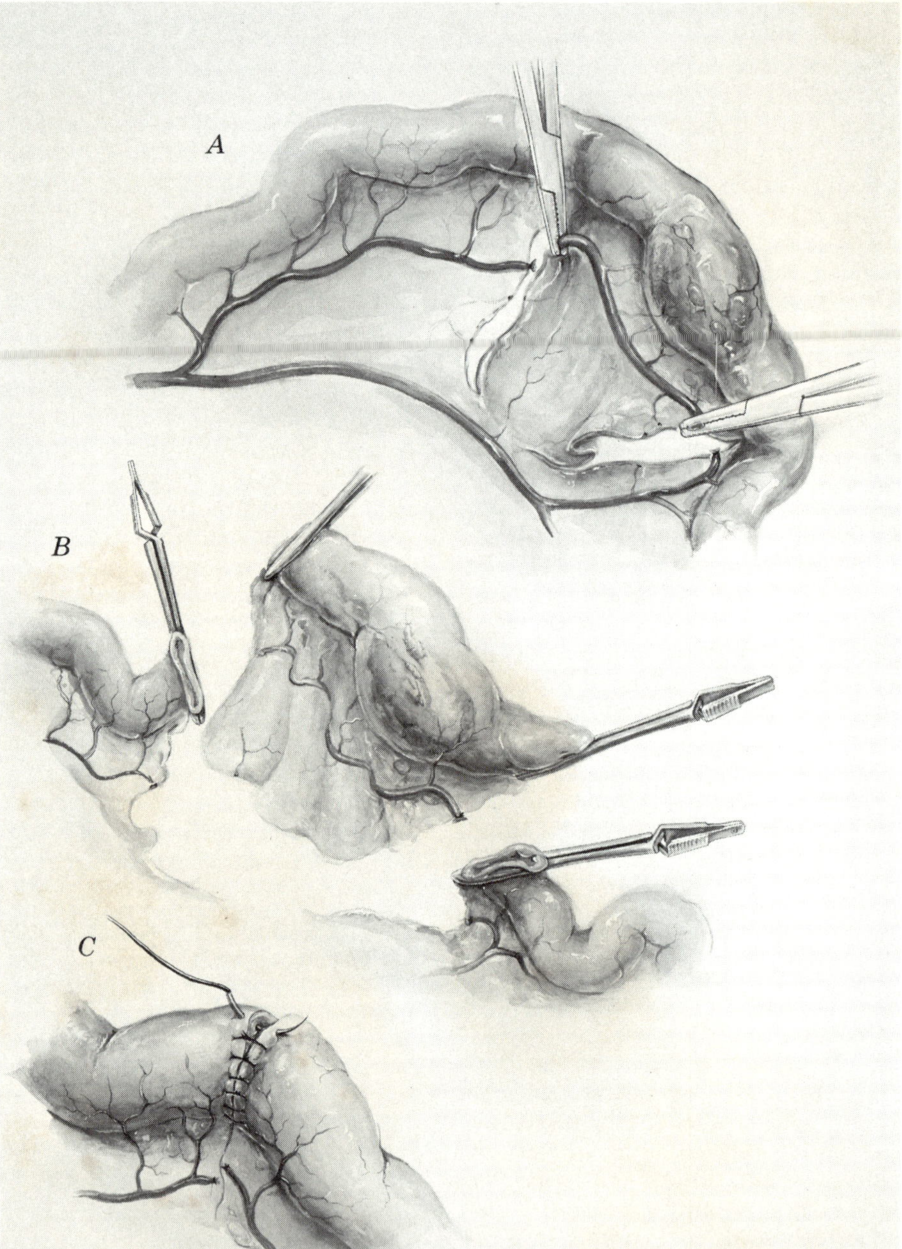

Figure 10–7 ABC. Colectomy procedure.

single or multiple, and pedunculated or sessile; they are usually friable and bleed easily.

Surgery. The surgical prognosis is good for singular or isolated small groups of polyps.[72] Multicentric polyps, which grossly resemble human familial polyposis, have a more guarded prognosis because of the increased difficulty in removing the affected segment of bowel. Single, pedunculated polyps in the rectum can be removed through the anus by using an anal speculum and either clamping and ligating the stalk or by excision with cutting cautery. Hemorrhage can be controlled by direct pressure or by applying a clamp to twist the pedicle.[4] Cryosurgery can be used for accessible lesions as well. Colonic polyps may be removed with an electrocautery snare through a proctoscope by an experienced surgeon, but the disastrous consequences of bowel perforation eliminate this option for the novice. A colotomy or colectomy is indicated for polyps that are not readily accessible through the anus. Multiple polyps necessitate extensive resection by segmental colectomy.[34] Either a Swenson-type pull-through or a rectal pull-through procedure can be used, depending on the location of the lesion. The tissue should be submitted for histopathological examination to check for intraepithelial carcinomatous changes and invasive tendencies.[72] In humans, polyps are usually situated several centimeters from the anal verge, and the majority of malignant polyps are located in the left colon.[5, 15] Fortunately, in the dog, polyps are less common in the colon than in the rectum and usually have a good prognosis.[72] Postoperative care is adjusted according to the severity of the lesion and the extent of the surgery.

Lesions of the Rectum

Lesions of the proximal, mid, and distal sections of the rectum can readily be removed by a modified pull-through resection.[8, 32] The disadvantage of this technique is the elimination of the abdominal phase; the surgeon does not have an opportunity to survey the abdomen for metastatic lesions. The advantage is the reduction in anesthetic and surgery time, which may be critical in the poor-risk patient. The author has successfully done this procedure using a narcotic and epidural anesthesia in lieu of general anesthesia for excision of multiple polyps.

Surgery. Preoperative management includes giving cleansing enemas and antibiotics and withholding food for 24 hours. General anesthesia is preferred, but sedation and an epidural block are adequate for selected cases. The latter regimen can be supplemented with a mixture of oxygen and halothane administered through a face mask. If the dog is intubated and assisted ventilation is being provided, the animal is placed on a well-padded perineal stand in sternal recumbency. The dog is placed in lateral recumbency if spontaneous ventilation governs respiration. The tail is positioned over the dog's back, and the perineum is clipped and scrubbed. Three-corner or fenestrated draping can be used. Four stay sutures are placed just inside the anal verge at the anorectal junction equal distances apart to provide gentle traction on the rectum and to enlarge the anal orifice. The rectum is incised circumferentially through all layers approximately 6 to 8 mm cranial to the stay sutures (Fig. 10–8*A*). The free, proximal rim of the rectum is grasped with Allis tissue clamps and gentle traction is applied. A dissection plane is established between the serosal surface of the rectum

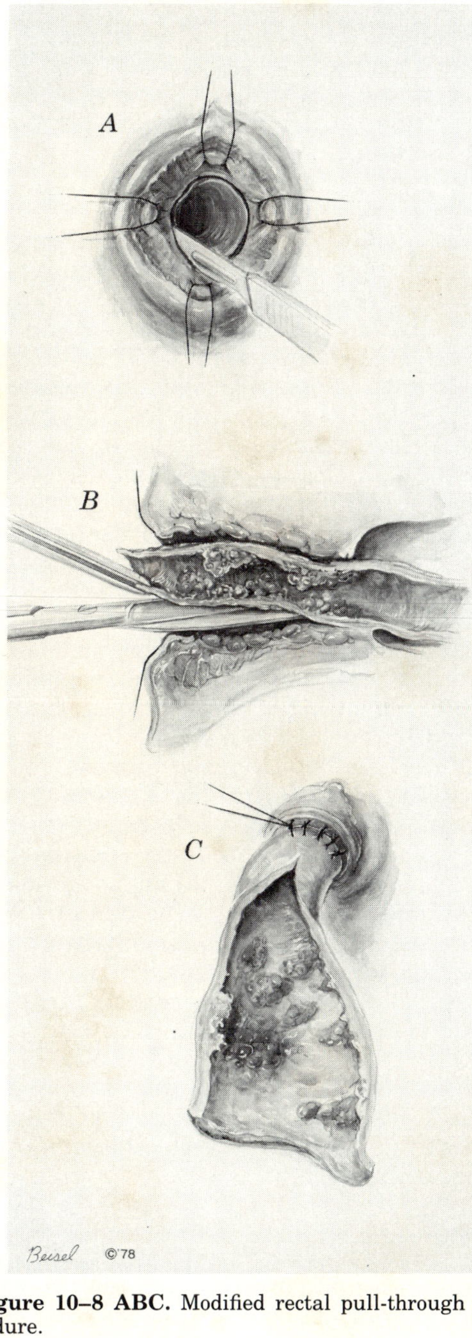

Figure 10–8 ABC. Modified rectal pull-through procedure.

and the external anal sphincter. By blunt dissection and caudal traction, the rectum and distal colon can be exteriorized to the level of the caudal mesenteric lymph node and cranial rectal artery (Fig. 10–8*B*). Dissection is continued until a margin of healthy tissue that is cranial to the lesion is available for anastomosis. Discrete lesions can be palpated through the rectal tube. Disseminated lesions, such as occur with multiple polyposis, are difficult to palpate, and the rectum should be incised cranially on the dorsal surface to provide direct observation of the cranial extent of the lesion.

The anastomosis is effected by first placing a simple, interrupted pattern of 3/0 to 4/0 polyglycolic acid sutures or polyglactin 910 through the serosa muscularis around the circumference of the prolapsed segment and the anorectal cuff (Fig. 10–8*C*). The anorectal cuff is everted toward the surgeon in order to provide access to its serosal surface. The colorectal segment is then excised slightly distal to the first suture line, and the mucosal-submucosal layers are united with 4/0 polyglycolic acid sutures or polyglactin 910 in a continuous pattern. The author has done a single-layer, through-and-through closure with a satisfactory result; however, this method requires opening of the colorectal tube for accurate suture placement. Symmetrical placement of sutures is essential to avoiding a disparity in tension on the anastomotic line.

Caudal rectal lesions may be made accessible and amenable to surgical excision by eversion or prolapse of the rectum through the anus. Tension sutures and tissue clamps must be used judiciously because of the possibility of tissue trauma. For most cases, a rectal pull-through would be satisfactory and would facilitate accurate, adequate tissue resection. In humans, adenocarcinoma of the mid-anal region to the distal rectum most often requires an abdominoperineal resection for adequate tissue removal. Because of the attendant colostomy, this technique is not feasible in veterinary surgery.

Animals with malignant disease of the rectum and with coexisting pathology or positive evidence of metastasis may receive palliative support from electrocoagulation or cryosurgery.[43, 85]

Polypoid, or exophytic, lesions have a good chance of being cured by electrocoagulation. The goal of electrocoagulation is to destroy, by the use of coagulating current, the entire tumor and a margin of normal tissue both deep to and around it. As the tissue is destroyed, it is removed by scraping, until normal tissue is encountered. In one study, all exophytic lesions were assumed to be Dukes' type A and all ulcerative lesions to be Dukes' type B or C. Ninety-two per cent of the patients with exophytic lesions had successful treatment when evaluated for 5-year cure rates, compared with 33 per cent of patients with ulcerative lesions.[43]

Postoperative Management. Postoperative care is essentially the same as that for colectomy, although tenesmus may be more of a problem. If the dog strains excessively, it should be confined and kept under surveillance. The dog should be taken outside to defecate or urinate and should be returned to its cage immediately after eliminating. If it is left in a run, the animal will frequently strain repeatedly for variable periods. Stool softeners may help diminish the tenesmus. Bulky diets should be avoided.

PROGNOSIS

One must emphasize that only polyps warrant a good prognosis. Adenocarcinoma offers, at best, a guarded prognosis, as do the less frequently occurring sarcomas, and the client should be so advised.

References

1. Abcarian H, Lowe R: Colon and rectal trauma. Surg Clin North Am 58:519, 1978.
2. Ackerman NB: The influences of mechanical factors on intestinal lymph flow and their relationship to operations for carcinoma of the intestine. Surg Gynecol Obstet 138:677, 1974.
3. Anderson NV: Biopsy of the gastrointestinal system. Vet Clin North Am 4:317, 1974.
4. Anseline PF, Fazio VW: Management of massive postpolypectomy hemorrhage: Report of a technique. Dis Colon Rectum 25:251, 1982.
5. Appel F.: Distribution of malignant polyps in the colon. Dis Colon Rectum 25:427, 1982.
6. Arango A, Lester JL 3d, Martinez OV, et al.: Bacteriologic and systemic effects of intraoperative segmental bowel preparation with povidone iodine. Arch Surg 114:154, 1979.
7. Belliveau P, Goldberg SM, Rothenberger DA, Nivatvongs S: Idiopathic acquired megacolon: The value of subtotal colectomy. Dis Colon Rectum 25:118, 1982.
8. Betts CW: Rectal pull-through, resection and anastomosis. *In* Bojrab MJ (ed): *Current Techniques in Small Animal Surgery II*. Lea & Febiger, Philadelphia, 1983, p. 202.
9. Biggers OR, Ready RL, Beart RW Jr: Risk of additional intra-abdominal procedures at the time of colectomy. Dis Colon Rectum 25:185, 1982.
10. Blake KE, Dalbow MH, Concannon JP, et al: Clinical significance of the preoperative plasma carcinoembryonic antigen (CEA) level in patients with

carcinoma of the large bowel. Dis Colon Rectum 25:24, 1982.
11. Brodey RS, Cohen D: An epizootiological and clinicopathologic study of 95 cases of gastrointestinal neoplasms in the dog. Proc 101st Annual Meeting, Am Vet Med Assoc, 1964.
12. Bubrick MP, Rolfsmeyer ES, Schauer RM, et al: Effects of high-dose and low-dose preoperative irradiation on low anterior anastomoses in dogs. Dis Colon Rectum 25:406, 1982.
13. Canfield PJ, Bennett AM, Watson AD: Large intestinal biopsies from normal dogs. Res Vet Sci 28:6, 1980.
14. Carb A, Barret RB: Leiomyosarcoma of the cecum in the dog. J Am Anim Hosp Assoc 14:631, 1978.
15. Chapuis PH, Dent OF, Goulston KJ: Clinical accuracy in the diagnosis of small polyps using the flexible fiberoptic sigmoidoscope. Dis Colon Rectum 251:669, 1982.
16. Clarke JS, Condon RE, Bartlett JG, et al: Preoperative oral antibiotics reduce septic complications of colon operations: Results of prospective, randomized, double-blind clinical study. Ann Surg 186:251, 1977.
17. Condon RE: Prevention of sepsis in treatment of large bowel cancer. *In* DeCosse JJ (ed): *Large Bowel Surgery: Clinical Surgery International.* Churchill Livingstone, New York, 63, 1981.
18. Couch NP, Tilney NL, Moore FD: The cost of misadventures in colonic surgery. A model for the analysis of adverse outcomes in standard procedures. Am J Surg 135:641, 1978.
19. Deveney KE, Way LW: Effect of different absorbable sutures on healing of gastrointestinal anastomoses. Am J Surg 133:86, 1977.
20. Edwards NJ: Cecocolic invagination in the dog. Vet Med/Small Anim Clin 376, 1977.
21. Endres WA, Remondini DJ, Graber ER: A case report of torsion of the descending colon in a six-month-old female collie. Vet Med/Small Anim Clin 954, 1968.
22. Enker WE, DeCosse JJ: The evolving surgical treatment of rectum and colon cancer. CA 31:66, 1981.
23. Fain SN, Patin CS, Morgenstern L: Use of a mechanical suturing apparatus in low colorectal anastomosis. Arch Surg 110:1079, 1975.
24. Fellenbaum S: Partial colectomy in the treatment of recurrent obstipation/megacolon in the cat. Vet Med/Small Anim Clin 737–742, 1978.
25. Fitzgerald RH Jr: What is the Dukes' system for carcinoma of the rectum? Dis Colon Rectum 25:474, 1982.
26. Gerosa RM, deEstrada M: Colorectal resection in a cat with adenocarcinoma. Feline Pract 12:6, 1982.
27. Gilchrist RK, David VC: A consideration of pathological factors influencing five year survival in radical resection of the large bowel and rectum for carcinoma. Ann Surg 126:421, 1947.
28. Goldsmith, HS: Protection of low rectal anastomosis with intact omentum. Surg Gynecol Obstet 144:585, 1977.
29. Goligher JC, Riley TR, Dukes SE, Bussey HJR: Local recurrences after sphincter-saving excisions for carcioma of the rectum and rectosigmoid. Br J Surg 39:199, 1951.
30. Gray BN, Walker C, Barnard R, Bennett RC: Tennessee antigen: The predictive value of preoperative and postoperative assays in large-bowel cancer. Dis Colon Rectum 25:539, 1982.
31. Gray BN, Walker C, Barnard R, Bennett RC: Tennessee antigen: Its value in the monitoring of patients with colorectal cancer. Dis Colon Rectum 25:542, 1982.
32. Greene JA, Knecht CD: Pull-through resection of the rectum. Canine Pract 43, 1977.
33. Greiner TP, Johnson RG, Betts CW: Diseases of the rectum and anus. *In* Ettinger SJ (ed): *Textbook of Veterinary Internal Medicine,* 2nd ed. W. B. Saunders Company, Philadelphia, 1493, 1983.
34. Greiner TP, Christie T: The cecum, colon, rectum, and anus. *In* Bojrab MJ (ed): *Current Techniques in Small Animal Surgery.* Lea & Febiger, Philadelphia, 1975, p. 126.
35. Grinnell RS: Lymphatic block with atypical and retrograde lymphatic metastasis and spread in carcinoma of the colon and rectum. Ann Surg 163:272, 1966.
36. Guffy MM, Wallace L, Anderson NV: Inversion of the cecum into the colon of a dog. J Am Vet Med Assoc 156:183, 1970.
37. Gulati SM, Iyengar B, Thusoo TK, Pan Dey KK: Comparative study of free omental, peritoneal, Dacron velour, and Marlex mesh reinforcement of large-bowel anastomosis: An experimental study. Dis Colon Rectum 25:517, 1982.
38. Hayden DW, Nielsen SW: Canine alimentary neoplasia. Zentralbl Veterinaermed 20:1, 1973.
39. Hintz BL, Charyulu KK, Sudarsanam A: Anal carcinoma. Basic concepts and management. J Surg Oncol 10:141, 1978.
40. Höjer H, Wetterfors J: Systemic prophylaxis with doxycycline in surgery of the colon and rectum. Ann Surg 187:362, 1978.
41. Horney FS, Archibald J: Colon, rectum, and anus. *In* Archibald J (ed): *Canine Surgery,* 2nd ed. American Veterinary Publications. Santa Barbara, 603, 1974.
42. Howard ER: Hirschsprung's disease—Staining of ACH and adrenal nerves. Postgrad Med J 48:471, 1972.
43. Hughes EP: Electrocoagulation of rectal cancer. Dis Colon Rectum 25:215, 1982.
44. Jiborn H, Ahonen J, Zederfeldt B: Healing of experimental colonic anastomoses. III. Collagen metabolism in the colon after left colon resection. Am J Surg 139:398, 1980.
45. Jiborn H, Ahonen J, Zederfeldt B: Healing of experimental colonic anastomoses. IV. Effect of suture technique on collagen metabolism in the colonic wall. Am J Surg 139:406, 1980.
46. Jonsell G, Edelmann G.: Single-layer anastomosis of the colon—A review of 165 cases. Am J Surg 135:630, 1978.
47. Jubb KV, Kennedy PC: *Pathology of Domestic Animals.* Academic Press, New York, 1970.
48. Kasper JB, Chiapella AM: Gastrointestinal biopsy techniques. *In* Kirk RW (ed): *Current Veterinary Therapy VII.* W. B. Saunders Company, Philadelphia, 962, 1980.
49. Keane FB, Moore DJ, Byrne PJ, Hennessy TP: A comparison of circular stapling devices for rectal anastomoses. A study in dogs. Dis Colon Rectum 25:285, 1982.
50. Khubchandani M, Upson JF: Single-layer anastomosis of the colon and rectum. Dis Colon Rectum 25:113, 1982.
51. Lazorthes F, Legrand G, Monroies X, et al: Comparison between oral and systemic antibiotics and their combined use for the prevention of compli-

cations in colorectal surgery. Dis Colon Rectum 25:309, 1982.
52. Leff EI, Hoexter B, Labow SB, et al: The EEA stapler in low colorectal anastomoses: Initial experience. Dis Colon Rectum 25:704, 1982.
53. Lehr K, Schober O, Hundeshagen H, Pichlmayr R: Total body potassium depletion and the need for preoperative nutritional support in Crohn's disease. Ann Surg 196:709, 1982.
54. Leighton RL: Personal communication, 1983.
55. Levine SH: Ruptured cecum due to abscessation in a dog. A case report. J Am Anim Hosp Assoc 18:337, 1982.
56. Lord MG, Broughton AC, Williams HT: A morphological study on the effect of suturing the submucosa of the large intestine. Surg Gynecol Obstet 146:211, 1978.
57. Lorenz MD: Disease of the large bowel. *In* Ettinger SJ (ed): *Textbook of Veterinary Internal Medicine,* 2nd ed. W. B. Saunders Company, Philadelphia, 1346, 1983.
58. Maingot R: *Abdominal Operation,* 6th ed. Appleton-Century-Crofts Medical Books, New York, 1974.
59. Marks G, Gathright JB, Boggs HW, et al: Guidelines for use of the flexible fiberoptic sigmoidoscope in the management of the surgical patient. Dis Colon Rectum 25:187, 1982.
60. Martin LW, Fischer JE: Preservation of anorectal continence following total colectomy. Ann Surg 196:700, 1982.
61. Menaker GJ, Litvak S, Bendix R, et al: Operations on the colon without preoperative oral antibiotic therapy. Surg Gynecol Obstet 152:36, 1981.
62. Miller ME, Christensen GC, Evans HE: *Anatomy of the Dog.* W. B. Saunders Company, 1964.
63. Moesgaard F, Nielsen ML, Hansen JB, Knudsen JT: High-fiber diet reduces bleeding and pain in patients with hemorrhoids: A double-blind trial of Vi-Siblin. Dis Colon Rectum 25:454, 1982.
64. Moulton JE: *Tumors in Domestic Animals.* University of California Press, Berkeley, 1961.
65. Nivatvongs S, Gilbertsen VA, Goldberg SM, Williams SE: Distribution of large-bowel cancers detected by occult blood tests in asymptomatic patients. Dis Colon Rectum 25:420, 1982.
66. Reilly JC, Rusin LC, Theuerkauf FJ Jr: Colonoscopy: Its role in cancer of the colon and rectum. Dis Colon Rectum 25:532, 1982.
67. Richardson DC, Duckett KE, Krahwinkel DJ Jr, Shipman LW: Colonic anastomosis: Evaluation of an end-to-end crushing and inverting technique. Am J Vet Res 43:436, 1982.
68. Salsbury AJ, McKinna JA, Griffiths JD, et al: Circulating cancer cells during excision of carcinomas of the rectum and colon with high ligation of the inferior mesenteric vein. Surg Gynecol Obstet 120:1266, 1965.
69. Schauer RM, Burbick MP, Feeney DA, et al: Effects of low-dose preoperative irradiation on low anterior anastomosis in dogs. Dis Colon Rectum 25:401, 1982.
70. Scher KS, Scott-Conner C, Jones CW, Leach M: A comparison of stapled and sutured anastomoses in colonic operations. Surg Gynecol Obstet 155:489, 1982.
71. Schrock T, Cerra F, Hawley PR, et al: Wounds and wound healing. (Clinical conference) Dis Colon Rectum 25:1, 1982.
72. Seiler RJ: Colorectal polyps of the dog: A clinicopathologic study of 17 cases. J Am Vet Med Assoc 174:72, 1979.
73. Sharefkin J, Joffe N, Silen W, Fromm D: Anastomotic dehiscence after low anterior resection of the rectum. Am J Surg 135:519, 1978.
74. Silverberg SG: Carcinomas arising in adenomatous polyps of the rectum of a dog. Dis Colon Rectum 14:191, 1971.
75. Stearns MW Jr: Benign and malignant neoplasms of the colon and rectum. Diagnosis and Management. Surg Clin North Am 58:605, 1978.
76. Stone EA, Rawlings CA, Prasse KW, et al: Intraoperative biopsy and microscopy during exploratory laparotomies. Vet Surg 7:93, 1978.
77. Strombeck DR: Dietary management of gastrointestinal problems. *In* Kronfield DS, Low DG (eds): *Diet and Disease in Dogs.* Symposium published by the Continuing Education Medical Veterinary Dept. of California at Irvine, University of California, 1975, p. 36.
78. Stromberg BV, Klein L: Collagen formation during the healing of colonic anastomosis. Dis Colon Rectum 25:301, 1982.
79. Sugarbaker PH, Corlew S: Influence of surgical techniques on survival in patients with colorectal cancer. A review. Dis Colon Rectum 25:545, 1982.
80. Sullivan ES, Garnjobst WM: Advantage of initial transanal mucosal stripping in ileo-anal pull-through procedures. Dis Colon Rectum 25:170, 1982.
81. Swenson O, Bill AH: Resection of rectum and rectosigmoid with preservation of sphincter for benign spastic lesions producing megacolon; experimental study. Surgery 24:212, 1948.
82. Szymendera JJ, Nowacki MP, Szawlowski AW, Kaminska AW: Predictive value of plasma CEA levels: Preoperative prognosis and postoperative monitoring of patients with colorectal carcinoma. Dis Colon Rectum 25:46, 1982.
83. Turnbull RB, et al: Cancer of the colon: The no-touch isolation technique of resection. *In* Maingot R (ed): *Abdominal Operations,* 6th ed. Appleton-Century-Crofts Medical Books, New York, 2018, 1974.
84. Vargish T, Crawford LC, Stallings RA, et al: A randomized prospective evaluation of orally administered antibiotics in operations of the colon. Surg Gynecol Obstet 146:193, 1978.
85. Veidenheimer MC: Alternatives to surgery in the treatment of carcinoma of the rectum. Surg Clin North Am 51:815, 1971.
86. Vezeridis M, Evans JT, Mittelman A, Ledesma EJ: EEA stapler in low anterior anastomosis. Dis Colon Rectum 25:364, 1982.
87. Wilson GP, Burt JK: Intussusception in the dog and cat: A review of 45 cases. J Am Vet Med Assoc 164:515, 1974.
88. Yoder JT, Dragstet LR 2nd, Starch CJ: Partial colectomy for correction of megacolon in a cat. Vet Med/Small Anim Clin 63:1049, 1968.

CHAPTER

11

Surgical Diseases of the Anorectum

JONATHAN N. CHAMBERS

The intent of this section is to review and update the principles of anorectal surgery and those problems most often treated at least in part by surgery. The reader is directed to the reference list at the end of the chapter for additional descriptions of specific surgical techniques.

Anatomy

The anatomical and functional distinctions between the colon and rectum are more clearly defined in humans than in domestic animals. The division is placed, arbitrarily, at the pelvic inlet, at about the level of the 7th lumbar vertebra in animals.[38] The columnar epithelium of the rectum is surrounded by inner circular and outer longitudinal layers of smooth muscle. The outer longitudinal layer is prominent and consolidated dorsally to form the rectococcygeus muscles, which attach to the vental surfaces of the first few coccygeal vertebrae.[38] The inner circular layer is prominent and consolidated at the anorectal junction, constituting the involuntary internal anal sphincter.[13]

The innervation of the rectal smooth muscle, including the internal anal sphincter and the rectococcygeal muscles, is autonomic (involuntary). The contribution from the parasympathetic system originates in the sacral spinal nerves, emerging primarily in the S_2 nerve, with lesser contributions from the S_1 and S_3 spinal nerves. The sacral spinal nerves form the sacral plexus, and parts of this plexus converge to form the pelvic nerve. The short pelvic nerve then diverges to form the pelvic plexus and ganglia, with small (almost microscopic) terminal branches entering the rectal wall. The sympathetic innervation is similar, in that the nerves are sequentially derived from the lumbar spinal nerves L_2 through L_4 and L_5, sympathetic trunk, caudal mesenteric ganglion, hypogastric nerve, and the pelvic plexus.[14]

The blood supply to the rectum is segmentalized into cranial, middle, and caudal thirds. The cranial rectal artery is the most terminal branch of the caudal mesenteric artery; it supplies the cranial one-third and the dorsal surface of the middle one-third of the rectum. The middle and caudal rectal arteries are terminal branches of the internal pudendal artery and supply blood to the walls of the rectum and the anal canal, respectively.[13, 14] Venous drainage is into both the systemic and portal systems via the caudal rectal and cranial rectal veins, respectively.

The terminal large bowel is difficult to deal with surgically. The pertioneal cavity as a real and potential space ends as the rectal (visceral) pertioneum reflects cranially to line the interior of the pelvis laterally, the sacrum dorsally, and the other pelvic organs ventrally (Fig. 11–1). This reflection is at the level of the levator ani muscle as it crosses the rectum laterally. Abdominal exposure of the rectum is restricted by this limiting membrane caudally, by the pelvis and urogenital tract ventrally, by the sacrum dorsally, and by the levator ani muscles, which are tightly associated, laterally.

Several structures, including the perito-

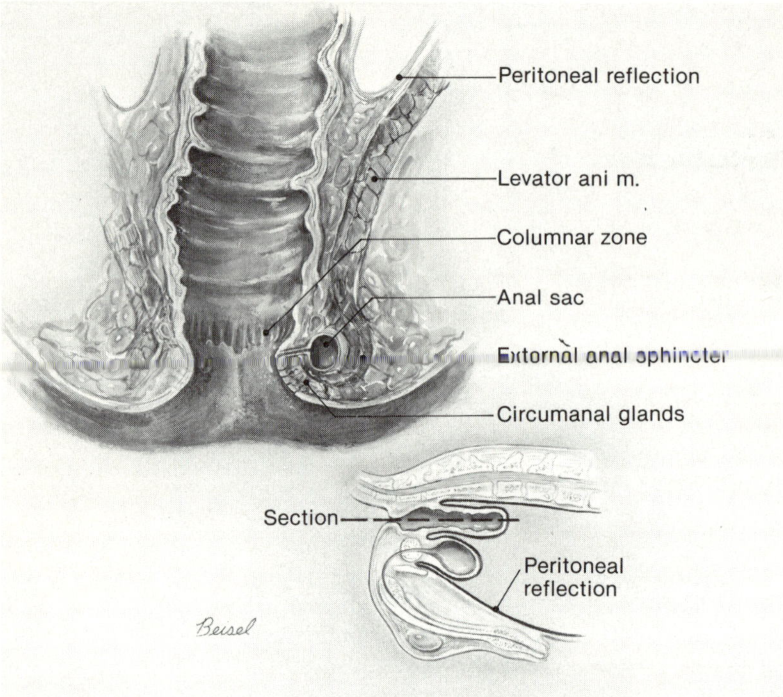

Figure 11–1. Median and dorsal sections through the anorectal region. (Reprinted with permission from the University of Georgia © 1979.)

neal folds, the very short mesorectum (originating from the sacrum), the short fibrous attachments to the pelvis, and other interweaving muscle and connective tissue fibers, fix the rectum in its normal position and limit its exposure and mobilization through the anus.

The anus is the last 1 to 2 cm of the alimentary tract, and it is divided into zonal segments. Its cranial margin is the anorectal line, where the relatively smooth surface of the rectal epithelium is replaced by longitudinally oriented ridges of stratified squamous epithelium.[38] The ridges are several millimeters in length and end abruptly at the anocutaneous line. The epithelium becomes progressively more cornified and hair-bearing beyond the anocutaneous line. The circumanal and anal glands are a concentration of sebaceous, apocrine, tubuloalveolar, and sweat glands that lie beneath the anal epithelium. Many of the glands have ducts that open onto the epithelial surface. The paired anal sacs are approximately 1 cm in diameter and lie between the internal and external anal sphincter muscles at the ventrolateral aspects of the anus.[13] The ducts are approximately 5 mm long and are directed dorsomedially from the sacs, opening onto the hairless skin just outside the anocutaneous line. Large, coiled, apocrine, sudoriparous tubules and sebaceous acini line the sacs and ducts.[57]

The external anal sphincter completely surrounds the anal canal, with some fibers completing the ring dorsally and ventrally and others blending with the rectococcygeus muscles dorsally or with the muscles of the external genitalia ventrally. The craniolateral borders of the external anal sphincter are joined to the levator ani muscles by fascia. This fascial attachment is the primary site of weakness in perineal hernia.

The external anal sphincter is composed of striated muscle and is innervated by the sacral spinal nerves via the caudal rectal branch of the pudendal nerve. The pudendal nerve also supplies sensory innervation to the anus and perineal skin. The caudal cutaneous femoral nerve and the cutaneous branches from the sacral root plexus provide additional sensory innervation.[13] The caudal rectal and perineal arteries, which are branches of the internal pudendal artery, supply blood to the anus. The paired cranial rectal arteries further branch to create an arterial circle around the anal canal.[13] Lymphatic vessels from the anus and rectum drain into the left colic, internal iliac, and external iliac lymph nodes.

Preoperative Considerations

The size and character of a rectal lesion will somewhat determine whether an abdominal, an anal, or a combined surgical approach is needed. Digital palpation should be followed by visual examination. A self-retaining rectal retractor* works well for exposure in larger patients, and a nasal speculum† in small dogs and cats. Lesions that can be easily and completely exteriorized through the anus may be dealt with from an anal approach. Lesions that are further cranial or that are fixed in position, preventing exteriorization, should be operated through an abdominal approach or a combined abdominal and anal approach.

Sufficient exposure must be gained to enable precise dissection and suturing, assessment and control of contamination, and minimization of trauma to surrounding tissues. To operate on a lesion where accessibility by the anus alone is questionable is unwise considering the potentially disastrous consequences of dehiscence, localized or generalized sepsis, and incontinence.

The extent of preoperative cleansing that is necessary must also be determined. Ideally, the entire gastrointestinal tract should be empty of ingesta at the time of rectal surgery and for a sufficient period after surgery to allow undisturbed healing of the rectum. To wait for ideal conditions is not realistic or practical in most cases. An exhaustive routine of preoperative and postoperative control of feces should be instituted when an elective situation exists. Total parenteral alimentation might be considered. A wide variety of preoperative and perioperative broad-spectrum antibiotic regimens have been recommended.[52] Emergency situations call for intraoperative removal of feces by gentle irrigation and suction rather than by less controlled preoperative enemas.

Anal and perineal surgery can be performed with less preparation; a cotton tampon or a purse-string suture will often serve to prepare the area. Insufficient preparation of the bowel, a common mistake, is often worse than no preparation at all. Solid stool is relatively easy to isolate from the surgical field, whereas insufficient enemas or an enema that is given immediately before operation may result in the presence of voluminous liquid stool that obscures and contaminates the surgical field.

*Cook Sim Self Retaining Rectal Retractor, J. Sklar Mfg. Co., Inc., Long Island City, NJ.

†Killian Nasal Speculum, J. Sklar Mfg. Co., Inc., Long Island City, NJ.

Wound Healing

Because the majority of the rectum is extraperitoneal, relatively distant, and isolated from the omentum, rectal wounds must heal without the protection this fibrinoplastic serous membrane offers to help seal a dehiscence and to prevent dissemination from a contaminated or infected focus. Adequate drainage of the pelvic space, either from the abdomen or from the perirectal fossa to the perineum, will greatly enhance healing if contamination is present.

The procedure for suturing the rectum follows the same principles as for wounds elsewhere in the bowel. Interrupted stitches of 3/0 or 4/0 suture material are used and spaced 3 to 4 mm apart. The mucosal surface should be slightly inverted by using a single-layer Lembert pattern, or an inner layer of simple interrupted stitches followed by an outer layer of Lembert stitches. Simple interrupted stitches placed from inside the lumen will produce slight mucosal inversion. Monofilament non-absorbable* or synthetic absorbable† sutures are preferred because of the likelihood of contamination. Swaged-on tapered or reverse cutting needles are preferable.

Incised wounds of the anus, which should otherwise undergo uncomplicated primary union, often heal by granulation if the base is deeply scarred.[46] Peacock[46] suggests that failure to keep the tissue at rest is the primary cause, and that chronic spasm of the external anal sphincter due to irritation is an additional important factor in producing stenosis. Prudent conservative use of sutures, especially skin sutures, and central and local pain relief are suggested to aid in primary wound healing. Sterile, water-soluble, local anesthetic jelly†† that is used for urological examination works well to relieve anal irritation.

Anorectal Disorders

RECTAL TRAUMA

Crushing injuries to the pelvis such as those seen in automobile mishaps can pro-

*Prolene, Ethicon Inc., Somerville, NJ. Ethilon, Ethicon Inc., Somerville, NJ.

†Coated Vicryl, Ethicon Inc., Somerville, NJ.

††Xylocaine Jelly, Astra Pharmaceutical Products, Inc., Worcester, MA.

duce severe rectal trauma due to displacement of bone fragments. Fortunately, the incidence of rectal trauma from pelvic fracture is low. Penetrating abdominal injuries such as those caused by gunshots may also involve the rectum. All patients that are examined for trauma to the caudal abdomen or pelvis must be evaluated for rectal involvement. Iatrogenic trauma that occurs during diagnostic or therapeutic procedures is another possible cause of rectal perforation.

Because of the predominately intrapelvic, retroperitoneal position of the rectum, perforation there may go undiagnosed, often with disastrous consequences, unless it is specifically looked for.

After a thorough general physical examination, a gloved and well-lubricated finger is gently inserted into the rectum. The rectal wall and bony architecture are carefully palpated. Suspicion of a defect or finding even a small amount of blood warrants further investigation with a proctoscope.[50] The fecal mass is removed manually or by suction and gentle irrigation during the examination. No enemas should be given. If direct visual examination fails to disclose a perforation and one is still suspected, radiographs should be taken. A loss of soft tissue detail, especially of the sublumbar musculature, or the presence of free air in the abdomen and retroperitoneal space are signs of rectal perforation that can be detected on survey films. Positive-contrast studies should be performed using water-soluble contrast media; pertionitis caused by a mixture of feces and barium is often lethal.[1]

The prognosis and treatment for a rectal wound depends on its cause, its location, and the presence of concomitant injuries. Small wounds to the anus or caudal rectum caused by thermometers or enema tips may be treated by conservative débridement, hemostasis, antibiotics, and vigilant monitoring of the patient and wound. Deterioration of the patient's condition or evidence of complicated wound healing should prompt more aggressive treatment.[50]

Rectal perforation due to a crushing injury or a gunshot wound is a medical and surgical emergency. Patients that have sustained trauma of these types often have other severe or life-threatening injuries, which must be assessed and treated simultaneously.[30, 34, 50] Attention to a rectal perforation must take precedence. If a perforation is left untreated, it will usually prove fatal;[1] gram-negative sepsis with endotoxic shock will be the cause of death.

Pre-operative medical therapy should be instituted at the time of diagnosis or as the diagnostic procedures are carried out. Intravenous fluids and high doses of water-soluble corticosteroids* are used to support the cardiovascular system against impending endotoxemia. Antibiotics, preferably bactericidal, with a high degree of efficacy against gram-negative enterobacteria are given parenterally. The aminoglycosides (gentamicin,† kanamycin,‡ amikacin,§ tobramycin‖) are appropriate choices. The presence of anaerobic bacteria, particularly *Bacteroides fragilis,* causes a major problem in human colorectal surgery and therefore, clindamycin¶ is often used in combination with either gentamicin or kanamycin.[10, 35]

Cleansing of the rectum and surrounding tissues should be done by irrigation at the time of surgery. Preoperative enemas are contraindicated because they will undoubtedly disseminate the contamination.

Depending on the site and extent of the perforation, a perineal, abdominal, or combined approach is used. Feces are removed by gentle swabbing and irrigation with sterile lactated Ringer's solution. Necrotic tissue is débrided and the rectum is repaired. A variety of suture materials and patterns have been used. A two-layer approach is generally recommended; the inside layer is of simple interrupted stitches of fine chromic gut or synthetic absorbable material, and the outer layer is of interrupted Lembert or mattress stitches of 3/0 or 4/0 monofilament nylon or polyethylene. Adequate drainage is ensured by liberal use of Penrose drains or continuous suction ribbon drains.**

There is general agreement among experts in the field of colorectal surgery that all cases of major rectal perforation, even those in which fecal contamination is minimal, should be managed by total diversion of the stool during healing (colostomy).[10, 35, 50]

---

*Solu-Delta-Cortef, Upjohn Co., Kalamazoo, MI.

†Gentocin, Shering Veterinary, Shering Corporation, Kenilworth, NJ.

‡Kantrim, Bristol Laboratories, Syracuse, NY.

§Amikin, Bristol Laboratories, Syracuse, NY.

‖Nebcin Distra Products Co., Indianapolis, IN.

¶Cleocin Phosphate, Upjohn Co., Kalamazoo, MI.

**J-Vac Closed Wound Drainage System, Johnson & Johnson Products, Inc., New Brunswick, NJ.

Surgeons who now advocate primary repair in selected cases of colon perforation agree that rectal injury should be managed with colostomy.[34] Once the contamination has been cleared and the rectum has been repaired, the tissue can heal, at rest, without danger of further contamination.

The diverting colostomy is relatively easy to construct, but its creation must be treated as a major surgical procedure and attention must be paid to technical detail.[2] A ventral midline abdominal approach is used. The transverse colon provides a sufficiently long mesentery for mobilization to the ventral abdominal wall in the region of the umbilicus. The colon is divided and both ends are passed through holes in the abdominal wall that are created by full-thickness trephine-like resection (Fig. 11–2). The defects in the abdominal wall should be several millimeters larger than the diameter of the bowel to prevent obstruction or compromise of the mesenteric vasculature. The incised edge of the colon wall is sutured to the skin without tension. Alternatives are (1) to exteriorize and transversely open a loop of colon and (2) to over-sew the end of the distal limb and create a single stoma for drainage of the proximal bowel.[52] Regardless of the technique used, the distal colon must be temporarily but completely defunctionalized.

The implications of colostomy in the dog are many and are not to be taken lightly. Management of the stoma is difficult; it requires almost constant attention, cleansing, and possibly bandaging to prevent mutilation. Closure of the colostomy will necessitate major surgery a second time. Reconstruction of the bowel is performed only after sufficient healing of the rectum is assured. Healing takes at least 10 to 14 days, or longer, depending on the severity of the injury.

In the author's experience, the few temporary colostomies that have been used in clinical veterinary surgery have been less than gratifying to manage, but lack of experience probably contributed to the difficulty. Experience from human medicine indicates that colostomy is virtually the only way to manage severe disorders of the colorectum, such as a contaminated crushing injury, and must be given consideration. Ideally, severe colorectal disease is managed at a specialty practice or an institution where adequate personnel and facilities are available to deal with it. Unfortunately, immediate referral may not be possible. Even a few hours' delay in cleansing the damaged tissue and diverting the feces may result in fatal sepsis.

RECTAL PROLAPSE

The diagnosis of rectal prolapse is straightforward. The history of tenesmus is rarely necessary to arrive at the diagnosis, but it may be of some value in assessing the problem and in formulating a plan for management.

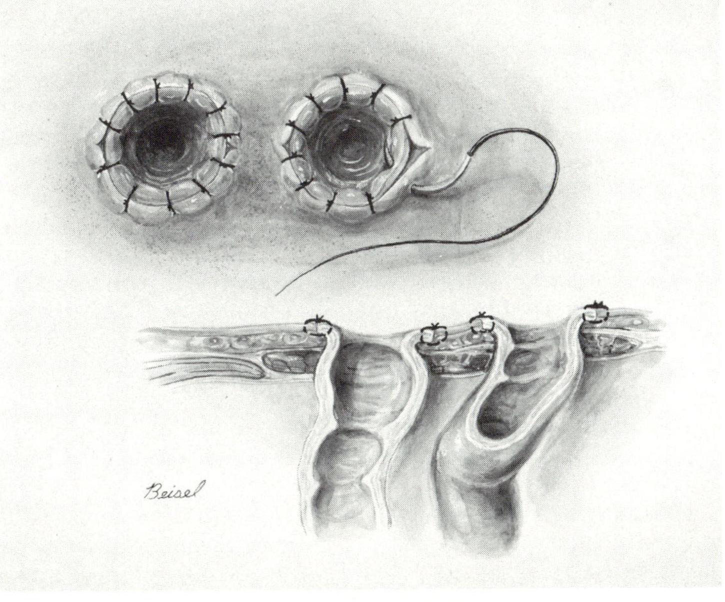

Figure 11–2. Technique for colostomy. See text for explanation of procedure. (Reprinted with permission from the University of Georgia © 1979.)

There are many degrees of rectal prolapse, varying from protrusion of the mucosa layer at the anorectal junction, to full-thickness extrusion of several centimeters, including the colorectal junction (procidentia). A mucosal prolapse assumes a swollen donut shape as it protrudes from the anus. If all the layers are involved, the prolapsed tissue will take on a more cylindrical shape. The only problem that might be mistaken for rectal prolapse is intussusception of a more proximal section of bowel through the anus, which is rare. Differentiation between rectal prolapse and intussusception is made by the unsuccessful attempt to insert a finger between the anal skin and the protruding bowel. The absence of the rectal cul-de-sac indicates an intussusception.

The color and character of the prolapsed mucosa should be noted. Edematous but viable tissue will appear moist and vary from pink to dark red. Mucosa that is irreversibly damaged or necrotic will appear leather-like and be purple or black.

Further examination of the awake dog should be done carefully; the examiner should keep in mind that the induction of excessive straining may result in additional prolapse. Serious consideration should be given to the use of deep sedation or anesthesia.

The rectum (lumen of the prolapse) should be examined digitally and feces should be collected for gross and microscopic examination. The descending colon should be examined proctoscopically. A barium enema should be considered if a higher lesion is suspected.

Rectal prolapse does not occur without cause, although the structural and functional origin may be hard to recognize. An almost universal sign is habitual or continual straining, and the clinician should concentrate on ruling out obvious causes of tenesmus.

Failure to identify and treat a primary cause of tenesmus may result in unsuccessful treatment of the prolapse. The common causes for straining, e.g., diarrhea, enteritis, masses, should be explored. The search for parasitic enteritis should be thorough. Irritation and structural damage following perineal hernia and anal sac surgery are other causes of prolapse.

An anatomical cause has been suggested for many of the otherwise unexplained cases of prolapse in humans.[19, 40, 42] Emphasis has been placed on the colorectal angle and its maintenance by the opposing pull of the levator ani and puborectalis muscles.[40] No analogous problem has been described in the dog.

The initial treatment of rectal prolapse should include symptomatic control of diarrhea and appropriate medication in the case of parasitic or bacterial enteritis.

A minor prolapse of healthy mucosa should be reduced manually. Desiccants such as hypertonic solutions of glucose or urea may help in reducing the edema.[18] Reduction is maintained by a purse-string suture in the anus, leaving an orifice of about 0.5 to 1 cm. The orifice is created by drawing the suture closed around a rectal thermometer or another instrument of similar diameter. A regimen that has been used in children but has not been tried to any extent in the dog is cauterization of the mucosa by injection with almond oil or phenol followed by mucosal replacement.[40]

Procidentia or prolapse with necrosis of the mucosa requires more radical surgical treatment. More aggressive procedures are also indicated for chronic problems.

The mucosal layer is the most susceptible to swelling and necrosis and presents the main problem in correction. Greiner has suggested full-thickness amputation and anastomosis as the preferred treatment in most cases.[16, 17] A technique that has been largely ignored in the more recent veterinary literature, but emphasized in the medical literature, is repair by mucosal resection (Fig. 11–3).[11]

Colopexy should be entertained as a prophylactic measure in any case of severe prolapse; it must be considered in cases of recurrent disease that are unresponsive to more conservative treatment. The descending colon is approached from the midline of the abdomen and is sutured to the left ventral wall. Several interrupted mattress stitches of non-absorbable suture material are used and incorporate the submucosal layer of the colon into the muscles of the abdominal wall.[17, 18, 52]

RECTAL DIVERTICULUM DUE TO PERINEAL HERNIA

Tenesmus and dyschezia are presenting complaints in 75 per cent of cases of perineal hernia, and more than 90 per cent of dogs with perineal hernia have a rectal diverticulum in which stool accumulates.[8] Rectal diverticulum as a separate disease entity is virtually non-existent, and it is generally agreed that the diverticulum is the result of the hernia.

There is some confusion over terminology. Some authors refer to the lesion as a pouch, diverticulum, or sacculation,[5, 16, 17] whereas others refer to it as a deviation or flexure.[29, 54] In medical terminology, a diverticulum involves a break in the muscular layer of the organ affected. This break is not an obvious finding with perineal hernia, although it may be more apparent on histological examination.[17] Whether it is a simple sac or a true diverticulum, the potential space for diversion and accumulation of feces is easily discerned by rectal palpation. The author has not observed the high incidence of rectal flexure that has been recorded by others.[54]

Prompt relief of tenesmus, dyschezia, and obstipation can be afforded by evacuating the feces from the diverticulum either man-

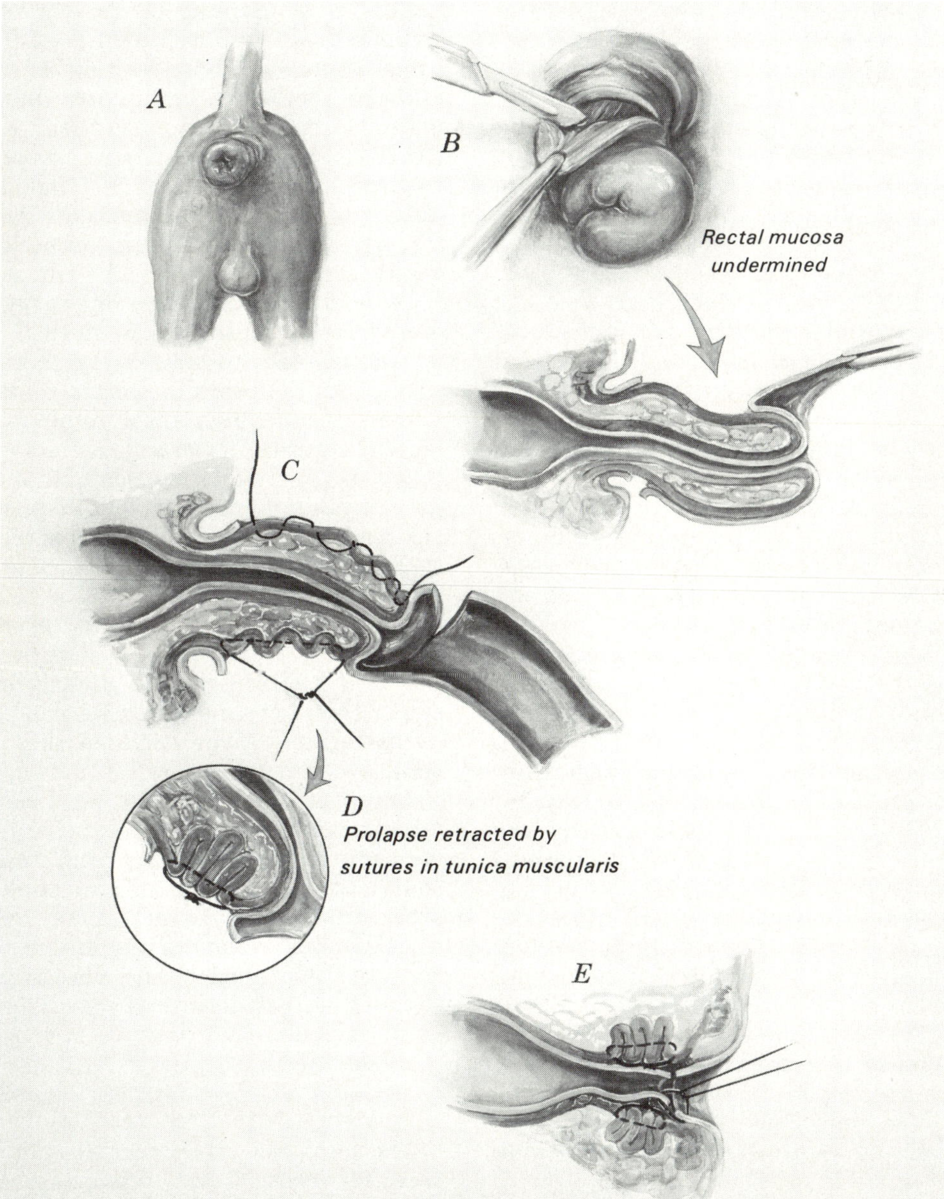

Figure 11–3. The surgical technique for mucosal resection for correction of rectal prolapse. See text for explanation of procedure. (Reprinted with permission from the University of Georgia © 1979.)

ually or with enemas. The repeated accumulation of feces can be partially controlled by use of a low-bulk diet* and stool softeners,† but this is only partially effective, whereas successful perineal herniorrhaphy is curative.

The classic approach to surgical repair of perineal hernia is reconstruction of the pelvic diaphragm by simple interrupted sutures, joining the caudal edges of the levator ani muscle, lateral coccygeal muscle, and sacrotuberous ligament to the external anal sphincter muscle.[1,6,8] The technique has not been uniformly successful either in permanently correcting the hernia or in alleviating the symptoms;[23] however, a recently reported modification shows promise in bringing reccurence levels down to less than 5 per cent at 1-year follow-up.[22,32] The internal obturator muscle is elevated from the floor of the pelvis, remaining attached only at its origin on the pubic symphysis. The lateral edge of the muscle is then transposed dorsally, filling the hernial defect with the muscle belly and supporting the rectal wall directly. The cranial edge of the internal obturator muscle is sutured to the superficial gluteal muscle and the sacrotuberous ligament with interrupted stitches of 0 monofilament nylon. The caudal edge of the internal obturator muscle is sutured to the external anal sphincter in a similar manner. The levator ani and coccygeus muscles are included in the repair, if they are strong enough to hold sutures.[22]

Persistence of the rectal diverticulum after surgery has been suspected as a cause of continued straining and recurrence of the hernia, and simultaneous obliteration or plication of large diverticula has been suggested.[5,6,16] A series of four or five stitches of 0 or 2/0 chromic gut is used to invert the rectal wall. Starting with the first stitch in the most cranial aspect of the sacculation, the suture needle is passed in and out of the rectal musculature in a dorsal to ventral direction. Three or four bites of tissue are included in each stitch.[16] Using a plastic syringe case (5-ml for small dogs, 10-ml for large dogs) as a rectal tampon during perineal herniorrhaphy is recommended. The syringe case helps identify the rectal wall and approximates the rectal diameter over which the preplaced plication stitches are to be tied. The rectum should be digitally palpated after operation to ensure that it has the proper diameter and that the hernia has been repaired. The herniorrhaphy alone may invert a smaller rectal lesion, either a diverticulum or a sacculation, and may prevent further accumulation of feces. To what degree the stretched and redundant tissue resolves is not known.

ANAL SAC DISEASE

Disease of the anal sacs is very common. The anal sacs are actually diverticula of the inner cutaneous, hairless zone of the anus, and the secretions of the apocrine and sebaceous glands that line their walls are discharged into them.[7] One report states that impaction, inflammation, infection, and abscess of the anal sacs account for approximately 2 per cent of the case load of a typical canine practice.[24]

Impaction occurs when defecation fails to empty the sac of secretions. If the impaction is not relieved, inflammatory changes take place; the epithelium becomes disrupted, bacteria replicate in high numbers, and infection occurs. As the inflammatory process proceeds, the body responds with an intense polymorphonuclear leukocyte response, and the region of the sac fills with bacteria-laden leukocytes (abscess). If the duct of the sac remained widely patent, the pus could drain at the surfaces of the anus. More often, inspissation of the combined secretion and pus and swelling of the ductal lining obstruct the duct, and drainage is established by disruption of the perianal skin over the sac.

The presenting signs of anal sac disease are characteristic, if not pathognomonic. In addition to the "scooting" and fixed attention to the anal region, one author described other signs in detail and placed great emphasis on them not only in diagnosis but in staging the disease.[20] The clinical presentation of anal sac disease is usually so typical as to exclude other diagnoses. Even so, the clinician needs to guard against diagnosis based on symptoms without objective findings.

The presence of characteristic signs in certain breeds of dogs suggests a diagnosis of anal sac disease. Studies have shown that small breeds are predisposed to this problem.[24,44] Overall pet hygiene and the envi-

*Science Diet, Hill's Pet Products, Inc., Topeka, KS. Eukanuba, Iams Co., Lewisburg, OH.

†Metamucil, Searle Laboratories, Chicago, IL.

ronment may also contribute to this disease. The sac is normally emptied when a well-formed stool is passed. Irregular bowel habits, loose stools, or anything that causes other than normal defecation may lead to anal sac disease.

No one physical finding is enough on which to base a diagnosis of anal sac disease. The size of the sac will vary even in health.[13] The normal gland should be empty or easily expressed between thumb and finger. The amount of displeasure displayed by the dog during the procedure must be assessed in light of the animal's temperament. Extreme discomfort exhibited by an otherwise calm and cooperative patient should be weighed heavily. An anal sac that is full of secretion is not necessarily diseased. However, if the sac is full and is not expressable, and the dog's presenting signs are consistent, then the diagnosis of impaction is justified.

There is some variation in normal anal sac secretion. In general, it should be serous with some flocculent cellular debris. The color may vary from straw to brown. A thick, pasty secretion, which is ribbon-like on expression, is most likely normal, but inspissated cellular debris is seen with impaction. An opaque, creamy material is most likely purulent exudate. The most accurate assessment of the secretion and the state of the sac is made microscopically. Desquamated epithelial cells, debris, and the presence of few bacteria indicate a normal sac or an impacted sac without inflammation. High numbers of polymorphonuclear leukocytes with many intra-cellular and extracellular bacteria are evidence for inflammation and infection. Culture of the exudate may be indicated.

Abscess of the sac is usually accompanied by extreme pain and swelling. In the peracute stage of infection there will be generalized heat, swelling, and erythema of the skin over the sac (cellulitis). As the infection becomes more organized, a discrete abscess forms, points, and eventually ruptures.

Recurrent Impaction

Impacted anal sacs should be expresssed as atraumatically as possible. There is little justification for further treatment other than to correct any obvious predisposing causes such as diarrhea. Client management with frequent expression may obviate recurrences or progression to infection.[16] Recurrent impaction of the anal sacs may be a problem for either medical or surgical management, depending on the chronicity of the problem and the wishes of the client. The same considerations apply to the management of infection, except that the morbidity is greater, and a permanent cure usually lies in surgical treatment.

Acute anal sac infection with surrounding cellulitis should be treated with systemic antibiotics. Hot packs may be used to encourage circulation in the area. It is unwise to manipulate the tissue excessively or to attempt to establish drainage. These techniques will be ineffective and will tend to cause more inflammation. Once the abscess has formed, liberal drainage should be established by lancing. Irrigation of the abscess cavity may encourage removal of the debris, but irrigation should be done gently with a non-caustic agent such as saline or dilute povidone-iodine. Caustic agents merely incite additional inflammation. Continuous drainage is the most important factor in resolving the infection.

The choice of antibiotic is based on culture and sensitivity testing of the causative organism. One study incriminated a variety of bacteria in anal sac infection; Chloramphenicol* exhibited the widest range of effectiveness *in vitro*.[20]

Anal sacculectomy should be done when the acute inflammation has subsided. Many techniques have been described and all are acceptable, if the general principles of anal surgery are applied. The dissection should be as gentle as possible; blood supply, nerves, and muscles should be preserved and suturing should be kept to a minimum. Adequate drainage should be ensured because of contamination, which is unavoidable. The author prefers the closed technique, in which the overlying external sphincter muscle is bluntly dissected rather than intentionally incised. A cotton tampon is placed in the rectum to prevent gross fecal contamination. A blunt probe in the duct may help delineate the sac, but its value will vary, depending on the chronicity of the disease. The intact sac can be filled with a commercial packing material† or with melted wax to help outline it during the dissection. Once the sac has been excised,

*Chloromycetin, Parke-Davis, Morris Plains, NJ.

†Vettec and Sac Gel, Vettec, Division of Cadco, Los Angeles, CA.

the dead space is closed with one or two stitches of absorbable suture material, and the remainder of the wound is left open.

PERIANAL FISTULAE

Perianal fistulization occurs almost exclusively in middle-aged or older German shepherds. This breed makes up about 90 per cent of the patients in several studies;[25, 27, 33] Irish setters, Labrador retrievers, and cocker spaniels were other affected animals. It is rare to see the disease in any but the preceding four breeds or crosses thereof. The diagnosis of the syndrome in a dog of a small or toy breed would be suspect and warrant substantiating, objective evidence.

Common presenting signs are tenesmus, dyschezia, hemorrhage, odoriferous mucopurulent discharge, and licking of the anus. Unfortunately, the disease is insidious and often advanced before professional help is sought. An average interval of 7.5 months from discovery of the problem to definitive treatment was noted in a recent study.[27] The clinician is fortunate to find the condition in the sub-clinical state and should examine every German shepherd over 2 years of age specifically for perianal fistulae on a routine basis. Clients with German shepherds should be informed to watch for signs of anal disease and to act promptly in seeking professional advice if signs are noted.

The cause of perianal fistulae remains elusive. It was originally proposed, and is still tempting, to incriminate the glandular elements of the anus as the site of origin. An early histological finding is suppurative inflammation of the perianal sweat glands.[7] Also, although a direct analogy may not be possible, a similar condition exists in humans, for which there is little doubt that the anal glands are the inciting cause.[21]

If the pus in the anal wall drains into the lumen, the proper term is perianal sinus; but if the drainage tract breaks through the perianal skin, a true fistula is formed. Both lesions occur in this disease.[25, 36] The fistulae first appear as small punctures in the perianal skin. The surrounding skin is usually inflamed and hyperpigmented. Occasionally, a thin layer of epidermis will cover the tract. As more tracts develop, they tend to coalesce, appearing as large ulcerations of the anoderm.

Chronic necrotizing pyogranulomatous dermatitis is the histopathological lesion seen once the disease is well developed. The dense fibrous connective tissue tracts are lined by a heavy infiltrate of plasma cells, macrophages, and neutrophils. Islands of necrosis are present in the zone of infiltration. This reaction extends to the level of the perianal glands and external anal sphincter muscle.

Perianal fistulation is a surgical disease because the majority if not all of the diseased tissue must be removed to effect a cure. Granulation tissue forms as a reaction to an improper environment for healing. The chronically colonized granulation tissue is very resistant to either systemic or local antibiotic therapy. Caustic cauterization of the tissue may produce some chemical débridement, but it also increases inflammation. A combined treatment of surgically débriding superficially involved tissues and flushing deeply involved tissues with 10 per cent Lugol's solution has been reported to be successful and to have a lower complication rate than more radical techniques.[12]

Complete excision of the diseased tissue allows for primary healing. Excision is accomplished by two concentric 360° incisions, one in the perineal skin peripheral to the disease, and the other at the anorectal junction. All of the diseased tissue in between, including skin, subcutaneous tissue, glands (including the anal sacs), and muscle, is excised. The rectal and skin margins are then united with simple interrupted stitches of 2/0 or 3/0 monofilament nylon suture, with as little tension as possible. Reduction of tension may require some undermining of the perineal skin or the placement of relief incisions in the region of the ischiatic tuberosities or at the skin folds at the base of the tail.

Treatment by complete excision has several drawbacks. The surgery is arduous; hemorrhage is profuse and difficult to control, and discerning diseased tissue from healthy tissue is also difficult.[25] The external sphincter muscle or its innervation is often mutilated. Approximately half of the patients require partial or complete excision of the external anal sphincter.[25] Dehiscence of the wound is common, and the length of hospitalization approaches a week. Complete resolution with primary healing and normal anal function is the exception, and the client should be apprised of this fact from the outset of treatment.

Cryosurgery (Fig. 11–4) has several ad-

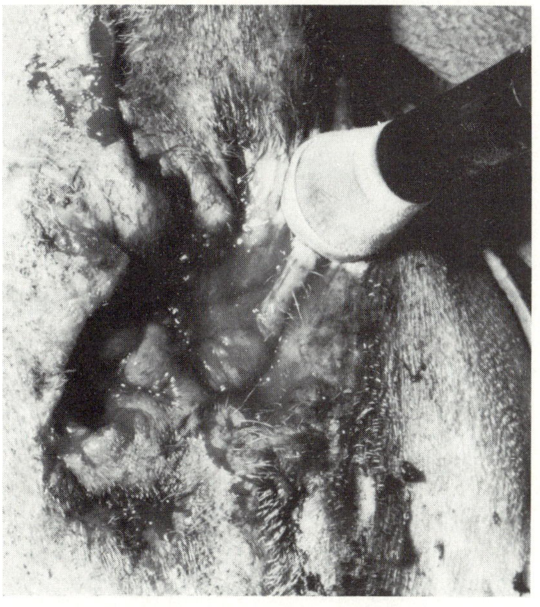

Figure 11–4. Cryosurgery for perianal fistulas.

vantages over conventional knife excision. Hemorrhage is minimal, and total operating time including preparation and anal sac excision is approximately 1 hour. The spincter can be somewhat protected by thermocouple monitoring. There is no suture line, postoperative discomfort is minimal, and the length of hospitalization can be as little as 24 hours.

Cryosurgery for perianal fistulae is no panacea. The client must deal with the odoriferous and messy slough of necrotic tissue. The recurrence rate after intial treatment is about the same as for knife excision, and multiple treatments are often necessary. The healing time after each treatment is about 6 weeks. The wounds heal by second intention. Contrary to initial reports,[33] anal stenosis can be seen in as many as 40 per cent of cases.[56] Other approaches that have been tried recently include electrosurgery[7, 27] and electrosurgery combined with cryosurgery.[28]

The key to a successful outcome is early diagnosis and treatment while the disease still is confined to the anoderm and can be eradicated without sacrificing external anal sphincter function. A better than 80 per cent success rate can be expected when a case is treated early, whereas neglected cases carry a guarded prognosis regardless of the method of treatment.

ANAL STENOSIS

Anal stenosis is often secondary to perianal fistulae or their treatment. Scarring after treatment for tumors, anal trauma, and advanced anal sac disease are also possible causes.[18] The signs of anal stenosis are tenesmus, dyschezia, and constipation or ribbon-like stools, depending on the hardness of the feces. Inspection of the anus may reveal evidence of the scarring, but palpation should be done to ascertain the degree of involvement.

The normal anal diameter varies, depending on the animal's size. The index finger can be inserted in even the smallest dog and in adult cats, two fingers can be inserted in medium-sized dogs, rarely more than three fingers can be inserted even in the giant breeds. The symmetry and pliability of the anus are as important to assess as the size. The normal anus is easily distensible, although some form of sedation or anesthesia may be needed to demonstrate distensibility or to overcome spasms of the sphincter. The shape should be slightly funnel-like, with the wider diameter caudal. Maximum stretching will reveal two limiting bands, the anorectal line and the anocutaneous line. Each is 1 to 2 mm wide with 1 to 2 cm of a columnar zone separating them. Any variation from normal warrants further investigation with an anoscope.

True stenosis is the result of unyielding scar tissue. The depth, cranial-caudal dimension, and the amount of anal circumference involved should be estimated. An attempt should be made to establish a primary cause for the stenosis before or at the time of primary correction. Biopsy should be done on suspicious lesions, as some neoplasms can take on a scirrhous character.

The surgical treatment of anal stenosis is based on the level and severity of the disease. Mild stenosis at the anorectal ring frequently can be corrected by simple digital dilation under anesthesia.[37] The canal must be gradually and gently dilated until the scar tissue is torn. Another approach, if the involvement is circumferential, is to make four or five small incisions through the fibrous ring, spacing them equal distances around the circumference of the anus.[17] The anus is then dilated. This would seem the better approach if the scar extends deeply into the external sphincter muscle. If the scarring has resulted in extensive loss of

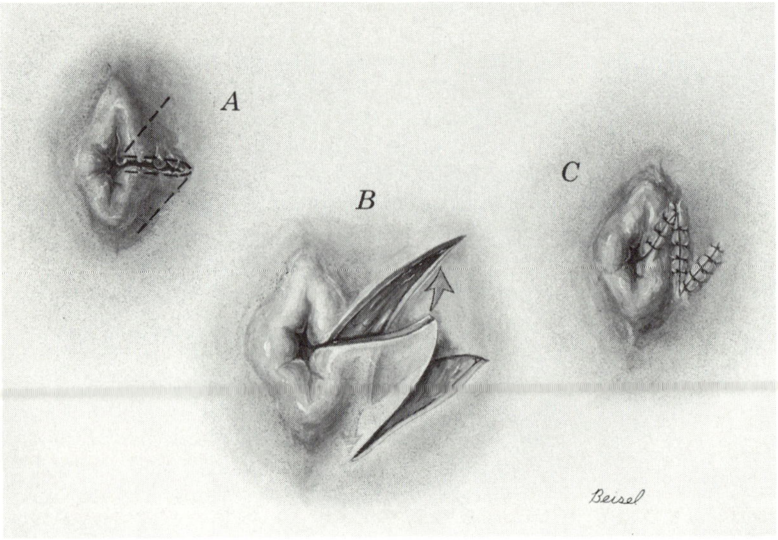

Figure 11–5. Anoplasty for treatment of anal stricture. (Reprinted with permission from the University of Georgia © 1979.)

anoderm, an even more radical treatment is necessary. Excision of the scar, sphincterotomy, and anoplasty such as the S-plasty, are often necessary to enlarge the circumference (Fig. 11–5).

IMPERFORATE ANUS

Imperforate anus encompasses several types of congenital deformity. The deformity may be as simple as failure of perforation of the anal membrane or as complex as complete anorectal agenesis.[18] The abnormalities may be associated with other malformations, especially of the genitourinary tract, with the terminal bowel opening into the vagina, urinary bladder, or urethra.[31, 43, 48] Excellent veterinary references are available describing the embryological development of these defects.[3, 38]

The client usually presents a puppy or kitten because of an obvious abnormality in the anatomy of the perineal structures, voiding of urine or feces through an inappropriate orifice, or absence of defecation has been noted. Tenesmus and a distended abdomen often accompany these problems if obstruction is present. The abnormalities may occasionally go unnoticed until the animal is several weeks old.

Anorectal anomalies of the dog are: (1) imperforate anal (cloacal) membrane, (2) atresia ani and rectum, (3) segmental aplasia, (4) rectovaginal fistula, (5) rectovestibular fistula, (6) anovaginal cleft, and (7) rectal urethreal fistula.[43, 47, 48, 58]

The character and severity of the anomaly may not be readily diagnosed from the apearance of the perineum. Often an anal dimple is present at the base of the tail, showing where the orifice should have been. The colon will be distended with feces and gas, if any degree of obstruction is present. Megacolon may be severe enough to cause abdominal distention. Contrast radiography is needed to establish the presence and position of fistulae between the anorectum and urogenital tracts (Fig. 11–6). A complete physical examination should be done on patients with imperforate anus to rule out congenital deformities in other systems.

The presence or absence of voluntary bladder function is a crude index of sacral plexus innervation of the lower urinary tract and of the muscles involved in defecation.[53] The presence and function of the external anal sphincter muscle can be evaluated by pinching the bulb of the penis or vulva and watching carefully for an anal "wink" (bulbourethral reflex).[41] The sphincter is present and functional in most cases, giving a much better prognosis for surgical correction.[3, 18]

Correction of a deformity that is predominately a cosmetic problem, such as anovaginal cleft, should be delayed until the puppy is 12 to 16 weeks old and is large enough to minimize the anesthetic risk.[58] Defects producing obstruction are an entirely different matter and should be considered surgical emergencies.

Imperforate anal membrane and atresia ani can be corrected by simply excising the membrane and suturing the mucous membrane to the skin. Often the excision can be accomplished without the aid of general anesthesia. A convenient way of excising the anal membrane and exposing the underlying rectum is to make two incisions at right angles to each other, forming a "+" centered on the anal dimple.[29] The four, angled skin flaps thus formed are undermined and excised. The subcutaneous tissue is bluntly separated and the blind-ended rectum is isolated and gently pulled caudally with forceps or stay sutures. The end of the rectum is then incised and the mucous membrane is apposed to the skin with simple, interrupted stitches of absorbable suture material.

Fistulae require lengthy dissection, and general anesthesia is required. The majority of these defects can be isolated through a vertical midline perineal incision from the ventral anus to the vulva. Gentle, blunt dissection is used to separate the areolar tissue between the rectum and urogenital tracts. Once isolated, the fistula is excised and the lumens of the anorectum and urogenital tracts are closed separately with simple interrupted stitches of 4/0 or 5/0 synthetic absorbable suture material. If it is malpositioned, the anorectum is relocated in the center of the external anal sphincter muscle, and the mucosa is joined to the skin circumferentially with simple interrupted stitches of the same suture material. The colonic distention is relieved manually and with judicious use of enemas. The colon often is atonic and may require intermittent decompression.

The age and size of dogs with imperforate anus make them poor anesthetic risks and surgical challenges. The ultimate prognosis is good if the condition is diagnosed early and if the animal survives the immediate postoperative period.[18] However, the client must be warned of the potential for incontinence.

Atresia of the rectum requires a pull-through procedure, for which a combined perineal and abdominal approach may be necessary.

TUMORS OF THE RECTUM AND ANUS

Rectal Tumors

Tumors of the rectum are relatively rare.[39] The two most commonly reported are benign polyps (adenomas) and adenocarcinomas.

Rectal polyps usually take the form of solitary or multiple, dark red, sessile or slightly pedunculated masses 0.5 to 3.0 cm.[51, 55] The usual presenting sign is hematochezia, but tenesmus and dyschezia also may be problems. Large polyps are palpable per rectum, but proctoscopy will be necessary for diagnosis when the polyps are small. The short stalk attaching a polyp to the deeper layers of the rectal wall may be apparent or may be obscured by adenomatous epithelium. Several histological forms of polyps have been described.[51]

Rectal polyps can be successfully treated through an anoscope or proctoscope, or by exposure with a rectal retractor. A thorough examination should be made to avoid missing multiple lesions. Several techniques have been described for removing polyps.[45] If the polyp stalk is relatively long, it may

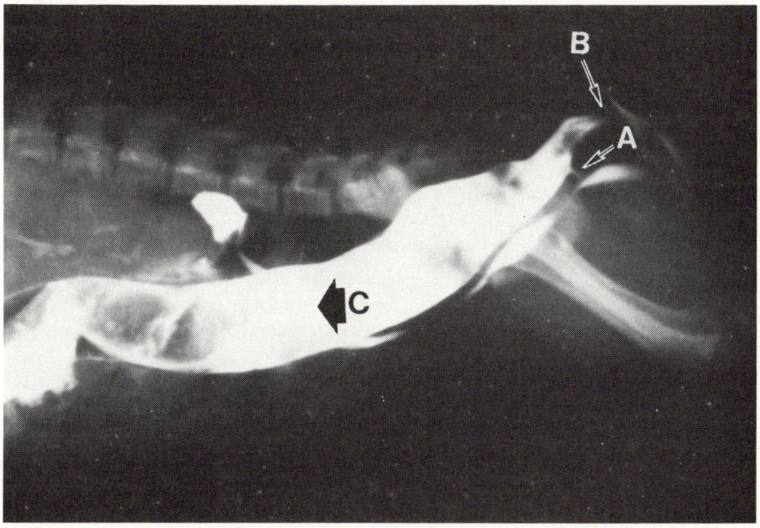

Figure 11–6. Lateral view vaginogram of a 4-week-old chihuahua with imperforate anus and dribbling of liquid stool from the vulva. Note the rectovaginal fistula *(A)*, imperforate anus *(B)*, and megacolon *(C)*.

be clamped with two hemostats, and the polyp may be excised by cutting between the clamps. A tonsil snare works well for removal, if the stalk is short. Electrocautery has also been used. The author has also found cryosurgery to be a safe and expeditious treatment for rectal polyps. A small (2 to 3 mm) cryosurgical probe is used. The probe is touched to the polyp to obtain cryoadhesion. Gentle traction with the probe will then allow easy monitoring of the freeze line as it extends to the base of the stalk.

Carcinoma in situ (malignant-appearing cells) within rectal polyps has been described in both humans and dogs.[49, 51] If the polyp is treated in a manner that preserves the lesion, the specimen should be submitted for histological evaluation.

Rectal adenocarcinomas are most often infiltrative and circumferential, forming a short obstructive "napkin ring" lesion.[39, 55] The clinical signs are tenesmus, dyschezia, and occasionally hematochezia, The bowel wall will become stiff as the tumor spreads into adjacent areas, and it may become attached to the surrounding structures if the serosal and peritoneal surfaces become infiltrated. Besides direct extension, the tumor spreads primarily by way of the lymphatics, and metastasis to the regional lymph nodes is often present at the time of diagnosis.[17] Definitive diagnosis is made by biopsy through an anoscope or a proctoscope.

Surgical treatment for rectal adenocarcinoma is difficult because of the limited ability to completely remove the cancer while maintaining a functionally acceptable pet. Complete abdominoperineal resection is the procedure most commonly used in humans.[52] Because abdominoperineal resection is a complex operation with many complications, its description is beyond the scope of this text.

Anal Tumors

Perinanal adenoma is one of the most common tumors in the dog. It is most often seen in older intact males.[18, 39, 55] It has been suspected for many years that these tumors are hormone-dependent because of the sex predilection and the apparent sensitivity to castration or exogenous estrogen therapy. Recent research has helped to confirm and to explain the role of sex hormones in the development and treatment of these tumors.[9, 26]

The tumors usually develop from the sebaceous or hepatoid-like cells of the perianal glands.[39, 55, 59] They can be solitary or multiple and are usually confined to the perianal region. These tumors may also develop on the dorsal and ventral midline from the tail to the base of the skull.[59]

Perianal adenomas are ovoid or spherical and vary in size. They are located in the anal dermis and frequently are firmly attached to the epidermis.[39] Ulceration with periodic bleeding is common and is often the presenting clinical sign, along with signs of anal irritation such as scooting and licking.[18, 39, 55]

These tumors have characteristic histological features.[39, 55] Lobules or strands of tumor cells extend from the main mass into the muscle bundles of the external anal sphincter.[39] This spread may partially account for the high recurrence rate when limited excision is used as the sole treatment.

Castration alone is an effective treatment for perianal adenomas,[59] although limited resection, cryosurgery, or radiation therapy is often used in conjunction with castration to hasten resolution of the clinical problem.[15, 18, 55, 59] Overzealous local treatment, which might harm or destroy the external anal sphincter, is unwarrented. Exogenous estrogen therapy has fallen into disfavor because of the undesirable side effects estrogens have on the bone marrow.[55, 59]

Adenocarcinoma of the anus cannot be positively differentiated from perianal adenoma on gross appearance,[18, 55] so biopsy of a perianal tumor is always indicated. Adenocarcinomas may develop from either the perianal or anal sac glands. These are aggressive tumors and metastasis to the regional lymph nodes is early and may be present at the time of diagnosis.[18, 59] Wide resection may effect a cure if the tumor is small.[18] Radiation, cryosurgery, and chemotherapy have been recommended for palliative treatment if the adenocarcinoma is advanced or if metastasis is evident, but the prognosis is poor.[15, 18, 55, 59]

Squamous cell carcinomas, melanomas, leiomyomas, and mast cell tumors[18, 55] occasionally originate in the perianal area and must be differentiated from the more common perianal tumors by biopsy.

References

1. Abcarian H, Lowe R: Colon and rectal trauma. Surg Clin North Am 58:519, 1978.
2. Abrahms BL, Alsikafi FH, Waterman NG: Colostomy: A new look at morbidity and mortality. Am Surg 45:462, 1979.
3. Amand, WB: Nonneurogenic disorders of the anus and rectum. Vet Clin North Am 4:535, 1974.
4. Archibald J, Sumner-Smith G: Abdomen. *In* Archibald J (ed): *Canine Surgery*, 2nd ed. American Veterinary Publications, Inc., Wheaton, IL 505, 1974.
5. Bellenger CR: Perineal hernia in dogs. Aust Vet J 56:434, 1980.
6. Berge E, Westhves M: *Veterinary Operative Surgery*. Medical Book Company, Copenhagen, Denmark, 239, 1977.
7. Bloomberg MS: The clinical management of perianal fistulas in the dog. Comp Cont Ed. 2:615, 1980.
8. Burrows CF, Harvey CE: Perineal hernia in the dog. J Small Anim Pract 14:315, 1973.
9. Chaisiri N, Pierrepoint CG: Steroid-receptor interaction in a canine anal adenoma. J Small Anim Pract 20:405, 1979.
10. Condon RE: Rational use of prophylactic antibiotics in gastrointestinal surgery. Surg Clin North Am 55:1300, 1975.
11. Ejaife JA, Elias EG: Delorme's repair for rectal prolapse. Surg Gynecol Obstet 144:757, 1977.
12. Elkins AD, Hobson HP: Management of perianal fistulae. A retrospective study of 23 cases. Vet Surg 11:110, 1982.
13. Evans HE, Christensen, GC: *Miller's Anatomy of the Dog*, 2nd ed. W. B. Saunders Company, Philadelphia, 1973.
14. Fletcher TF: Anatomy of the pelvic viscera. Vet Clin North Am 4:471, 1974.
15. Goldstein RS, Hess PW: Cryosurgery of canine and feline tumors. J Am Anim Hosp Assoc 12:340, 1976.
16. Greiner TP, Christie TR: The cecum, colon, rectum and anus. *In* Bojrab MJ (ed): Current Techniques in Small Animal Surgery. Lea & Febiger, Philadelphia, 126, 1977.
17. Greiner TP, Betts CW: Diseases of the rectum and anus. *In* Ettinger SJ (ed): *Textbook of Veterinary Internal Medicine*. W. B. Saunders Company, Philadelphia, 1307, 1975.
18. Greiner TP: Surgery of the rectum and anus. Vet Clin North Am 2:167, 1972.
19. Hagihara PF, Griffen WO: Transsacral repair of rectal prolapse. Arch Surg 110:343, 1975.
20. Halnan CRE: The diagnosis of anal sacculitis in the dog. J Small Anim Pract 7:527, 1976.
21. Hanley PH: Anorectal abscess fistula. Surg Clin North Am 58:479, 1978.
22. Hardie EM, Kolata RJ, Earley TD, Rawlings CA: Evaluation of internal obturator transposition in treatment of perineal hernia in dogs. Vet Surg 12:69, 1983.
23. Harvey CE: Treatment of perineal hernia in the dog—reassessment. J Small Anim Pract 18:505, 1977.
24. Harvey CE: Incidence and distribution of anal sac disease in the dog. J Am Anim Hosp Assoc 10:573, 1974.
25. Harvey CE: Perianal fistula in the dog. Vet Rec 91:25, 1972.
26. Hayes HM, Wilson GP: Hormone dependent neoplasms of the canine perianal gland. Cancer Res 37:2068, 1977.
27. Houlton JEF: Anal furunculosis: A review of seventy-five cases. J Small Anim Pract 21:575, 1980.
28. Houlton, JEF: Canine anal furunculosis: A modified approach. J Small Anim Pract 21:585, 1980.
29. Horney FD, Archibald J: Colon, rectum and anus. *In* Archibald J (ed): *Canine Surgery*, 2nd ed. American Veterinary Publications, Inc., Wheaton, IL 603, 1974.
30. Howel HS, Bartizal JF, Freeark RJ: Blunt trauma involving the colon and rectum. J Trauma 16:624, 1976.
31. Jubb KVF, Kennedy PC: *Pathology of Domestic Animals*, 2nd ed. Academic Press, New York, 1970.
32. Kolata RJ, Early TD: Perineal hernia in the dog: An alternative method of correction. *In* Bojrab MJ (ed): *Current Techniques in Small Animal Surgery*, 2nd ed. Lea & Febiger, Philadelphia, 405, 1983.
33. Lane JG, Burch DGS: The cryosurgical treatment of canine anal furunculosis. J Small Anim Pract 16:387, 1975.
34. LoCicero J 3rd, Tajima T, Dropanas T: A half-century of experience in the management of colon injuries: Changing concepts. J Trauma 15:575, 1975.
35. Lorber B: The bacteriology of intra-abdominal infections. Surg Clin North Am 55:1349, 1977.
36. Lowry CE: Perianal Fistulas. *In* Bojrab MJ (ed): *Current Techniques in Small Animal Surgery*. Lea & Febiger, Philadelphia, 159, 1977.
37. Mazier WP, De Moraes RT, Dignan RD: Anal fissure and anal ulcers. Surg Clin North Am 58:479, 1978.
38. Nickel R, et al: *The Viscera of the Domestic Mammals*. Springer-Verlag, New York, 1973.
39. Neilsen SW: Classification of tumors in dogs and cats. J Am Anim Hosp Assoc 19:13, 1983.
40. Nigro ND: Procidentia of the rectum. Surg Clin North Am 58:539, 1978.
41. Oliver JE, Selcer RR: Neurogenic disorders of the rectum and anal sphincter. Vet Clin North Am 4:551, 1974
42. O'Rourke DA: An anorectal sling in the treatment of rectal prolapse and incontinence. Aust NZ J Surg 44:144, 1974.
43. Osborne CA, Engen MH, Yano BL: Congenital urethrorectal fistula in two dogs. J Am Vet Med Assoc 166:999, 1975.
44. Palminteri A: Anorectal disease. *In* Kirk RW(ed): *Current Veterinary Therapy IV*. W. B. Saunders Company, Philadelphia, 554, 1971.
45. Palminteri A: The surgical management of polyps of the rectum and colon of the dog. J Am Vet Med Assoc 148:771, 1966.
46. Peacock EE: *Wound Repair*, 3rd ed. W. B. Saunders Company, Philadelphia, 1984.
47. Rawlings CA: Anovaginal and rectovaginal fistulas. *In* Bojrab MJ (ed): *Current Techniques in Small Animal Surgery*. Lea & Febiger, Philadelphia, 161, 1977.
48. Rawlings CA, Capps WF: Rectovaginal fistula and imperforate anus in a dog. J Am Vet Med Assoc 159:320, 1971.
49. Rittenhouse MC, Copeland EM: Carcinoma in situ of the distal part of the colon and of the rectum. Surg Gynecol Obstet 146:225, 1978.

50. Robertson HD, Ray JE, Ferrari BT, Gathright JB: Management of rectal trauma. Surg Gynecol Obstet 154:161, 1982.
51. Seiler RJ: Colorectal polyps of the dog: A clinicopathologic study of 17 cases. J Am Vet Med Assoc 174:72, 1979.
52. Shackelford RT, Zuidema GD (eds): Operative techniques. *In*: *Surgery of the Alimentary Tract*, Vol. 3, 2nd ed. W. B. Saunders Company, Philadelphia, 197, 1982.
53. Smith EI, Tunell WP, Williams GR: A clinical evaluation of the surgical treatment of anorectal malformations (imperforate anus). Ann Surg 187:583, 1978.
54. Spreull JSA, Frankland AL: Transplanting the superficial gluteal muscle in the treatment of perineal hernia and flexure of the rectum in the dog. J Small Anim Pract 21:265, 1980.
55. Theilen GH, Madewell, BR: *Veterinary Cancer Medicine*. Lea & Febiger, Philadelphia, 321, 1979.
56. Vasseur, PB: Perianal fistulae in dogs: A retrospective analysis of surgical techniques. J Am Anim Hosp Assoc 17:177, 1981.
57. Walshaw R, Harvey CE: The rectum and anus. *In* Bojrab MJ (ed): *Pathophysiology In Small Animal Surgery*. Lea & Febiger, Philadelphia, 118, 1981.
58. Wilson CF, Clifford DH: Perineoplasty for anovaginal cleft in a dog. J Am Vet Med Assoc 159:871, 1975.
59. Wilson GP, Hayes HM: Castration for treatment of perianal gland neoplasms in the dog. J Am Vet Med Assoc 174:1301, 1979

CHAPTER

12

Diseases of the Pancreas

FREDERICK H. DRAZNER

The pancreas is a unique organ possessing both exocrine (digestive) and endocrine (hormonal) functions. Because of its multiple physiological functions, pancreatic disease may cause varied symptoms. In addition, the pancreas lies deeply nestled within the abdominal cavity, making physical and radiographic examination difficult. Thus, precise and early detection of pancreatic disease (especially exocrine) presents the clinician with a true diagnostic challenge. In the case of acute necrotizing pancreatitis, early diagnosis is essential if the patient is to be successfully treated, particularly if shock is present.

This chapter concerns itself with both exocrine and endocrine diseases of the pancreas and their relationships to the rest of the alimentary tract. A strong emphasis is placed on normal and abnormal physiology. Relevant comparisons to human pancreatic disease are made. The prospects of future diagnostic and therapeutic techniques are also discussed.

ANATOMY AND PHYSIOLOGY OF THE PANCREAS

GENERAL, GROSS, AND TOPOGRAPHICAL ANATOMY

The pancreas is located in the anterior right abdominal quadrant caudal to the liver and the diaphragm. The color of the pancreas varies from a light pink to a brownish red, depending upon its physiological activity and amount of congestion. Its relative weight is approximately 0.2 per cent of the body weight. When hardened *in situ,* it forms a "V," with the apex extending cranially. The gland is lobulated, consisting of a long, slender right lobe and a shorter, thicker left lobe.[11]

The right lobe of the pancreas is situated within the mesoduodenum, lying in close contact with the duodenum. It extends from the pylorus, often reaching as far posterior as the cecum. The caudal portion of the right lobe comes in contact with the sublumbar fat and is adjacent to the right ureter, the ventral surface of the right kidney, and the caudate process of the liver (Fig. 12–1).[11]

The left lobe of the pancreas is encased in the dorsal sheet of the greater omentum and originates at the pancreatic angle, running caudally to the left. The dorsal surface comes in contact with the portal vein, postcava, aorta, spleen, and left kidney (from cranial to caudal), while the ventral surface is close to the stomach and the transverse colon (from cranial to caudal).[11]

These intimate anatomical relationships readily explain the effects of acute pancreatitis on the adjacent viscera, including the duodenum, stomach, left and right kidneys, transverse colon, and proximal portion of the small intestine. Pancreatic necrosis and subsequent peritonitis can cause extensive damage to the organs through direct contact with pancreatic ferments.[30] Injury can occur to the numerous large vascular structures that course through the pancreatic area; hemorrhage or thrombosis and ischemic necrosis result from this type of injury.

The dog nearly always has two pancreatic ducts—one beginning dorsally at the duodenum and the other ventrally at the end of

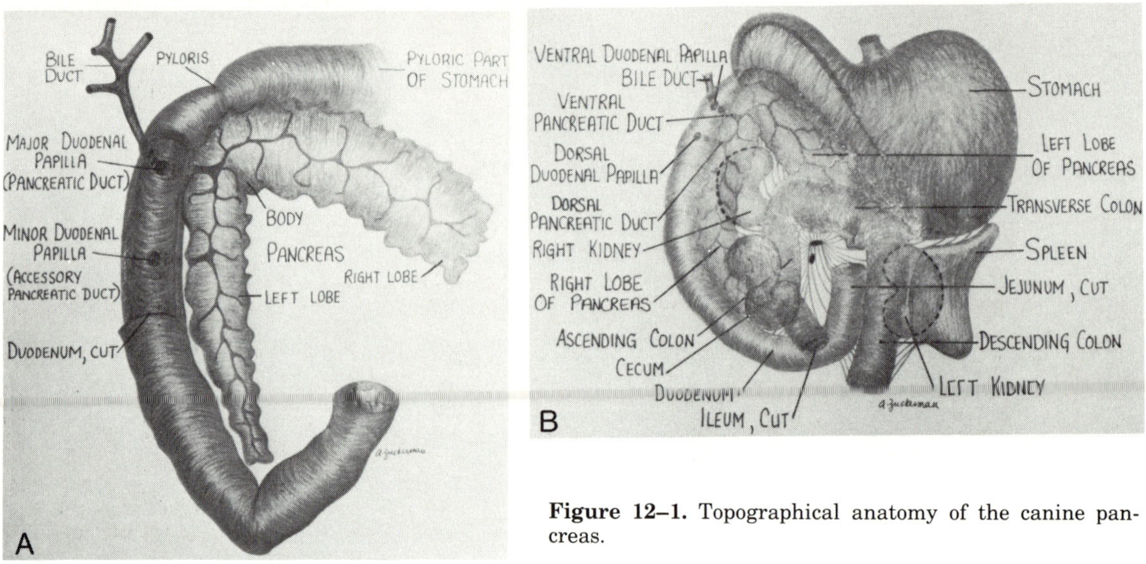

Figure 12–1. Topographical anatomy of the canine pancreas.

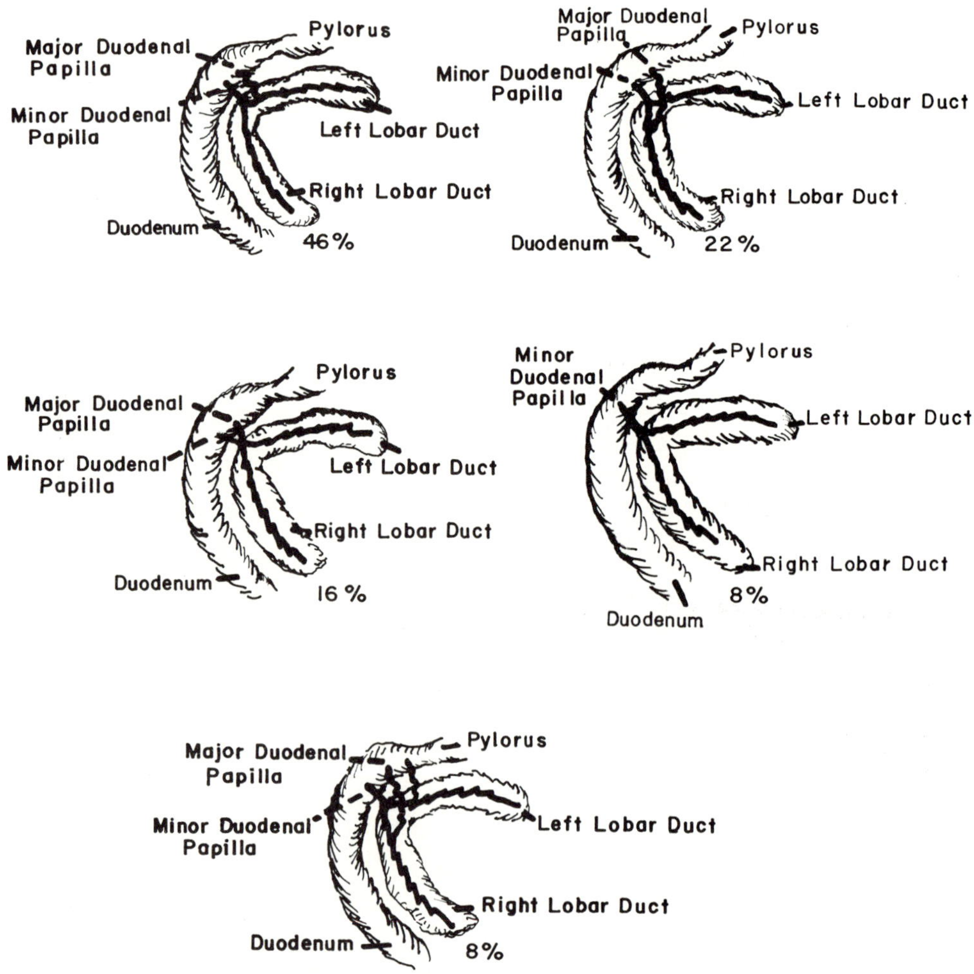

Figure 12–2. Variations of the duct system of the canine pancreas.

the bile duct.[11] Usually, these ducts run side-by-side within the gland and intercommunicate.[11] In those animals whose pancreatic ducts do not intercommunicate within the gland, the ventral duct drains the right pancreatic lobe and the dorsal duct drains the left lobe.[11] In 75 per cent of canine specimens the two pancreatic ducts individually enter the duodenum.[11] In the dog, five main ductal arrangements have been described (Fig. 12–2), whereas in the cat, the common bile duct enters the pancreas, an arrangement similar to that seen in humans, and then travels with the dorsal pancreatic duct to the major duodenal papilla where they both enter the duodenum.[11, 31] The ventral or accessory pancreatic duct is sometimes absent in the cat.[31] The configuration with the dorsal pancreatic ducts being intimately related to the common bile duct explains the finding of icterus in the feline patients with acute necrotizing pancreatitis.

The majority of the arterial blood supply of the right lobe of the pancreas arises from the celiac artery via the cranial and caudal pancreaticoduodenal arteries (Fig. 12–3). The pancreatic branch of the splenic artery supplies the left side of the pancreas. Venous drainage of the right lobe of the pancreas is provided by the caudal pancreaticoduodenal vein, where the left lobe is drained by two veins that terminate in the splenic vein. Lymphatic drainage is by vessels that course into the duodenal, hepatic, splenic, and mesenteric lymph nodes.[11]

It is important to consider pancreatic innervation because one consistent clinical sign of patients suffering from pancreatic inflammatory or neoplastic disease is pain.[10] In humans, the pain can be referred to the thoracolumbar area.[10] The author has seen several cases of acute canine pancreatitis in which the primary veterinarian had ordered a work-up for thoracolumbar disc disease because the chief clinical sign was back pain. The most common area of hyperesthesia is in the upper right abdominal quadrant. It has been found that pain pathways are mediated by both parasympathetic and sympathetic nerve fibers.[10] The sympathetic innervation arises from the celiac and cranial mesenteric plexuses.[11] The celiac plexus innervates the majority of the gland and travels with the cranial pancreaticoduodenal artery, whereas the caudal portion of the right pancreatic lobe is innervated by sympathetic fibers of the mesenteric plexus, which run beside the caudal pancreaticoduodenal artery.[11] In the dog, parasympathetic innervation is provided by the vagal fibers, which are quite filamentous and traverse with the caudal pancreaticoduodenal artery, the splenic branch of the celiac artery, and the cranial mesenteric artery.[11]

MICROSCOPIC ANATOMY

Being both an endocrine and exocrine gland, the pancreas develops from the dorsal and ventral outgrowths of the primitive gut.[10, 16] The dorsal and ventral diverticula arise from the endodermal lining of the developing duodenum and are transformed into mesoderm.[10, 16, 53] In the canine, the two separate diverticular buds persist in the neonate as separate pancreatic ducts, each opening separately into the duodenum and

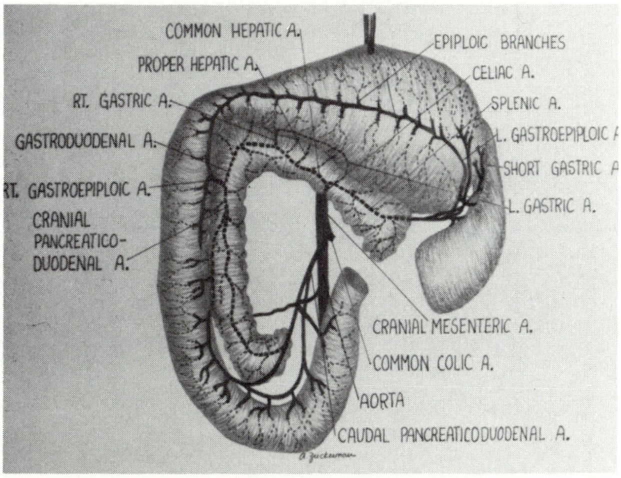

Figure 12–3. Arterial supply to the pancreas. The ventral, mesenteric aspect of the celiac and cranial arteries is shown. The stomach is reflected cranially.

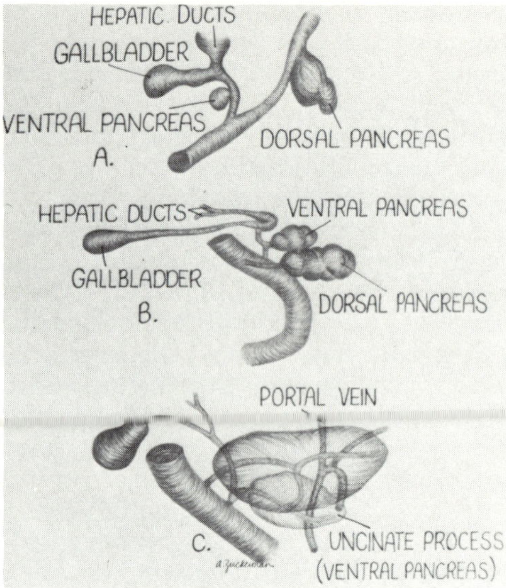

Figure 12–4. Pancreatic embryogenesis.

each draining the part of the pancreas that originates from the specific diverticulum with which that duct is associated (Fig. 12–4).[16, 53]

The mesoderm or mesenchymal factor in the embryonic development of the pancreas appears to play a part in cytodevelopment by interacting with the cellular membrane or the precursor cells.[50] This factor has the ability to affect the differentiation of the precursor epithelial cells. It is made up of at least two functional components, a heat-stable component that may be substituted by cyclic AMP derivatives, which freely cross cell membranes and a high molecular-weight component that is not interchangeable with cyclic AMP, cyclic GMP, or their analogues.[53] This multiple developmental system may be found in the physiological activity of mesenchymal cells in other organ systems because nearly all organ systems are characterized by interactions between epithelial and mesenchymal cell derivatives.[53]

The pancreas is a compound tubuloacinar gland resembling the structure of a salivary gland.[5, 16] The terminal sections of the two ductal systems develop into exocrine secretory units. The clusters of cells that form around the intralobular ducts resemble grapes dangling on stems and are thus called acini.[5] Parasympathetic nerves are

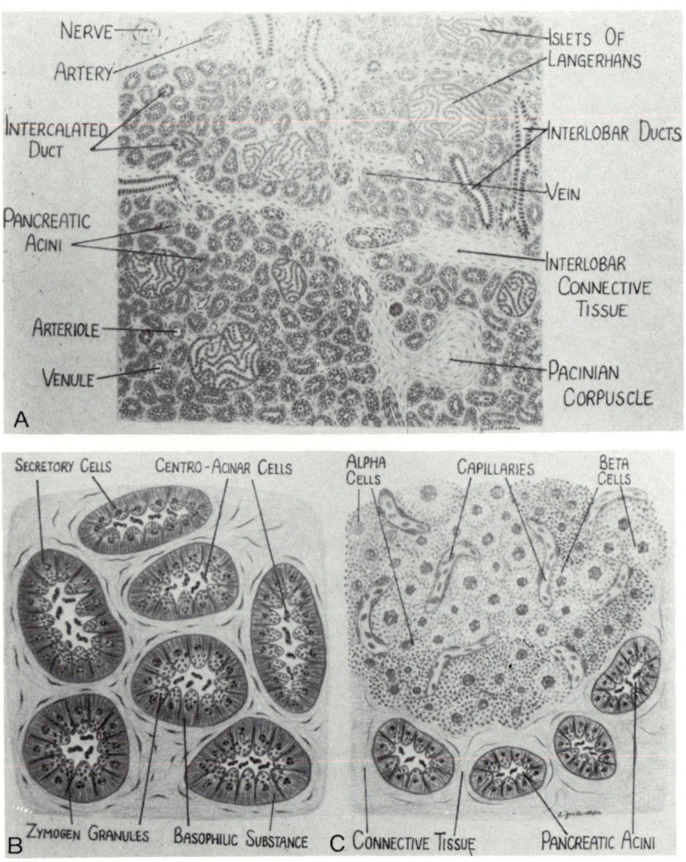

Figure 12–5. A diagrammatic scheme of the microscopic structure of the pancreas. *A*, Sectional view of the pancreas. *B*, Pancreatic acini. *C*, Islets of Langerhans.

found in contact with the base of the acinar cells where they regulate secretory activity.[16] Some clumps of cells that arise from a developing duct system fail to develop a lumen and become islets of Langherhans, which are endocrine in function (Figs. 12–5 and 12–6).[5]

The pancreas of the canine, and especially of the feline, is also interspersed with pale-staining concentrically layered structures called pacinian corpuscles that function in mediating sensory and proprioceptive impulses.[3, 16]

The morphology of the acinar cell is influenced by its function.[5, 16] The acinar cells are pyramidal, with the apexes directed toward the lumen.[5, 16] The purpose of these cells is to synthesize enzymes and secrete them into the ductal system.[5, 16] Acinar cells are large and contain elaborate nuclei and an abundantly granular cytoplasm.[16] The cytoplasmic packets, zymogen granules, have acidophilic-staining material.[5] Zymogen granules are released from the apical region of sensory cells into the lumen of the secretory unit.[16] The number and elaborate

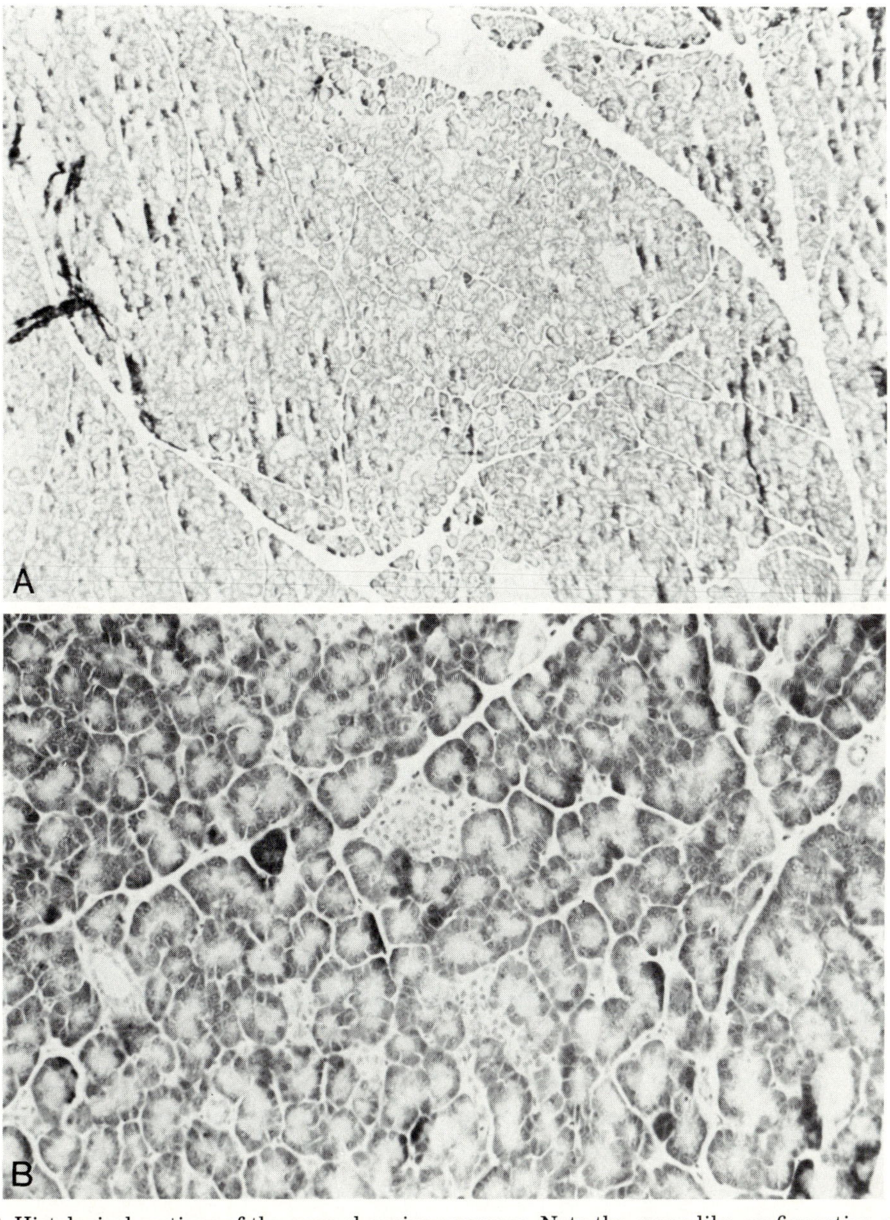

Figure 12–6. Histological sections of the normal canine pancreas. Note the grape-like configuration of the acinar tissue, which is exocrine in function (*B*), and pale-staining islet tissue, which is endocrine in function (*A*). *A*, ×100; *B*, ×250.

structure of the organelles within the pancreatic acinar cells reflect the dynamic metabolic activity of the gland in the production of digestive enzymes, fluid, and electrolytes.[10]

The islets of Langerhans are vital centers for the production of hormones.[16, 55] In addition, a significant number of endocrine cells are found in the acinar structures and in the walls of excretory ducts. The existence of alpha and beta islet cells that secrete glucagon and insulin, respectively, has been known for many years; however, recent studies employing both light and electron microscopy and involving various animal species have revealed four additional types of islet cells (C, D, E, and F cells).[10] Some researchers have termed these non–beta islet cells amine precursor uptake and decarboxylation (APUD) cells.[21] These cells arise embryologically from the neural crest, like those cells that produce the catecholamines epinephrine and norepinephrine as well as 5-hydroxytryptamine (serotonin).[21] APUD cells function to synthesize the preceding vasoactive amines and, in addition, the peptide hormones gastrin, somatostatin, antidiuretic hormone (ADH), adrenocorticotropic hormone (ACTH), parathormone, vasoactive intestinal peptide (VIP), enterogastrone, insulin, and glucagon.[21] Besides residing in the pancreas, these specialized cells are found in the intestinal tract, the pituitary gland, the thyroid gland, and the adrenal glands.[21] In humans, tumors of the islet cells and the organs where these cells are located sometimes have been found to produce excessive quantities of peptide hormones, leading to a variety of bizarre clinical symptoms;[21] similar findings have been recently reported in dogs.[21] Some of the syndromes that result are discussed later in this chapter.

NORMAL PANCREATIC PHYSIOLOGY

Greater than 90 per cent (by weight) of the canine pancreas is devoted to exocrine function, delivering pancreatic juice to the duodenum.[3] The enzymes in pancreatic juice have the ability to split starch (amylase), fats (lipase), and proteins (trypsin, chymotrypsin, carboxypeptidase, elastase, ribonuclease, deoxyribonuclease, and collagenase.[5] Secreting at its maximum capacity, the pancreas transports a quantity of sodium bicarbonate that is more than ample to neutralize the gastric acid.[5, 32] The alkalinization of the duodenal area is vital for proper digestion, since all the enzymes of the pancreas function optimally in an alkaline environment.[5, 32]

Pancreatic secretory activity is not a steady process but a rapid response to appropriate digestive stimuli.[5, 32, 52] Pancreatic juice is colorless and odorless and has a specific gravity of approximately 1.010 to 1.040, which increases with increased enzyme secretion.[5, 32, 52] When the rate of secretion is minimal, the viscosity of the pancreatic juice increases owing to a higher concentration of mucus produced by the goblet cells that line the ductal system and respond to parasympathetic vagal or sympathetic stimulation.[5, 32, 52] Canine pancreatic juice has a pH of 8.0 to 8.3 and is produced at the rate of 70 ml/kg daily.[3, 7] The most significant difference between pancreatic juice and blood plasma is the high concentration of pancreatic bicarbonate (60 to 148 mEq/1 *vs* 24 mEq/1). Concentrations of the remainder of the ionic components (Na^+, K^+, H_2O) are similar to those of the plasma.[10, 32, 52]

The proteolytic enzymes are produced, stored, and secreted in an inactive form (trypsinogen, chymotrypsinogen, procarboxypeptidase, and proelastase).[5, 32, 52] The action of enterokinase, an enzyme secreted by the duodenal mucosa, activates trypsinogen into proteolytically active trypsin.[5, 32, 52] Trypsin will then activate the rest of the proteases.[5, 32, 52] It has been shown that zinc is essential for the catalytic activity of carboxypeptidase (Tab. 12–1).[56]

Because these potentially damaging enzymes are present in pancreatic juice, some self-protective mechanism must also be present. Actually, three protective mechanisms are utilized. The first is that the proteolytic enzymes are not activated until they enter the duodenum.[10, 38, 56] The second is that trypsin, ribonuclease, and deoxyribonuclease inhibitors are secreted by the pancreatic acinar cells.[56] These protease inhibitors are proteins which are similar to although chemically distinct from the inhibitors present in the bloodstream.[56] The third protective mechanism is the presence of circulating protease inhibitors that prevent the activation of any proteolytic enzymes that may slip into the extracellular fluid (ECF) or plasma.[38, 56] These inhibitors are essential because approximately 1 to 2 per cent of the proteases that are normally secreted by the pancreatic acinar cells do not enter the ducts and migrate into the duodenal lumen.[56] Instead, these proteases diffuse back into the ECF and plasma.[56] The protease inhibitors found in the canine plasma include: (1) α-1-antitrypsin, which inhibits trypsin, chymotrypsin, and elastase as well as plasmin, and thrombin; (2) alpha-2-macroglobulin, which prevents trypsin from digesting proteins; and (3) complement (C_1) esterase inhibitor, which inhibits C_1 esterase, chymotrypsin, plasma, and kallikrein). All of these protease inhibitors are manufactured by the liver. Thus, it is apparent that in patients with hepatic impairment (e.g., cirrhosis) there would be a deficiency of these circulating protease inhibitors in the plasma and an increased incidence of pancreatitis. With pancreatic acinar damage, the production of these inhibitor substances is blocked, allowing intracellular and intraductal activation of the proteolytic enzymes.

Pancreatic amylase is secreted in its active form and splits polysaccharides (glycogen and amylopectin) to form a mixture of disaccharides and monosaccharides.[3,4,5,32] Its work is supplemented by the disaccharidases produced by the intestinal mucosa. The normal serum amylase activity in the dog has been shown to be derived from the intestinal brush border. In patients with enteritis (without pancreatic inflammatory disease) serum amylase activity will sometimes double.[7] Thus, a technique for differentiating the sources of serum amylase activity via electrophoresis would be a useful tool in the diagnosis of acute pancreatitis.

Pancreatic lipase (glycerol ester hydrolase) is also secreted in its active form.[32,56] It hydrolyzes neutral fat to glycerol and fatty acids optimally at an alkaline pH.[32] This enzyme acts by cleaving the alpha ester bonds of emulsified, water-insoluble carboxylic esters (e.g., the glycerol esters).[5,10,32] This cleavage results in the splitting of triglyceride to yield fatty acids (FA) from the two primary (alpha) positions and 2-(beta) monoglyceride.[32] In addition, lipase binds the water-soluble side of the molecule to triglyceride particles, which are also hydrophobic.[32] It is apparent that emulsifying substances for water-insoluble substrates are needed for lipase activity.[32] Previously, it was thought that bile salts enhance lipase activity, but recent evidence now shows that bile salts shift the optimal intraluminal duodenal pH of between 8 and 9 to between 6 and 7.[4] It has now been shown that a small (MW, 10,000 daltons) protein, and co-lipase, which is secreted in pancreatic juice, forms a 1-1 complex with lipase.[56] Co-lipase shields lipase from the inhibitory effects of bile salts and protects the enzyme from denaturation.[56] It is imperative for calcium ions to be present (they are bonded to bile salts) to permit the binding of lipase to water-insoluble substrates.[56] Another ill-defined form of lipase that does require bilt salts for its activation exists in mammalian pancreatic juice.[56] This enzyme has been termed non-specific lipase-esterase.[56] An example of its function is in the cleaving of vitamin A esters to vitamin A alcohol and fatty acids.[56] A third enzyme with lipolytic activity splits ingested cholesterol and has been called cholesterol esterase.[56] Cholesterol esterase requires the bile salt, taurocholic acid, as a co-factor.[56] Pancreatic juice also contains two phospholipases, A and B, which produce lysolecithin, and lysocephalin and glyceryl-phosphorylcholine, respectively.[54]

The pancreas, like the stomach, manufactures a minimal concentration of juice at rest.[5,10,32] Pancreatic secretion is controlled by both nervous and hormonal mechanisms

Table 12–1. DIGESTIVE ENZYMES IN PANCREATIC JUICE

Secreted Form	Activator	Active Form	Inhibitor
Trypsinogen	Enterokinase + Ca^{++}	Trypsin	Trypsin inhibitor
Chymotrypsinogen A	Trypsin + Ca^{++}	Chymotrypsin A	Trypsin inhibitor
Chymotrypsinogen B	Trypsin + Ca^{++}	Chymotrypsin B	Trypsin inhibitor
Procarboxypeptidase	Trypsin + Zn^{++}	Carboxypeptidase	None
Leucine aminopeptidase	None	Same	None
Ribonuclease	None	Same	Specific inhibitor
Deoxyribonuclease	None	Same	Specific inhibitor
Proelastase	Trypsin + Ca^{++}	Elastase	Elastase inhibitor
Prophospholipase-A	Trypsin + Ca^{++}	Phospholipase A	None
Collagenase	None	Same	None
2-Amylase	None	Same	None
Lipase	Co-lipase + Ca^{++}	Same	None

that are affected by the cephalic, gastric, and intestinal phases of digestion.[5, 30]

The cephalic phase is influenced by the sight, smell, and anticipation of food and by the presence of food in the oral cavity. This phase, mediated entirely by the efferent vagal fibers, produces a pancreatic secretion that is small in volume and concentrated in enzymes.[10] Vagal stimulation liberates not only acetylcholine but also the peptide hormone gastrin from the antrum of the stomach. Gastrin is similar in structure to cholecystokinin/pancreozymin (CCK/PZ) and causes a considerable flow of pancreatic enzymes.[10] The vagal stimulation of gastrin is about five times as potent as the vagal release of acetylcholine in producing pancreatic enzyme release.[10] In addition, gastrin release stimulates acid secretion; the acid enters the duodenum, thereby causing the release of secretin, another potent pancreatic exocrine stimulus.[10] Vagal impulses have only a slight influence on water and electrolytes.[10]

The gastric phase of digestion is influenced both neurally and hormonally.[10] The neural mechanism is known as the gastropancreatic reflex (vagovagal reflex); mechanical distention of the stomach evokes an afferent vagal impulse to the brain and a subsequent efferent vagal motor response to the pancreas, causing it to secrete an enzyme-rich fluid.[10] The hormonal component is activated by release of gastrin in response to gastric distention.[10]

The intestinal phase appears to be entirely influenced by humoral factors.[10] The release of secretin is stimulated by the presence of acid in the duodenum and produces a voluminous flow of pancreatic juice that is high in bicarbonate and other electrolytes, but low in enzymes.[10] A definitive study has shown that the two classic duodenal hormones, cholecystokinin (CCK) and pancreozymin (PZ), are in reality the same chemical substance, a peptide of 33 amino acid residues; thus, CCK/PZ is called CCK for the remainder of this discussion.[10, 56] Cholecystokinin secretion is enhanced greatly by amino acids and long-chain fatty acids and causes secretion of a pancreatic fluid that is very rich in enzymes. In addition, another peptide hormone termed vasoactive intestinal peptide (VIP) has been isolated and seems to be similar in structure and activity to secretin.[56] CCK's effects upon pancreatic secretion when given intravenously may be blocked by infusion of somatostatin, a hormone that is found in the central nervous system and gastrointestinal tract.[56] Somatostatin has been shown to block the release of growth hormone, insulin, glucagon, secretin, and pancreatic polypeptide.[56] Although it has been isolated from a variety of mammalian pancreases, the physiological role of pancreatic polypeptide is ill-defined.[56] Plasma levels of pancreatic polypeptide rise post-prandially, because of the entrance of gastric HCl into the duodenal lumen or because of vagal stimulation.[30] It is curious that large concentrations of infused pancreatic polypeptide block secretin responses and pancreatic enzyme secretion, but minute concentrations will augment enzyme secretion.[56] A peptide hormone, chymodenin, has been isolated and has been shown to augment the secretion of chymotrypsinogen in the rabbit pancreas (Tab. 12–2).[56]

An important co-factor in pancreatic secretion is calcium.[56] Calcium activates certain pancreatic lipases and proteases and acts as a second messenger for acetylcholine, gastrin, and CCK.[56] Approximately one-fifth of the intrapancreatic calcium is enzyme-bound, whereas the remaining four-fifths is in the ionized state.[56] Ionized calcium may migrate into the pancreatic juice through the intracellular tight junctions.[56] The increased incidence of acute pancreatitis in human patients with hypercalcemia is of clinical importance.[56]

Inhibition of pancreatic secretion can be achieved by infusions of hypertonic glucose, glucagon, antidiuretic hormone, catecholamines, and belladonna derivatives.[3, 56] Knowledge of this phenomenon may be useful in clinical management of pancreatitis.

Pancreatitis

INCIDENCE AND ETIOLOGY

Acute pancreatitis and chronic relapsing pancreatitis account for the majority (approximately 66 per cent) of clinical cases of pancreatic disease in dogs.[2, 3] Strombeck reports an incidence of 3.2 per 1,000 cases of canine acute pancreatitis in a six-year period at the Veterinary Medicine Teaching Hospital (VMTH), University of California, Davis, with an approximately equal distribution between males and females.[63] The data also indicates that the dachshund has a higher breed incidence. However, in the

Table 12–2. HORMONAL CONTROL OF PANCREATIC SECRETION

Hormone*	Origin	Stimuli for Release	Pancreas Target Cells	Second Messenger	Effects on Exocrine Pancreas
CCK	Duodenum, jenunum, I cells	Essential amino acids; HCl released to duodenum (pH < 3); fatty acids; soaps; Ca^{++}, K^{+}, Mg^{++}. Bile salts inhibit release (may be clinically useful)	Acinar cells	Ca^{++}	Increases enzyme secretion (+ + +) and synthesis; potentiates secretin; stimulates acinar hyperplasia
Gastrin	Stomach antrum, duodenum, G cells	Antrum or duodenum pH < 3; postganglionic vagal stimulation	Acinar cells	Ca^{++}	Increases enzyme secretion (+); potentiates secretin
Secretin	Duodenum, S cells	Duodenal pH < 4.5; bile in the duodenum	Acinar cells, centroacinar cells pancreas; ductal cells pancreas; bile ducts	cAMP	Bicarbonate and water secretion (+ + +); potentiates CCK
(VIP)	Intestine, ?H cells, pancreas, D_1 cells	Physiological release mechanisms unknown; possible local tissue hormone	Ductal cells, acinar cells	cAMP	Bicarbonate and water secretion (+); in large doses, vasodilation, smooth muscle relaxation; augments CCK effect
Glucagon	A cells, pancreatic islet cells	Hypoglycemia; secretin, CCK, gastric inhibitory polypeptide	Ductal cells, acinar cells	cAMP	Inhibits enzyme secretion and volume output (may be clinically useful)
Acetylcholine	Postganglionic cholinergic fibers	CNS stimulation to vagal nucleus; smell, taste; hypoglycemia; local reflexes like gastric distention	Acinar cells	Ca^{++}	Increases enzyme secretion (+ + +) and synthesis
(Somatostatin)	Pancreatic islet cells, stomach antrum, upper intestine, D cells	Probable local tissue hormone; release factors unknown	?	?	Inhibits secretin and CCK release, and volume response to secretin (may be clinically useful)
(Pancreatic polypeptide)	Non-islet D_2 cells, acinar cells, ductal cells	Mixed gastric meal and duodenal HCl; probably CCK, secretin; insulin, hypoglycemia	Acinar cells	?	Suppresses enzyme secretion; low doses augment and high doses inhibit secretin responses
(Chymodenin)	?	Unknown	Acinar cells	?	Specific stimulation of chymotrypsinogen secretion

*Hormones in brackets ( ) have not been proved to have a physiological role in pancreatic secretion.

Adapted from Snodgrass PJ: Pathophysiology of the pancreas. *In* Sodeman WA, Sodeman TM (eds): Pathologic Physiology. W. B. Saunders Company, Philadelphia, 1979.

author's experience, the miniature schnauzer has been most frequently diagnosed as having acute pancreatitis, followed by the dachshund.[3, 63] Non-inflammatory diseases (e.g., juvenile atrophy, neoplasia, and primary diabetes mellitus) constitute the remaining 33 per cent of cases of canine pancreatic disease.[63] Pancreatic inflammatory disease has been documented less frequently in the cat. It appears that many cases of feline pancreatic disease may progress as subclinical interstitial processes that are frequently incidental findings at necropsy.[46] However, the subclinical nature of feline pancreatic disease may be misleading and may reflect the outdoor habits of some cats or a lack of observation by clients.[46] Even though the usual configurations of the pancreatic and biliary ducts of cats and humans are similar, it is the dog that has an incidence of pancreatitis similar to that of humans.

The etiology of naturally occurring canine and feline acute pancreatitis is obscure. Most often the small animal clinician must be content to advise the client that the cause of the animal's acute pancreatitis is unknown. Much of the confusion regarding the etiology of acute pancreatitis can be attributed to (1) the confusion between naturally occurring disease and the methods that may be used to experimentally produce acute pancreatitis, (2) the confusion, which is due to a paucity of pathological studies, of simple acute interstitial edematous pancreatitis with acute necrotizing pancreatitis, and (3) the confusion among small animal clinicians in the establishment of an ante-mortem diagnosis of acute pancreatitis.

Nutrition imbalance appears to be an important factor in the development of the canine disease.[63] Experimentally, acute pancreatitis can be produced by feeding dogs a diet containing more than 60 per cent fat. Dogs that are fed a low-fat diet and are exercised at frequent intervals rarely develop acute necrotizing pancreatitis.[63] Indeed, a lack of exercise and the "privilege" of eating high-calorie table scraps are often part of the history.[63] It has been shown that CCK is optimally stimulated by ingestion of foods that are high in fats and proteins, thereby increasing synthesis and release of pancreatic enzymes.[63] Experimental data suggests that the stability of acinar cell membranes against the lytic effects of trypsin and bile salts is reduced by a high-fat diet, perhaps because the lipid structure of these membranes is changed.[15, 63]

Abdominal trauma is another cause of acute pancreatitis. It has been seen in dogs that have been hit by cars and in cats that have fallen or jumped from high altitudes ("high rise syndrome").[46] In addition, abdominal surgery may result in acute pancreatitis due to trauma to the organ (spearing the pancreas with a spay hook) or excessive manipulation.

Hypercalcemia has been incriminated as a cause of acute pancreatitis in humans.[14, 57] There has been a case report of pancreatitis in a dog that was given excessive parenteral calcium supplementation.[45] The pathological processes involved in pancreatitis due to hypercalemia are hypothesized to be the production of a vasculitis in the pancreatic microcirculation, the precipitation of protein plugs in the pancreatic ducts, and the intrapancreatic activation of trypsin by the excessive concentration of calcium.[45] Hypercalcemia can be caused by hyperparathyroidism, vitamin D intoxication, excessive parenteral calcium supplementation, metastatic bone tumors, and lymphoreticular tumors that manufacture a parathormone-like hormone.[22]

Drugs have long been incriminated in the production of human pancreatitis. Iatrogenic pancreatitis has been reported secondary to the administration of sulfamethizole, thiazide, morphine, salicylazosulfapyridine,* chlorpromazine,† isoniazid, and corticosteroids.[15, 24, 57] The author has seen several acute cases of acute pancreatitis that were thought to be precipitated by hyperadrenocorticism (Cushing's syndrome) due to adrenal hyperplasia. All of these patients eventually became insulin-dependent diabetics. It is thought that glucocorticoids cause proliferation of pancreatic ductal epithelium, increased enzyme production, increased viscosity of secretions, and occlusive angiopathy of the pancreatic microcirculation.[63] It is interesting to note that earlier veterinary texts advocated the use of corticosteroids in acute pancreatitis to relieve inflammation.

Hyperlipidemia may play a role in the pathogenesis of acute pancreatitis in some dogs.[63] Some miniature schnauzers appear

*Azulfidine, Pharmacia Laboratories, Piscataway, NJ.

†Thorazine, Smith Kline Corporation, Philadelphia, PA.

to have abnormal lipoprotein patterns (types IV and V). It is thought that high levels of plasma lipids may produce fat emboli and subsequent pancreatic ischemia.[63] In addition, high levels of circulatory fatty acids may injure pancreatic capillaries. In humans, a familial lipidemia with recurrent pancreatitis has been described, and in another variant (type I-hyperchylomicronemia) an elevated plasma triglyceride level is thought to be responsible for a reduction of lipoprotein lipase activity.[57]

Infectious agents are thought to cause pancreatitis in some cases, with viral organisms such as cytomegaloviruses, picornaviruses, herpesviruses, and reoviruses causing experimentally induced acute pancreatitis.[15, 57] Recently, the author has found pancreatic necrosis at post-mortem examination in a few dogs afflicted with canine parvovirus CPV.[23] It is unknown whether CPV is directly cytotoxic against pancreatic tissue or whether pancreatitis develops secondarily to the reflux of enterokinase into the pancreatic ducts as a result of profound duodenal paralytic ileus. The canine pancreas contains a resident population of bacteria such as *Clostridium perfringens* that may proliferate secondarily to pancreatic ischemia.[30, 63] In addition, gram-negative enteric bacteria present in the duodenum may reflux into the pancreas. However, the role of bacteria as a cause of acute necrotizing pancreatitis appears to be either as a secondary complication of pancreatic ischemia with the establishment of an anaerobic environment or as the extension of a primary cholecystitis through connecting lymphatics into the pancreas.[63]

Vascular impairment may account for a considerable number of cases of acute pancreatitis.[24, 57] In hypovolemic shock, the body releases a high level of catecholamines (epinephrine and norepinephrine) in an attempt to divert blood from the splanchnic viscera to areas that are more vital to survival (e.g., brain and coronary circulation), thus producing pancreatic ischemia.[10] A classic example of secondary acute pancreatitis may be seen in dogs with gastric volvulus. The author has noted the presence of acute necrotizing pancreatitis with disseminated intravascular coagulation in several terminal cases of gastric volvulus. It is thought that the hypovolemic shock associated with gastric volvulus creates profound pancreatic ischemia.

Pancreatitis has been observed in some dogs that have undergone thoracolumbar neurosurgery.[44, 63] Most thoracolumbar myelopathies (especially intervertebral disc syndrome) are treated with glucocorticoids; this treatment may lead to the development of pancreatitis. Manipulation of the spinal cord will sometimes result in a severe reflex hypotensive episode.[63] With a reduction of pancreatic blood flow, the level of α-trypsin inhibitors is greatly diminished; the likelihood of intraorgan activation of trypsin, which catalyzes the activation of the other proteases is increased.[10] Vagotonia may be another mechanism of insult to the pancreas; the innervation of the intestine and pancreatic sphincter is altered, resulting in stasis of pancreatic secretions and pancreatitis.[44]

Some investigators believe that chronic relapsing pancreatitis may be the result of immune-mediated disease. According to one hypothesis, the initiation of acute necrotizing pancreatitis causes the release of various intracellular organelles (e.g., Golgi apparatus, endoplasmic reticulum).[13, 63] An antigenic response from the body results with the subsequent production of antibody.[13, 63] Immunofluorescent studies have detected antibody formation against the acinar cytoplasmic organelles.[13, 63] This hypothesis is similar to the belief that some patients with chronic active hepatitis progress to a cirrhotic state because of immune-mediated disease. Thus, the seemingly subclinical progression of acute pancreatitis to pancreatic fibrosis and exocrine insufficiency may be the result of a combination of a type III immunological (Arthus) reaction and cell-mediated lymphocyte cytotoxicity, a type IV immunological reaction.[13, 63]

Two causes of naturally occurring acute pancreatitis in humans cannot be considered important in the dog.[63] The influence of cholecystitis[10, 63] upon the development of acute pancreatitis is due to the connection of the lymphatic vessels of the gallbladder with those of the pancreatic subacinar spaces.[15] Infectious agents or toxic products may migrate into the pancreas. However, cholecystitis is uncommon in the dog.[63] Human, but not canine, acute pancreatitis is also caused by the reflux of duodenal contents into the pancreatic duct secondary to duodenitis.[15] Acute pancreatitis may be experimentally produced by closure of the proximal and distal duodenum and injection of enterokinase into the pancreatic duct.[10, 63] The activation of trypsin that results will activate the other proteolytic enzymes. Duodenal reflux is not a factor in naturally occurring canine acute pancreatitis because the pressure of the fluid within the duodenum must be greater than that within the pancreatic duct.[63] This pressure relationship is not possible because the canine duodenum is a hollow tube that is open at both ends.[63] Any increase in duodenal fluid pressure at one end would cause the fluid to be moved toward the opposite end.[63] The only instances in which naturally occurring acute pancreatitis may be explained by duodenal reflux are the presence of a duodenal obstruction and severe duodenal paralytic ileus, which may occur with severe canine parvovirus.[63]

PATHOGENESIS OF ACUTE PANCREATIC ACINAR INFLAMMATION

The pancreas may be regarded as a sac of potentially lethal proteolytic enzymes. The basic pathological process is autodigestion due to the destruction of cell membranes and the premature activation and release of these proteolytic and lipolytic enzymes.[2, 3, 15, 54] The classic forms of pancreatitis are the interstitial endematous form and the highly fatal necrotizing form.[2, 3, 15, 30]

Many theories have been proposed regarding the factors that trigger the inflammatory process. Three inciting factors usually must be present (1) an actively secreting or stimulated gland, (2) pancreatic ductal obstruction, and (3) degeneration and lysis of the cell membrane with a subsequent activation of enzymes.[10, 15, 30] The exact cause of the cytolytic process within the pancreatic cellular membranes is unknown; however, activation of the complement system may be a contributory step.[15, 57] It has been shown experimentally that fixation of complement components five to nine ($C_5{}^1$ to $C_9{}^1$) produces cellular membrane degeneration, permitting extracellular fluid to permeate the cell and to cause its destruction.[10, 15, 57] It is currently accepted that acute pancreatitis begins as an interstitial process that may progress to a necrotizing parenchymatous form.[10, 15, 30]

Previously, the protease trypsin had been incriminated as the sole destructive enzyme in pancreatic autodigestion.[10] Inactivated pancreatic trypsinogen can be experimentally activated by calcium ions and bile salts as well as by enterokinase.[10] It is believed that trypsin initiates the autodigestive process by activating two additional potent and destructive enzymes (proelastase to elastase and prophospholipase A to phospholipase A).[10, 30] Elastase causes digestion of the elastic fibers within arterioles and may transform the pancreatic inflammation from an edematous state to a hemorrhagic or thrombolic state.[10, 30] Because it is a protease, elastase may also break down proteins within the pancreatic interstitial tissue.[10, 30, 47] Phospholipase A is indirectly responsible for the destruction of acinar cell membranes by the conversion of lecithin to lysolecithin and cephalin to lysocephalin.[10, 30, 47]

With the activation and liberation of pancreatic proteolytic enzymes, the localized inflammatory process can catalyze the development of profound secondary hypotension and shock.[10, 54] Trypsin will convert kallikreinogen into kallikrein.[10, 15] Kallikrein, an enzyme, will then activate bradykininogen (which is bound to an alpha-globulin in the serum) to bradykinin.[10, 15] Bradykinin is a potent vasoactive peptide that produces marked vasodilation with a subsequent drop in vascular resistance in the general microcirculation.[10, 15] A drop in vascular resistance will produce a reduction in mean arterial pressure and depress venous return to the heart, complicating the hypovolemia that usually occurs as a result of protracted vomition.[2, 10, 15] The combination of severe vasodilation and hypovolemia can produce shock.[10, 15] In addition, it is thought that bradykinin is partly responsible for the pain and leukocyte migration seen in acute pancreatitis.[10] Locally, bradykinin is instrumental in creating a vicious circle, in that it produces pancreatic arteriole vasodilation, resulting in an edematous and exudative state in the pancreas.[15] The exudation will liberate more activated trypsin, which will, in turn, release more bradykinin.[10] The clinician must be aware that death due to acute pancreatitis results not from destruction of the gland, but from profound hypotension and subsequent vascular collapse caused by kinin activation.[54] Thus, the therapeutic goal must be the maintenance of vascular integrity and adequate venous return to the heart[54] (Fig. 12–7).

Amylase and carboxypeptidase are released into the pancreatic interstitial spaces; however, they do not appear to play an important part in the pathogenesis of acute pancreatitis.[10, 24] Lipase can migrate to the peritoneal and retroperitoneal surfaces during enzymatic leakage, causing fat necrosis.[15, 24]

To protect the pancreas from autodigestion after very minimal trauma or inflammation, varous proteinase inhibitors are present in alpha-globulins, in tissue fluids (α-1-antitrypsin, alpha-2-macroglobulin, and C_1-esterase inhibitor), and in pancreatic tissue (pancreatic secretory trypsin inhibitor).[15, 38] In massive inflammation these intrapancreatic protease inhibitors are consumed, and the remaining free, activated enzymes appear in pancreatic interstitial tissue, peritoneal effusive fluid, and thoracic lymph.[15, 38] In addition, because of hypovolemia and hypotension, the arterial blood flow to the pancreas is greatly reduced, thus diminishing the supply of circulatory proteinase inhibitors to the gland.[15, 38]

Because of the actions of lysolecithin and lysocephalin and subsequent cell membrane necrosis, the other proteolytic enzymes and pancreatic lipase are released upon the peritoneal surface, producing a localized chemical peritonitis.[10, 15] As the degree of pancreatic ischemia intensifies and persists, a hypoxic state is produced in the pancreatic tissue.[15] This state favors the proliferation of various anaerobic bacteria, especially *Clostridium perfringens,* a normal inhabitant of the canine pancreatic ducts.[3] Reflux of the duodenal fluid with its usual gram-negative bacterial flora can occasionally occur during acute pancreatitis and duodenal paralytic ileus. With loss of pancreatic compartmentalization due to cell membrane necrosis, these bacterial organisms may migrate to the peritoneal and retroperitoneal surfaces, thus transforming a chemical peritonitis into a septic one.

Also, in response to tissue ischemia, the pancreas is thought to release a peptide known as myocardial depressant factor (MDF), which has a negative inotropic effect upon the heart, lowering cardiac output with a subsequent additional reduction of mean arterial blood pressure.[10] This phe-

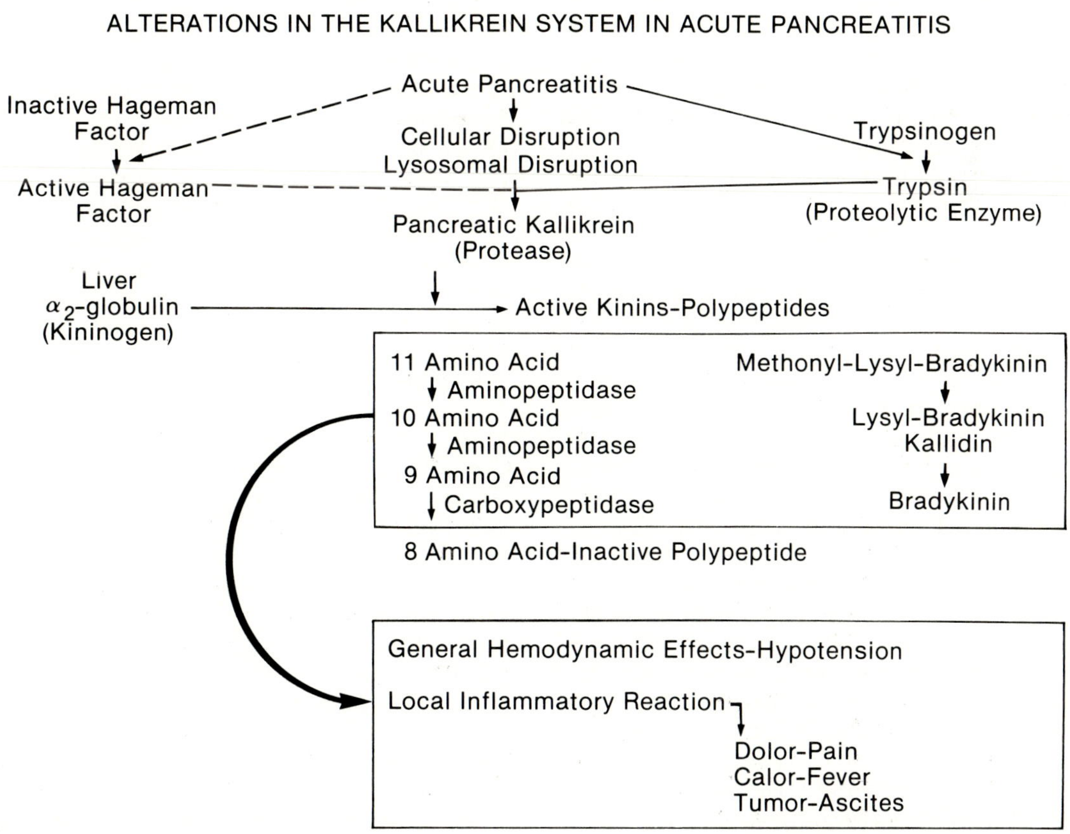

Figure 12–7. Alterations of the kallikrein system in the pathogenesis of acute pancreatitis. Hageman factor = coagulation factor XII.

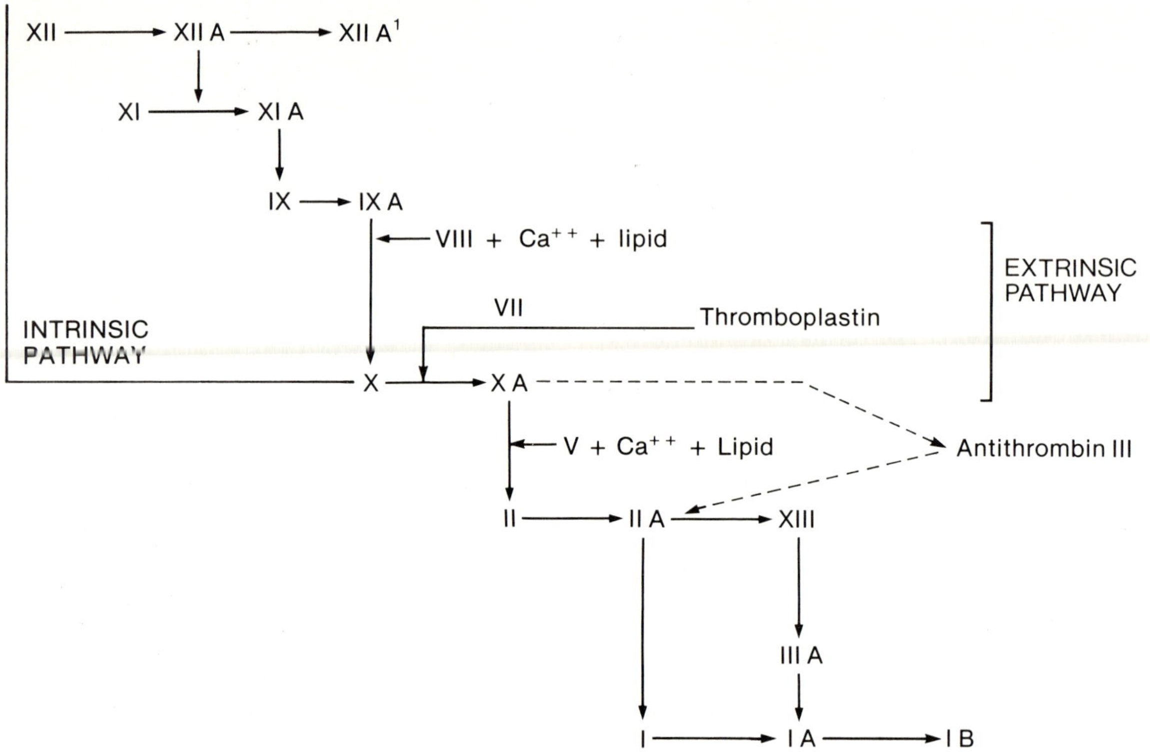

Figure 12–8. BLOOD COAGULATION. Activated forms of coagulation factors are designated A. Broken lines denote inhibitory activity. Stable fibrin polymer is designated IB.

nomenon will further complicate the hypovolemic shock that has been developing.[10]

Human patients suffering from acute pancreatitis often have accompanying hypocalcemia (serum calcium 7 mg/dl or less) that may be severe enough to manifest signs of tetany.[10] The exact significance of the phenomenon in the dog and cat is uncertain because the utilization of automated biochemical surveys has become widespread only recently. The author has treated several patients with acute pancreatitis with accompanying hypocalcemia that were referred for neurological evaluation and electroencephalography owing to the presence of tetany. An old theory proposed that hypocalcemia was caused by the deposition of calcium salts on necrotic adipose tissue.[24] Recent findings indicate that the diseased pancreas releases large concentrations of glucagon from the alpha cells within the islets of Langerhans.[63] Glucagon stimulates the release of calcitonin from the parafollicular cells of the thyroid gland, thus lowering serum calcium levels.[63] In addition, it has been found that human patients with secondary hypocalcemic tetany may have inadequate parathormone secretion.[63] Magnesium deficiency resulting from deposition of magnesium soaps may also be responsible for hypocalcemia.[63] Magnesium deficiency can interfere with parathormone release or with its action upon osteoid tissue.[63]

Terminal cases of hemorrhagic pancreatitis may be the result of disseminated intravascular coagulation (DIC).[20] Stimulation of the intrinsic pathway in the clotting mechanism, which is due to activation of the Hageman factor (factor XII), and release of massive amounts of tissue thromboplastin appear to be the two most influential pathogenetic mechanisms in the production of DIC.[20] The mechanisms by which acute necrotizing pancreatitis propagates DIC include the release of massive amounts of tissue thromboplastin (the pancreas is a rich source of this clotting factor) and the activation and liberation of trypsin.[20] In small amounts trypsin, the inciting enzyme of pancreatic autodigestion, will activate prothrombin and activate the fibrinolytic system.[21] The effect of trypsin liberation upon DIC is twofold; it initiates microthrombi production and it promotes bleeding tendencies through thrombin inactivation and massive secondary fibrinolysis.[20] The progression of mild interstitial edematous pancreatic inflammation to acute fulminant necrosis has been generally attributed to the activation of the complement system (C_5 to C_9).[20] In addition, activation of the alternate complement pathway will, in turn, potentiate Hageman factor activation.[21] Another consequence of the liberation of trypsin into the systemic circulation is the activation of the kinin system (principally the vasoactive amine, bradykinin), which produces vasodilation, increased capillary permeability, and marked neutrophilic migration. An intermediary effect of kinin system activation is the potentiation of Hageman factor.[20] Another important part played by Hageman factor in the pathogenesis of DIC is the activation of the fibrinolytic system.[20] The inactive precursor of plasmin, plasminogen, is activated by Hageman factor, causing the breakdown of fibrin into fibrinogen degradation products (FDPs) and augmenting bleeding tendencies in DIC (Figs. 12–8 to 12–11).

The end-result of acute fulminant hemorrhagic pancreatitis is irreversible shock due to profound hypovolemia from vomition and diarrhea, severe hypotension due to kinin activation, potential enterotoxemia and sepsis, and uncontrollable hemorrhage due to DIC.[20] It is easy to see why this condition is responsible for such high mortality and morbidity rates (Fig. 12–12).

If the patient is fortunate enough to survive acute necrotizing pancreatitis, exacerbation of the disease (chronic relapsing pancreatitis) may occur.[24, 25] Thus, some patients will be presented with a history of repeated "gastrointestinal tract disturbances," including vomition and abdominal pain and distention.[24, 25] It is now believed that the necrotizing process may smolder continuously, producing clinical flareups, and then later asymptomatically, resulting in a scarred, fibrotic gland.[24, 25] In late stages of chronic relapsing pancreatitis the patient may exhibit clinical signs of exocrine (maldigestion and steatorrhea) and endocrine (diabetes mellitus) insufficiency (Tab. 12–3).[24, 25]

PATHOLOGICAL FEATURES

Because of the friability of the pancreas and the likelihood of shock's developing as a result of acute necrotizing pancreatitis, pancreatic biopsies are not routinely performed unless an exploratory celiotomy is done.

On gross examination, in cases of fatal pancreatic necrosis there is usually a small quantity of peritoneal effusion, which may be blood-tinged or contain fat droplets.[4, 36] The omental fat contains petechial and ecchymotic hemorrhages as well as many foci of chalky fat necrosis.[4, 36] Fat necrosis may

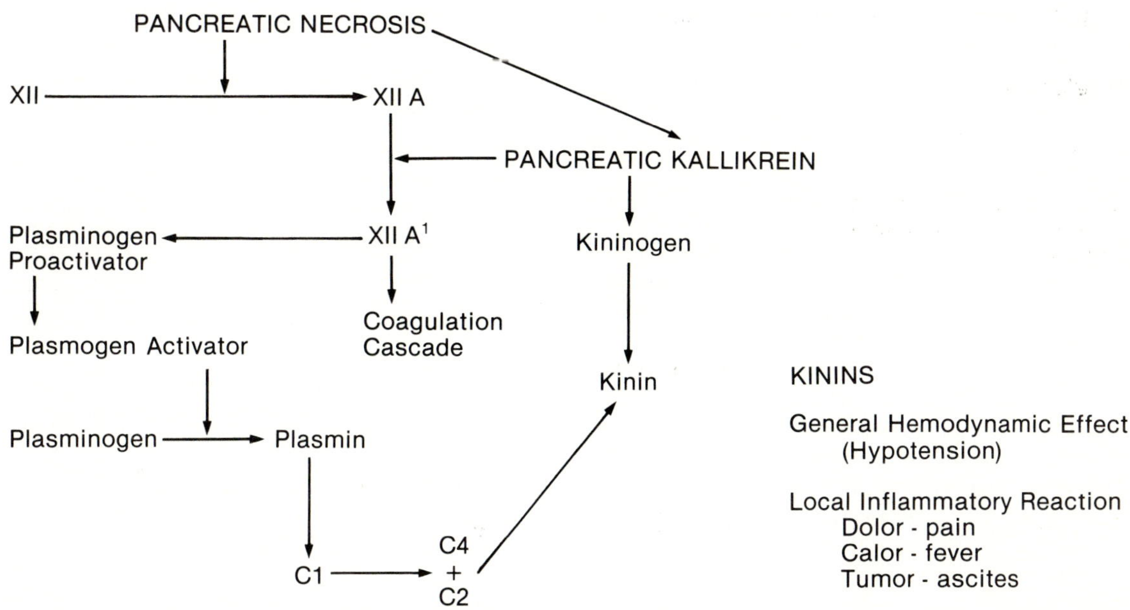

Figure 12–9. The link between pancreatic necrosis and the coagulation cascade, the fibrinolytic mechanism, the activation of the complement system (C1, C4 + C2), and the kinin system.

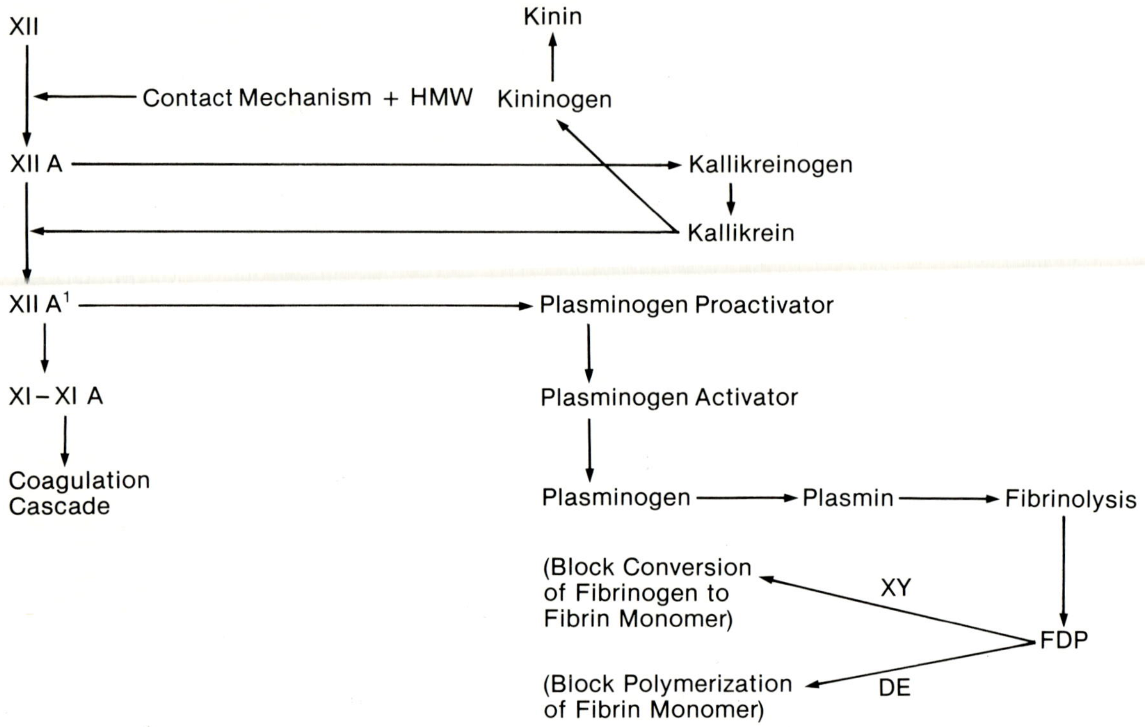

Figure 12–10. The interrelationship between the intrinsic pathway (contact mechanism) and the fibrinolytic system. HMW = high molecular weight; FDP = fibrinogen degradation products.

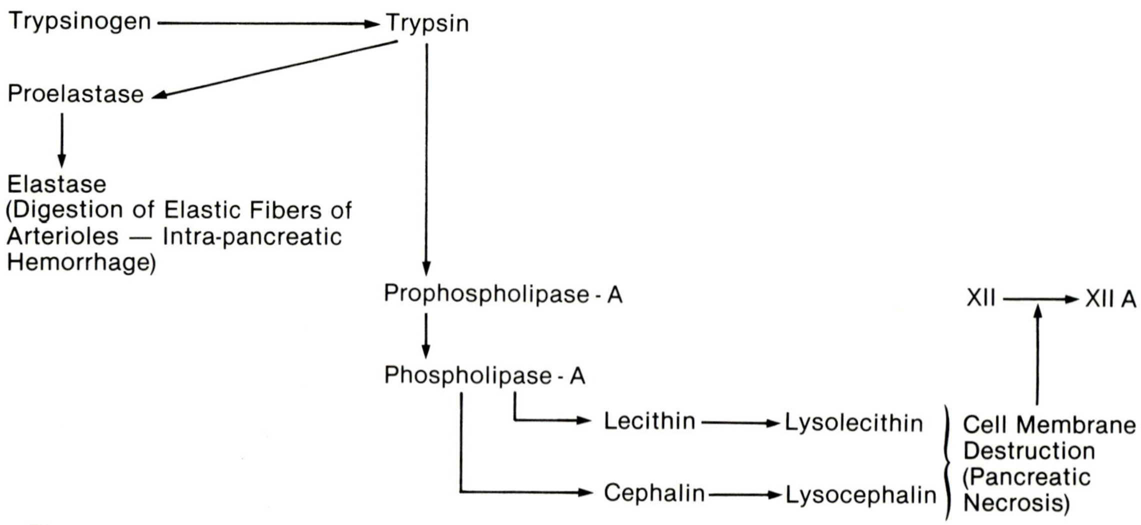

Figure 12–11. The interrelationship between pancreatic necrosis and activation of Hageman factor (XII A).

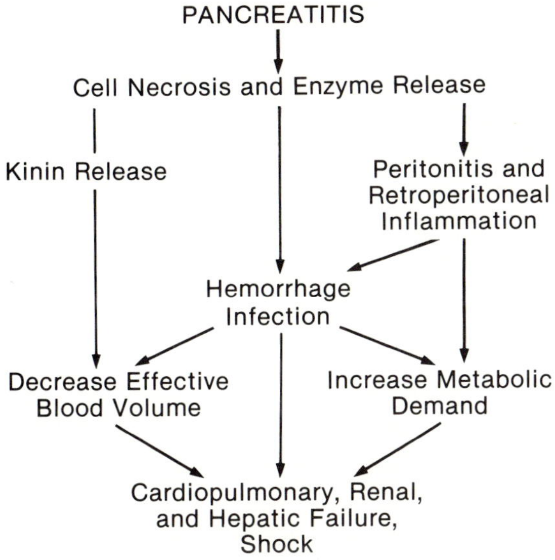

Figure 12–12. Pathogenesis of acute pancreatitis.

be seen in regions that are a great distance from the pancreas, including the pleural surface and the mediastinal areas.[4, 36] It is thought that the necrotizing enzymes are carried to these regions via lymphatic drainage.[4, 36] The pancreas appears to be grossly swollen and edematous, with the midsection of the organ containing grayish-yellow, greasy areas of fat and parenchymal necrosis.[4, 36] The gland may be knobby and irregular, with a loss of its normal lobular architecture.[4, 36] If secondary bacterial infection has occurred, there may be abscess, with a secondary purulent exudate (Figs. 12–13 to 12–15).[4, 36]

On microscopic examination, the gland has areas of fat and parenchymal necrosis, and an edematous process within the stroma.[4, 36] Considerable polymorphonuclear leukocyte infiltration separates the necrotic tissue from the unaffected tissue.[4, 36] Pancreatic vascular changes include fibrin deposition within the capillaries and venous thrombosis secondary to a necrotizing phlebitis (Fig. 12–16).[4, 36]

It is thought that the necrotizing process within the pancreas persists even if the pancreatitis is subclinical.[10] The continuation of the necrotizing process is perhaps due to a secondary immune-mediated process that occurs in response to the release of intracellular organelles that act as antigens during the initial phases of necrosis. The term relapsing pancreatitis may be only a clinical one because the necrotizing process appears to smolder and to worsen progressively, causing periodic bouts of vomiting, abdominal pain, and diarrhea, until the gland is reduced to a shrunken, fibrotic, adhesive piece of tissue.[10] If the patient has survived these repeated clinical exacerbations, then signs of exocrine and endocrine insufficiency may ensue.

Subacute interstitial edematous pancreatitis is often seen in animals, usually as an incidental finding at necropsy.[3] This disease is far more common in the feline than acute pancreatic necrosis.[36, 46] The pancreas may be enlarged or reduced.[36, 46] There is considerable replacement of the normal parenchymal fibrous, connective tissue.[36, 46] The ducts may become dilated and tortuous and may contain a tenacious, mucopurulent exudate.[36, 46]

Microscopically, the ducts are surrounded by extensive fibrosis and may have squamous metaplasia of their epithelial surfaces.[36, 46] Segmental stenosis of the ducts may occur.[36, 46] There is atrophy of the parenchymal tissue, with a mixture of polymorphonuclear and mononuclear leukocyte infiltration.[36, 46]

Table 12–3. COMPLICATIONS OF ACUTE PANCREATITIS

Localized	Chemical peritonitis Septic peritonitis Pancreatic abscess Necrosis of adjacent organs (transverse colon, duodenum) Jaundice (obstructive) Ascites
Systemic	Hypovolemic shock
Cardiovascular	ECG changes (PVCs, ventricular tachycardia, changes in QT interval due to hypocalcemia)
Gastrointestinal	Hematemesis Hemorrhagic diarrhea
Renal	Prerenal azotemia with oliguria Associated renal parenchymal necrosis
Metabolic	Diabetic ketoacidosis Hypocalcemia Hyperlipemia
Hematological	Disseminated intravascular coagulation (DIC)
Pulmonary	Pneumonia Pleural effusion Respiratory distress syndrome
Central and nervous system	Cerebral vascular accident (secondary to DIC) Septic meningoencephalitis

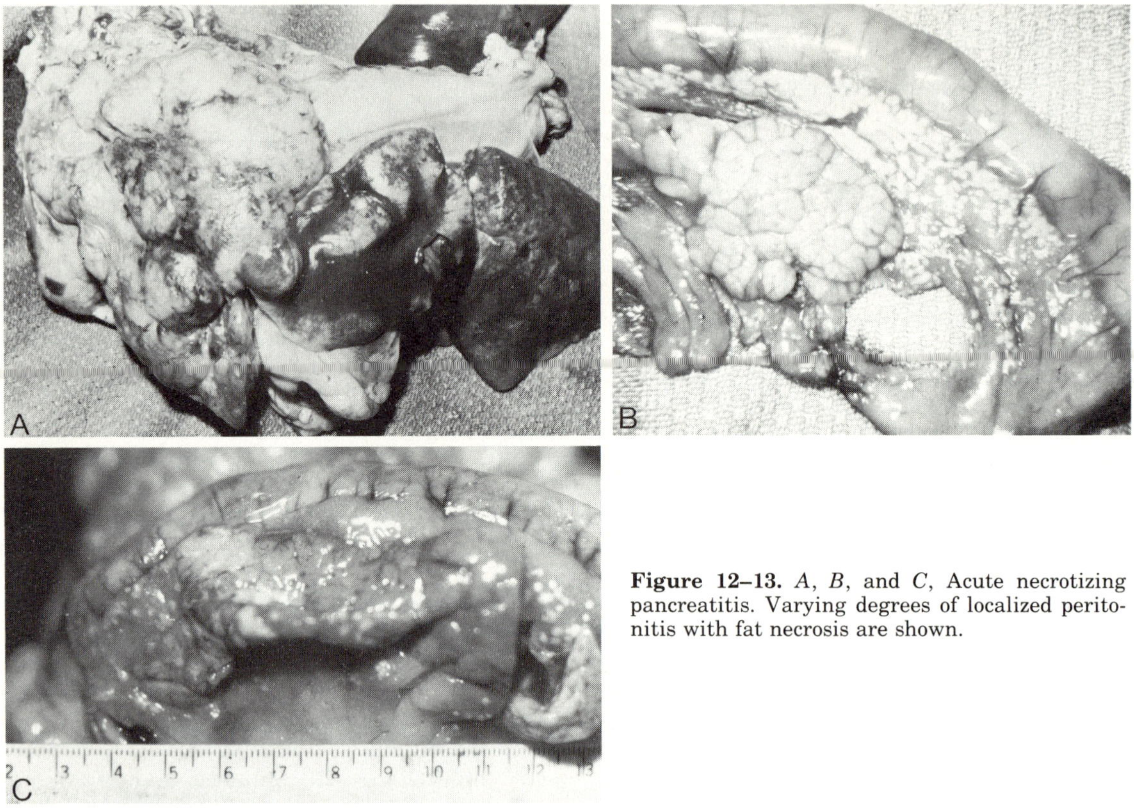

Figure 12–13. *A*, *B*, and *C*, Acute necrotizing pancreatitis. Varying degrees of localized peritonitis with fat necrosis are shown.

ACUTE PANCREATITIS

History and Physical Examination

Because this disease may intimately involve several body systems and may have varying degrees of severity, acute pancreatitis may be described by clients using a variety of chief complaints and clinical signs. Vomiting is probably the most consistent sign and is thought to be caused by afferent stimulation of the vomiting center due to distention, irritation, and pain involving the duodenum, peritoneum, or stomach.[2, 3, 30] The author has seen acute pancreatitis in several animals with massive hyperlipasemia and hyperamylasemia that never exhibited vomition. Often included in the history is the fact that the dog has recently been given a large amount of fatty table scraps.[30] Arching of the back and a forced expiratory grunt due to pain are sometimes described by the client.[30, 47] In addition, marked abdominal distention and bloating due to a localized peritonitis and secondary paralytic ileus may be noted.[47, 63] With the presence of intestinal ileus, overgrowth of the intraluminal microflora develops, producing a diarrhea that is often hemorrhagic. A history of recent abdominal surgery (e.g., ovariohysterectomy), abdominal trauma, or recent administration of high levels of corticosteroids may sometimes be given by the client.

Physical examination of the patient may reveal a wide variety of clinical findings. Pain can usually be elicited upon palpation of the anterior right quadrant of the abdomen.[6] The accompanying localized peritonitis stimulates pain receptors that produce intense stimulation of the sympathetic nervous system.[6] The release of high levels of catecholamines results in a loss of intestinal motility and subsequent paralytic ileus.[6]

Patients that have been vomiting profusely exhibit varying degrees of dehydration.[30] The percentage of dehydration can be assessed by testing integumentary elasticity, recession of the eyeballs within the orbits, and dryness of the oral mucous membranes.[30] Those patients with extensive dehydration may be extremely weakened and depressed owing to accompanying electrolyte and acid-base imbalances.[47] In fulminant necrotizing pancreatitis the patient may be presented in lateral recumbency and suffering from shock.[6] If pure hypovolemic shock is present, the extremities will feel cold, and the oral mucous membranes will appear blanched, with an extremely delayed capillary refill time.[6] If secondary bacteremic shock with enterotoxemia occurs, the oral mucous membranes may appear flushed and hyperemic with poor capillary perfusion.[6]

Icterus is often encountered in cats with acute necrotizing pancreatitis, possibly because the pancreatic ducts and the common bile duct are joined proximal to the duodenal orifice.[46] In dogs, icterus is not as commonly seen because the pancreatic duct and the common bile duct enter separately; however, when icterus does occur it is usually the result of massive pancreatic necrosis, either with resultant obstruction of bile flow or with accompanying cholangiohepatitis (Fig. 12–17).[63]

The patient's body temperature may be quite variable. Fever may be present if there is extreme abdominal pain that is causing excitement and agitation, chemical peritonitis with inflammation, tissue destruction and bradykinin activation, secondary septic peritonitis with polymorphonuclear leukocyte infiltration, and pyrogen release.[30] Often, patients suffering from hypovolemic shock will be severely hypothermic.[30]

A number of secondary pathological complications can occur in severe necrotizing pancreatitis. In fact, these secondary events may produce symptoms that obscure the "classic" picture of pancreatitis, making the condition difficult to diagnose.

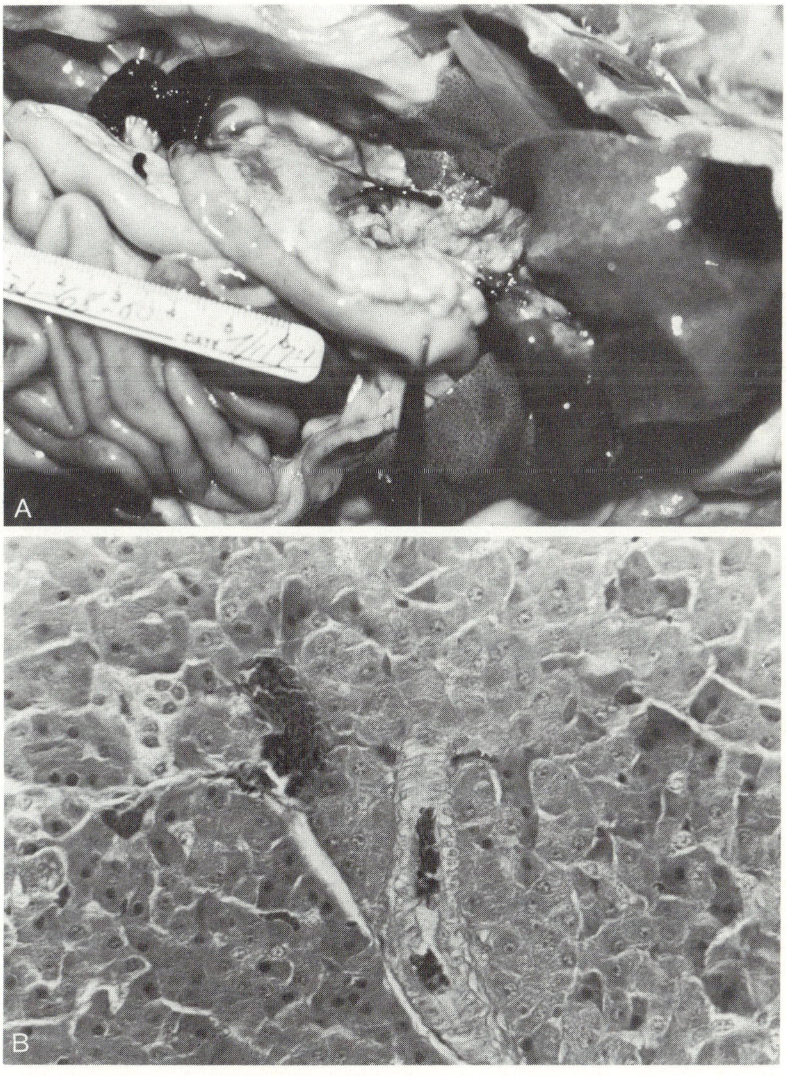

Figure 12–14. *A*, Gross specimen from a cat that fell from an apartment window ("high rise syndrome") and suffered traumatic pancreatitis. Note severe hemorrhage and clotted blood on the surface of the pancreas. *B*, Microscopic section. Note the aggregations of red blood cells and the absence of inflammatory leukocytes (×250).

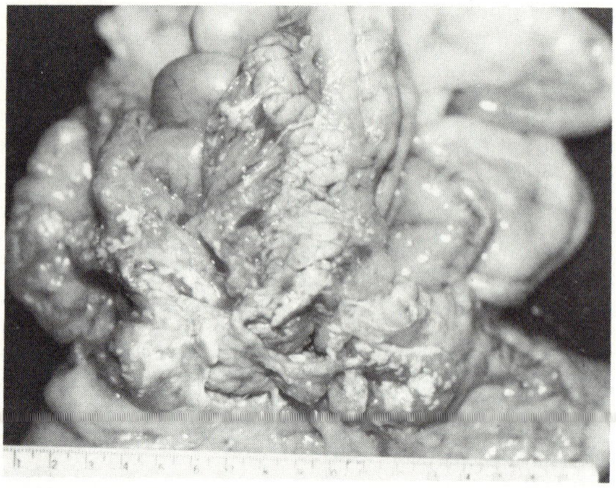

Figure 12–15. Acute necrotizing pancreatitis with secondary abscess formation.

Hypocalcemic tetany is often found in human patients and is beginning to be recognized in canine patients with pancreatitis.[6] With increased utilization of automated multichannel biochemical blood tests, the incidence of documented secondary hypocalcemia should increase. When the serum calcium level falls below 6 mg/dl, tetany usually occurs and is considered a poor prognostic sign.

Animals with acute necrotizing pancreatitis can be presented for acute respiratory distress.[42] Clinical signs include dyspnea, tachypnea, and cyanosis. The respiratory embarrassment seen in these patients may be attributed to pulmonary edema, pleural effusion, and interstitial pneumonitis. It is theorized that elevated plasma levels of phospholipase A and free fatty acids (FFA) break down the phospholipid-rich, alveolar cell membranes and surfactant.[63] In addition, liberated bradykinin may contribute to the edema and effusion by causing increased capillary permeability and subsequent fluid extravasation.[63]

If the islets of Langerhans have also been destroyed during the necrotizing process, fulminant diabetes mellitus with ketoacidosis may be encountered. Sometimes the patient is presented in a semi-comatose state with rapid, deep respiration (Kussmaul's respiration) that has occurred in response to the accompanying metabolic acidosis. The hyperglycemia that occurs must be distinguished from the transient hyperglycemia that results from the expulsion of large concentrations of glucagon from the inflamed pancreas, which stimulates hepatic glycogenolysis, and from the high levels of circulating catecholamines, which block insulin release.

In the terminal condition, patients may show signs of external as well as internal hemorrhage. There may be fulminant, bloody diarrhea.[20] The skin and mucous membranes may reveal petechiation, ecchymoses, and suffusive hemorrhages.[20] These signs may be due to the presence of disseminated intravascular coagulation and intravascular defibrination (DIC with secondary fibrinolysis) (Fig. 12–18).[20]

It is apparent that a number of conditions that manifest acute abdominal signs must be considered in the differential diagnosis of acute pancreatitis. These conditions include simple gastroenteritis, hemorrhagic gastroenteritis (HGE), gastrointestinal foreign body, cholangiohepatitis, pyelonephritis, ruptured intestine, ruptured prostatic abscess, rupture of uterus due to pyometra, retained torsed testicle, and ruptured thoracolumbar intervertebral disc.[2,6] Thus, only through careful history taking and physical examination and judicious use of ancillary diagnostic tests can the diagnosis of this complex syndrome be accurately established.

Diagnosis (Table 12–4)

Laboratory confirmation of acute pancreatitis is sometimes difficult to achieve owing to the lack of consistent correlation between abnormal laboratory results and pancreatic morphological findings. If the history and physical findings warrant the consideration of acute pancreatitis, an extensive data base is indicated as part of the initial diagnostic plan and should include: a complete blood count, urinalysis, automated biochemical blood survey, serum amylase and lipase determinations, and radiographs of the thorax and abdomen.[2,6]

Initially, the contents of the microhematocrit tube should be examined for evidence of fasting hyperlipidemia and icteric serum, which often accompany acute pancreatitis (Fig. 12–19).[14] The hemogram will often reveal an elevated hematocrit and an increased total serum protein level due to hemoconcentration resulting from profound vomition and fluid loss.[14] If hemorrhage has occurred owing to hematoemesis, hemorrhagic diarrhea, or with secondary DIC fibrinolysis, the hematocrit may still be

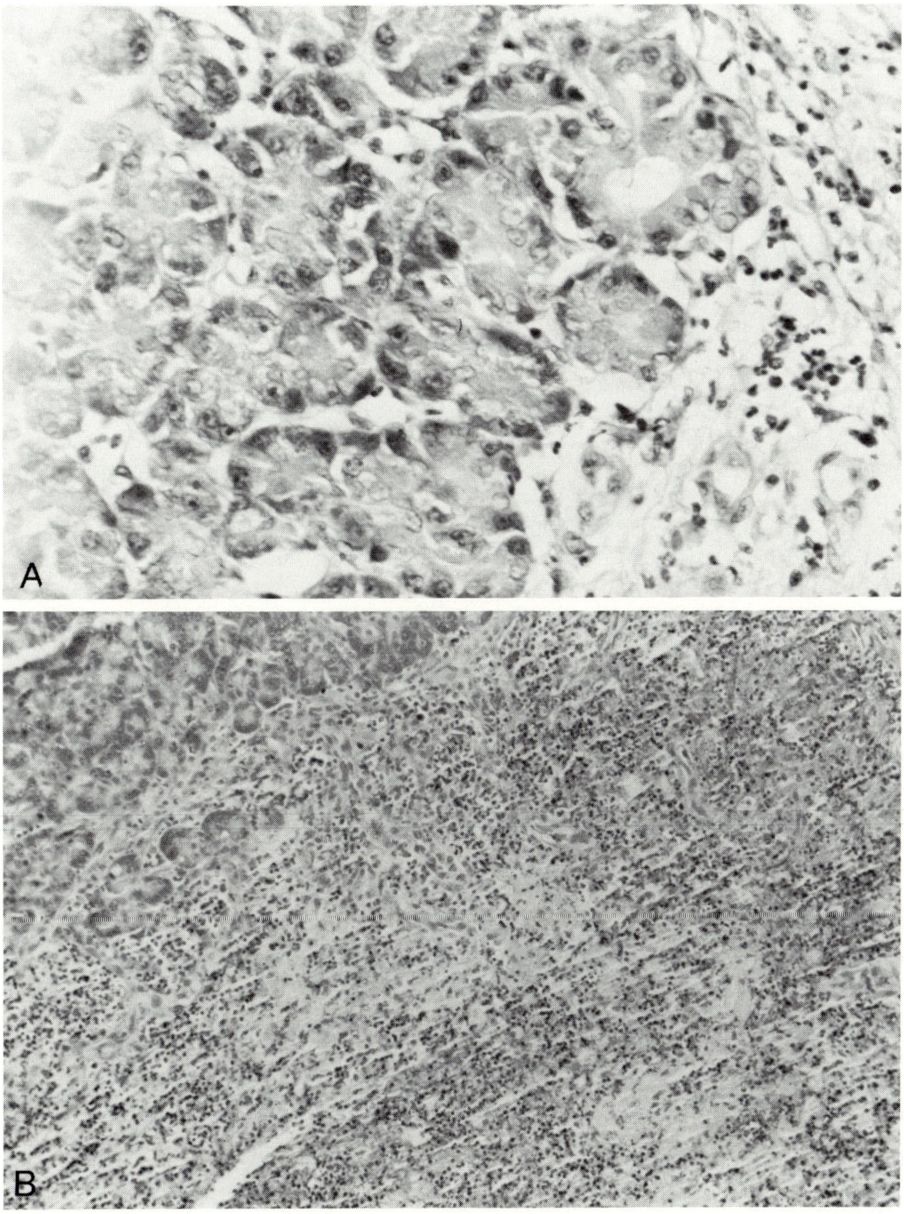

Figure 12–16. Microscopic sections from a dog with acute necrotizing pancreatitis. Note the intense neutrophilic infiltration. *A*, ×100; *B*, ×250.

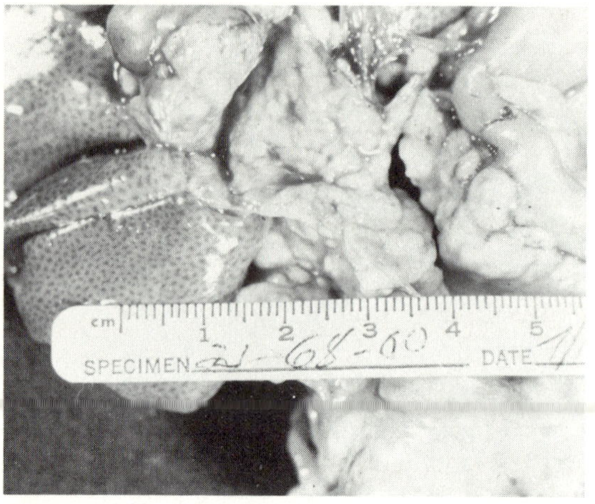

Figure 12–17. Acute necrotizing pancreatitis with secondary jaundice in a cat. Jaundice is a common sequel to pancreatitis because the common bile duct often joins the pancreatic duct before entering the duodenum.

normal because of the profound hemoconcentration resulting from dehydration.[14]

The total and differential white blood cell counts may be variable, depending upon the degree of pancreatic necrosis and the presence or absence of a secondary septic peritonitis.[14] If extensive inflammation has occurred, a neutrophilic leukocytosis (WBC greater than 20,000/mm^3) is often present.[2, 6, 14] If the bone marrow is responding well to the inflammatory stimulus, a regenerative left shift will be present; sometimes stab cells, metamyelocytes, and myelocytes are seen in the differential WBC count (Fig. 12–20).[14] An unfavorable sign is a degenerative left shift (decrease of the WBC count with many immature neutrophil forms in the peripheral smear), which may indicate overwhelming infection, enterotoxemia, or shock.[14] It is important to order serial hemograms to assess the bone marrow's response to the inflammatory process.[14]

The author has seen several cases of acute pancreatitis in cats that have initial leukopenia and granulocytopenia. These findings are similar to those in human patients with acute pancreatitis caused by Coxsackie B virus or mumps virus.

A urinalysis prior to the administration of parenteral fluids is a valuable part of any complete general workup, especially if acute pancreatitis is being considered.[14, 30] If the patient has an accompanying azotemia (elevated blood urea nitrogen or creatinine concentration), the urine specific gravity affords the clinician the ability to determine whether the azotemia is prerenal or primary renal in origin.[14, 30] If the urine specific gravity is greater than 1.025, indicating adequate tubular function, the azotemia is of prerenal origin and is due to profound dehydration and shock with subsequent renal hypoperfusion.[14, 30] If the urine specific gravity is less than 1.020, in spite of marked clinical dehydration, indicating little tubular ability to conserve body water, the azotemia is primary renal in origin.[14, 30]

The presence of glycosuria and ketonuria indicates diabetes mellitus, whereas a large concentration of conjugated bilirubin indicates secondary post-hepatic (common bile duct) obstructive jaundice.[14, 30] In addition, the urinary sediment should be examined for evidence of pyuria resulting from secondary pyelonephritis. In the author's experience, pyelonephritis may occur as a result of bacterial peritonitis and septicemia.

An automated biochemical survey offers the clinician a relatively inexpensive and accurate screening procedure to assess the patient's body systems. The blood urea nitrogen and creatinine concentrations in conjunction with the urine specific gravity may reveal concurrent renal disease.[14] Like many humans with acute pancreatitis, many dogs with the disease have hypercholesterolemia.[14] A blood glucose level higher

Table 12–4. DIAGNOSTIC FEATURES OF ACUTE PANCREATITIS

Physical findings	Abdominal pain
	Fever
	Tachycardia
	Vomition/dehydration
	Diarrhea (often hemorrhagic)
	Jaundice
	Hypovolemic shock
Laboratory findings	Leukocytosis
	↑ Serum lipase
	↑ Serum amylase
	↓ Serum calcium
	↑ Serum alkaline phosphatase
	↑ SGPT
	↑ Peritoneal amylase
	↑ Peritoneal lipase
	Presence of methemalbuminemia
	Hyperlipemia
Radiographic abnormalities	Gas ileus (duodenum, transverse colon)
	Truncation and craniosinistral displacement of the gastric silhouette
	Abdominal effusion
	Pleural effusion (rare)

than 200 mg/dl along with glycosuria and ketonuria is indicative of secondary diabetes mellitus. Most canine or feline patients with acute pancreatitis will have an elevated alkaline phosphatase level, which may be caused by one of the following factors: (1) cholestasis due to common bile duct obstruction, (2) pre-existing cholecystitis or choloangiohepatitis with lymphatic spread to the pancreas, (3) pre-existing hepatic lipidosis with hypercholesterolemia, and (4) pre-existing hyperadrenocorticism causing the pancreatic inflammatory process.[14, 30] An elevation of directly read bilirubin occurs if the patient is exhibiting jaundice, the hyperbilirubinemia being due to obstruction of the bile duct and regurgitation of conjugated bilirubin.[14, 30] If the patient is exhibiting tetany or if the abdominal radiographs reveal calcification of omental fat, hypocalcemia may be present.[30]

If an elevated level of plasma methemalbumin is seen, hemorrhagic pancreatitis may be suspected. Methemalbumin is a pigment produced by proteolytic action upon hemoglobin. The heme molecule is released and subsequently binds to albumin. The presence of an elevated methemalbumin level may be valuable in distinguishing hemorrhagic pancreatitis from interstitial edematous pancreatitis.[2]

To confirm the actual presence of pancreatic acinar inflammation, measurement of serum amylase and lipase concentrations is necessary.[7, 14] Although measurement of serum amylase concentration has historically been the most important laboratory aid in the diagnosis of acute pancreatitis in humans, the following shortcomings limit its use in dogs:

1. There seems to be little correlation between the degree of hyperamylasemia and the severity of the pancreatic lesion.[14]
2. Since the canine kidney is a major site of filtration and degradation of serum amylase, the level of serum amylase can be falsely elevated in renal impairment.[14]
3. The mucosa of the canine small intestine secretes amylase, and moderate hyperamylasemia can be seen in dogs with acute enteritis.[14]
4. Because canine serum has a high concentration of maltase, a falsely elevated serum amylase level may be seen if Somog-

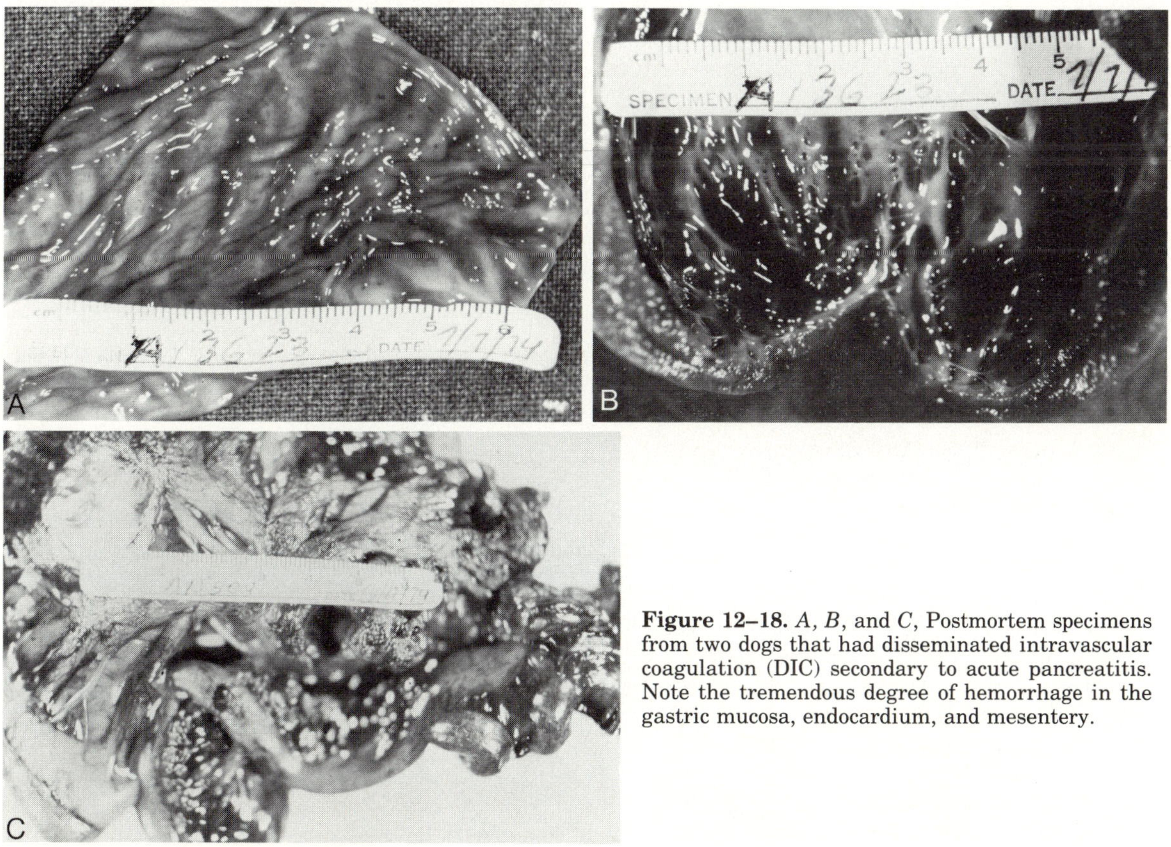

Figure 12–18. *A, B*, and *C*, Postmortem specimens from two dogs that had disseminated intravascular coagulation (DIC) secondary to acute pancreatitis. Note the tremendous degree of hemorrhage in the gastric mucosa, endocardium, and mesentery.

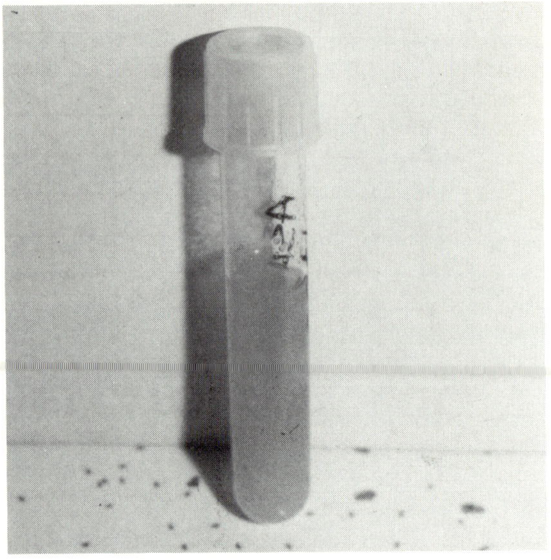

Figure 12–19. A serum sample from a dog with acute pancreatitis shows fasting hyperlipemia.

yi's saccharogenic method (measuring the appearance of glucose in the assay) is used.[7, 14] Thus, serum amylase concentration should be determined by an amyloclastic method (measuring the disappearance of starch in the assay).[7]

5. Lipemia that occurs with acute pancreatitis can yield falsely lowered levels of amylase.[7]

A serum amylase level of three times the upper normal limit in the presence of normal renal function may help to confirm the occurrence of pancreatic ductal obstruction with disruption of acinar cells.

In humans, an elevation of urinary amylase concentration has been used to diagnose acute pancreatitis.[10, 29] Levels of 6,000 units per 24 hours or 300 units per hour can be seen in afflicted patients.[10, 29, 40] A more precise method of diagnosing acute pancreatitis is to calculate the ratio of amylase clearance to creatinine clearance using the following equation.[10, 29, 40]

$$\frac{C_{am}}{C_{cr}}(w) = \frac{\text{Amylase (urine)}}{\text{Amylase (serum)}} \times \frac{\text{Creatinine (serum)}}{\text{Creatinine (urine)}} \times 100$$

Normal people have a ratio of 2.3 per cent ± 0.1 per cent, whereas patients with acute pancreatitis have ratios of 6.5 to 7.0 per cent.[10, 29, 40] Urinary amylase determination in the dog seems to be of little value; even though amylase appears in the renal glomerular filtrate, it is thought to be degraded and reabsorbed in the proximal convoluted tubule, and thus only 1 per cent is present in the urine.[63] In humans, serum amylase levels reach a peak 12 to 24 hours following an attack of acute pancreatitis, gradually returning to normal in two to six days.[27, 40] However, researchers have demonstrated the persistence of hyperamylasemia for three to five weeks in some subjects.[27, 40]

Because the primary source of serum lipase in the dog is the pancreas, with only a fraction originating from the gastric mucosa, a serum lipase elevation in the presence of normal renal function is more reliable than hyperamylasemia as documentation of acute pancreatitis.[7] Owing to the presence of lipoprotein lipase in the plasma, use of a heparinized sample to determine lipase concentrations may yield a false ele-

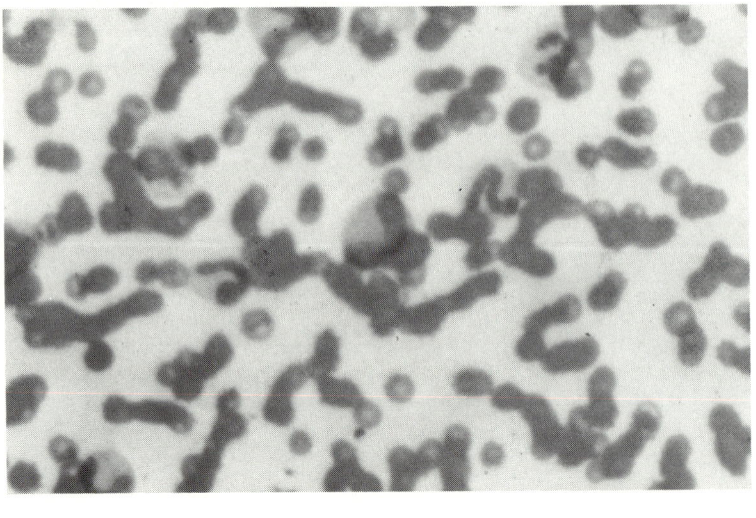

Figure 12–20. Peripheral-blood smear from a cat with acute pancreatitis, illustrating a marked leukocytosis with a regenerative left shift.

vation.[14] As with hyperamylasemia, the degree of hyperlipasemia does not correlate well with the severity of the pancreatic lesion.[7] Lipase elevation in dogs appears to occur approximately as rapidly as, and does not remain elevated appreciably longer than, the serum amylase level.[7]

From recent retrospective studies on dogs that had clinical signs consistent with acute pancreatitis, it appears that increased serum amylase activity had little correlation with the documentation of pancreatic necrosis at necropsy. Thus, an increase in serum amylase activity may lead the clinician to falsely diagnose acute pancreatitis. On the other hand, markedly elevated serum lipase activity (> 500 IU/L) usually correlates very well with the presence of pancreatic inflammatory disease.[61]

In humans, the diagnosis of acute pancreatitis may in the future be aided by the determination of serum concentrations of pancreatic cationic trypsinogen by radioimmunoassay (RIA).[50] It has been shown that the average normal human serum trypsinogen level was 25 ng/ml with a range of 12 to 41 ng/ml.[50] Patients with acute pancreatitis had at least a 15-fold increase in concentrations of this protease precursor in their sera.[50] The correlation of pancreatic cationic trypsinogen elevation in the sera of dogs with acute pancreatitis is currently being studied.

Abdominal radiographs are an integral part of the workup for a patient presented for an acute abdomen.[63] An ill-defined radiopacity in the right anterior quadrant accompanied by duodenal gas ileus is often seen in patients with acute pancreatitis.[63] The transverse colon may have a thickened wall with segmental gas retention due to the spread of the inflammatory process.[30, 63] If the inflammatory process has spread extensively to the omental fat, with saponification and calcium salt deposition, areas of radiopaque densities may be seen.[63] If the patient is suffering from an exudative peritonitis, abdominal radiographs may reveal a loss of abdominal detail with an overall hazy appearance ("ground-glass" appearance).[2, 30, 63] In cases of chronic relapsing pancreatitis with acute exacerbations, the anterior duodenal segment may be corrugated, constricted, and in a fixed position owing to fibrous adhesions and scarring of the organ.[63] This radiographic sign may be illustrated by the use of oral barium sulfate to help delineate the rigid portion of the duodenum.[63] Hypotonic duodenography, a human medicine technique, utilizing duodenal intubation, vagal blockade, fluoroscopy, and positive-contrast radiography, may be useful in veterinary medicine to diagnose pancreatitis (Figs. 12–21 to 12–24).[10]

If there is a suggestion of peritoneal effusion, an abdominocentesis should be performed.[6] The fluid should be checked to determine whether it is a transudate (specific gravity less than 1.013), modified transudate (specific gravity 1.021 to 1.052), or inflammatory effusion (greater than 1.032).[6] The amylase and lipase contents of the fluid may be determined and the fluid may be examined cytologically for inflammatory cells. If fluid findings are suggestive of an inflammatory process, culture and sensitivity tests should be performed (Fig. 12–25).[6]

If there is evidence of a secondary bleeding disorder, it is important to document disseminated intravascular coagulation with secondary fibrinolysis.[20] In DIC most coagulation parameters (platelet count, whole blood clotting time, prothrombin time, plasma fibrinogen concentration, and partial thromboplastin time) will be abnormal and fibrinogen degradation products will be present.[20]

If the diagnosis of acute pancreatitis is still uncertain or if the patient is not responding to therapy, possibly because of pancreatic abscesses or a pseudocyst, an exploratory celiotomy may be performed.[10]

Treatment

Regardless of the severity of clinical signs, the one basic principle that should be followed in the management of the patient with acute pancreatitis is prevention of further pancreatic secretory activity.[10] If the organ is not further stimulated, it will not release the proteolytic enzymes and the lipase that are instrumental in the pathogenesis of acute pancreatitis.

The two most important hormones that influence pancreatic enzyme production and secretion are cholecystokinin (CCK) and gastrin. These two peptide hormones are in the same family and are structurally similar. Gastric gastrin is released in response to the presence of gastric distention and protein breakdown products, whereas CCK is stimulated by the presence of peptide chains and medium-chain fatty acids in the

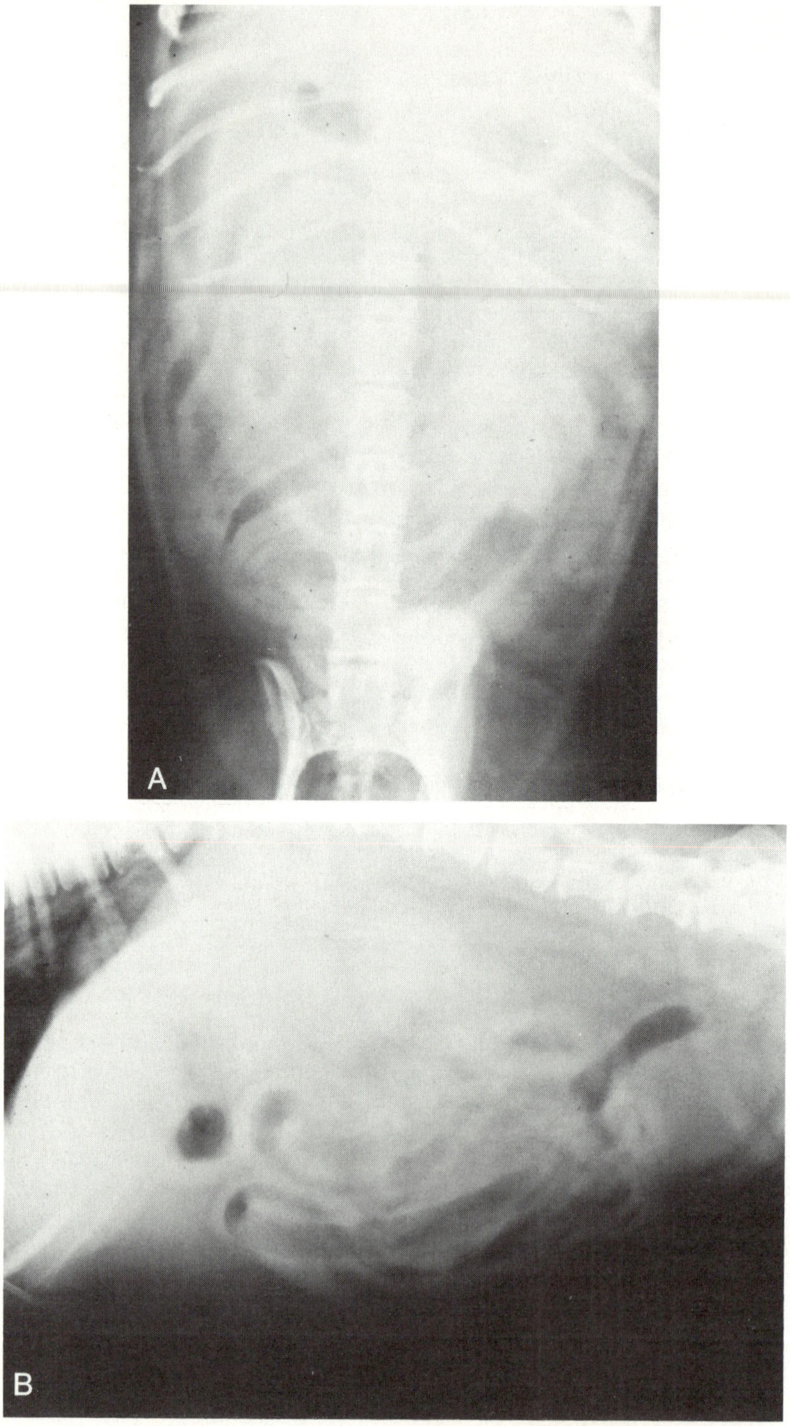

Figure 12–21. Ventrodorsal *(A)* and lateral *(B)* abdominal radiographs of a dog with acute pancreatitis. Note the markedly dilated anterior duodenal segment and the diffuse gas in the intestinal loops.

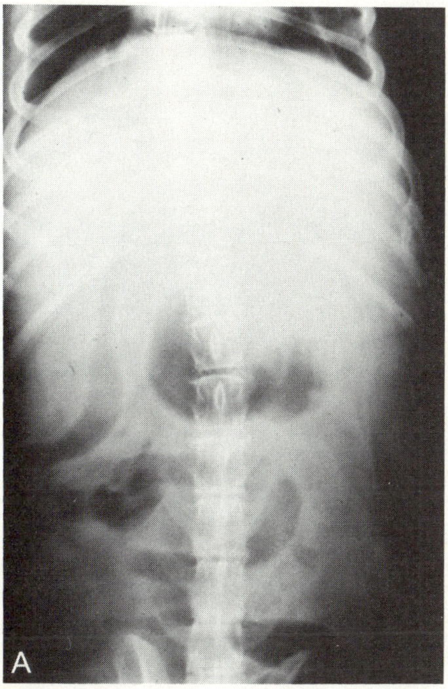

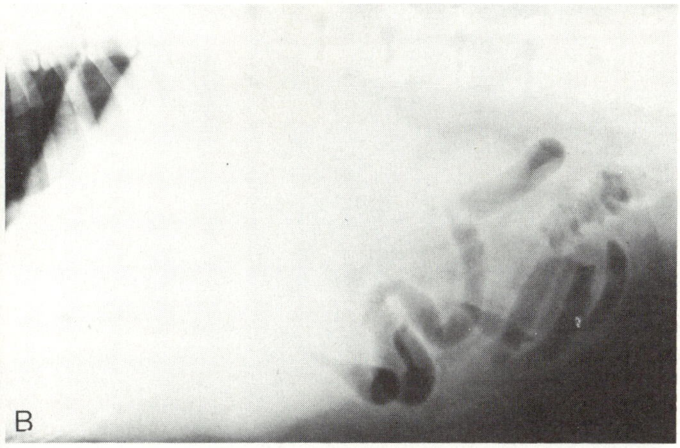

Figure 12–22. Ventrodorsal *(A)* and lateral *(B)* abdominal radiographs of a dog with acute pancreatitis and secondary peritonitis. Note the lack of abdominal detail, the dilated intestinal bowel loops, the deviation of the gastric shadow caudally and toward the mid-line, and the markedly dilated cranial duodenal segment.

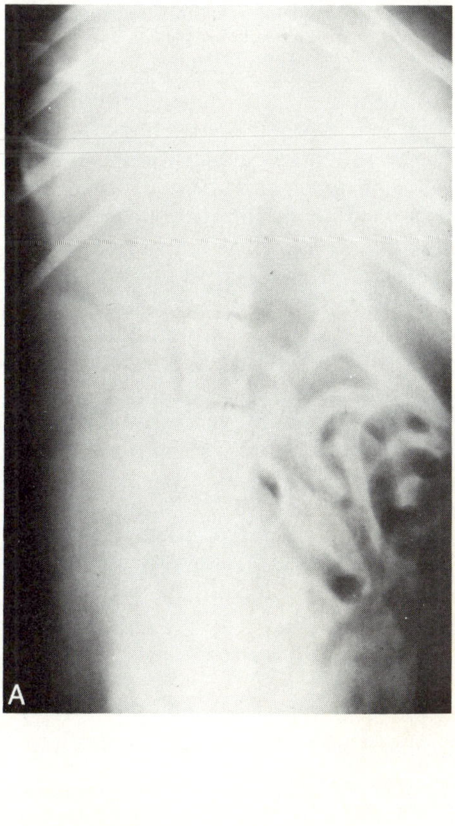

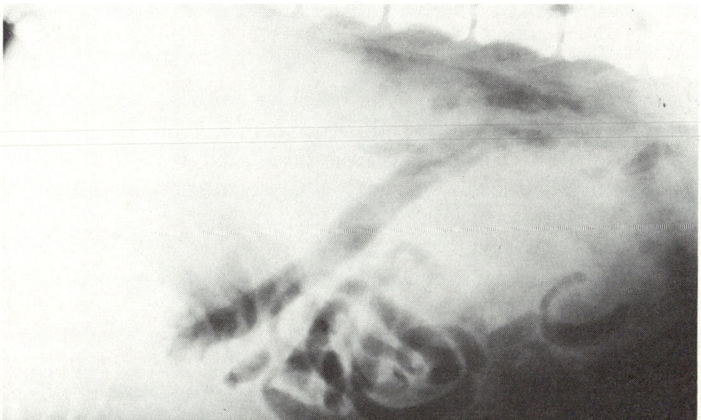

Figure 12–23. Ventrodorsal *(A)* and lateral *(B)* abdominal radiographs of a dog with acute pancreatitis and bowel necrosis due to a stagnant loop and peritonitis. Note the free gas near the retroperitoneal region on the lateral view and the marked gas ileus in the intestines.

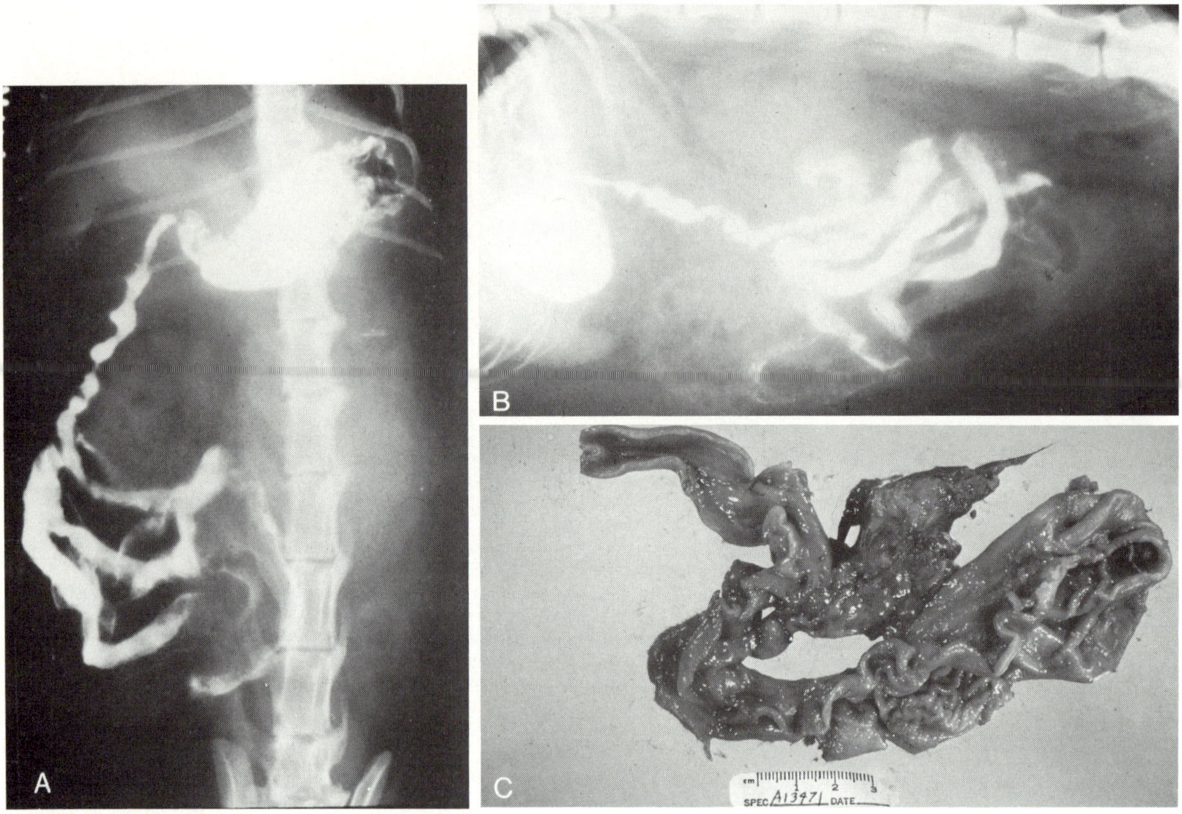

Figure 12–24. *A* and *B*, An upper GI series from a cat with chronic relapsing pancreatitis reveals a markedly corrugated descending duodenum, which was a result of pancreatic fibrosis and adhesions. *C*, Postmortem specimen reveals corrugation of the duodenum and severe adhesions, the result of recurrent peritonitis.

duodenum. It has been shown that CCK is a much more potent stimulator of pancreatic enzyme production and release than gastrin. Thus, complete denial of any oral substance (foods, liquids, and medication) for two to five days is mandatory.

In the past, treatment of human patients with acute pancreatitis has included the placement of a nasogastric suction tube to minimize secretin release by inhibiting the delivery of acidic gastric fluid to the duodenum.[10] However, secretin has little effect upon pancreatic enzyme release, causing the pancreas to secrete mainly HCO_3^-, water, and electrolytes. In addition, if the acid content of the stomach is continually removed, there is no negative feedback upon gastrin release. Gastrin has a considerable effect upon pancreatic enzyme release. Recent studies have shown that nasogastric suction is probably beneficial only in the amelioration of pain by reducing gastrointestinal ileus.[10] Also, insertion of a nasogastric suction tube may not be technically practical in canine and feline patients.

Another practice in the management of patients with acute pancreatitis is anticholinergic therapy.[10] The most widely used drugs are atropine sulfate and propantheline bromide.[10]* The rationale for their use is that they suppress gastric acidity (a stimulus for secretin release), and they inhibit the vagal influence upon pancreatic secretion. However, these pharmacological agents will inhibit only pancreatic secretion of an organ that has been already stimulated to secrete, and they have little effect upon an organ that is at rest in a fasted animal.[10] In addition, these drugs may do more harm than good through suppression of gastrointestinal motility, and they are contraindicated in those patients with radiographic evidence of intestinal ileus because of the threat of producing a stagnant bowel loop with subsequent bacterial overgrowth and enterotoxemia.[10]

Two other pharmacological agents that have been used experimentally and clini-

*Pro-Banthine, Searle & Co., San Jaun, PR.

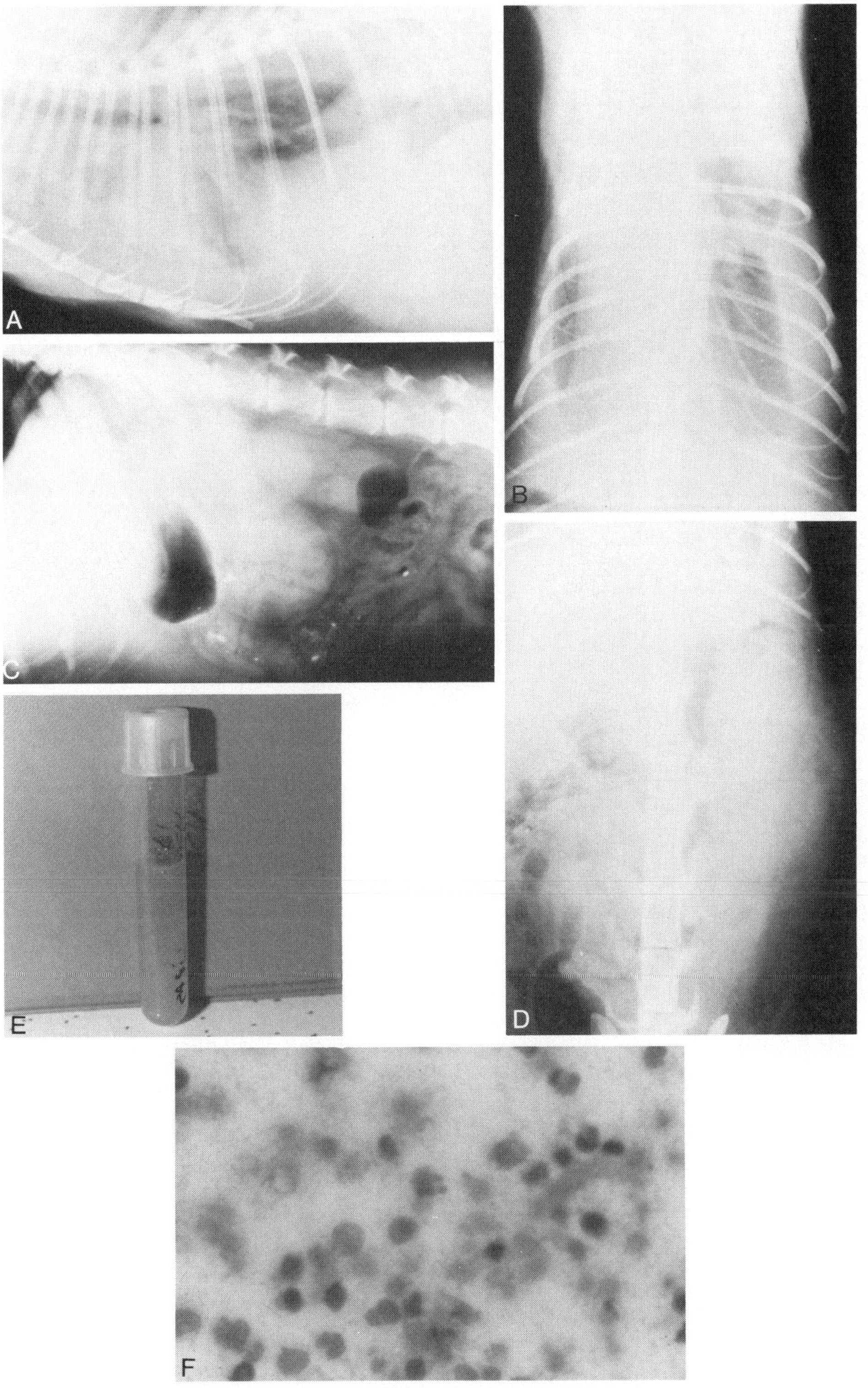

Figure 12–25. Thoracic (*A* and *B*) and abdominal (*C* and *D*) radiographs from a cat with acute pancreatitis reveal a marked pleural effusion, a mild peritoneal effusion, marked hepatomegaly, and diffuse gas in the intestines. *E*, The thoracic fluid from the same cat. Analysis revealed amylase activity to be 4,500 dye units/1 and lipase activity to be 5 Cherry Crandall Units. *F*, Cytological specimen revealing a mixed-cell population of neutrophilic, lymphocytic and mesothelial cells.

Table 12–5. CONCENTRATIONS OF SODIUM BICARBONATE ADDED TO IV FLUIDS

Degree of Acidosis	Venous CO_2 (approx.)	HCO_3^- Required (mEq/1/kg)
Mild	18	3
Moderate	14	6
Severe	10	9

cally in an attempt to inhibit enzyme secretion are glucagon and insulin.[10, 41] Glucagon may be of benefit because it is in the same peptide family as secretin and may compete with secretin for the pancreatic receptor sites.[10, 41] Of far greater importance is the fact that glucagon, having a positive inotropic effect upon the myocardium, improves pancreatic arterial perfusion, thus minimizing pancreatic ischemia.[10, 41] Clinically, the administration of 1 mg of glucagon (0.3 mg/kg intravenously) in normal saline every few hours has resulted in relief of pain and a fall in serum amylase concentrations in people with acute pancreatitis.[10, 41] Insulin (0.5 U/kg IV) has been shown to be beneficial in those patients suffering from pain due to omental fat necrosis.[10] A hormone-sensitive lipase that is inhibited by insulin is believed to be responsible for the lipolysis.

Since most patients suffering from acute pancreatitis have persistent vomiting with secondary dehydration and impending hypovolemic shock, intravenous fluid administration is mandatory.[6, 39] In addition, increased survival rates in humans have been achieved when adequate pancreatic arterial perfusion is maintained.[6, 39]

An ideal initial fluid is normal saline with potassium supplement, since a patient with an uncomplicated case usually exhibits a hypochloremic alkalosis with accompanying hyponatremia and hypokalemia.[39] With secondary hypovolemic shock and accompanying poor capillary perfusion and ischemia, a state of metabolic acidosis may develop.[39] In patients with metabolic acidosis a balanced electrolyte fluid such as lactated Ringer's solution may be of benefit.[39] One must be certain that hepatic failure is not present, because the liver converts lactate into bicarbonate. If blood gases are being monitored, the base deficit may be determined and the appropriate quantity of sodium bicarbonate may be added to the fluids. If blood gases are not being monitored the concentration of sodium bicarbonate necessary may be determined from Table 12–5.

Low molecular weight dextrans* (20 ml/kg/hr IV) have been shown to be effective in expanding plasma volume, improving peripheral blood flow, and decreasing blood viscosity.[10] These dextrans can aggravate hemorrhagic tendencies and thus are contraindicated in hemorrhagic pancreatitis. The use of vasopressin† (2 to 5 units IM) to improve blood flow to the inflamed pancreas has been shown to improve survival rates in humans.[10, 20]

In acute fulminant pancreatitis that is refractory to the conventional therapy for shock just described, soluble intravenous corticosteroids such as prednisolone sodium succinate†† may be indicated.[39] Corticosteroids improve survival rates in experimentally induced shock because they stabilize lysosomal and cellular membranes, helping the cells to resist bacterial endotoxins.[39] In addition, glucocorticoids have been shown to increase vascular tone, thereby improving venous return to the heart, and to exert a positive inotropic effect upon the myocardium.[39] These physiological properties increase cardiac output.[39] The dosage for prednisolone sodium succinate is 6 to 20 mg/kg as an intravenous bolus. It should be emphasized that glucocorticoids are indicated only in shock conditions and only for one or two administrations. They have been shown to cause proliferation of pancreatic ductal epithelium and to increase the viscosity of secretions, thus increasing intraductal pressure.[63] Glucocorticoids have been shown experimentally to induce pancreatitis in rabbits.[63] The author has documented several cases of iatrogenic, steroid-induced pancreatitis in dogs and cats following long-term glucocorticoid administration.

Although antibiotics have not been demonstrated to significantly reduce mortality rates in human patients with acute pancreatitis, prophylactic administration of antibiotics is indicated.[39, 63] The rationale behind their use is that the necrotized, poorly perfused tissue is an excellent medium for the growth of gram-negative enteric and anaerobic bacteria.[39, 63] The combination of intravenous potassium penicillin (10,000 u/kg IV TID) against the anaerobes and an amino-

*LMD 10% IV in sodium chloride 0.9%, Abbott Laboratories, North Chicago, IL.

†Pitressin, Parke-Davis, Morris Plains, NJ.

††Solu-Delta Cortef, Upjohn Pharmaceuticals, Kalamazoo, MI.

glycoside (kanamycin, 5 mg/kg IV BID or gentamicin, 1.8 mg/kg IV TID) against the gram-negative microorganisms (if renal function is adequate) should be used.[63] An adequate substitute antibiotic is intravenous chloramphenicol.[63]

Miscellaneous therapeutic measures such as the use of meperidine hydrochloride* (2 mg/kg SC q6h) for pain and heparin (600 units/kg SC TID) for hemorrhagic diathesis due to DIC may be indicated. Meperidine hydrochloride is favored over morphine sulfate because it does not produce spasms of Oddi's sphincter, which would increase intraductal pressure.[10, 39] Hypocalcemic tetany should be treated with calcium gluconate 10% (10 to 30 ml IV, slowly or mixed in fluids).

Drugs that have been used both clinically and experimentally in acute necrotizing pancreatitis and in acute hemorrhagic pancreatitis are the trypsin inhibitor fibrinolysin and the antihyperthyroid agent propylthiouracil.[10, 27, 39] Fibrinolysin has been used extensively in humans in both Europe and the United States, with most studies indicating increased survival rates for treated patients.[10, 27, 39] Propylthiouracil† (50 to 150 mg/day) has been studied in dogs with experimentally induced hemorrhagic pancreatitis, with impressive results.[10, 27, 64] Fibrinolysin is quite expensive and is not clinically available in this country, but it may offer promise in the future.

The possibility of surgical intervention should be considered in those patients exhibiting fulminant effusive peritonitis or pancreatic abscess.[13, 50] The area around the pancreas should be thoroughly explored and any abscesses should be decompressed, lanced, and drained.[13, 50] Recently, the utilization of a combination of peritoneal lavage with a balanced electrolyte solution and an aminoglycoside antibiotic has improved survival rates.[13, 48, 50] The clinician should monitor the patient for hypokalemia and hypoproteinemia and should replenish both potassium and protein when necessary.[13, 48, 49, 50]

Prognosis

Patients with acute interstitial edematous pancreatitis usually recover with or without supportive therapy and often are not presented to the veterinarian. When treating a patient for acute necrotizing pancreatitis the clinician should give the client both a short-term and a long-term prognosis. Both prognoses usually are guarded. On a short-term basis, if the patient can survive the accompanying hypovolemic shock, its chances for recovery from the acute clinical episode greatly improve. Complications that commonly occur in acute necrotizing pancreatitis include: endotoxic or septic shock, hypocalcemic tetany, DIC, and acute renal failure.[6, 30] Any of the preceding sequelae warrants a poor prognosis.[6, 30] On a long-term basis, the client should be advised of the smoldering pathological process occurring in the pancreas, the possibility of reexacerbations of acute illness, and the eventual development of exocrine or endocrine insufficiency.

Client Education

As part of the long-term prognosis, the client should be advised of the possible development of malassimilation due to pancreatic exocrine insufficiency and should be instructed to look for weight loss and bulky voluminous stools. Signs of diabetes mellitus (polyuria, polydipsia, weight loss, etc.) should be reported to the veterinarian immediately.

The most important facet of client education is emphasis on strict adherence to dietary restrictions to minimize the possibility of relapse of acute symptoms. The cause of relapse is an overly active secreting gland, whose stimulus is excessive CCK release as a result of ingesting large quantities of amino acids and medium-chain fatty acids. Thus, it is imperative that foods containing large concentrations of proteins and fats be avoided. Prescription diets* that are low in fat and excessive amounts of protein may be implemented. Specially prepared table foods such as lean chicken, turkey, beef, and lamb, macaroni, rice, and a variety of vegetables are acceptable. The patient should be fed small amounts at frequent intervals to minimize excessive exocrine secretory activity.

CHRONIC RELAPSING PANCREATITIS

Chronic relapsing pancreatitis is the most common clinical form of chronic pancreati-

*Demerol, Winthrop Laboratories, New York, NY.
†Propylthiouracil, Eli Lilly Co., Indianapolis, IN.

*Prescription Diet i/d, Hills Pet Products, Topeka, KS.

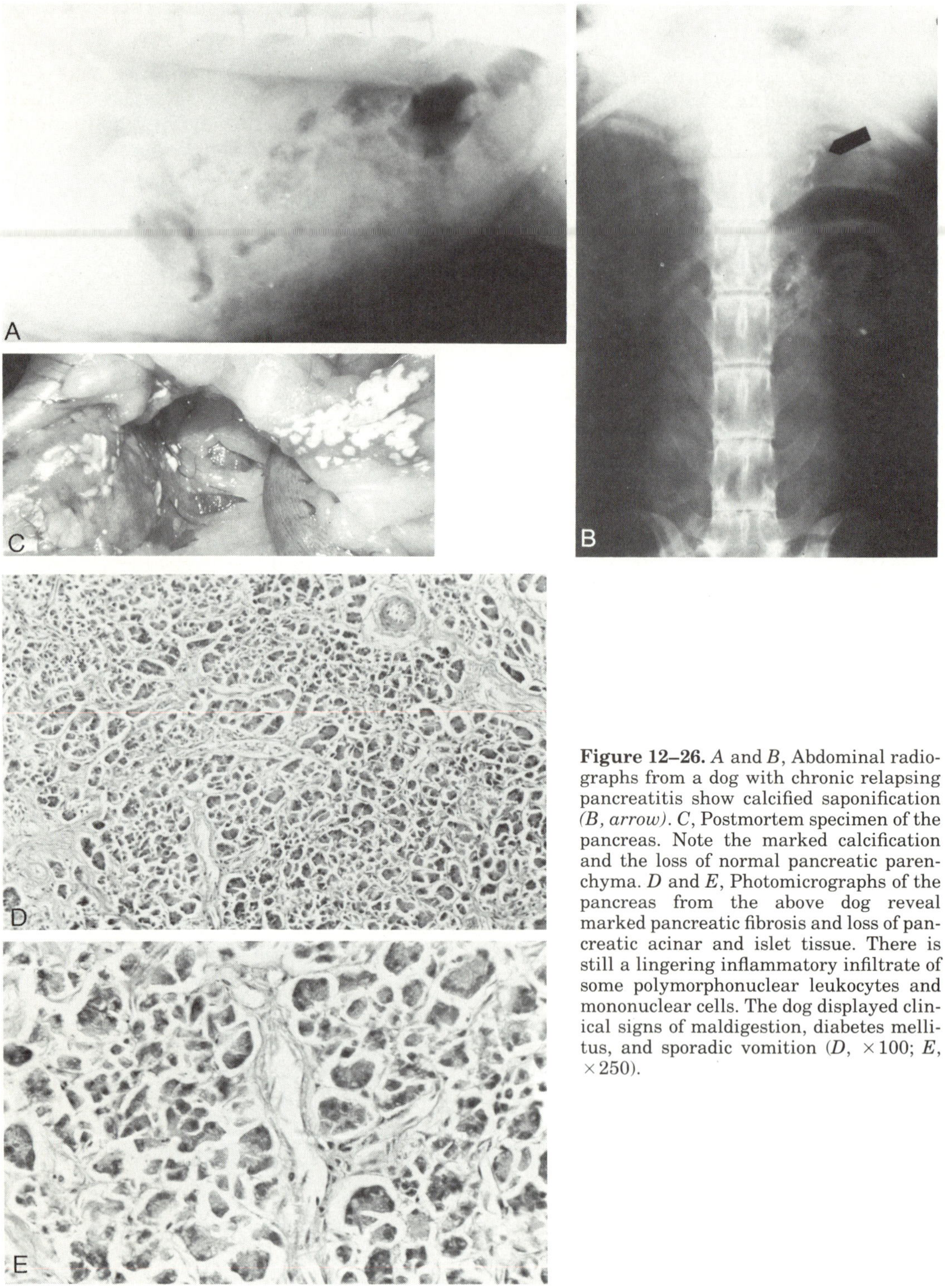

Figure 12–26. *A* and *B*, Abdominal radiographs from a dog with chronic relapsing pancreatitis show calcified saponification (*B, arrow*). *C*, Postmortem specimen of the pancreas. Note the marked calcification and the loss of normal pancreatic parenchyma. *D* and *E*, Photomicrographs of the pancreas from the above dog reveal marked pancreatic fibrosis and loss of pancreatic acinar and islet tissue. There is still a lingering inflammatory infiltrate of some polymorphonuclear leukocytes and mononuclear cells. The dog displayed clinical signs of maldigestion, diabetes mellitus, and sporadic vomition (*D*, ×100; *E*, ×250).

tis, suggesting that it is caused by exacerbations of acute disease upon a previously injured gland.[63] This suggestion is consistent with the current belief that acute pancreatic necrosis is a progressively smoldering process with repeated cycles of fat necrosis, edema, and calcification.[63] Eventually, the gland is replaced by fibrotic tissue, with extensive loss of both acinar and islet tissue.

The clinical signs reflect the frequency, intensity, and stage of the acute flareups. Often the clinical signs are similar, if not identical, to those of acute pancreatitis; abdominal pain, nausea, vomition, diarrhea, dehydration, and hypovolemic shock all are seen.[3, 10] After repeated acute exacerbations, which are often initially diagnosed as acute gastritis, signs of pancreatic exocrine insufficiency and diabetes mellitus are encountered.[3, 10]

Laboratory findings during acute exacerbations will be similar to those in acute necrotizing pancreatitis, except that there is less likelihood of hypocalcemia.[10, 63] Radiographs may be helpful in revealing areas of omental saponification and calcification.[63] A barium swallow may reveal constriction and corrugation of the duodenal segment.[63]

The duration of the pathological process will dictate the amount of fibroblastic infiltration throughout the parenchymal tissue; varying degrees of subacute to chronic inflammation (mixed neutrophilic and mononuclear cellular infiltration) are present.[4, 36] In severe cases the acinar ducts become extremely dilated with a purulent exudate, forming a pancreatic abscess (Fig. 12–26).[4, 36]

Pancreatic Exocrine Disease

PANCREATIC EXOCRINE INSUFFICIENCY

Pancreatic exocrine insufficiency may be congenital or may be acquired as a result of repeated bouts of chronic relapsing pancreatitis leading to fibrotic atrophy. Congenital pancreatic hypoplasia (juvenile atrophy) has been seen in certain genetic lines of German shepherd puppies, with clinical signs beginning prior to one year of age. These puppies usually have enough of a reservoir of insulin and do not exhibit diabetes mellitus due to hypoinsulinism (Fig. 12–27).

In congenital and acquired pancreatic exocrine insufficiency the subsequent clinical symptoms will be similar. The patient is usually presented with signs of weight loss in spite of exhibiting a good to voracious appetite. Varying degrees of frequent (six to ten stools per day), foul-smelling, bulky, greasy, loose stools are described by the client.[19] The diarrhea is an osmotic type, with undigested sugars and fats being fermented by intestinal bacteria to become osmotically active particles.[19] In addition, the undigested fatty acids inhibit colonic water absorption ("castor oil" effect).[19]

Because the pancreas is unable to deliver adequate concentrations of lipase and phospholipase A (to split fats) and alpha amylase (to split starches and polysaccharides) to the intestinal lumen, there is an overabundance of osmotically active particles within the lumen.[19] Owing to a marked increase in these osmotically active particles and a subsequent efflux of water into the lumen of the alimentary canal, the colon is unable to reabsorb the increased volume, and diarrhea ensues.[19] The volume of unabsorbed intraluminal water produces marked intestinal distention and hypomotility, which at times may be severe enough to cause intestinal and colonic bacterial overgrowth.[19] In addition, unabsorbed fatty acids may impair the absorptive capacity of the small intestine by damaging the brush border and blunting the villi.[19]

It is apparent that, left unchecked, chronic osmotic diarrhea with steatorrhea will produce a chronic deterioration of nutritional homeostasis.[19] Previously, pancreatic exocrine insufficiency was referred to as a maldigestive syndrome and chronic intestinal mucosal disease was referred to as a malabsorption syndrome (Tab. 12–6). For convenience, the term malassimilation syndrome has been proposed to encompass both subclasses of chronic osmotic diarrhea.[19] Besides having a voluminous diarrhea, patients with malassimilation syndrome exhibit signs of secondary polysystemic involvement, including a roughened seborrheic-like haircoat, marked weight loss, listlessness, anemia, coagulation abnormalities, bone pain, and tetany (Tab. 12–7).[19]

In puppies with congenital pancreatic hypoplasia, the chief clinical sign may be coprophagia. In both the congenital and acquired forms of the disease, a general picture of poor condition (dull, dry haircoat, and loss of muscle mass) is usually encountered. Although approximately 85 per cent of the functional parenchymal tissue must

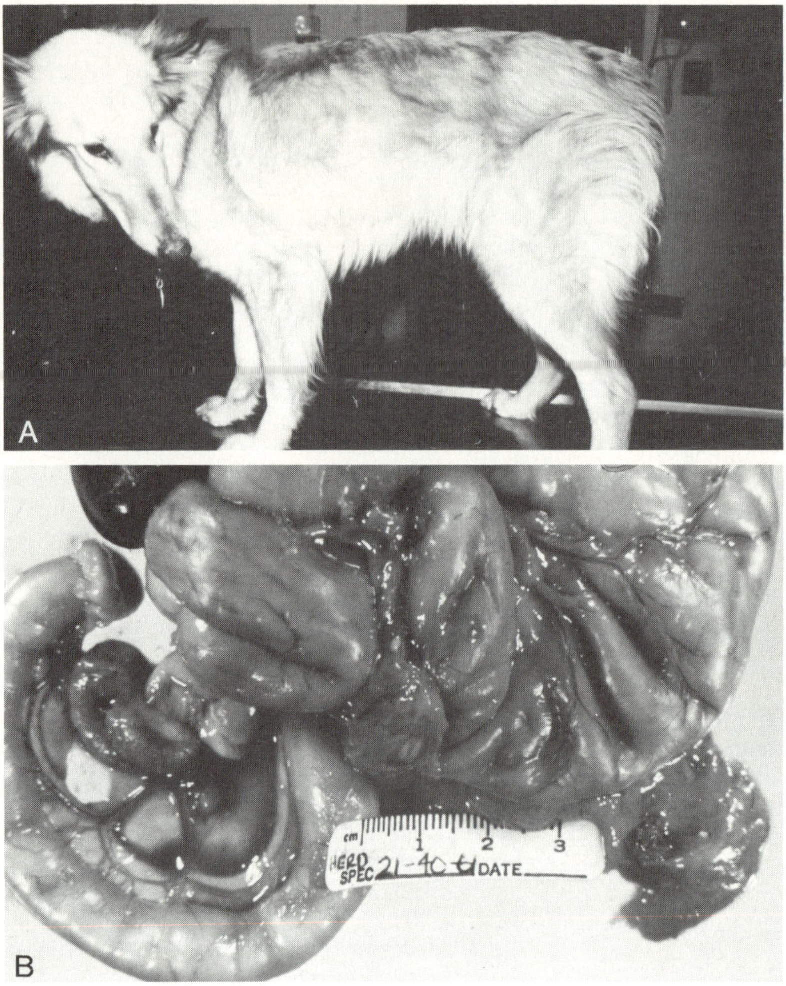

Figure 12–27. *A*, A 10-month-old collie with pancreatic exocrine insufficiency. Note the thin, emaciated condition of the pup. *B*, Postmortem specimen of the pancreas, duodenum, and stomach reveals a small rim of pancreatic tissue above the duodenum.

be lost before signs of pancreatic exocrine insufficiency occur, congenital pancreatic hypoplasia is still the most common cause of malassimilation in the dog.[2]

The diagnostic workup of patients with pancreatic exocrine insufficiency should be designed to differentiate this disease from intestinal mucosal malabsorption and from biliary tract disease with impaired bile salt production and release.[19] Since diarrhea is the most common clinical sign, a complete fecal examination is mandatory.[19] Routine examination of the feces for parasites and ova is advised to rule out severe endoparasitism, especially chronic giardiasis with secondary atrophy of the intestinal villi.[19] Staining the stool with Sudan III and iodine will qualitatively document the presence of steatorrhea and amylorrhea, respectively.[19] If the patient has been fed a canned meat product, undigested muscle fibers may be seen microscopically. The gelatin digestion test for fecal trypsin is routinely performed; however, this test may produce false-negative results in normal patients. In some cases, the absence of fecal trypsin activity becomes apparent only after acinar destruction is nearly complete.[2, 63]

A recent study indicated that the quantitative release of trypsin into the feces varies markedly according to the type of diet the dogs are fed, with a meat-based diet evoking a five-fold greater release of trypsin into the feces than a cereal-based diet.[8, 43] A number of other non-pancreatic factors may alter the amount of trypsin recovered in the feces, including fecal pH, intestinal transit time, and protein decomposition by intestinal flora.[8] In dogs with pancreatic exocrine insufficiency, the quantity of 24-hour fecal trypsin was approximately one-tenth that in normal dogs (approximately 0.50 gm/kg/24 hrs vs 5.0 gm/kg/24 hrs).

A simple, yet helpful, screening test for

Table 12–6. ETIOLOGY OF MALDIGESTION AND MALABSORPTION (MALASSIMILATION)

Maldigestion
Pancreatic exocrine insufficiency
Congenital
Acquired-relpasing chronic pancreatitis
Inactivation of pancreatic enzymes
Pyloroplasty
Canine gastrinoma
Mastocytosis
Chronic uremia with inadequate excretion of gastrin
Bile acid deficiency
Intrahepatic biliary obstruction (advanced cirrhosis)
Extrahepatic biliary obstruction
Cholelithiasis
Biliary flukes in cats *(Eurytrema* sp. *Opisthorcus felineus)*
Relapsing pancreatitis
Pancreatic carcinoma
Chronic ileal disease
Regional ileitis
Lymphoma
Ileal resection (secondary to ileocolic intussusception)
Stagnant bowel loop syndrome
Drug induced (sequestration of bile salts)
Tumors of common bile duct
Brush border enzyme deficiency
Disaccharidase deficiency
Protease deficiency
Malabsorption
Villous atrophy and derrangement
Canine parvovirus (CPV)
Canine coronavirus (CCV)
Canine rotovirus (CRV)
Chronic giardiasis
Chronic coccidiosis
Gluten enteropathy
Infiltration of lamina propria
Inflammatory cells
Lymphocytic-plasmacytic enteritis
Eosinophilic enteritis
Gluten enteropathy
Histoplasmosis
Amyloidosis
Neoplastic cells, lymphoma
Lymphangectasia

fat absorption ability is the administration of 6 ml/kg of corn oil.[19]* Plasma samples using edetate disodium calcium (CaEDTA) are collected at 1, 2, and 3 hours and are centrifuged.[19] The failure of turbidity to appear is indicative of either pancreatic maldigestion or intestinal malabsorption.[19] The test may be repeated by mixing desiccated pancreatic enzyme powder† with the corn oil and 1½ tsp of baking soda (to alkalinize the suspension for maximal lipase activity). The mixture should be allowed to stand at room temperature for 30 minutes.[19] The appearance of plasma turbidity (lipemia) is highly suggestive of pancreatic exocrine insufficiency and maldigestion.[19]

For quantitative documentation of steatorrhea, one may feed the patient a controlled diet that contains a known percentage of fat. After a 72-hour acclimation period, stool is collected for 24 hours; the exact amount of fat in the sample is determined.[19] Recent data indicate that normal dogs excrete much less fecal fat than was previously thought (approximately 0.25 gm/kg/24 hrs) and that dogs with pancreatic exocrine insufficiency excrete approximately eight times more fecal fat (approximately 2.1 gm/kg/24 hrs) than normal dogs.[8]

The ability of the patient to absorb monosaccharide compounds may yield valuable information regarding the degree of small intestinal absorptive capabilities. The oral glucose tolerance test (OGTT) is simple to perform and is relatively inexpensive. The transport of glucose, a hexose monosaccharide, requires no pancreatic or brush border enzymatic activity; glucose is transported across the brush border of the epithelial cells. A 20 per cent solution of glucose is given orally at a concentration of 2 gm/kg, and plasma glucose levels are measured every 30 minutes for 180 minutes. Blood glucose levels in patients with normal intestinal absorptive functions reach maximum concentrations between 30 and 60 minutes after glucose ingestion, and the plasma concentration rarely exceeds 160 mg/dl. The return to glucose levels comparable to those found in the fasting dog should be achieved within 180 minutes. Patients with intestinal malabsorption have a "flattened" curve, with blood glucose levels rarely exceeding 115 mg/dl. Patients with pancreatic exocrine insufficiency and maldigestion will have a normal OGTT curve, but they may exhibit prolonged hyperglycemia, indicating previous relapsing pancreatitis with some degree of islet cell destruction and a prediabetic state.[19]

A more sensitive but technically more difficult and far more expensive monosaccharide absorption test employs D-xylose as the sugar source.[19] D-xylose is a pentose monosaccharide that is not utilized for energy by mammalian species but is passively absorbed through the intestinal mucosa and requires almost no transport via intestinal lymphatics to be absorbed.[19] The patient is fasted for at least 12 hours prior to the

*Lipomul, the Upjohn Company, Kalamazoo, MI.
†Viokase, A. H. Robins Co., Richmond, VA.

Table 12–7. PATHOPHYSIOLOGICAL CORRELATIONS OF CLINICAL SIGNS SEEN IN MALASSIMILATION DISORDERS

Clinical Sign	Pathophysiological Correlation
Weight loss; poor nutritional state	Inadequate absorption of proteins, fats, and carbohydrates; negative caloric state
Diarrhea (bulky, voluminous, and frothy)	Absorptive capacity of the colon is far exceeded because (1) dehydroxylation of fatty acids and bile acids increases colonic secretion of electrolytes and water and (2) carbohydrate malabsorption produces osmotically active particles
Weakness, listlessness	Depletion of electrolytes (K^+ and Mg^{++}); anemia
Petechiae and ecchymoses	Malabsorption of vitamin K (fat-soluble vitamins) leads to hypoprothrombinemia
Integumentary changes (seborrhea, eczema, alopecia)	Impaired absorption of vitamin A
Anemia	Impaired absorption of iron, folate, and Vitamin B_{12}
Tetany	Vitamin D (calcium) and magnesium malabsorption
Bone pain	Vitamin D (calcium) malasorption leads to osteomalacia
Nocturia, polyuria	Hyposthenuria due to hypokalemia
Edema	Malabsorption of amino acids leads to hypoproteinemia

administration of D-xylose (500 mg/kg of a 10 per cent solution via stomach tube). Blood samples for determination of D-xylose levels are taken every half hour for 3 hours. Within 90 minutes, normal animals will have reached a maximal serum level of D-xylose (> 45 mg/dl). Patients with intestinal malabsorption will have a "flattened" D-xylose curve with blood levels of substantially less than 45 mg/dl. The major advantage of the D-xylose absorption test over the OGTT is that blood levels of D-xylose are not affected by insulin or glucagon or by the stress induced by venupuncture. Both the D-xylose test and the OGTT may yield false-negative results owing to delayed gastric emptying or impaired intestinal circulation.[19]

Evaluation of pancreatic protease activity may be achieved by the para-aminobenzoic acid (PABA) test.[19, 62] In this test, a synthetic peptide composed of n-benzoyl-1-tyrosine and PABA is given by stomach tube at a dosage of 16.7 mg (0.25 ml)/kg after an 18-hour fast.[19, 62] The patient is then placed in a metabolic cage.[62] After 6 hours urine is collected to determine the concentration of PABA.[62] The ingested synthetic peptide stimulates the release of pancreatic chymotrypsin, which cleaves the compound and allows the freed PABA to be absorbed into the systemic circulation and excreted in the urine.[62] Dogs that have urinary PABA excretion levels of less than 16 per cent require pancreatic enzyme replacement.[19, 62] Spurious results may occur in patients that have renal failure because the clearance rate of plasma PABA into the glomerular filtrate would be impaired, or who have received sulfonamides, other antibiotics, or furosemide.[21, 62]

Miscellaneous tests employed in the evaluation of patients with possible pancreatic exocrine insufficiency include a determination of blood glucose level and urinalysis to document co-existing diabetes mellitus and abdominal radiographs to reveal radiopaque calcium soap deposits.

Treatment of patients with pancreatic insufficiency depends upon supplementation with pancreatic enzymes, fat- and water-soluble vitamins, daily NPH or PZI insulin administration if diabetes mellitus is present, and feeding a low-fat diet.[19] Researchers working with human patients with pancreatic exocrine insufficiency have shown that giving eight tablets of pancreatic enzyme with meals resulted in much higher intraduodenal lipase activity than giving two tablets hourly.[18] It has been thought that in humans with pancreatic exocrine insufficiency, steatorrhea and creatinorrhea could be blocked if the ingested pancreatic enzymes could attain intraduodenal concentrations equal to approximately 10 per cent of normal physiological pancreatic enzyme release.[18] The eight tablets administered to these patients achieved intraduodenal concentrations of only 22 per cent of the trypsin and 8 per cent of the lipase that were contained in the tablets and represented 2 per cent of the enzyme levels achieved with normal pancreatic secretion.[18] Thus, this study illustrates how only small percentages of ingested enzymes reach the duodenum in an active form.[18] Possible explanations for this phenomenon include: (1) delayed gastric emptying, (2) decomposition of enzymes by the highly acidic gastric juice, (3) dispersion of the tablets into the ingested chyme, and (4) dilution of the enzymes in the total intragastric volume.[18] It is quite remarkable that minute concentrations of active enzymes such as that reaching the proximal small intestine would cause amelioration of steatorrhea and creatinorrhea.[18]

Desiccated pancreatic powder (1 tsp/20 kg) mixed with canned or well-moistened dry food and incubated for 20 minutes before feeding appears to give the best clinical results. Pancreatin tablets have not been shown to be as efficacious as the desiccated powder. The author has had limited experience with Pancrease,* a capsule containing individually enteric coated microspheres of pancrealipase. Because pancreatic lipase is optimally activated in an alkaline pH and in the presence of bile salts, one-half to one teaspoon of baking soda (sodium bicarbonate) and 150 mg of bile salts† and desiccated pancreatic powder mixed with the food may give an improved clinical response.[19] It has been shown that cimetidine,†† an H_2 receptor antagonist that inhibits gastric acid secretion, was effective in human patients who, because of the inactivation of lipase and trypsin by gastric acid and pepsin, did not respond to conventional pancreatic enzyme replacement therapy.[18, 51] Thus, cimetidine (5 mg/kg TID) may prove useful in the treatment of refractory disease in canine patients. Neomycin may be a helpful adjunctive treatment for the bacterial overgrowth in the small intestine that often accompanies maldigestion. In addition, the patient should be fed small amounts at frequent intervals to prevent dietary overload and subsequent osmotic diarrhea.[19]

The prognosis depends upon the success of pancreatic exocrine replacement therapy. Pancreatic exocrine insufficiency is never curable, but it is often manageable. Of equal importance in this condition is the presence or absence of diabetes mellitus with subsequent ketoacidosis and hepatic lipidosis.

At necropsy, the pancreas of a patient with acquired pancreatic insufficiency is grossly shrunken and fibrotic with saponification of the omentum and mesentery.[4, 36] Often there are adhesions of adjacent visceral structures.[4, 36] Patients with pancreatic juvenile atrophy exhibit no evidence of preexisting inflammation, just a hypoplastic rim of pancreatic tissue with an intact ductal system.[4] On microscopic examination, the parenchymal cells are small, have an indifferent staining character, and do not assume an acinar arrangement (Fig. 12–28).[4]

*Pancrease, Johnson & Johnson, Shillman, NJ.
†Bilron, Eli Lilly & Co., Indianapolis, IN.
††Tagamet, Smith Kline & French Lab Co., Carolina, PR.

NEOPLASIA OF THE EXOCRINE PANCREAS

Neoplastic conditions of the exocrine pancreas are infrequently diagnosed in dogs and cats. Benign epithelial tumors are much rarer than carcinomas of acinar tissue or excretory ducts.[28] Carcinomas in dogs and cats tend to originate from the central section or the duodenal wing of the pancreas.[36] Those carcinomas that arise from the central area may soon cause clinical icterus by impinging upon the common bile duct.[36] Because they have a tendency toward early metastasis, pancreatic carcinomas locally invade the duodenum and spread to the liver and peritoneum.[4, 36]

Later in the course of the disease, pulmonary metastases are usually found.[4, 36]

On microscopic examination these tumors are adenocarcinomas that often incite a considerable fibrous tissue reaction with secondary pancreatitis.[4, 36] The biological behavior of the tumors cannot be correlated with the degree of differentiation of cellular morphology.[4, 28, 36] Some well-differentiated pancreatic carcinomas may metastasize extensively (Fig 12–29).[1, 4, 28, 36]

The insidious clinical signs and the tendency toward early metastasis make adenocarcinomas most difficult to correctly diagnose early enough for successful treatment. Clinical signs include weight loss due to anorexia, prolonged and relentless abdominal pain (especially when the tumor invades the celiac nerves), vomiting, diarrhea with bulky malabsorptive stools, and icterus if the tumor invades or compresses the common bile duct or metastasizes to the liver.[1]

Special radiographic techniques including an upper GI series and pneumoperitoneography may be valuable in establishing an ante-mortem diagnosis.[1] Hypotonic duodenography may be useful in diagnosing carcinomas involving the duodenal wing of the pancreas because it reveals corrugation and nodularity along the medial aspect of the

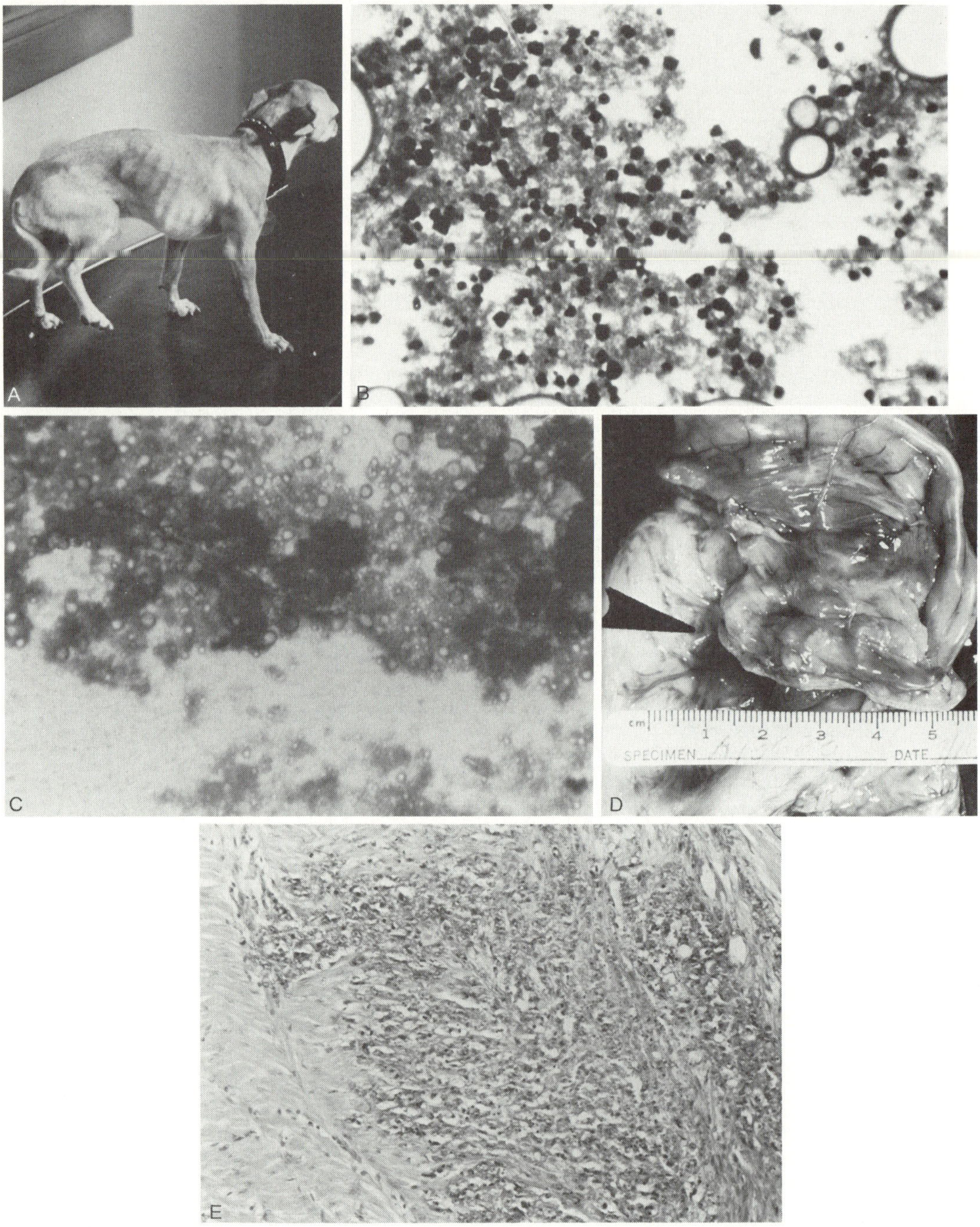

Figure 12–28. *A*, A chihuahua with severe acquired chronic pancreatitis with exocrine and endocrine insufficiency. Note the extreme cachectic appearance of the dog. *B*, Lugol's iodine stain of a stool sample reveals numerous starch granules. *C*, Sudan III stain of a stool sample shows numerous fat droplets. *D*, Postmortem specimen reveals marked pancreatic fibrosis. *E*, Photomicrograph of the pancreas shows marked infiltration of the acinar and islet parenchyma by fibrotic tissue.

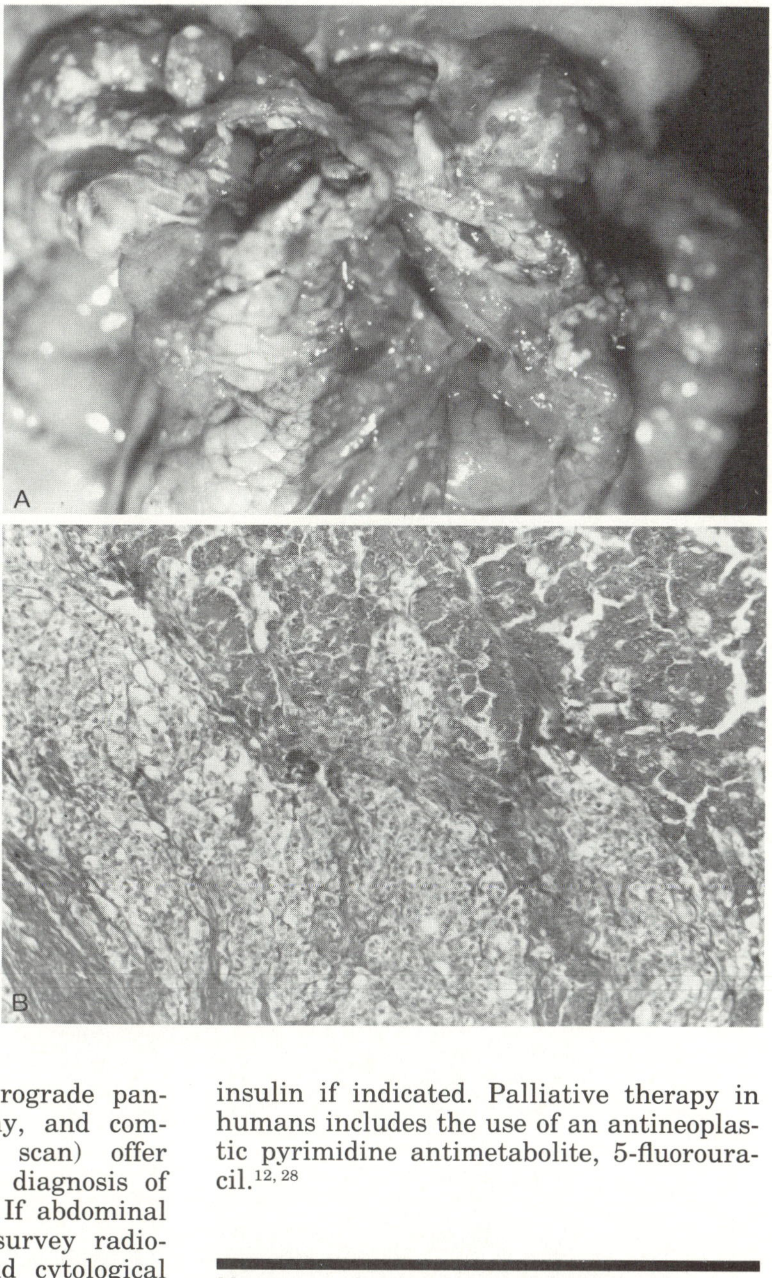

Figure 12–29. *A*, Postmortem specimen from a dog with pancreatic adenocarcinoma with secondary necrosis. *B*, Photomicrograph from the pancreas. Note the marked proliferation and infiltration of bizarre pancreatic acinar tissue with secondary fibrosis *(lower left)*.

duodenum.[28] In humans, retrograde pancreatography, ultrasonography, and computerized tomography (CT scan) offer greater promise of an early diagnosis of pancreatic adenocarcinoma.[28] If abdominal effusion is present on the survey radiographs, abdominocentesis and cytological examination of the fluid may aid in establishing the presence of carcinomatous pancreatic cells.[14, 28]

In the vast majority of patients exploratory laparotomy is necessary to confirm the presence of pancreatic neoplasia.[1] In most instances the tumor has metastasized to the duodenum, liver, or regional lymph nodes by the time exploratory surgery is performed.[4] If the condition is diagnosed before metastasis has occurred, then partial or complete pancreatectomy is feasible, with supplementation of pancreatic enzymes and insulin if indicated. Palliative therapy in humans includes the use of an antineoplastic pyrimidine antimetabolite, 5-fluorouracil.[12, 28]

Hormonal Aspects of Pancreatic Disease

The most common disorders associated with endocrine malfunction in the canine and feline are hypoinsulinism resulting in diabetes mellitus and hyperinsulinism resulting in hypoglycemia and associated neuromuscular symptoms. Recently, several cases of an ulcerogenic condition of the upper gastrointestinal tract due to a gastrin-secreting, non–beta islet cell tumor have been described in the dog.

DIABETES MELLITUS

Post-mortem studies indicate that the most common cause of diabetes mellitus in the dog is progressive necrosis with subsequent fibrosis of the pancreas that occurs during acute exacerbations of chronic relapsing pancreatitis.[36, 52] There may be no clinical evidence of acute flareups, and the patient may be suddenly presented with signs of diabetes mellitus (polyuria, polydipsia, depression, anorexia, and an acute onset of bilateral cataract formation). If the previous history of the patient is carefully traced, the occurrence of a single episode that was clinically compatible with acute pancreatitis may be noted.[36] In a patient with this history the original pathological process has progressed subclinically toward a constricting pancreatic fibrosis, with subsequent destruction of the islets of Langerhans.[36]

Pathological Features

In some canine and feline diabetics, no gross or histological evidence of progressive pancreatic necrosis and fibrosis is evident; however, on microscopic examination sclerosis and vacuolar degeneration of the islets are seen.[36] In some diabetic cats, a pathological finding is nodular hyperplasia causing constriction, fibrosis, and degeneration of the islets.[36] Diabetic feline patients most commonly develop the disease as a result of amyloidosis of the islets (Fig. 12–30). The amyloid deposition is found only in the islets of Langerhans, causing them to become greatly swollen.[36] Since amyloid has been shown to be the denatured light chains of

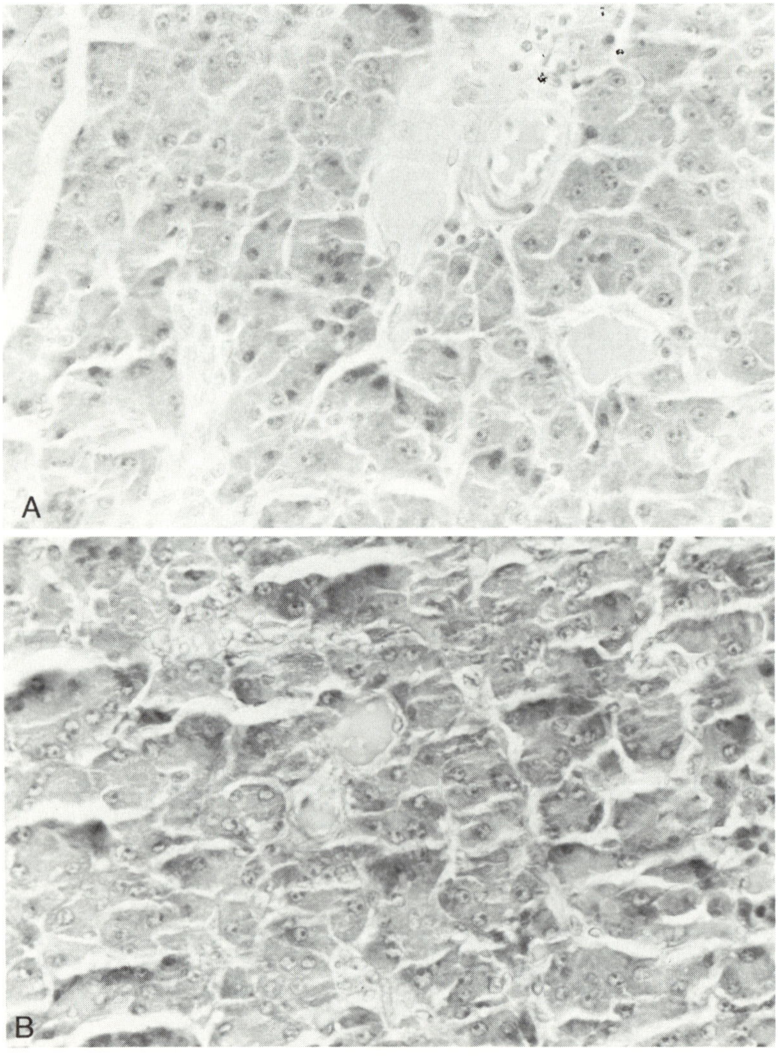

Figure 12–30. Micrographs from a cat with clinical diabetes mellitus. There is a marked infiltration of amyloid into the islets of Langerhans. *A*, H & E, ×250. *B*, Congo Red, ×250.

immunoglobulins G and A (IgG and IgA), an immune-mediated process may be implicated.

Regardless of the pathological lesion, the clinical signs encountered in canine and feline diabetic patients are the result of hypoinsulinism and hyperglucagonemia.[55] Feline and canine diabetes mellitus is clinically similar to juvenile diabetes mellitus, with ketoacidosis being a common clinical finding.[26] However, most dogs and cats are older, with the majority of cases seen in animals more than 8 years of age. The clinical signs observed are due to an inability of muscle and adipose tissue to use glucose, with subsequent hyperglycemia.[26,55] The resultant hyperglycemia produces an osmotic diuresis with the characteristic polyuria and compensatory polydipsia.[24,55] The osmotic diuresis results in a loss of sodium, chloride, and potassium in the urine, producing serous fluid and electrolyte imbalances.[26,54] Because the cells can no longer utilize glucose as an energy source for metabolic functions, lipolysis (the breakdown of triglycerides to form free fatty acids) occurs at an accelerated rate.[26] These free fatty acids are converted by the hepatocyte mitochondria to acetylcoenzyme A (acetyl CoA), which then combines with pyruvate to form citric acid; ultimately ATP and energy are produced.[26] However, if there is an excess of acetyl-CoA substrate, ketone bodies (acetoacetic acid, acetone, and beta-hydroxybutyric acid) will be formed.[26] The resultant ketonemia produces a metabolic acidosis, leading to severe depression, dehydration, and hypotension.[26] A characteristic rapid and deep respiratory pattern (Kussmaul's respiration), an attempt by the lungs to expire large amounts of CO_2 in order to raise the pH, is seen.[26,54] If untreated, diabetic ketoacidosis results in coma and death.[24]

It has been shown that not only insulin insufficiency but also hyperglucagonemia play an important part in the pathogenesis of diabetes mellitus ("bi-hormonal hypothesis").[26,41,55] Glucagon is a peptide hormone that is found in the alpha cells of the islets of Langerhans, the gastric fundus, and duodenum.[55] Excessive secretion by this extrapancreatic source of glucagon is thought to be responsible for hyperglycemia in diabetes mellitus.[26,55] Glucagon produces accelerated glycogenolysis, gluconeogenesis, and lipolysis.[26,41,55] Somatostatin, a potent glucagon inhibitor, is able to lower the elevated blood sugar in diabetic patients, making this peptide hormone a consideration for future therapeutic use.[55] Other peptide hormones, including cortisol, growth hormone, and catecholamines, which are insulin antagonists, have been shown to be present in elevated plasma concentrations in human ketoacidotic diabetic patients.[55]

The routine evaluation of patients with overt diabetes mellitus should consist of a CBC, urinalysis, biochemical blood survey, serum amylase and lipase determinations, and abdominal radiographs.[55] If ketonemia is present and the patient is exhibiting signs of metabolic acidosis, a blood gas determination may be helpful.[55]

Treatment

Therapeutic principles for diabetes mellitus with ketoacidosis include: (1) restoration of fluid and electrolyte balances, (2) correction of acid-base disturbances, and (3) use of supplemental insulin injections.[54] Fluid and electrolyte imbalances are corrected by the intravenous administration of isotonic saline.[54] Since most diabetic patients are geriatric and may have compromised cardiac function, parenteral fluids should be administered via an intravenous jugular catheter in order to monitor central venous pressure.[54] Usually, diabetic patients have hypokalemia due to vomiting and osmotic diuresis, and since insulin will drive potassium ions into the cells, supplemental potassium chloride (KCl) should be added to the parenteral fluids.[54] In the presence of adequate urine output, 20 to 40 mEq/day of KCl may be used.[54] In cases of metabolic acidosis due to ketonemia that is refractory to fluid and insulin therapy, 3 to 6 mEq of $NaHCO_3$ (sodium bicarbonate) may be added to the parenteral fluids daily if blood gas determinations have not been performed.[54] Because diabetic ketoacidosis is a medical emergency, the patient requires continuous monitoring, and treatment should include the judicious use of short-acting regular insulin 1–2 IU/kg SC or IM at hourly intervals until ketoacidosis is abolished.[54] The patient may be monitored utilizing plasma or urine glucose levels and ketone concentrations. Intermediate-acting isophane (NPH) insulin is begun as soon as plasma and urinary ketones clear.[54]

Some diabetic patients that do not have ketoacidosis may still develop stupor, obtundation, and coma (non-ketotic hyperosmolar encephalopathy). In these patients the degree of hyperglycemia is profound, often greater than 1000 mg/dl. The massive elevation of blood glucose levels along with severe dehydration and occasional hypernatremia elevates the plasma osmolality to greater than 330 mOsm/kg (normal value is approximately 295 mOsm/kg). The resultant hyperosmolality of the plasma and cerebrospinal fluid tends to drive water out of the neuronal cells, causing intracellular dehydration and subsequent coma. Clinically, these patients do not exhibit ketonemia or acetone breath odor. Therapy should include vigorous administration of hypotonic (0.45 per cent) sodium chloride and small amounts of regular insulin at frequent intervals, since this type of diabetes mellitus is extremely responsive to insulin administration.

Maintenance therapy of diabetes mellitus includes the determination of urinary glucose and ketone levels and the administration of isophane (NPH) insulin or protamine zinc insulin (PZI) daily.[54] Ideally, the urine glucose concentration should be maintained at a trace level to prevent hypoglycemic reactions.[54] Patients should be fed immediately after insulin administration and approximately 8 hours later (the beginning of NPH insulin peak) to prevent hypoglycemia. If signs of hypoglycemia (weakness, truncal ataxia, stupor, convulsions, and coma) develop, the client should administer oral corn syrup* if the animal can swallow.

Secondary complications in poorly controlled diabetic patients include bilateral cataract formation, emphysematous cystitis, nodular glomerulosclerosis, hepatic lipidosis, and microangiopathy of the retina (Figs. 12–31 to 12–33).

INSULINOMA

Overproduction of insulin resulting in overt hypoglycemia has been well-documented in dogs with islet (beta) cell neoplasms (insulinoma).[34, 59] As opposed to human tumors, canine insulinomas are usually malignant (69 per cent carcinomas vs. 31 per cent adenomas).[9, 34] Clinical signs are extremely variable and include truncal ataxia, paraparesis, neuromuscular fasciculations, convulsions, and coma.[9, 34] These signs are most commonly seen in older dogs (greater than 7 years); however, a study of the patient's previous history may reveal the onset of clinical signs 2 to 3 years prior to the time of diagnosis.[9, 34] The severity of the neurological signs does not directly correlate with the degree of hypoglycemia.[34] Often patients with insulinomas are initially evaluated for seizure disorders and are treated with various anticonvulsant

*Karo Syrup, CPC International, Inc., Englewood Cliffs, NJ.

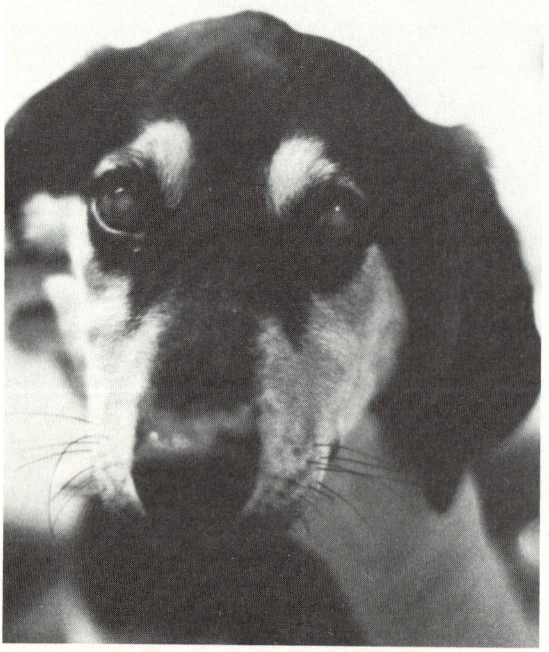

Figure 12–31. A dachshund with diabetes mellitus and bilateral cataracts.

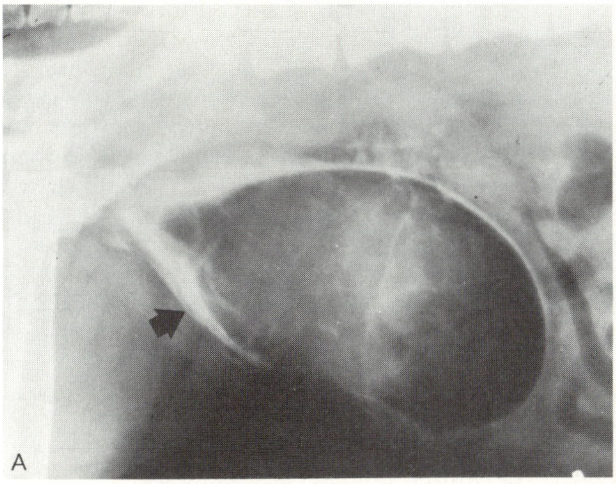

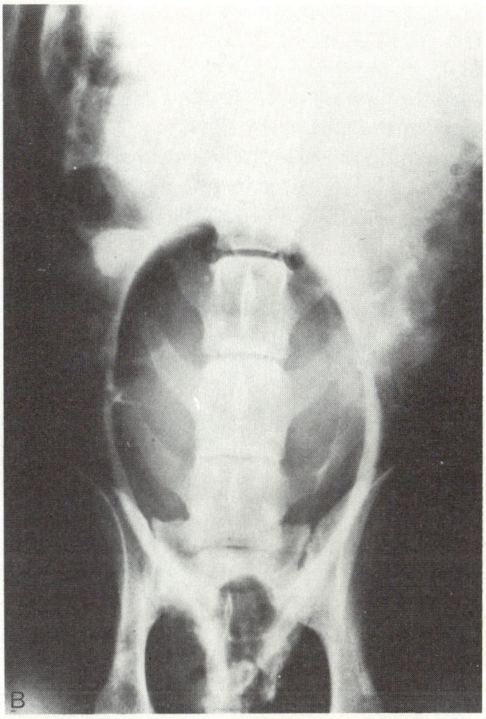

Figure 12–32. *A* and *B*, A double-contrast cystogram from a diabetic dog shows emphysematous cystitis. The bladder wall is thickened and distended with air *(arrow)*.

drugs, with little success in ameliorating the convulsions.[34]

Diagnosis

Diagnosis of the condition is based on the documentation of hypoglycemia and hyperinsulinemia.[34] Patients with insulinoma frequently give the clinical picture known as Whipple's triad (a typical clinical episode with neuromuscular signs caused by the documented hypoglycemia and relief of all symptoms by administration of glucose).[34] Clinical signs may occur early in the morning, during the longest fasting period, or 2 to 5 hours after feeding owing to massive insulin release due to stimulation from the meal.[9] Fasting blood glucose levels (12- to 18-hour fast) are usually subnormal (less than 65 mg/dl). Sometimes a 24- to 48-hour

Figure 12–33. Postmortem specimen from a dog with diabetes mellitus reveals marked hepatic lipidosis.

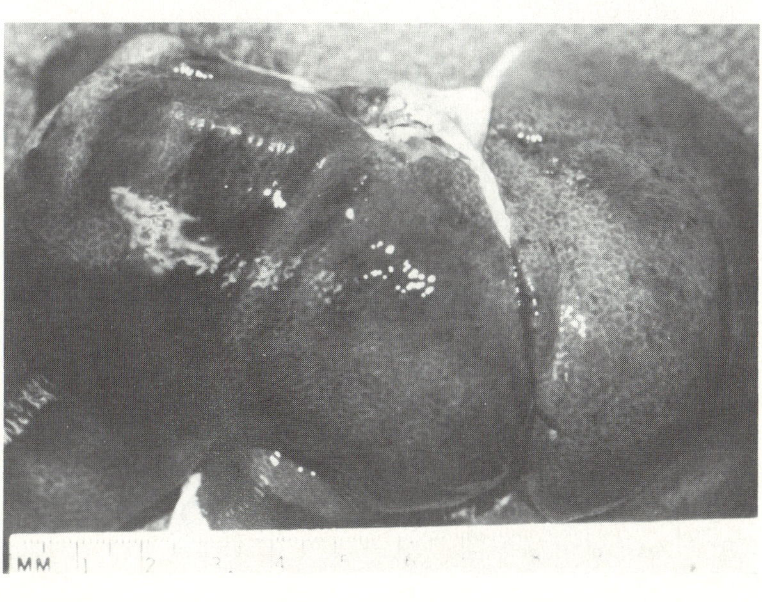

fast may be necessary to reveal hypoglycemia.[34] The advent of radioimmunoassay (RIA) determination of fasting plasma insulin levels has facilitated the diagnosis of insulinomas; levels of greater than 50 mg/dl are considered significant.[34] However, the documentation of a functional insulinoma is achieved by an amended insulin to glucose ratio (AIGR) of greater than 30, as determined by:

$$\frac{(\text{serum insulin} \times 100)}{(\text{plasma glucose} \times 30)}$$

Alternatively, functional insulinoma is demonstrated by a positive response to provocative challenge(s) with beta islet cell secretogogues.[34] Potent insulin stimulators such as intravenous tolbutamide, leucine, and glucagon (0.03 mg/kg IV) may all be effectively utilized to produce a characteristic marked fall in blood glucose concentration.[32] Besides monitoring of the fall in blood glucose levels, an RIA determination of plasma insulin levels is indicated.[32]

Disease entities that may manifest with clinical signs similar to those of insulinoma include: hepatic encephalopathy, adrenal insufficiency, cardiac dysrhythmias, organic brain lesions that cause seizures, polymyopathic syndromes, and hypocalcemia.

Treatment

Ultimately, an exploratory celiotomy is indicated to attempt to locate the neoplasm.[34, 65] In some instances, the tumor can be found and extirpated (Fig. 12–34).[65] If the tumor cannot be grossly visualized, the pancreatic tail and then the head may be excised.[65] Dogs with visible metastases will remain hypoglycemic even after subtotal or

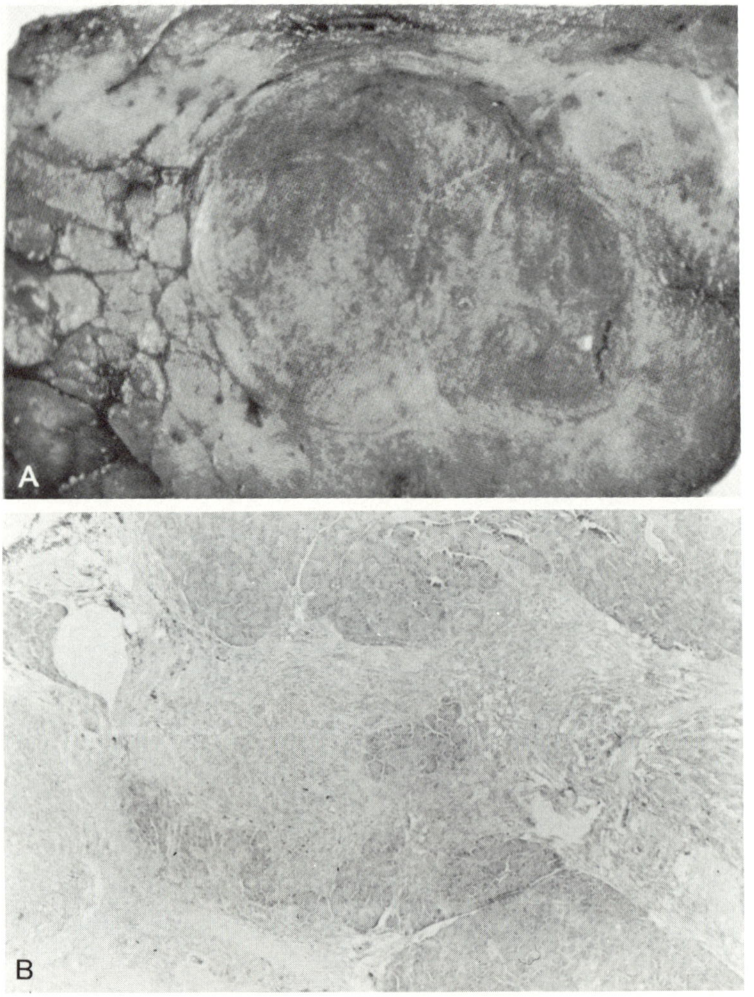

Figure 12–34. *A*, This specimen from a dog with an insulinoma was taken during surgery. *B*, A photomicrograph reveals a marked proliferation of islet cells.

total pancreatectomy.[65] For these patients and for patients that are considered poor surgical risks, amelioration of hypoglycemia may be achieved by the administration of 10 to 40 mg/kg/day of diazoxide,* a benzothiadiazine diuretic that inhibits insulin secretion.[34] In human patients with non-resectable malignant insulinomas, palliative therapy may be attempted with streptozocin, a broad-spectrum antimicrobial with specific cytotoxic action upon the islet cells.[12]

NON–BETA ISLET CELL TUMORS OF THE PANCREAS

Another islet cell tumor of non–beta islet cell origin that has been well-documented in humans and recently has been reported in the dog is the gastrinoma (Zollinger-Ellison syndrome).[17,66] Prior to 1955, there were isolated reports of human patients, presenting with symptoms of fulminant peptic ulceration, who at autopsy were found to have pancreatic non-beta islet cell tumors.[17] In 1955 Drs. Robert Zollinger and Edward Ellison described two patients with these clinical signs and correlated the marked gastric hypersecretion and severe ulceration of the upper gastrointestinal tract to an unknown secretogogue produced by the pancreatic tumors.[21,66] In 1960 it was shown that extracts of the pancreatic islet cell tumors from Zollinger-Ellison (ZE) patients stimulated gastric acid secretion when infused into laboratory animals.[21,66] By 1968, radioimmunoassay and chemical peptide mapping techniques identified the ulcerogenic secretogogue as gastrin.[17,66] To further emphasize the analogy to insulin-secreting beta islet cell tumors (insulinomas) these gastrin-secreting, non–beta islet cell tumors have been termed gastrinomas.[66]

In the past decade a relationship between gastrinomas and other polypeptide-secreting tumors located throughout the body (e.g., in the foregut, adrenal medulla, pituitary gland, pancreatic islet cells, mast cells, melanotrophic cells, and thyroid C cells) has been established.[21] These tumors have now been termed apudomas.[21] The concept of APUD (amine, precursor, uptake, decarboxylation) cells developed from ultrastructural and histochemical studies and linked the cells from the aforementioned sites embryologically, structurally, and biochemically.[21] APUD cells appear to arise from neuroectodermal cells of the neural crest, to contain membrane-bound secretion vesicles, and to secrete polypeptide hormones.[21] Apudomas may produce clinical signs by secreting excessive levels of normally occurring hormones (orthoendocrine syndrome).[21] An example of such a syndrome is the insulinoma. Because of the relatively simple (and interchangeable) polypeptide structure of these hormones, apudomas may secrete hormones that are not characteristically produced in the cell of origin but that are secreted by other APUD cells (paraendocrine syndrome).[21] Examples of paraendocrine syndromes include ACTH-secreting islet cell tumor, ACTH-secreting medullary thyroid carcinoma, and gastrin-secreting melanoma. None of the preceding paraendocrine syndromes has been documented in small animal practice.

Diagnosis

Clinical data from human ZE patients indicate that 90 per cent of them develop recalcitrant peptic ulcer disease that is unresponsive to antacid, dietary, and conventional surgical therapy.[21,35,66] Because 75 per cent of these patients have an ulcer located in either the proximal duodenum or the stomach (less common), the most common clinical sign is persistent epigastric pain.[21,35,66] Most patients have a single ulcer; however, some patients develop multiple lesions that are located distal to the original ulcer, usually in the distal duodenum or jejunum.[21,35,66]

Another common sign is diarrhea; 40 per cent of ZE patients exhibit this sign; seven per cent manifest it in the absence of detectable peptic ulcerations.[21,66] The pathogenesis of the diarrhea appears to involve hypergastrinemia, the production of excessive gastric acid.[21,66] The duodenum becomes overwhelmed with acid, which lowers the intraluminal pH, causing inactivation of pancreatic lipase and bile salts.[21,66] In addition, gastrin inhibits absorption of sodium and water and increases gastrointestinal motility.[21,66] Thus, the end result of hypergastrinemia is diarrhea accompanied by steatorrhea. Because of the excessive amount of gastric acid delivered through the intestinal tract to the terminal ileum, absorption of vitamin B_{12} may be impaired, resulting in a macrocytic anemia (Fig. 12–35).

Greater than 90 per cent of human ZE patients have tumors within either the head

*Proglycem, Schering Corp., Kenilworth, NJ.

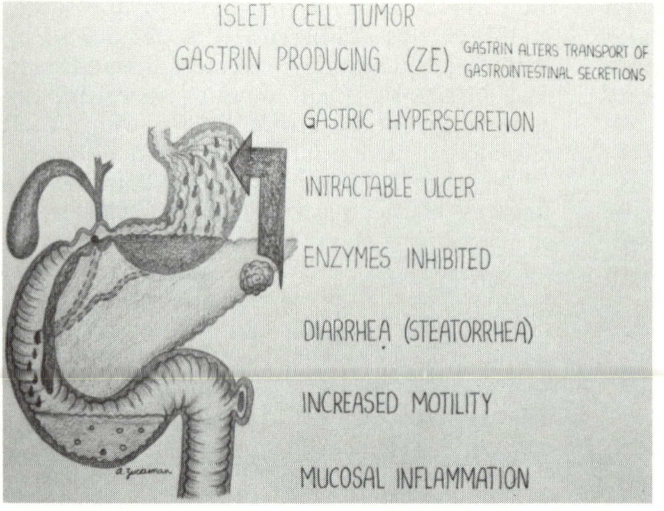

Figure 12–35. The pathogenesis of canine gastrinoma.

or the tail of the pancreas.[21,66] The vast majority (67 per cent) of these tumors are both histologically and biologically malignant and have metastasized by the time surgical exploration is performed.[21,66] The remainder of gastrinomas may be found in the distal duodenum, hilus of the spleen, gastric mucosa, parathyroid gland, or ovary.[21,66] Pancreatic gastrinomas may also be found to secrete other polypeptide hormones, including vasoactive intestinal peptide (VIP), the principal causative hormone of pancreatic cholera, pancreatic polypeptide, ACTH, glucagon, and insulin.[21,66]

Laboratory diagnosis of gastrinoma may be confirmed by elevation of serum gastrin as determined by RIA.[21,35,66] Most normal humans have fasting serum gastrin levels of 60 to 150 pg/ml, whereas most ZE patients have a wide range of 200 to 450,000 pg/ml.[21,66] Most authorities agree that values of greater than 1000 pg/ml are diagnostic for gastrinoma.[21,60,66] It must be noted that other syndromes, including chronic gastritis, gastric atrophy, pernicious anemia, achlorhydria, and chronic renal failure, may cause a mild fasting hypergastrinemia (in the range of 200 to 400 pg/ml).[21,66]

In the event that a patient suspected of having ZE does not have a fasting gastrin level of greater than 1000 pg/ml, several provocative serum gastrin tests may be utilized.[21] The intravenous calcium infusion test is usually the first such test performed.[21] Calcium gluconate (5 mg/kg/hr) is infused into the patient for 3 hours. Serum gastrin levels are measured immediately and every half-hour for 4 hours. Gastrinoma patients usually exhibit an increase of greater than 50 per cent of pre-infusion serum gastrin levels.[21] Another provocative test is to feed the animal a standard meal and to measure gastrin levels at 0 time and at 15-minute intervals for 90 minutes.[21] Most ZE patients exhibit little or no increase in serum gastrin concentrations.[21] The most specific provocative test is the intravenous administration of secretin which stimulates a paradoxical increase in serum gastrin levels in ZE patients. Most normal patients and those with a common duodenal ulcer will exhibit either no increase or a decrease in serum gastrin levels after the administration of secretin, whereas gastrinoma patients have an increase of more than 200 pg/ml.[21] A canine patient diagnosed as having gastrinoma by the author had a dramatically elevated fasting serum gastrin level compared with the level in a normal control dog (1084 pg/ml vs 39 pg/ml).[21]

Like other polypeptide hormones, gastrin is present in the serum in a variety of molecular forms.[21,66] In 1964, the first configuration of gastrin was described as a 17 amino acid chain (heptadecapeptide).[21,66] Later another form of gastrin, a peptide containing 34 amino acid residues, was found in higher concentrations than those of the heptadecapeptide form. The smaller chain has been designated G-17 or "little gastrin," and the larger form has been termed G-34 or "big gastrin."[21,66] It has been shown that G-17 is approximately six times more potent in stimulating gastric acid secretion than G-34.[21] By the use of chromatographic separation techniques, a variety of other molecular forms of gastrin have been found in the serum and in tumors of human ZE patients. These forms include component I gastrin, a very large molecule (molecular weight 20,000 daltons), which has been designated "big, big gastrin."[21] Big, big gastrin has not been detected in the sera of non-gastrinoma patients.[21]

Treatment

Gastrin exerts its activity upon the oxyntic or parietal cells of the gastric mucosa.[63] Three receptors located in the oxyntic cell initiate hydrochloric acid (HCl) secretion.[63, 66] These receptors respond to histamine (H_2 receptors), acetylcholine, or gastrin.[63, 66] Although gastrin exerts activity upon its own receptor site, it will not cause hydrochloric acid secretion unless the acetylcholine and histamine sites are occupied at the same time.[63, 66] This knowledge of the mechanics of HCl secretion by the oxyntic cells has been valuable in the development of drugs that suppress HCl secretion. One histamine analogue, cimetidine, will occupy the H_2 receptor site instead of histamine, thereby blocking HCl secretion.[63] This drug has been quite useful in lowering gastric acid secretion in patients with simple peptic ulcer, ZE syndrome, and disseminated mastocytoma, and also in preventing de-activation of supplemental pancreatic enzymes in patients with pancreatic exocrine insufficiency.[21, 63] The canine gastrinoma patient seen by the author was a 7-year-old, female, spayed German shepherd that had been referred for intractable diarrhea accompanied by abdominal pain, hematemesis, and weight loss (7.5 kg). The fasting serum gastrin level was markedly elevated (1084 pg/ml) compared with the level in a normal control dog (39 pg/ml). Fiberoptic examination revealed a large ulcer in the pyloric antrum of the stomach, with gastric hypertrophy. The dog made objective, temporary improvement while being treated with cimetidine; abdominal pain and diarrhea ceased and the animal regained some weight.[21]

Besides stimulating copious gastric secretion, chronic hypergastrinemia results in edema of the gastric wall with hypertrophy of the rugae.[21, 60, 66] This phenomenon may be detected on plain abdominal radiographs or on a barium study.[66]

The treatment of gastrinoma patients remains controversial. If the tumor is solitary and is located in the pancreas or duodenum, with no visible metastases, surgical removal may be attempted.[21, 66] However, since most gastrinoma patients have multiple tumors and micrometastases, total gastrectomy is usually the procedure of choice.[21, 60, 66] Removal of the target organ of the hypergastrinemia alleviates the subsequent hazards of hemorrhage, perforation, and peritonitis.[21, 66] In contrast, the simple resection of a visibly isolated tumor results in the recurrence of symptoms in one-half of ZE patients.[21, 66] Most sources report a 75 per cent survival rate with total gastrectomy; some patients may survive for longer than 5 years even with visible metastases to the regional lymph nodes and liver.[21, 66] Some investigators suggest that removal of the target organ via gastrectomy produces atrophy of the metastatic tumors.[66] Adjunctive therapy of tumor metastases has been attempted with streptozocin, a potentially nephrotoxic antibiotic derived from *Streptomyces achromogenes* that is specifically cytotoxic for islet cell tumors (Fig. 12–36).[12, 58]

Veterinarians should consider the possibility of a gastrinoma in any dog that exhibits a chronic malabsorptive diarrhea accompanied by abdominal pain with or without hematemesis. Documentation of hypergastrinemia via RIA and exploration of the pancreas, stomach, and liver confirm the diagnosis. Palliative therapy may be achieved with cimetidine (5 mg/kg TID). If a solitary pancreatic tumor exists, surgical extirpation may be attempted. Total gastrectomy in a dog that is a house pet is impractical and ill-advised.

PANCREATIC CHOLERA

Pancreatic cholera is a syndrome characterized by watery diarrhea, hypokalemia, and achlorhydria (WDHA); the disease was named because of its similarities to *Vibrio cholerae* infection.[17, 66] Pancreatic cholera is also caused by a functional non–beta islet cell tumor that some investigators believe produces an excessive amount of vasoactive intestinal peptide, vipoma.[17] It has been found that VIP has a secretin-like activity and thus inactivates and antagonizes gastrin. This activity results in severe achlorhydria, which inhibits proper gastric chymification.[62] The material delivered to the small intestine is not sufficiently hydrolyzed to allow proper digestion by pancreatic enzymes and bile salts.[66] In addition, VIP pro-

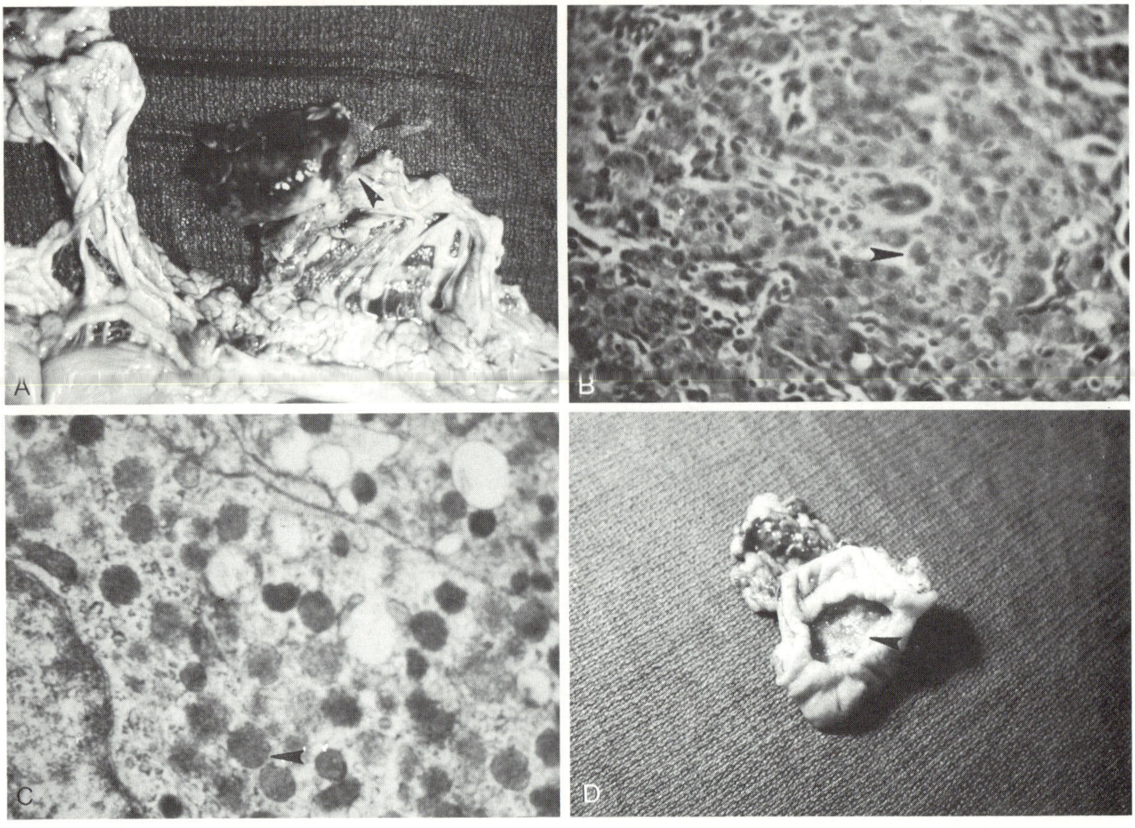

Figure 12–36. *A*, Postmortem specimen from a dog reveals a large gastrinoma *(arrow)* originating from the left lobe of the pancreas. *B*, Photomicrograph of the specimen. The arrow indicates a marked proliferation of islet cells. *C*, Electronmicrograph illustrating typical G-cell (gastrin-secreting) granules *(arrow*, Karnovsky fixation). *D*, Examination of a postmortem specimen from the same dog shows a large gastric ulcer *(arrow)*.

duces severe intestinal vasodilation and efflux of fluid into the intestinal lumen.[66] The end result is a profuse, watery, osmotic diarrhea with hypokalemia (Figs. 12–37 and 12–38).

Recently, the role of VIP as the causative agent of pancreatic cholera has been challenged.[33] Some researchers have described elevations in plasma levels of prostaglandin E and decreases in levels of VIP in patients that clinically respond to indomethacin, a potent prostaglandin inhibitor.[33, 37]

Since both the Zollinger-Ellison syndrome and pancreatic cholera have a cellular basis in the APUD cells of the islets of Langerhans, and since APUD cells have been found in other organs (thyroid, parathyroid, pituitary, and adrenal glands as well as the small intestine) multiple hormonal release by these tumors may be clinically detected.[17, 66] Pancreatic cholera has been frequently associated with hypercalcemia because of the production and release of a parathormone-like peptide hormone and with hypocal-

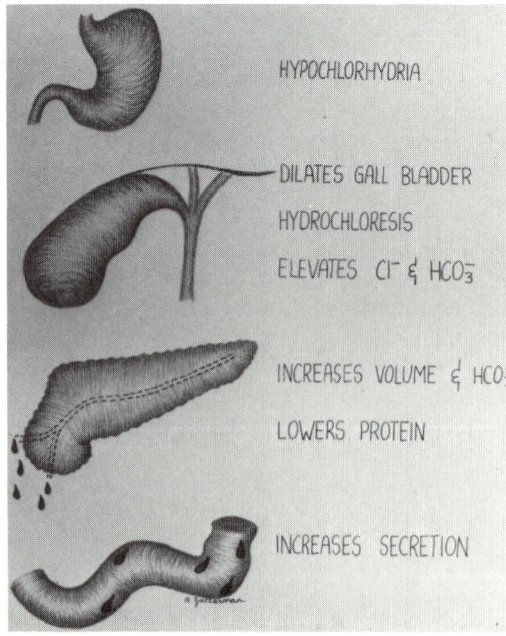

Figure 12–37. The effects of vasoactive intestinal peptide (VIP).

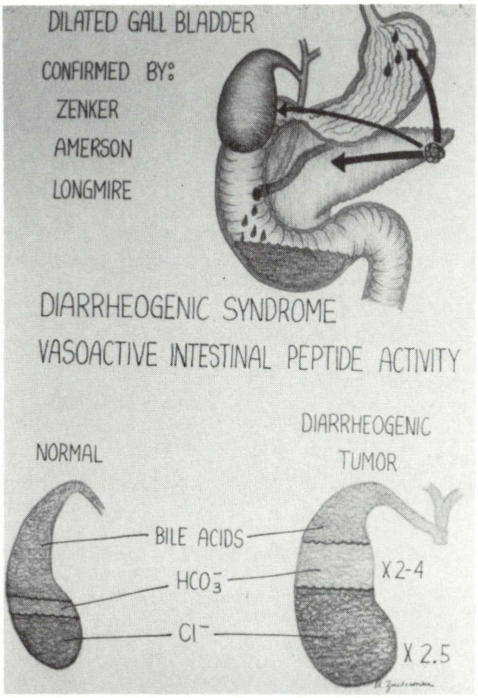

Figure 12–38. The pathogenesis of pancreatic cholera.

cemia because VIP will stimulate calcitonin release.[17] The Zollinger-Ellison syndrome is sometimes associated with hypercalcemia, and on occasion the delta islet cells may release insulin and ACTH.[66]

Finally, both Zollinger-Ellison syndrome and pancreatic cholera may be associated with simultaneously occurring tumors in any of the APUD cell organs (MEA or Multiple Endocrine Adenomatosis).[66] The discovery of naturally occurring cases of Zollinger-Ellison syndrome in a dog has stimulated interest in these curious gastrointestinal hormonal syndromes, and the author believes that in time they will also be documented in canine and feline patients.

References

1. Anderson NV, Johnson KH: Pancreatic carcinoma in the dog. J Am Vet Med Assoc 150:286, 1977.
2. Anderson NV: Pancreatitis in dogs. Vet Clin North Am 2:79, 1973.
3. Anderson NV: Review of literature: Pancreas. J Am Anim Hosp Assoc 9:89, 1973.
4. Anderson WA, Scotti TM: *Synopsis of Pathology,* 8th ed. C. V. Mosby Co., St. Louis, 676, 1976.
5. Beck IT, Sinclair DG: *The Exocrine Pancreas.* Williams & Wilkins, Baltimore, 1971.
6. Botsford TW, Wilson RE: *The Acute Abdomen,* 2nd ed. W. B. Saunders Company, Philadelphia, 1977.
7. Brobst DF: Pancreatic function. *In* Kaneko JJ, Cornelius CE (eds): *Clinical Biochemistry of Domestic Animals.* Academic Press, New York, 231, 1970.
8. Burrows CF, Merritt AM, Chiapella AM: Determination of fecal fat and trypsin output in the evaluation of chronic canine diarrhea. J Am Vet Med Assoc 174:62, 1979.
9. Capen CC, Martin SL: Hyperinsulinism in dogs with neoplasia of the pancreatic islets. Vet Pathol 6:309, 1969.
10. Carey LC: *The Pancreas.* C. V. Mosby Co., St. Louis, 1973.
11. Christensen GC, Evans HE: *Miller's Anatomy of the Dog,* 2nd ed. W. B. Saunders Company, Philadelphia, 1979.
12. Cline MJ, Haskell CM: *Cancer Chemotherapy.* W. B. Saunders Company, Philadelphia, 1975.
13. Cooperman AM: Chronic pancreatitis. Surg Clin North Am 61:71, 1981.
14. Cornelius LM: Laboratory diagnosis of acute pancreatitis and pancreatic adenocarcinoma. Vet Clin North Am 6:671, 1976.
15. Creutzfeldt W, Schmidt H: Aetiology and pathogenesis of pancreatitis (current concepts). Scand J Gastroenterol 5:Suppl 6:47, 1970.
16. Dellman HD: *Veterinary Histology.* Lea & Febiger, Philadelphia, 171, 1971.
17. Demling L, Ottenjann R: *Non-Insulin Producing Tumors of the Pancreas.* Grune & Stratton, New York, 1969.
18. Di Magno EP, Malogelada JR, Go VL, et al: Fate of orally ingested enzymes in pancreatic insufficiency: Comparison of two dosage schedules. N Engl J Med 296:1318, 1977.
19. Drazner FH: Mechanisms of diarrheal disease. *In* Kirk RW (ed).: *Current Veterinary Therapy VIII.* W. B. Saunders Company, Philadelphia, 773, 1983.
20. Drazner FH: Clinical implications of disseminated intravascular coagulation. Comp Cont Ed 4:974–986, 1982.
21. Drazner FH: Canine gastrinoma, a condition analogous to the Zollinger-Ellison syndrome in man. Calif Vet 35:6–13, 1981.
22. Drazner, FH: Hypercalcemia in the dog and cat. J Am Vet Med Assoc 12:1252, 1981.
23. Drazner, FH. Unpublished data. 1977–1980.
24. Dreiling DA, Janowitz HD, Perrier CV: *Pancreatic Inflammatory Disease.* Harper & Row, New York, 1964.
25. Dworken HJ: *The Alimentary Tract.* W. B. Saunders Company, Philadelphia, 233, 1974.
26. Fajans SS: What is diabetes? Med Clin North Am 55:793, 1971.
27. Geokas MC, Van Lancker JL, Kadell BM, et al: Acute pancreatitis. Ann Intern Med 76:105, 1972.
28. Grage TB, Ferguson RM, Simmons RL: Gastrointestinal tract cancer. *In* Horton J, Hill GJ II (eds): *Clinical Oncology.* W. B. Saunders Company, Philadelphia, 259, 1977.
29. Gyr N: *Tests of Exocrine Pancreatic Function.* Hans Huber, Stuttgart, 1975.
30. Hardy RM, Stevens JB: Exocrine pancreatic disease. *In* Ettinger SS (ed): *Textbook of Veterinary Internal Medicine.* W. B. Saunders Company, Philadelphia, 1247, 1975.
31. Harrison BB: *Dissection of the Cat & Comparisons with Man.* C. V. Mosby Co., St. Louis, 1966.
32. Hightower NC Jr, Janowitz HD: Pancreatic secretion. *In* Brobeck JR (ed). *Best & Taylor's Physio-*

logical Basis of Medical Practice, 9th ed. Williams & Wilkins, Baltimore, 2, 49, 60, 1973.
33. Jaffe BM, et al: Indomethacin-sensitive pancreatic cholera. N Engl J Med. 294:1440, 1976.
34. Johnson RK: Hypoglycemia in the dog. *In* Kirk RW (ed): *Current Veterinary Therapy VI.* W. B. Saunders Company, Philadelphia, 1010–1016, 1975.
35. Jones BP, Nichols MR, Badman R: Peptic ulceration in a dog associated with an islet cell carcinoma of the pancreas and an elevated plasma gastrin level. J Small Anim Pract 17:593, 1976.
36. Jubb, KVF, Kennedy PC: *Pathology of Domestic Animals.* Academic Press, New York, 225, 1963.
37. Kahn CR, Levy AG, Gardner JD, et al: Pancreatic cholera: Beneficial effects of streptozocin. N Engl J Med 292:941, 1975.
38. Kelly TR, Bratcher EP, Falor WH: Trypsin inhibitor in acute hemorrhagic pancreatitis. Arch Surg 89:317, 1964.
39. Kinzie JL: Acute pancreatitis. *In* Rosenfeld MG (ed): *Manual of Medical Therapeutics.* 20th ed. Little, Brown & Co., Boston, 291, 1972.
40. Kowlessar OD: Disease of the pancreas. *In* Beeson PB, McDermott W (eds): *Textbook of Medicine.* W. B. Saunders Company, Philadelphia, 1243, 1975.
41. Lawrence AM: Glucagon in medicine: New ideas for an old hormone. Med Clin North Am 54:183, 1970.
42. Laees GE, Suter PF, Johnson CC: Pulmonary edema in a dog with acute pancreatitis and cardiac disease. J Am Vet Med Assoc 172:690, 1978.
43. Merritt AM, Burrows CF, Cowgill L, Street W: Fecal fat and trypsin in dogs fed a meat-base or cereal-base diet. J Am Vet Med Assoc 174:59, 1979.
44. Moore RW, Withrow SJ: Gastrointestinal hemorrhage and pancreatitis associated with intervertebral disc disease in the dog. J Am Vet Med Assoc 180:1443, 1982.
45. Neuman NB: Acute pancreatic hemorrhage associated with iatrogenic hypercalcemia in a dog. J Am Vet Med Assoc 166:381, 1975.
46. Owens JM, Drazner FH, Gilbertson SR: Pancreatic disease in the cat. J Am Anim Hosp Assoc 11:83, 1975.
47. Parks JL: Acute pancreatitis. *In* Kirk RW (ed): *Current Veterinary Therapy VI.* W. B. Saunders Company, Philadelphia, 973, 1977.
48. Parks JL: Peritoneal drainage. J Am Anim Hosp Assoc 10:289, 1974.
49. Parks JL, Gahring D, Greene RW: Peritoneal lavage for peritonitis and pancreatitis in twenty-two dogs. J Am Anim Hosp Assoc 9:442, 1973.
50. Ranson JHC: Acute pancreatitis—where are we? Surg Clin North Am 61:55, 1981.
51. Regan PT, Malagelada JR, DiMagno EP, et al: Comparative effects of antacids, cimetidine and enteric coating on the therapeutic response to oral enzymes in severe pancreatic insufficiency. N Engl J Med 297:854, 1977.
52. Rudnick J: Physiology of pancreatic secretion. Surg Clin North Am 61:47, 1981.
53. Rutter WJ: The development of the endocrine and exocrine pancreas. *In* Fitzgerald PJ, Morrison AB (eds): *The Pancreas,* Williams & Wilkins, Baltimore, 30, 1980.
54. Schaer M: The pancreas. *In* Bojrab MJ (ed): *Pathophysiology for the Surgeon.* Lea & Febiger, Philadelphia, 292–303, 1981.
55. Siegel ET: *Endocrine Diseases of the Dog.* Lea & Febiger, Philadelphia, 97, 1977.
56. Snodgrass PJ: Pathophysiology of the pancreas. *In* Sodeman WA Jr, Sodeman TM (eds): *Pathologic Physiology,* 6th ed. W. B. Saunders Company, Philadelphia, 928, 1979.
57. Snodgrass PJ: Disorders of the pancreas. *In* Wintrobe MM (ed): *Harrison's Principles of Internal Medicine,* 6th ed. McGraw-Hill Book Company, New York, 1575, 1970.
58. Stadil F, Stage G, Rehfeld JF, et al: Treatment of Zollinger-Ellison Syndrome with stroptozocin. N Engl J Med 294:1440, 1976.
59. Strafuss AC, Njoku CO, Blauch B, et al: Islet cell neoplasm in four dogs. J Am Vet Med Assoc 159:1008, 1971.
60. Strauss E, Johnson GF, Yallow RS: Canine Zollinger-Ellison syndrome. Gastroenterology 72:380, 1977.
61. Strombeck DR, Farver TF, Kaneko JJ: Serum amylase and lipase activities in the diagnosis of pancreatitis in dogs. Am J Vet Res 42:1966, 1981.
62. Strombeck DR: New method for evaluation of chymotrypsin deficiency in dogs. J Am Vet Med Assoc 173:1319, 1978.
63. Strombeck DR: The Pancreas. *In* Strombeck DR (ed): Small Animal Gastroenterology. University of California Press, Davis, 301, 1975.
64. Thompson BW, Lip RJ, Clark RL: Propylthiouracil in acute hemorrhagic pancreatitis. Arch Surg 88:966, 1964.
65. Wilson JW: Surgical correction of islet cell adenocarcinoma in a dog. J Am Vet Med Assoc 164:603, 1974.
66. Zollinger RM, Coleman DW: *The Influences of Pancreatic Tumors on the Stomach.* Charles C Thomas, Springfield, Il, 1974.

CHAPTER

13

Diseases of the Liver

WILLIAM A. ROGERS

The liver is the center of metabolic activity for the body and as such is of great interest to the veterinarian practicing internal medicine.[119] The liver may be the primary site of a disease process, as in cirrhosis, or it may be disturbed in a secondary fashion, as in diabetes mellitus.

Functional and Anatomical Considerations[96]

Knowledge of gross and microscopic anatomy of the liver is of practical importance to the veterinary clinician for: (1) performance of safe and accurate biopsy, (2) performance of surgery, (3) understanding of developmental and acquired hepatic malformations, (4) detection of hepatic diseases associated with disease of adjacent organs, (5) radiographic examination, (6) interpretation of histopathological descriptions (liver biopsy reports), and (7) understanding of the functional significance of the distribution of lesions within the liver. The gross and microscopic anatomy is discussed to provide information applicable to these objectives.

ANATOMICAL CONSIDERATIONS

The liver is the largest parenchymal organ in the body, weighing 0.45 to 0.50 kg in the medium-sized dog (3.4 per cent of the body weight).[34] The organ is multilobed in the dog and cat, is located caudal to and contiguous with the diaphragm, and is cranial to the stomach and other abdominal viscera (Fig. 13–1). It is close to the esophagus, caudal vena cava, stomach, spleen, pancreas, duodenum, and kidneys.[34]

Major vessels of the liver include the portal vein, which supplies venous blood obtained from the stomach, intestines, pancreas, and spleen, and the hepatic artery, a branch of the celiac artery that supplies

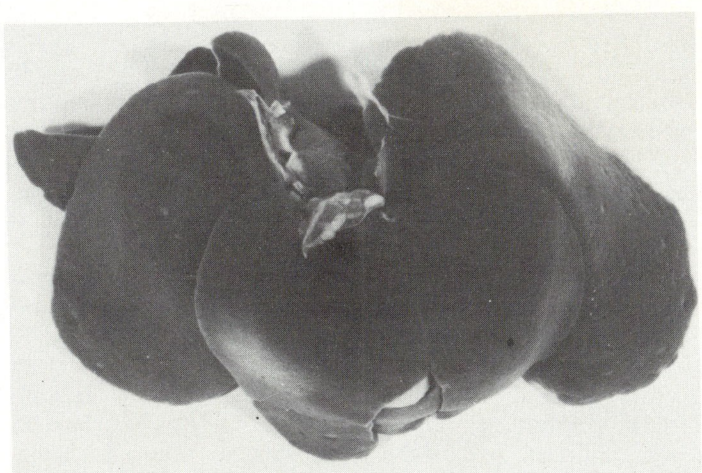

Figure 13–1. Diaphragmatic surface of a dog's multilobed liver.

arterial blood to the liver. This organ is drained by the hepatic veins, which return blood to the caudal vena cava.

The portal vein and hepatic artery deliver about 20 per cent of the total cardiac output to the liver. Portal vein blood must circulate through the liver to be detoxified prior to entering the systemic circulation. If portal blood is not processed by the liver, serious intoxication, e.g., portosystemic encephalopathy, results.[57, 107, 110] The portal vein supplies 70 per cent of the hepatic blood flow and the hepatic artery supplies the remaining 30 per cent. The well-oxygenated hepatic artery blood is vital to the survival of the liver. If the hepatic artery is ligated, the liver usually dies, whereas if the portal vein is ligated the hepatic artery can dilate to deliver more blood, and the liver survives.[34, 79]

In the fetus, blood is shunted from the umbilical vein to the hepatic venous system by way of the ductus venosus, which normally closes at birth. If the ductus venosus fails to close at birth, a portacaval shunt results.[74]

The hepatic artery and the portal vein empty into the sinusoids of the liver. These vessels are accompanied by infoldings of Glisson's capsule, the connective tissue covering of the liver. The bile ducts also follow these vessels to their finest ramifications. On microscopic examination, the small vessels in the portal triads—the adjacent portal venule, hepatic arteriole, and bile ductule—that are coursing through the parenchyma, can be identified. The portal blood and the arterial blood empty into endothelium-lined spaces called sinusoids. The sinusoids are drained by the hepatic veins.

The parenchymal mass that is supplied by the terminal ramification of the afferent vessels (e.g., portal venules and hepatic arterioles) is called an acinus. "Acinus" indicates a grape-like cluster; in this case, a cluster of hepatocytes around the terminal branches of afferent vessels.

The sinusoidal endothelium and the hepatocytes are separated by the space of Disse. Plasma filters from the sinusoids into the space of Disse, where it is made available to the hepatocytes. Products of hepatocyte metabolism are sent back to the space of Disse and returned to the sinusoids. Fluid in the space of Disse drains into the hepatic lymph system and leaves the liver via the hilar lymphatics.

In addition to releasing substances into the space of Disse, the hepatocytes actively secrete bile into the bile canaliculi. Bile canaliculi are spaces formed between adjacent hepatocytes by invaginations of their cell membranes. The bile flows from bile canaliculi into bile ductules and eventually enters the hepatic bile ducts. Bile is then stored and concentrated in the gall bladder. Upon contraction of the gall bladder, bile is secreted into the duodenum via the common bile duct (Fig. 13–2). Bile formed by hepatocytes exits the liver by way of bile ductules that travel the same path as the portal veins and hepatic arteries, but bile flow is directed opposite to the direction of blood flow. The acini are functional units, i.e., bile from one acinus must exit via its own bile ductules.

Histologically, lesions may affect selected regions of the acinus. In general, the periphery of the acinus is most susceptible to disease because it has the lowest oxygen tension. This relative hypoxia of the acinar periphery occurs because much of the oxygen is removed by the hepatocytes of the central acinus, which have first contact with the entering blood. However, other regions of the acinus are prone to injury; e.g., in some hepatotoxicities periportal hepatocytes are predisposed.

The distribution of lesions within the acinus may determine their effect on liver function. For example, if the center of the acinus is most severely affected, the disorder is more likely to be characterized by icterus (cholestasis) than if the lesions are at the acinar periphery.[45]

FUNCTIONAL CONSIDERATIONS[25]

Because it is impossible and unnecessary to discuss all of the hepatic functions, attention will be concentrated on those that are clinically important.

Assimilation of absorbed nutrients (carbohydrates, fats, proteins, vitamins, etc.) requires adequate liver function, so that malnutrition is an important facet of liver disease.[81] Many of the body proteins are synthesized by the liver (Table 13–1).[67] Essentially all of the albumin is made by the liver. Albumin is important because it contributes to normal blood oncotic pressure and because it functions as a carrier protein. It is the most abundant plasma protein.

Reports on the serum half-life of albumin in the dog have been inconsistent (as short as 1 week to as long as 3 weeks).[22, 25] Regardless of the correct value, hypoalbuminemia caused by liver failure (lack of al-

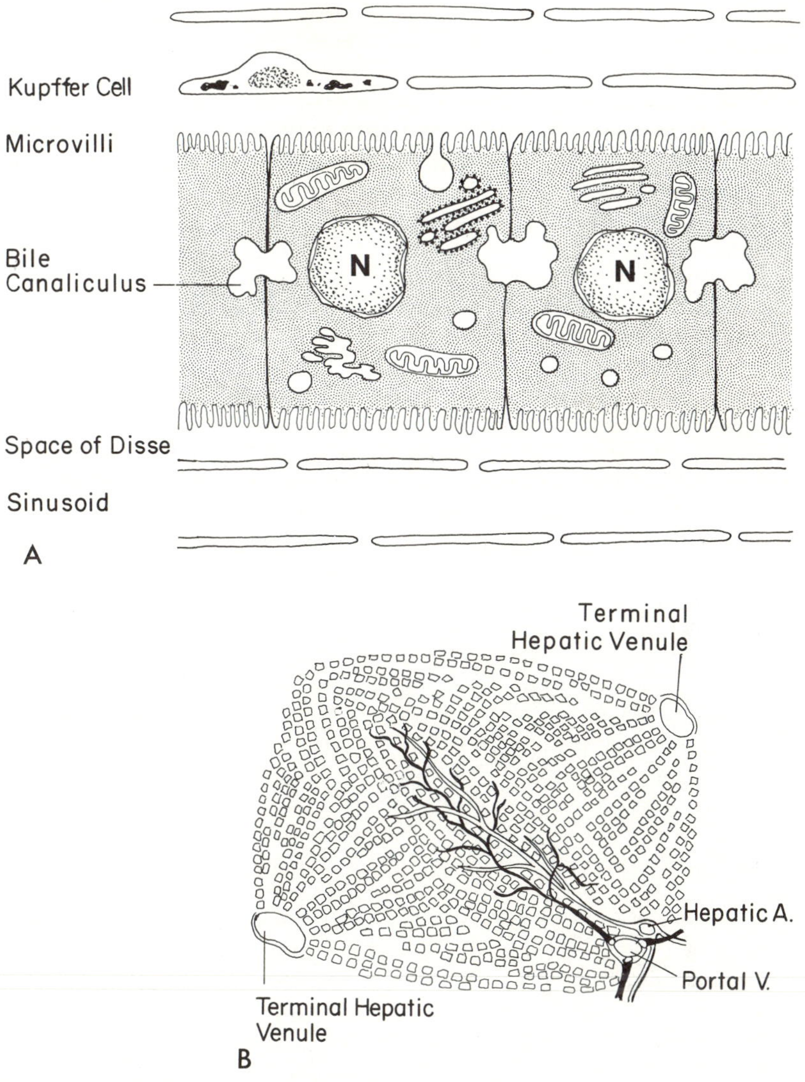

Figure 13–2. *A*, Microscopic anatomy of the liver. The relationship between permeable sinusoidal membranes, interstitial space of Disse, Kupffer's cells lining the sinusoid, and bile canaliculi formed by adjacent invaginations of hepatocyte membranes is demonstrated. *B*, The hepatic acinus is composed of the portal triad, which supplies afferent blood vessels and drains the bile ductule to the center of the acinus, and the terminal venule, which drains the periphery of the acinus. The acinus is the functional unit of the liver.

bumin production) represents relatively chronic disease, as compared with deficient production of short-lived proteins such as prothrombin, which can occur in acute disease. This concept can be used to assess chronicity of liver disease.[20]

Liver function is important for proper carbohydrate homeostasis. Liver failure can result in energy deficits and hypoglycemia. Glycogen (starch) is formed and stored in the liver during periods of positive energy balance, e.g., the postprandial state. Later, when energy is required, the glycogen is broken down and released from the liver to supply the body, and the liver itself, with glucose to be used for energy. Blood glucose levels are maintained by gluconeogenesis, the production of glucose from noncarbohydrates in the liver. In addition to forming, storing, and breaking down of carbohydrates, the liver metabolizes important hormones, such as insulin and glucagon, that are involved in glucose metabolism.

The liver plays a central role in lipid metabolism. Lipoproteins are formed in and released from the liver. The production of lipoproteins makes the lipids miscible, enabling them to be transported in the aqueous plasma. Lipids are transported to other tis-

Table 13–1. IMPORTANT PROTEINS MANUFACTURED BY THE LIVER

Albumin
Lipoproteins
Hormone transport proteins
Haptoglobin—carries hemoglobin
Transferrin—carries iron
Ceruloplasmin—carries copper
Alpha- and beta-globulins
Fibrinogen (factor I)
Prothrombin (factor II)
Clotting factors (III, V, VIII, IX, X, XI)

sues to be used as body fuel (fatty acid and triglyceride) or as structural components of cell membranes (cholesterol and phospholipid). Liver failure can result in energy imbalances and structural defects in cell membranes throughout the body. Failure of the liver to package and release lipoproteins properly results in a fatty liver (hepatic lipidosis).[58]

Bile salts are formed by the liver from cholesterol (Fig. 13–3). The bile salts are excreted in bile and released into the duodenum after a meal. These bile salts are essential for proper absorption of fat from the small intestine, where they emulsify fat and form micelles when combined with fatty acids. Insufficient secretion of bile salts can result in malabsorption of fat, which is manifested clinically as weight loss and steatorrhea. In addition to bile salts, bile contains

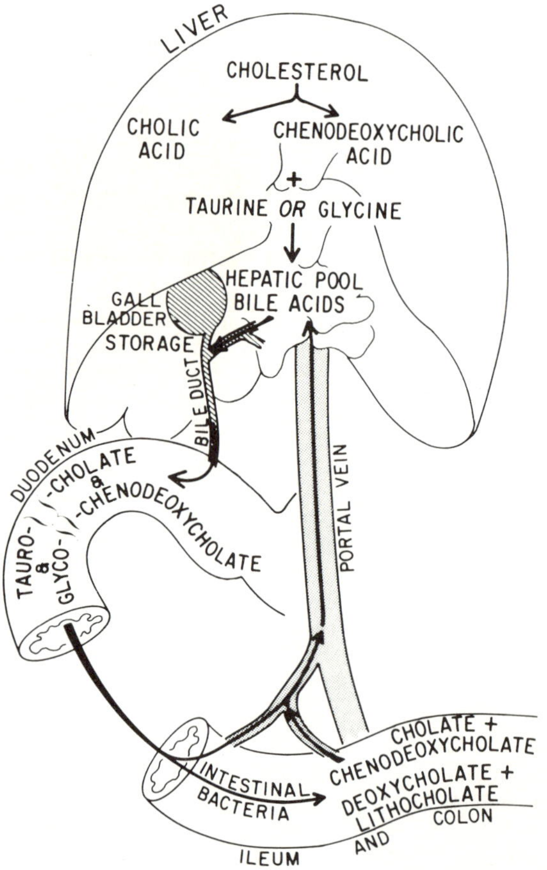

Figure 13–3. Bile acid synthesis, secretion, release into the intestine, bacterial degradation, absorption from intestine, and resecretion by the liver. (Reprinted with permission from Strombeck DR: *Small Animal Gastroenterology*. Davis, CA, Stonegate Publishing, 1983.)

water, bicarbonate, other electrolytes, and substances such as drugs are excreted.

Detoxifying portal blood before it enters the systemic circulation is an important function of the liver.[57, 107] The toxins removed from portal blood include ammonia, short-chain fatty acids, mercaptans, and biogenic amines. The ammonia is removed from portal blood and enters the hepatic urea cycle, resulting in the production of urea. If the portal blood bypasses the liver and contaminates systemic blood, the toxins interfere with cerebral function and cause portosystemic encephalopathy (hepatoencephalopathy).[57, 107]

The liver is an important part of the reticuloendothelial (RE) system.[100] RE cells are derived from circulating monocytes and then develop into phagocytes, which populate the sinusoids. The phagocytes, called Kupffer cells, remove toxic substances, microorganisms, and cellular debris from the portal blood. They also remove endotoxins; if the RE system of the liver fails, endotoxemia may ensue.[39]

Hepatocytes have a tremendous regenerative capacity (turnover rate of 50 to 75 days in humans), but new hepatocytes are functionally immature. The maturation process requires vitamin B_{12}, folic acid, and a considerable amount of protein. These substances should be supplied to diseased livers that are undergoing regeneration, to ensure that deficiencies do not delay healing. Besides these vital nutrients, the liver needs hepatotrophic factors that are present in portal blood. Lack of these portal factors, as occurs in portacaval shunting, results in liver atrophy. The most important hepatotrophic factor in portal blood appears to be insulin.[116, 117]

History and Clinical Signs

History taking is very important when a clinician is dealing with patients with liver disease. In addition to the usual questions, the clinician should ask about the possibility of drug or toxin exposure, the presence of neurological signs and their association with diet, and the presence of polydipsia or polyuria.

The effects of liver failure on the patient are often subtle and nonspecific. The clinical signs of acute and chronic liver disease are listed in Table 13–2. Liver disease can smol-

Table 13–2. CLINICAL SIGNS OF ACUTE AND CHRONIC LIVER DISEASE

Acute	
Mild	Anorexia Vomiting Diarrhea ± Hepatomegaly
Severe	Anorexia Vomiting Diarrhea Icterus Ascites PSE Bleeding Hepatomegaly or microhepatica
Chronic*	Anorexia Vomiting Diarrhea Weight loss or stunted growth Weakness Ascites PSE Acholic stools PU/PD Hepatomegaly or microhepatica Intolerance to drugs Pruritus

*Signs are often intermittent.

der for a long time without producing any clinical signs. For this reason, geriatric patients that appear healthy should nevertheless be tested for liver disease during routine check-ups, and any patient with signs of anorexia, depression, vomiting, or weight loss should be investigated for liver disease.

Jaundice, ascites, hepatomegaly, and acholic stools are clinical signs that should engender strong suspicion of liver disease (Fig. 13–4).[87, 135] Jaundice can be caused by an acute hemolytic episode (prehepatic jaundice), but it is not as common as jaundice caused by hepatic disease. When mucous membranes are not pale or when jaundice is chronic, acute hemolysis is a less likely diagnosis. Jaundice appears when the total serum bilirubin content reaches about 2.8 mg/dl (normal is less than 0.6 mg/dl); therefore, significant hyperbilirubinemia can occur without jaundice. Acholic stools lack normal coloration because of the absence of bile pigments and are thus indicative of biliary obstruction.

Hepatomegaly can be detected by abdominal palpation or by radiography (Fig. 13–5). Variation in liver size and position in relation to the rib cage from one breed to another makes detection of abnormalities of liver size a subjective evaluation. Hepatomegaly may be caused by infiltration of the liver by fat, inflammatory cells, neoplastic cells, or amyloid.[132]

A small liver (microhepatia) is difficult to detect by palpation, but it may be suspected when the free edges of the liver are not palpable in relaxed dogs, in dogs under general anesthesia, or in cats, in which the liver should be easily palpated. When palpating the liver, the clinician should be patient and gentle, allow the abdominal wall to relax, and perform the procedure with the animal in a variety of positions.

Ascites is another hallmark of liver disease (see Figure 13–4*A*).[48] In some cases, abdominal distention may be the only reason that the client seeks medical attention for the animal. Ascites is often accompanied by muscle wasting, which is associated with deficient protein synthesis and increased tissue catabolism. The pathogenesis of ascites is complex, but hypoalbuminemia and portal hypertension are the most important factors. Ascites can usually be detected by ballottement of the abdomen. Occasionally, sagging abdominal muscles or hepatomegaly causes abdominal distention, giving the appearance of ascites. Ascites due to liver disease must be differentiated from that due to right-sided cardiac failure, hypoproteinemic states of nonhepatic origin (e.g., nephrotic syndrome), and other causes of abdominal effusions.

Polydipsia and polyuria are common clinical signs of hepatic disease.[119] The cause is not understood; however, theoretically, blood urea nitrogen levels, which are needed for the counter-current multiplier system of the kidney, are low because of a lack of hepatic urea synthesis. The lowering of BUN levels could lead to a loss of the normal corticomedullary concentration gradient.[51] The polydipsia and polyuria may also be neurological manifestations of portosystemic encephalopathy (PSE), a psychogenic disorder.[51]

Portosystemic encephalopathy can evoke a variety of neurological signs.[110] The client may describe grand mal seizures, blindness, circling, viciousness, and episodes of coma. An important historical clue is worsening of the neurological sign after eating, followed by gradual improvement, and then recurrence after the next meal. This postprandial association is caused by hyperammonemia and by the presence of elevated levels of other metabolic toxins. Normally, dietary protein is converted to ammonia by enteric

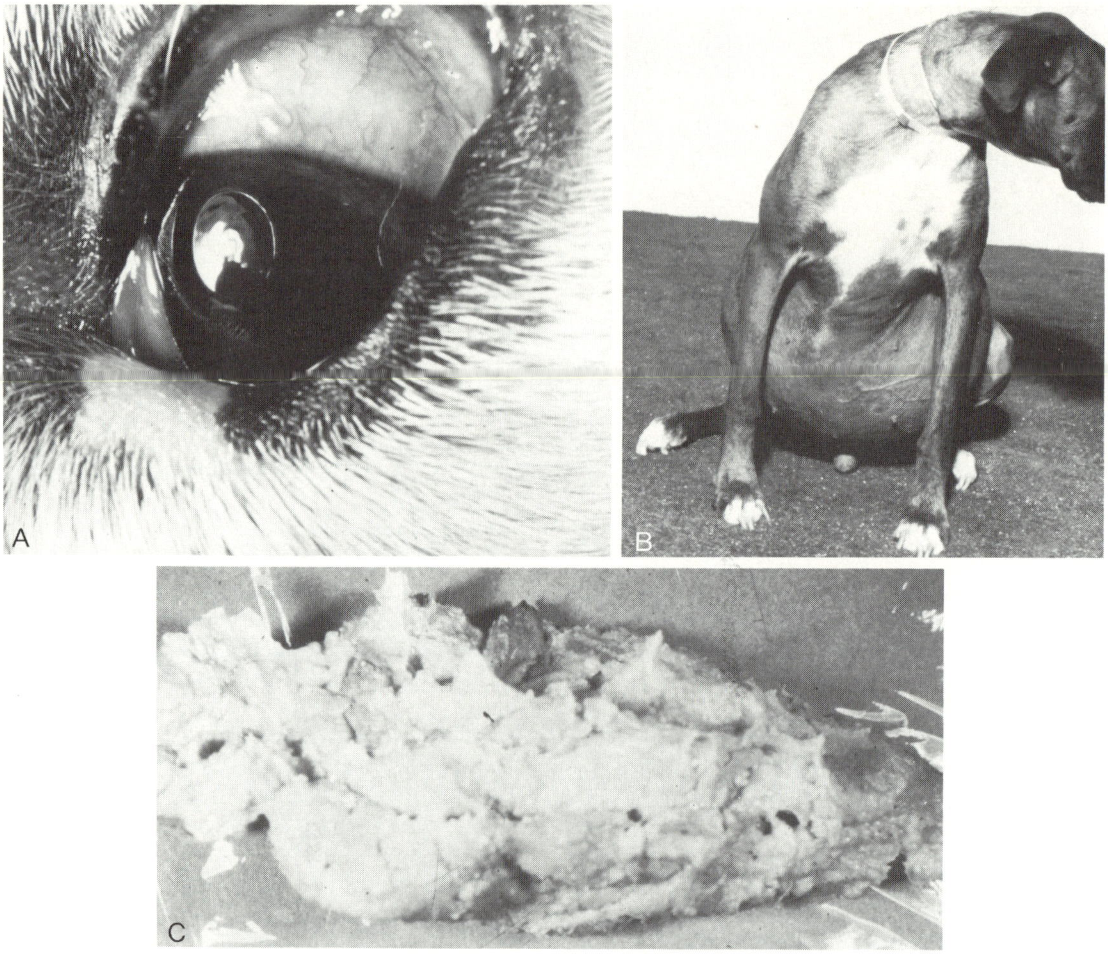

Figure 13–4. Common signs of liver disease in the dog and cat. *A*, Icterus. *B*, Ascites. *C*, Acholic feces, which are characteristic of patients with complete biliary obstruction.

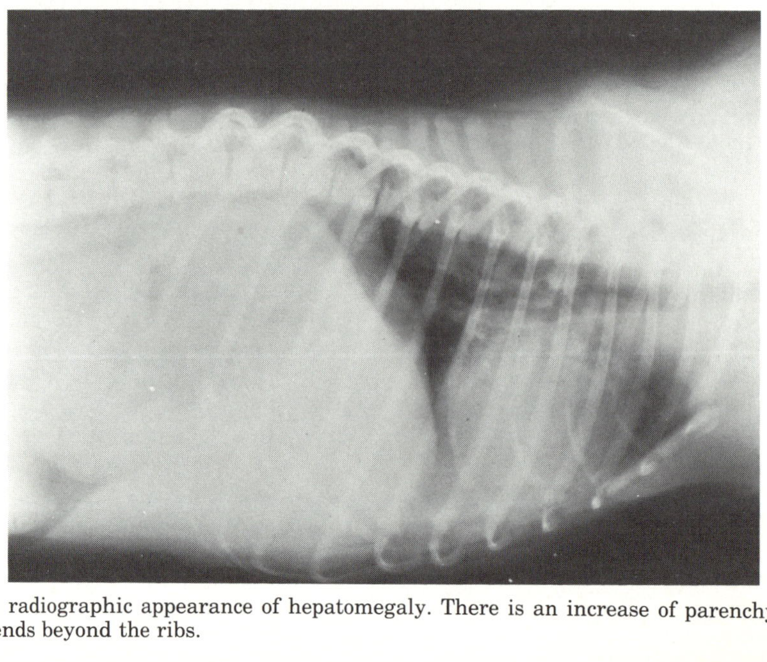

Figure 13–5. The radiographic appearance of hepatomegaly. There is an increase of parenchyma mass and the caudal border extends beyond the ribs.

bacteria, and the ammonia is subsequently absorbed into portal blood. If disease impairs the ability of the liver to process portal blood, the ammonia and other toxins gain access to the systemic circulation, where they precipitate neurological signs. The signs may abate as ammonia levels drop during fasting. Absence of this postprandial association in no way rules out hepatoencephalopathy. If portosystemic encephalopathy occurs in a young dog, the clinician should suspect a congenital vascular anomaly (e.g., portacaval shunt), whereas if it occurs in older dogs, cirrhosis is the more likely cause, since acquired portacaval shunting is common in cirrhosis. Neurological signs caused by liver failure should be differentiated from those caused by epilepsy, distemper encephalitis, lead poisoning, hydrocephalus, brain tumors, and other central nervous system diseases. Of assistance in the differential diagnosis is the history of worsening neurological disease after administration of anticonvulsants or sedatives, because these drugs enhance cerebral sensitivity in patients with PSE.

Most clinicians are familiar with the anterior uveitis and interstitial keratitis (blue eye) that are seen in infectious canine hepatitis or as a post-vaccination reaction. Anemia is also detected in some dogs with chronic hepatic disease.

Diagnostic Aids

Diagnostic procedures most easily available to the veterinary clinician include: determinations of serum enzyme activity (e.g, SGPT, SAP), serum levels of bile acid and total protein, blood glucose levels, and bilirubin levels; dye excretion tests; urinalysis; radiography; electrophoresis; and liver biopsy. These procedures are used to make a diagnosis, assess progression of liver disease, and evaluate the effectiveness of therapy. This section will concentrate on readily available, practical diagnostic aids. Newer techniques such as ultrasonography and liver scanning are promising diagnostic procedures for the future.[19]

Because the liver has many functions, no single liver function test or biochemical test is adequate for evaluating or detecting liver disease. Therefore, a liver profile consisting of a battery of tests is usually used to evaluate the liver. A minimal liver profile for the dog and cat should include serum enzyme determinations, measurements of bilirubin, glucose, total serum protein and albumin, and a urinalysis. A bromsulphalein (BSP) dye excretion test, total serum bile acid assay, or ammonium chloride tolerance test should be performed if liver disease is suspected and the profile yields negative results.

ENZYMES[105, 112]

Serum Glutamic Pyruvic Transaminase (SGPT)

SGPT, or serum alanine aminotransferase (SALT), activity is indicative of hepatocyte necrosis or increased cell membrane permeability in the dog, cat, and primate. Significant liver disease may be present even if SGPT activity is normal. The SGPT value is increased in cases of liver disease accompanied by hepatic necrosis or by increased hepatic cell membrane permeability caused by toxic insult, viral infection, inflammation, or severe lipidosis of the liver. SGPT levels increase markedly in dogs with biliary obstruction. Thus, it cannot be used to differentiate cholestatic liver disease from hepatitis. The degree of increased SGPT activity correlates not necessarily with the severity of hepatic disease, but rather with the amount of leakage of cell contents from the hepatocytes or the degree of necrosis. An increased SGPT value may persist for several days after hepatic injury.

Serum Glutamic Oxaloacetic Transaminase (SGOT)

The principles of serum glutamic oxaloacetic transaminase, or aspartate aminotransferase (SAST) activity are similar to those that apply to SGPT activity. However, the SGOT measurement is not as specific for liver dysfunction because other tissues contain enough GOT to cause increased SGOT activity when they are damaged. For instance, increased SGOT activity may occur in myositis, in which muscle GOT is released into the serum.

Serum Alkaline Phosphatase (SAP)

Alkaline phosphatase is present in many tissues, but increased serum alkaline phosphatase activity (SAP) is usually caused by liver disease in the dog.[98, 104, 143] SAP is bound to microsomes within hepatocytes, unlike GPT, which is soluble in cell cytoplasm.

Therefore, tissue necrosis does not release enough AP into the serum to significantly increase the SAP value. The SAP value is high when hepatocytes produce increased amounts of AP, such as occurs in cholestasis or with the induction of enzyme activity by drugs. Most notably, drug-induced increases in SAP occur with the administration of glucocorticoids, phenobarbital, primidone, and phenytoin.[29, 83, 97, 128] If there is no history of the use of these drugs, an increased SAP value is a reliable indicator of liver disease with cholestasis. Occasionally, bone diseases, such as osteosarcoma, or bone surgery can cause an increased SAP.[98] SAP activity is also higher in young dogs than in adults, because growing dogs have greater osteoblastic activity and thus release more bone AP into the blood.

Alkaline phosphatase isoenzyme determination may be of diagnostic value in selected cases.[54, 55] Isoenzyme detection requires a very proficient laboratory and the utmost care in laboratory techniques. Differentiation of the origin of the SAP increase (bone, liver, or drug-induced) may help to differentiate the presence of liver disease, bone disease, Cushing's disease, and iatrogenic hyperadrenocorticism.

Interpretation of increased SAP activity in the cat differs from that in the dog because the cat tends to have lower normal SAP values and a less pronounced increase in SAP values during cholestatic liver disease.[65] This difference may occur because of lower hepatic content of AP and shorter half-life of AP in the cat.[55] Therefore, increase in SAP activity should be considered clinically significant in the cat, and normal SAP values should not be considered to rule out cholestatic liver disease.[35, 56, 80]

Other Enzymes

Other enzyme tests less commonly used in assessing the condition of the liver include: the serum gamma glutamyl transpeptidase (SGGT), serum arginase, sorbitol dehydrogenase (SDH), and lactate dehydrogenase (LDH) test. SGGT is not liver specific, but its activity in serum is increased in cholestatic liver disease.[16, 111, 115] Like high SGPT values, a high serum arginase value indicates active necrosis or increased cell membrane permeability.[86] Serum arginase activity decreases more rapidly than SGPT activity. Thus, a high SGPT value and a concommitant normal serum arginase value may indicate that previous necrosis has subsided.

LDH determination can be substituted for the SGPT test. The LDH is not specific for liver disease, and isoenzyme determination must accompany LDH measurement to pinpoint liver disease.

BROMSULPHALEIN (BSP) DYE EXCRETION TEST[24]

The BSP dye excretion test is a very effective means of detecting hepatic disease. The test is performed by administering BSP dye* intravenously (5 mg/kg) and measuring its concentration or calculated percentage retention in plasma collected 30 minutes after the injection (normal is less than 5 per cent retention). Normal enzyme activity does not preclude the presence of liver disease, and BSP dye retention will often be increased even if enzyme activity is not. BSP is taken up by hepatocytes, conjugated, and excreted into the bile like bilirubin. One difference is that bilirubin is conjugated mainly with glucuronic acid, whereas BSP is conjugated with glutathione.

Hyperbilirubinemia interferes with BSP excretion, potentially altering BSP dye excretion values. More importantly, little is learned by doing a BSP dye excretion test in an icteric dog or cat, since the excretion of dye will be predictably impaired. Although it is an uncommon occurrence, BSP excretion can be normal in the presence of hepatic disease. BSP excretion is enhanced by feeding, exercise, certain enzyme-inducing drugs, and hypoalbuminemia.[46] Fever and decreased blood flow in the hypovolemic patient may delay BSP excretion. Otherwise, decreased ability to excrete BSP indicates liver disease. Other dye excretion tests offer few advantages over the BSP excretion test. ICG† (indocyanine green) differs from BSP in that it is not conjugated for excretion. Thus, a combination of BSP and ICG could be used to differentiate lesions involving the conjugation step from those that do not. However, ICG is quite expensive and therefore has not attained widespread clinical acceptance.

---

*Bromsulphalein, Hynson, Westcott & Dunning, Baltimore, MD.

†Cardio-Green, Hynson, Westcott & Dunning, Baltimore, MD.

SERUM BILE ACID

Total serum bile acid determination is a new and useful test for liver disease in the dog.[60] It has the advantage over the BSP dye excretion test of not requiring administration of an exogenous test substance. Rather, a serum sample taken after an 18-to-24 hour fast is submitted for bile acid assay.

The basis for the test is that peripheral blood contains low levels of bile acids (0 to 6 μM/l), and portal blood has very high levels (42 to 60 μM/l).[60] This difference in concentrations is caused by the very efficient extraction of bile acids from the portal blood by the liver. Therefore, whenever the liver fails to process portal blood normally or when portosystemic shunting occurs, peripheral blood bile acid levels rise precipitously.

Total serum bile acid (fasting) concentrations are consistently increased in dogs with cirrhosis, hepatitis, hepatic neoplasia, and portacaval shunts.[60] Values are also increased in most dogs with glucocorticoid-induced hepatopathy and biliary obstruction, although overlap with normal values occurs.[60] The degree of bile acid increase correlates with the severity of liver disease as judged by biopsy.[60]

Future studies of postprandial serum bile acid levels or fractionation of individual bile acids (e.g., cholic acid versus chenodeoxycholic acid) will probably demonstrate further diagnostic or prognostic uses.

AMMONIA AND AMMONIA TOLERANCE TEST

When disease impairs the ability of the liver to process ammonia (urea cycle) or when there is profound shunting of blood, the fasting blood ammonia content may rise. However, some patients with significant liver disease have normal fasting blood ammonia values (<50 μg/dl).[119] In these patients, the impairment may be detected by the ammonia tolerance test. This test is performed by measuring the blood ammonia content before and after giving ammonium chloride orally or by enema.[12, 30, 84] The laboratory should be consulted in advance to obtain instructions concerning specimen collection and handling. In the author's opinion, the bile acid assay can usually be substituted for blood ammonia testing.

MEASUREMENT OF SERUM AND PLASMA PROTEINS

Measurement of serum (or plasma) proteins is helpful in the evaluation of hepatic disease.[24] The plasma content of all proteins normally produced by the liver may decrease in hepatic failure. Most commonly, hypoalbuminemia is associated with hepatic failure due to impaired albumin synthesis. Dilutional hypoalbuminemia can also occur if the patient tends to retain water. Hypoalbuminemia seen in chronic or diffuse liver disease is often associated with an increased globulin value, i.e., a decreased albumin-globulin ratio. Protein electrophoresis reveals changes in plasma protein content, but these changes are not specific for liver disease.

Other proteins that may be easily evaluated include prothrombin and fibrinogen. In liver failure, production of clotting factors may be decreased.[20] Hypoprothrombinemia may be detected by a prolonged prothrombin time.[6] The activated clotting time (ACT) can be used clinically to screen for clotting disorders in dogs with liver disease.[18] Plasma fibrinogen content (normal 100 to 500 mg/dl) may be increased in inflammatory diseases or may be decreased in hepatic failure. Fibrinogen content may change in many other disorders besides liver disease. Thus fibrinogen levels are very nonspecific.

BLOOD GLUCOSE

Blood glucose levels may decrease in hepatic failure because hepatic glycogen, which is needed to maintain blood glucose content, is depleted. Hypoglycemia may also be caused by depressed gluconeogenesis that may occur in endotoxemia.[72] Poorly defined hypoglycemic diseases in which enzyme deficiency impairs release of glycogen from the liver (so-called glycogen storage diseases) have been detected in dogs. Tumor-associated hypoglycemia also occurs in patients with hepatoma.[104]

BILIRUBIN AND BILE PIGMENTS

Although evaluation of bile pigments may be helpful in the icteric patient, bile pigment assays are usually more helpful in patients who are not icteric. Figure 13–6 outlines the normal bilirubin metabolism. Many dogs and cats with liver disease have im-

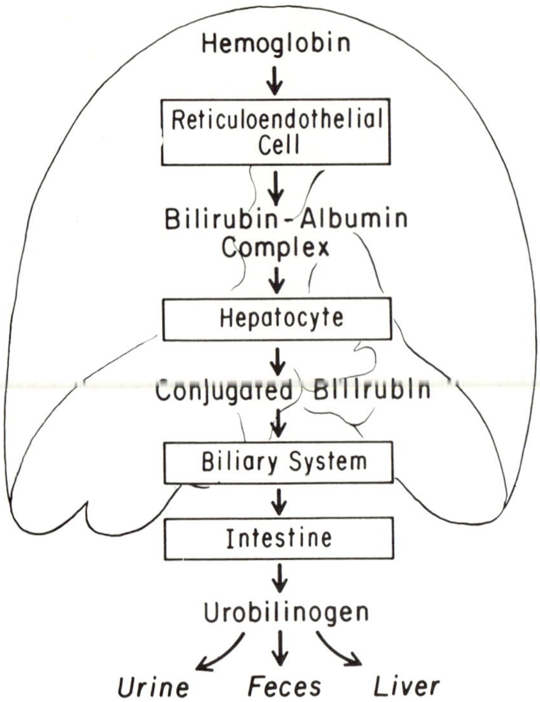

Figure 13–6. Bile pigment metabolism from its formation from heme to its conversion to various metabolites in the intestine. (Reprinted with permission from Strombeck DR: *Small Animal Gastroenterology*. Davis, CA, Stonegate Publishing, 1983.)

paired bilirubin metabolism but do not have high enough serum bilirubin values to cause icterus. In the dog, there is a low threshold for urinary excretion of bilirubin, and the possibility of high bilirubin levels without icterus is very important.[87] In the dog, it is not unusual to have severe liver failure, absence of icterus, and a normal total serum bilirubin value. However, in an animal with these signs, the result of the urine bilirubin determination is strongly positive for bilirubin. The high rate of urinary bilirubin excretion keeps the serum bilirubin content low. The process of bilirubin excretion is better developed in the male dog than in the female. Icterus is usually detected in dogs with severe, generalized, acute liver disease or as a late manifestation of chronic hepatic failure.

Significant bilirubinuria (bilirubin level = ++, urine specific gravity = 1.015 to 1.035) suggests that liver disease is present and is an indication that further investigation is necessary. Normal dogs do have some bilirubin in their urine because of their low renal threshold, but strong positive test results are significant. Conversely, low urine bilirubin values or an absence of bilirubinuria is unusual in dogs with liver failure.[91]

Cats do not normally have positive urine bilirubin test results. Therefore, any animal with positive bilirubin results on urinalysis should be evaluated for liver disease.[91]

The urobilinogen content of the urine can be used to evaluate patency of the biliary system. Absence of urobilinogenuria may occur in the normal dog but is unusual in dogs with hepatic failure unless complete biliary obstruction is present. If biliary obstruction is total, no urobilinogen is present in the urine. Bilirubin does not reach the gut and, therefore, is not acted upon by the intestinal bacteria that convert bilirubin to urobilinogen. Thus, the detection of urobilinogen in the urine of dogs and cats with liver disease implies that complete biliary obstruction is not present. Conversely, absence of urine urobilinogen suggests that complete bilirubin obstruction is present when other liver function tests indicate hepatic failure or when the patient is jaundiced. Important clinical decisions should not be based solely on urobilinogen measurements, since many variables, such as urine pH, urine concentration, and the amount of urobilinogen breakdown by ultraviolet light, may affect the urobilinogen value.[119]

In addition to abnormal pigment content, urinalysis may reveal ammonium biurate crystals in urine from patients with liver failure (see Fig. 13–16).[77] The presence of these crystals is usually an indication of hyperammonemia. Further testing of liver function is necessary when crystals are detected in patients without known liver disease.

The total serum bilirubin content is valuable in detecting liver disease.[87] It may be significantly increased (>0.6 mg/dl in dogs or >0.3 mg/dl in cats) without causing jaundice, thus providing evidence of hepatic disease. The serum bilirubin can be further analyzed chemically to yield indirect (unconjugated) and direct (conjugated) reacting bilirubin (van den Bergh's test). Bilirubin that has been acted upon by the liver to make it more soluble for excretion is called conjugated or direct reacting bilirubin. Unconjugated or indirect reacting bilirubin has not been made soluble for excretion by the liver. In hemolytic jaundice, greater than 80 per cent of the total bilirubin is usually indirect reacting (bilirubin that has not been conjugated by the liver). In extrahepatic obstructive jaundice, such as occurs when a mass lesion obstructs the bile duct, the total bilirubin is almost all direct reacting (bilirubin that has been conjugated by the liver). In intrahepatic cholestasis there is an approximately 50 to 50 ratio of conjugated to unconjugated bilirubin. Since there are more helpful tests for determining the cause of jaundice, the van den Bergh test is of limited value. Also, the ratio of direct reacting to indirect reacting bilirubin may change as the disease progresses, making interpretation of test results difficult.

LIVER BIOPSY, LAPAROSCOPY, AND LAPAROTOMY

Liver biopsy is one of the most important tools available for the diagnosis of liver disease.[15, 18, 38, 69, 108] Other diagnostic aids, such as serum enzymes or BSP dye excretion tests, provide evidence for the presence of hepatic disease, but usually a biopsy is needed to make a definite diagnosis. A liver biopsy specimen can be obtained by the blind percutaneous puncture, by the keyhole technique, by laparoscopic examination, or by direct guidance of the biopsy instrument via laparotomy.[69] When available, ultrasound scanning can be used to direct the biopsy needle into the liver. The author recommends the use of the Menghini needle for obtaining liver biopsy specimens in all methods (Fig. 13–7). The Menghini needle is a thin-walled needle with a 45° bevel and a cutting edge that makes up the entire circumference of the tip. Suction is applied to the needle with a saline-filled 6- or 12-ml syringe, and the needle is rapidly plunged into and out of the liver, cutting a core of liver tissue that remains in the needle shaft. The specimen is then expelled into formalin by pushing saline through the needle with the syringe. The author feels strongly that the Menghini needle is superior to the Vim-Silverman and Tru-cut needles for obtaining liver specimens because it is used at a higher speed and makes a smaller puncture.

The indications and contraindications for liver biopsy are listed in Table 13–3. One should not delay in obtaining a liver biopsy specimen when a definitive diagnosis is needed to plan therapy. However, a biopsy should not be performed unless the clinician is confident of the safety of the technique. Generally, the author prefers the percutaneous Menghini needle technique using local anesthesia because it is safe and inexpensive, and there is a high rate of client compliance. When done with local anesthesia, laparoscopy is superior to percutaneous Menghini needle because it has the tremendous advantage of visual inspection

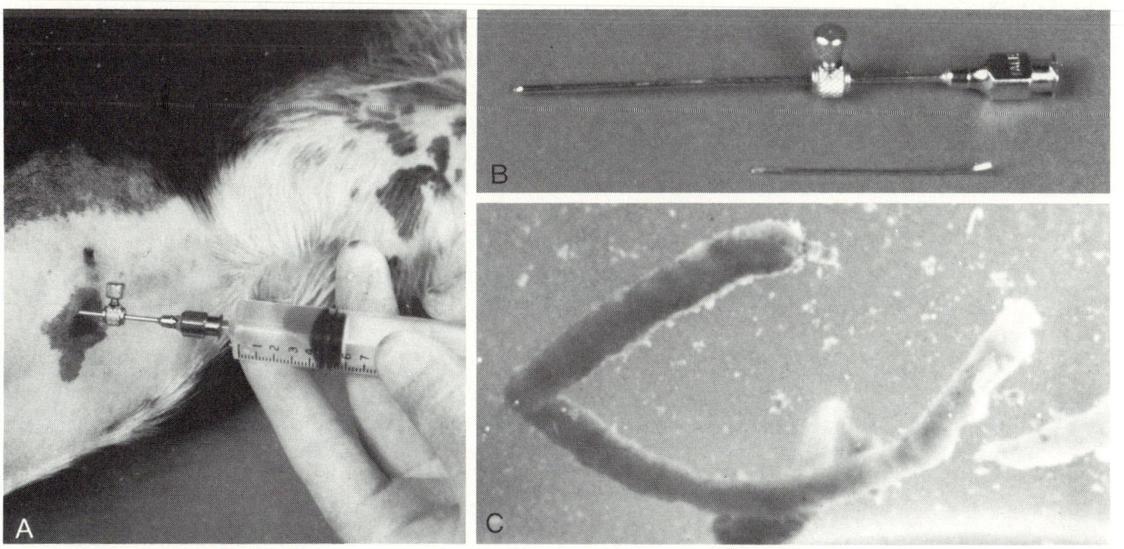

Figure 13–7. *A*, Menghini needle biopsy of a dog's liver is a percutaneous technique. The dog lies on his right side, and the needle is inserted behind the last rib and to the left of the xiphoid cartilage. The procedure is performed under local anesthesia. Practice is needed to perform this technique safely. *B*, The Menghini needle. A blocking pin *(beside the needle)* keeps the specimen within the needle shaft, and a "stop" on the needle shaft can be adjusted to limit the depth of the puncture. *C*, The biopsy specimen obtained by Menghini needle aspiration biopsy.

Table 13–3. INDICATIONS AND CONTRAINDICATIONS FOR PERCUTANEOUS LIVER BIOPSY

Indications	Abnormal laboratory values indicating hepatic disease
	Enzymes
	BSP dye excretion
	Abnormal liver size
	Heptomegaly
	Microhepatica
	Assessment of progression of hepatic disease
	Evaluation of response to therapy
	Detection of cause of ascites
	Evaluation of hepatic involvement in systemic disease
	Hepatodynia
Contraindications	Lack of operator confidence
	Microhepatica
	Inexperienced operator
	Uncooperative patient
	Bleeding disorder
	Marked anemia
	Extrahepatic cholestasis
	Infection along biopsy pathway
	Hepatic abscess
	Ascites
	Pleuritis
	Hepatic cyst
	Vascular tumor

of the liver and of directing the biopsy instrument. Laparoscopy is quite safe and accurate. The use of heavy sedation or general anesthesia should be avoided in patients with serious liver disease. The advantage of the keyhole technique is that it enables the clinician to direct the needle into the liver by finger palpation; however, the disadvantages of the technique are that it causes greater trauma (invasive), it takes longer to perform, and there is frequent need for sedation. These disadvantages outweigh the advantages of the keyhole technique over the percutaneous Menghini needle technique. The laparotomy offers little advantage over other techniques and is not generally indicated for the sole purpose of obtaining a liver specimen.

The prebiopsy preparation should include an evaluation of clotting ability and radiographic evaluation of liver size. Minimal clotting tests should include a platelet count and bleeding time. Activated clotting time is an additional valuable screening test.[18] A complete clotting profile (prothrombin time, activated partial thromboplastin time, platelet count) may be advisable in some cases. It is also advisable to fast the dog and to give it a small, fatty meal (e.g., corn oil) 30 minutes prior to biopsy, in order to empty the gall bladder.

Postbiopsy care should include observation for anemia and abdominal pain for 2 to 4 hours. Marked abdominal pain may indicate bile peritonitis, a serious complication that usually requires surgical intervention.

Analysis of the biopsy specimen requires evaluation of the sections by an experienced examiner. The findings must be correlated with the clinical data. The detection of pathological alterations in a biopsy specimen requires knowledge of the normal hepatic appearance, and an understanding of the nonspecific histological changes that are commonly encountered in nonhepatic disorders and are of little clinical importance (Fig. 13–8).[134]

Specific Liver Diseases

The most commonly encountered hepatopathies, rather than all of the diseases that may affect the liver, will be discussed.

CHRONIC ACTIVE LIVER DISEASE

Inflammatory diseases of the liver of unknown etiology occur in dogs and cats; however, little is known about them. They will receive more attention and recognition in the future as liver biopsy becomes more commonplace.

Chronic active liver disease (CALD), an inflammatory disease of the liver, has been described in the dog.[28, 32, 84, 121, 126] It has various causes including drug reaction, viral infection, and leptospirosis.[11, 42, 43] Immunological injury is probably a feature in all cases. Other causes will probably be discovered. Infection by the canine hepatitis virus in partially immune dogs may persist as CALD.[42, 43]

CALD often is undetected in the early stages because the dogs frequently are asymptomatic. A chronic stage of the disease, with a wide range of clinical signs such as vague illness, jaundice, ascites, and portosystemic encephalopathy, follows. Often, the client reports that the signs wax and wane. CALD is more common in the female than the male dog and may occur at any age.[28, 62, 121]

Laboratory testing usually reveals increased SGPT level and BSP dye retention. The SAP level may also be increased. Di-

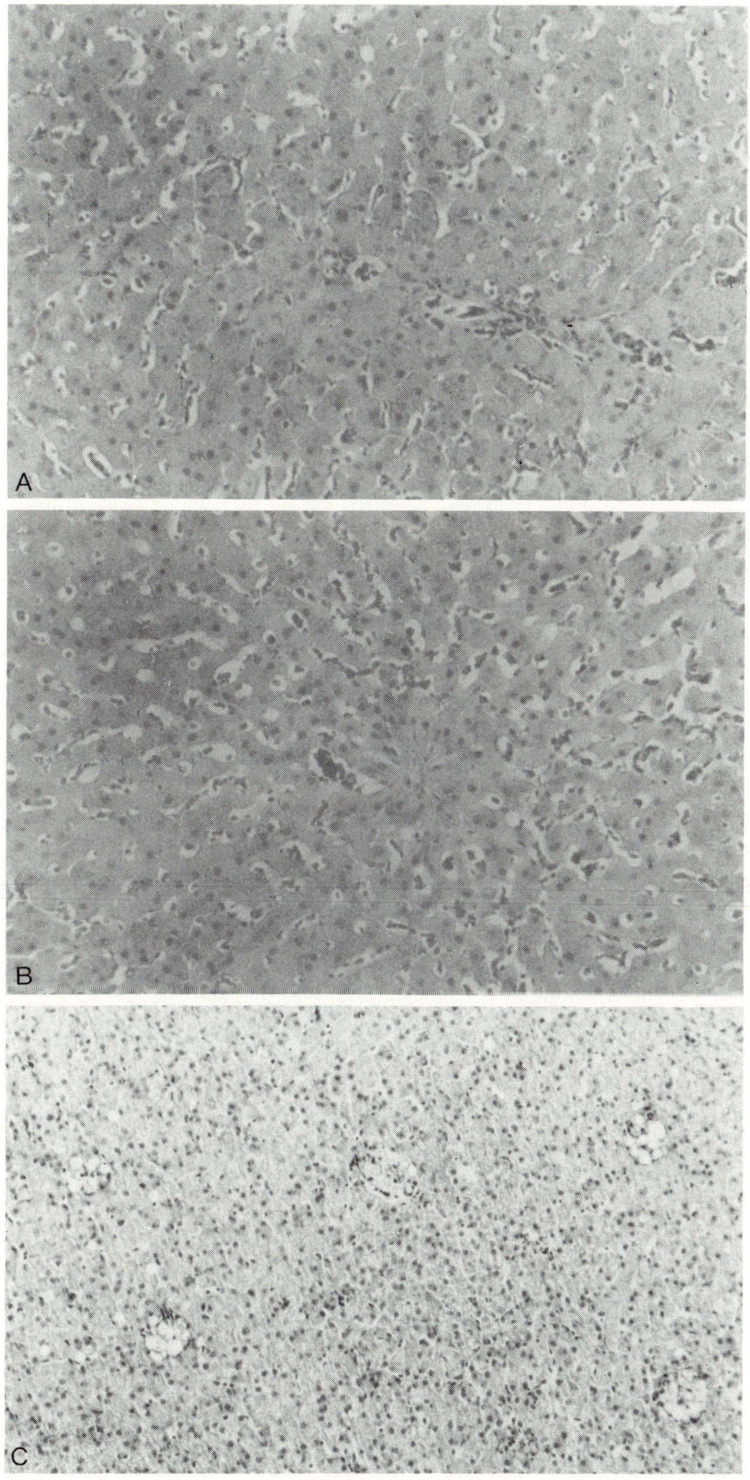

Figure 13–8. Histologic appearance of a normal liver biopsy specimen stained by hematoxylin and eosin; *A*, Centroacinar (periportal) region. *B*, Pericentral area (H&E, ×42). *C*, A liver biopsy specimen such as occurs in reactive hepatitis showing focal necrosis and mild increase in mononuclear cell population. These nonspecific lesions are common in dogs and cats with extrahepatic diseases, such as acute pancreatitis, uremia, and infections (H&E, ×16).

agnosis is based on biopsy findings and a history of chronicity, usually of longer than 2 months.

On histological examination, periportal infiltration of inflammatory cells, primarily mononuclear cells, is detected. This infiltrate extends into the adjacent parenchyma where it is gradually surrounded by small groups of hepatocytes, eventually causing cell death. This process is called piecemeal necrosis (Fig. 13–9). A variable degree of fibrosis accompanies the damage caused by inflammation and piecemeal necrosis. The necrosis accounts for the increased SGPT level. As the lesion becomes more severe, it causes cholestasis and an increased SAP level.

If chronic active liver disease is allowed to progress, it results in portal cirrhosis. Prior to this stage, CALD may be severe enough to cause ascites, icterus, or PSE.

The possibility that CALD is present in asymptomatic dogs with increased SGPT activity and the dire consequence of progression to cirrhosis are justifications for early liver biopsy in patients with chronic asymptomatic hepatitis.

Personal experience and empirical evidence suggest that prednisolone or prednisone therapy is effective in controlling or curing CALD.[121] Dosages of 0.5 to 1 mg/kg given daily may be used. If prednisolone alone is ineffective, azathioprine* may be added to the regime at a dosage of 1 mg/kg per day. In addition to these drugs, good supportive care (nutrition, avoidance of stress) and control of PSE, if present, are indicated. Therapy should be monitored by appropriate laboratory data or by serial biopsies to ensure resolution of the hepatitis.

*Imuran, Burroughs Wellcome Co, Research Triangle Park, NC.

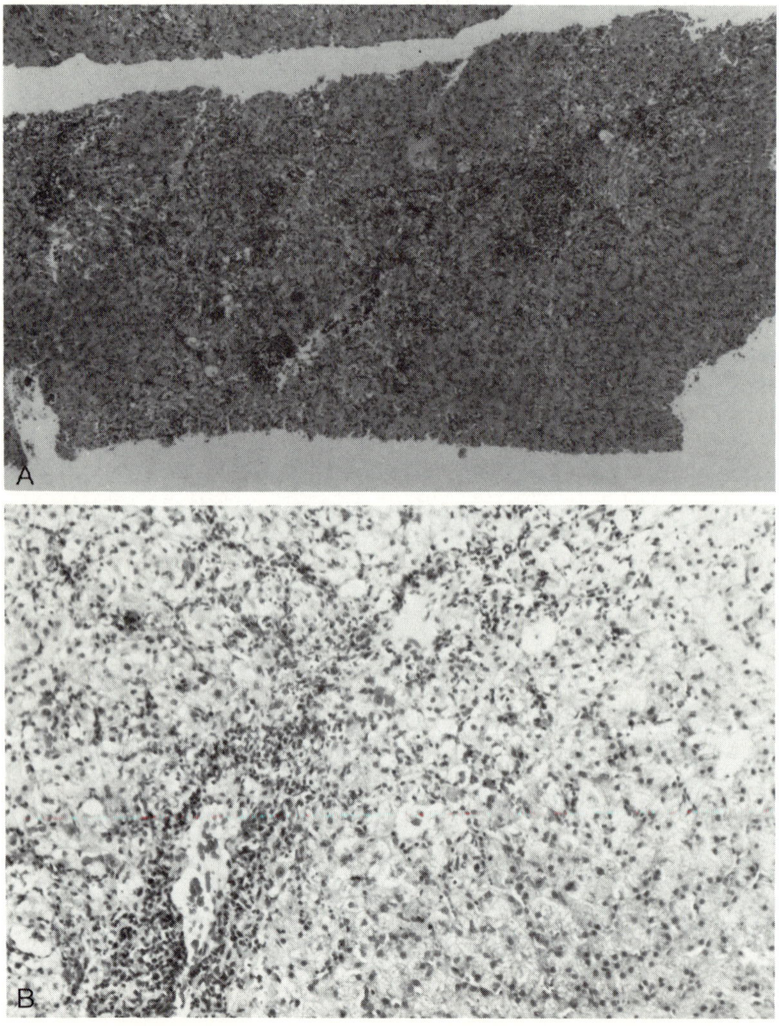

Figure 13–9. Histological appearance of chronic active liver disease (CALD) in the dog. *A*, Periportal inflammation by mononuclear cells. *B*, Extension of the inflammation into adjacent parenchyma tissue causing piecemeal necrosis (H&E, ×42).

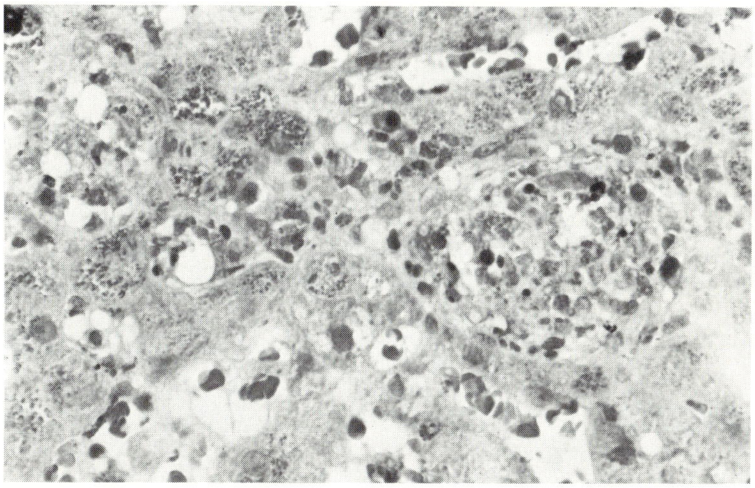

Figure 13–10. A biopsy specimen from a Doberman pinscher with a form of chronic active liver disease peculiar to the breed (H&E, ×42).

Chronic active liver disease has been described in female Doberman pinschers as a disease entity peculiar to those animals.[62] Doberman pinschers with CALD that the author has observed have had peculiar intracytoplasmic granules (Fig. 13–10).

PYOGRANULOMATOUS HEPATITIS

Another inflammatory disease that occurs in the dog but has not been well described is pyogranulomatous hepatitis.[119] As with CALD, the cause of this disease is unknown. The degree of liver failure is usually pronounced, causing signs that are associated with failure (ascites, icterus, and PSE). In making a diagnosis, infections such as histoplasmosis, blastomycosis, and others that cause granulomatous inflammation should be ruled out. Therapy should consist of immunosuppression with steroids such as prednisone (2 mg/kg, initial dose). A biopsy specimen demonstrating the typical granulomatous inflammation is required for diagnosis (Fig. 13–11).

FELINE CHOLANGIOHEPATITIS

Cholangiohepatitis is a disease of unknown etiology that affects adult domestic cats of all ages, breeds, and sexes. The cats are usually anorexic, depressed, and icteric, although some cats are anicteric throughout the course of illness. Clinical signs may be either acute or chronic and commonly may wax and wane.

Laboratory testing reveals increased SAP levels, total bilirubin concentration, and BSP dye retention. The SGPT level is variably increased. Cats with prolonged illness are often moderately anemic. Toxoplasmosis and feline infectious peritonitis (FIP) may

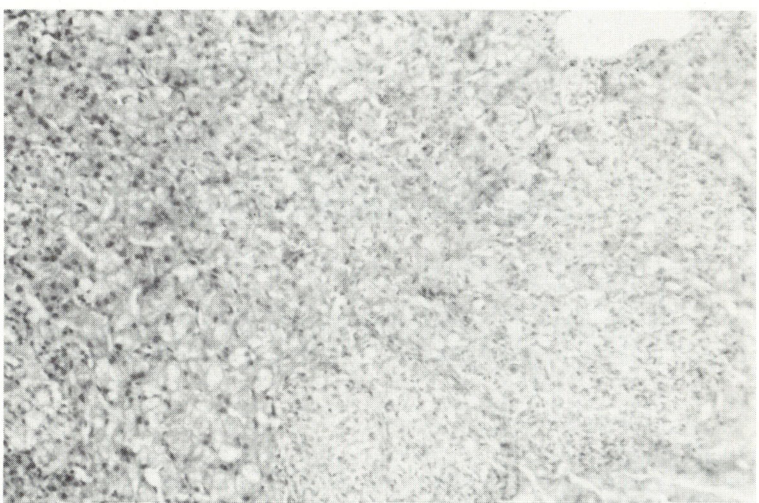

Figure 13–11. Pyogranulomatous hepatitis in the dog. Severe hepatitis with extensive pyogranulomatous inflammation of the hepatic parenchyma (H&E, ×39).

cause similar clinical signs and should be included in the differential diagnosis.[90, 114] An associated pancreatitis has been described, thus a serum amylase test may also be indicated.[62]

The liver is icteric and moderately enlarged; the gall bladder and biliary tree are dilated and thickened. Biopsy of the liver reveals nonspecific inflammation of the bile ductules and adjacent parenchyma. Cultures of the bile and biliary tree are usually negative. The biliary tree is usually clogged with thick, inspissated bile that is causing the obstruction. This "sludged bile" probably forms secondary to cholangiohepatitis (personal speculation).

Specific treatment for feline cholangiohepatitis is unknown. In some cases, surgical relief of the biliary obstruction is effective. The gall bladder and common bile duct should be flushed to remove inspissated bile. However, the proximal biliary tree may also be clogged, and removal of sludged bile from the gall bladder and common duct will not result in bile flow in such cases. Furthermore, the stress of laparotomy and biliary surgery may not be well tolerated by the cat. Complications from biliary surgery, especially leakage of bile with bile peritonitis, are potential hazards.

Several antibiotics such as ampicillin and chloramphenicol are secreted into the bile by healthy patients. However, it is unlikely that they are secreted into the bile when the biliary tree is diseased as in cholangiohepatitis.[5] Antibiotics are indicated to protect the cat from systemic infections, rather than as specific therapy for cholangiohepatitis.

Cholerectics (bile salts) were once recommended for cholestatic disorders to stimulate flow of watery bile. However, bile salts are choleretic only in the healthy patient and probably have no effect on the diseased liver.

Since cholangiohepatitis does not appear to be an infectious disease, a trial of glucocorticoids seems rational, and some cats seem to benefit from this treatment (empirical evidence). The clinician may try steroids prior to an attempt at surgical correction, to avoid the potential complications of surgery.

LIVER DISEASE OF THE BEDLINGTON TERRIER

An inherited form of liver disease characterized by the accumulation of copper in the lysosomes, inflammation resembling CALD, and a progressive course leading to cirrhosis has been described in Bedlington terriers.[50, 52, 61, 75, 118, 136] The disease appears to be quite common in this breed, and it affects both sexes and all ages. The dogs have variable clinical signs; some animals are asymptomatic, and others have signs of liver failure.

Liver profiles usually reveal an increased SGPT value, although normal SGPT results do not rule out the disorder. Later in the disease, the results of the SAP test and other tests of liver disease are abnormal.

Definitive diagnosis requires liver biopsy and histological demonstration of characteristic copper-containing intracytoplasmic granules (Fig. 13–12). Measurement of liver copper content may also be advisable in some cases. The liver copper content of affected dogs is 5 to 50 times greater than that of a normal dog (mongrel) liver (91 to 377 μg/gm).

Early diagnosis is very important in order to prevent liver failure and cirrhosis. D-penicillamine* (125 to 250 mg) given 30 minutes before meals may control the disease. The whole dose may be given at once or it may be divided and given two or three times a day if vomiting is a problem. If the disease is left untreated, there is usually a progression from focal necrosis to chronic active hepatitis and finally to cirrhosis. Feeding diets with lower copper content (noncommercial dog food) and enhancing urinary copper excretion with oral ascorbic acid (500 to 1000 mg/day) may help to reduce liver copper levels.[50]

Further investigation of this syndrome, including its genetic transmission, is needed.[61] Prevention by routine testing and selective breeding of Bedlington terriers will be needed to rid the breed of this insidious disease.

CIRRHOSIS

Cirrhosis is a chronic disease of the liver in which diffuse destruction and regeneration of hepatic parenchymal cells have occurred and in which diffuse increase in connective tissue has resulted in disorganization of the lobular architecture. (Fig. 13–13).[23] Various classification schemes have been proposed to describe types of cirrhosis, and these have been universally

*Cuprimine, Merck Sharp & Dohme, West Point, PA.

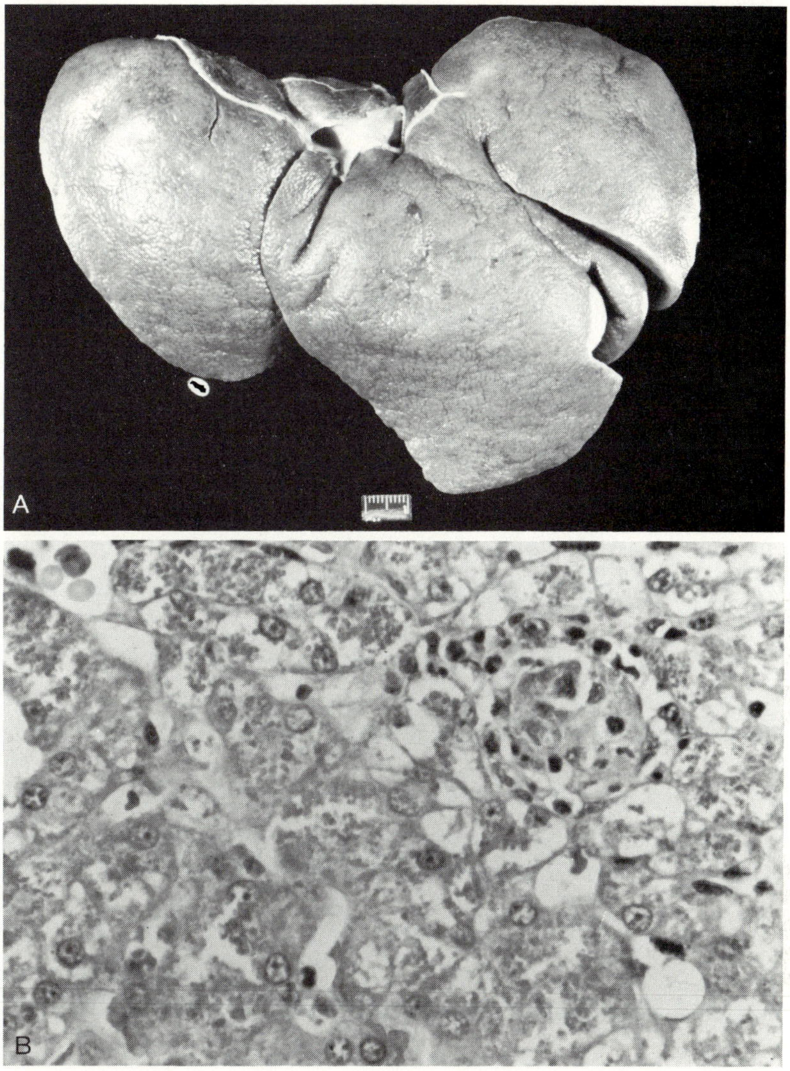

Figure 13–12. The liver from a Bedlington terrier with a form of liver disease peculiar to the breed. *A*, The liver is swollen and more tan than normal. *B*, Focal necrosis and characteristic intracytoplasmic granules (H&E, ×104).

adopted for the dog. However, the following descriptions are useful. In portal cirrhosis, the connective tissue appears to emanate from portal areas toward central areas. In postnecrotic cirrhosis, there is extensive deposition of connective tissue with disorganization of normal architecture. Fibrosis and disorganization occur secondary to lobular collapse that is caused by extensive necrosis. Postnecrotic cirrhosis may be a sequel to severe toxic or viral hepatitis. Biliary cirrhosis is caused by chronic biliary obstruction (secondary biliary cirrhosis). There is marked bile stasis with bile plugs and proliferation of interlobar bile ducts within the scarred portal areas. Associated with scarring, biliary hyperplasia, and bile stasis is nonspecific inflammation of the portal areas. Cardiac cirrhosis results from chronic passive congestion of the liver, which is caused by congestive heart failure. This type of cirrhosis is uncommon, probably because dogs and cats do not live long enough to acquire it. Fibrosis begins centrally and may join adjacent central areas while sparing the portal regions. The pattern of fibrosis in cardiac cirrhosis is the reverse of that in portal cirrhosis.

Cirrhosis usually occurs in an older animal, although younger animals may be affected.[133] When cardiac cirrhosis is detected clinically, the liver is usually shrunken, and difficult to palpate and it appears small on radiographs, although this sign may not be present early in cirrhosis. Early in cirrhosis, severe lipidosis may cause increased liver size.

The dog or cat is depressed and usually has gastrointestinal upsets, e.g., vomiting and diarrhea. Jaundice may be present, and in the nonicteric animal, hyperbilirubinuria usually occurs. The animal may also exhibit

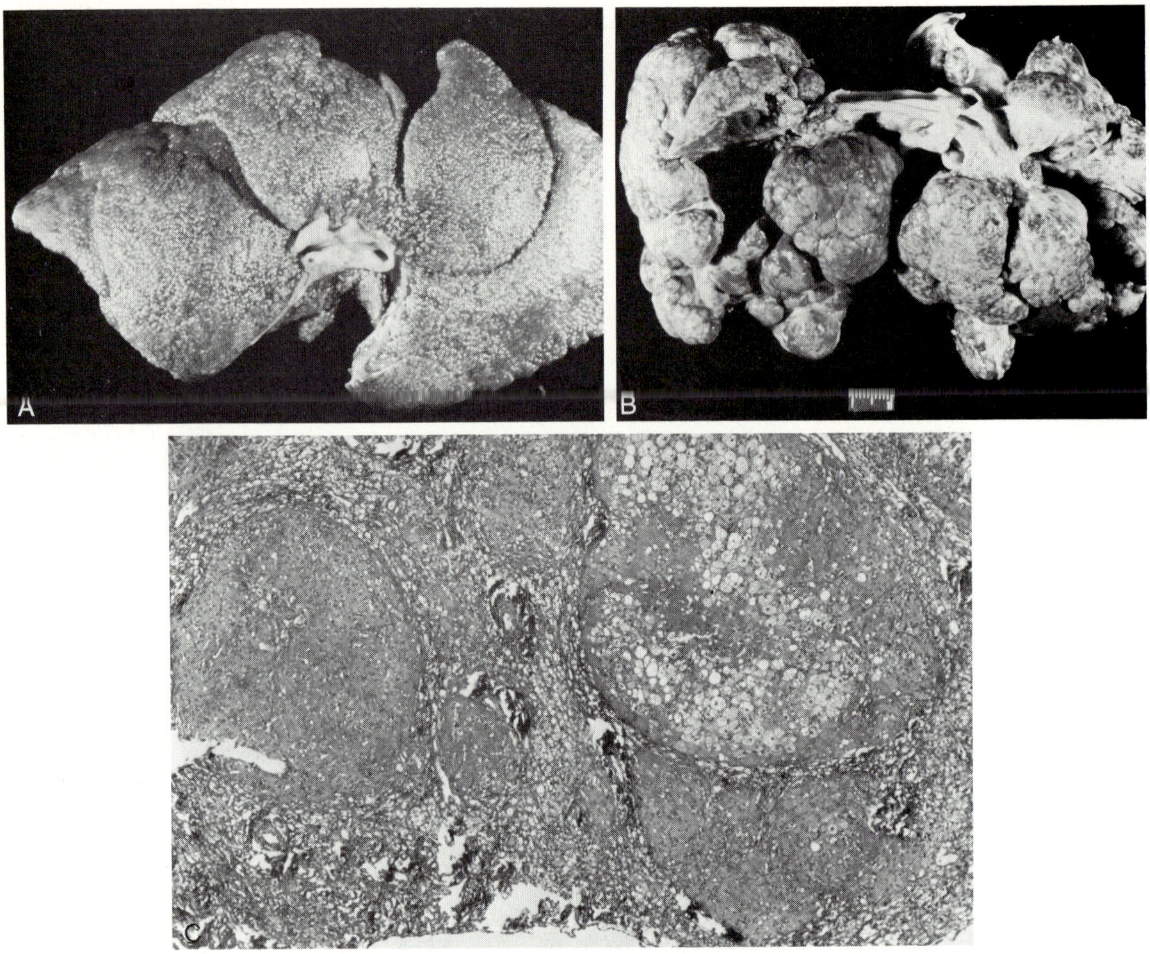

Figure 13–13. The gross appearance of cirrhosis in the dog. *A*, Micronodular. *B*, Macronodular. *C*, Histological appearance of cirrhosis in the dog, demonstrating nodule formation and marked fibrosis with destruction of normal architecture of the liver.

signs of portosystemic encephalopathy. Laboratory data often reveal a high SAP level, a normal or an increased SGPT level, a marked increase in BSP dye retention, or an increase in total serum bile acid content. The diagnosis is confirmed by biopsy.

The causes of postnecrotic and portal cirrhosis include viral infections, toxins, drug reactions, malnutrition, chronic biliary obstruction, and CALD. However, once cirrhosis is diagnosed, the cause is usually difficult to determine, and therapy is usually supportive. New drugs that may reduce the collagen content of the liver, such as colchicine, offer some hope for future therapy.[64]

DRUG-INDUCED HEPATOPATHIES

Although many drugs (toxins) can cause hepatic disease,[76] this discussion concerns those that are of clinical importance.

The most common hepatopathy is the steroid hepatopathy induced by glucocorticoid administration to dogs.[27, 131] This type of hepatopathy occurs in many dogs given steroids in routine doses for pruritus or lameness, as well as in shock doses. Steroid hepatopathy is characterized by hepatomegaly, by increased SAP and SGPT levels, and in some cases, by BSP dye retention (Table 13–4, Fig. 13–5).[97] A morphological lesion, consisting of hepatocyte ballooning and mild necrosis, also occurs (Fig. 13–14). This ballooning degeneration apparently is a hydropic change. The lesion is also present in hyperadrenocorticism (Cushing's disease). The lesion is reversible upon withdrawal of steroid therapy or treatment of hyperadrenocorticism. The effect on the liver of long-term steroid administration is unknown. The knowledge that steroid hepatopathy occurs in the dog is clinically

Table 13–4. LABORATORY FINDINGS IN DOGS WITH STEROID-INDUCED HEPATOPATHY*

Factor	No. of Dogs Evaluated	No. (%) of Dogs Affected	Abnormal Values *Median*	Abnormal Values *Range*
Increased SGPT activity (>55 IU/L)	18	13 (72)	168	79–2,238
Increased SAP activity (>123 IU/L)	17	16 (94)	1,140	238–3,235
Increased SGGT activity (>6 IU/L)	8	6 (75)	35	6–191
Increased BSP retention (>5% in 30 min)	15	11 (73)	11	6–43
Increased resting blood ammonia (>180 mg/dl)	7	0 (0)	—	—
Hepatomegaly†	20	11 (55)	—	—
Presence of additional hepatic lesions	22	5 (23)	—	—
Polydipsia and polyuria‡	11	7 (64)	—	—

*From Rogers WA, Ruebner BH: A retrospective study of probably glucocorticoid-induced hepatopathy in dogs. J Am Vet Med Assoc 170:603, 1977.
†Hepatomegaly was detected by palpation or radiography or at necropsy.
‡Polydipsia and polyuria were considered to be present, according to the client's descriptions.

important. Steroids should be used sparingly. Increased values for SAP and SGPT tests should be correctly interpreted; the presence of steroid hepatopathy should be considered in order to avoid unnecessary treatments or expense (e.g., liver biopsy). Finally, the detection of steroid hepatopathy without a history of steroid administration is an indication of hyperadrenocorticism (Cushing's disease).

Anticonvulsant drugs can also cause increased SAP levels and liver disease.[17, 83, 128] A distinctive morphological lesion may not exist, although an increase in liver glycogen content may be detected (personal observation). Long-term administration of primidone is associated with permanent hepatic damage (cirrhosis).[17] Whether or not there is an increased risk of liver disease in dogs or cats given other anticonvulsant drugs is unclear.[89]

An association between mebendazole administration as an anthelmintic and development of a toxic hepatitis also has been made.[93, 130] Experimental studies of the effects of mebendazole on the liver failed to demonstrate toxicity. Further studies are needed to explain the clinical association between hepatitis and mebendazole therapy.[136] Many other drugs are capable of causing hepatic disease in either a predictable or an idiosyncratic fashion (e.g., O'p'DDD, arsenamide, methoxyflurane) but further clinical studies of these are needed.

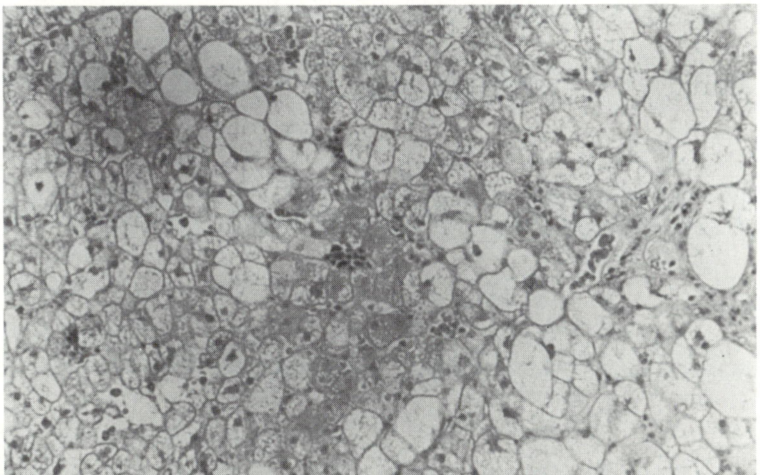

Figure 13–14. The biopsy specimen is characteristic of steroid hepatopathy. Note marked swelling (ballooning) of hepatocytes, which is caused by hydropic degeneration.

PORTACAVAL SHUNTS

Shunting of venous blood from the portal vein into the general circulation can result from acquired or congenital vascular communication between the portal circulation and the systemic circulation.[4, 7, 26, 31, 32, 36, 53, 95, 99, 113] The most common communications are venovenous shunts e.g., from the portal vein to the caudal vena cava. The most common shunt is the patent ductus venosus, which is apparently a congenital malformation. Acquired shunts may form in response to portal hypertension; these shunts are collateral vessels that bypass the liver. Therefore, portacaval shunts may be congenital malformations or they may be collateral vessels that form in response to portal hypertension, such as occurs in cirrhosis.[139, 140]

Portacaval shunts may be single or multiple and may take various pathways. For instance, there may be a connection between the splenic and renal veins (a splenorenal shunt) or there may be connection between the portal and the azygos veins (a portoazygos shunt). Any shunt that allows portal vein blood to bypass the liver will have two important effects: (1) atrophic changes will occur in the liver as a result of shunting of hepatotrophic factors, namely insulin; and (2) portosystemic encephalopathy, caused by "hepatotoxins" that are not cleared from the portal blood, will occur.[57]

Knowledge of the pathophysiology of portacaval shunts allows an understanding of the clinical findings in affected dogs and cats. In patients with congenital portacaval shunts, hepatic hypoplasia results in retarded growth, a stunted dog (Fig. 13–15). The patients also have neurological signs of portosystemic encephalopathy, such as coma, circling, convulsions, blindness, and aggression.[36] Some animals also have polydipsia and polyuria, possibly a neurological manifestation of PSE or the result of low blood urea nitrogen (BUN) levels.[36, 129] Feeding may exacerbate signs of PSE by increasing the content of ammonia and other toxins in the blood. In addition to neurological signs, affected dogs and cats usually have gastrointestinal upsets, which are manifested by vomiting and diarrhea. In patients with acquired shunts, signs of PSE are accompanied by signs of primary liver disease (e.g., weight loss, jaundice, ascites.)[36]

The laboratory findings in dogs with congenital portacaval shunts are often unre-

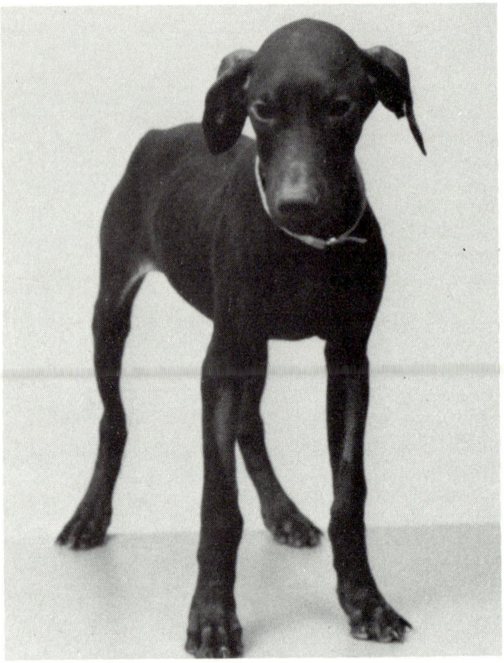

Figure 13–15. A patient with a patent ductus venosus. This six-month-old Doberman pinscher showed stunted growth and had episodes of blindness, head pressing, and convulsions.

markable.[49] The SGPT, SGOT, and SAP values are normal or slightly increased.[36] The blood glucose level is often normal, although hypoglycemia is a problem in some cases. BSP dye excretion is usually impaired, although a normal result of the BSP dye test does not rule out the presence of congenital shunts. The total serum bile acid content is increased, indicating contamination of systemic blood by portal blood. Urinalysis may reveal ammonium biurate crystals (Fig. 13–16), which indicate the presence of hyperammonemia. Blood ammonia levels and ammonia tolerance test results are usually abnormal; however, the blood ammonia assay may not be available to the general practitioner. Blood ammonia levels may be within normal limits in affected dogs.[85] The plasma protein content is often mildly decreased.

On radiographic examination, a small (hypoplastic) liver and enlarged kidneys are good indications of portacaval shunts (Fig. 13–16*C*).[4, 129] Urinary calculi composed of urates may also be observed radiographically (see Fig. 13–16). Ascites is not usually present and when detected can be explained in many cases by hypoalbuminemia.

Congenital vascular anomalies of the liver have been detected in cats.[65, 68, 70, 141] The

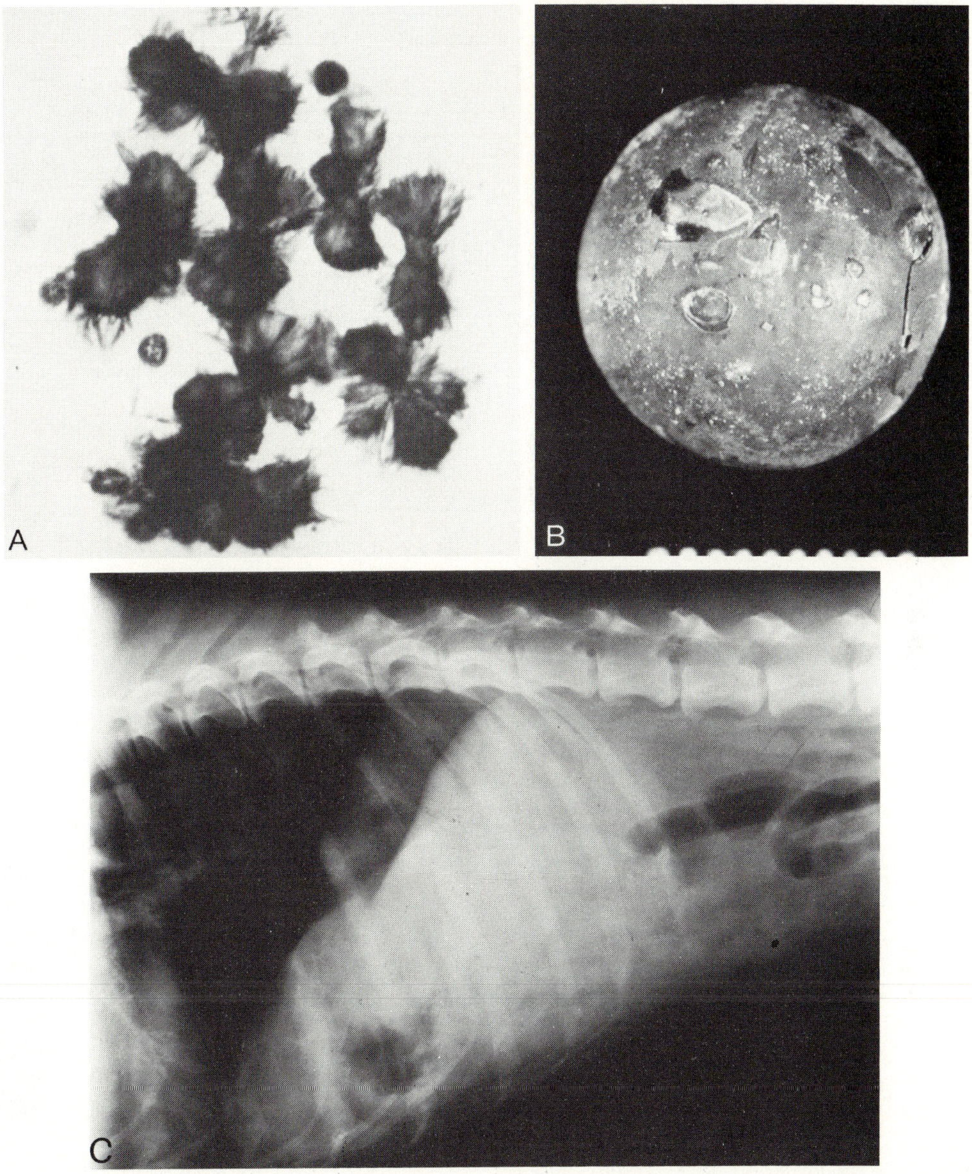

Figure 13–16. Indications of congenital portacaval shunt. Biurate crystalluria *(A)* and urate urolithiasis *(B)* may be detected in dogs with hyperammonemia and are common in dogs with congenital portacaval shunts. *C*, Microhepatica.

clinical signs, diagnosis, and treatment of feline vascular anomalies are similar to those in dogs. Ptyalism, an additional clinical sign that has been observed in cats with portacaval shunts, may be a diagnostic clue.

Confirmation of portacaval shunting requires angiographic evaluation.[129] Angiography can be performed by injecting contrast material into the anterior mesenteric artery, the splenic pulp (splenoportography) or mesenteric vein. Anterior mesenteric artery injection is performed under fluoroscopic control by inserting a catheter into the anterior mesenteric artery via the femoral artery. Splenoportograms can be obtained by injecting contrast medium into the spleen by percutaneous puncture or by direct visualization (laparotomy) (Figs. 13–17 to 13–19). Mesenteric vein catheterization and injection are performed by direct visualization at laparotomy.

Splenoportograms demonstrate the shunting veins so that a plan for surgical correction can be devised. General treatment for portosystemic encephalopathy should be instituted in the meantime. Partial ligation of

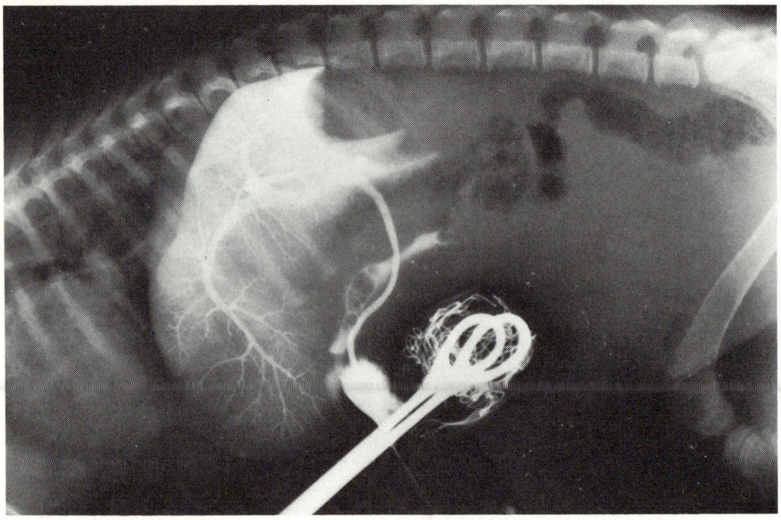

Figure 13–17. *A*, Splenoportagram in a normal dog shows perfusion of the liver and arborization of the portal blood vessels.

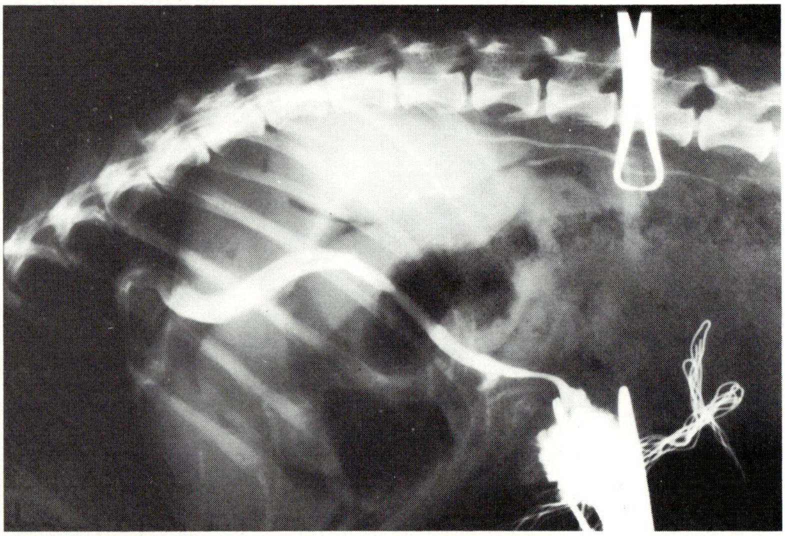

Figure 13–18. Splenoportagram shows a portacaval shunt.

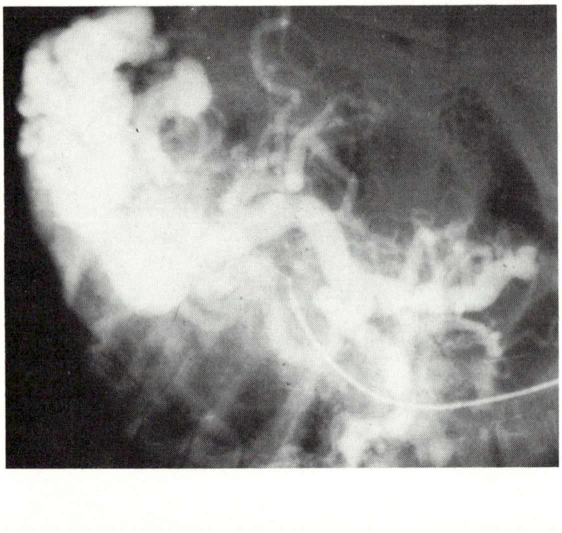

Figure 13–19. Angiogram of the hepatic artery shows intrahepatic arteriovenous shunts and hepatofugal blood flow.

the shunting vessel directs blood into the liver, causing regeneration of the liver and relief of PSE.[13, 14, 44, 123] The shunt should not be completely ligated because of the danger that blood will back up into the splanchnic circulation and cause pooling of blood, shock, and hemorrhagic enteritis.[109] Partial ligation is a difficult operation that requires assessment of portal vein pressure; it is best performed by an experienced surgeon. If surgery is impractical, medical management of PSE should be attempted. An evaluation of the effectiveness of long-term medical management has not been reported. When shunting occurs as a result of portal hypertension in primary hepatic disease such as cirrhosis, both the primary disease and PSE should be treated.

FELINE HEPATIC LIPIDOSIS[9, 21]

In the author's experience, feline hepatic lipidosis is one of the most common causes of liver failure in cats (along with feline cholangiohepatitis and lymphosarcoma). In this disorder a remarkable accumulation of lipid within the hepatocytes is accompanied by liver failure (Fig. 13–20*A*). The cause of feline hepatic lipidosis is unknown. Attempts to identify a hormonal or toxic cause have been unsuccessful. Anorexia may be an important factor although sick cats with profound anorexia do not necessarily develop hepatic lipidosis. Barium contrast radiography has revealed delayed gastric emptying but the significance of this finding is not clear.[21]

Clinical signs are the same as those in cats with other causes of liver failure, except that hepatic lipidosis may be more common in females than in males.[21] Obesity is often a historical finding. Anorexia then becomes evident and is followed by marked weight loss.

Diagnosis is made by detection of liver disease (icterus, abnormal laboratory test results) and by liver biopsy. On histological examination, marked accumulation of fat within hepatocytes, variable degrees of cholestasis, and little, if any, inflammation are found (Fig. 13–20*B*).

The prognosis is grave inasmuch as most treatments have failed. Treatments that have been tried include administration of thyroid hormone and insulin and hyperalimentation. At present, treatment of liver failure (PSE) and supportive nutritional care are recommended. However, most cats with hepatic lipidosis died soon after diagnosis.

PRIMARY INFECTIONS OF THE LIVER[37]

Many infectious diseases, such as feline infectious peritonitis, Rocky Mountain spotted fever, salmonellosis, and histoplasmosis, involve the liver (Fig. 13–21).[73] In this discussion, primary infections of the liver are included.

Infectious Canine Hepatitis[2, 22]

Infectious canine hepatitis (ICH) is an adenovirus hepatitis that affects young dogs and varies in severity from subclinical to peracute. Although the virus is ubiquitous, overt hepatitis is uncommon, probably because of effective vaccination programs. Infected animals usually have a high body temperature (105 to 106°F). Dogs with mild cases have anorexia, fever, and depression. Moderately affected puppies also have vom-

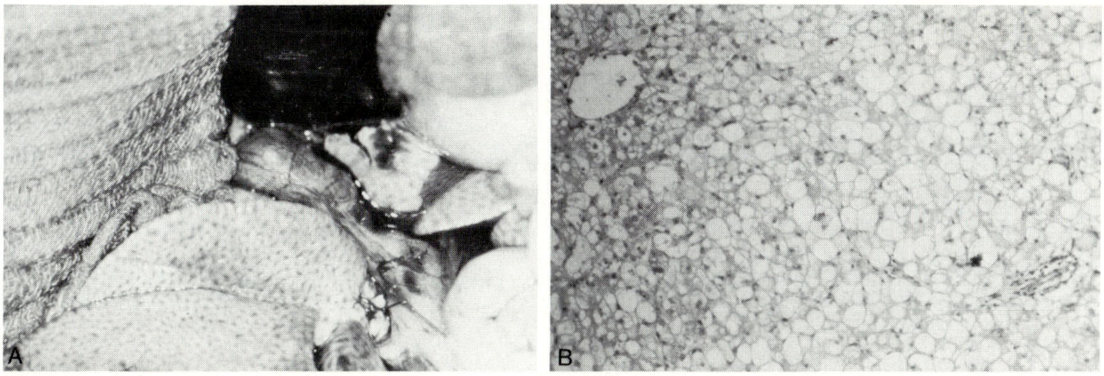

Figure 13–20. *A*, Gross appearance of the fatty liver of a cat with hepatic lipidosis. *B*, Microscopic appearance of the liver from a similarly affected cat.

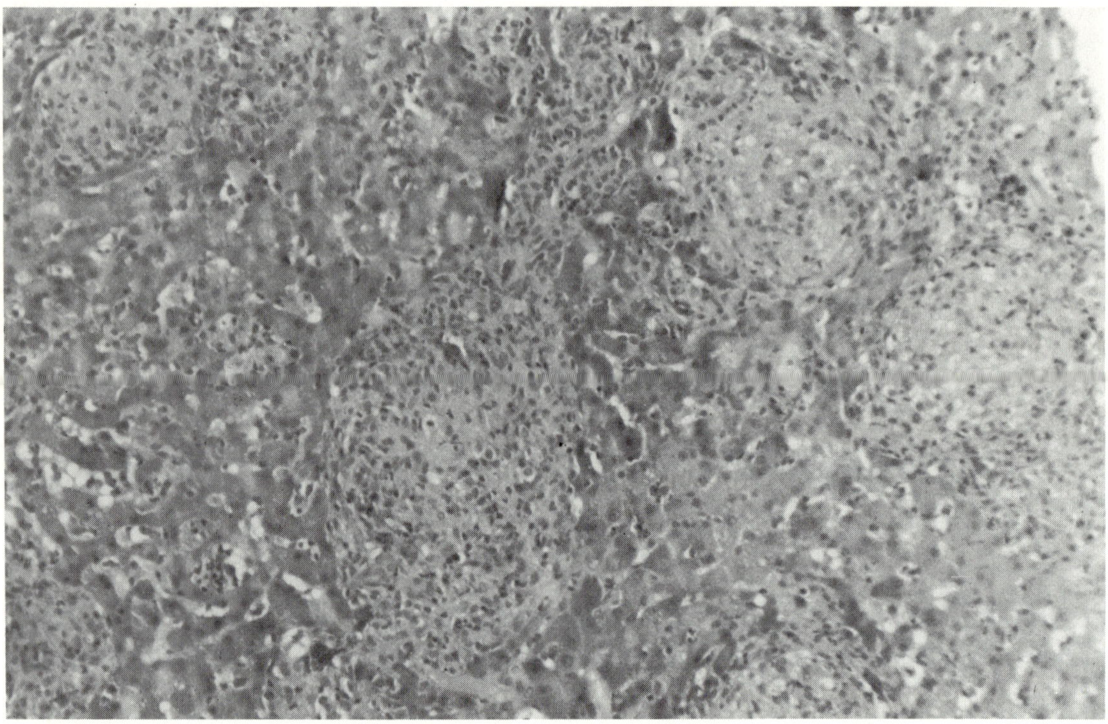

Figure 13–21. Granulomatous hepatitis caused by histoplasmosis (H&E, ×42).

iting and abdominal discomfort. Animals with peracute cases have severe abdominal pain and fever and die within 12 to 24 hours. The dogs usually are not icteric. They often have petechial hemorrhages of the mucous membranes.

The hemorrhages are a result of vasculitis and a bleeding tendency that is due to disseminated intravascular coagulopathy (DIC).[142] The virus infects endothelial cells, precipitating vasculitis. The blood platelet count is decreased, and prothrombin time and partial thromboplastin time are prolonged.

The complete blood count reveals leukopenia in the uncomplicated case of ICH. Biochemical evaluation by protein electrophoresis reveals increased SGOT, SAP, and γ-globulin concentrations.

Affected dogs have enlarged, swollen livers with necrosis and intranuclear inclusion bodies. The gall bladder is edematous. The kidneys are swollen, and gastrointestinal bleeding is often apparent. Anterior uveitis and the typical "blue eye," or corneal cloudiness, caused by viral damage to the corneal endothelium with subsequent arthus reaction may be detected.

Vaccination is very effective in preventing infectious canine hepatitis. The modified live adenovirus, type I, vaccine is capable of causing the "blue eye" and renal lesions. Because "blue eye" is common in the Afghan hound, and therefore the killed vaccine or adenovirus, type II, vaccine should be used in that breed. Adenovirus, type II, modified live vaccine is generally preferred over other vaccines because it offers protection against ICH without causing "blue eye" or renal lesions.

Experimental information indicates that partial or passive immunity to infectious canine hepatitis with subsequent exposure to virulent ICH virus may cause chronic hepatitis, which could lead to cirrhosis.[94] Thus, the clinician should probably vaccinate dogs annually using full doses of vaccine to maintain a good level of immunity to ICH.

Treatment of infectious canine hepatitis includes supportive care (fluids and antibiotics) and management of disseminated intravascular coagulopathy, if needed.

Leptospirosis[22, 37]

Leptospirosis is a bacterial infection of dogs that often involves the liver. Affected

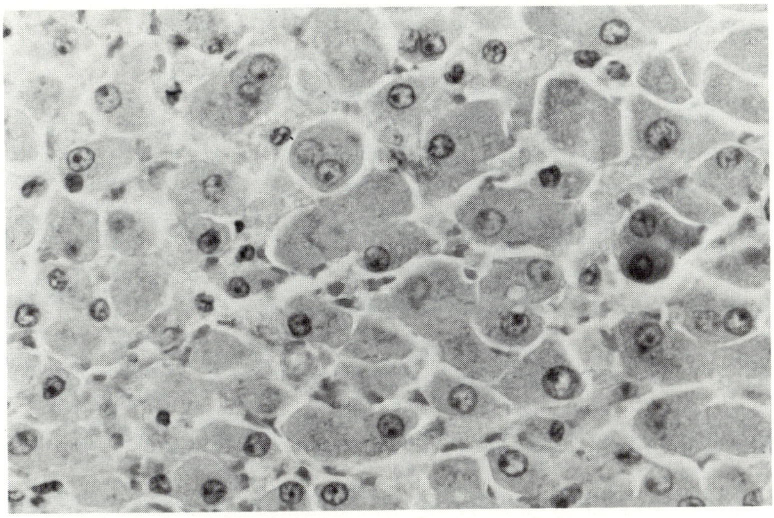

Figure 13–22. Liver specimen from a dog with leptospirosis shows individualization of hepatocytes (H&E, ×42).

dogs are often uremic and have leukocytosis and fever. About 15 per cent of the dogs have jaundice. The common serotypes in the dog are *Leptospira canicola* and *L. icterohaemorrhagiae*. *L. icterohaemorrhagiae* infection is much more likely to cause jaundice (70 per cent of cases) than *L. canicola* infection.

The liver biopsy specimen is usually unremarkable. There may be a peculiar "individualization" of hepatocytes accompanied by marked cholestasis (Fig. 13–22), and liver enzyme values are increased. In spite of the minimal morphological changes within the liver, liver function may be severely impaired. Diagnosis is based on clinical signs and the detection of rising antibody titers against *L. icterohaemorrhagiae* or *L. canicola*.

Treatment of leptospirosis should include administration of antibiotics that are effective against leptospires, such as streptomycin combined with penicillin. Tetracycline is effective in treating the carrier state. Good supportive care, e.g., the administration of fluids and electrolytes, is important.

Feline Liver Flukes

Liver flukes that cause biliary obstruction and hepatitis have been observed in the cat, and their presence should be considered in the differential diagnosis of a cat that is presented for liver disease.[8, 71, 103] *Amphimerus pseudofelineus* and *Platynosomum concinnum* are two flukes of importance in the cat.[8, 71]

DISEASES OF THE BILIARY TREE

Three disorders of the biliary tree that are not very common nevertheless deserve limited discussion.

Rupture of the Biliary Tree[10]

Rupture of the biliary tree due to trauma occurs primarily in the dog. The cause is usually a concussion to the abdomen. Rarely, a penetrating wound lacerates the biliary tree.

The location of the rent is usually the common bile duct. Initially, a sterile chemical peritonitis occurs, and the dog is presented for jaundice, abdominal distress, and sometimes ascites (Fig. 13–23). In some cases, the rent heals spontaneously, but usually once diagnosed, the leakage persists.

The prognosis in dogs with ruptured common bile ducts is guarded. The treatment is surgical, involving repair of the rent and various procedures involving intubation of the biliary tree or cholecystoduodenostomy (after ligation proximal and distal to the rent).

Strict aseptic technique is critical, since septic peritonitis is a common postoperative complication (see Fig. 13–23). Routine doses of prophylactic antibiotics (e.g., penicillin and gentamicin) are indicated before surgery. If surgical correction can be accomplished without secondary sepsis, the prognosis is favorable. The second most common postoperative complication is formation of new leaks.

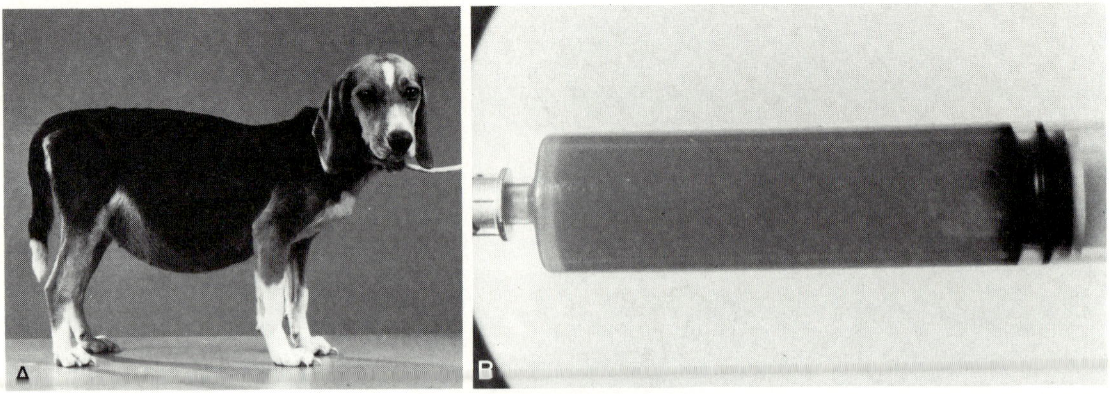

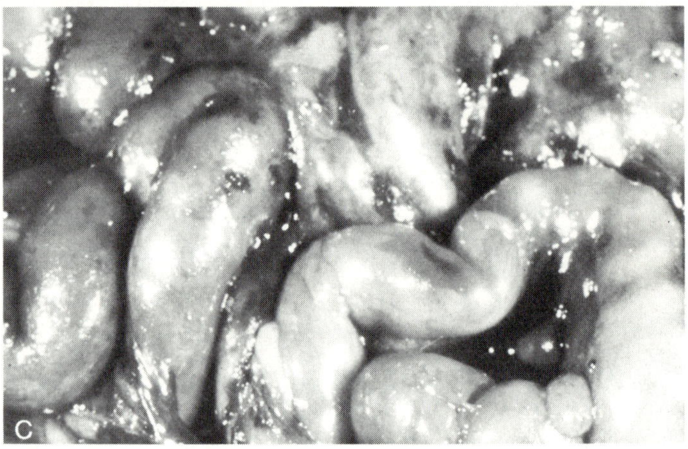

Figure 13–23. *A*, Ascites in a dog with a ruptured bile duct. *B*, Characteristic ascitic fluid from a dog with a ruptured common bile duct. *C*, The gross appearance of the peritoneum, showing severe bile peritonitis.

Canine Cholelithiasis[106]

Choleliths themselves are not rare, but cholelithiasis as a cause of obstruction is uncommon in the dog (Fig. 13–24). Intermittent jaundice should suggest the diagnosis.[106]

Choleliths are pigment stones composed of bile salts, calcium bilirubinate, and other substances found in bile. Cholelithiasis can be induced in dogs by feeding a diet that is deficient in the amino acid, taurine.[33] Bile acids are conjugated primarily to taurine in the dog; therefore, it is speculated that taurine deficiency may alter solubility of canine bile and may cause pigment stone formation.

In the dog, asymptomatic cholelithiasis that is detected on radiographic examination probably should not be treated. If obstructive jaundice develops, removal of the cholelith should be considered.

Cystic Malformations of the Biliary Tree

Congenital cystic disease of the biliary tree, which is similar to Caroli's disease in human beings, occurs in the dog (Fig. 13–25). The clinical signs of cystic biliary disease include jaundice, increased SAP

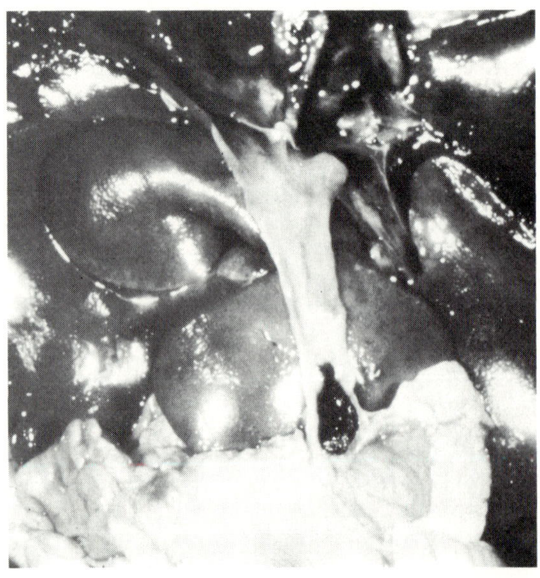

Figure 13–24. Liver specimen shows a pigment cholelith lying in the common bile duct, which has been opened longitudinally.

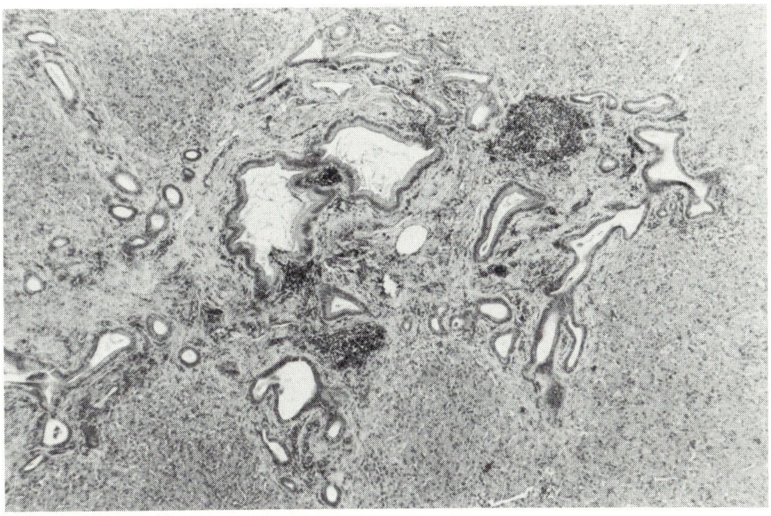

Figure 13–25. Cystic dysplasia of the biliary tree in a dog with congenital malformation of the biliary tree resembles Caroli's disease of human beings (H&E, ×42).

level (e.g., evidence of biliary obstruction), and fever and leukocytosis caused by secondary biliary infection. The signs may wax and wane. Cystic disease of other organs, e.g., polycystic kidney disease, may also be present and should be sought in the clinical work-up.

Diagnosis is confirmed by exploratory laparotomy or by finding characteristic ectasia of the bile ductules on liver biopsy. Treatment includes antibiotics to control secondary bacterial infection, and the prognosis is guarded.

NEOPLASMS OF THE LIVER

Neoplasia commonly invades the liver of older dogs or cats either as a primary tumor or frequently as a metastasis. Common tumors include hepatocellular carcinoma, cholangiocellular carcinoma, carcinoid, lymphosarcoma (Fig. 13–26), and pancreatic adenocarcinoma.[92, 120] Primary tumors usually cause liver function tests to be abnormal, and hepatomegaly is often detected (Fig. 13–27). If the liver is infiltrated by metastatic neoplasia, the dog or cat is often presented for signs of liver disease rather than for signs related to the primary tumor.

Hepatomas (hepatocellular carcinomata) may cause hypoglycemia.[124] These tumors may be very active, consuming large amounts of glucose. They may also invade adjacent parenchyma to the extent that there is insufficient normal liver parenchyma to support the blood glucose content. Hepatomas have

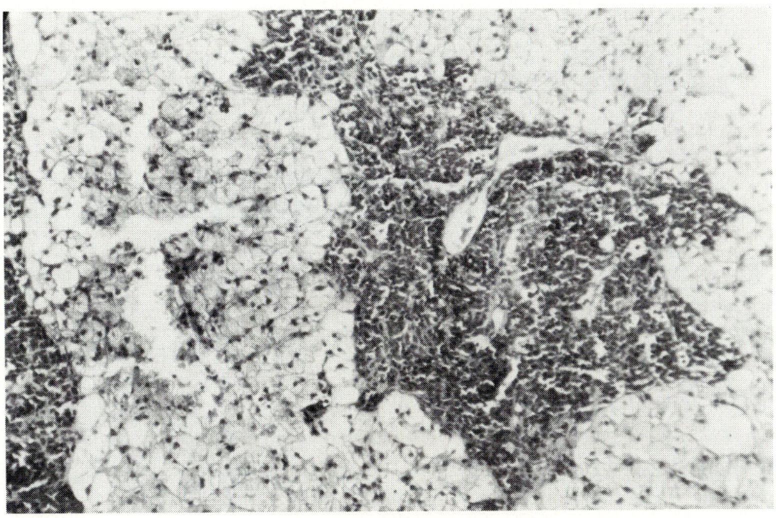

Figure 13–26. Characteristic periportal infiltration of the liver by neoplastic lymphocytes (H&E, ×42).

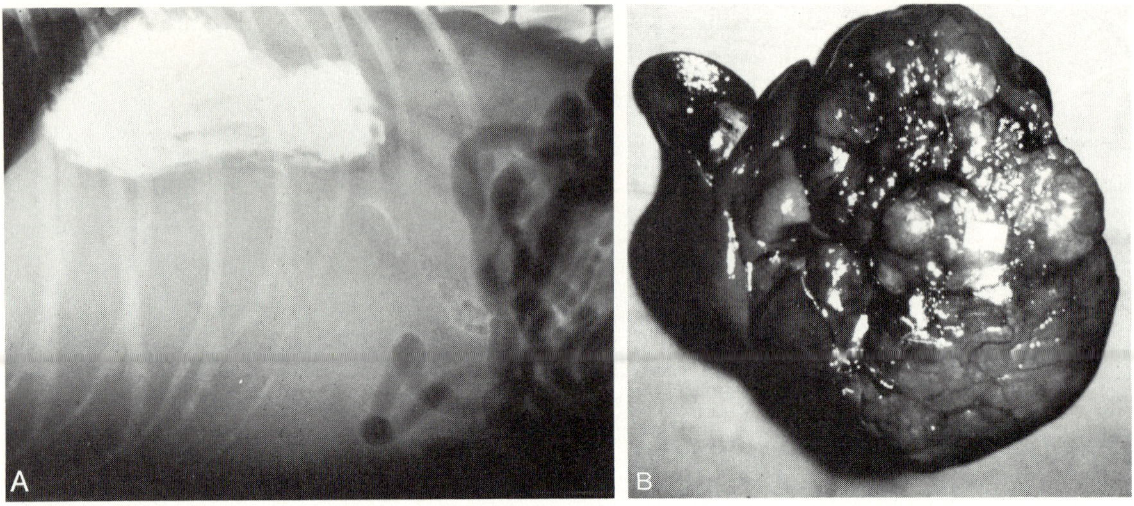

Figure 13–27. Hepatoma in the dog. *A*, Radiograph shows marked hepatomegaly. Barium has been given to demonstrate displacement of the stomach. *B*, Large hepatoma consuming the left side of the liver.

also been suspected of producing an insulin-like substance that causes hypoglycemia (para-neoplastic syndrome).[78, 124]

It is worthwhile to resect hepatomas that have not metastasized, but a guarded prognosis is warranted inasmuch as new hepatoma formation occurs frequently. Insulinoma may also cause hypoglycemia and may have hepatic metastases, making differentiation of this tumor from hepatoma difficult. In cases in which the identification of the tumor is difficult, liver biopsy, glucose tolerance test, glucagon tolerance test, insulin/glucose ratio, or exploratory laparotomy may be necessary (alone or in combination) to make a diagnosis.

Of clinical importance is the fact that hepatic neoplasms may easily be missed owing to errors in sampling with the blind percutaneous biopsy technique. In the author's experience, about one-third of the hepatic neoplasms are overlooked.[32] Thus, a negative biopsy result does not rule out the presence of neoplasia. In cases in which neoplasia is suspected visual inspection of the liver via laparoscopy or laparotomy is required.

Treatment of Liver Disease

GENERAL PRINCIPLES

Because the liver is the major site of drug metabolism, it is important to consider some of the factors that affect hepatic drug metabolism as well as to discuss specific therapy for liver diseases. Several factors that determine the degree to which hepatic drug metabolism is altered by the liver include diet, previous drug therapy, hepatic blood flow, and serum albumin content. Other factors include species, breed, and individual variations, as well as age and sex of the patient.

It is usually impossible, on a clinical basis, to predict with confidence the pharmacological effect of a particular drug in a body in which hepatic function is impaired, because all of the factors that affect the drug's metabolism cannot usually be assessed. For instance, altered hepatic blood flow markedly affects the metabolism of lidocaine,* a frequently used antiarrhythmic agent. A dog with an arrhythmia or with congestive heart failure may have a reduced hepatic blood flow. The clinician must be able to assess hepatic blood flow or measure serum lidocaine content in order to predict the effect of a given dose of lidocaine on the heart. The important conclusion is that potentially toxic drugs should be used with extreme caution in the presence of hepatic disease. Furthermore, drug dosages cannot be altered on the basis of results of liver function tests such as a BSP dye excretion test. In fact, enhanced excretion of a drug can actually occur with hepatic disease and abnormal liver function test results.

*Xylocaine, Astra Pharmaceutical Products, Inc., Westboro, MA.

PORTOSYSTEMIC ENCEPHALOPATHY (PSE)

Portosystemic encephalopathy (hepatoencephalopathy) is most commonly recognized in patients with congenital portacaval shunts or with liver failure. In these patients, substances that originate in the gut and that are normally extracted from portal blood by the liver are delivered instead to the systemic circulation. These "toxins" cause the PSE. Ammonia that originates from the gut appears to be a significant toxin. Ammonia is normally converted to urea in the liver by the urea cycle, and the urea produced is subsequently excreted in urine.

When ammonia escapes metabolism by the liver, it reaches the brain, where it exerts a toxic influence. In the brain, glutamine is formed from the combination of glutamate and ammonia in an attempt to lower cerebrospinal fluid ammonia content. Cerebrospinal fluid glutamine content increases in hepatoencephalopathy.[107] In the kidney, this reaction is reversed; glutamine is converted to glutamate and ammonia, and the ammonia is delivered to the urine.

When the ability of the liver to convert blood ammonia into urea and the compensatory mechanisms in the brain and kidney are insufficient to keep blood ammonia levels in the safe range, PSE with hyperammonemia results.[127] Short-chain fatty acids, amino acids and amino acid imbalances, and the formation of biogenic amines that affect neurotransmission also have been blamed for hepatoencephalopathy.[41]

The following measures are designed to prevent hepatoencephalopathy, but they should also be instituted in patients that already have hepatic coma.

1. Sedatives, tranquilizers, hypnotics, anesthetics, and anticonvulsants, which are all cerebral depressants, should not be given to patients with PSE or with liver disease capable of causing PSE. It may be tempting for the clinician to use these agents, especially the anticonvulsants, because many patients exhibit neurological signs. However, the patients have increased cerebral sensitivity to cerebral depressants; the activity of these drugs is prolonged because of decreased hepatic clearance.

2. Diuretics should be avoided in patients with potential hepatoencephalopathy. The clinician may be tempted to use diuretics to treat ascites or edema caused by liver disease. Diuretics may cause hypovolemia and prerenal azotemia. The increased BUN level will raise blood ammonia content, because the urea will circulate to the gut, where it will be converted to ammonia by bacteria. This ammonia is subsequently absorbed. Diuretics may also induce hypokalemia and metabolic alkalosis. Alkalosis is associated with trapping of ammonium ions within the intracellular fluid compartment, which accentuates hepatoencephalopathy. Diuretics may also cause hyperammonemia by increasing renal production of ammonia. The carbonic anhydrase inhibitor diuretics, such as acetazolamide, increase renal vein ammonia production.

3. Hypokalemia and alkalosis of any cause should be avoided. For instance, hypokalemia caused by decreased oral intake of potassium should be prevented. Hypokalemia may cause intracellular trapping of ammonia.[107]

4. Gastrointestinal bleeding should be controlled immediately. Blood is a rich source of protein; hence, blood ammonia content increases when gastrointestinal bleeding occurs. It is important to control hookworm infestation, simple gastroenteritis, gastrointestinal (peptic) ulcers, and bleeding disorders.[88, 119] If colonic bleeding is present, cleansing enemas may be administered. Whole blood also contains high concentrations of ammonia and may cause hyperammonemia when given to patients with hepatic disease. Blood's ammonia content increases as it is stored.[30]

5. Clinical observations in human patients with hepatic coma indicate that infections may worsen PSE. Therefore, it is rational to control infections with appropriate antibiotics in animals with PSE.

Once PSE has developed, certain general measures can be instituted to reduce or abolish the neurological signs. Restriction of dietary protein is of utmost importance.[47] The diet of patients with PSE should consist mostly of carbohydrate and fat. Vegetables and cottage cheese are good foods for these patients; some prescription diets* may be helpful. Affected animals should never be given red meat, which will worsen hepatic encephalopathy. In fact, hepatic encephalopathy has been called "meat intoxication." The human patient is restricted to from one-third to one-half of the daily protein allow-

*k/d Prescription Diet, Hill's Pet Products, Topeka, KS.

ance. In dogs, this degree of restriction equals 1.4 to 2.2 gm of protein/kg daily. The administration of commercial parenteral amino acid solutions that have high ammonia contents should also be avoided. This precaution is consistent with the restriction of proteins. If these amino acid solutions are given intravenously, they enter the systemic circulation rather than the portal circulation; thus, blood ammonia levels may rise precipitously. Products with methionine, which is often an ingredient of the so-called lipotrophic drugs, should also be avoided. Methionine is converted in the gut to mercaptans, which act synergistically with ammonia in the production of the PSE.[82, 144] Vitamins should also be supplied.

Oral antibiotics are important in controlling PSE, and the drug of choice is oral neomycin (Table 13–5).[3] Neomycin is given to decrease the intestinal population of the urea-splitting bacteria that produce ammonia. After oral neomycin has been instituted, it may be possible to increase dietary protein without precipitation of hepatoencephalopathy. Neomycin should be used on a short-term basis, since prolonged use may alter the gut flora and may allow for mycotic overgrowth.

Enemas and cathartics can be used to decrease contact time of ammonia with the intestinal mucosa, thus decreasing intestinal ammonia absorption. Neomycin can be added to the enema. It is important not to cause electrolyte imbalances or dehydration by overzealous use of enemas or cathartics.

Lactulose is a non-absorbed disaccharide that is hydrolyzed by anaerobic bacteria in the gut to form lactic acid and acetic acid (see Table 13–5).[3] Given orally, lactulose results in the acidification of the colon and causes an osmotic catharsis. Acidification of intestinal contents with lactulose decreases absorption of ammonia by favoring the formation of the less diffusible ammonium ion. There is increased uptake of nitrogen by the colonic bacteria and increased loss of nitrogenous substances in the feces. Lactulose is very effective and is given as long as needed.

Besides these standard therapeutic measures, several new treatments have appeared on the horizon.[137] These new modes of therapy await confirmation of efficacy by clinical testing.

Imbalances in plasma amino acid concentrations have been measured in humans and in animals with hepatoencephalopathy.[59, 102, 122] When portacaval shunting is present, there is an increase in plasma aromatic amino acid content and a decrease in branched-chain amino acid content.[2] This imbalance, which is accentuated by the catabolic state, is caused by impaired hepatic clearance of aromatic amino acids and increased peripheral utilization of branched-chain amino acids for energy. The neurological manifestations of hepatoencephalopathy can be abolished by intravenous infusion of an amino acid mixture that corrects the amino acid imbalance. In the future, it may be possible to obtain an aminogram, i.e., a measurement of the levels of various amino acids, and then to correct imbalances with intravenous administration of tailored amino acid mixtures.[40]

Recently, partial ligation of a shunting vessel in dogs and cats with portacaval shunts caused hepatic regeneration and improved hepatic function.[13, 14] These case reports suggest that further evaluation of surgical correction of portacaval shunts should be done.

L-Dopa is a precursor of dopamine. Dopamine and norepinephrine are normal neurotransmitters in the brain. It has been postulated that there is an accumulation of false neurotransmitters, such as octopamine and β-phenylethanolamine in the brain in hepatoencephalopathy.[107] L-Dopa and bromocriptine (dopamine agonist) have been administered to stimulate formation of normal neurotransmitters that can override the effects of the false neurotransmitters. This treatment needs further clinical evaluation.

Table 13–5. DRUGS IN THE MANAGEMENT OF PORTOSYSTEMIC ENCEPHALOPATHY

Drug	Dosage	Action
Neomycin	10–20 mg/kg, Q6H, orally for 5 days; can be given as a retention enema	Decreases ammonia production by urea-splitting, colonic bacteria
Lactulose	5–30 ml, Q6H, orally; can be used indefinitely. Can be given as a retention enema	Increased fecal nitrogen excretion

Two drugs have been recommended to increase uptake and metabolism of ammonia. Sodium glutamate combines with ammonia to form glutamine, thus decreasing ammonia concentration. Arginine has been administered to stimulate the urea cycle, thus enhancing conversion of ammonia to urea. Neither of these drugs has had notable clinical success to date.[119]

ACUTE HEPATIC FAILURE

Therapeutic principles used in the treatment of PSE due to chronic liver failure apply to the treatment of hepatoencephalopathy secondary to acute liver failure. Treatment of acute hepatic failure differs in that the objective is to minimize the immediate systemic effect of liver failure until the episode has subsided. In most cases of acute hepatic failure, a toxin (e.g., aflatoxin) or infectious agent (e.g., leptospire) is suspected of causing the problem.

Fluids tailored to meet the patient's water and electrolyte needs are given intravenously. Usually, a balanced solution such as lactated Ringer's solution is adequate, but the serum electrolyte content must be measured, and the hydration (fluid balance) status must be determined on an individual basis in order to select proper solutions. Glucose (5 to 10 per cent) is added to the fluid to ensure maintenance of blood glucose levels and to increase uptake of ammonia by glutamate. Broad-spectrum antibiotic therapy may be indicated to prevent septicemia.

Acute hepatic failure is often accompanied by endotoxemia and shock. Impaired function of the reticuloendothelial system (Kupffer cells) may allow endotoxin to enter the systemic circulation. The effects of endotoxin include disseminated intravascular coagulopathy, hypoglycemia (depressed gluconeogenesis), hypotension, renal failure, and gastrointestinal bleeding.[72, 125, 144] Endotoxins are also directly hepatotoxic. The clinician must be on the alert for these complications and must treat them as they develop.

Glucocorticoid treatment may be indicated if endotoxic shock is present. Otherwise, glucocorticoids have not been of value in the treatment of acute hepatic failure.

HEPATIC LIPIDOSIS[10]

The clinical significance of hepatic lipidosis is often difficult to assess. It is probably of little consequence in simple obesity, in which hepatic lipid represents an overall increase in body lipid stores. Hepatic lipidosis may be severe in toxic hepatitis, in which intrahepatic lipoprotein formation and excretion is deranged. For example, hepatic lipidosis develops in diabetics as free fatty acids enter the liver to be formed into lipoprotein; because lipoprotein synthesis and excretion are impaired, the lipoproteins accumulate. This lipidosis is fully reversible by insulin therapy. Similarly, the lipidosis detected in dogs with hypothyroidism can be treated by proper thyroid hormone replacement. The etiology and treatment of idiopathic feline hepatic lipidosis are not known, and the prognosis is grave.

Dietary deficiency of choline results in hepatic lipidosis and cirrhosis. Choline is a precursor of phosphorylcholine, which is important in lipoprotein formation. Therefore, choline use has been advocated in treatment of hepatic lipidosis. It is often used in combination with methionine because methionine (also cystine) can replace choline as a precursor of phosphorylcholine. There is no good evidence that methionine or choline is useful in treating hepatic lipidosis that is not caused by a choline deficiency, and oral methionine can be harmful if hepatoencephalopathy is present or potential.[12]

CIRRHOSIS

There is no known specific therapy for cirrhosis; however, good supportive care and management of PSE are important. Colchicine has been used to decrease accumulation of hepatic collagen in experimental and naturally occurring cirrhosis.[101] Colchicine acts by impairing formation of new collagen and by enhancing collagen degradation in the liver. Colchicine could be used (with the informed consent of the client) as a last resort in dogs with hepatic failure due to cirrhosis.

SUMMARY OF TREATMENTS OF LIVER DISEASES

The liver is the center of drug metabolism and is therefore subject to damage by toxic compounds. Predictability of therapeutic response to drugs is poor when liver function is altered; hence, clinicians cannot make confident extrapolations from observations made in normal animals. Marked species and individual variations further impair predictability of drug response. Problems exemplifying these principles include precipitation of hepatic coma by sedatives or diuretics in dogs with portacaval shunts.

Treatment of liver disease is often supportive. Drugs may be useful in some cases; for example, oral neomycin or lactulose can be used in patients with hepatic coma and glucocorticoids can be used in dogs with chronic active liver disease. Promising new treatments, such as tailored amino acid solutions for use in animals with hepatic coma and colchicine in patients with cirrhosis, are on the horizon. All of these therapeutic techniques need careful clinical evaluation before they can be recommended with confidence.

References

1. Ackerman N, Silverman S: Radiographic interpretation: Liver enlargement. Mod Vet Pract 58:949, 1977.
2. Aguirre A, Yoshimura N, Westman T, Fischer HE: Plasma amino acids in dogs with two experimental forms of liver damage. J Surg Res 16:339, 1974.
3. Atterbury CE, Maddrey WC, Conn HO: Neomycin-sorbitol and lactulose in the treatment of acute portal-systemic encephalopathy. A controlled, double-blind clinical trial. Am J Dig Dis 23:398, 1978.
4. Audell L, Jonsson L, Lannek G: Congenital portacaval shunts in the dog: A description of three cases. Zentralbl Veterinarmed (A) 21:797, 1974.
5. Babb RR: The use of antibiotics in biliary tract disease. Am J Gastroenterol 63:37, 1975.
6. Badylak SF, Dodds WJ, Van Fleet JF: Plasma coagulation factor abnormalities in dogs with naturally occurring hepatic disease. Am J Vet Res 12:2336, 1983.
7. Barrett RE, Delahunta A, Roenick WJ, et al: Four cases of congenital portacaval shunts in the dog. J Small Anim Pract 17:71, 1976.
8. Barriga OD, Caputo CA, Weisbrode SE: Liver flukes *(Platynosomum concinnum)* in an Ohio cat. J Am Vet Med Assoc 179:901, 1981.
9. Barsanti JA, Jones, BD, Spano JS, Taylor HW: Prolonged anoexia associated with hepatic lipidosis in three cats. Feline Pract 7:52, 1977.
10. Berson JL: Surgical repair of traumatic injuries of the biliary system. J Am Anim Hosp Assoc 17:421, 1981.
11. Bishop L, Strandberg JD, Adams RJ, et al: Chronic active hepatitis in dogs associated with leptospires. Am J Vet Res 40:839, 1979.
12. Branam JE: Suspected methionine toxicosis associated with a portacaval shunt in a dog. J Am Vet Assoc 181:929, 1982.
13. Breznock EM, Berger B, Pendray D, et al: Surgical manipulation of intrahepatic portacaval shunts in dogs. J Am Vet Med Assoc 182:798, 1983.
14. Breznock EM: Surgical manipulations of portosystemic shunts in dogs. J Am Vet Med Assoc 174:819, 1979.
15. Brobst DF, Schall, WC: Needle biopsy of the canine liver and correlation of laboratory data with histopathologic observations. J Am Vet Med Assoc 161:382, 1972.
16. Brunson DB, Stevens JB, McGrath CJ: Preoperative liver screen selection: Comparison of serum glutamic-pyruvic transaminase and serum alkaline phosphatase. J Am Anim Hosp Assoc 16:209, 1980.
17. Bunch SE, Castleman WL, Hornbuckle WE, et al: Hepatic cirrhosis associated with long-term anticonvulstant drug therapy in dogs. J Am Vet Med Assoc 181:357, 1982.
18. Byars TD, Ling GV, Ferris NA, Keeton KS: Activated coagulation time (ACT) of whole blood in normal dogs. Am J Vet Res 37:1359, 1976.
19. Carte RE: Diagnostic real time ultrasonography of the liver of the dog and cat. J Am Anim Hosp Assoc 17:731, 1981.
20. Center SA, Baldwin BH, King JM, Tennant BC: Hematologic and biochemical abnormalities associated with induced extrahepatic bile duct obstruction in the cat. Am J Vet Res 44:1822, 1983.
21. Chiapella A: Personal communication, 1982.
22. Cornelius CE: Biochemical evaluation of hepatic function in dogs. J Am Anim Hosp Assoc 15:259, 1979.
23. Conn HO: Cirrhosis. *In* Schiff L (ed): *Diseases of the Liver,* 4th ed. J. B. Lippincott Co., Philadelphia, pp. 833–924, 1975.
24. Cornelius CE, Himes JA: New concepts in canine hepatic function. J Am Anim Hosp Assoc 9:147, 1973.
25. Cornelius CE: Liver function. *In* Kaneko JJ, Cornelius CE (eds): *Clinical Chemistry of Domestic Animals,* 2nd ed, Vol I. Academic Press, New York, p. 161, 1970.
26. Cornelius LM, Thrall DE, Halliwell WH, et al: Anomalous portosystemic anastomoses associated with chronic hepatic insufficiency in six young dogs. J Am Vet Med Assoc 167:220, 1975.
27. Dillon AR, Sprano JS, Powers RD: Prednisolone-induced hematologic biochemical and histologic changes in the dog. J Am Anim Hosp Assoc 16:831, 1980.
28. Doige DE, Lester D: Chronic active hepatitis in dogs—a review of fourteen cases. J Am Anim Hosp Assoc 17:725, 1981.
29. Dorner JJ, Hoffman WE, Long GB: Corticosteroid induction of an isoenzyme of alkaline phosphatase in the dog. Am J Vet Res 35:1457, 1974.
30. Drazner FH: Hepatic encephalopathy in the dog. *In* Kirk RW (ed): *Current Veterinary Therapy VIII.* W. B. Saunders Company, Philadelphia, p. 831, 1983.
31. Easley JC, Carpenter JL: Hepatic arteriovenous fistula in two Saint Bernard pups. J Am Vet Med Assoc 166:167, 1975.
32. Edwards DF: Blind percutaneous liver biopsy: A safe diagnostic procedure. Calif Vet 31:9, 1977.
33. Englert E, Harman CG, Freston JW, et al: Studies on the pathogenesis of diet-induced dog gall stones. Am J Dig Dis 22:305, 1977.
34. Evans HE, Christensen GC: *Miller's Anatomy of the Dog,* 2nd ed: W. B. Saunders Company, Philadelphia, p. 492, 1980.
35. Everett RM, Duncan JR, Prasse KW: Alkaline phosphatase, leucine aminopeptidase and alanine

aminotransferase activities with obstructive and toxic hepatic disease in cats. Am J Vet Res 38:963, 1977.
36. Ewing, GO, Suter PF, Bailey CS: Hepatic insufficiency associated with congenital anomalies of the portal vein in dogs. J Am Anim Hosp Assoc 10:463, 1974.
37. Farrow BRH, Love DN: Bacterial, viral, and other infectious problems. *In* Ettinger SJ (ed): *Textbook of Veterinary Internal Medicine,* 2nd ed., W. B. Saunders Company, Philadelphia, p. 269, 1975.
38. Feldman EC, Ettinger SJ: Percutaneous transthoracic liver biopsy in the dog: A review of 75 cases. J Am Anim Hosp Assoc 13:17, 1977.
39. Filkins JP, Buchanan BJ: In vivo vs. in vitro effects of endotoxin of glycogenolysis, gluconeogenesis, and glucose utilization. Proc Soc Exp Biol Med 155:216, 1977.
40. Fischer JE, Rosen HM, Ebeid AM, et al: The effect of normalization of plasma amino acids on hepatic encephalopathy in man. Surgery 80:77, 1976.
41. Fischer JE, Funovics JM, Aguirre A, et al: The role of plasma amino acids in hepatic encephalopathy. Surgery 78:276, 1975.
42. Gocke DJ, Morris TQ, Bradley SE: Chronic hepatitis in the dog: The role of immune factors. J Am Vet Med Assoc 156:1700, 1970.
43. Gocke DJ, Preisig R, Morris TQ et al: Experimental viral hepatitis in the dog: Production of persistent disease in partially immune animals. J Clin Invest 46:1506, 1967.
44. Gofton N: Surgical ligation of congenital portosystemic venous shunts in the dog: A report of three cases. J Am Anim Hosp Assoc 14:728, 1978.
45. Gopinath C, Ford EJH: Location of liver injury and extent of bilirubinaemia in experimental liver lesions. Vet Pathol 9:99, 1972.
46. Grausz H, Schmid R: Reciprocal relation between plasma albumin level and hepatic sulfobromophthalein removal. New Engl J Med 284:1401, 1972.
47. Greenberger NJ, Carley J, Schenker S, et al: Effect of vegetable and animal protein diets in chronic hepatic encephalopathy. J Dig Dis 22:845, 1977.
48. Greene CE: Ascites: Diagnostic and therapeutic considerations. Comp Cont Ed 1:712, 1979.
49. Griffiths GL, Lumsden JH, Valli VEO: Hematologic and biochemical changes in dogs with portosystemic shunts. J Am Anim Hosp Assoc 17:705, 1981.
50. Hardy RM: Copper-associated hepatitis in Bedlington terriers. *In* Kirk RW (ed): *Current Veterinary Therapy VIII.* W. B. Saunders Company, Philadelphia, p. 834, 1983.
51. Hardy RM: Diseases of the liver. *In* Ettinger SJ (ed): *Textbook of Veterinary Internal Medicine,* 2nd ed. W. B. Saunders Company, Philadelphia, p. 1372, 1983.
52. Hardy RM, Stevens JB, Stowe L: Chronic progressive hepatitis in Bedlington terriers associated with elevated liver copper concentrations. Minn Vet 15:13, 1975.
53. Hickman J, Edwards JE, Mann FD: Venous anomalies in a dog. Anat Rec 104:137, 1949.
54. Hoffman WE: Diagnostic value of canine serum alkaline phosphatase and alkaline phosphatase isoenzymes J Am Anim Hosp Assoc 13:237, 1977.
55. Hoffman WE, Dorner JL: Disappearance rates of intravenously injected canine serum alkaline phosphatase isoenzymes. Am J Vet Res 38:1553, 1977.
56. Hoffman WE, Renegar WE, Dorner JL: Serum half-life of intravenously injected intestinal and hepatic alkaline phosphatase isoenzymes in the cat. Am J Vet Res 38:1637, 1977.
57. Hoyumpa AM Jr, Desmond PV, Avant JR, et al: Hepatic encephalopathy (clinical conference). Gastroenterology 76:18, 1979.
58. Hoyumpa AM, Greene HL, Dunn GD, Schenker S: Fatty liver, biochemical and clinical considerations. Am J Dig Dis 20:1142, 1975.
59. Iob V, Mattson WJ Jr, Sloan M, et al: Alterations in plasma-free amino acids in dogs with hepatic insufficiency. Surg Gynecol Obstet 130:794, 1970.
60. Johnson SE: Determination of fasting serum bile acids in normal dogs and in dogs with spontaneous hepatobiliary disease. Master's thesis. Ohio State University, 1982.
61. Johnson GF, Sternlieb I, Twedt DC, et al: Inheritance of copper toxicosis in Bedlington terriers. Am J Vet Res 41:1865, 1980.
62. Johnson GF, Zawie DA, Gilbertson SR, et al: Chronic active hepatitis in Doberman pinchers. J Am Vet Med Assoc 180:1438, 1982.
63. Kelly DF, Baggot DG, Gaskell CJ: Jaundice in the east associated with inflammation of the biliary tract and pancreas. J Small Anim Pract 16:163, 1975.
64. Kerschenobich D, Uribe M, Suares GI, et al: Treatment of cirrhosis and colchicine: A double-blind, randomized trial. Gastroenterology 77:532, 1979.
65. Khan IR, Vitums A: Portosystemic communications in the cat. Res Vet Sci 12:215, 1971.
66. Kramer JW, Sleight SD: The isoenzymes of serum alkaline phosphatase in cats. Am J Vet Clin Pathol 2:87, 1968.
67. Kukral JC, Sporn J, Louch J, Winzler RJ: Synthesis of alpha- and beta-globulins in normal and liverless dogs. Am J Physiol 204:262, 1963.
68. Legendre AM, Krahwinkel DJ, Carris CB, Michel RL: Ascites associated with intrahepatic arteriovenous fistula in a cat. J Am Vet Med Assoc 168:589, 1976.
69. Lettow VF: Die blends leberpunktion nach Menghini beim hund. Ber Munch Tierarztl Wochensch 76:273, 1963.
70. Levesque DC, Oliver JE Jr, Cornelius LM, et al: Congenital portacaval shunts in two cats: Diagnosis and surgical correction. J Am Vet Med Assoc 181:143, 1982.
71. Levine ND, Beamer PD, Maksic D: Hepatitis due to *Amphimerus pseudofelineus* in a cat. Ill Vet 1:45, 1958.
72. Liehr H, Grün M, Brunswig D: Endotoxinämie bei Leberzirrhose. Gastroenterol 14:23, 1976.
73. Lissman BA, Benach JL: Rocky Mountain spotted fever in dogs. J Am Vet Med Assoc 176:994, 1980.
74. Lohse CL, Suter PE: Functional closure of the ductus venosus during early postnatal life in the dog. Am J Vet Res 38:839, 1977.
75. Ludwig J, Owen CA, Barham SS, et al: The liver in the inherited copper disease of Bedlington terriers. Lab Invest 43:82, 1980.
77. Maretta SM, Pask AJ, Greene RW, Liu SS: Urinary calculi associated with portosystemic shunts in six dogs. J Am Vet Med Assoc 178:133, 1981.

78. Marks LJ, Steinke J, Podolsky S, Egdahl RH: Hypoglycemia associated with neoplasia. Ann NY Acad Sci 230:147, 1974.
79. Markowitz J, Rappaport A, Scott AC: The function of the hepatic artery in the dog. Am J Dig Dis 16:344, 1949.
80. McLain DL, Nagode LA, Wilson GP, Kociba GL: Alkaline phosphatase and its isoenzymes in normal cats and in cats with biliary obstruction. J Am Anim Hosp Assoc 14:94, 1978.
81. Megey E: Liver disease and nutrition, progress in hepatology. Gastroenterology 74:770, 1978.
82. Merino GD, Jetzer T, Doizaki WMD, Najarian JS: Methionine-induced hepatic coma in dogs. Am J Surg 130:11, 1075.
83. Meyer DJ, Noonan NE: Liver tests in dogs receiving anticonvulsant drugs (diphenylhydantoin and primidone). J Am Anim Hosp Assoc 17:261, 1981.
84. Meyer DJ, Iverson WO, Terell TG: Obstructive jaundice associated with chronic active hepatitis in a dog. J Am Vet Med Assoc 176:41, 1980.
85. Meyer DJ, Strombeck DR, Stone EA, et al: Ammonia tolerance test in clinically normal dogs and in dogs with portosystemic shunts. J Am Vet Med Assoc 173:377, 1978.
86. Mia AS, Koger HD: Comparative studies on serum arginase and transaminase in hepatic necrosis in various species of domestic animals. Vet Clin Pathol 8:9, 1979.
87. Murdoch DB: Jaundice in the dog. J Small Anim Pract 17:119, 1976.
88. Murray M, Robinson PB, McKeating FJ, Lauder IM: Peptic ulceration in the dog: A clinicopathological study. Vet Rec 91:441, 1972.
89. Nash AJ: Phenytoin toxicity: A fatal case in the dog with hepatitis and jaundice. Vet Rec 1:280, 1977.
90. Neufeld JL, Brandt RW: Case report: Cholangiohepatitis in a cat associated with a coccidia-like organism. Can Vet J 15:156, 1974.
91. Osborne CA, Stevens JB, Lees GE, et al: Clinical significance of bilirubinuria. Comp Cont Ed 2:897, 1980.
92. Patnaik AK, Hurvitz AI, Lieberman PH: Canine hepatic neoplasms: A clinicopathologic study. Vet Path 17:553, 1980.
93. Polzin DJ, Stowe CJ, O'Leary TP, et al: Acute hepatic necrosis associated with the administration of mebendazole. J Am Vet Med Assoc 179:1013, 1981.
94. Preisig R, Gocke DC, Morris TQ, Bradley SE: Chronic hepatic injury following experimental viral hepatitis in the dog. Experientia 22:701, 1966.
95. Prouty DL: Hepatoencephalopathy due to portacaval shunt in a dog. J Am Vet Med Assoc 167:756, 1975.
96. Rappaport AM: Anatomic Considerations. *In* Schiff L (ed): *Diseases of the Liver,* 4th ed., J. B. Lippincott Co., Philadelphia, pp. 1–43, 1975.
97. Rogers WA, Ruebner BH: A retrospective study of probably glucocorticoid-induced hepatopathy in dogs. J Am Vet Med Assoc 170:603, 1977.
98. Rogers WA: Source of serum alkaline phosphatase in clinically normal and diseased dogs: A clinical study. J Am Vet Med Assoc 168:934, 1976.
99. Rogers WA, Suter PF, Breznock EM, Reubner BH: Intrahepatic arteriovenous fistulae in a dog resulting in portal hypertension, portacaval shunts and reversal of portal blood flow. J Am Anim Hosp Assoc 13:470, 1975.
100. Rogoff TM, Lipsky PE: Role of the Kupffer cells in local and systemic immune responses. Gastroenterology 80:854, 1981.
101. Rojkind M, Kershenobich D: Hepatic Fibrosis. Prog Liver Dis, 5:294, 1976.
102. Rosen HM, Yoshimura N, Hodgman JM, Fischer JE: Plasma amino-acid pattern in hepatic encephalopathy of differing etiology. Gastroenterology 74:483, 1977.
103. Rothenbacker H, Lindquist WD: Liver cirrhosis and pancreatitis in a cat infected with *Amphimerus pseudofellneus*. J Am Vet Med Assoc 143: 1099, 1963.
104. Saini PK, Saini SK: Origin of serum alkaline phosphatase in the dog. Am J Vet Res 39:1510, 1978.
105. Schall WD: Laboratory diagnosis of hepatic disease. Vet Clin North Am 6:679, 1976.
106. Schall WD, Chapman WL, Finco DR, et al: Cholelithiasis in dogs. J Am Vet Med Assoc 163:469, 1973.
107. Schenker S, Breen JJ, Hoyumpa AM: Hepatic encephalopathy, current status. Gastroenterology 66:131, 1974.
108. Scheuer PJ: *Liver Biopsy Interpretation,* 2nd ed., Williams & Wilkins, Baltimore, 1973.
109. Schmidt S, Suter PF: Indirect and direct determination of the portal vein pressure in normal and abnormal dogs and normal cats. Am J Vet Rad Soc 21:246, 1980.
110. Sherding RG: Hepatic encephalopathy in the dog. Comp Cont Ed 1:55, 1979.
111. Shull RM, Hornbuckle W: Diagnostic use of serum gamma glutamyltransferase in canine liver disease. Am J Vet Res 40:1321, 1979.
112. Shull RM, Tasker JB, Hiltz FL: A computerized retrospective study of liver enzyme concentrations in dogs. Vet Clin Pathol 7:13, 1978.
113. Simpson ST, Hribernik TN: Portosystemic shunt in the dog: Two case reports. J Small Anim Pract 17:163, 1976.
114. Smart ME, Downey RS, Stockdale PHG: Toxoplasmosis in a cat associated with cholangitis and progressive pancreatitis. Can Vet J 14:313, 1973.
115. Spano JS, August JR, Henderson RA, et al: Serum γ-glutamyl transpeptidase activity in healthy cats and cats with induced hepatic disease. Am J Vet Res 44:2049, 1983.
116. Starzl TE, Porter KA, Watanake K, Putna CW: Effects of insulin, glucagon and insulin/glucagon infusions on liver morphology and cell division after complete portacaval shunt in dogs. Lancet 1:821, 1976.
117. Starzl TE, Porter KA, Putnam CW: Intraportal insulin protects from the liver injury of portacaval shunt in dogs. Lancet 2:1741, 1975.
118. Sternlieb I, Twedt DC, Johnson GF, et al: Structural changes in inherited hepatic copper toxicity in Bedlington terriers. Gastroenterology 71:930, 1976.
119. Strombeck DR: *Small Animal Gastroenterology.* Stonegate Publishing Co., Davis, 1979.
120. Strombeck DR: Clinicopathologic features of primary and metastatic neoplastic disease of the liver in dogs. J Am Vet Med Assoc 173:267, 1978.

121. Strombeck DR, Gribble D: Chronic active hepatitis in the dog. J Am Vet Med Assoc 173:380, 1978.
122. Strombeck DR, Rogers Q: Plasma amino acid concentrations in dogs with hepatic disease. J Am Vet Med Assoc 173:93, 1978.
123. Strombeck DR, Breznock EM, McNeel S: Surgical treatment for portosystemic shunts in two dogs. J Am Vet Med Assoc 170:1317, 1977.
124. Strombeck DR, Krum S, Meyer D, Kappesser RM: Hypoglycemia and hypoinsulinemia associated with hepatoma in a dog. J Am Vet Med Assoc 169:811, 1976.
125. Strombeck DR, Krum S, Rogers Q: Coagulopathy and encephalopathy in a dog with acute hepatic necrosis. J Am Vet Med Assoc 169:813, 1976.
126. Strombeck DR, Rogers W, Gribble D: Chronic active hepatic disease in a dog. J Am Vet Med Assoc 169:802, 1976.
127. Strombeck DR, Weiser MG, Kaneko JJ: Hyperammonemia and hepatic encephalopathy in the dog. J Am Vet Med Assoc 166:1105, 1975.
128. Sturtevant F, Hoffman WE, Dorner JC: The effect of three anticonvulsant drugs and ACTH on canine serum alkaline phosphatase. J Am Anim Hosp Assoc 13:754, 1977.
129. Suter PF: Portal vein anomalies in the dog: Their angiographic diagnosis. J Am Vet Radiol 16:84, 1975.
130. Swanson JF, Breider MA: Hepatic failure following mebendazole administration to a dog. J Am Vet Med Assoc 181:72, 1982.
131. Thompson SW, Sparano BM, Diener RM: Vacuoles in the hepatocytes of cortisone-treated dogs. Am J Pathol 63:135, 1971.
132. Thornburg LP, Moody GM: Hepatic amyloidosis in a dog. J Am Anim Hosp Assoc 17:721, 1981.
133. Tuzhilin SA, Podolsky AE, Dreilling DA: Hepatic lesions in pancreatitis: Clinicoexperimental data. Am J Gastroenterol 64:108, 1975.
134. Twedt DC: Jaundice, hepatic trauma, and hepatic encephalopathy. Vet Clin North Am 11:121, 1981.
135. Twedt DC, Sternlieb I, Gilbertson DR: Clinical, morphologic and chemical studies in copper toxicosis of Bedlington terriers. J Am Vet Med Assoc 175:269, 1979.
136. Uribe M, Farca A, Marquez MA, et al: Treatment of chronic portalsystemic encephalopathy and bromocriptine: A double-blind controlled trial. Gastroenterology 76:1347, 1979.
137. Van Canteren H, Marsboom R, et al: Safety studies evaluating the effect of mebendazole on liver function in dogs. J Am Vet Med Assoc 183:93, 1983.
138. Vitums A: Portosystemic communications in animals with hepatic cirrhosis and malignant lymphoma. J Am Vet Med Assoc 138:31, 1961.
139. Vitums A: Portosystemic communications in the dog. Acta Anat 39:271, 1959.
140. Vulgamott JC, Tumwald GH, King CK, et al: Congenital portalcaval anomalies in the cat: Two case reports. J Am Anim Hosp Assoc 16:915, 1981.
141. Wigton DH, Kociba GJ, Hoover EA: Infectious canine hepatitis: Animal model for viral-induced disseminated intravascular coagulation. Blood 47:287, 1976.
142. Young JT: Source, fate and possible significance of elevated serum alkaline phosphatase in nonicteric animals with partial biliary obstruction. J Am Anim Hosp Assoc 10:415, 1975.
143. Zieze L, Doizaki WM, Zieve FJ: Synergism between mercaptans and ammonia or fatty acids in the production of coma: A possible role for mercaptans in the pathogenesis of hepatic coma. J Lab Clin Med 83:16, 1974.

CHAPTER

14

Radiology of the Gastrointestinal System

EVERETT ARONSON
COLIN B. CARRIG
JIMMY C. LATTIMER

Radiography of the gastrointestinal system should not be exclusively relied on to arrive at a definitive diagnosis. However, in conjunction with the patient's history, physical examination, blood tests, and other diagnostic procedures such as ultrasonography, endoscopy, and biopsy, radiography has an important role in establishing the final diagnosis.

Survey radiographs of the head can be used to diagnose radiopaque pharyngeal foreign bodies, pharyngeal tumors and abscesses, dental caries, periapical abscesses, periodontal disease, and oral neoplasia. Special radiographic studies can be performed to evaluate the salivary glands and the normal swallowing mechanism. Esophageal abnormalities such as megaesophagus, persistent right aortic arch, esophageal foreign body, perforation, diverticulum and gastroesophageal intussusception can be diagnosed by survey radiographs and contrast studies of the esophagus.

Abdominal radiography is indicated to confirm or differentiate suspected clinical disease, determine the extent of involvement of known clinical disease, and seek evidence of tumor metastases; it is also useful as a screening procedure for diseases with obscure clinical signs.[67] Abdominal radiography involves the evaluation of abdominal organs based on their location, size, shape, and density.[67]

In this chapter, the normal radiographic anatomy of the gastrointestinal system will be described. Examples of gastrointestinal abnormalities that can be diagnosed by survey radiography will be presented. The indications, contraindications, complications, and techniques for performing special procedures including sialography, esophagography, upper and lower gastrointestinal studies, and portography will be discussed in detail.

The Oral Cavity

SURVEY FILMS

Because of the wide variation in the conformation of the heads of different breeds of dogs it is imperative to have good positioning when radiographing the head. To ensure proper positioning and to prevent patient motion during the exposure, all animals radiographed should be anesthetized.

A complete dental study can be performed with six radiographs, utilizing a combination of extraoral and intraoral film placement.[92, 104] Four films are needed for the lateral open-mouth oblique projections of the right and left maxillary and mandibular dental arcades, for evaluation of the canine, premolar, and molar teeth. The incisors are evaluated with oblique dorsoventral (DV) and ventrodorsal (VD) radiographs of the maxilla and mandible, using regular film placed intraorally in a cardboard holder

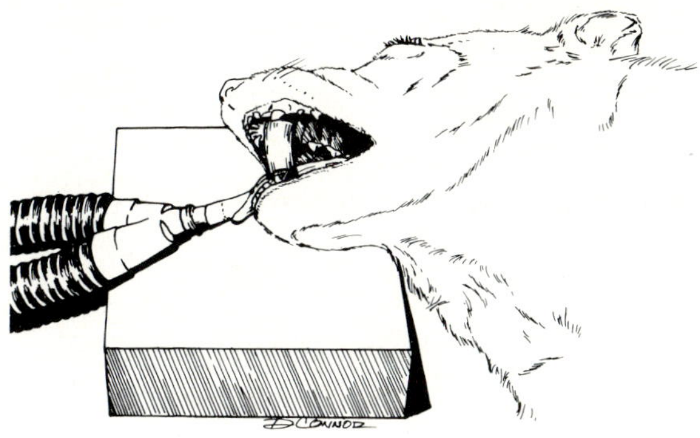

Figure 14–1. Proper position for radiography of maxillary dental arcade. The animal is placed in lateral recumbency with the affected side down. The mandible is elevated and the animal's mouth is held open and rotated 30° along its longitudinal axis. A wedge sponge may be used to elevate the mandible.

rather than a radiographic cassette. The exposure factors must be increased to compensate for the absence of screens.

For radiography of the maxillary dental arcade, the patient is placed in lateral recumbency with the mouth held open by wedging radiolucent material, such as a cork, sponge, or roll of bandage, between the teeth. A radiopaque metal mouth speculum should not be used because the image will be superimposed over the dental arcades. The animal's head is rotated on its long axis by lifting the mandible away from the film so that the maxillary dental arcade closest to the film is clearly projected onto the film without superimposition of overlying structures. The animal's head is kept in this position by using a foam wedge under the elevated mandible (Fig. 14–1). Tabletop technique using fine screens and par-speed x-ray film will produce satisfactory radiographs. The x-ray beam is centered over the fourth premolar. To avoid confusion when identifying the maxillary arcades, both right (R) and left (L) film markers are used.[58, 104] The appropriate marker is placed below the dental arcade being x-rayed, and the other marker is placed above the nose to indicate the opposite maxillary arcade in silhouette (Fig. 14–2). The mandibular arcade is radiographed in a similar manner by elevating the maxilla off the film (Figs. 14–3 and 14–4). For radiography of the maxillary incisors, the patient is positioned in sternal recumbency and par-speed or high-speed x-ray film in a cardboard holder is placed in the animal's mouth. The animal's mouth is closed gently on the film to keep it in place. The dorsal ventral beam is centered on the central incisors and directed caudad at a 20° to 30° angle, which is roughly perpendicular to the long axis of

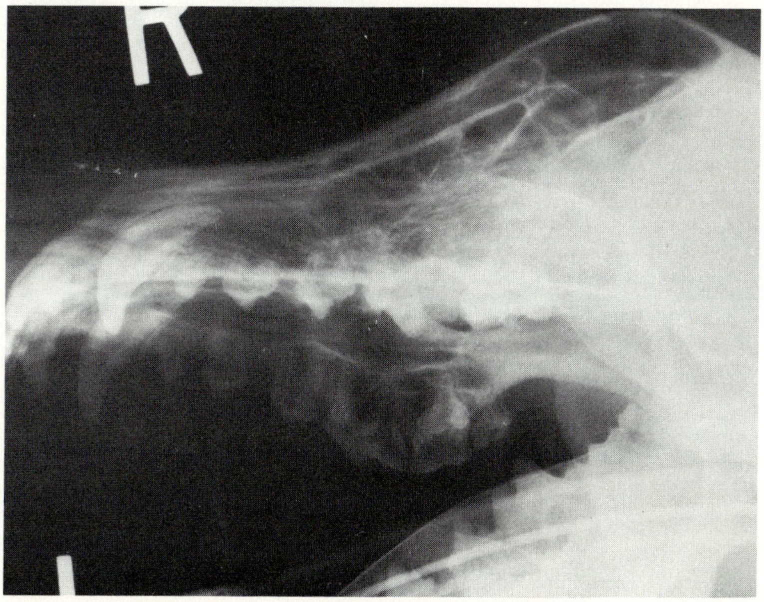

Figure 14–2. Normal radiograph of oblique projection of maxillary dental arcade.

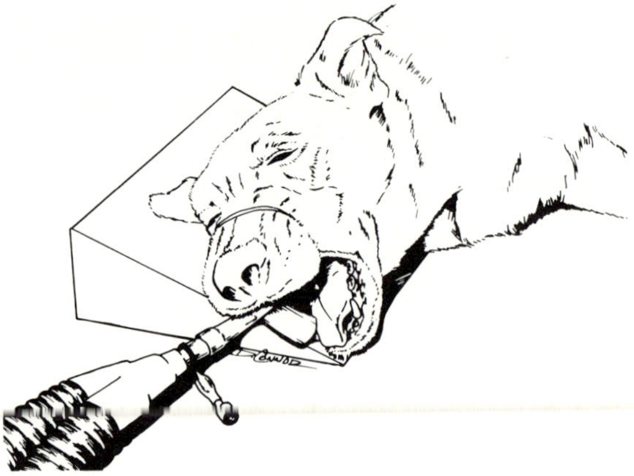

Figure 14–3. Proper position for radiography of mandibular dental arcade. The animal is placed in lateral recumbency with the affected side down. The maxilla is elevated, and the animal's mouth is held open and rotated 30° along its longitudinal axis. A wedge sponge may be used to elevate the maxilla.

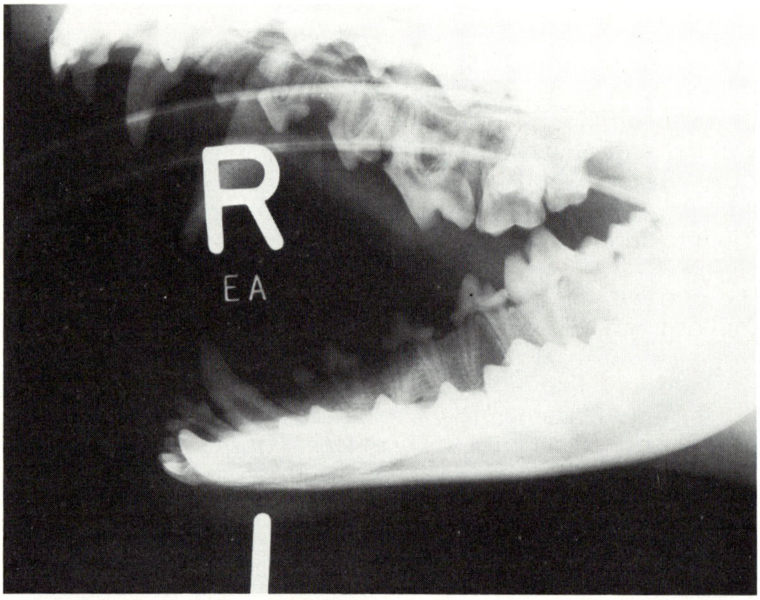

Figure 14–4. Normal radiograph of oblique projection of mandibular dental arcade.

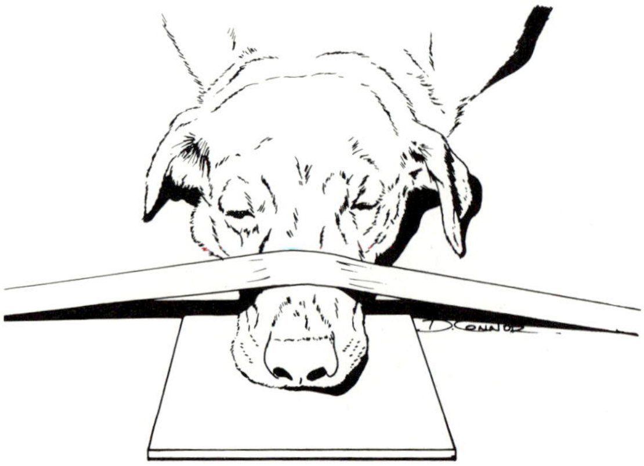

Figure 14–5. Proper position for radiography of maxillary incisors. The animal is placed in sternal recumbency. A film in a cardboard holder is placed in the animal's mouth, and the x-ray beam is centered on the central incisors directed at a 20° caudad angle.

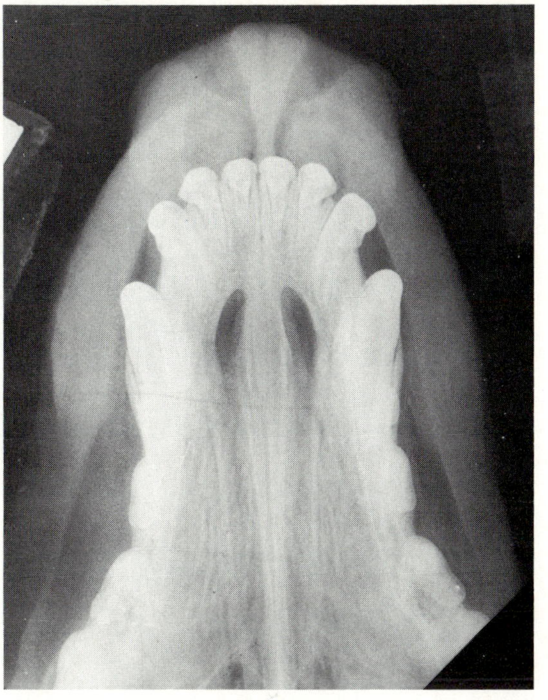

Figure 14–6. Normal intraoral radiograph of maxillary incisors.

the incisors (Figs. 14–5 and 14–6). For radiography of the mandibular incisors the animal is positioned in dorsal recumbency. Film placement, beam centering, and angulation are the same as was described for the maxillary incisors. The radiographs are marked with the appropriate DV or VD and R or L markers (Figs. 14–7 and 14–8).

NORMAL ANATOMY

The dog has 28 deciduous teeth, including three incisors, one canine, and three premolar teeth in each side of the mandibular and maxillary dental arcades. Calcification of the tooth crowns occurs at 20 days while calcification of the tooth roots is complete between 40 and 50 days.[104] The permanent teeth develop in a crypt immediately below the deciduous teeth (Fig. 14–9). The crowns of the permanent teeth begin to calcify at six weeks of age except for the last molar teeth of the mandibular and maxillary arcades which calcify at 15 and 16 weeks, respectively.[40] Following calcification of the crowns, the roots calcify and the roots of the deciduous teeth are resorbed. These changes occur as early as nine weeks of age in the incisor teeth, whereas it takes approximately 13 weeks in the case of second, third and fourth premolar teeth.[40] Eruption of the permanent teeth begins at 14 weeks for the lower incisor teeth and ends at 7 months with the eruption of the last molar teeth.[40]

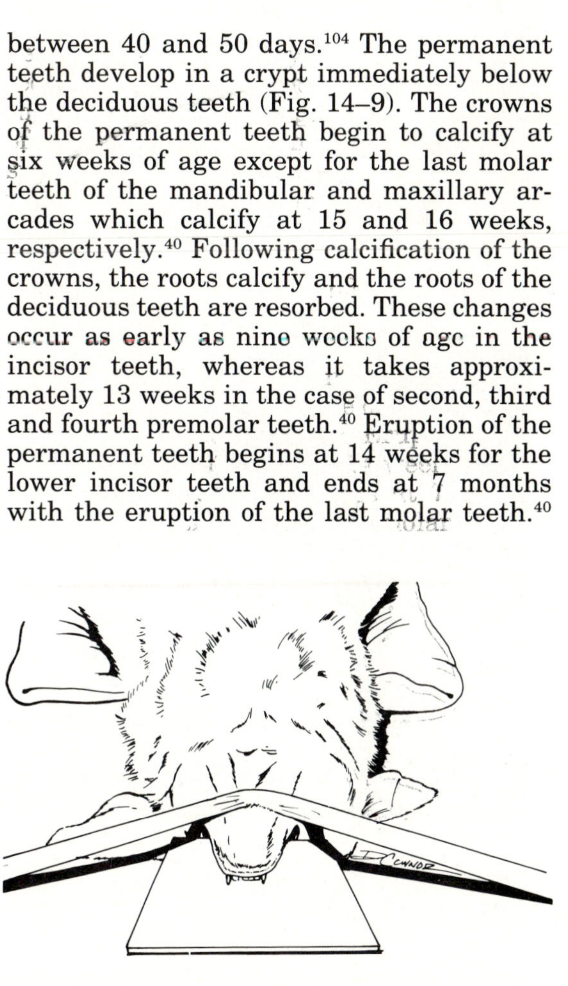

Figure 14–7. Proper position for radiography of mandibular incisors. The animal is placed in dorsal recumbency. A film in a cardboard holder is placed in the animal's mouth, and the x-ray beam is centered on the central incisors directed at 20° caudad angle.

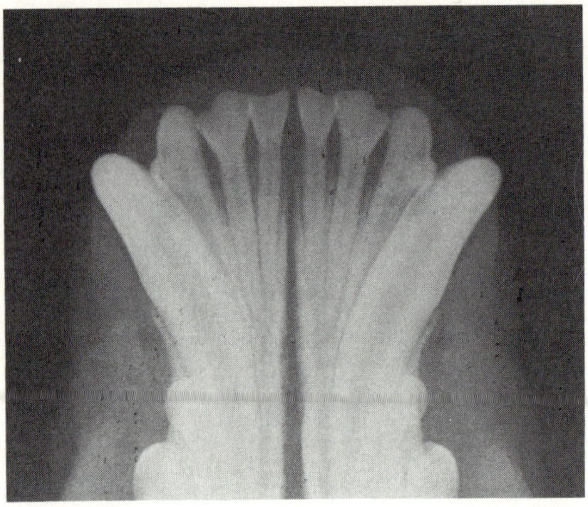

Figure 14–8. Normal intraoral radiograph of mandibular incisors.

The dog's permanent dental formula, consisting of 42 teeth, is

$$2 \times \frac{3\text{-}1\text{-}4\text{-}2}{3\text{-}1\text{-}4\text{-}3}.$$

Features of the permanent teeth that can be identified radiographically include the enamel, tubercle, amelocemental junction, periodontal membrane (represented by the radiolucent zone between the tooth root and the adjacent dense bone lining the tooth socket), lamina dura, cementum, dentin, and pulp cavity (Fig. 14–10).[104] At the base of the pulp cavity is the apical foramen. It is wide in young dogs but gets smaller as the dog ages. Other changes that occur in the teeth as the dog ages include narrowing of the pulp cavity and regression of the alveolar crest; also, the lamina dura becomes less distinct.

The cat has 26 deciduous and 30 permanent teeth. The dental formulas are, respectively,

$$2 \times \frac{3\text{-}1\text{-}3}{3\text{-}1\text{-}2}$$

and

$$2 \times \frac{3\text{-}1\text{-}3\text{-}1}{3\text{-}1\text{-}2\text{-}1}.$$

DENTAL DISEASE

Caries

Caries appear as radiolucent defects that can occur in any area of the enamel. They can vary in size from a small dot to a large ragged crater and must be differentiated from tooth fractures (Figs. 14–11 and 14–12).[103]

Periodontal Disease

Since periodontal disease involves the gingiva, a structure that cannot be evaluated radiographically, the diagnosis is primarily

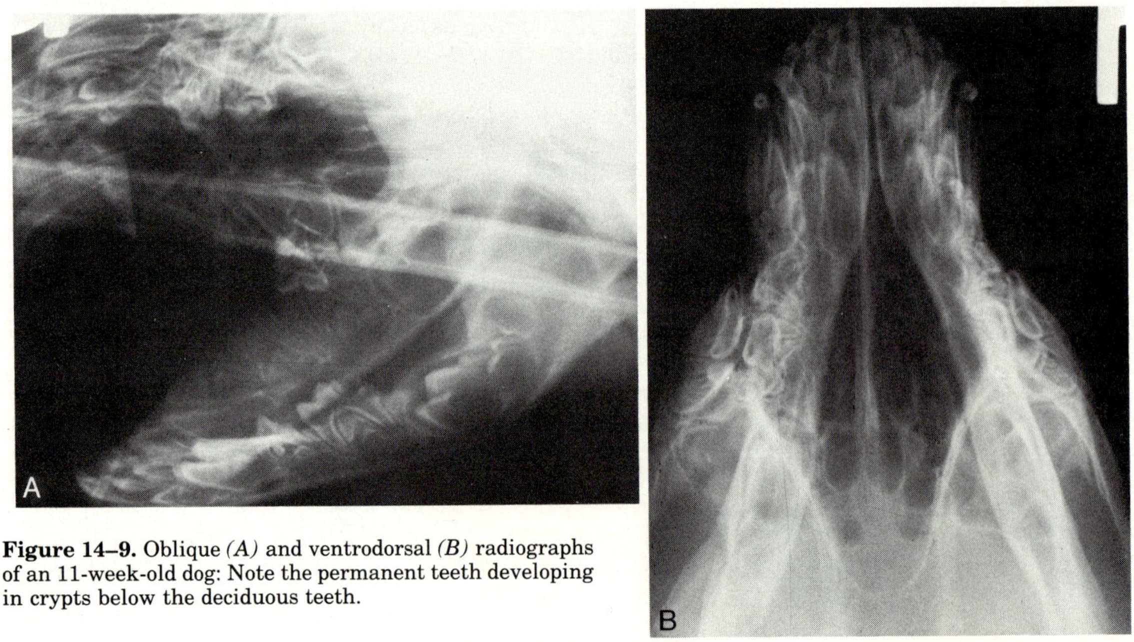

Figure 14–9. Oblique *(A)* and ventrodorsal *(B)* radiographs of an 11-week-old dog: Note the permanent teeth developing in crypts below the deciduous teeth.

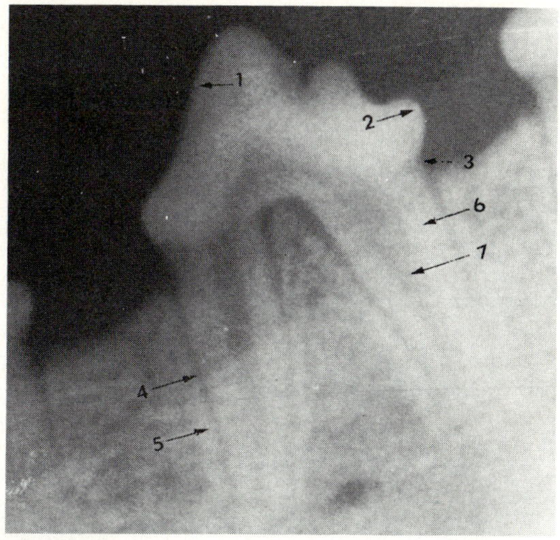

Figure 14–10. Radiographic features of a normal tooth include (1) enamel, (2) tubercle, (3) amelocemental junction, (4) periodontal membrane, (5) lamina dura, (6) dentin, and (7) pulp cavity.

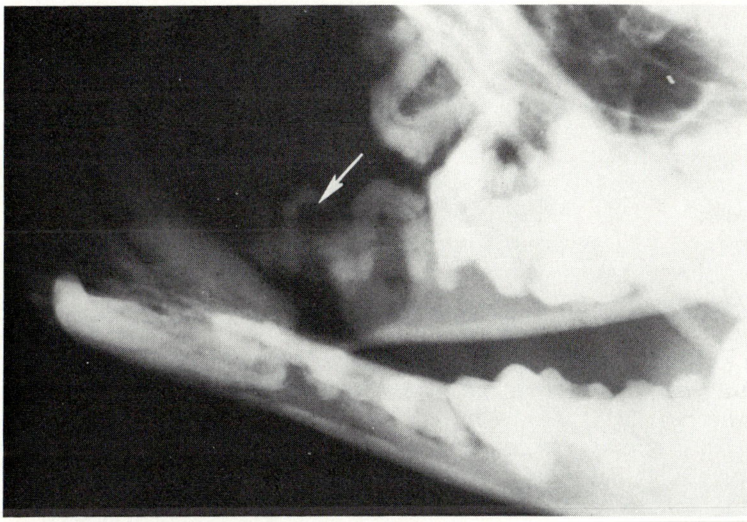

Figure 14–11. Dental caries. There is a radiolucent defect *(arrow)* in the enamel of the crown of the second mandibular premolar.

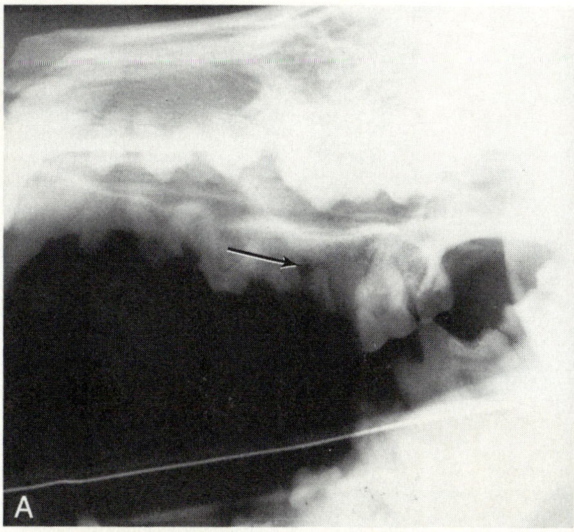

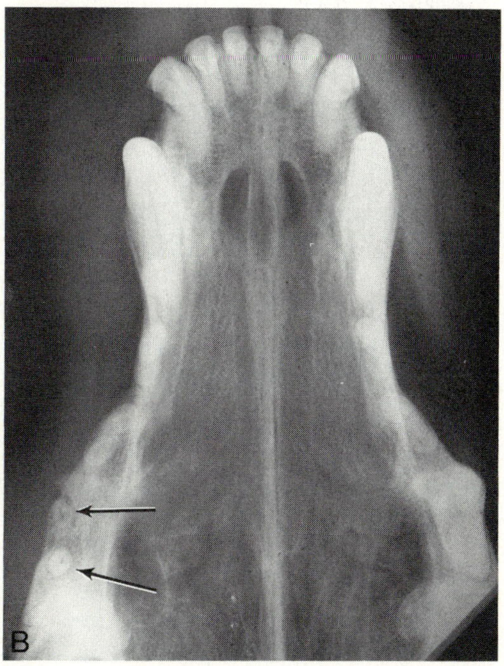

Figure 14–12. Lateral *(A)* and ventrodorsal *(B)* radiographs of a fractured tooth. Note the fractured roots of the upper right fourth maxillary premolar *(arrows)*. There is a periapical abscess associated with the caudal root.

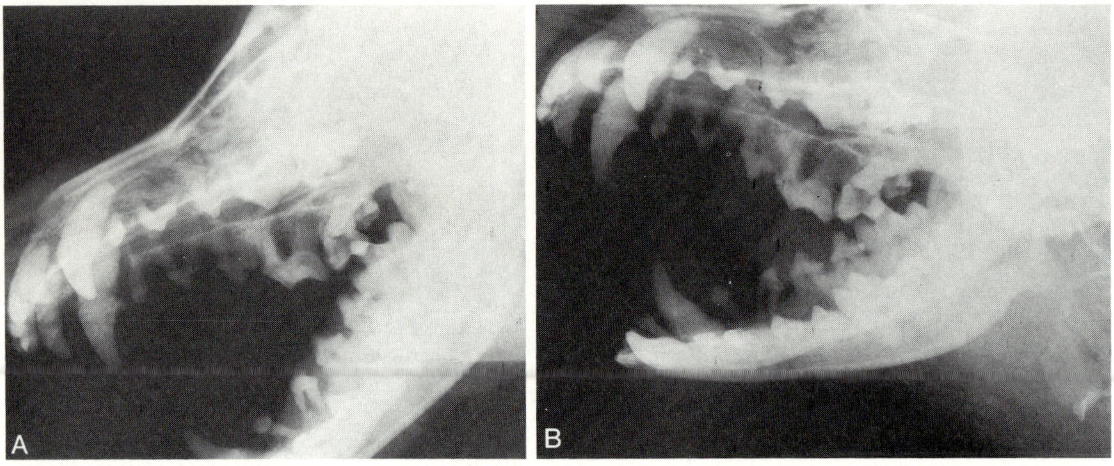

Figure 14–13. *A,* Periodontal disease of the maxilla; note the marked rarefaction and resorption of the supporting bone around the canine tooth, and the first, second, and third premolars. *B,* Periodontal disease of the mandible; there is marked rarefaction and resorption of the supporting bone around the first, second, and third premolars.

a clinical one, with radiography utilized to determine the extent of the disease and whether it has progressed into the periodontal space or around the root of the tooth.[103]

Radiographic signs of periodontal disease include rarefaction and rounding of the amelocemental junction, changes in the width of the periodontal space around the tooth root, and changes in density of the supporting bone. Changes in the bone due to infection include rarefaction, destruction, or an increase in density (sclerosis) of the bone (Fig. 14–13).[103]

Rarefaction is the easiest change to recognize and is the best indicator of the lesion's aggressiveness. The prognosis of the disease depends largely on the amount and distribution of the alveolar bone remaining around the tooth and the apposition of the remaining bone to the root.[103]

The most common systemic diseases affecting the teeth and the supporting bone are nutritional and secondary renal hyperparathyroidism.[103] Early in the course of the disease a symmetrical radiolucent area is seen surrounding the tooth roots with resorption of the lamina dura. As the disease

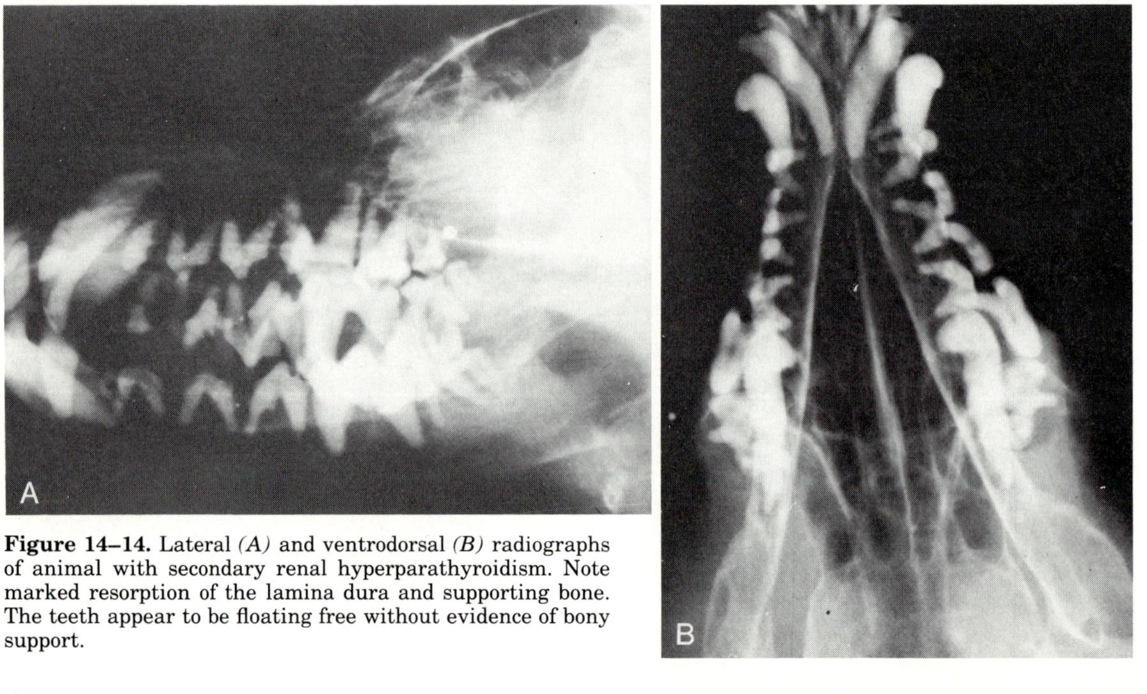

Figure 14–14. Lateral *(A)* and ventrodorsal *(B)* radiographs of animal with secondary renal hyperparathyroidism. Note marked resorption of the lamina dura and supporting bone. The teeth appear to be floating free without evidence of bony support.

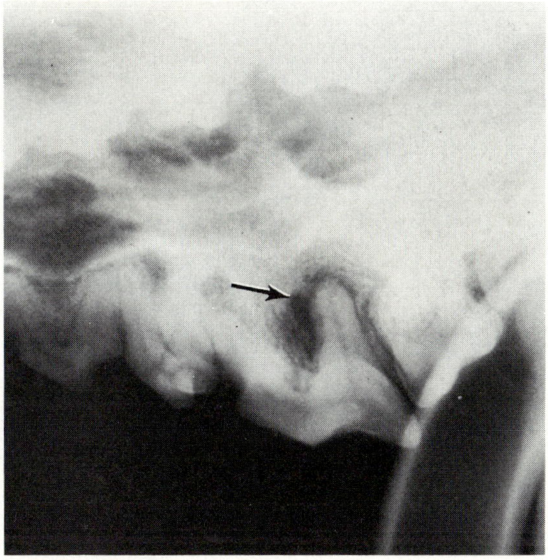

Figure 14–15. Periapical abscess. Note the large radiolucent area surrounding the caudal root of upper fourth premolar (arrow).

progresses, there is further demineralization of the bone and the teeth appear to be floating free without evidence of the bony support (Fig. 14–14).[59, 103]

Periapical Disease

Periapical disease is a pathological process surrounding the apex of one or more roots of the tooth, which can occur as an extension of periodontal disease, from trauma, cysts, hematogenous infections, tumors, or inflammation or necrosis of the pulp cavity.[103] The radiographic changes are consistent with signs of chronic infection and are characterized by a radiolucent zone with a sclerotic border surrounding the root of the tooth, with or without root resorption (Fig. 14–15).[103] It is not uncommon for an abscess of the upper fourth premolar tooth or the first molar tooth to form a draining fistulous tract cranial to the eye on the dorsum of the nasal bone.

ORAL NEOPLASIA

When neoplasia is present, lateral, ventrodorsal, lateral open-mouth oblique, and ventrodorsal open-mouth projections are necessary to properly evaluate the oral cavity. The proper positioning for these views, except for the ventrodorsal open-mouth projection, has been previously described. The ventrodorsal open-mouth projection is performed with the animal in dorsal recumbency, with the maxilla parallel to the film. The mandible is pulled distally, opening the mouth as wide as possible. The beam is centered at the level of the third premolar teeth perpendicular to the film (Fig. 14–16). This view allows visualization of the maxilla without superimposition of the mandible (Fig. 14–17).[58, 92]

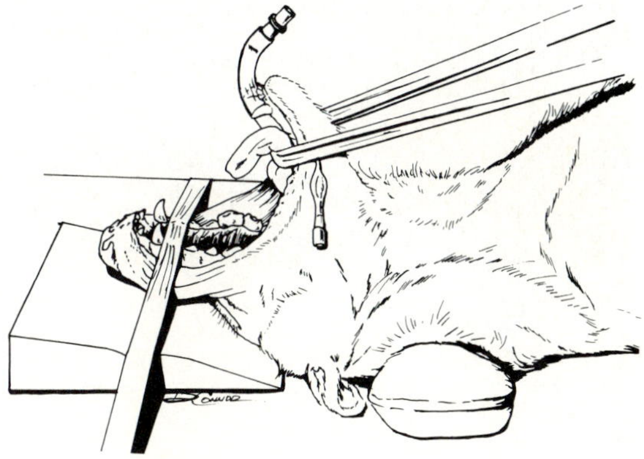

Figure 14–16. Correct position for open-mouth ventrodorsal projection. The animal is placed in dorsal recumbency with the maxilla parallel to the film. The mandible is pulled distally and the beam is centered at the level of the third premolar.

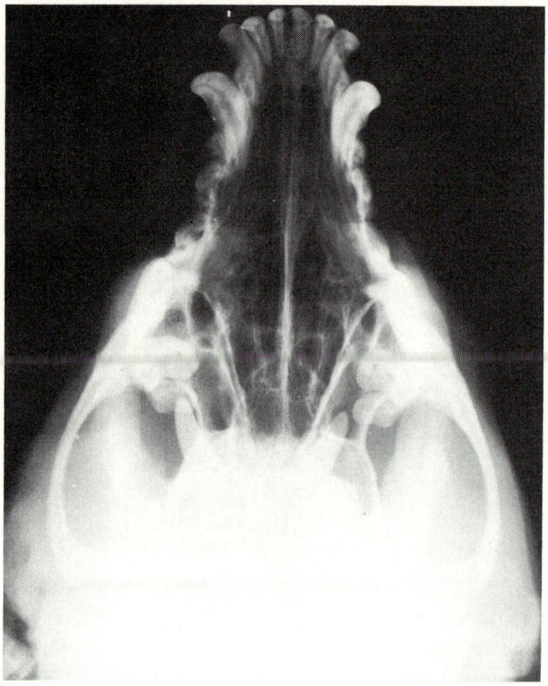

Figure 14–17. Normal radiograph of open-mouth ventrodorsal projection of the maxilla.

Common benign oral pharyngeal tumors seen in the dog include epulis and oral papilloma. Malignant melanoma, squamous cell carcinoma, and fibrosarcoma are the three most common malignant oral tumors found in dogs.[11, 96] In the cat the most common oral tumors are squamous cell carcinoma and fibrosarcoma.[10, 22] Radiography can be used to help differentiate malignant tumors from benign tumors. Benign tumors are usually well-marginated, soft-tissue masses which lack the bony destruction and invasiveness associated with malignant tumors (Fig. 14–18).

Malignant tumors affecting the gingiva and teeth, such as malignant melanoma, squamous cell carcinoma, fibrosarcoma and ameloblastoma, often appear radiographically as soft-tissue dense masses that are locally invasive with poorly defined margins causing marked lysis and destruction of the supporting bony structures. Teeth in the

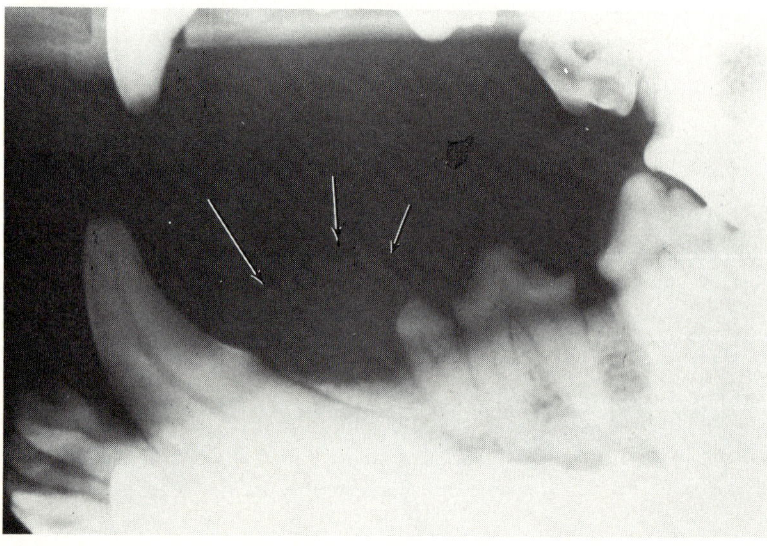

Figure 14–18. Epulis. Note the soft-tissue mass between the canine and first premolar tooth (arrows). There is slight bony erosion of the mandible. (Courtesy Dr. Linda Konde, Colorado State University.)

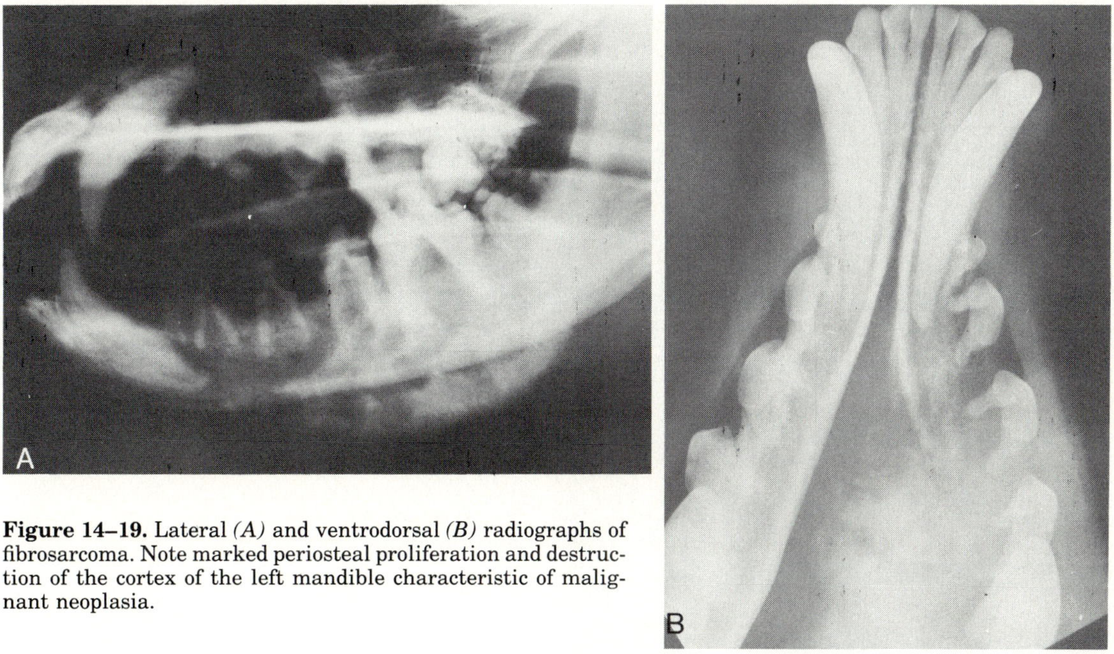

Figure 14–19. Lateral *(A)* and ventrodorsal *(B)* radiographs of fibrosarcoma. Note marked periosteal proliferation and destruction of the cortex of the left mandible characteristic of malignant neoplasia.

vicinity of the tumor may be displaced or absent (Figs. 14–19, 14–20, and 14–21).

An odontoma is a non-neoplastic hamartoma consisting of a mixture of enamel, dentin, and cementum. Radiographically it can appear as an expansile soft-tissue mass containing hundreds of irregularly shaped calcified densities resembling small teeth (Fig. 14–22).[60]

Pharynx

The pharynx is the common passage of the respiratory and digestive systems. It can be subdivided into the oropharynx, nasopharynx, and laryngopharyngeal and pharyngeal isthmus. On a lateral radiograph when there is good air contrast in the pharynx, the soft palate, epiglottis, hyoid apparatus, and cricoid cartilage can be identified (Fig. 14–23).[66] Plain film radiographic signs of pharnygeal disorders include changes in the contrast, size, shape, and location of the pharynx.[67]

Disorders of the pharynx that can be recognized radiographically include mass lesions, salivary cysts, inflammation, elongation of the soft palate, and foreign bodies (Figs. 14–24, 14–25, and 14–26). The location of the larynx is useful in determining the etiology of pharyngeal disorders.[67] The larynx is located on the midline and slightly cranial to the third cervical vertebra. The distance between the dorsal aspect of the larynx and the ventral body of the axis in most cases should not exceed the length of the body of the third cervical vertebra.[67] Dogs with short well-muscled necks are exceptions to this rule. Ventral displacement of the larynx and increased density in the pharynx are signs of neoplasia or abscessation in the pharyngeal or retropharyngeal region (Fig. 14–27). Squamous cell carcinoma, lymphosarcoma, thyroid adenocarcinoma, retropharyngeal lymphadenopathy due to metastasis are some of the more common neoplasms that affect this area.[67] Radiographic findings in abscessation or cellulitis secondary to a penetrating foreign body may include the presence of gas shadows in the surrounding soft tissue.

The dynamic action of swallowing and the disorders associated with it cannot be seen on plain film or contrast studies of the pharynx. Cinefluorography or videofluorography is necessary to study the complete act of swallowing. The normal oropharyngeal phase of swallowing, which begins with the formation of a bolus in the mouth and ends with its passage through the cricopharyngeal region, can be divided into oral, pharyngeal and cricopharyngeal stages.[89] The oral stage begins after food has been prehended and the stripping action of the tongue organizes a bolus in the oropharynx.

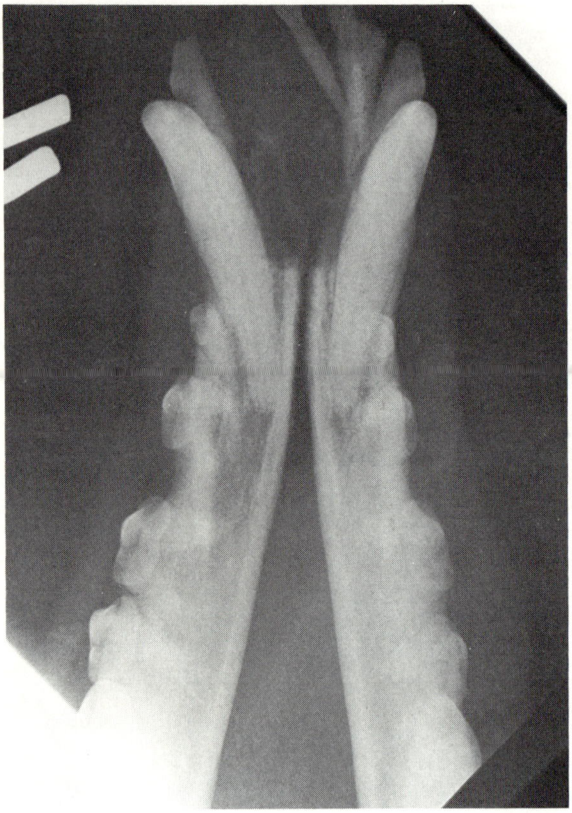

Figure 14–20. Squamous cell carcinoma. Note large soft-tissue dense mass causing marked lysis of the mandibular symphysis, soft tissue calcification, and displacement of the incisors. (Courtesy Dr. Linda Konde, Colorado State University.)

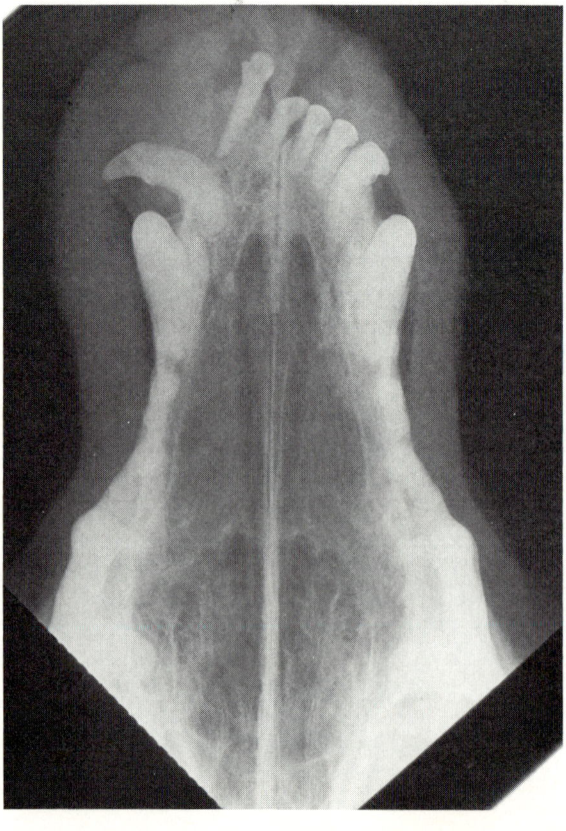

Figure 14–21. Malignant melanoma. Note soft-tissue dense mass displacing the right incisors and causing marked lysis of the right incisive bone. (Courtesy Dr. Linda Konde, Colorado State University.)

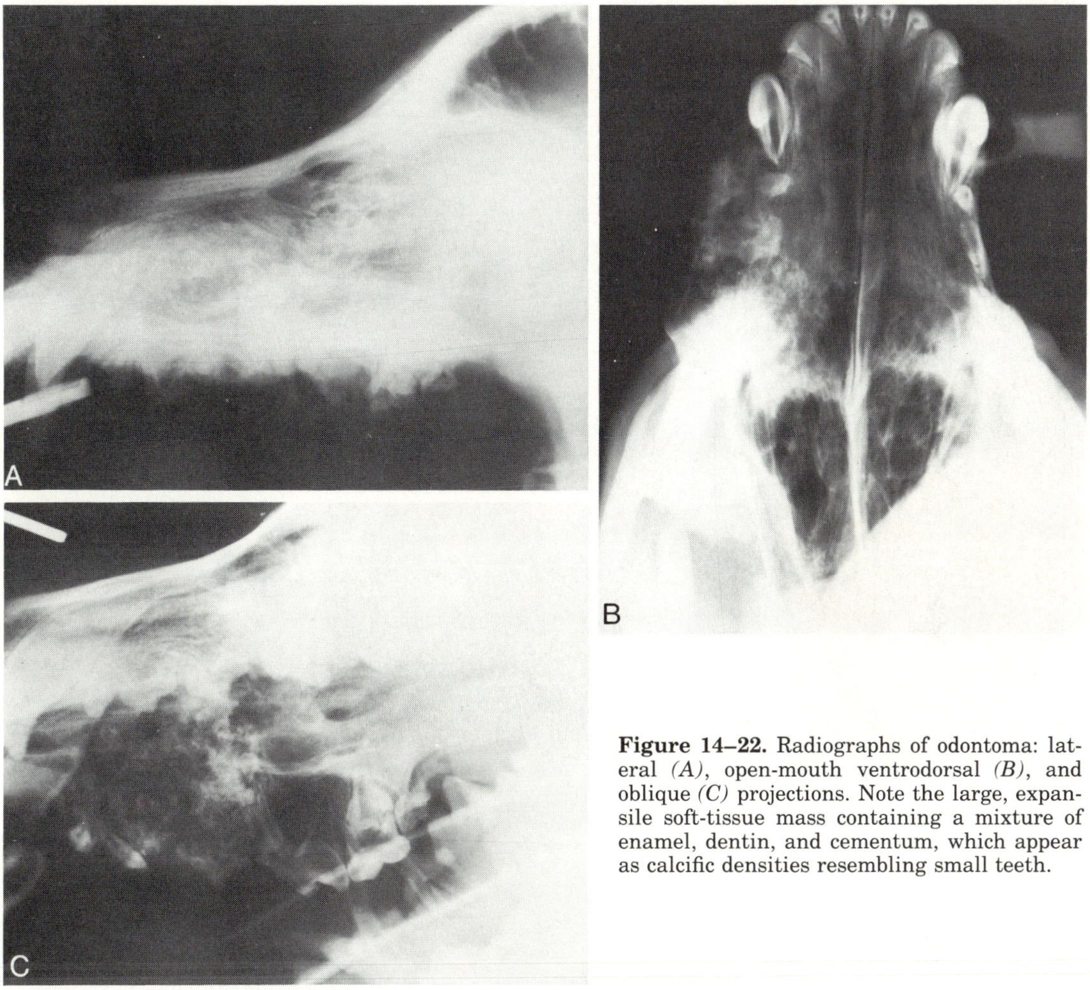

Figure 14–22. Radiographs of odontoma: lateral *(A)*, open-mouth ventrodorsal *(B)*, and oblique *(C)* projections. Note the large, expansile soft-tissue mass containing a mixture of enamel, dentin, and cementum, which appear as calcific densities resembling small teeth.

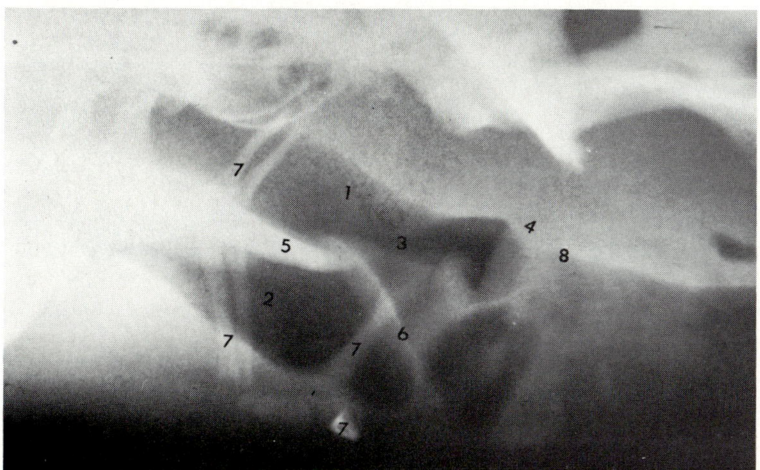

Figure 14–23. Regions of the pharynx: (1) nasopharynx, (2) oropharynx, (3) isthmus, (4) laryngopharynx, (5) soft palate, (6) epiglottis, (7) hyoid apparatus, and (8) cricoid cartilage.

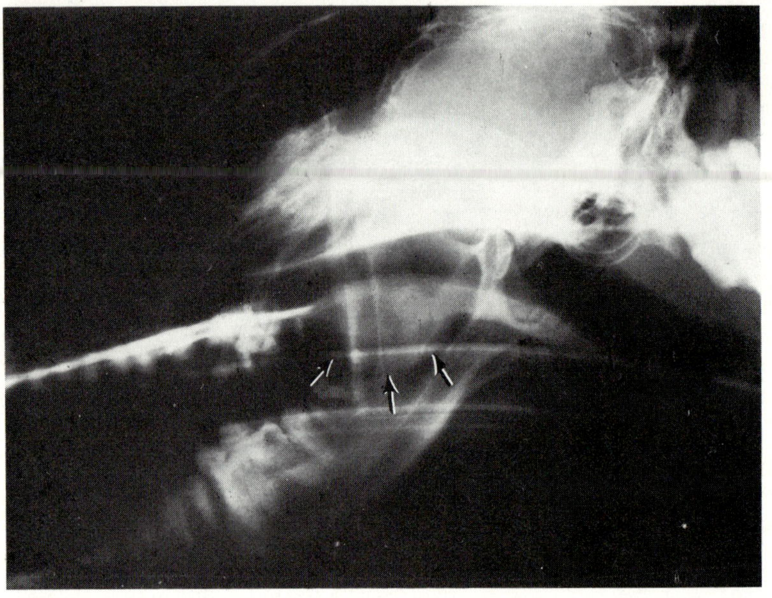

Figure 14–24. Fibrosarcoma of soft palate. Note dense soft-tissue mass in soft palate caudad to the last molar, causing narrowing of the oropharynx *(arrows)*.

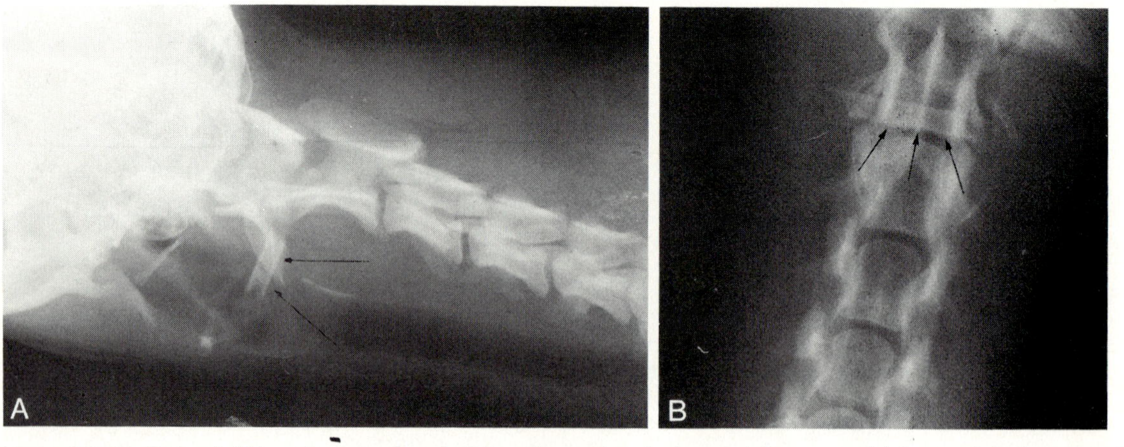

Figure 14–25. Lateral *(A)* and ventrodorsal *(B)* radiographs of pheasant bone caught in caudal pharyngeal isthmus *(arrows)*.

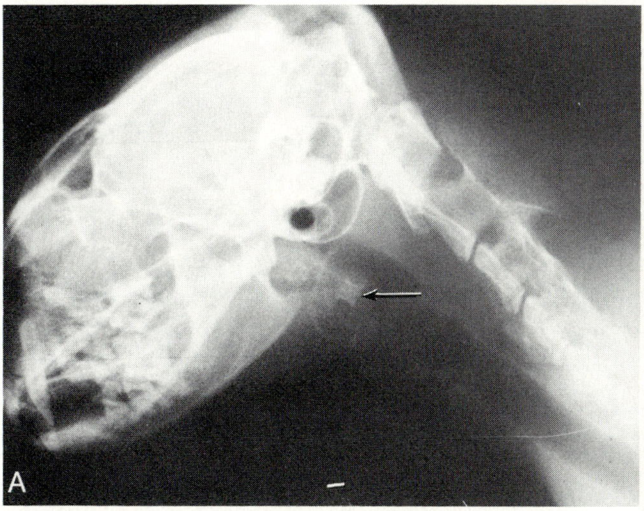

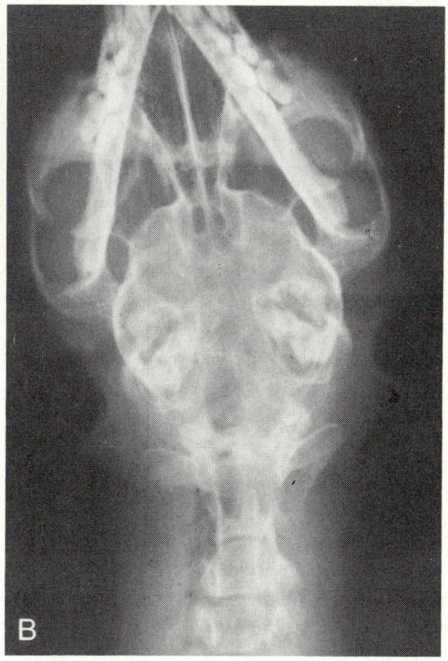

Figure 14–26. *A*, Lateral radiograph of radiopaque foreign body lodged in pharyngeal isthmus *(arrow)*. *B*, The foreign body is not well-visualized in this ventrodorsal projection.

The bolus is then propelled aborally to the base of the tongue. The pharyngeal phase consists of peristaltic contraction of the pharynx and propulsion of the bolus from the base of the tongue to the laryngopharynx. The cricopharyngeal stage begins with the opening of the cricopharyngeal sphincter and is coordinated with contraction of the pharynx allowing the bolus to pass into the esophagus. This stage ends with closure of the cricopharyngeal sphincter and relaxation of the pharynx.[89]

Survey films and contrast studies should be made in cases of oropharyngeal dysphagias to rule out gross structural abnormalities such as foreign bodies and extrinsic or intrinsic masses. However, these studies are inadequate to differentiate between the different types of oropharyngeal dysphagias. Dynamic studies such as videofluorography or preferentially, cinefluorography are essential to evaluate for functional disorders of the oropharyngeal swallowing phase.[89]

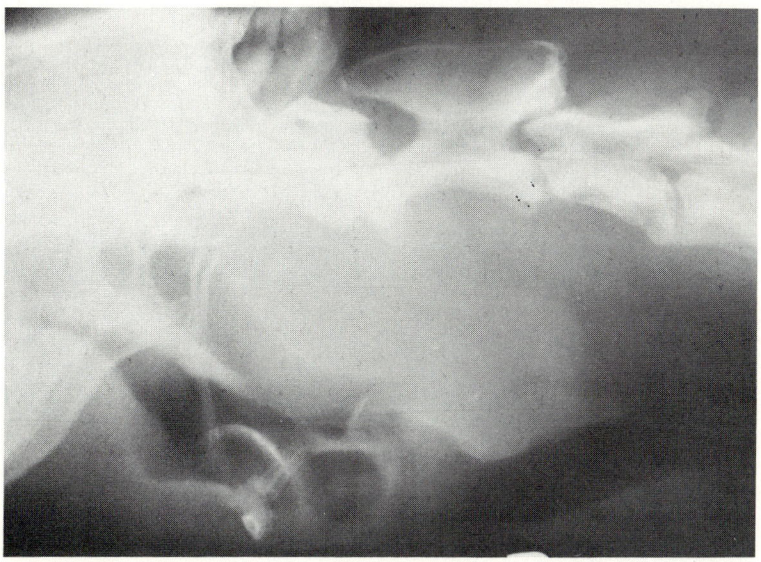

Figure 14–27. Thyroid adenocarcinoma. Note large, dense soft-tissue mass causing marked ventral displacement of the pharynx and larynx.

Oropharyngeal Dysphagias

Oropharyngeal dysphagias have been classified as three basic types of disorders: (1) oral stage dysphagias with deficits mainly due to a reduction of the tongue function; (2) pharyngeal dysphagias with poor contractility and transport function of the cranial and caudal pharyngeal constrictors; and (3) cricopharyngeal dysphagias with an absolute deficit in cricopharyngeal opening or closure, that is, incoordination between cricopharyngeal sphincter relaxation and pharyngeal contraction.[89] Table 14–1 describes radiographic signs useful for differentiation of these three basic types.

The major cineradiographic findings in dogs with oral dysphagias include poor bolus accumulation at the base of the tongue and diminished rostral and caudal movement of the tongue markedly reducing the efficiency of dorsal transport of food. Other findings include absence of a plunger-like action of the tongue during the pharyngeal stage, with failure to deliver contrast media to the larynopharynx resulting in the retention of contrast media in the oropharynx.[89]

The major cinefluorographic finding of pharyngeal dysphagias is incomplete pharyngeal contraction indicated by residual gas and contrast medium in the pharynx despite normal-appearing cricopharyngeal relaxation, with slow induction and slow progression of the peristaltic-like contraction from the rostral to the caudal pharynx. Other findings include retention of contrast medium in the intrapharyngeal opening and in the piriform recesses, and laryngotracheal inhalation of residual contrast media.[89]

Survey radiographs often show an abnormally large gas shadow in the cranial esophagus due to associated reduced esophageal motility; in contrast studies, some contrast medium is returned immediately caudal to the cricopharyngeal passage. Pharyngeal dysphagias often lead to aspiration pneumonia.[89]

Cricopharyngeal dysphagia is the most common oropharyngeal dysphagia.[100] Cinefluorography is often necessary to definitely demonstrate the disease and to differentiate it from pharyngeal dysphagia and mixed oropharyngeal dysphagias. The major cinefluorographic finding is failure of the cricopharyngeal muscle to relax in a coordinated sequence with the onset of pharyngeal contraction. Other findings include retention of contrast media in the pharynx, incomplete transport of bolus through the cricopharyngeal passage, misdirection of contrast into the nasopharynx, and aspiration of contrast media retained in the pharynx.[100] Cricopharyngeal dysphagias are differentiated from pharyngeal dysphagias cinefluorographically by the appearance of the pharyngeal wall during swallowing. In cricopharyngeal dysphagia the vigorous pharyngeal contraction distorts the pharyngeal

Table 14–1. RADIOGRAPHIC SIGNS FOR DIFFERENTIATION OF OROPHARYNGEAL DYSPHAGIAS

	Survey/Contrast Films	Cinefluorography
Oral	Retention of contrast medium in oropharynx No aspiration pneumonia	Poor bolus accumulation at base of tongue Diminished rostral and caudal movement of the tongue
Pharyngeal	Aspiration pneumonia Large gas shadow in cervical esophagus Contrast medium retained immediately caudal to the cricopharyngeal passage Retention of contrast medium in oropharynx, pharynx and piriform recesses	Residual gas or contrast in the pharynx with normal cricopharyngeal sphincter function Incomplete pharyngeal contraction Slow progression of the peristaltic-like contraction from the rostral to the caudal pharynx
Cricopharyngeal	Aspiration pneumonia Gas cervical esophagus Pharyngeal stasis of contrast medium Contrast medium in nasopharynx	Failure of the cricopharyngeal muscle to relax in a coordinated sequence with the onset of pharyngeal contraction Incomplete transport of the bolus through the cricopharyngeal passage Misdirection of contrast medium into the nasopharynx

passage and/or forces the bolus into the caudal pharyngeal wall, causing the formation of transient pharyngeal outpouchings. In pharyngeal dysphagia no deformation of the cricopharyngeal passage occurs.[89]

Radiographic findings on survey films and contrast studies that suggest cricopharyngeal dysphagia are retention of moderate amounts of gas in the cervical esophagus with a normal intrathoracic esophagus, pharyngeal stasis of contrast media, misdirection of a contrast medium bolus into the nasopharynx, and signs of aspiration pneumonia (Fig. 14–28).[100]

Sialography

Sialography is the radiographic examination of the salivary glands and ducts performed by the injection of positive contrast media retrograde through the salivary ducts. It is useful in detecting abnormalities of the salivary glands and ducts, including determining of the origin of saliva from mucoceles prior to surgery,[36] and in detecting obstruction of the salivary ducts due to infection, tumor, sialolithiasis, or dental disease.[39, 58, 83]

TECHNIQUE

The patient should be anesthetized for the procedure. Atropine should not be used as a preanesthetic agent because it inhibits salivary secretion, making it more difficult to cannulate the ducts.[58] Blunt 22- and 26-gauge cannulas made from shortened hypodermic needles, lacrimal cannulas or 25- to 27-gauge lymphography needles* can be used to cannulate the ducts. A water-soluble iodinated contrast agent† (1 to 3 ml) is used for the injection. Lateral and ventrodorsal radiographs of the head should be taken immediately following each injection.

The parotid duct opens into the mouth on a papilla located on the labial oral mucosa opposite the upper fourth premolar tooth (Fig. 14–29). The duct enters the mouth perpendicular to the oral mucosa but bends caudally 90° beneath the duct papilla.[56] To make cannulation of the duct easier, the oral mucosa caudal to the papilla is grasped with fine forceps and retracted rostromedially.[36] A 22-gauge cannula is then directed into the duct and the contrast medium injected.

The zygomatic duct has one major and several minor ducts. The major duct opens into the mouth slightly dorsal and caudal to the parotid duct papilla on a ridge of oral mucosa that runs lateral to the upper molar teeth.[36] The zygomatic duct is smaller than the parotid duct; therefore a 25- to 26-gauge cannula 1 cm long is needed to cannulate the duct (Fig. 14–30).

*Cook Inc., Box 489, Bloomington, IN.

†Renografin, E. R. Squibb & Sons, Inc., Georges Rd., New Brunswick, NJ; Hypaque Sodium 50%, Winthrop Labs, 90 Park Avenue, New York, NY.

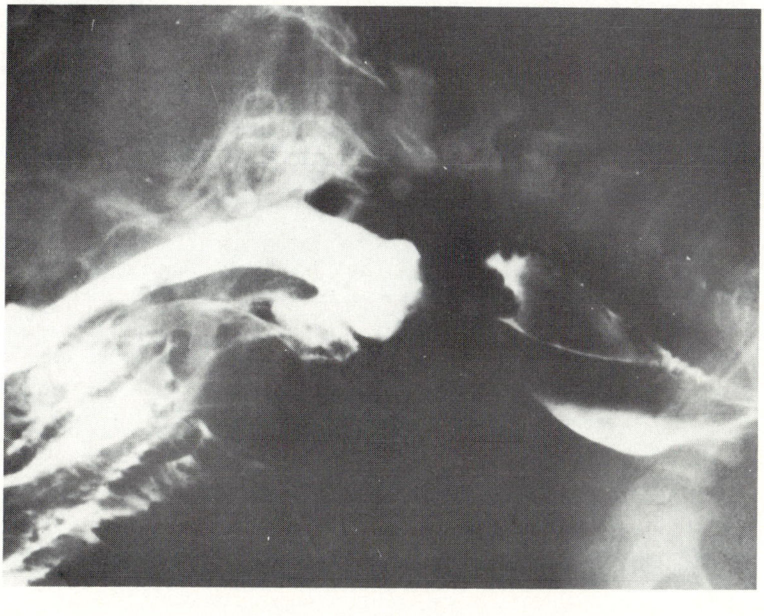

Figure 14–28. Cricopharyngeal achalasia. Note the contrast medium filling the nasopharynx and adhering to the wall of the trachea.

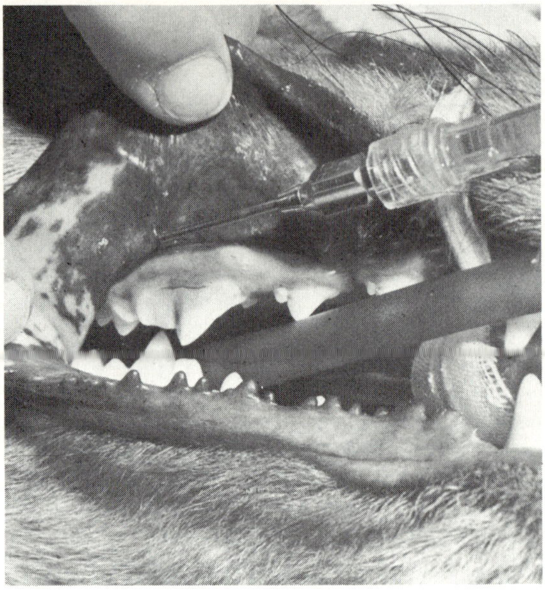

Figure 14–29. Cannulation of the parotid duct. The duct opens into the mouth on a papilla located on the labial oral mucosa opposite the upper fourth premolar tooth.

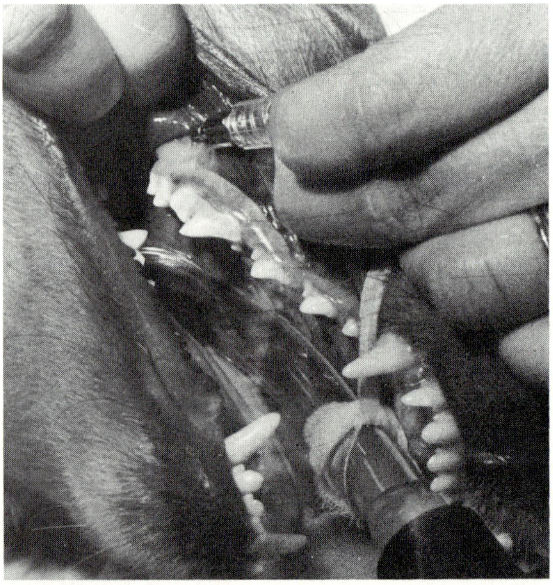

Figure 14–30. Cannulation of the zygomatic duct. The duct opens on a ridge of oral mucosa slightly dorsal and approximately one centimeter caudal to the parotid duct papilla.

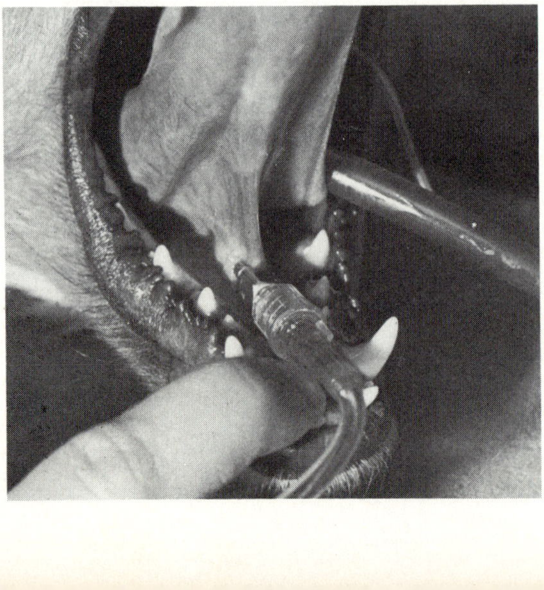

Figure 14–31. Cannulation of the mandibular duct. The duct opens on the lateral surface of the lingual caruncles.

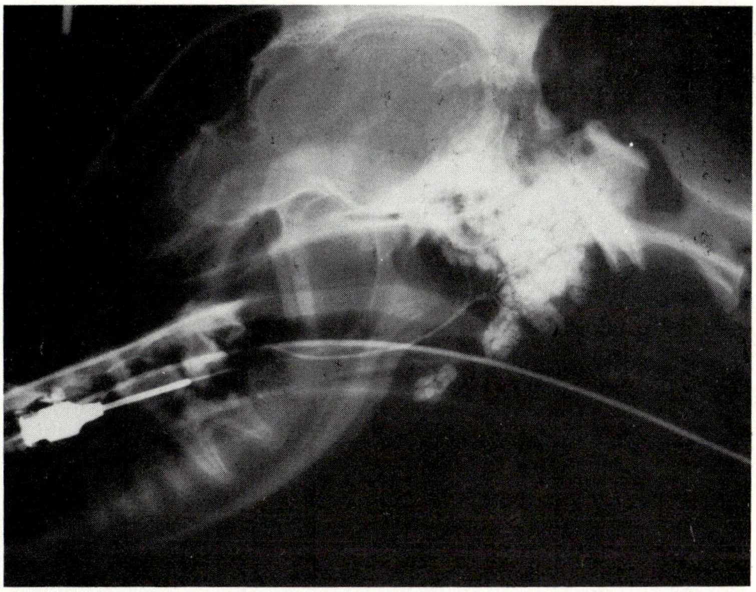

Figure 14–32. Normal parotid sialogram.

The mandibular and sublingual ducts are located on the lateral surface of the lingual caruncles. In the majority of dogs the sublingual duct lies 1 to 2 mm caudal to the mandibular duct and appears as a small red dot.[36] Approximately one-third of all dogs have a common opening of the mandibular and sublingual ducts either unilaterally or bilaterally.[36] It is important to visualize the position of the ducts prior to excessive manipulation or application of forceps since marks left on the mucosa may be confused with duct openings. A 22-gauge cannula is used for the mandibular duct and a 26-gauge cannula for the sublingual duct (Fig. 14–31).

NORMAL APPEARANCE

On a lateral radiograph of the head the parotid duct passes caudally from the cannula to the angle of the jaw, where it splits into several small ductules before each enters the irregularly lobulated parotid gland (Fig. 14–32). The course of the parotid duct is influenced by the position of the jaws. The zygomatic duct runs in a dorsocaudal direction from the cannula to a large single-lobed structure situated ventral to the rostral end of the zygomatic arch (Fig. 14–33). The mandibular duct runs caudally parallel to the horizontal ramus of the mandible to the

Figure 14–33. Normal zygomatic sialogram.

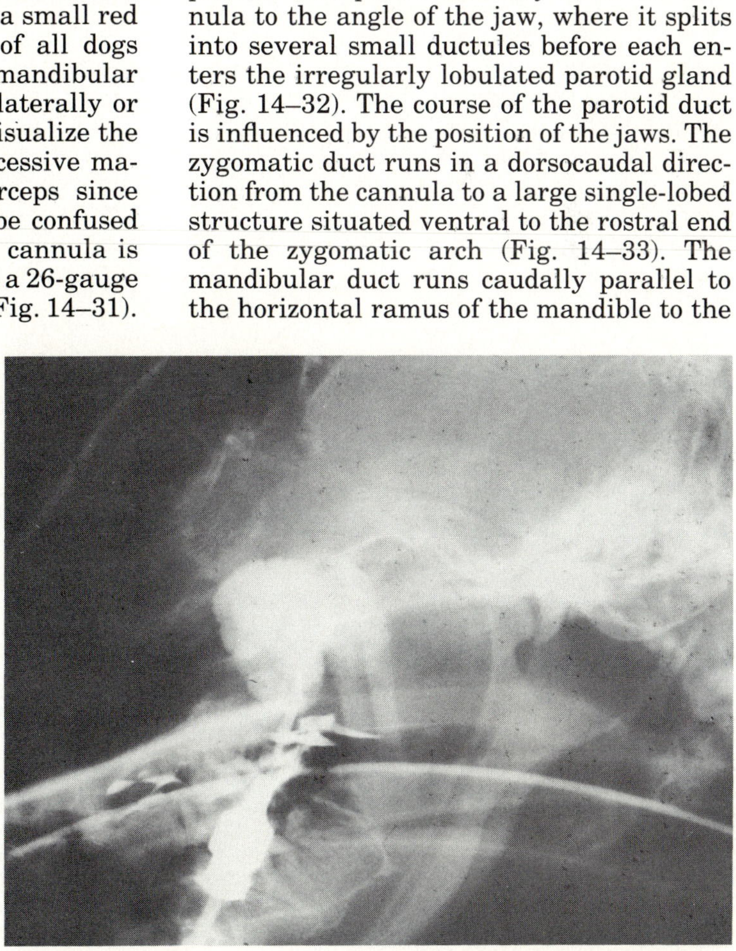

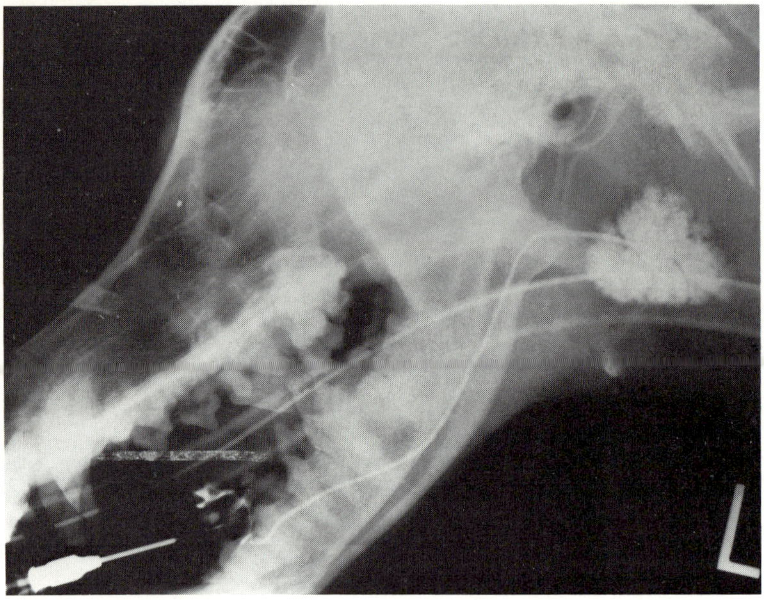

Figure 14–34. Normal mandibular sialogram.

angle of the jaw, where it courses ventrally to a smooth unilobar gland (Fig. 14–34). The sublingual duct runs caudally parallel to the horizontal ramus similar to the mandibular duct; however, it encounters several lobules of the sublingual gland along its path before it reaches the main gland at the level of the lower second molar tooth. The sublingual gland is divided into a bilobed cranial section and a single-lobed caudal section (Fig. 14–35).

Diseases of the Salivary Glands

Sialadenitis and tumors of the salivary glands are rare in the dog and cat.[37] Salivary mucocele is the most frequent clinical condition affecting the salivary glands.[37] The sublingual and the mandibular salivary glands are most often involved.[37] Sialography is used to confirm the presence of a mucocele and to identify the affected salivary gland or duct (Fig. 14–36).

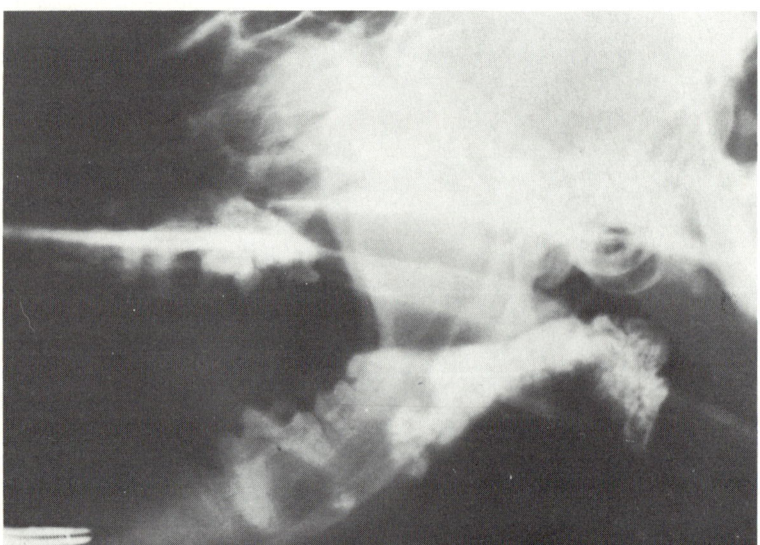

Figure 14–35. Normal sublingual sialogram.

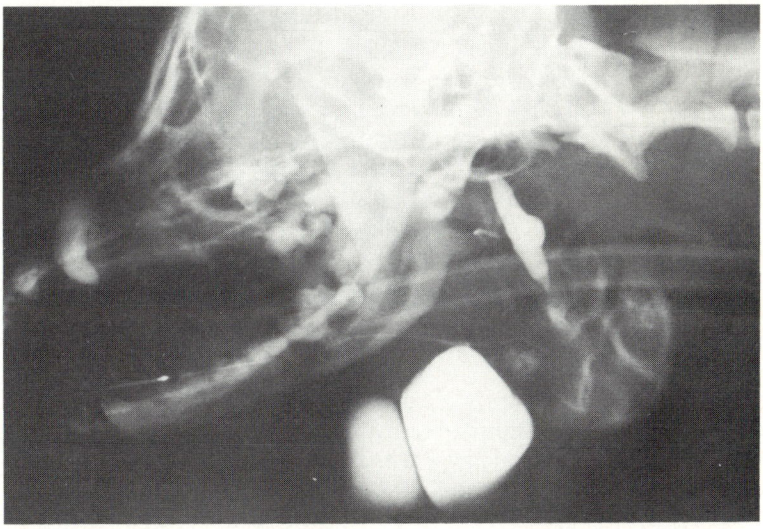

Figure 14–36. Bilateral mandibular mucocele. Both mandibular ducts were cannulated. Note the enlarged mandibular duct and extravasation of contrast medium into the soft tissues.

Esophagus

NORMAL ANATOMY

The normal esophagus extends from the posterior pharynx at the level of the second cervical vertebra to the cardia of the stomach at the eleventh or twelfth rib. The position of the esophagus in relation to the trachea varies. In the cervical region the esophagus is dorsal to the trachea, while at the thoracic inlet it lies to the left of the trachea and may be slightly ventral to it. It then rises and courses toward the midline where it becomes dorsal to the tracheal bifurcation at the base of the heart. The esophagus remains midline as it enters the esophageal hiatus and ends at the cardia of the stomach (Fig. 14–37).[33, 56]

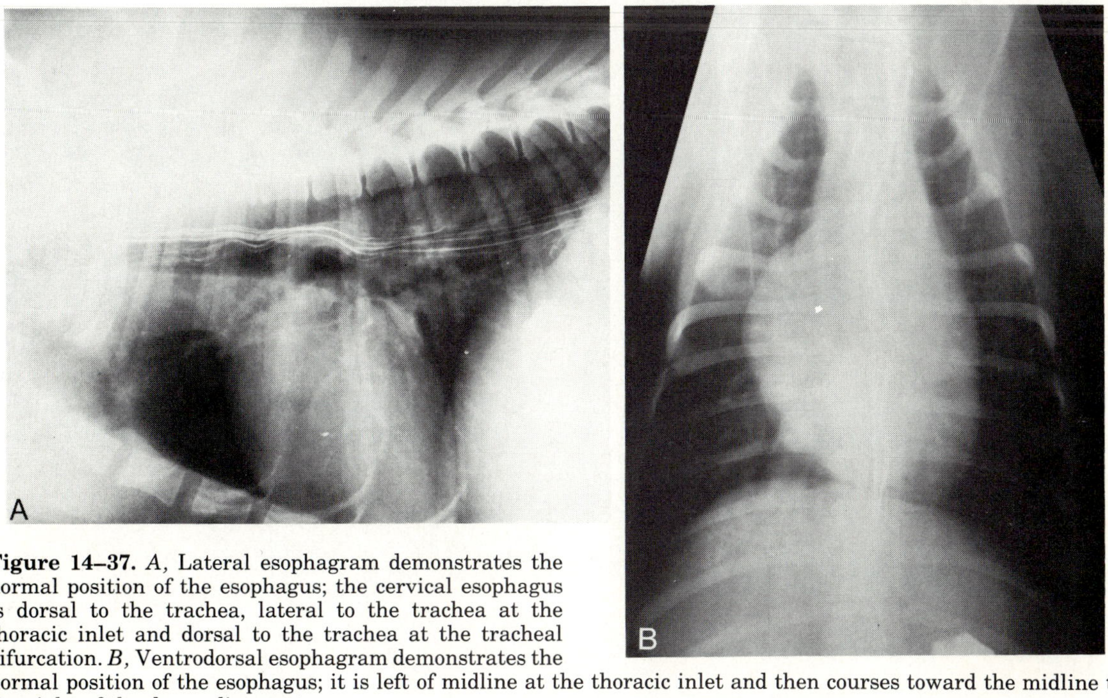

Figure 14–37. *A*, Lateral esophagram demonstrates the normal position of the esophagus; the cervical esophagus is dorsal to the trachea, lateral to the trachea at the thoracic inlet and dorsal to the trachea at the tracheal bifurcation. *B*, Ventrodorsal esophagram demonstrates the normal position of the esophagus; it is left of midline at the thoracic inlet and then courses toward the midline to the right of the descending aorta.

SURVEY FILMS

The normal esophagus is collapsed and is not visualized on survey radiographs because it lies within the mediastinum and is of the same density as the surrounding structures (Fig. 14–38).[67, 74] However survey radiographs can provide valuable information in the presence of esophageal disease. Esophageal diseases can be recognized as they often cause alterations in the density in or around the esophagus that allow it to be visualized, or they can cause displacement of other thoracic structures such as the trachea.[67] Radiographs of the neck and thorax should be taken in the standard lateral and ventrodorsal projections to demonstrate the cervical, thoracic, and abdominal esophagus. A right ventrodorsal oblique projection that projects the esophagus away from the thoracic vertebra may also be useful.[92]

CONTRAST STUDIES

Esophagography is the contrast examination of the esophagus used to evaluate its function, location, and morphology. It is indicated in patients with persistent regurgitation or vomition, dysphagia, or suspected esophageal foreign body. A dynamic study of the esophagus can be obtained using fluoroscopy to evaluate esophageal function and motility.

The location and morphology of the esophagus is best demonstrated with esophagography. No special patient preparation is necessary prior to performing the study. Survey films should be taken before esophagography to ensure proper technique and positioning and to serve as reference films for the special study. Barium sulfate is the contrast medium of choice.

Both micropulverized barium sulfate suspension*, which has a viscosity similar to that of light cream, and a barium suspension that has the consistency of thick paste† are used for the study. The liquid barium is used to evaluate sufficient esophageal motility to propel the barium through the esophagus and into the stomach and to estimate the size of the esophageal lumen. The thick barium suspension adheres well to the esophageal folds and provides good detail of the esophageal mucosa.[58]

To demonstrate a partial esophageal obstruction or stricture, liquid barium mixed with food can be given.[58] If esophageal perforation is suspected a water-soluble iodinated oral contrast agent‡ should be used because it is absorbed from the body tissues and does not cause the severe tissue reaction

*Redi-flow, Burns Pharmaceuticals, Oakland, CA.
†Esophotrast, Barnes-Hind, Sunnyvale, CA.
‡Hypaque Sodium Oral, Winthrop Lab., 90 Park Ave., New York, NY; Gastrografin, Squibb & Sons, Inc., Georges Rd., New Brunswick, NJ.

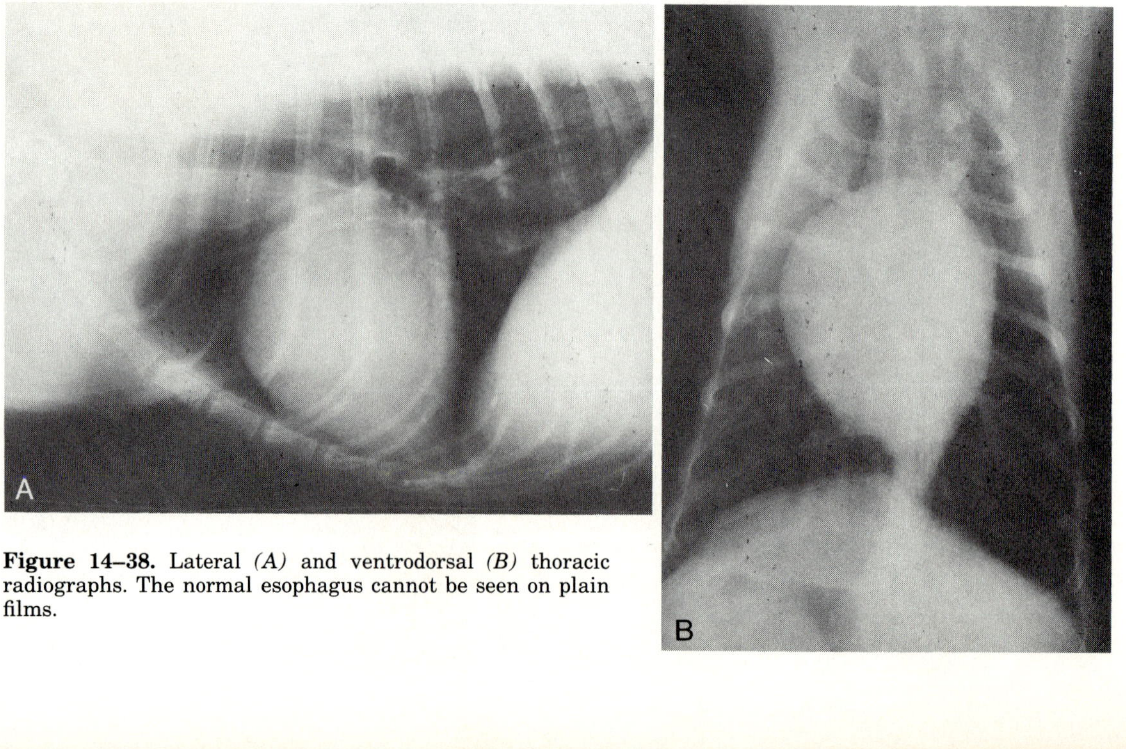

Figure 14–38. Lateral *(A)* and ventrodorsal *(B)* thoracic radiographs. The normal esophagus cannot be seen on plain films.

in the periesophageal tissues caused by barium.[67]

The procedure for esophagography is the same in the dog and cat. Chemical restraint is usually not necessary. Survey films should be taken prior to performing the study for the reasons previously mentioned and to assure that the esophagus is empty. Liquid barium (3 to 5 ml/kg) is administered with a catheter tip syringe into the buccal pouch of an awake animal in right lateral recumbency. The contrast medium must be given slowly enough to allow normal swallowing and prevent aspiration of the medium into the trachea and lungs. Recumbent right lateral ventrodorsal and oblique right ventrodorsal radiographs are then taken. One to three fluid ounces of the barium paste is then placed on the animal's hard palate with a tongue depressor, and the radiographic sequence is repeated. If there are no abnormalities seen on these initial radiographs, liquid barium mixed with food should be given per os and the radiographic series should be repeated. If water-soluble iodinated oral contrast agents are used, they are administered into the buccal pouch via a catheter tip syringe at a dosage of 1 ml/lb body weight.

The normal esophagram in a dog given thick barium paste appears as a series of parallel longitudinal folds extending the en-

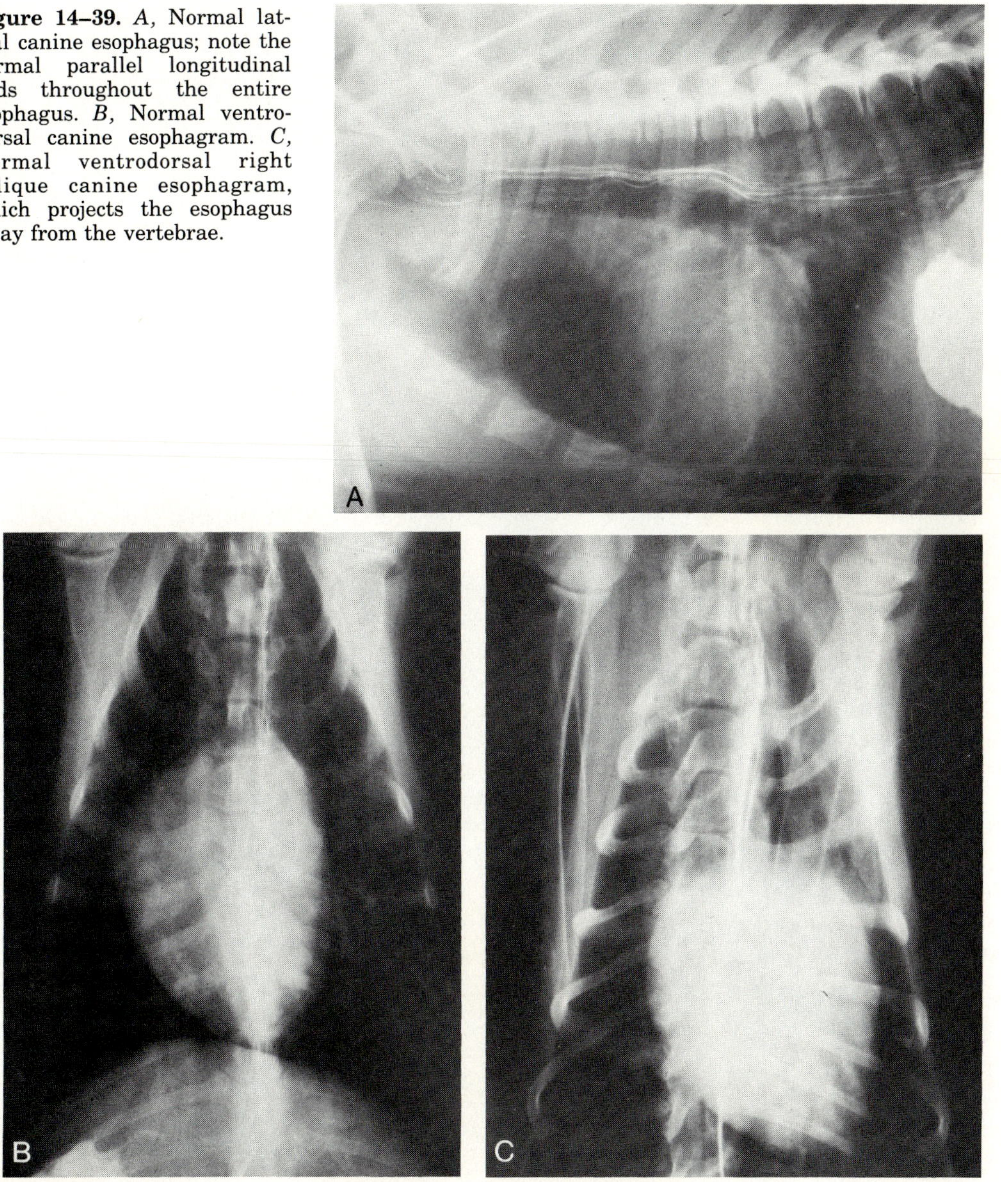

Figure 14–39. *A,* Normal lateral canine esophagus; note the normal parallel longitudinal folds throughout the entire esophagus. *B,* Normal ventrodorsal canine esophagram. *C,* Normal ventrodorsal right oblique canine esophagram, which projects the esophagus away from the vertebrae.

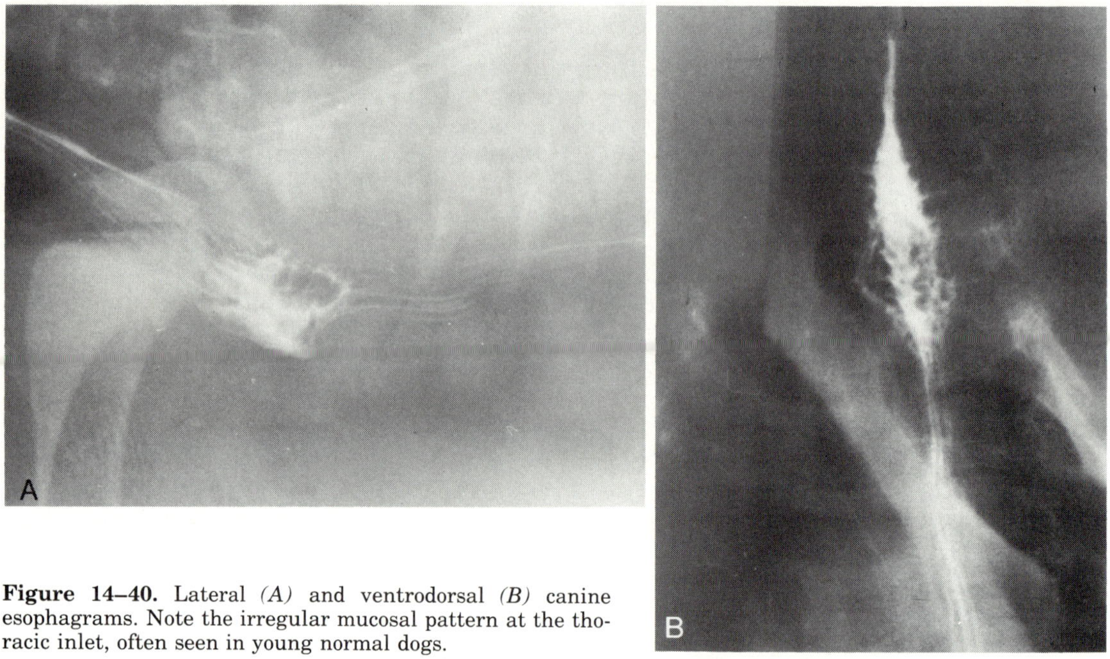

Figure 14–40. Lateral *(A)* and ventrodorsal *(B)* canine esophagrams. Note the irregular mucosal pattern at the thoracic inlet, often seen in young normal dogs.

tire length of the esophagus (Fig. 14–39). However, at the thoracic inlet the esophagus may deviate ventrally and have an irregular mucosal pattern (Fig. 14–40). This represents a normal variation in the esophagus of young dogs and should not be diagnosed as an esophageal diverticulum (Fig. 14–41).[44, 67]

In cats, only the cranial two-thirds of the esophagus has the characteristic parallel longitudinal folds. The transverse striations of the caudal third of the esophagus give it the characteristic "herringbone" appearance (Fig. 14–42); this should not be mistaken for inflammatory disease.[44]

ESOPHAGEAL ABNORMALITIES

Any significant amounts of air seen in the esophagus on plain film radiographs should be considered pathologic unless proven otherwise. Some non-pathologic causes of air in

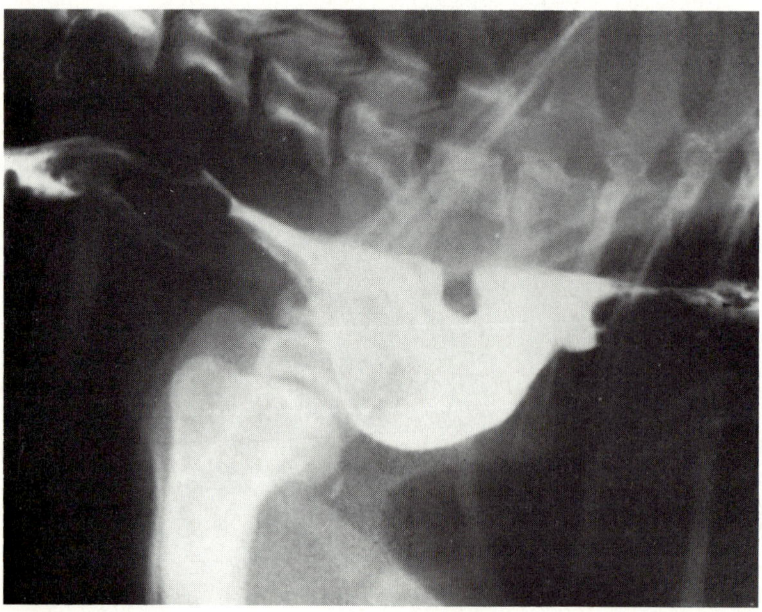

Figure 14–41. Lateral esophagram demonstrating large diverticulum at the thoracic inlet.

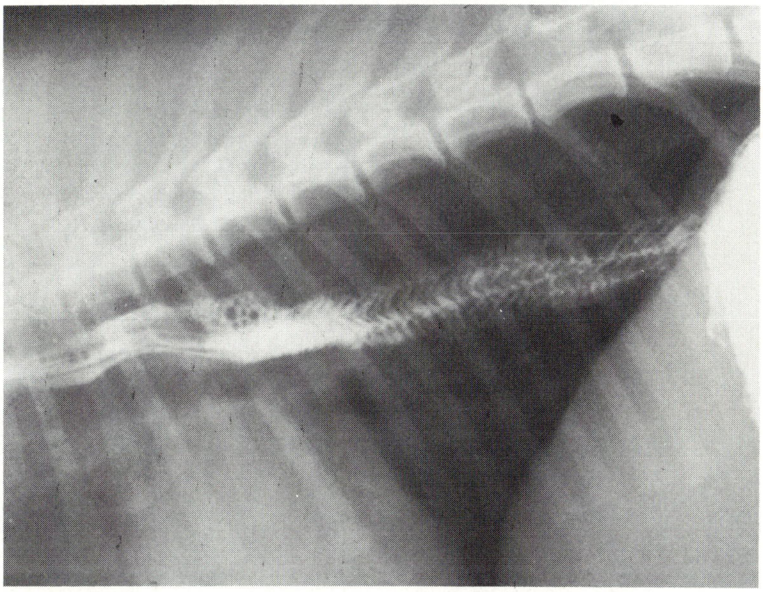

Figure 14–42. Normal feline lateral esophagram. Note normal transverse striations in caudal third of esophagus that give the esophagus a "herringbone" appearance.

the esophagus include aerophagia due to excitement, struggling, and anesthesia. In aerophagia due to excitement or struggling gas will usually be present in the stomach, and it will tend to be transient. In the esophagus it will often appear differently or disappear altogether between radiographic examinations. Aerophagia following anesthesia is generalized and uniform and outlines normal mucosal borders of the pharynx and esophagus (Fig. 14–43). Air in the esophagus may be associated with pathological conditions including inflammation, obstruction, foreign body, granuloma, stricture, and neurogenic disorders.[67] Differentiation regarding the amount, location, and contour of the gas pattern is often helpful in determining the cause of the gas accu-

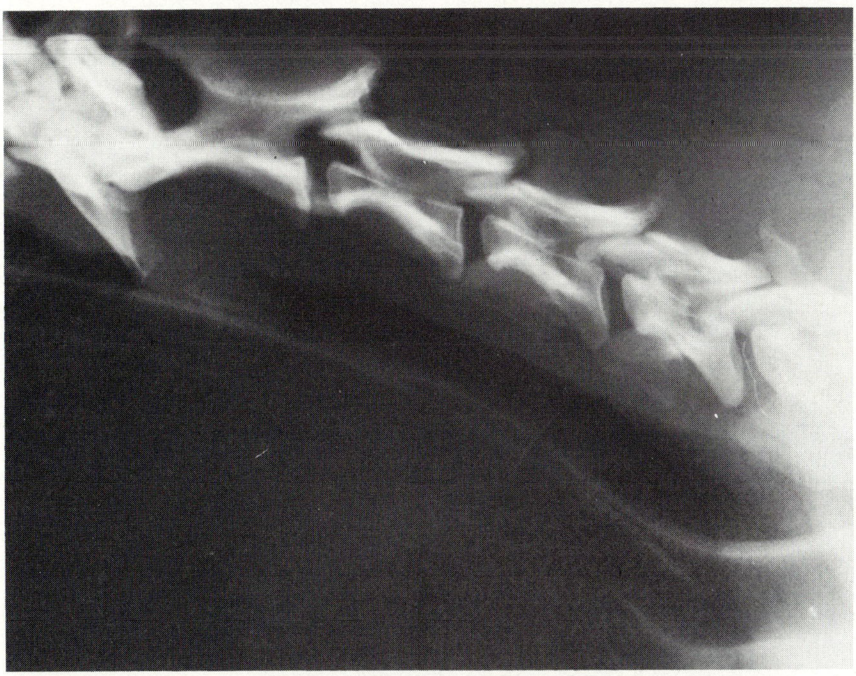

Figure 14–43. Aerophagia due to anesthesia. Note the generalized gas-distended esophagus commonly seen following general anesthesia.

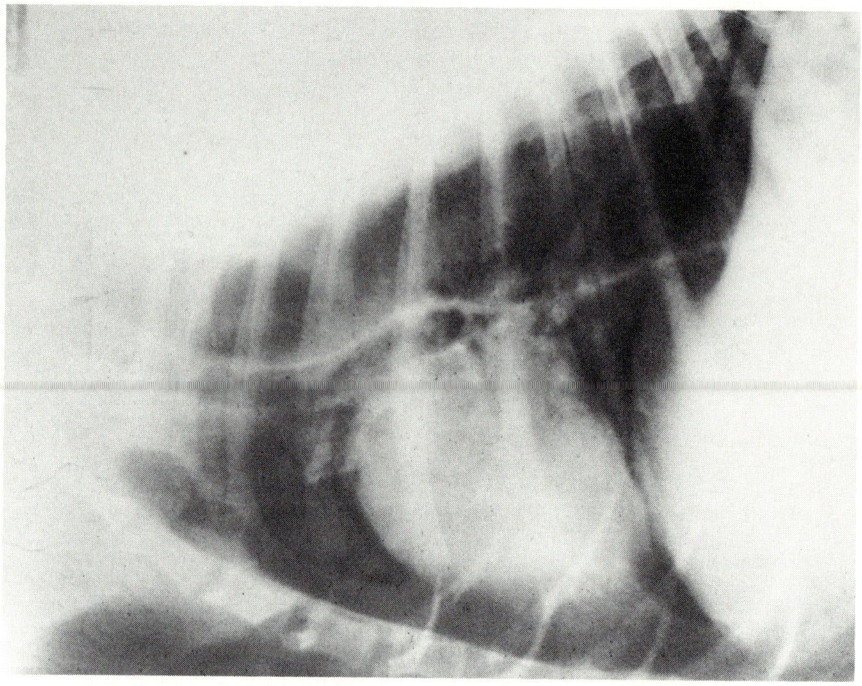

Figure 14–44. Generalized gas-filled megaesophagus. Note the ventral displacement of the trachea.

mulation. Gas normally accumulates orally to a lesion. A generalized, large, dilated gas-filled esophagus suggests an obstructive lesion at the cardia or a neurogenic disorder of the esophagus (Fig. 14–44).[67] A localized, mottled gas accumulation is suggestive of a focal inflammatory lesion or an obstructive lesion due to foreign body, stricture, granuloma, or tumor (Fig. 14–45).[67]

Gas is seen around the esophagus when there is a pneumomediastinum (Fig. 14–46). It is important to differentiate the cause of a pneumomediastinum between rupture of the respiratory system and perforation of the esophagus. A perforated esophagus is often associated with an increased density in the pleural space and mediastinum from secondary infection. A perforated esophagus

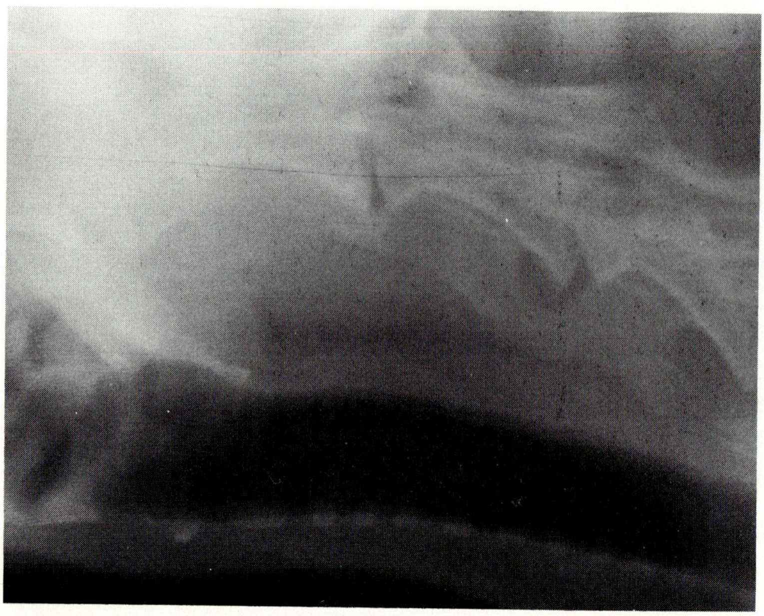

Figure 14–45. Localized, mottled gas accumulation in the esophagus suggestive of focal esophageal inflammatory or obstructive lesion.

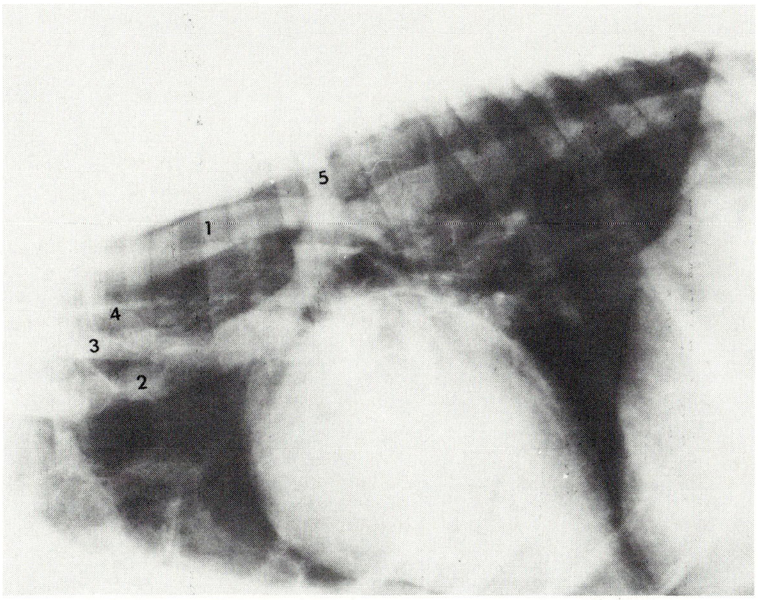

Figure 14–46. Pneumomediastinum. The soft-tissue dense esophagus is clearly visualized because it is surrounded by air (1). Other structures visualized include cranial vena cava (2), brachiocephalic trunk (3), left subclavian artery (4), and azygos vein (5).

should be confirmed by performing an esophagram with a water-soluble iodinated oral contrast agent.*

MEGAESOPHAGUS

The survey radiographs demonstrate a dilated gas and/or fluid filled esophagus with ventral displacement of the trachea (Fig. 14–47). Gas in the dilated esophagus causes the walls of the esophagus to appear as thin, dense, white lines (Fig. 14–48). Aspiration pneumonia may often be seen secondary to megaesophagus (Fig. 14–49). An esophagram outlines a dilatation of the entire esophagus (Fig. 14–50). Esophagrams should be performed with the animal in right lateral recumbency rather than in left lateral recumbency. In left lateral recum-

*Hypaque Sodium Oral, Winthrop Lab., 90 Park Ave., New York, NY.

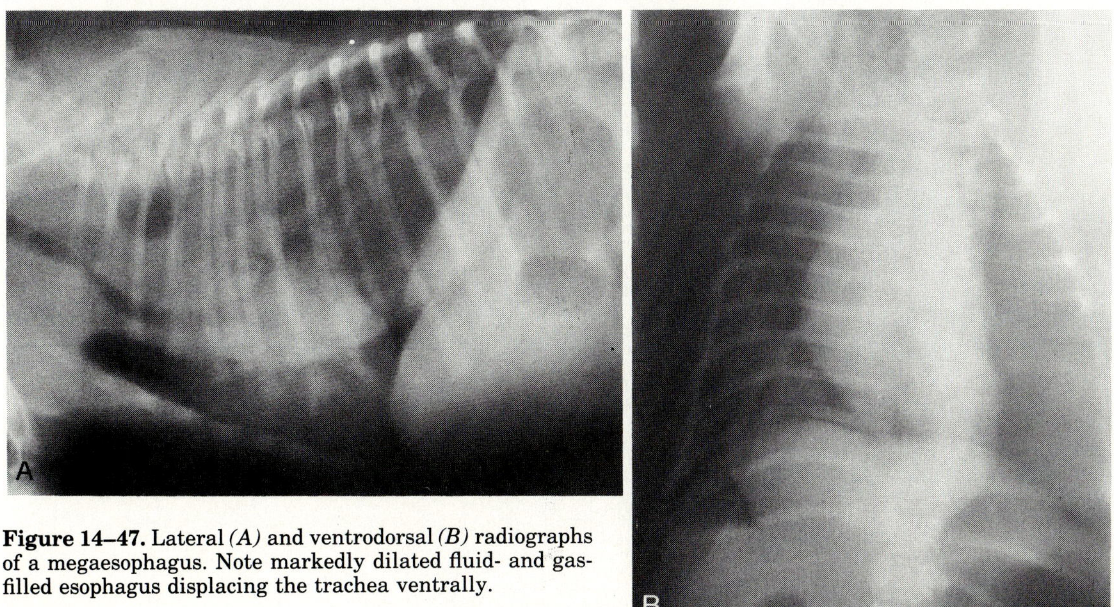

Figure 14–47. Lateral *(A)* and ventrodorsal *(B)* radiographs of a megaesophagus. Note markedly dilated fluid- and gas-filled esophagus displacing the trachea ventrally.

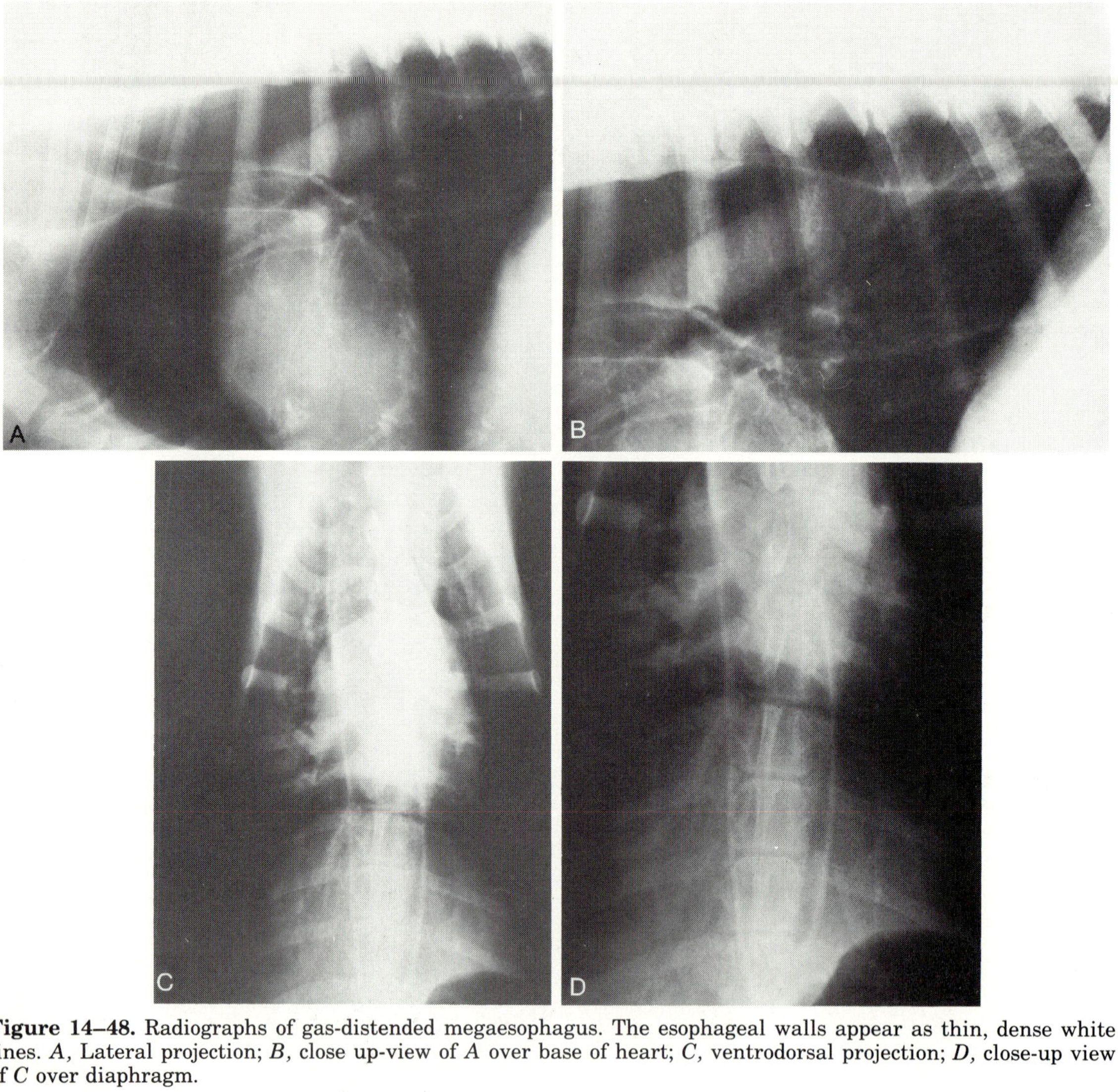

Figure 14–48. Radiographs of gas-distended megaesophagus. The esophageal walls appear as thin, dense white lines. *A*, Lateral projection; *B*, close up-view of *A* over base of heart; *C*, ventrodorsal projection; *D*, close-up view of *C* over diaphragm.

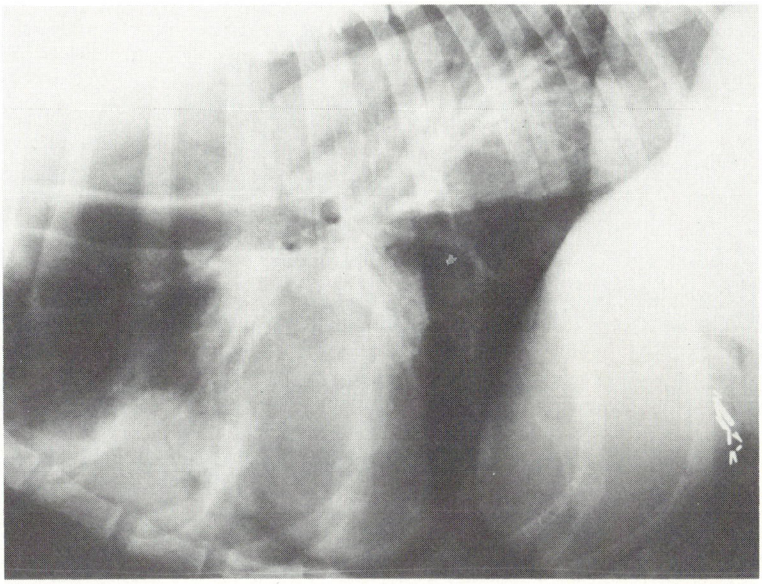

Figure 14–49. Megaesophagus with aspiration pneumonia. Note the consolidation of the cranial ventral lung lobes.

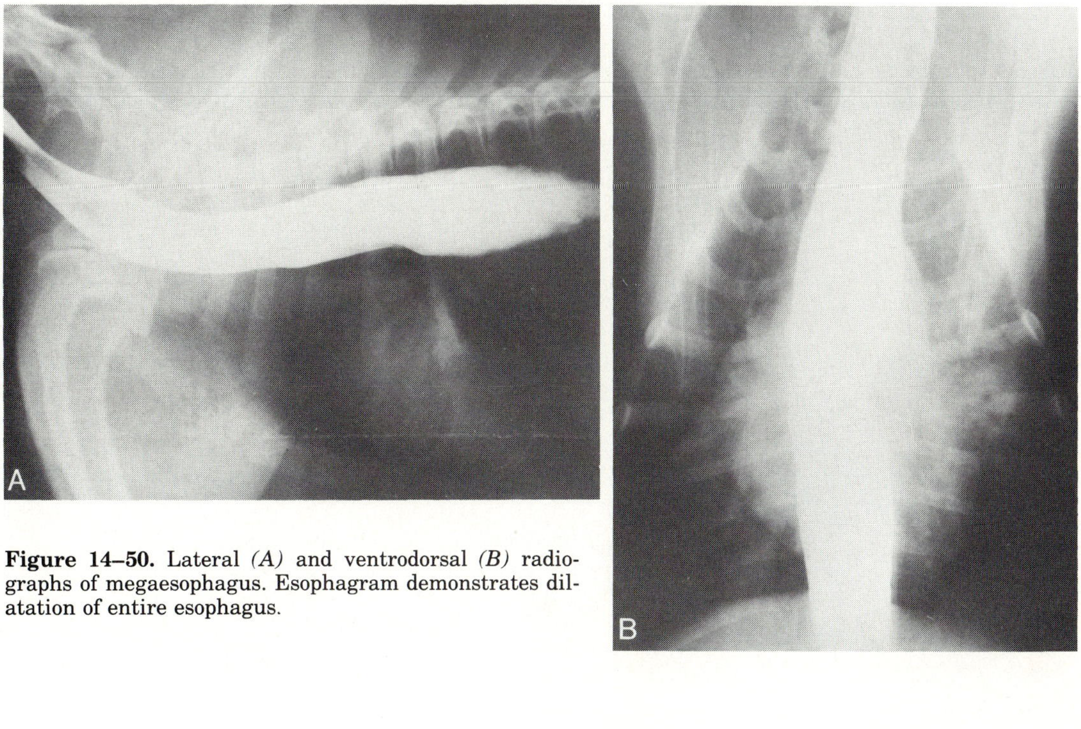

Figure 14–50. Lateral *(A)* and ventrodorsal *(B)* radiographs of megaesophagus. Esophagram demonstrates dilatation of entire esophagus.

bency the aorta, which is to the left of the esophagus, lies underneath the esophagus. A megaesophagus may drape over the aorta, causing contrast medium to pool in the cranial thoracic esophagus rather than fill the caudal thoracic esophagus. This could mimic the appearance of a vascular ring anomaly (Fig. 14–51).

VASCULAR RING ANOMALY

A vascular ring anomaly causes dilatation of the cervical and cranial thoracic esophagus. It is due to an abnormal embryonic development of the great vessels that constrict the esophagus at it passes over the base of the heart. The caudal thoracic esophagus often remains normal, which differentiates it from a megaesophagus. The condition is readily diagnosed on an esophagram (Fig. 14–52). Occasionally a megaesophagus will be present concurrently with a vascular ring anomaly.

ESOPHAGEAL DIVERTICULUM

Esophageal diverticulum is an outpouching of the esophageal wall that is usually seen at the thoracic inlet or cranial to the diaphragm. It is a relatively uncommon condition. It may be seen on survey radiographs as a gas-filled or fluid-filled rounded density associated with the esophageal wall. However, a contrast study is often necessary to outline the diverticulum and visualize the lesion (Fig. 14–53).

FOREIGN BODIES

Esophageal foreign body is a common problem in the dog and cat. Foreign bodies tend to lodge at the thoracic inlet, at the base of the heart, or in the distal hiatal esophageal region (Figs. 14–54, 14–55, and 14–56). If they are radiopaque, they are readily visualized on survey radiographs, whereas if they are radiolucent, a contrast study must be performed to visualize them. Air can be introduced into the esophagus to outline a foreign body and is harmless in cases of esophageal perforation.[44] On survey radiographs gas or fluid will usually accumulate orally to an esophageal foreign body. Gas or areas of increased density in the mediastinum surrounding a foreign body suggest esophageal perforation.

ESOPHAGEAL STRICTURES

Esophageal strictures can result from either extraluminal sources or intraluminal lesions. Gas or fluid will often accumulate orally to the stricture and be visible on survey radiographs. However, a contrast study is usually necessary to differentiate between extraluminal and intraluminal lesions. Although both lesions cause narrowing of the esophageal lumen, intraluminal lesions cause irregular mucosal borders, whereas with extraluminal lesions there will be smooth esophageal mucosal borders (Figs. 14–57 and 14–58).[67]

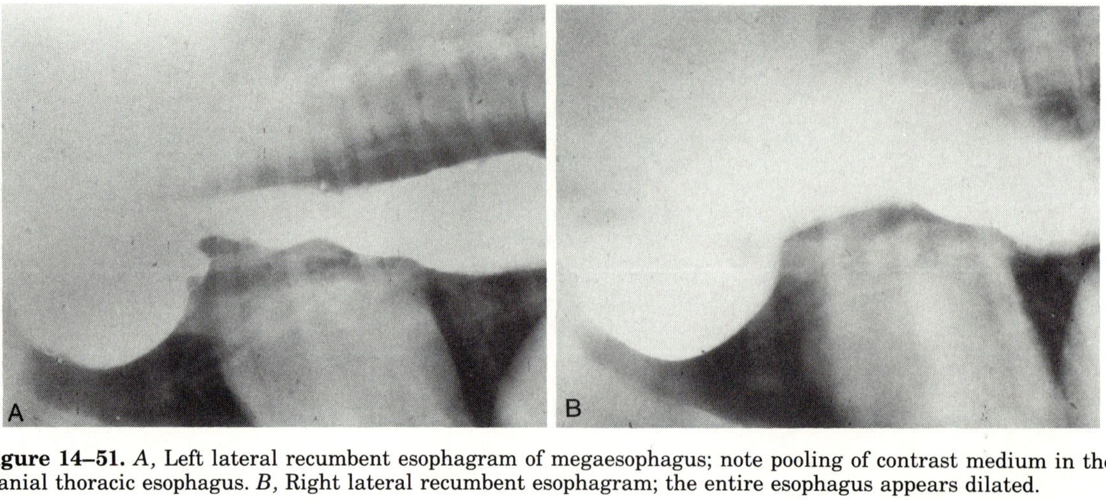

Figure 14–51. *A,* Left lateral recumbent esophagram of megaesophagus; note pooling of contrast medium in the cranial thoracic esophagus. *B,* Right lateral recumbent esophagram; the entire esophagus appears dilated.

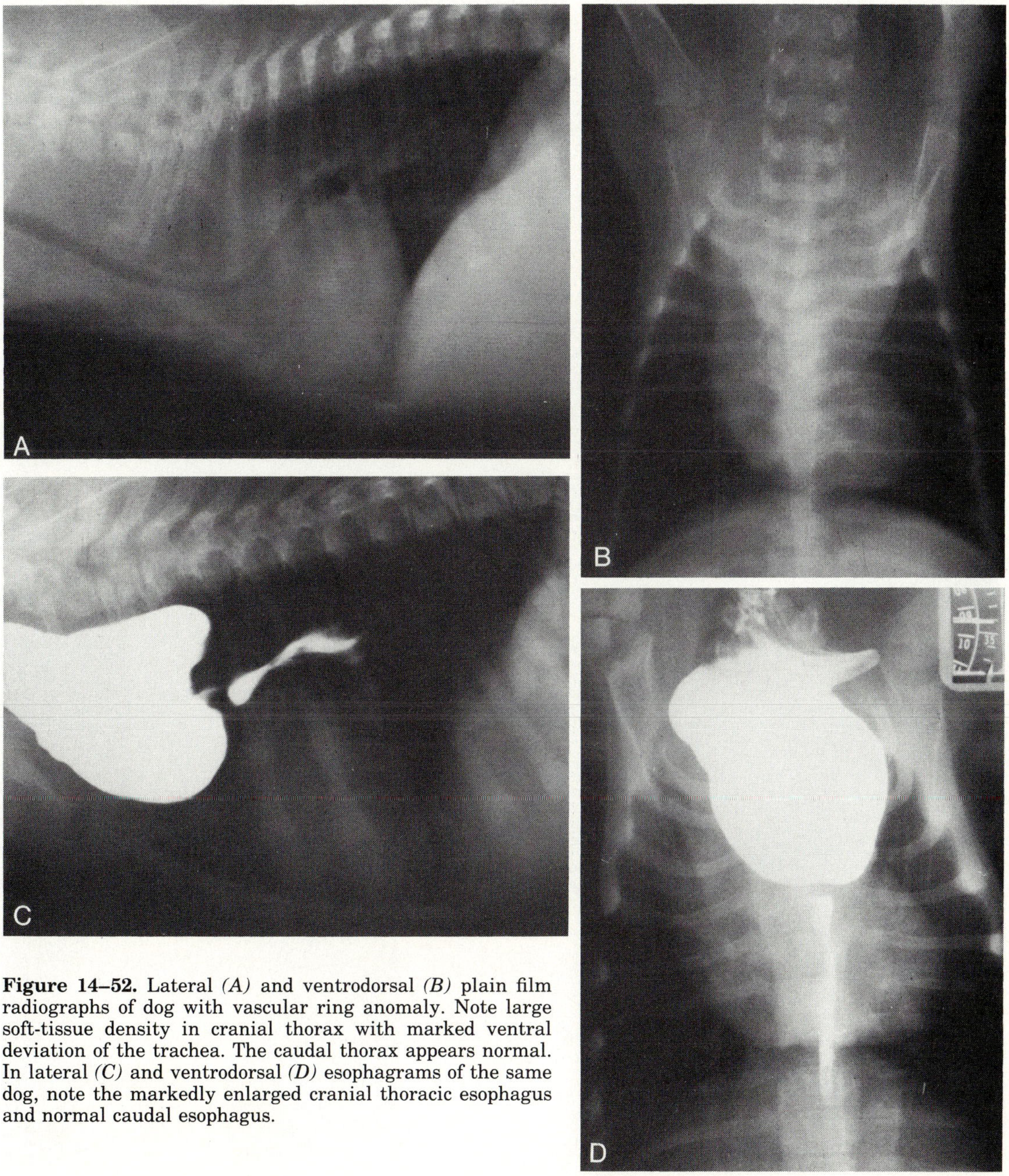

Figure 14–52. Lateral *(A)* and ventrodorsal *(B)* plain film radiographs of dog with vascular ring anomaly. Note large soft-tissue density in cranial thorax with marked ventral deviation of the trachea. The caudal thorax appears normal. In lateral *(C)* and ventrodorsal *(D)* esophagrams of the same dog, note the markedly enlarged cranial thoracic esophagus and normal caudal esophagus.

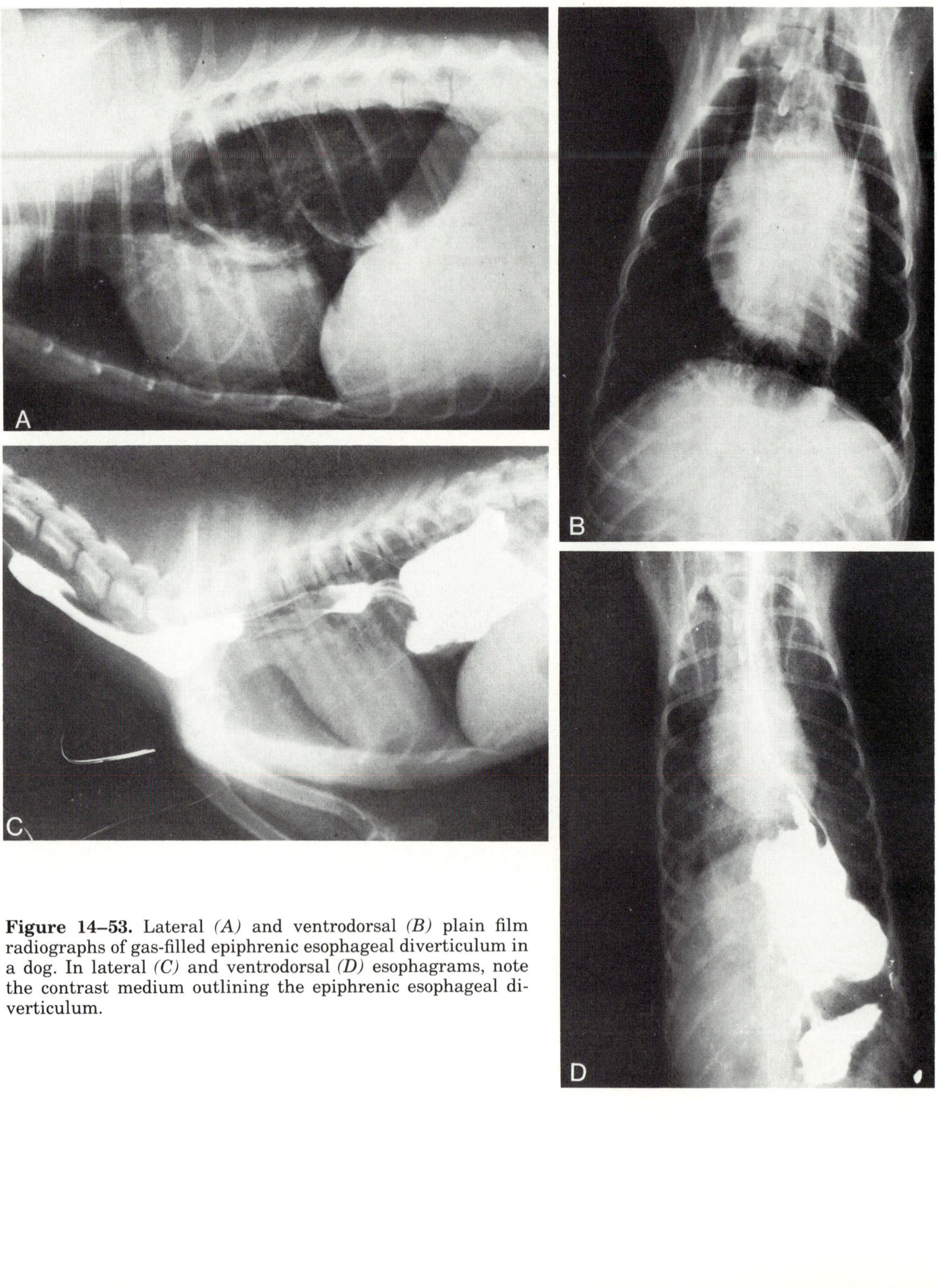

Figure 14–53. Lateral *(A)* and ventrodorsal *(B)* plain film radiographs of gas-filled epiphrenic esophageal diverticulum in a dog. In lateral *(C)* and ventrodorsal *(D)* esophagrams, note the contrast medium outlining the epiphrenic esophageal diverticulum.

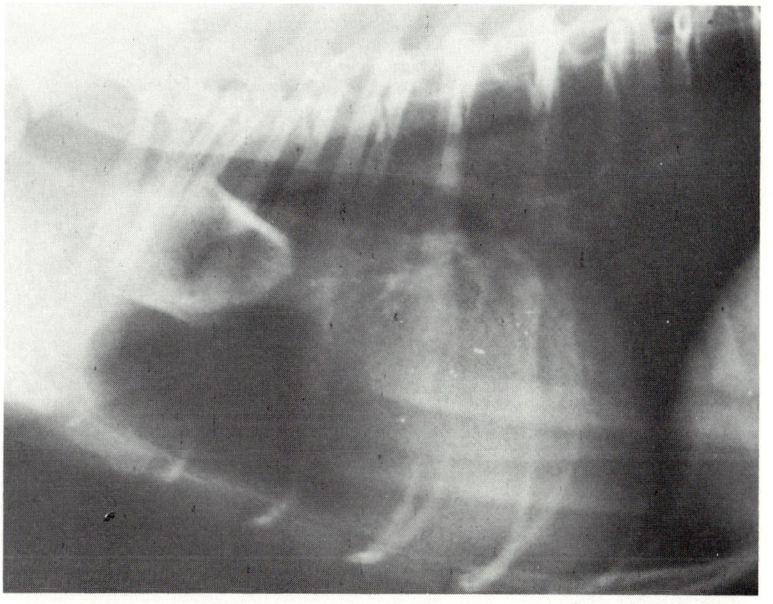

Figure 14–54. Esophageal foreign body. Bone lodged at thoracic inlet.

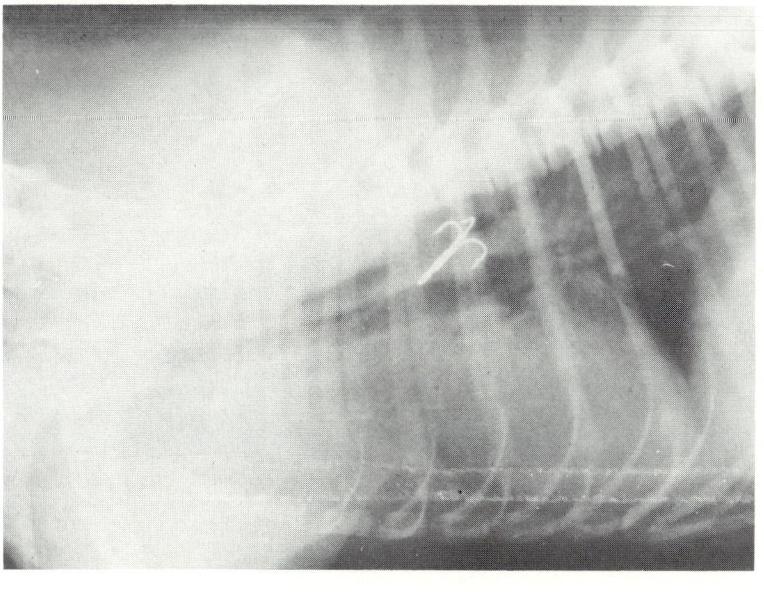

Figure 14–55. Esophageal foreign body. Fish hook lodged over the base of the heart. Note gas present in the cranial thoracic esophagus.

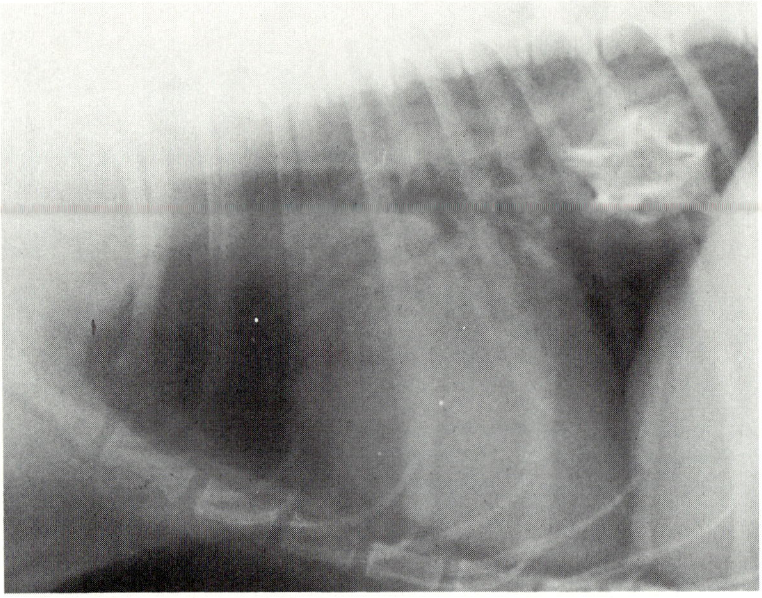

Figure 14–56. Esophageal foreign body. Bone lodged in esophagus in the caudal thorax near the diaphragm.

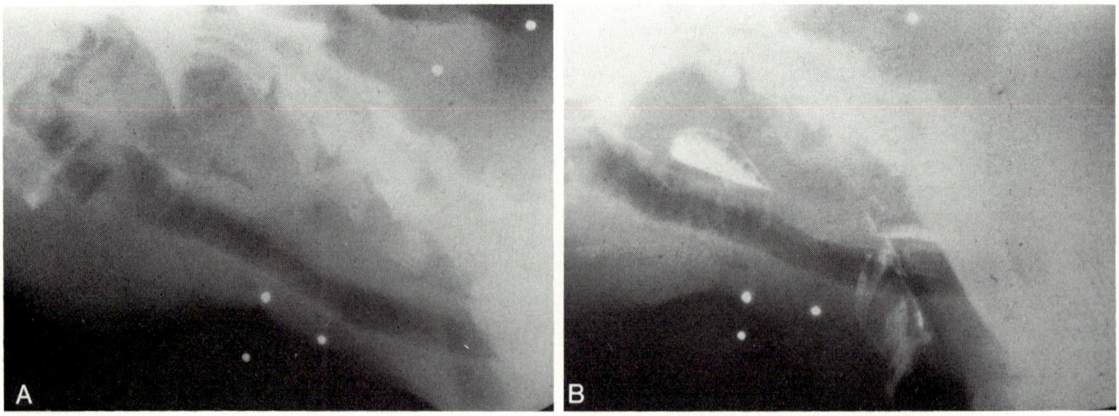

Figure 14–57. Esophageal stricture in dog. *(A)* Plain film radiograph; note soft-tissue swelling around the larynx and the irregular accumulation of gas in the cranial cervical esophagus. *B*, Esophagram; note marked extraluminal stricture of the esophageal lumen at the level of C_4.

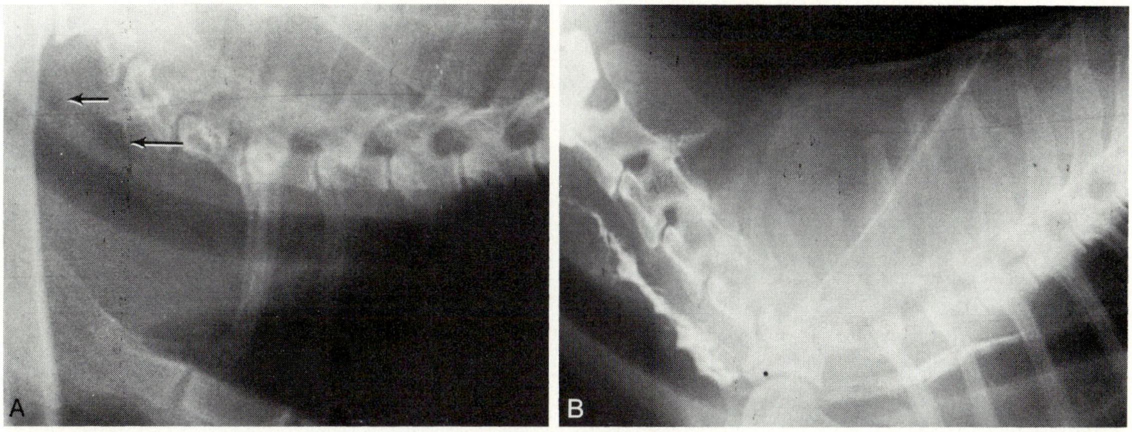

Figure 14–58. Esophageal stricture due to an esophageal squamous cell carcinoma in a cat. *A*, Plain film lateral radiograph; note the irregular accumulation of gas in the cervical esophagus *(arrows)*. *B*, Esophagram; there is stricture of the esophageal lumen with irregular mucosal borders indicative of an intraluminal lesion.

ESOPHAGEAL NEOPLASIA

Primary or secondary neoplasia of the esophagus in the dog or cat are rare. Fibrosarcomas and osteosarcomas do occur secondary to granuloma formation caused by the parasite *Spirocerca lupi,* which invades the esophageal wall during its larval stage. It forms a granuloma that appears as an area of increased density in the caudal thoracic area. An esophagram demonstrates an intramural, intraluminal space-occupying mass with irregular mucosal borders. Ossification of the granuloma may be present. Ventral spondylitis of T_6 and T_7 is often associated with the esophageal mass (Fig. 14–59).[33]

GASTROESOPHAGEAL INTUSSUSCEPTION

Gastroesophageal intussusception occurs most commonly in young dogs when the stomach invaginates into the esophagus. Plain film radiographic findings include dilatation of the esophagus with a well-circumscribed area of increased density in the caudal thoracic esophagus. If sufficient air is present in the stomach, the gastric rugae can be visualized in the caudal esophagus. The gas-filled fundus of the stomach is not seen in its normal location. An esophagram demonstrates a dilated esophagus with restriction of the flow of contrast media into the abdomen (Fig. 14–60).

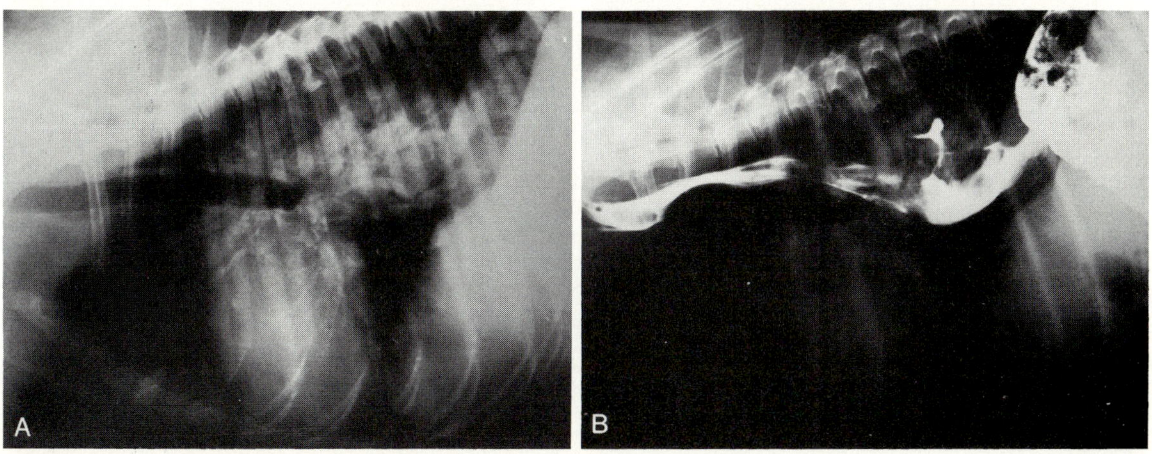

Figure 14–59. *Spirocerca lupi* in a dog. *A*, Plain film lateral radiograph; note large irregular soft-tissue density in the caudal thoracic area. There is spondylitis of T_5-T_6-T_7-T_8. *B*, Esophagram; note large intramural, intraluminal space-occupying mass with irregular mucosal borders. (Courtesy of Dr. J. Burns, Mississippi State University.)

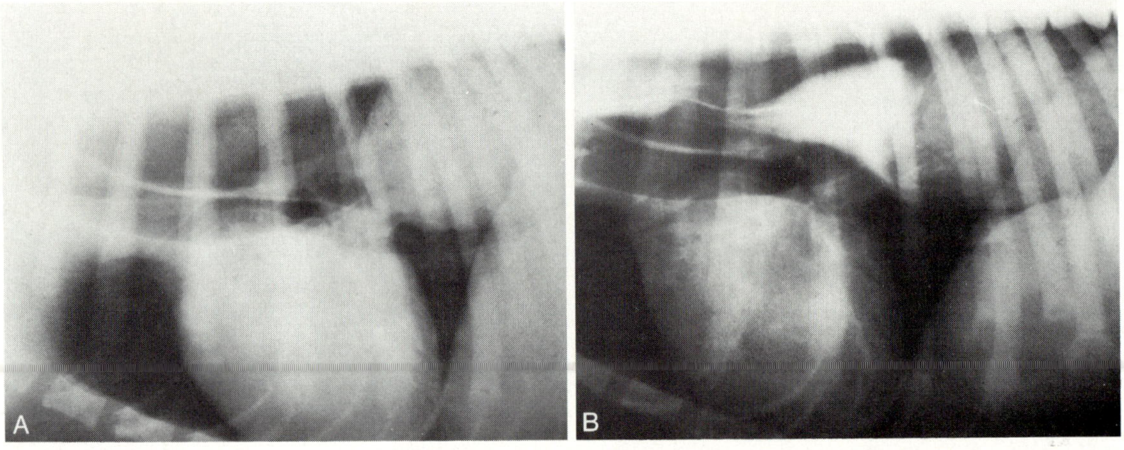

Figure 14–60. Gastroesophageal intussusception in a dog. *A*, Plain film lateral radiograph; note gas-distended dilated esophagus with a well-circumscribed area of increased density representing the stomach in the caudal esophagus. The trachea is displaced ventrally. *B*, Esophagram; note that the flow of contrast is restricted by the displaced stomach.

Abdomen

Routine examination of the abdomen consists of lateral and ventrodorsal radiographs.[95] The lateral radiograph is commonly made with the patient lying on the left side. This will encourage any gas present in the stomach to locate in the pyloric portion of the stomach, and therefore the position of the pylorus will be more easily determined on the radiograph.

Optimal interpretation of abdominal radiographs in the dog and cat depends on optimal radiographic technique. A grid should be used in animals with over 10 cm in abdominal thickness to minimize scattered radiation.[95]

Visualization of structures within the abdomen is dependent on the inherent contrast between the various tissues. The majority of tissues in the abdomen are composed of water-density tissue or fat-density tissue. The ability to identify the various water-density tissues is dependent upon their separation from one another by interposed fat-density tissue. To maximize the contrast between these water and fat densities, it is preferable to use a kVP setting that is in the lower ranges available on the machine.[95] Lower kVP settings result in enhanced radiographic contrast. Any situation that interferes with this fat-soft tissue interface will result in a reduced ability to identify intra-abdominal structures. Hence, poor abdominal detail will result when there is a reduction in the amount of intra-abdominal fat. This situation exists in the cachetic animal and in the very young animal. Loss of detail is also seen when there is increased fluid-density tissue in the abdomen. This separates the fat from the soft tissues, and the serosal surfaces of the organs, intestines, and abdominal wall become obscured.

The increase in abdominal fluid that leads to indistinctness or loss of detail can be generalized or confined to a certain region of the abdomen. Generalized fluid in the abdomen is mostly due to the presence of ascites following congestive heart failure, ruptured bladder, rupture of the cisterna chyli, severe generalized peritonitis, and massive hemorrhage. Commonly, the loss of detail is confined to a particular region of the abdomen, and in these cases the cause can be localized peritonitis, hemorrhage, or diffuse spread of tumor in that region. For instance, localized increase in density and indistinctness of bowel loops in the right upper quadrant could be due to the presence of peritonitis involving the region of the pancreas, and in this case a diagnosis of acute pancreatitis would be suspected. It is important to understand how fluid is distributed in the abdomen so that ascites can be diagnosed radiographically. There is no tendency for the fluid to pool in the abdomen; rather it is distributed uniformly around the various bowel loops, organs, and abdominal wall. Because the abdominal radiograph is taken with the animal recumbent, there are never fluid lines on the plain radiograph. Even on radiographs of an animal with ascites taken using a horizontal x-ray beam, no distinct fluid line is seen; rather there is a generalized impression that the lower aspects of the abdomen are increased in density. No line is seen because the bowel loops tend to float on the top of the fluid and the fluid dissects up around the serosal surfaces, and therefore no distinct separation between fluid and nonfluid zones can be appreciated.

Abdominal gas is also distributed in the abdomen in a similar manner to the fluid and is usually recognized as triangular accumulations of increased radiographic density (i.e., black) between bowel loops. This is an important difference that allows differentiation from intraluminal intestinal gas, which has more parallel-type borders. Free abdominal gas is frequently associated with ruptured bowel and, if present in sufficient quantity, can result in clear visualization of structures not normally seen on the radiograph, such as serosal surfaces of the intestine and the peritoneal surface of the diaphragm (Fig. 14–61). To detect small amounts of free abdominal gas, it is recommended that an exposure be made utilizing a horizontal x-ray beam with the animal positioned in left lateral recumbency. Under these circumstances, the free gas will rise to the upper levels of the abdomen and accumulate between the abdominal wall or diaphragm and the liver shadow.[67] Because of the tendency for the bowel to fall away from this region or not be present in this region, free abdominal gas can be easily detected and will not be confused with intraluminal bowel gas.

The following structures are normally identifiable on routine abdominal radiographs: stomach, small bowel, large bowel, cecum, spleen, liver, kidneys, urinary bladder, prostate gland, diaphragm, abdominal wall, sublumbar musculature, thoracolumbar and lumbar vertebral column, caudal thoracic ribs, and portions of the bony pelvis (Fig. 14–62). The most important landmarks are the liver, stomach, spleen, kidneys, urinary bladder, colon, cecum, and small bowel. Normally one does not identify the adrenal glands, mesenteric lymph nodes, omentum, pancreas, abdominal vena cava, abdominal aorta, gallbladder, uterus, or ovaries.

To satisfactorily interpret the abdominal radiograph, it is important to be aware of the normal location of the various abdominal organs on the radiograph. On the lateral radiograph, the cranial abdomen contains the liver, stomach, spleen, duodenum, pancreas, ascending and transverse colon, and cecum. The caudal abdomen contains the bladder, prostate gland, uterus, descending colon, and rectum. The small intestine normally occupies the area between the bladder and stomach. On the ventrodorsal radiograph, the right cranial region contains the right liver lobe, gallbladder, cranial portions of the duodenum, pancreas, and the pyloric portion of the stomach. The left cranial region contains the body and the fundus of the stomach, left liver lobes, and the spleen.

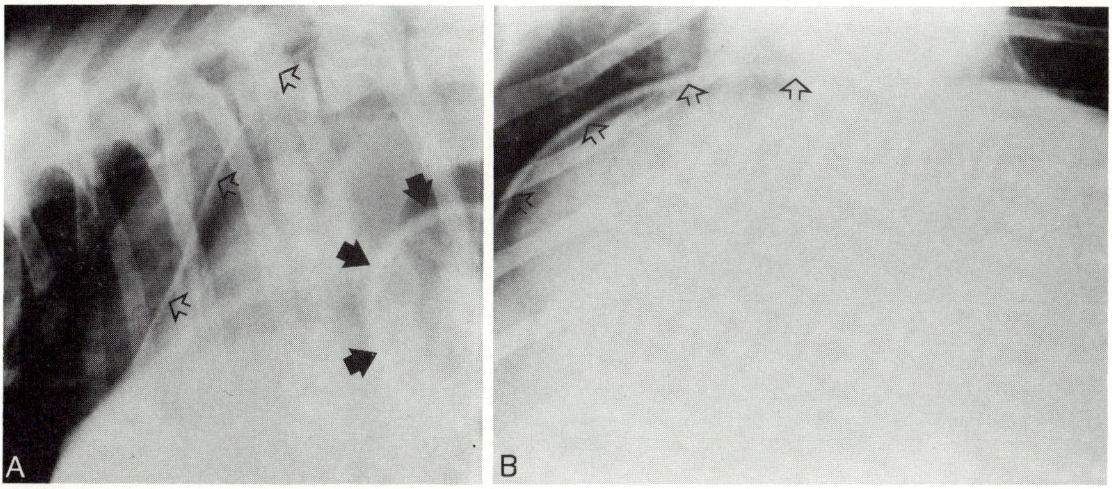

Figure 14–61. Lateral *(A)* and ventrodorsal *(B)* radiographs of the cranial abdomen of 3-year-old Great Dane with a ruptured stomach. The peritoneal surface of the right crus of the diaphragm is seen *(open arrows)* together with the serosal surfaces of the intestines *(closed arrows)*, indicating the presence of free peritoneal gas.

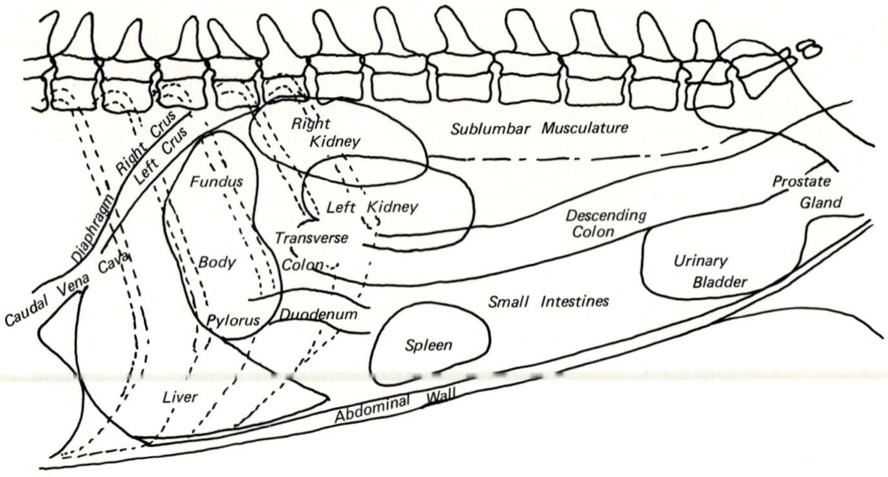

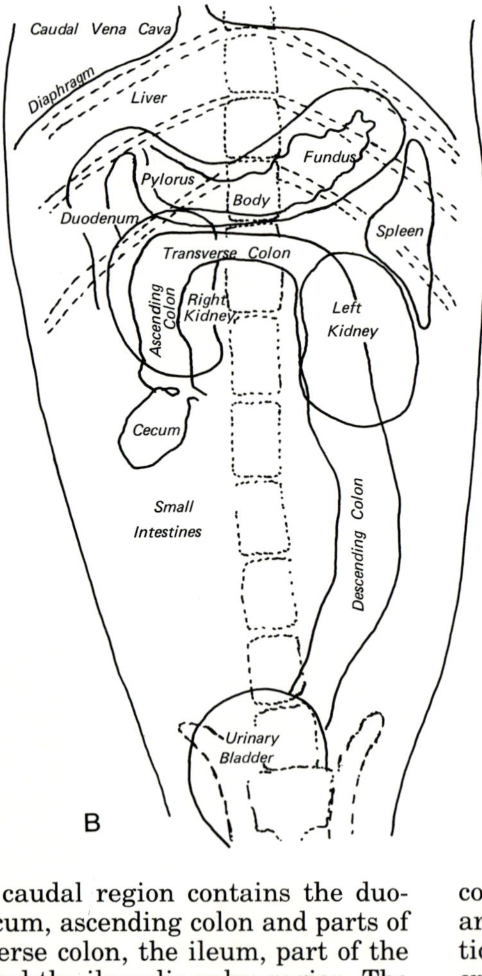

Figure 14–62. Diagrams indicating location of anatomic structures that are usually seen in lateral *(A)* and ventrodorsal *(B)* radiographs of normal canine abdomen.

The right caudal region contains the duodenum, cecum, ascending colon and parts of the transverse colon, the ileum, part of the jejunum, and the ileocolic valve region. The left caudal region contains the main portions of the jejunum, descending colon, and part of the transverse colon, and portions of the spleen.

The regional approach to radiographic interpretation is important to establish a complete list of potential diagnoses for an area of increased density and loss of definition between organs; for example, the right cranial or upper quadrant may lack definition and have an increased density in the following conditions: hemorrhage of the right liver lobes, trauma to the gallbladder, pancreatitis, pancreatic tumors or abscesses, perforated duodenal or pyloric foreign bodies and ulcers, and pyloric masses.

Abdominal Wall

The density of the abdominal wall can be separated from the density of adjoining organs by fat deposited in the subserosal areas and around the organs. Fat is deposited between the various muscles in the fascial planes and this allows their identification. The lack of visualization of the fascial planes and the subserosal fat line can be caused by emaciation or by the accumulation of fluid of any sort. The disappearance of the peritoneal surface of the abdominal wall is often a sign indicating peritoneal effusion or peritonitis. In very obese animals, the abdominal wall can be particularly well outlined.

Sublumbar Musculature

The sublumbar muscles include the psoas minor, iliopsoas, and quadratus lumborum muscles. These are often surrounded by large lumbar fat deposits providing a lucent background for the shadows of the kidneys. Any increase in the amount of fluid in the sublumbar region will cause a lack of definition in the fascial planes of the sublumbar musculature; therefore, as the kidneys are retroperitoneal organs, some interference with visualization of the renal shadows would be expected. It is important to realize that the ventral borders of the second, third, and fourth lumbar vertebrae are often indistinctly outlined. This is the region in which the diaphragmatic crura are attached. The appearance should not be mistakenly interpreted as an area of bone destruction. The same appearance on the ventral border of the fifth, sixth, or seventh lumbar vertebrae would make one suspicious of a destructive lesion due to osteomyelitis or a metastatic neoplastic process.

Kidneys

The kidneys are located retroperitoneally and the right kidney is located cranial to the left. The left kidney is more mobile than the right kidney and so has a variable location on the radiograph. It is usually ventral to the level of the right kidney. The length of the kidneys vary from two and a half to three times the length of the second lumbar vertebra in the dog. In the cat the length of each kidney is approximately two times the length of the fourth lumbar vertebra.

Liver

The liver is the main organ of the hypochondriac region of the abdomen and underlies the diaphragm, from which it cannot be separated under normal circumstances. The position of the diaphragm varies depending on the respiratory phase and the depth of inspiration. As the diaphragm varies so does the position of the liver. In animals with respiratory distress the liver will tend to move more caudally into the abdomen; conversely, in obese, pregnant, or tympanic animals the diaphragm will tend to be pushed cranially and be more within the rib cage. On the lateral projection the ventral border of the liver lobe stops at about the level of the costal arch. In the dog the liver extends down to the ventral abdominal wall, whereas in the cat the ventral border of the liver is separated from the ventral abdominal wall by a large fat pad. The size of the liver normally can be judged by the position of the stomach, because the liver is the main structure separating the stomach from the diaphragm. In the ventrodrosal projection the liver is more difficult to identify. The pylorus is affected by the size of the liver, and when there is massive liver enlargement the pylorus will be displaced caudally and toward the midline. When a small liver is present, the body and fundic portions of the stomach appear close to the cupula of the diaphragm. If the stomach shadow is not plainly noted on the plain radiograph, a small amount of barium sulfate can be given per os to identify the position of the stomach and hence indirectly obtain information on the size of the liver.

Spleen

The spleen is usually identified on both the lateral and ventrodorsal radiographs in the dog. It is identified as a triangular shadow, and on the ventrodorsal radiograph it is located between the fundic region of the stomach and the abdominal wall. In the lateral projection the free end of the spleen is seen at various distances caudoventrally to the pylorus and the liver. It also is represented as a triangular shape in this projection. The normal spleen varies considerably in size. It will increase in size in the anesthetized and tranquilized patient. The spleen of the cat is inconsistently seen radiographically because of its small size.

Pancreas

The normal pancreas is not identified on the plain radiograph. The pancreas can only be detected by its effect on the stomach and duodenum, which are intimately associated with it. In acute pancreatitis a localized increase in density and indistinctness of the intestinal outlines is noted in the upper right quadrant.

Stomach

The stomach is usually seen on survey radiographs because it contains gas and/or food material. It can be divided into four portions: the fundus, body, pyloric antrum, and pyloric canal.[31] The presence of rugae makes the appearance of the mucosal surfaces irregular in appearance, especially in the fundus. The fundus is present on the left side of midline. In the dog, the body of the stomach is located approximately on the midline and the pyloric antrum and pyloric canal are located to the right of midline. In the cat, the pyloric canal is located close to the midline (Fig. 14–63).[95] The stomach usually contains gas and fluid and, because of the distribution of these contents, the way in which the animal was positioned for radiography can be determined. If the animal is lying in left lateral recumbency, the gas in the stomach would be expected to be located in the pyloric region of the stomach. Conversely, when the animal is positioned in right lateral recumbency, the stomach gas bubble will be located in the fundic region, and the pyloric region will contain fluid.[95] This fluid-filled pyloric region can sometimes be misinterpreted as a mass lesion. On the dorsoventral radiograph the gas bubble is located in the fundic region on the left of the midline, whereas in the ventrodorsal radiograph the gas shadow is located to the right of midline in the body and pyloric regions of the stomach. The thickness of the stomach wall is difficult to assess from survey radiographs, because it will often be difficult to see its serosal surface and the mucosal surface will not be seen if there is fluid present in the adjacent lumen. The degree of distention of the stomach also influences stomach wall thickness.[95]

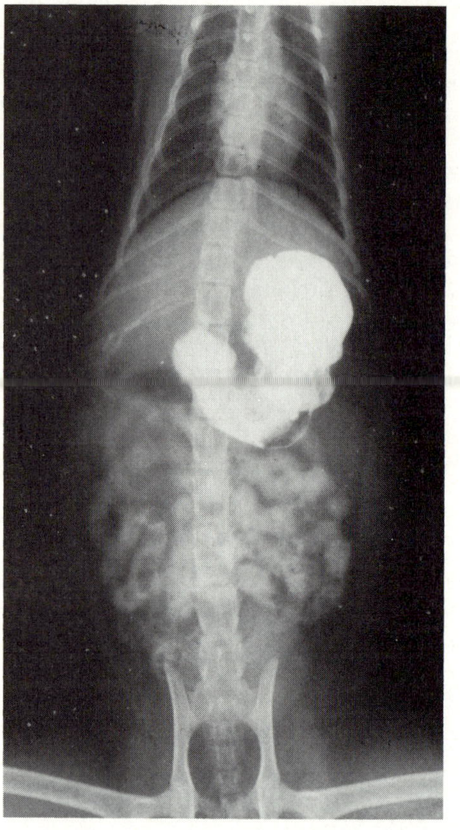

Figure 14–63. Ventrodorsal radiograph of feline abdomen following oral administration of water-soluble contrast agent. Notice that, in the cat, the pyloric antrum lies close to the midline. The density of the contrast agent in the small intestine is less than that in the stomach because it is hypertonic and is diluted as it draws fluid into the intestinal lumen.

Duodenum

The duodenum is located on the right side of the midline. It originates at the pylorus, and the descending duodenum traverses down the right abdomen parallel to the abdominal wall. On the lateral radiograph the position of the duodenum varies considerably. It should be realized that the normal duodenum contains areas of lymphoid tissues that have the form of a crater and that occasionally will be outlined by the presence of intraluminal gas. These will have the radiographic appearance of an ulcer on an upper GI and should be recognized as normal structures; a diagnosis of a duodenal ulcer should not be considered. These areas of lymphoid tissue have been referred to as pseudoulcers (Fig. 14–64).[68]

Jejunum and Ileum

The small intestines are usually spread out uniformly between the stomach and the bladder. They are relatively mobile and eas-

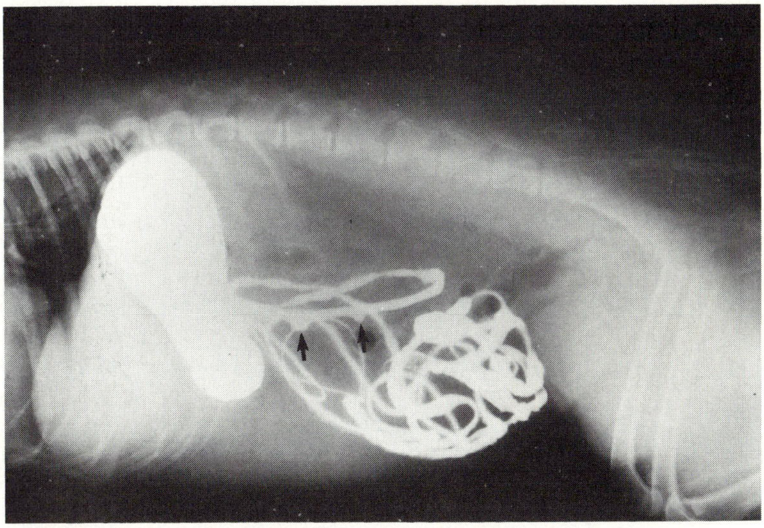

Figure 14–64. Lateral abdominal radiograph of 4-year-old Sheltie, taken 30 minutes following the oral administration of barium sulfate. Pseudoulcers are present in the descending duodenum *(arrows)*.

ily displaced by adjacent abdominal structures. Any tendency for the small intestines to clump in one region of the abdomen should be regarded as abnormal. Fluid or gas present in the small intestinal loops is visualized with good radiographic technique. The serosal surfaces of the small intestines can also be visualized. On the ventrodorsal radiograph the majority of the small intestines are located to the right midline. The normal diameter of the small intestinal loops should be less than two and a half times the width of a rib. Increased size of the small intestine usually indicates the presence of ileus (mechanical or paralytic).

Cecum and Large Intestines

The cecum and large colon are usually identified on plain radiographs by the presence of gas and fecal material. The cecum is located in the dorsal half of the abdomen on the lateral radiograph; on the ventrodorsal radiograph it is seen at the level of the second, third, or fourth lumbar vertebra to the right of the midline. The colon can be divided into ascending, transverse, and descending portions and their connecting flexures. On the lateral radiograph, the ascending colon and descending colon are located in the middle of the abdomen and are usually superimposed. On the ventrodorsal view, the colon has the general shape of a question mark. The ascending colon is located to the right of the midline, and the descending colon passes caudally on the left side of the midline. The descending colon usually enters the pelvic canal from the left of the midline, but can enter from the right, especially when the bladder is distended. The ileocolic and cecocolic junctions are located ventral to the right transverse process of the second to fourth lumbar vertebrae. The ascending colon is related to the mesoduodenum and the right limb of the pancreas dorsally where it lies ventral to the right kidney. The descending part of the duodenum bounds it on the right. The small intestinal mass lies adjacent to the ascending colon ventrally and on the left. The transverse colon forms an arc that runs from right to left, cranial to the cranial mesenteric artery and the dorsal part of the mesojejunoileum or root of the mesentery. It is related cranioventrally to the stomach and craniodorsally to the left limb of the pancreas. Ventrally and caudally it lies in contact with the small intestines. The descending colon is the longest segment of the colon. It extends from the left colic flexure on a transverse plane passing through the pelvic inlet, where it continues as the rectum. It lies in contact with the ventral surface of the left kidney. The uterus and the bladder lie ventral to its terminal part. In the male the prostate gland replaces the uterus as a ventral boundary.

Rectum

The rectum is the continuation of the descending colon caudal to the pelvic inlet. The rectum is bounded dorsally by the right and left ventral sacrococcygeal muscles. Laterally it is bounded primarily by the levator ani muscle. Ventrally the rectum is bounded by the vagina in the female and the urethra in the male. When the prostate gland is small, it lies within the pelvis or at the pelvic rim and bounds the rectum at that place. When it is enlarged, the prostate lies largely cranially to the pelvic inlet.

TECHNIQUES FOR IMPROVING ABDOMINAL DETAIL

Compression

Compression can be utilized as an aid to improve visualization of abdominal organs during routine radiography. The technique of abdominal compression is performed easily and causes little discomfort to the patient. It can be employed to obtain additional information on various abdominal structures besides that obtained from the survey radiograph. In many instances, abdominal compression will eliminate the necessity for a special contrast study; its use in association with contrast studies will increase the information obtained from the study. Compression can be applied to the abdomen so that a reduction in thickness of the entire abdomen is achieved, or compression can be applied to a more localized area to improve detail in a particular region of the abdomen.

For a generalized application of compression to the abdomen, a compression band is utilized. This band is made of thin radiolucent material which is passed from one edge of the radiographic examination table to the other; tension is then applied. An example of this apparatus is illustrated in Figure 14–65. The use of radiolucent triangular sponges under the compression band can be employed to provide a more uniform application of the compression over areas of varying thickness.

Regional applications of compression to the abdomen can be achieved using a variety of equipment. A commercial compression apparatus is available in which an inflatable rubber bladder is used to apply compression. The round outline of the inflated bladder enhances detail of adjacent or overlapping structures, as these structures will be separated when compression is applied. Readily available sources of equipment that can be used to apply localized pressure to the abdomen include mixing spoons made of wood and paddles constructed from plywood, lucite, or other thin radiolucent materials with reasonable rigidity (Fig. 14–66).

As the thickness of the part to be radiographed is significantly reduced, improved definition of the underlying structures is obtained because the amount of scattered radiation is reduced (Figs. 14–67 and 14–68). Another advantage of abdominal compression is that adjacent structures are separated from one another. This minimizes the confusion resulting from overlying radiographic densities. This effect is particularly helpful in the evaluation of uterine enlargement. Often on the survey radio-

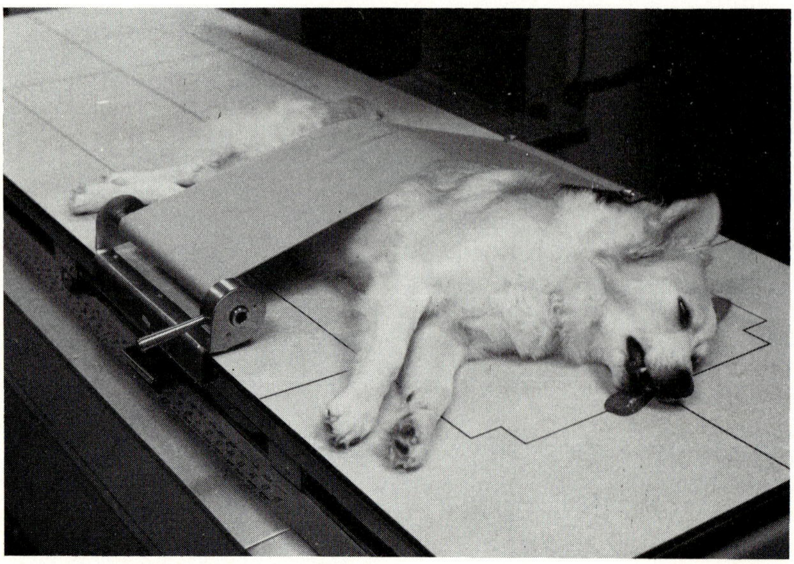

Figure 14–65. Application of compression band to the abdomen of a dog. To even out the compression on the abdominal organs, a wedge-shaped radiolucent sponge can be placed under the compression band.

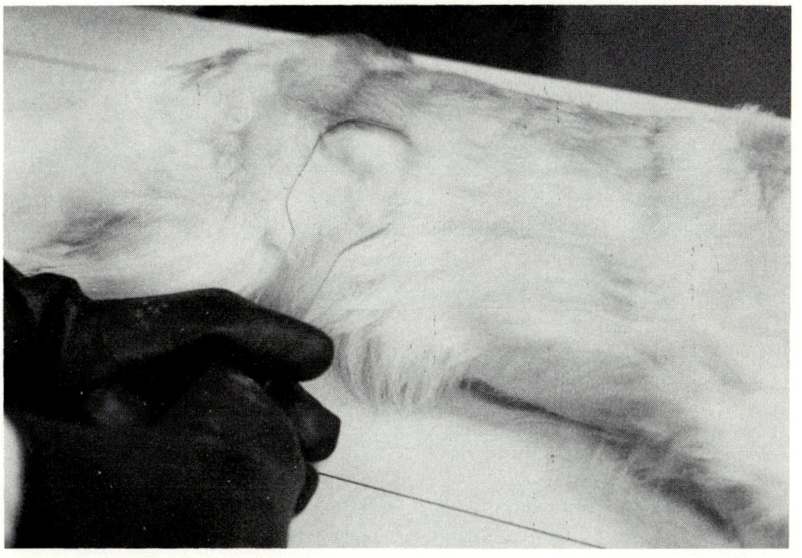

Figure 14–66. Application of a plexiglass compression paddle to the caudal abdomen of a dog. The paddle is placed over an area where enhanced detail is required.

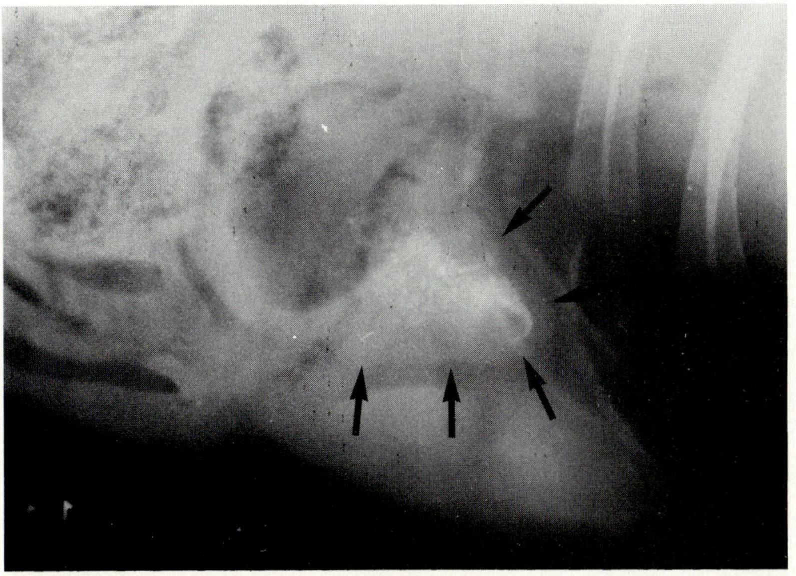

Figure 14–67. Lateral radiograph of cranial abdomen of 3-year-old Saint Bernard following application of compression band. Note that details of the ribs and pyloric region of stomach *(arrows)* enhanced. The calcific densities can be clearly identified as bone fragments within the stomach lumen.

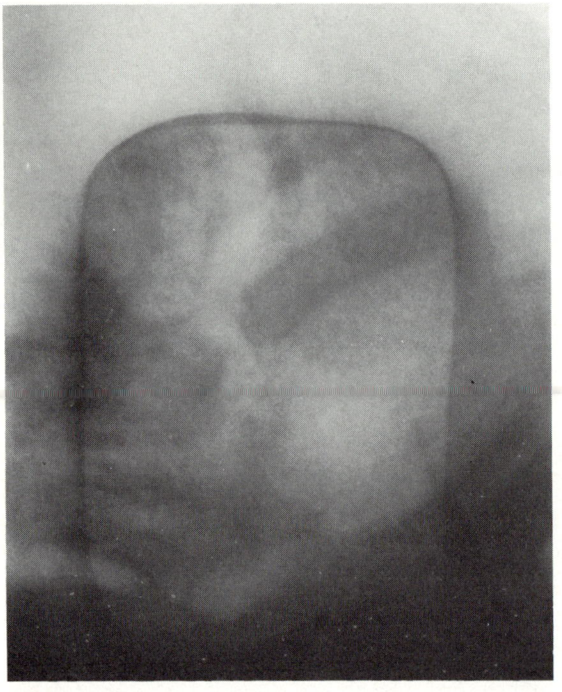

Figure 14–68. Radiograph of caudal abdomen of 8-year-old dog with early carcinomatosis. The serosal borders of the bladder and descending colon are clearly seen; however, the serosal surfaces of the small intestines cranial to the bladder are indistinct, indicating the presence of small amounts of fluid in the peritoneal cavity.

graph, the uterine shadow is obscured by overlapping densities of the rectum and/or urinary bladder. The application of compression separates the three structures and results in improved visualization of the uterine shadow. A third advantage of the use of a compression band is that the compression apparatus significantly aids in the restraint of patient and thus minimizes the risk of blurring of the radiograph due to movement. Personnel holding the animal for radiography are able to stand further from the source of x-rays; therefore the technique also contributes to radiation safety.

Compression is useful when used in conjunction with contrast studies of the gastrointestinal tract. The significance of space-occupying lesions of filling defects in the gastrointestinal tract can be resolved by the application of localized compression to the abdominal wall over the suspected site of disease. This will allow a more accurate determination of whether a lesion is luminal or extraluminal in location and will assist in diagnosis and prognosis (Fig. 14–67). False positive results associated with the imperfect preparation of the intestinal tract prior to contrast examination will also be minimized, as food or fecal material adhering to the mucosal surface of the intestines will usually dislodge or move following the application of the compression.

Several situations exist, however, in which the application of abdominal compression is contraindicated. The presence of a large, pus-filled uterus, an enlarged spleen suggestive of hemangiosarcoma, or any other enlarged viscus organ would dictate caution in the use of this technique, as rupture of the organ could result. Compression should not be used in animals with severe respiratory distress or on animals suspected of having diaphragmatic hernias. Fractures of ribs and vertebrae can result if generalized abdominal compression is applied to animals with severe depletion of skeletal mineralization.

Pneumoperitoneum

An appropriate gas (air, N_2O, or CO_2) is injected intraperitoneally to enhance radiographic visualization of the abdominal viscera. The intraperitoneally injected gas acts as a negative contrast agent. By varying the position of the patient and the direction of the x-ray beam, it is possible to evaluate the size, shape, contour, and position of selected abdominal organs. Pneumoperitoneography is ideal for evaluation of the liver, spleen, stomach, distal colon, kidneys, urinary bladder, uterus, and abdominal wall. However, the small bowel, proximal portion of the colon, mesenteric root, and pancreas are poorly evaluated with pneumoperitoneography.

Room air can be used as the contrast agent, but it is absorbed slowly and may produce an air embolus. Either CO_2 or N_2O (commercially available in pressurized cylinders) is preferred to air as the contrast medium because of their more rapid absorption from the abdominal cavity and lesser probability of causing a gas embolus. The technique of pneumoperitoneography has been described previously.[58]

Contraindications to the use of pneumoperitoneum include the following:

1. *Diaphragmatic hernia.* A pneumothorax is usually created when pneumoperitoneography is performed in the presence of a diaphragmatic hernia. If a small amount of rapidly absorbable gas such as CO_2 or N_2O is used, this is not an extremely

hazardous procedure. However, if air is used as the contrast agent, a longer-lasting iatrogenic pneumothorax results.

2. *Peritonitis and abdominal abscesses.* Pneumoperitoneum can result in extension of local abdominal infections.

3. *Abdominal fluid.* The quality of the examination is compromised by large amounts of free abdominal fluid. The fluid should be removed before injecting the negative contrast material.

4. *Respiratory difficulties.* If the patient is experiencing respiratory problems, distention of the abdomen with gas will result in increased respiratory difficulty.

Radiology of the Upper Gastrointestinal Tract

Stomach

The location of the stomach can yield important information about the size of the liver (Figs. 14–69 and 14–70); also it frequently will be displaced when a diaphragmatic hernia is present. Mass lesions involving the spleen, pancreas, and duodenum will also result in an alteration to the normal location of the stomach.

Stomach wall lesions such as stomach wall thickening and increased size of rugal folds sometimes can be assessed on the plain radiograph if considerable gas is present in the lumen, but usually these lesions require a contrast examination of the stomach for precise definition.[95] In the normal stomach, the width of rugal folds should not exceed the distance between adjacent rugae and they should be approximately parallel to one another.[74]

Intrinsic lesions in the stomach can reflect the presence of either local or systemic disease. Renal dysfunction can result in hypertrophy of rugal folds and thickening of the stomach wall due to uremic gastritis (Fig. 14–71). Calcification of submucosal tissues can also be seen with uremia (Fig. 14–72). Intrinsic lesions of the stomach include gastritis and gastric ulcers (Fig. 14–71), foreign bodies (Fig. 14–73), tumors (Figs. 14–74 and 14–75) and outflow obstruction due to pyloric hypertrophy or spasm (Fig. 14–76). Usually a contrast study will be necessary for accurate diagnosis. Gastric dilatation and volvulus also occur (Figs. 14–77 and 14–78).

Gastric volvulus and gastric dilatation are associated with acute onset of clinical signs and usually present as a greatly distended, fluid- and gas-filled stomach. When gastric volvulus is present, the pylorus is often identified dorsal to the fundus and to the left midline, and this allows differentiation from gastric dilatation.[46] Frequently a soft-tissue line can be seen across the distended

Text continued on page 429

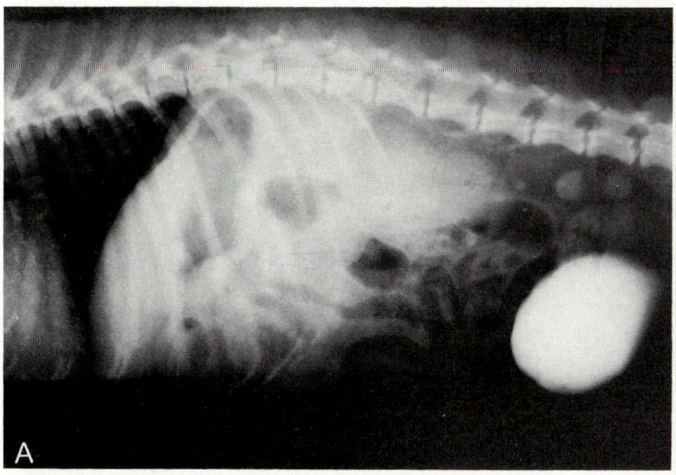

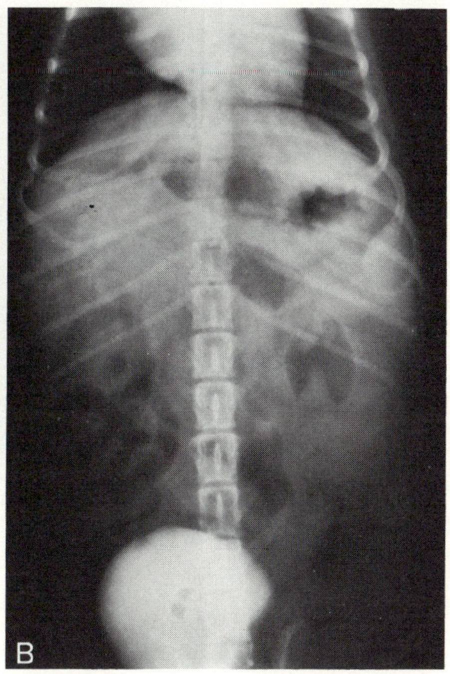

Figure 14–69. Lateral *(A)* and ventrodorsal *(B)* radiograph of 2-year-old miniature schnauzer with hepatoencephalopathy associated with a portacaval shunt. Note that on the lateral radiograph the stomach is vertical, indicating that the liver is smaller than normal. On the ventrodorsal view this is confirmed by the decreased distance between the stomach and the diaphragm. There is radiodense contrast agent in the urinary bladder.

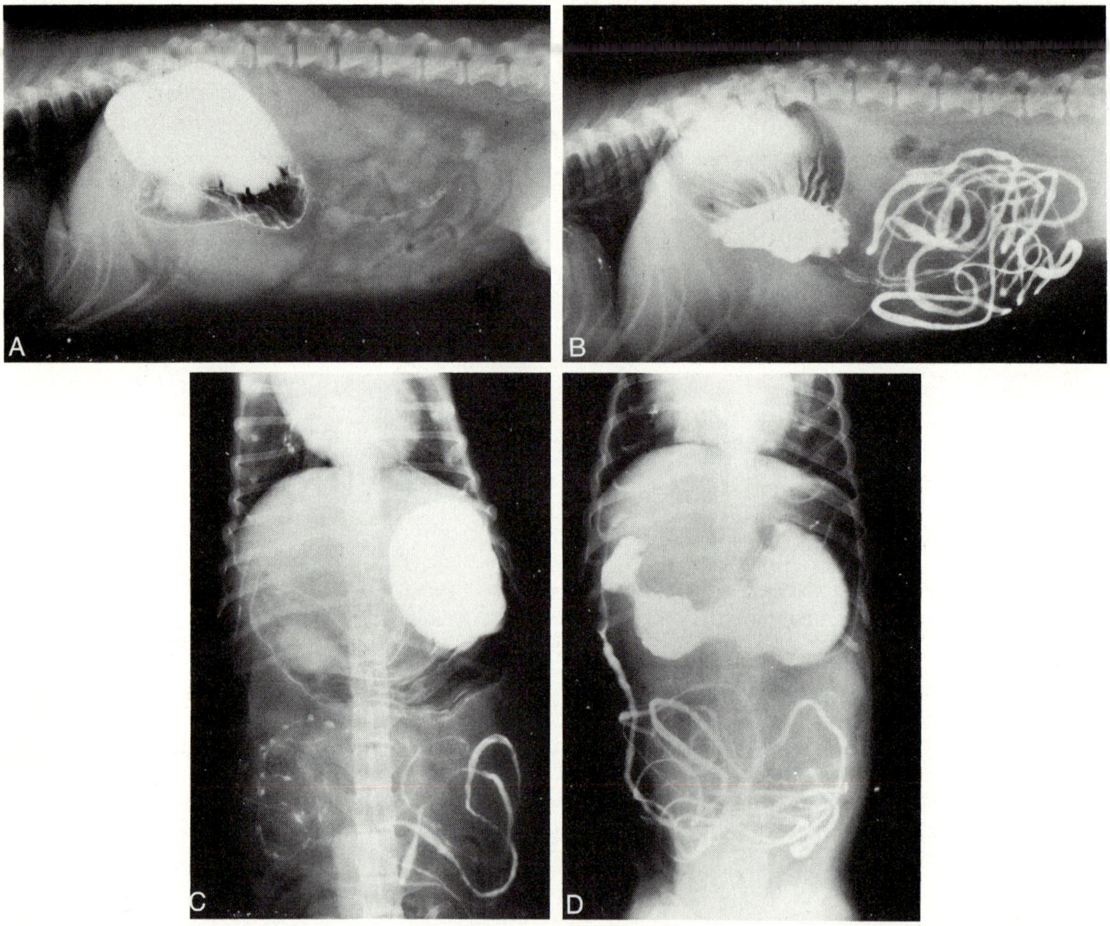

Figure 14–70. Abdominal radiographs, following oral administration of barium sulfate, of a 12-year-old male dachshund with an enlarged liver. *A,* Left lateral radiograph; *B,* right lateral radiograph; *C,* ventrodorsal radiograph; and *D,* dorsoventral radiograph. Note that the distribution of the barium sulfate and gas in the stomach changes with the different positions of the patient. Alteration of the plane of the stomach on the lateral views confirms the liver enlargment.

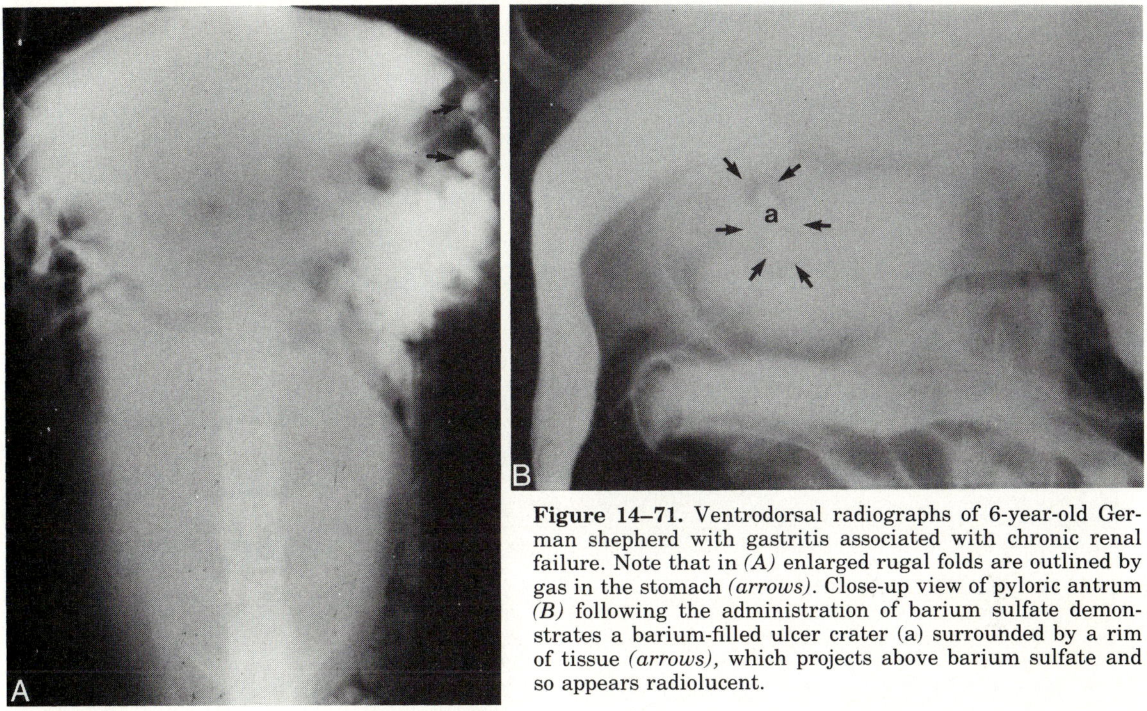

Figure 14–71. Ventrodorsal radiographs of 6-year-old German shepherd with gastritis associated with chronic renal failure. Note that in *(A)* enlarged rugal folds are outlined by gas in the stomach *(arrows)*. Close-up view of pyloric antrum *(B)* following the administration of barium sulfate demonstrates a barium-filled ulcer crater (a) surrounded by a rim of tissue *(arrows)*, which projects above barium sulfate and so appears radiolucent.

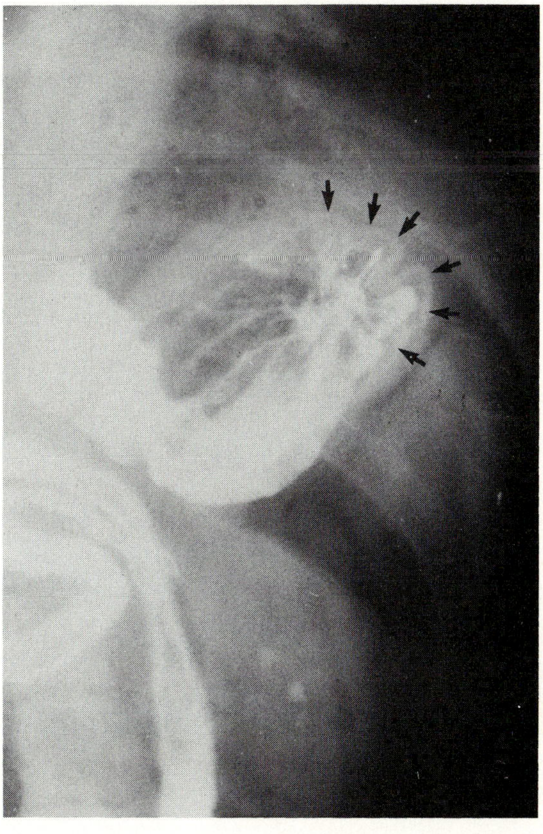

Figure 14–72. Ventrodorsal radiograph, following oral administration of barium sulfate, of 8-year-old sheltie with chronic renal failure. Calcification of the stomach wall was noted on plain radiographs, and the studies indicated that the calcification was in the submucosal layer of the stomach wall *(arrows)*. Notice also that calcification is also present in the left kidney.

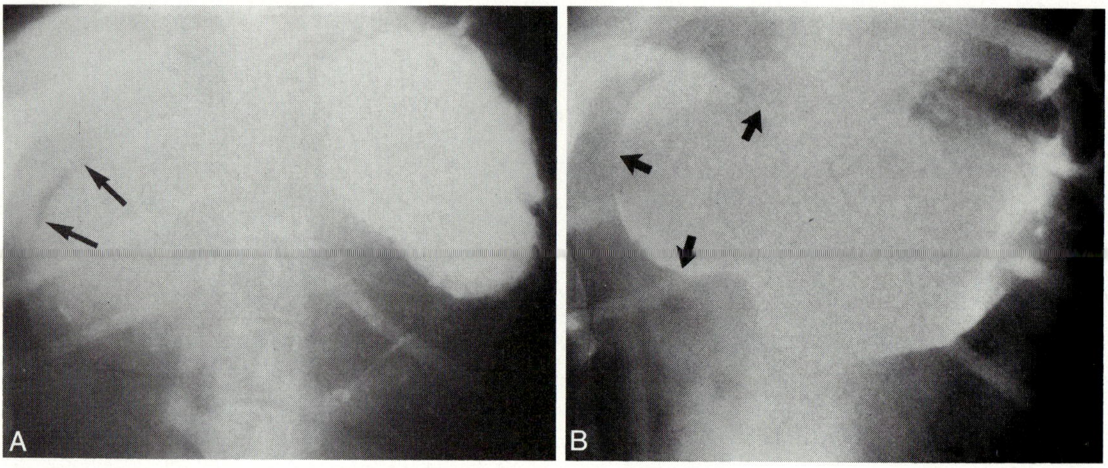

Figure 14–73. Radiographs, following oral administration of barium sulfate, of 2-year-old Doberman pinscher with a gastric foreign body (rubber ball). In the ventrodorsal view *(A)*, a small amount of gas in the pyloric region of the stomach surrounds the foreign body *(arrows)* and suggests its presence. The dorsoventral view *(B)* demonstrates the foreign body better, because the barium sulfate gravitates to the pyloric region of the stomach and the ball creates a filling defect in the contrast agent *(arrows)*.

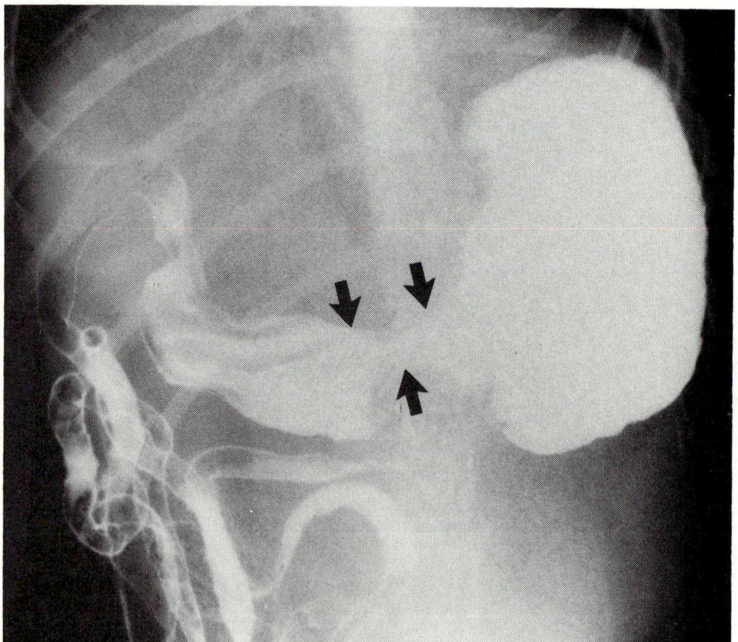

Figure 14–74. Ventrodorsal radiograph, following oral administration of barium sulfate, of 12-year-old golden retriever with gastric adenocarcinoma. Note annular constriction of the body of the stomach *(arrows)*.

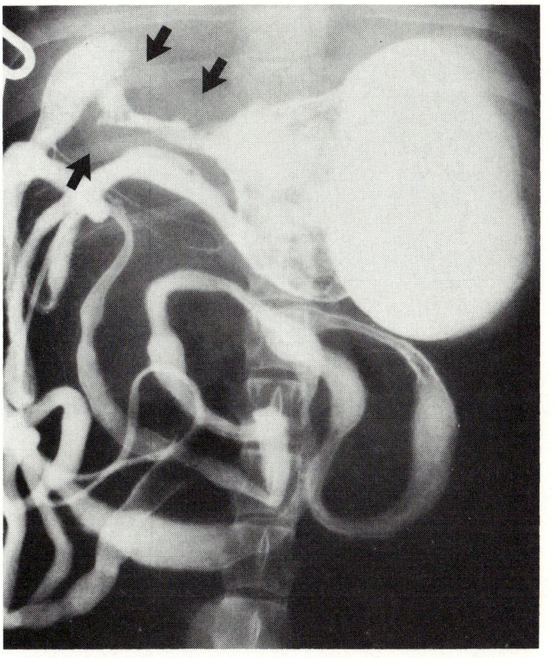

Figure 14–75. Ventrodorsal radiograph of 9-year-old Scottish terrier with adenocarcinoma of the pyloric portion of the stomach. Note lack of filling of the pyloric antrum and irregular mucosal–barium sulfate interfaces in this region. Thickening of the stomach wall is also seen *(arrows)*.

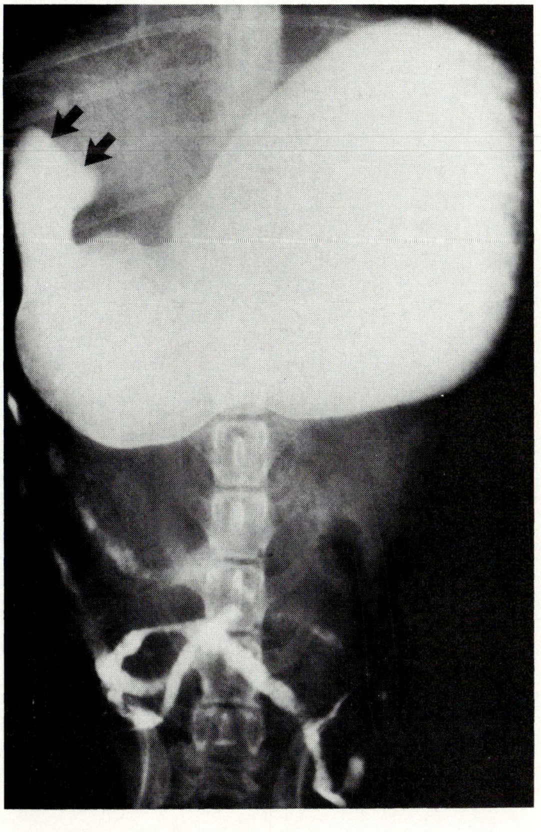

Figure 14–76. Ventrodorsal radiograph of 16-month-old boxer with a history of chronic vomiting secondary to hypertrophy of the pyloric sphincter. Barium sulfate was administered one hour previously. Notice enlarged stomach and delayed gastric emptying. The broad imprint of a hypertrophied pyloric sphincter on the pyloric antrum can be identified *(arrows)*.

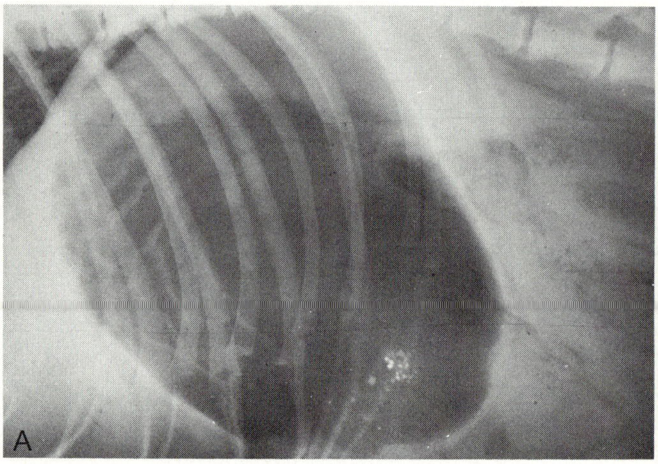

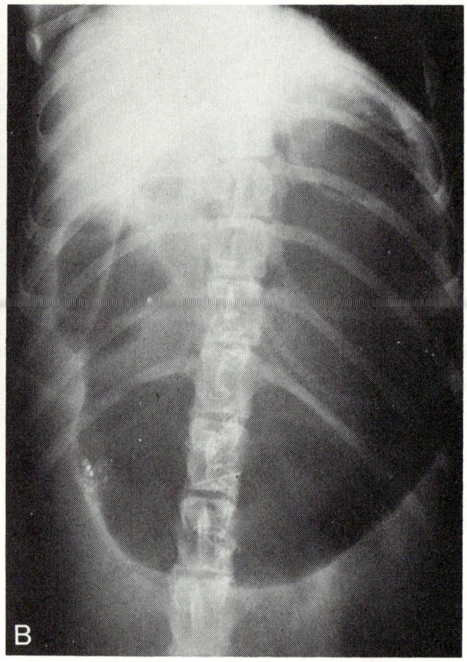

Figure 14–77. Lateral (*A*) and ventrodorsal (*B*) radiograph of 9-month-old Labrador retriever with gastric dilatation. Notice that although the stomach is greatly distended with gas, the relationships of the stomach within the abdomen remain normal.

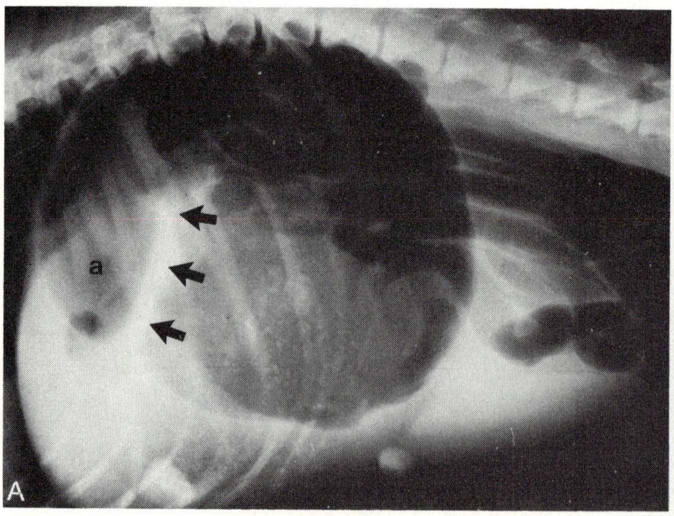

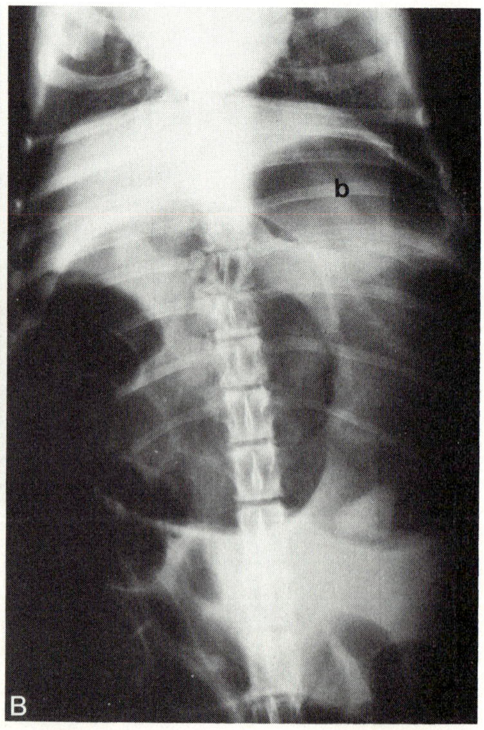

Figure 14–78. Lateral *(A)* and ventrodorsal *(B)* radiographs of nine-year-old boxer with gastric volvulus. There is marked distention of the stomach with gas and fluid. Note on the lateral view that the pyloric antrum (a) is displaced dorsally, and a soft-tissue dense band *(arrows)* suggests compartmentalization of the stomach. On the ventrodorsal view, the pyloric antrum (b) is present in the left cranial abdomen. On both radiographs, the small intestines are enlarged and gas filled, suggesting ileus.

stomach, and this confirms that twisting of the stomach has resulted in compartmentalization (Fig. 14–78). Paralytic gas ileus commonly accompanies gastric volvulus. With gastric enlargement secondary to pyloric sphincter hypertrophy, the enlarged stomach frequently will contain fluid and food material with less gas than is usually seen with gastric volvulus, and orientation of the stomach within the abdomen is normal (Fig. 14–76). Identification of the hypertrophic pyloric sphincter usually will require the oral administration of barium sulfate.

Small Intestines

The small intestines will exhibit disease by changes in the caliber, mucosal pattern, and motility of bowel loops. Abnormalities of motility and mucosal pattern are elusive and are most easily documented by fluoroscopy and/or barium sulfate contrast examinations.[30]

Frequently the intestinal tract is examined on the plain radiographs for evidence of obstruction. Intestinal obstruction has been defined as a condition in which there is partial or complete cessation of the normal forward motion of the intestinal contents for a period long enough to produce general and local pathologic changes. The contents of an obstructed small intestine consist of fluid alone or fluid and gas in varying amounts. The classic roentgenographic description of a simple, nonstrangulated small intestinal obstruction is that of moderate to severe distention of the small intestines cranial to the site of obstruction. If the obstruction is complete and has been present for several hours, there will be relatively little or no gas in the large intestine.[101] The diagnosis of obstruction is not difficult when gaseous distention of bowel loops is present and the small intestines can be seen to be larger than their normal diameter. On films taken using a horizontal x-ray beam, gas–fluid interfaces (fluid levels) are often seen (Fig. 14–79). These often appear as "hairpin" loops in cases of mechanical obstruction and result when the ascending and descending limbs of an obstructed bowel segment are filled with air and have fluid levels on either side but at different levels.[85] This indicates that rushes of peristalsis are dumping fluid from one side of the "hairpin" into the other. They do not have to always appear on the film, however, because frequently little or no gas accompanies the obstruction, especially in cases where the obstruction is due to strangulation of the bowel. In these cases the correct radiographic diagnosis will depend on the recognition of fluid in distended bowel loops rather than on the appearance of gas and the radiographic findings correlated with the history and physical examination.[101] Common causes of obstruction of the small intestines include foreign bodies, intussusception, tumors, adhesions, and incarceration from diaphragmatic or other peritoneal hernias. In cases of paralytic ileus and decreased peristalsis, the fluid levels in hairpin loops will tend to be at similar levels. The loops will appear to be flaccid

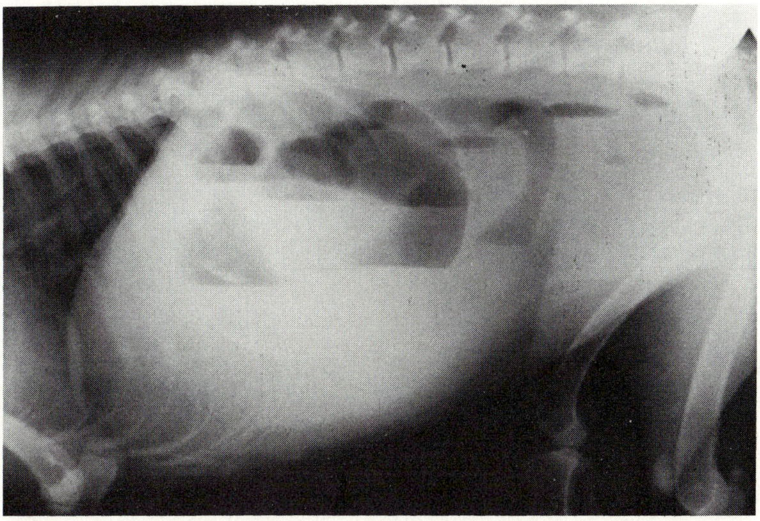

Figure 14–79. Standing lateral abdominal radiograph, using a horizontal x-ray beam, of 4-year-old boxer dog with intestinal obstruction. Note multiple gas-fluid levels in the distended small intestinal loops. The varying levels of the gas-fluid interfaces suggest an obstructive ileus.

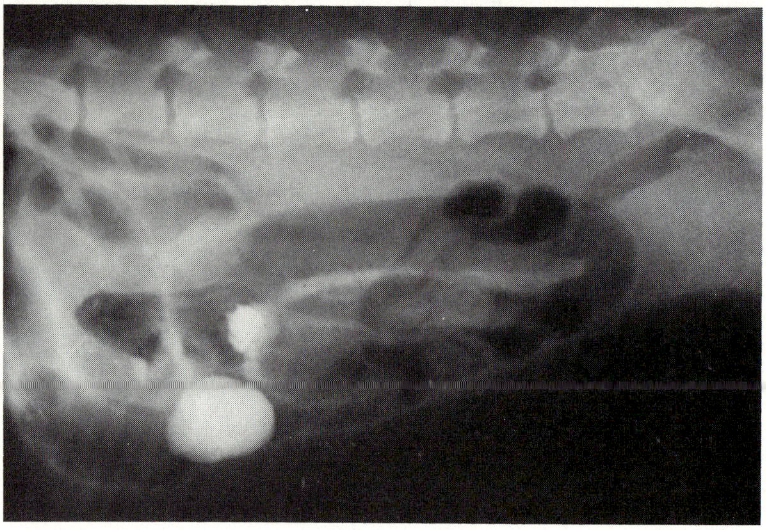

Figure 14–80. Lateral abdominal radiograph of 2-year-old Australian shepherd with intestinal obstruction due to a stone. Note the distended, gas-filled bowel loops proximal to the obstruction, indicating ileus.

and of wide caliber; in addition, on standing lateral radiographs the fluid levels are longer compared with the loops seen with mechanical obstruction.[85] Causes of paralytic ileus include peritonitis, uremia, vascular accidents and spinal cord injury.[31] It can also occur following surgery.

Radiodense foreign bodies are easily detected on the plain radiograph (Fig. 14–80). Occasionally radiolucent foreign bodies can be identified because they contain gas or because of their uneven texture. Linear foreign bodies frequently will be suggested on plain radiographs by clumping of the small intestines in the mid-abdominal region and the presence of increased numbers of "end-on" bowel loops (Fig. 14–81).

Intussusception most frequently occurs at the ileocolic junction but may involve any segment of the intestine. The recognition of the intussuscepted portion of bowel on the plain radiograph will frequently depend on gas accumulating in the lumen of the bowel cranial to the obstruction. Occasionally a sausage-shaped mass in the mid-abdominal region is observed.

In most instances, the presence of disease involving the small intestine will only be revealed following the administration of radiodense contrast agents. The presence of

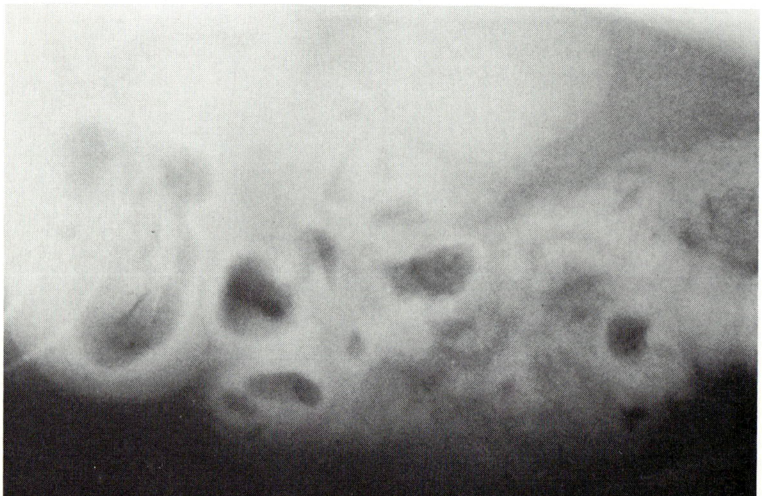

Figure 14–81. Lateral abdominal radiograph of a 3-year-old domestic short-haired cat with a linear foreign body. Note the abnormal gas pattern in the small intestines, which are clumped in the mid-abdominal region. Indistinctness of the serosal surfaces of the intestines suggests localized peritonitis, possibly secondary to bowel perforation caused by the foreign body.

small intestinal disease is frequently suggested on the plain radiographs, however, by the presence of increased amounts of gas and/or fluid in the intestinal loops (Fig. 14–82).

CONTRAST RADIOGRAPHIC EXAMINATION OF THE STOMACH AND SMALL INTESTINES (UPPER GASTROINTESTINAL STUDY)

Contrast media is administered orally and radiographs are made during the passage of contrast through the stomach and small intestines into the colon. Both positive and negative contrast agents can be used to evaluate the physiological and morphological characteristics of the gastrointestinal tract.[31] Most studies are performed using positive contrast agents; however, double-contrast techniques have been described to study the stomach specifically.[24] Following are some indications for a gastrointestinal contrast study:

1. Any conditions that alter the size, shape, or position of the stomach and small bowel and that cannot be sufficiently characterized by plain radiographs or physical examination.
2. Any suspected total or partial obstruction of the flow of gastric or intestinal contents.
3. Radiopaque foreign bodies noted on plain abdominal survey films; or a foreign body detected by physical examination.
4. Evaluation of the mucosal surface of the intestinal tract when specific clinical signs suggesting disease are present but the cause cannot be characterized on the plain radiographs.

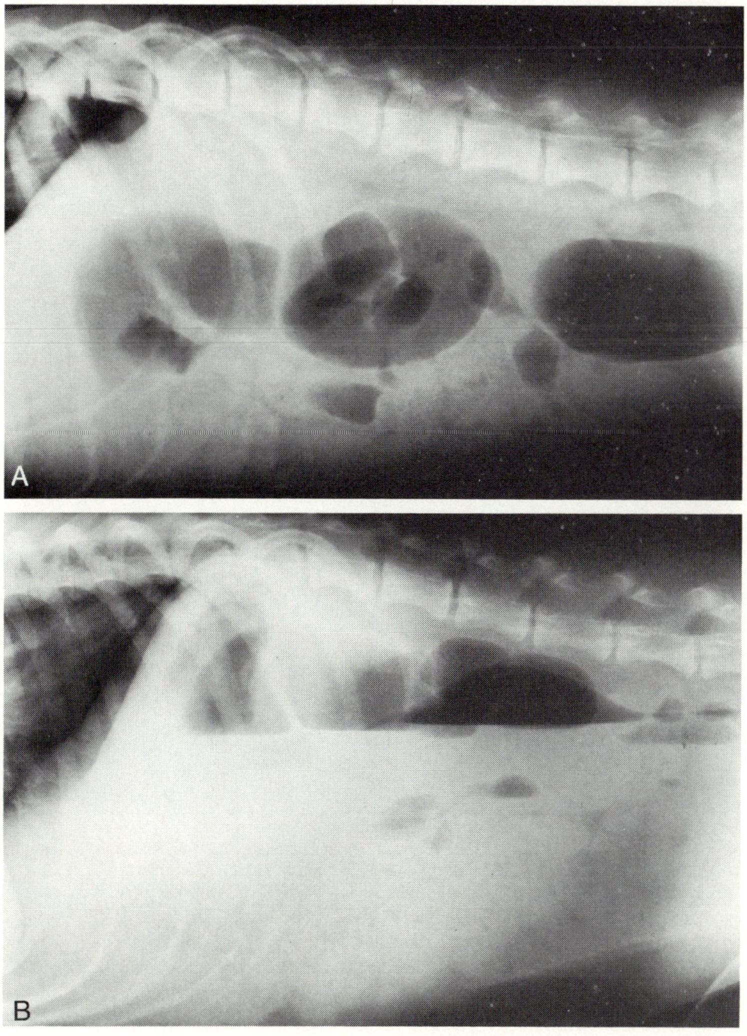

Figure 14–82. Lateral *(A)* and standing lateral *(B)* radiographs of 8-month-old female Doberman pinscher with acute enteritis. On the lateral radiograph the small intestines can be seen filled with fluid and, to a lesser extent, gas. The cecum and large colon are gas filled. On the standing lateral radiograph, gas-fluid lines are seen in the large colon and stomach but are not seen in the fluid-filled small intestine.

Contrast studies of the upper gastrointestinal tract are specifically used:

1. To outline the stomach and small bowel to confirm or prove displacement by an extrinsic mass—e.g., hepatic or splenic tumor (see 14–70).
2. To outline the stomach and confirm dilatation or abnormal shape of this organ—e.g., hypertrophy of the pyloric sphincter (Fig. 14–76).
3. To demonstrate a delayed passage of contrast and confirm a gastric or small bowel obstruction or partial obstruction—e.g., foreign body (Fig. 14–83 and 14–84) or tumor (Fig. 14–85).
4. To demonstrate a defect in the wall of the stomach or small bowel—e.g., tumor (Figs. 14–74, 14–86, and 14–87).
5. To demonstrate mucosal disease (Figs. 14–88 and 14–89).

Contraindications

The use of osmotically active contrast agents (e.g., water-soluble iodide compounds) in patients in cases in which fluid balance is critical, can cause shock; barium compounds are contraindicated when the possibility of gastrointestinal rupture exists. Barium sulfate can elicit a severe reaction if it passes into the peritoneal cavity.

Preparation of the Patient

The upper intestinal tract should be empty prior to the contrast study. This may require withholding food for a variable amount of time prior to the study and/or enemas or cathartics. The large bowel should be evacuated prior to the initiation of the contrast study. Tranquilizers or other drugs may affect the peristaltic activity of the stomach and bowel and should be used with caution. Acetylpromazine maleate* (0.05 mg/kg IV) has been found to be a suitable tranquilizer to use in conjunction with gastrointestinal studies.[105]

Technique

Survey abdominal radiographs (lateral and ventrodorsal) should be made prior to the initiation of the contrast study. This will enable an adequate check to be made of the preparation of the patient and will identify the normal position of the abdominal organs. The contrast agent can be administered by placing it in the cheek pouch by syringe, after which the animal is made to swallow, or else a stomach tube can be utilized. The dosage should be approxi-

*Acepromazine, Ayerst Laboratories, New York, NY.

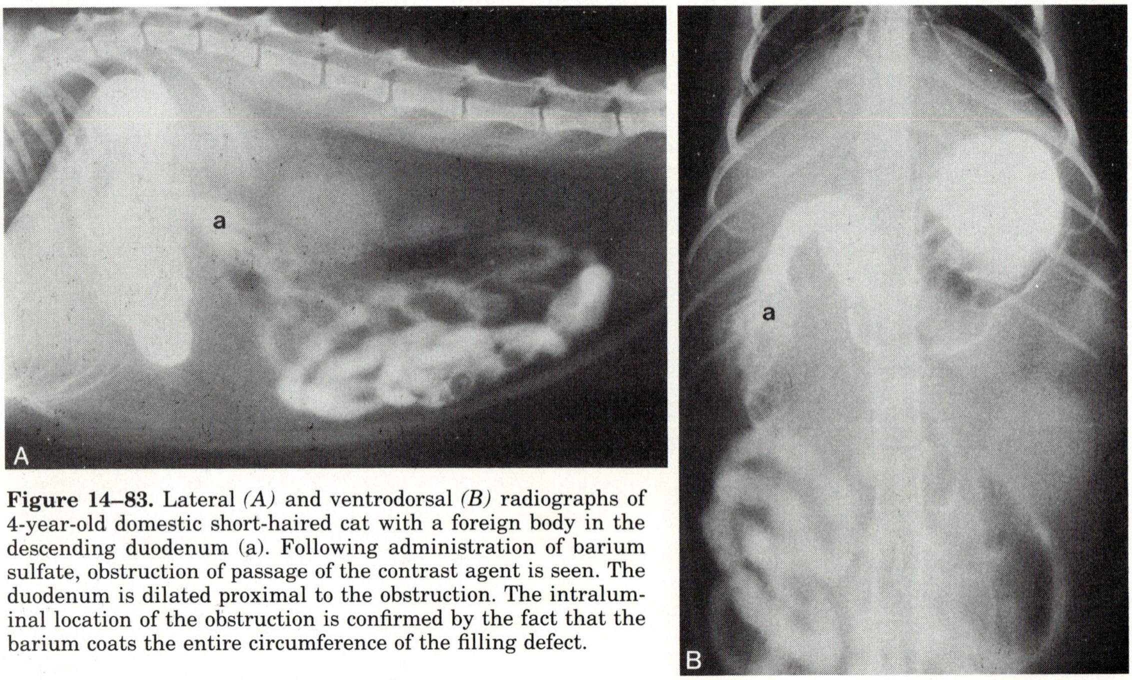

Figure 14–83. Lateral *(A)* and ventrodorsal *(B)* radiographs of 4-year-old domestic short-haired cat with a foreign body in the descending duodenum (a). Following administration of barium sulfate, obstruction of passage of the contrast agent is seen. The duodenum is dilated proximal to the obstruction. The intraluminal location of the obstruction is confirmed by the fact that the barium coats the entire circumference of the filling defect.

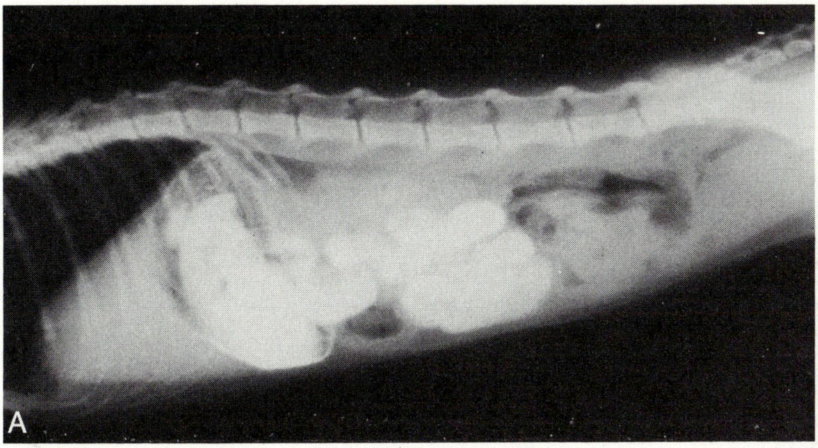

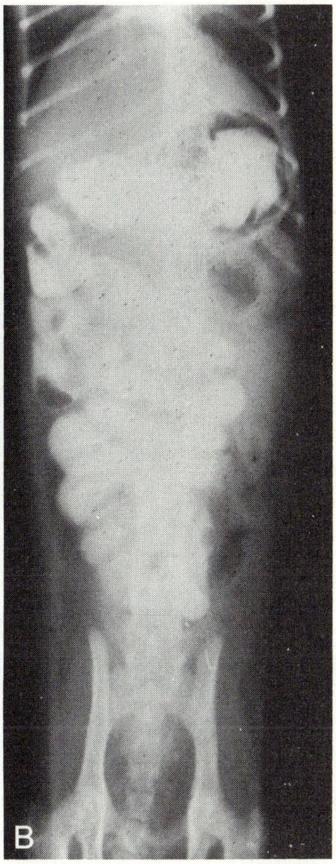

Figure 14–84. Lateral *(A)* and ventrodorsal *(B)* radiographs of 1-year-old domestic short-haired cat with linear foreign body. The radiographs were taken one hour after oral administration of barium sulfate. Note the pleating of the small intestines. The rate of passage of the barium sulfate is slower than normal.

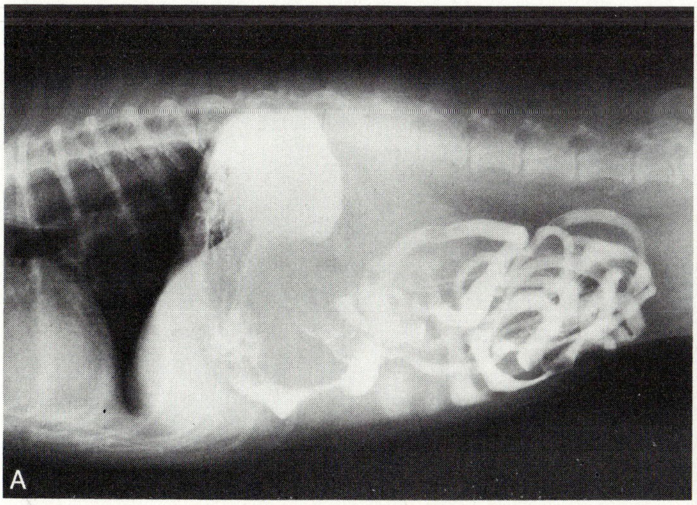

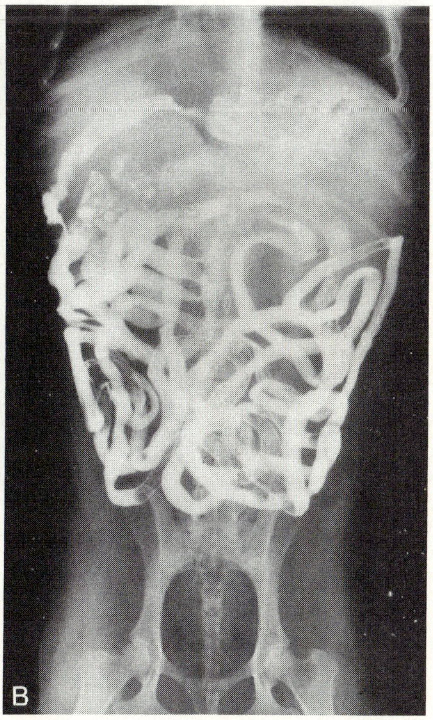

Figure 14–85. Lateral *(A)* and ventrodorsal *(B)* radiographs, taken 2 hours after oral administration of barium sulfate, of abdomen of 5-year-old wheaten terrier with duodenal neoplasm. Notice ventral displacement and irregular lumen size of the duodenum on the lateral radiograph. On the ventrodorsal radiograph, displacement of the stomach to the left is seen, together with distortion of the first part of the descending duodenum.

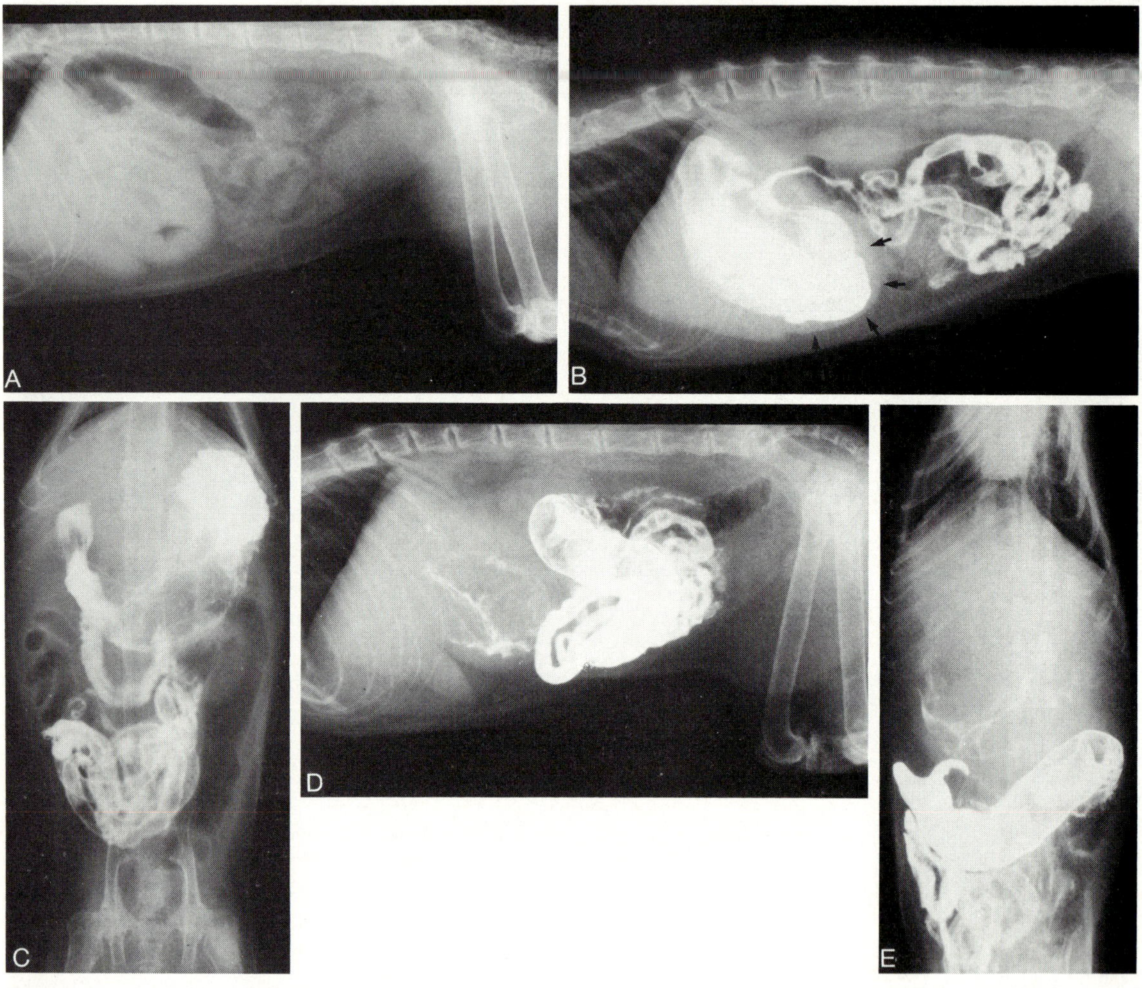

Figure 14–86. Lateral radiograph *(A)* of 6-year-old female Himalayan cat with gastric lymphosarcoma. Note enlarged stomach with markedly thickened walls. Following oral administration of barium sulfate *(B* and *C)*, the thickening of the stomach wall is confirmed *(arrows, B)*. On the films taken one hour after the administration of contrast agent (*D* and *E*), retained barium is noted in the stomach.

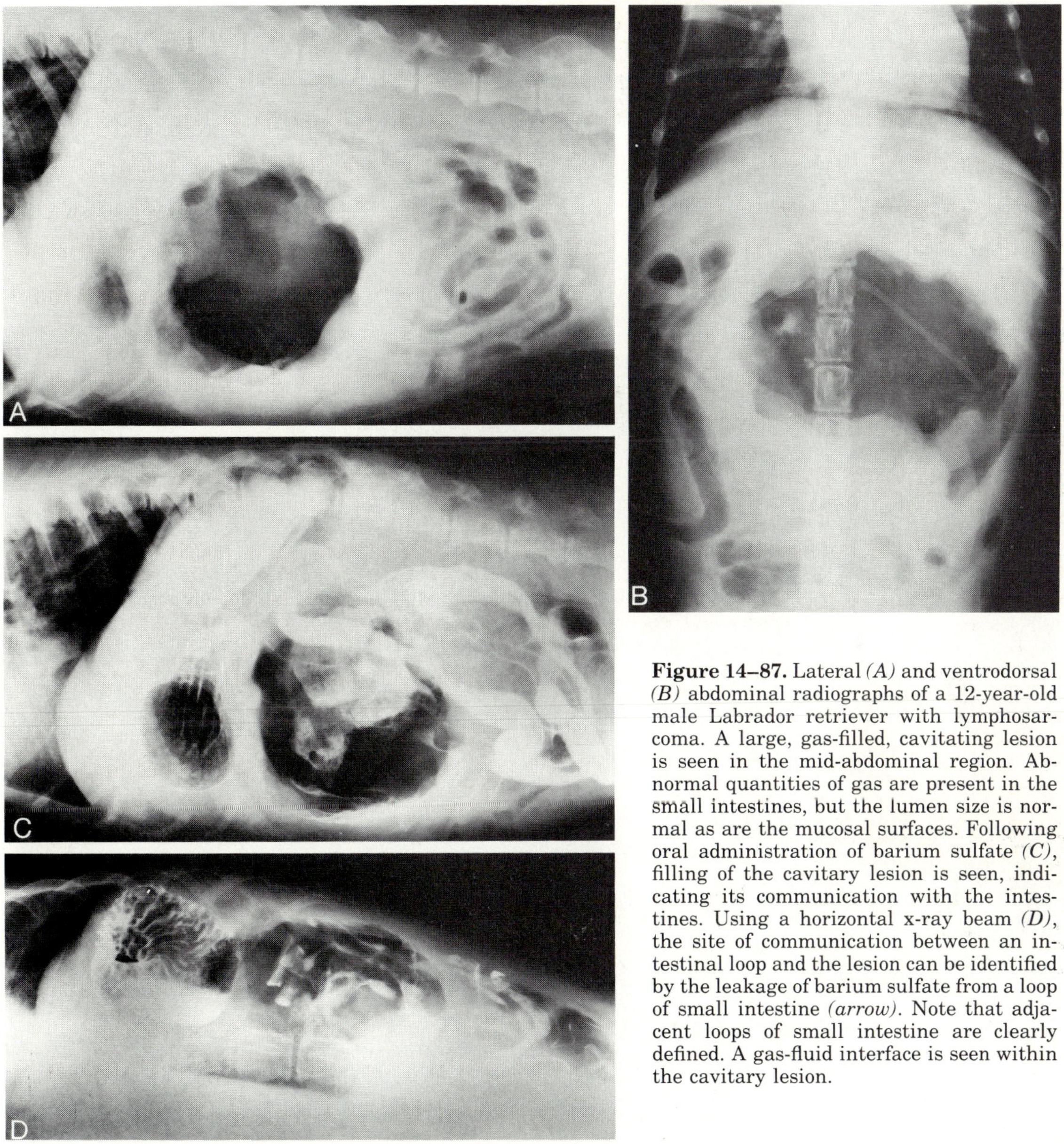

Figure 14–87. Lateral *(A)* and ventrodorsal *(B)* abdominal radiographs of a 12-year-old male Labrador retriever with lymphosarcoma. A large, gas-filled, cavitating lesion is seen in the mid-abdominal region. Abnormal quantities of gas are present in the small intestines, but the lumen size is normal as are the mucosal surfaces. Following oral administration of barium sulfate *(C)*, filling of the cavitary lesion is seen, indicating its communication with the intestines. Using a horizontal x-ray beam *(D)*, the site of communication between an intestinal loop and the lesion can be identified by the leakage of barium sulfate from a loop of small intestine *(arrow)*. Note that adjacent loops of small intestine are clearly defined. A gas-fluid interface is seen within the cavitary lesion.

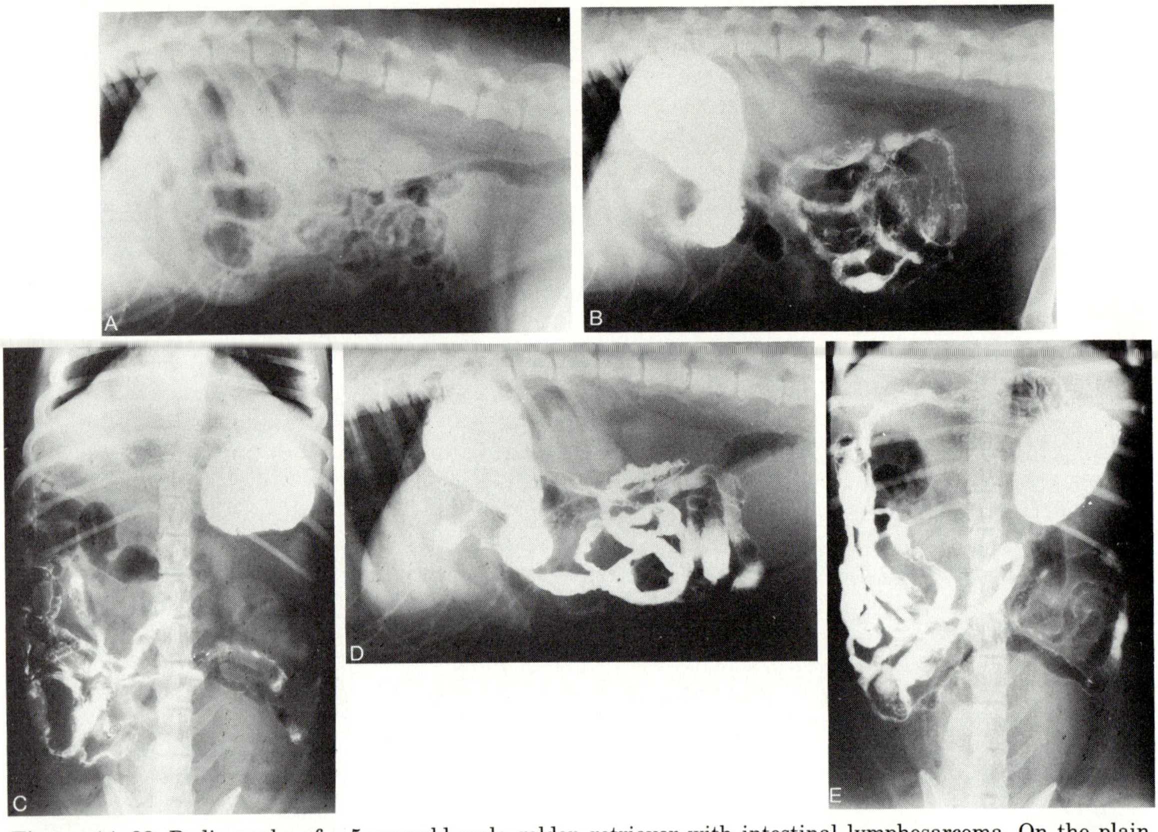

Figure 14–88. Radiographs of a 5-year-old male golden retriever with intestinal lymphosarcoma. On the plain radiograph *(A)*, increased amounts of gas are present in the intestines. Following oral administration of barium sulfate *(B* through *E)* uneven caliber of the intestines is seen, together with irregularity of the mucosal surfaces and thickening of the intestinal walls.

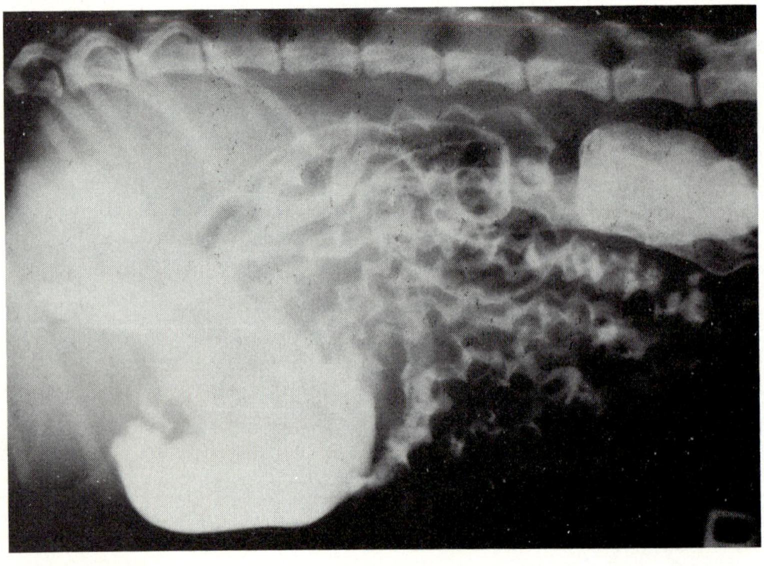

Figure 14–89. Lateral abdominal radiograph of a 2-year-old border collie with eosinophilic enteritis, taken 30 minutes after the oral administration of barium sulfate. Notice extensive thickening and distortion of small intestinal walls secondary to cellular infiltration and inflammation.

mately 8 to 10 cc of 30 per cent micropulverized barium sulfate per kilogram of body weight.[31] It is essential to distend the stomach so that meaningful evaluation of its mucosal surfaces can be made. It is important to characterize changes in the stomach and small intestine only when those segments of the bowel are fully distended with contrast agent, as irregular mucosal patterns may be seen in normal segments of the gastrointestinal tract that are only partially filled.[30] At a minimum in the dog, films should be exposed immediately following the administration of the contrast agent, and then 15 minutes, 60 minutes, and 2 to 3 hours following administration.[58] The series should be continued until the contrast agent reaches the colon. In the cat, films should be exposed immediately following contrast administration, and then every 15 minutes. It is often necessary to compare the presence of suspicious changes of the intestinal study on multiple films to add weight to the significance of any changes noted. Delayed emptying of the stomach can be due to a foreign body at the pyloric canal, hypertrophy of the pyloric canal of a congenital or acquired nature, a tumor mass (intrinsic or extrinsic), or a graulomatous lesion (extrinsic or intrinsic). Pancreatitis or bowel rupture can lead to an extrinsic granulomatous mass. It is essential to realize that there is a great variation in the normal time that the stomach commences to empty. In the normal, relaxed animal, emptying of the stomach commences almost immediately, whereas in an animal that is scared or apprehensive, emptying can be delayed for a considerable time. It is considered that if emptying of the stomach has not commenced within one-half hour after the administration of the contrast agent, then an abnormality exists. In the dog, barium sulfate normally will reach the ileocolic region approximately two to two and one-half hours after administration. In the cat, progression of the contrast agent through the small intestine is more rapid. Water-soluble gastrointestinal contrast agents are used when perforation of the bowel wall is suspected. Because of their hypertonic nature, dilution of the contrast agent occurs as it passes through the intestines. This results in poor definition of the mucosal surfaces of the small intestines (Fig. 14–63). Dehydration of the patient can also result.

Filling defects in the lumen of the stomach can be related to the presence of a foreign body or tumor. Alteration in the appearance of the rugal pattern is seen in various conditions including gastritis and tumors; it may also be due to failure to give the animal enough contrast agent to cause distention of the organ. Alteration in the position of the stomach can occur with hepatic enlargement (see Fig. 14–70), diaphragmatic hernia or pericardial–diaphragmatic herniation (Fig. 14–90), and in animals with portocaval shunts. A small liver will cause the stomach to attain a more upright position, while hepatic enlargement will result in the plane of the stomach becoming more horizontal. Alteration of the size of the stomach can be due to gastric volvulus or gastric dilatation and also can be secondary to pyloric obstruction. Pyloric obstruction secondary to hypertrophy of the pyloric sphincter will result in an enlarged stomach, frequently with exaggerated peristaltic activity. The hypertrophied pyloric sphincter will be confirmed by its effect on the adjacent pyloric antrum, where the impression of the thickened sphincter can often be observed (see Fig. 14–76). Filling defects in the stomach wall can be secondary to gastric ulceration and gastric tumors.

The normal barium sulfate–mucosa interface varies from smooth and well defined (Fig. 14–91), to noticeably fimbriated.[95] The lumen size is regular except for segmentation of the bowel that causes intermittent narrowing of the lumen. Causes of alteration in the appearance of the small intestines following barium sulfate administration are illustrated in Figure 14–92. In the normal cat it is not uncommon to see increased segmentation of the upper small intestine (Fig. 14–93); this may also be seen with duodenitis.[67]

The presence of dilated gas- and fluid-filled loops of small bowel usually signifies a partial or complete obstruction, and this can be due to foreign bodies, tumors, intussusception, volvulus, or adhesions. The radiographic appearance of mechanical bowel obstruction following contrast agent administration is characterized by delayed gastric emptying or delayed small bowel transit time. With long-standing obstructions there is often moderate to marked luminal distention of intestinal segments proximal to the obstruction and this will result in delay in the contrast agent reaching the site of obstruction. In addition, con-

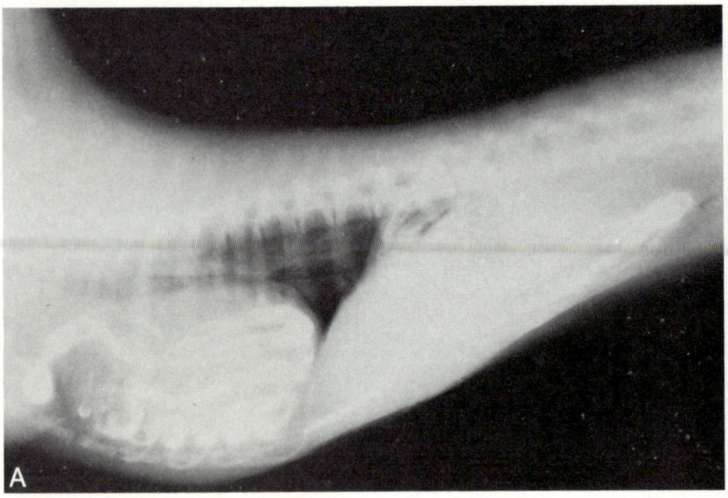

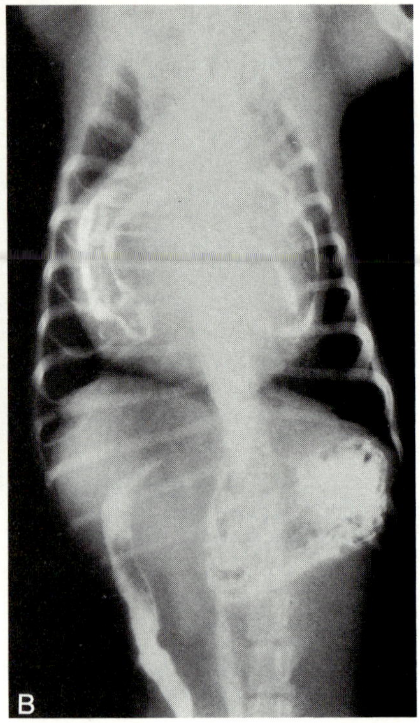

Figure 14–90. Lateral *(A)* and ventrodorsal *(B)* radiographs of 6-month-old beagle with pericardial-diaphragmatic hernia which was confirmed by the oral administration of barium sulfate. Notice the reduction in size of the abdomen because most of the small intestine is located in the pericardial sac.

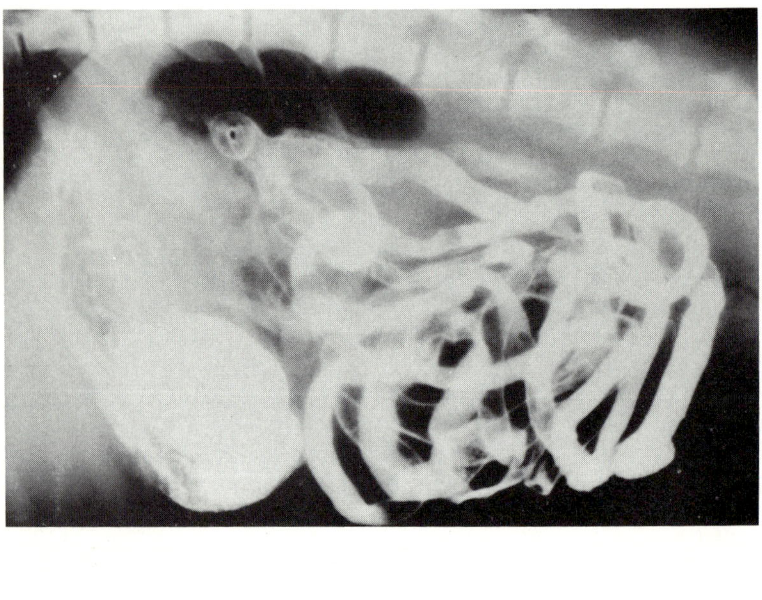

Figure 14–91. Lateral radiograph of 4-year-old cocker spaniel, taken one hour after the oral administration of barium sulfate. Notice the smooth mucosal–barium sulfate interface of the normal small intestine.

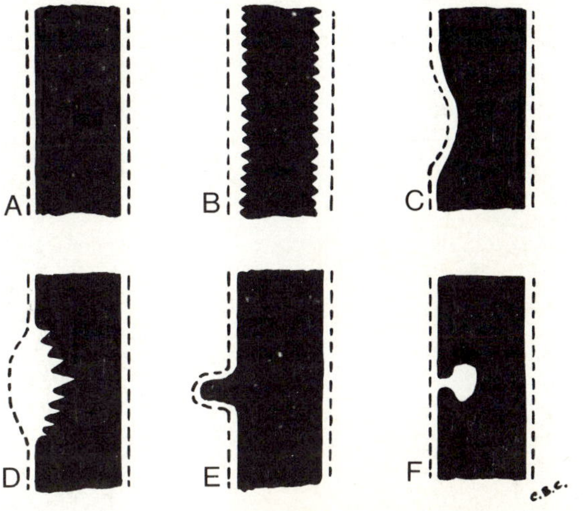

Figure 14–92. Diagrams of small intestine following filling of lumen with barium sulfate *(black)*. *(A)* Normal appearance with smooth barium-mucosal interface; *(B)* irregular barium-mucosal interface seen with enteritis; *(C)* narrowing of lumen caused by an extrinsic mass (notice that the barium-mucosal interface is smooth); *(D)* narrowing of lumen caused by an intramural mass (The barium-mucosal interface is likely to be irregular and the serosal surface displaced); *(E)* appearance of ulcer; and *(F)* appearance of polypoid lesion. The serosal surfaces are represented by the broken lines.

trast agent filling the distended bowel loops can obscure the lesions. For this reason, obstruction at the ileocolic level (for example, intussusception) can frequently be more efficiently identified using the barium enema examination.

With linear foreign bodies there is usually clumping of the intestines, and increased numbers of bowel loops seen "end-on." Sometimes serosal surfaces in the area are indistinct, indicating peritonitis secondary to the penetration of the bowel wall by the string-like foreign body. Contrast studies will confirm the pleating of the intestines (see Fig. 14–84). Water-soluble contrast agents are indicated if bowel perforation is suspected.

The radiographic appearance of small intestinal lesions can vary depending on the degree of obstruction produced and also on their relationship to the bowel wall. Mass lesions may originate from any portion of the small intestines but are most common in the duodenum and distal ileum. Intramural lesions frequently are irregular in outline and produce either eccentric or annular luminal narrowing with thickening or rigidity of the bowel wall. Pedunculated, intraluminal masses can be recognized as filling defects in barium contrast studies. Extraluminal masses will result in a gradual narrowing of the lumen of the intestine and the mucosal surface will be normal (Fig. 14–94). Diffuse abnormal mucosal patterns in the small bowel are often related to the presence of viral, bacterial, or fungal enteritis, eosinophilic enteritis, or intestinal lymphosarcoma (see Figs. 14–88 and 14–89).

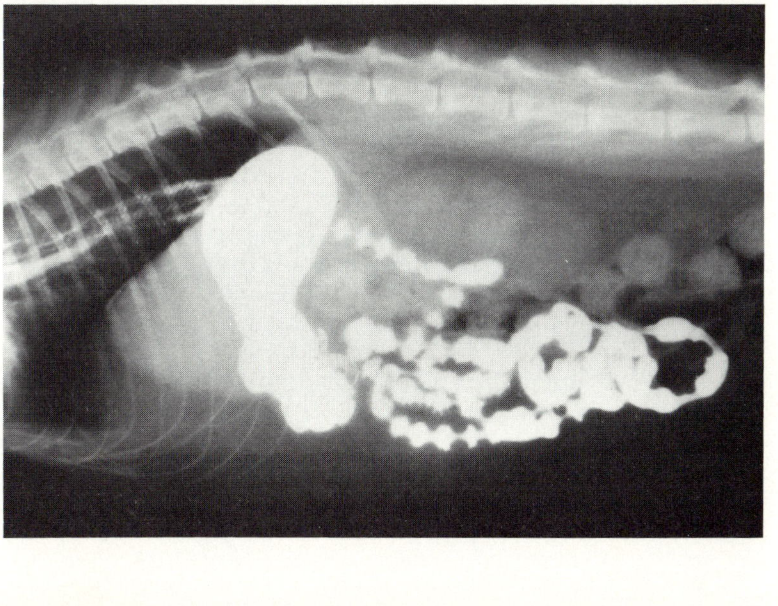

Figure 14–93. Lateral abdominal radiograph of 2-year-old domestic short-haired cat, taken 15 minutes after the oral administration of barium sulfate. Segmentation of the duodenum and jejunum as shown is commonly seen in the normal cat. Notice also the "herringbone" pattern in the caudal thoracic esophagus, which is also a normal radiographic finding in the cat.

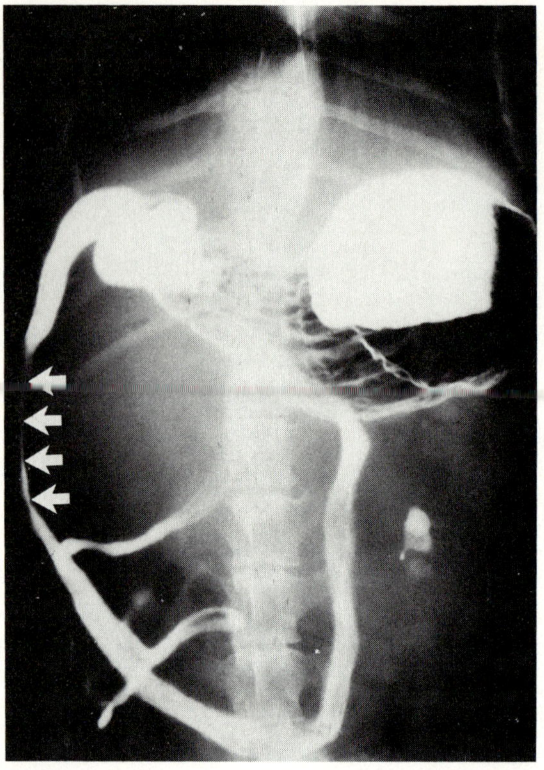

Figure 14–94. Ventrodorsal radiograph of 6-year-old beagle with a mass lesion on the tail of the spleen. The mass is compressing the descending duodenum against the right abdominal wall, creating an extraluminal effect on the contrast agent within the duodenum *(arrows)*. Note the smooth mucosal–barium sulfate interface in the compressed segment of bowel.

Radiology of the Large Intestine

On plain radiographs the large intestine can usually be seen because of the presence of gas and fecal material. Alteration in size or position will frequently be assessed from the plain radiographs. Increased size of the large intestine will be seen with constipation and colonic or rectal obstruction and can be also due to neurological dysfunction. Obstruction of the large intestine can result from strictures, tumors, inversion of the cecum, foreign bodies, rectal prolapse, and perineal diverticuli. These causes of obstruction are usually best demonstrated by barium enema. Intramural gas can also be identified in cases of emphysematous colitis (Fig. 14–95).

Displacement of the large bowel can occur with enlargement of organs or structures adjacent to it as the large intestine is readily displaced by external pressures. Although abnormal location of parts of the large intestine can frequently be determined on the plain abdominal radiographs, the introduction of a radiodense contrast agent into the large intestine will enhance the examiner's ability to recognize displacements.

CONTRAST RADIOGRAPHIC EXAMINATION OF THE LARGE INTESTINE (BARIUM ENEMA)

The examination of the large bowel cannot be satisfactorily performed by administering contrast material per os. Attempts to do so will result in errors such as incomplete filling of the colon and rectum together with the transport of food material from the small bowel, which will result in artifacts and misleading, inconclusive studies. For the complete evaluation of the large colon and rectum, a barium enema examination must be performed. However, it should be recognized that the barium examination of the lower colon and rectum is incomplete and should not be substituted for digital or endoscopic examinations of the colon. Clinical signs that suggest the need for a barium enema examination usually include protracted diarrhea with or without blood and sustained straining in an attempt to defecate. The barium enema is a time-consuming procedure and care must be exercised to obtain a diagnostic study. It is essential that the bowel be prepared adequately to minimize artifacts due to the presence of fecal material. Occasionally the introduction of a small amount of barium sulfate or air into the rectum and terminal colon will be sufficient to demonstrate displacement of these structures without the need for a complete barium enema examination.

Preparation of the Patient for Barium Enema

Food should be withheld for 24 hours. Mineral oil (0.5 ml/lb) may be given 24 hours prior to the examination. Three to six hours before the examination, lukewarm tap water or saline enemas should be administered until the large bowel is clean, as evidenced by the lack of fecal material in the return. Soapy water enemas should be avoided because of their potential irritating effect on the mucosa of the large bowel.

As with all contrast studies, preliminary radiographs should be taken to determine if

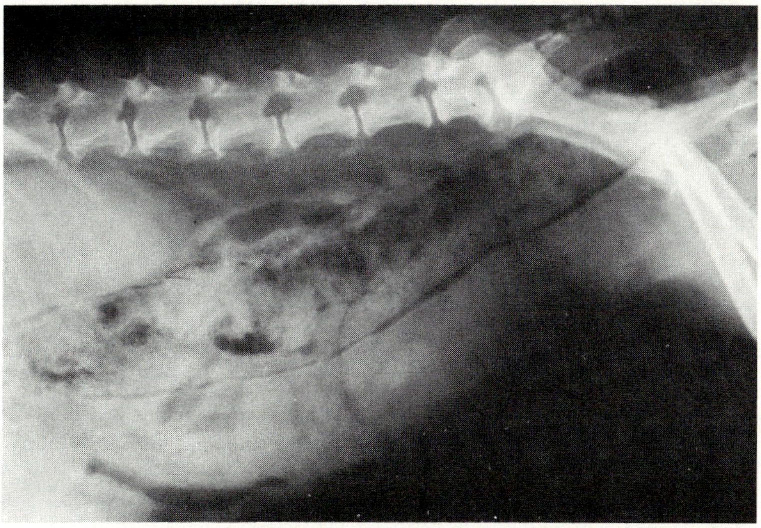

Figure 14–95. Lateral abdominal radiograph of 14-year-old Pomeranian with emphysematous colitis. Note gas accumulation within the wall of the large intestine.

the animal is adequately prepared. These films will have additional benefits, namely, as a check that the technique is adequate and to ensure that the positioning of the animal is optimal. With the use of positive contrast agents for the examination, the technique should be increased approximately 6 to 8 kVp over the adequate plain film technique to achieve more contrast between the barium-mucosa interface.

The barium enema is best carried out in animals under general anesthesia. Tranquilization is often inadequate because the increased pressure in the rectum will cause most patients to strain and become restless.

Technique for Barium Enema

The barium enema examination consists of two stages. First, the rectum and colon are filled with a radiodense material (usually barium sulfate) and films are exposed. Following this, the barium sulfate is evacuated from the colon and the colon is filled and distended with air. The latter stage constitutes a double-contrast study of the large bowel. The double-contrast examination has the advantage that extremely fine detail of the mucosal surfaces of the rectum and colon are obtained.

Contrast agents that can be used for the large bowel examination include various commercial forms of barium sulfate. The concentration of barium sulfate is approximately 20 per cent.[31] Water-soluble contrast agents can also be used in 15 to 20 per cent concentrations.

The water-soluble organic iodide compounds have several advantages:

1. They are less reactive than barium, should any medium enter the peritoneal cavity following perforation of the bowel wall.
2. They mix with fluid remaining in the colon to form a more homogeneous contrast column.
3. They coat the mucosa evenly without excessive distention.

Disadvantages include the higher cost of these agents and the fact that, in the young debilitated patient, the hypertonicity of the contrast material may have a detrimental effect on the patient's fluid balance. The dosage of contrast agent used to examine the colon is 16 to 20 ml/kg. Using this calculation, a dog weighing 10 kg would require 160 to 200 ml of contrast material. Possibly a more accurate way of estimating the volume of contrast material can be arrived at by measuring the diameter *(d)* and the length *(l)* of the colon on the preliminary radiographs. Using these measurements, the following formula can give an estimate of contrast material required:

$$\tfrac{3}{4}\, d^2 \times l = \text{Volume of contrast agent}$$

According to this formula, an average dog with a 3-cm diameter colon that is 25 cm long would require approximately 175 cc of contrast.

Bardex or Foley catheters are used to facilitate entry of the contrast material into the rectum and to minimize leaking of the contrast agent from the anus. It is advisable to cut the tip of the Bardex catheter close to the inflatable cuff so that irritation of the rectal wall will be minimal, thus lessening the resulting spasticity that is associated with rectal irritation. Because the descending colon is on the left side of the abdomen, it is best to commence the filling of the colon with the animal in left lateral recumbency. The catheter is introduced just anterior to the anal sphincter, the cuff is inflated, and the warm barium or water-soluble contrast material is infused at a slow rate. If fluoroscopy is available, the passage of the contrast agent should be observed using this method. Slow filling of the colon allows the bowel wall to distend evenly and will minimize the passage of contrast agent through the ileocolic junction into the small intestine.

After the descending colon is observed fluoroscopically to be filled, or when two-thirds of the estimated volume of contrast agent has been introduced, the animal can then be turned so that it is in right lateral recumbency. This will allow filling of the transverse and ascending portions of the colon. When adequate filling has been achieved, radiographs are taken. The objective of the positive-contrast study is to fill and distend the bowel wall so that mucosal irregularity and ulceration, intraluminal filling defects, diverticulum, spasms, and strictures can be seen. Post-evacuation radiographs, which are taken routinely in human radiology, are not widely used in veterinary radiology and do not appear to add a great deal to the interpretation of the study.

After obtaining adequate positive-contrast radiographs, the barium sulfate suspension is evacuated by removing the clamp on the Bardex catheter and utilizing gravity to encourage the back flow of contrast agent from the colon. Gentle manipulation of the colon through the abdominal wall is often beneficial in aiding removal of the contrast material. Initially, during removal of the barium sulfate, the animal should be in left lateral recumbency, toward the end of removal the head should be elevated while the animal is in right lateral recumbency.

Following adequate removal of barium from the colon, the next step is the introduction of air to distend the rectum and colon. The introduction of air should be done while the animal is in right lateral recumbency, at a slow, controlled rate, and should continue until the bowel is distended. The main advantage of the double-contrast study is that it provides the opportunity to study fine alterations from normal in the mucosal pattern.

Indications for Use of Barium Enema

Indications for the use of the barium enema examination include (1) intrinsic lesions, (2) extrinsic lesions displacing the colon, (3) intussusception, and (4) the need to determine the position of a gastrointestinal foreign body, that is, whether the location of the foreign body is in the small or large bowel.

Intrinsic Lesions. The normal colonic mucosal surface should be quite smooth and free from irregularities (Fig. 14–96). Inflammatory bowel disease (e.g., ulcerative colitis) is visualized radiographically by an irregularity to the mucosal-barium interface. Often this is associated with spasticity of the wall of the colon. Other intrinsic lesions that can be identified are intramural lesions not involving the mucosal surface. These lesions are characterized by an indentation into the contrast column, with the mucosal surface remaining relatively smooth, in contrast to mucosal or intramural lesions with mucosal involvement, in which an irregular mucosal-barium interface is seen. Deep ulcerative lesions and diverticula can be recognized by an extension of the barium column beyond the normal level of the mucosal-barium interface and polypoid lesions in which a filling defect is recognized in the barium column and a small discontinuity is present on the mucosal contrast interface. It is apparent that recognition of the sometimes subtle changes in the mucosal surface is dependent on optimal radiographic technique and proper preparation of the patient.

Extrinsic Lesions Displacing or Encroaching on the Colon. Because of the intimate relationship between the colon and rectum and various abdominal organs located in close proximity to the colon, changes in position of the colon and rectum will often allow identification of pathology in adjacent organs. To accurately predict the cause of displacement, it is essential to be conversant with the relationships between the various adjacent organs and the colon and rectum. Structures that commonly cause displacement of the large intestine are illustrated in Figures 14–97 through 14–101.

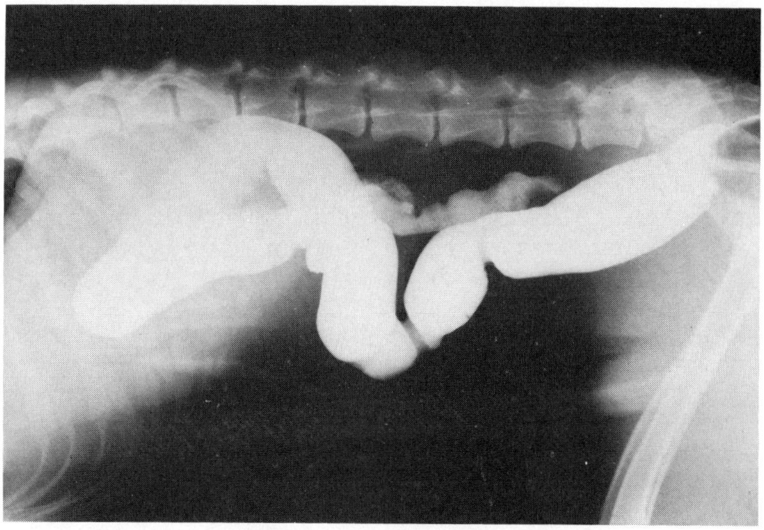

Figure 14–96. Barium enema contrast radiograph of 3-year-old Australian shepherd. There is a smooth barium-mucosal interface of the normal large intestine.

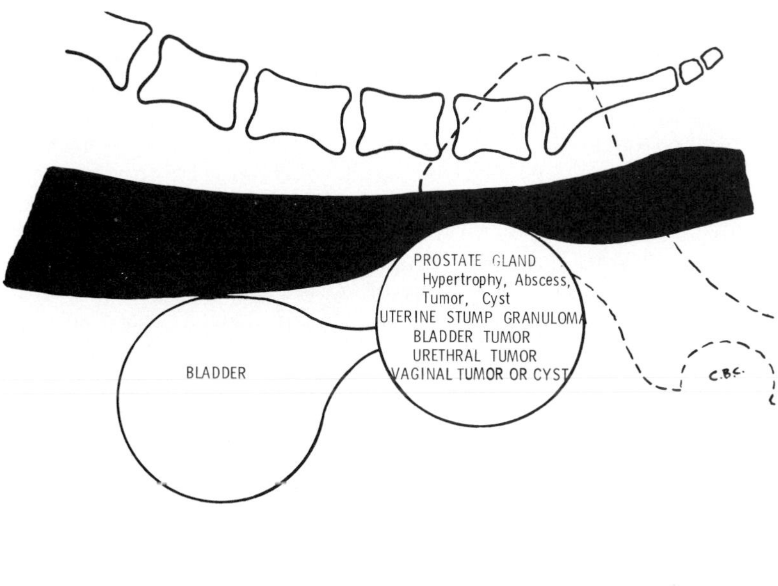

Figure 14–97. Diagram of lateral radiograph of caudal abdomen, illustrating causes of elevation of the descending colon and rectum. Disease processes involving the prostate gland, uterus, bladder neck, urethra, and vagina would be possible causes. Frequently cranial displacement of the bladder will also be seen.

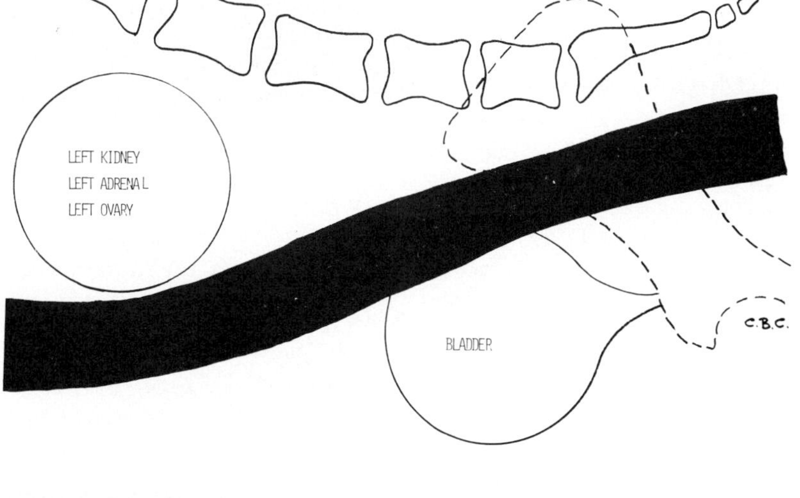

Figure 14–98. Diagram of lateral radiograph of caudal abdomen, illustrating causes of ventral displacement of the cranial portion of the descending colon. Mass lesions involving the left kidney, adrenal, and ovary would warrant consideration.

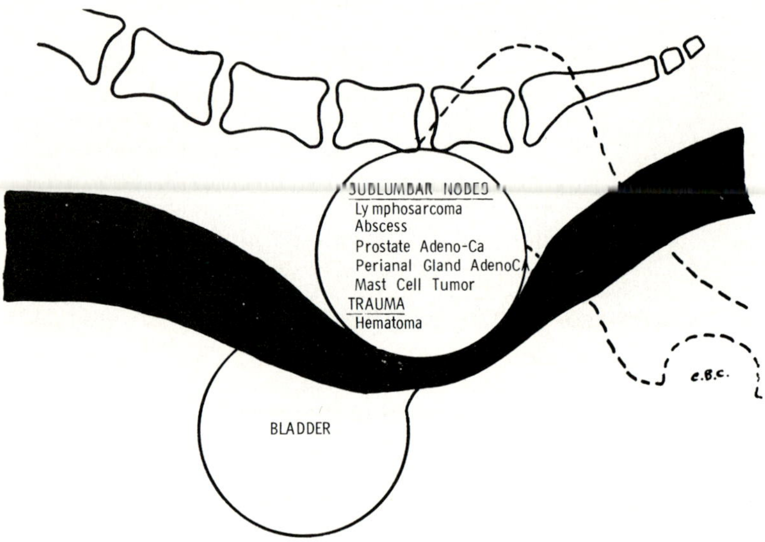

Figure 14–99. Diagram of lateral radiograph of caudal abdomen, illustrating causes of ventral displacement of the caudal portion of the descending colon. Enlargement of lymph nodes in the sublumbar region due to primary or metastatic neoplasia, abscess formation, and hematoma secondary to trauma would be possible causes.

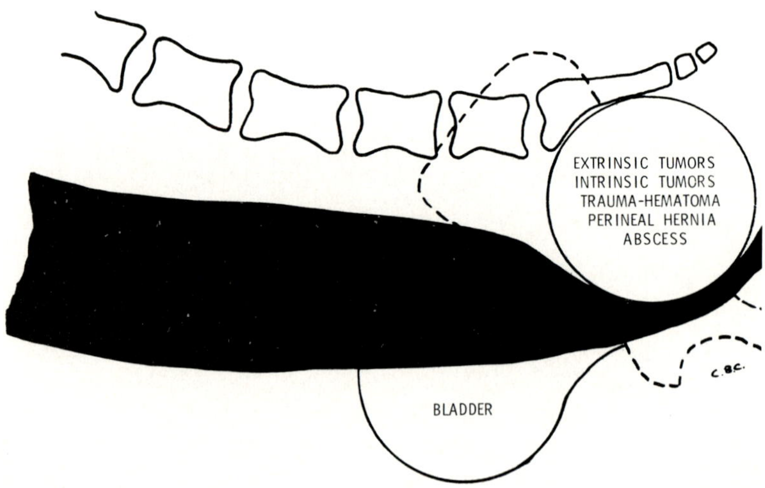

Figure 14–100. Diagram of lateral radiograph of caudal abdomen illustrating the radiographic appearance caused by mass lesions within the pelvic canal. Note that along with displacement of the rectum, enlargement of the descending colon usually results.

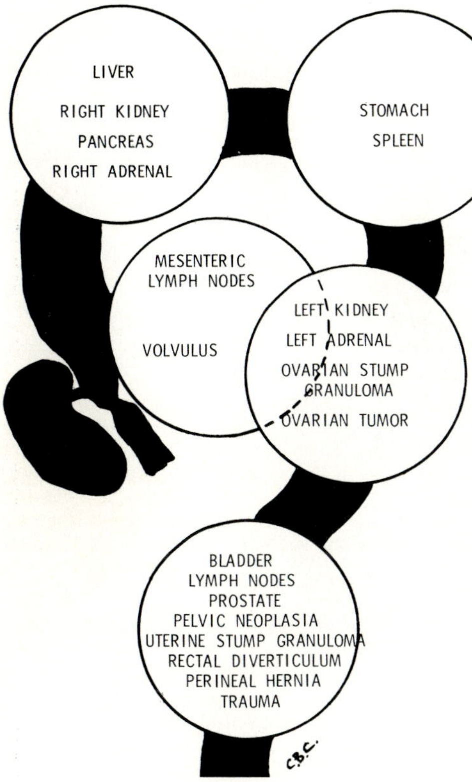

Figure 14–101. Diagram of ventrodorsal radiograph of abdomen illustrating the sites of influence of various enlargements of abdominal structures on the large intestine.

Intussusception. Intussusception in the dog and cat most commonly occurs at the ileocolic junction. When the intussusception leads to a complete intestinal obstruction, acute clinical signs will be present and a rapid diagnosis will be needed for optimal treatment of the patient. When the intussusception does not lead to a complete obstruction, but rather to a partial obstruction, massive dilatation of the small intestines anterior to the site of the intussusception is usual. Because of the preceding two facts, often the barium enema is the most satisfactory way of obtaining a radiographic diagnosis of intussusception (Fig. 14–102).[31]

In the acute situation often the time required for barium given per os to reach the site of the intussusception means intolerable delay in surgical treatment of the animal. When the intussusception is chronic and there are dilated loops cranial to it, the passage of contrast material is retarded as it passes through these dilated loops; furthermore, the contrast-filled dilated loops often will obscure the site of obstruction and so preclude adequate evaluation and accurate diagnosis.

The radiographic appearance of an intussusception will vary depending on the amount of edema and swelling in the intussuscepted portion of the bowel. On plain

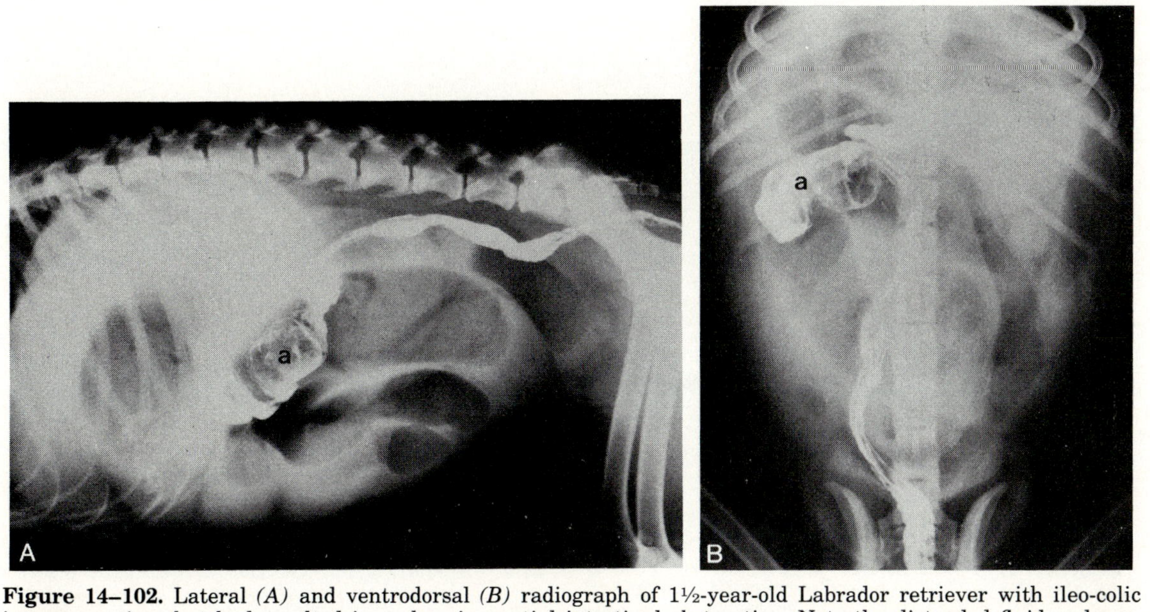

Figure 14–102. Lateral *(A)* and ventrodorsal *(B)* radiograph of 1½-year-old Labrador retriever with ileo-colic intussusception that had resulted in a chronic, partial intestinal obstruction. Note the distended fluid and gas-filled small intestines. Barium sulfate introduced into the large intestine outlines the intussusception, which appears as a filling defect.

films, signs of partial or complete obstruction will be evident: namely, dilated gas- and fluid-filled bowel loops. The barium enema will demonstrate a stoppage of the contrast column cranial to the normal location of the ileocolic junction, and barium will be seen dissecting through the luminal portion or around the peripheral area of the intussuscepted bowel loop (Fig. 14–103).

Cecal inversion is also best demonstrated by the barium enema and is characterized by a filling defect in the ascending colon associated with a normal-appearing ileocolic junction (Fig. 14–104).

Differentiation between Small and Large Intestinal Locations of Foreign Bodies. Often when a foreign body is noted on the plain film, it is necessary to determine whether the foreign body is located in the small or large intestine. Because the ileocolic junction is the narrowest part of the gastrointestinal tract caudal to the pyloric canal, once a foreign body passes beyond this junction it is usually capable of passage through the rest of the intestinal tract. However, if the foreign body is located in the small intestine, a decision for surgical removal is necessary. The quickest way to determine whether such a foreign body is in the small or large bowel is to perform a barium enema examination. If, on filling the large colon, the foreign body is determined to be unassociated with the barium-filled viscus, it can be concluded that it has a small intestinal location.

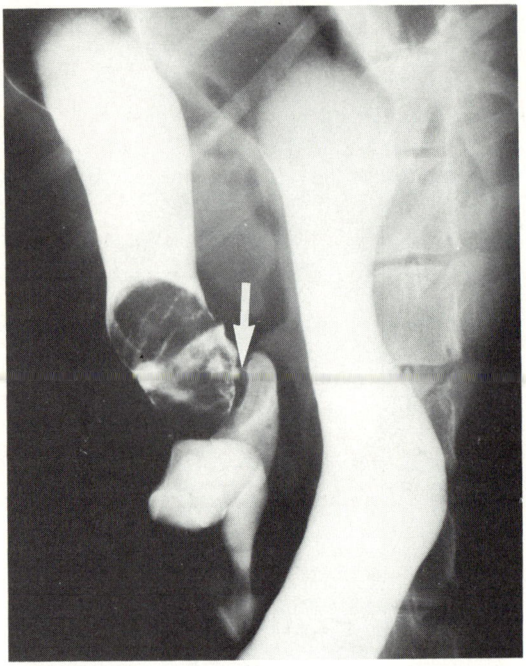

Figure 14–104. Ventrodorsal oblique radiograph of 18-month-old mixed-breed dog with cecal inversion following a barium enema. Note the filling defect in the ascending colon, representing the inverted cecum. The normal ileocolic valve is seen *(arrows)*.

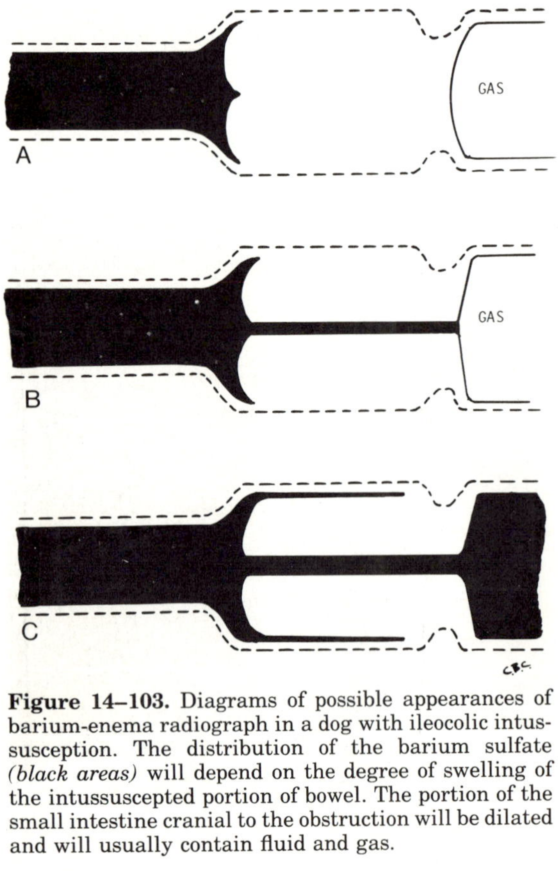

Figure 14–103. Diagrams of possible appearances of barium-enema radiograph in a dog with ileocolic intussusception. The distribution of the barium sulfate *(black areas)* will depend on the degree of swelling of the intussuscepted portion of bowel. The portion of the small intestine cranial to the obstruction will be dilated and will usually contain fluid and gas.

Liver

NORMAL APPEARANCE

The radiographic appearance of the normal liver varies with body conformation, age, condition, stage of respiration, and posture.[2, 29, 69, 93] Awareness of these normal variations in appearance is necessary for accurate evaluation of the liver silhouette.

The position of the stomach is an important indicator of both liver size and shape. Since a full stomach will distort the position of the liver and obscure part of it in both the lateral and ventrodorsal views, the stomach should be empty. In non-emergency situations, food should be withheld for at least 12 hours and water for 2 hours prior

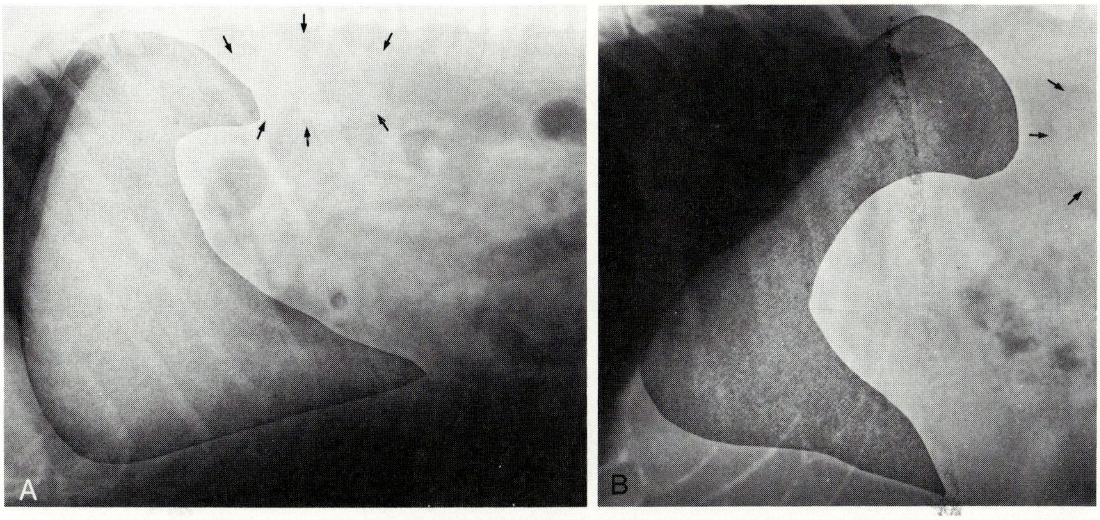

Figure 14–105. *A,* Approximate normal radiographic limits of the canine liver. The shaded area represents the area of density attributable to the liver and does not necessarily represent the true anatomical limits of the liver. Note that the caudoventral margin of the liver is sharp and extends just beyond the costal arch. The dorsocaudal limit of the liver is in contact with the right kidney *(arrows)*. *B,* Approximate normal radiographic limits of the feline liver. The shaded area represents the area of density attributable to the liver and does not necessarily represent the true anatomical limits of the liver. The caudoventral margin of the liver is somewhat thinner than that of the dog in Part *A*. This margin extends further beyond the costal arch than usual because the film was exposed during inspiration. The caudodorsal limit does not contact the right kidney *(arrows)*.

to radiography. Because sick animals are often anorexic, a fasting period while the animal is in the hospital may not be necessary if the history is reliable.

On the lateral view the liver extends from the spine to the ventral floor of the abdomen (Fig. 14–105). The cranial margin is indistinguishable from the diaphragm in the normal animal, whereas the caudoventral margin usually projects slightly beyond the margin of the costal arch.[29, 69] The caudoventral border of the liver is usually triangular in shape and sharply pointed. The liver may lie directly on the abdominal floor or be separated from the ventral abdominal stripe by fat in the falciform ligament, especially in cats (Fig. 14–106). The dorsal limits of the liver are difficult to define. The

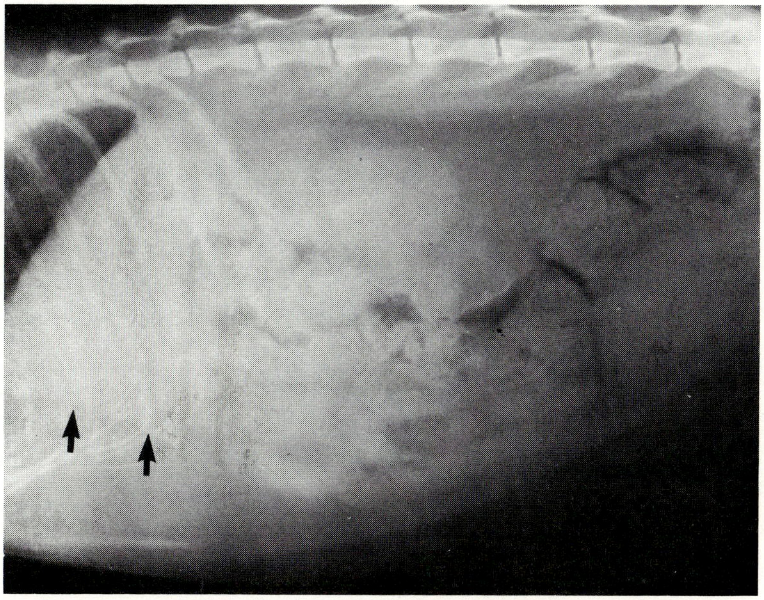

Figure 14–106. Normal radiographic appearance of the abdomen in an obese cat. There is marked elevation of the liver *(arrows)* from the ventral abdominal wall by a large accumulation of fat in the falciform ligament. The large amount of perirenal fat has displaced the right kidney caudally away from the liver shadow.

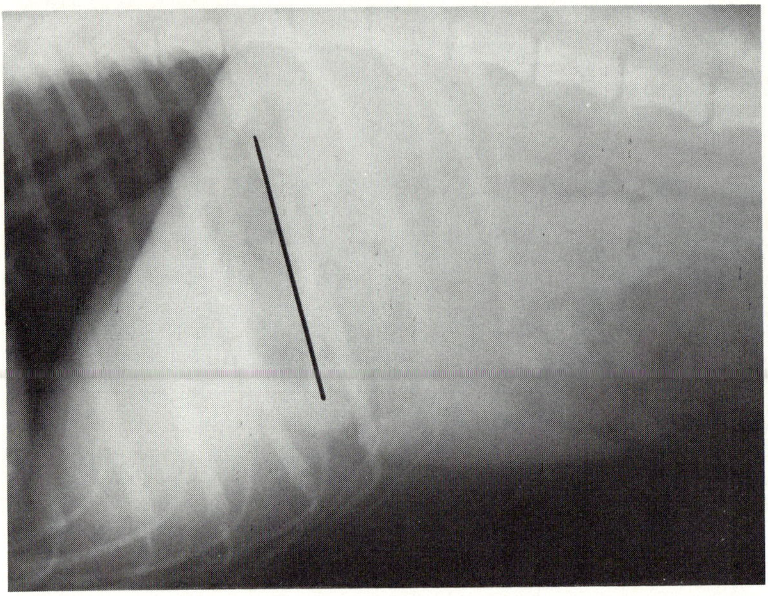

Figure 14–107. Normal position of the stomach shadow in the right lateral recumbent position. The long axis of the stomach *(line)* lies parallel to the overlying ribs. This is the average position of the stomach, but the position of the axis is subject to relatively marked changes in orientation with changes in position, stage of respiration, breed, and so forth.

caudate process of the caudate lobe is the most dorsal caudal limit of the liver. The right kidney is embedded in the renal fossa of this process in all but the most obese dogs.[55, 69, 93] The close contact of these two organs produces a mutual silhouette sign preventing appreciation of either organ margin. A clear separation of the liver and kidney is much more commonly seen in the cat than the dog.

Midway between the spine and the floor of the abdomen, the liver is directly opposed to the fundus of the stomach on the left side. However, on the right side of the abdomen, the right lateral and caudate lobes extend more caudally and are thus superimposed over the fundus of the stomach. The lateral radiograph therefore will show the caudal extent of the left dorsal aspect of the liver, but it does not accurately indicate the caudal limit of the right side of the liver. On the right lateral view the long axis of the stomach should roughly parallel the ribs that overlie it (Fig. 14–107); however, this is somewhat variable, depending on the animal's body conformation and position.[29]

The limits of the liver are not easily defined on the ventrodorsal projection (Fig.

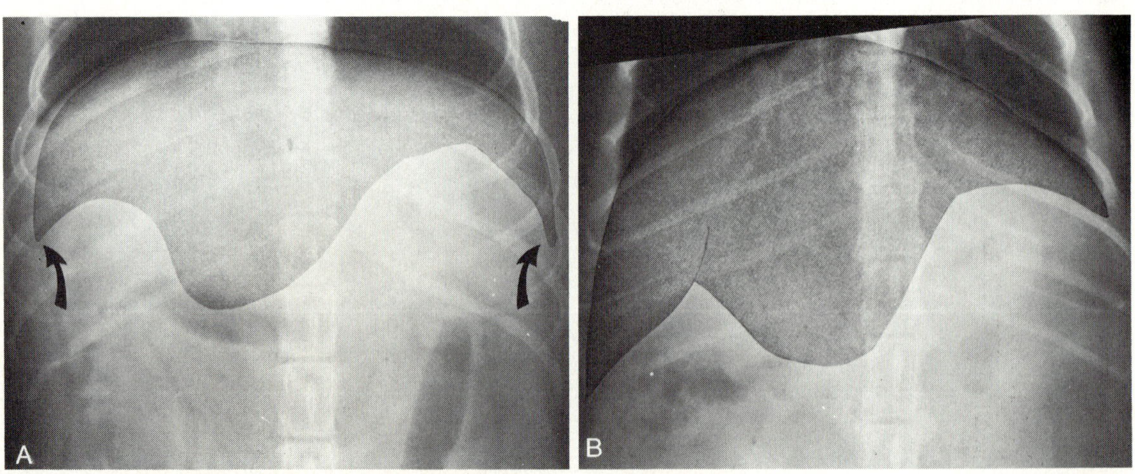

Figure 14–108. Approximate radiographic limits of the liver in an average conformation dog *(A)*. The shaded area represents the area to which the liver contributes density. Most of these margins are not visible as distinct borders except at the extreme lateral edges *(arrows)*. Note that in the cat *(B)* a greater proportion of the liver lies to the right of the midline than in the dog (see Fig. 14–105).

14–108). The only margins that are commonly identifiable on this projection are the caudolateral limits of the right and left lateral lobes. The remainder of the liver's limits can be inferred by the position of the organs directly adjacent to it. These organs are the right kidney, spleen, proximal duodenum, and the pylorus and fundus of the stomach.[2, 55, 69, 93] It should be realized that, because of the angle of this projection and the location of the bulk of the liver mass ventrocranial to the stomach on the left side, the fundus of the stomach may appear to be directly contiguous with the diaphragm, especially if dilated. The right kidney should normally lie with its center at approximately the level of the first lumbar disc space. The pylorus, when visible, will generally lie in the same plane as the empty fundus in the dog and at about the level of the thirteenth rib in the cat.[55, 93] The spleen is located opposite the eleventh intercostal space on the left side of the abdomen. Displacement of any or all of these organs may occur when the liver is of abnormal size.[2, 70, 78]

Body conformation has a marked effect on the appearance of the liver.[29, 70] Dogs that have a deep-chested conformation will often appear to have a small liver on the lateral view (Fig. 14–109). Since many of the deep-chested breeds have small, tight caudal abdomens, a greater proportion of the abdominal volume lies within the rib cage. In animals with this conformation, the liver may not extend caudally to the margin of the costal arch; the long axis of the stomach will lie at a more vertical angle than the overlying ribs and may even appear angulated cranially. The apparent smaller size of the liver is probably a combination of the greater proportion of the abdominal contents being present within the rib cage and the relatively large diaphragm. The large diaphragm provides a larger area over which the liver is distributed. Therefore, the liver does not appear as thick as it does in a dog with average conformation.

An animal with a barrel-chested conformation, such as a bulldog, may have a liver that protrudes further caudal to the costal arch than that of the "average" dog (Fig. 14–110). These animals have a proportionately smaller intrathoracic abdominal volume and a smaller diaphragmatic surface area for the liver to contact. Therefore, the liver appears thicker. Because the liver extends well caudally to the costal arch, the stomach will be angulated more caudally than the overlying ribs.[29, 70]

Cats have virtually constant body conformation and therefore little variation in appearance of the normal liver due to differences in body comformation.

The age of an animal can also have a marked effect on the appearance of the liver. Very young animals have livers that are larger on the basis of a percentage of body

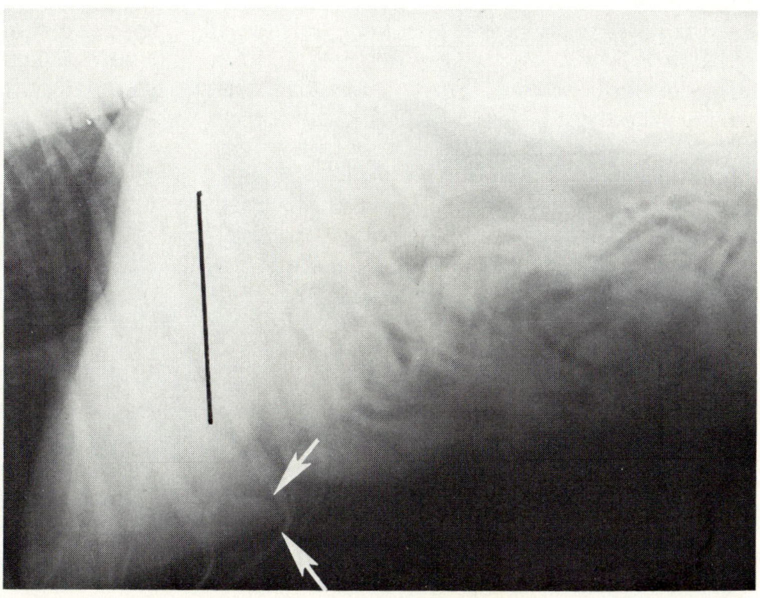

Figure 14–109. Normal position of the liver in a deep-chested dog. The caudoventral limit of the liver *(arrows)* is well within the costal arch. The long axis of the stomach *(line)* is at a more vertical angle than the overlying ribs.

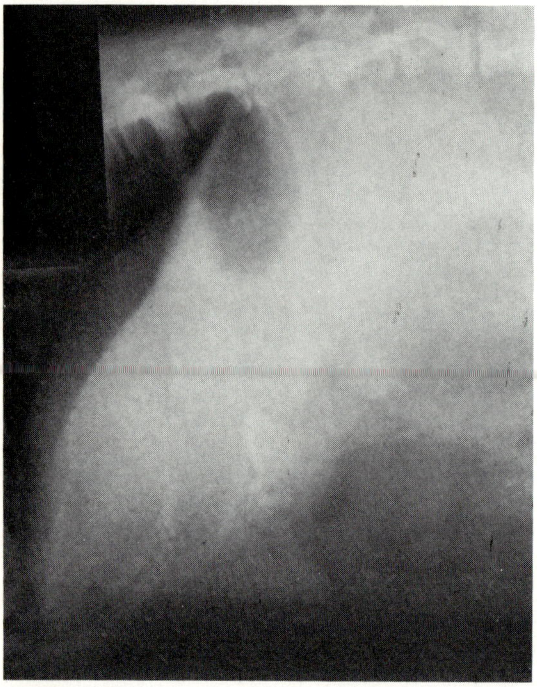

Figure 14–110. Normal shallow-chested dog. The caudoventral limit of the liver protrudes well beyond the costal arch. The long axis of the stomach is much more caudally oriented and is less vertical than the overlying ribs.

weight than those of adult animals.[55] The liver will appear to be much larger in small puppies and kittens than in adult animals (Fig. 14–111). Once the animal reaches maturity, the liver size should remain constant throughout the rest of life.

If an animal is obese, there will often be fatty deposition in the liver. This causes generalized enlargement of the liver, resulting in an appearance similar to that of infiltrative disease.[71] The degree of liver enlargement varies. Some animals with large amounts of body fat have relatively little enlargement of the liver while others show considerable enlargement. Enlargement of the liver due to fatty infiltration may also be a sign of a metabolic abnormality.[14, 29, 34, 71] Therefore, a moderately enlarged liver in an obese animal should not be dismissed as normal but this finding should be correlated with the physical and clinical pathology findings.

The stage of respiration affects the position of the liver. The normal criteria that have been published for evaluation of the position of the cranial abdominal viscera in the dog and cat are based on radiographs taken with the animal in expiration.[69] During the expiratory phase of respiration the diaphragm relaxes and moves forward into the thorax, drawing the liver with it. Thus, the liver appears smaller on expiration than on inspiration (Fig. 14–112). Conversely, if the film is exposed during inspiration the liver appears larger because it moves caudally with the diaphragm. When the diaphragm is maximally contracted, the liver may protrude well beyond the costal arch, giving the false impression of enlargement (Fig. 14–113).[2, 69, 93]

The effect of posture on the appearance of the liver may be difficult to assess. The caudoventral margin of the liver as seen on a radiograph can be either the right medial or left lateral lobe. If the animal is positioned with the left side down, gravity forces the abdominal contents toward the left side of the abdomen. This results in greater pressure on the left side of the diaphragm and it moves forward in relation to the right side. Thus, the right medial liver lobe is more likely to be projected as the caudal border of the liver. Conversely, if the animal is placed with the right side down, the left hemidiaphragm moves caudally in relation to the right, and the left lateral or quadrate lobe is more likely to be projected as the caudalmost margin of the liver. Since each of these lobes of the liver are differently shaped, the apparent shape of the caudal margin of the liver may change (Fig. 14–114).[69]

Another postural influence on the appearance of the liver is that of rotation. If the animal is rotated, the x-ray beam will pass through it at a slightly oblique angle, with the result that the liver lobe appears thicker than it actually is; the margins appear rounded rather than sharp.

Gravity also plays a role in the appearance of the liver in the ventrodorsal and dorsoventral projections. In the ventrodorsal projection, the weight of the viscera holds the stomach caudal and dorsal. Because of this and the angle at which the x-ray beam intersects the diaphragm, the stomach, particularly the fundus, is projected away from the cupola of the diaphragm (Fig. 115*A*). This is especially common in the deep-chested breeds with deep diaphragmatic recesses in their abdomens. The effect is a visual perception of the liver as larger than it should be (Fig. 14–116*A*). Examination of the lateral lobes will help determine the true liver size. In the dorsoventral projec-

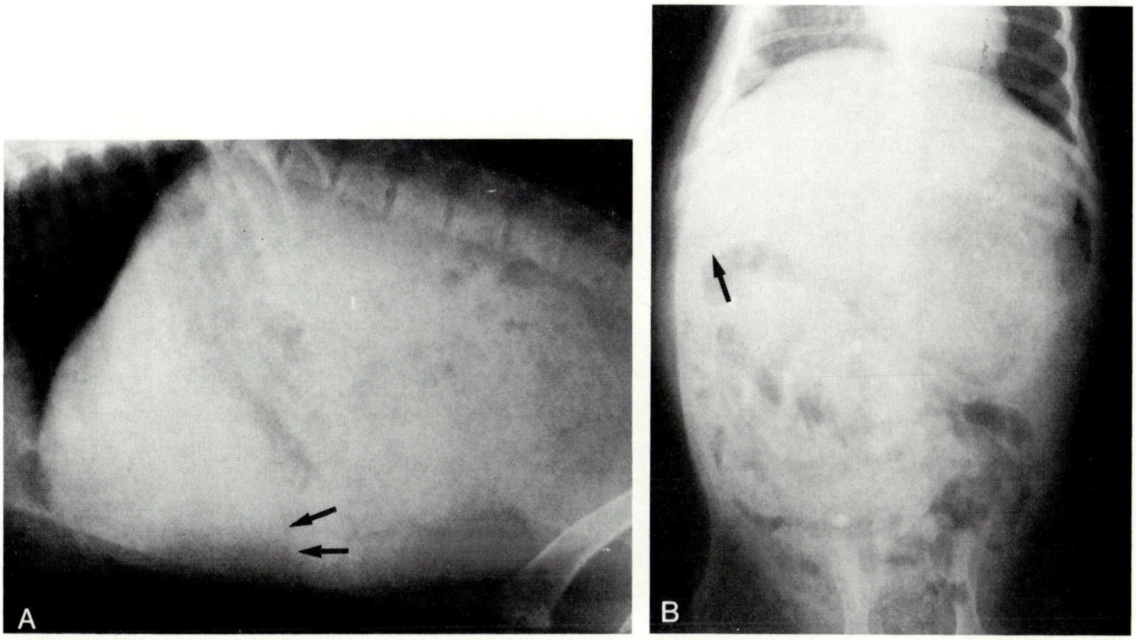

Figure 14–111. Normal abdomen in a young puppy: *(A)* lateral view, *(B)* ventrodorsal view. Note that the liver shadow appears much larger than it would in an adult animal. The caudal margin of the liver extends well back into the abdomen *(arrows)*. The normally larger size of the liver in the puppy is visually enhanced by the lack of calcification in the costal arch. This apparent organomegaly can easily be misinterpreted as a pathological process if the age of the animal is not taken into account.

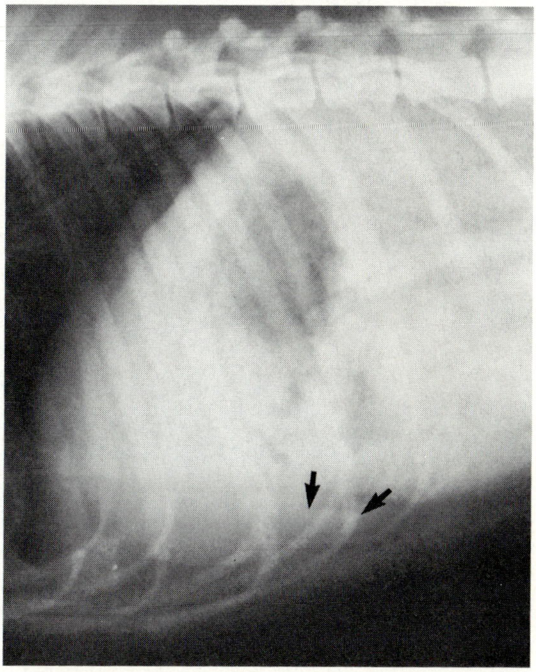

Figure 14–112. Normal liver shadow. This radiograph was exposed during the expiratory phase of respiration, and the liver lies completely within the rib cage. The caudoventral margin *(arrows)* is just within the rib cage.

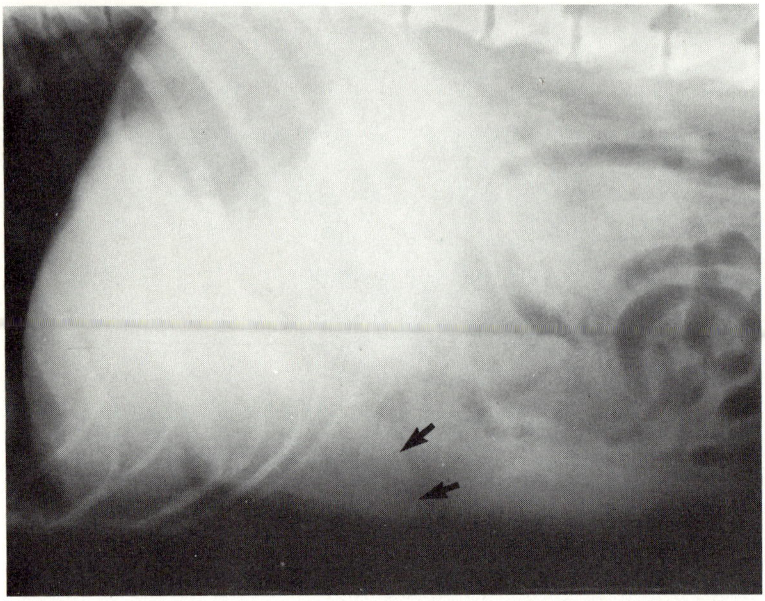

Figure 14–113. Normal liver shadow. This radiograph was exposed during the inspiratory phase of respiration. The caudoventral margin of the liver is well beyond the costal arch. Note the change in the appearance of the stomach shadow, compared with Figure 14–112.

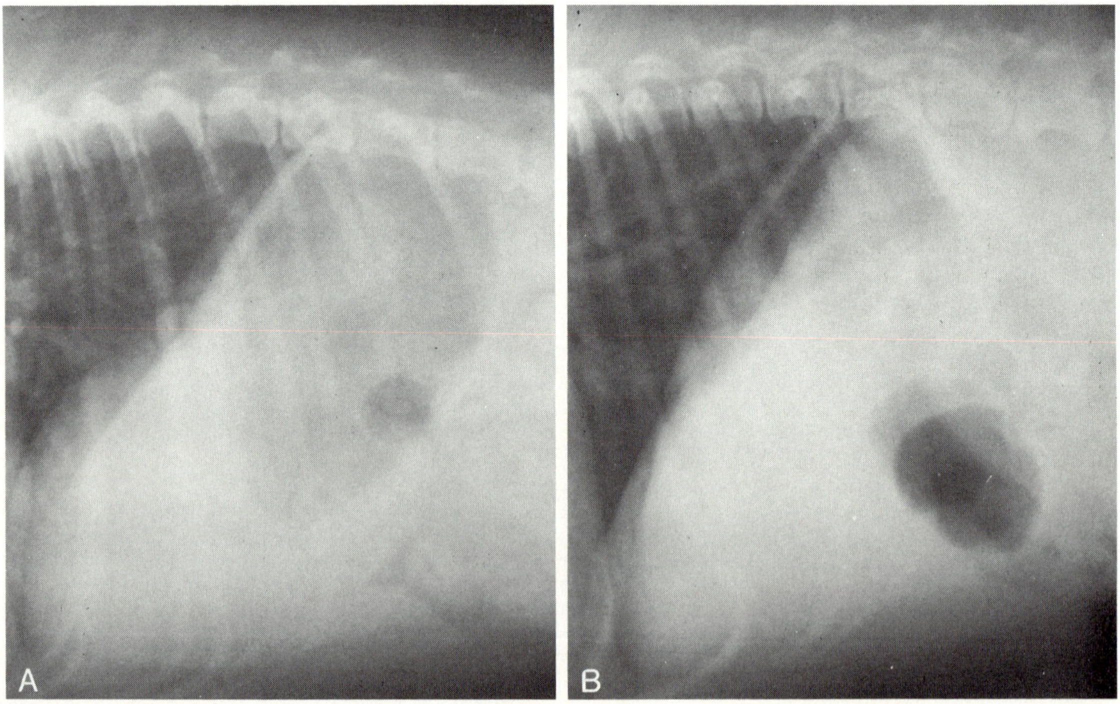

Figure 14–114. Normal liver shadows in right lateral *(A)* and left lateral *(B)* recumbent radiographs. The lobe of the liver extending caudally beneath the stomach is much thicker in *B* than in *A*. The change in posture of the animal has resulted in a marked change in the shape of the caudoventral margin of the liver, even though the distance that the liver extends beyond the costal arch is about the same in both cases. Note also the marked change in the position and orientation of the stomach shadow; in *A*, the long axis of the stomach is oriented in a cranial direction, whereas in *B*, it is parallel to the ribs.

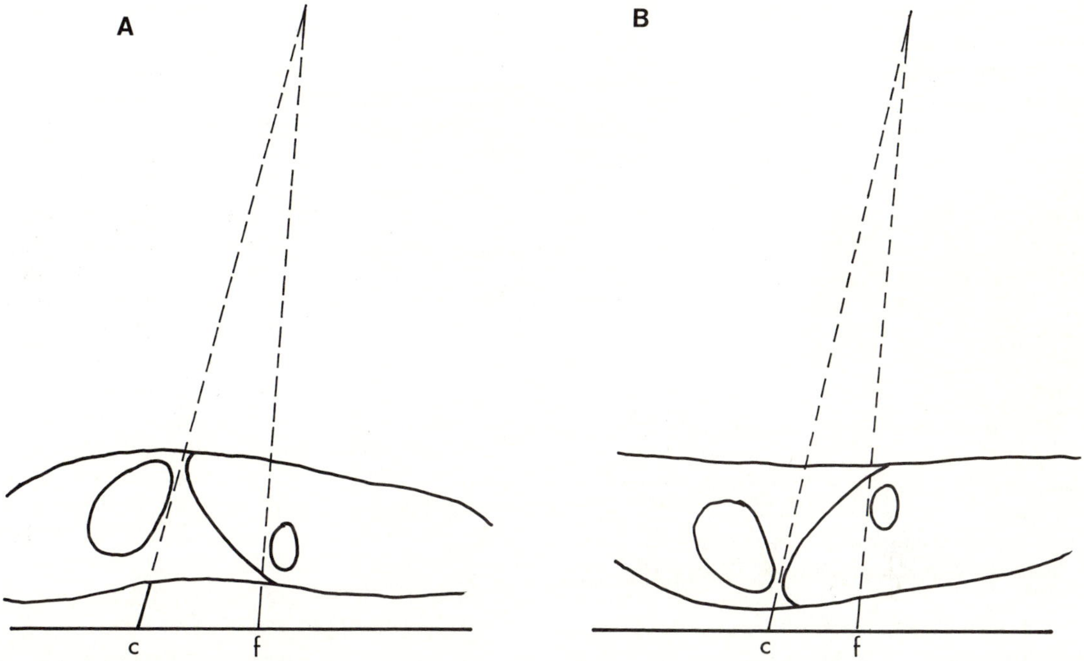

Figure 14–115. Effect of ventrodorsal *(A)* and dorsoventral *(B)* positioning on the relative projection of the gastric fundus (f) and the diaphragmatic cupola (c). In the ventrodorsal position the c–f distance is increased over the c–f distance in the dorsoventral position because of the greater arc that the diaphragm intercepts on this view. This effect is enhanced in larger dogs and in dogs with very deep chest cavities. This is a mechanical effect only and does not take into account the movement of the viscera due to gravity.

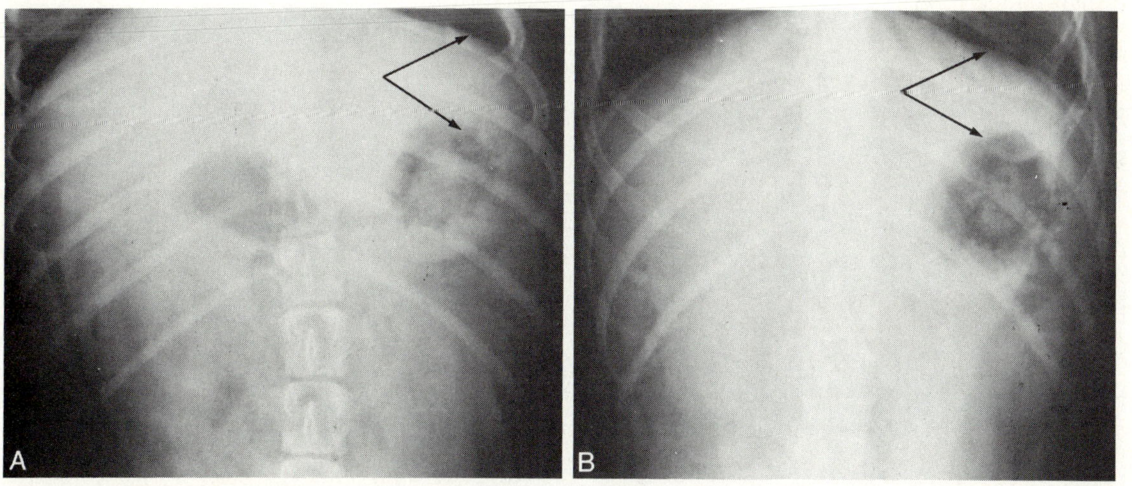

Figure 14–116. Ventrodorsal and dorsoventral views of the abdomen. On the ventrodorsal view *(A)*, the stomach is well within the rib cage and the spleen lies at the level of the 11th intercostal space. On the dorsoventral view *(B)*, both the fundus and the spleen appear to have moved approximately one space further caudal in the abdomen; this is an effect of the projection. Note that despite the further caudal position of the stomach in *B*, the distance between the stomach and the diaphragm *(arrows)* is less in *A* than in *B*.

tion, the cupola of the diaphragm is being held forward by the weight of the animal resting on the abdomen. However, the angle at which the x-ray beam strikes the abdomen is now radically different from that in the ventrodorsal view (Fig. 14–115*B*). The angle of the beam much more nearly parallels that of the diaphragmatic cura on the dorsoventral view than on the ventrodorsal projection. This results in less apparent separation of the stomach shadow from that of the diaphragm (Fig. 14–116*B*). The liver also slides slightly ventrally allowing the fundus of the stomach to shift slightly forward. The liver thus appears somewhat thinner on the dorsoventral projection than on the ventral dorsal (Fig. 14–116*B*).

The changes in liver position are also dependent on factors previously discussed governing the appearance of the liver shadow. Pathological changes in the liver may also influence the way in which the position of the liver is affected by posture. It is sometimes difficult to determine whether or not the perceived abnormality in the liver is due to a pathological change or to some effect of positioning.[94]

LIVER ENLARGEMENT

Liver enlargement can be symmetrical or asymmetrical. Symmetrical enlargement refers to equal enlargement of the whole liver. Asymmetrical enlargement refers to preferential enlargement of one portion of the liver. In asymmetrical enlargement the remainder of the liver may be normal in size or symmetrically enlarged for another or related reason.[2, 29, 71, 78]

Radiographic signs of symmetrical liver enlargement fall into two categories: increased size of the identifiable liver shadow itself and displacement of the surrounding organs away from their usual positions. Increased size of the liver shadow is usually judged by the distance it extends beyond the rib cage and the thickness of that part of the liver. If the liver extends a significant distance beyond the costal arch, it is said to be enlarged (Fig. 14–117).[2, 19, 29] To determine this, one must be familiar with the expected appearance of the liver in that breed of animal. Mild enlargements of the liver may be detected by increased thickness and rounding of the caudoventral margin of the liver.[2, 19, 29, 94] The caudolateral margins of the liver seldom extend caudal to the rib cage on the ventrodorsal view except in case of marked enlargement (Fig. 14–118).

The indirect signs of liver enlargement are displacements of the adjacent organs. Symmetrical enlargement displaces the stomach, spleen, duodenum, and right kidney caudally (Fig. 14–118).[78] The stomach may also be displaced dorsally. Caudal displacement of the transverse colon may be a secondary effect of gastric displacement. Due to the larger size of the liver lobes on the right side, marked symmetrical enlargement may also displace the stomach and

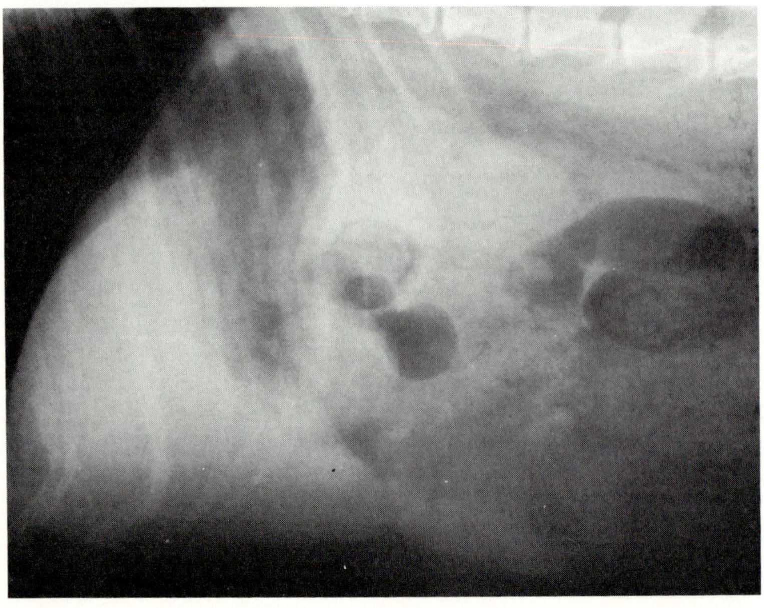

Figure 14–117. Mild enlargement of the liver. Although the stomach is still in its normal position, the liver extends a significant distance beyond the costal arch. The caudoventral margin of the liver is also somewhat thicker than normal. This degree of enlargement is not unusual in dogs, such as this one, that are moderately obese and is not usually associated with any clinical or clinicopathological evidence of liver disease.

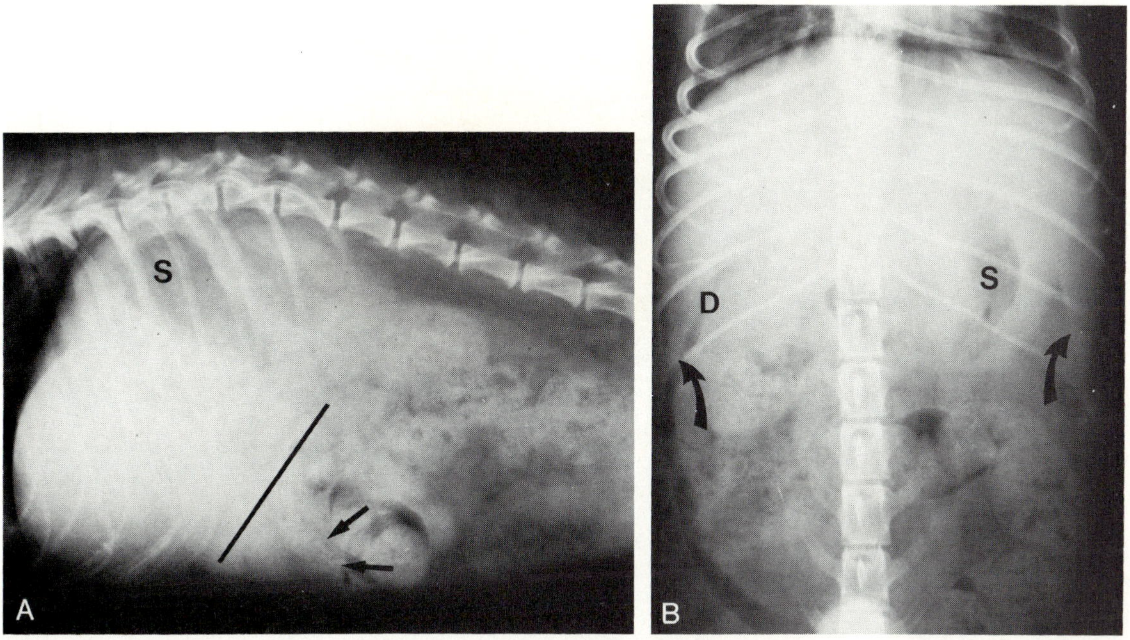

Figure 14–118. Symmetrical hepatomegaly. *A*, On the lateral projection, the caudoventral margin of the liver *(arrows)* extends well beyond the costal arch *(line)*; the stomach (S) is displaced caudally and dorsally and the feces-filled colon is displaced caudally. *B*, On the ventrodorsal projection, the stomach (S) and the duodenum (D) are displaced both caudally and medially; the caudolateral margins of the liver *(arrows)* are thickened and extend caudally (much farther than normal) to the margin of the costal arch.

duodenum toward the left side (Fig. 14–118).[55, 78] Mild enlargement of the liver may not result in any detectable displacement of adjacent organs.

The indirect signs of liver enlargement are very important in cases in which the detail in the abdomen is so poor that the liver margins cannot be seen, as in ascites. The stomach and duodenum are very important in this regard. They can always be visualized either by the swallowed air within them or by giving barium sulfate to identify the location of the gastrointestinal tract.[78] Thus, a positive diagnosis of liver enlargement may be made even though all abdominal detail is obscured (Fig. 14–119).

With the exception of primary hepatitis of either toxic or infectious origin, symmetrical enlargement of the liver is usually caused by disease processes that originate outside the liver.[2, 14, 23, 29, 71, 94] Common extrahepatic causes of liver enlargement include: metastatic neoplasia, metabolic abnormalities, cardiac insufficiency, lymphosarcoma, and fatty infiltration.[1, 71, 78] Other causes of symmetrical enlargement, such as obstructive bile duct disease and amyloidosis, are less common.[34, 38]

The degree of liver enlargement seen with inflammatory or toxic hepatitis is usually mild. It may be difficult to appreciate that the liver is enlarged unless film detail is sufficient to show rounded liver margins (Fig. 14–120). Rounding is usually the only appreciable radiographic evidence of hepatitis.[19, 29] Rarely inflammation of the biliary tree that is sufficient to cause obstruction of the ducts produces enough liver swelling to be detected radiographically. Animals so affected usually show severe clinical signs of liver disease.

Metastatic neoplasia may cause mild symmetrical liver enlargement. Neoplasms of the digestive tract and organs such as the spleen and pancreas, which have venous drainage via the portal vein, commonly metastasize to the liver early in the course of the disease.[88] Extraportal neoplasms also diffusely metastasize to the liver, as in cases of renal, mammary, and adrenal neoplasia. Although metastasis may occur simultaneously to the liver and lungs, extraportal neoplasia and portal system neoplasia will often exhibit radiographic evidence of pulmonary metastasis before significant liver enlargement occurs. Pulmonary metastases are usually recognized first radiographically because of the great differential contrast between the metastatic nodules and the lung parenchyma; this degree of contrast is

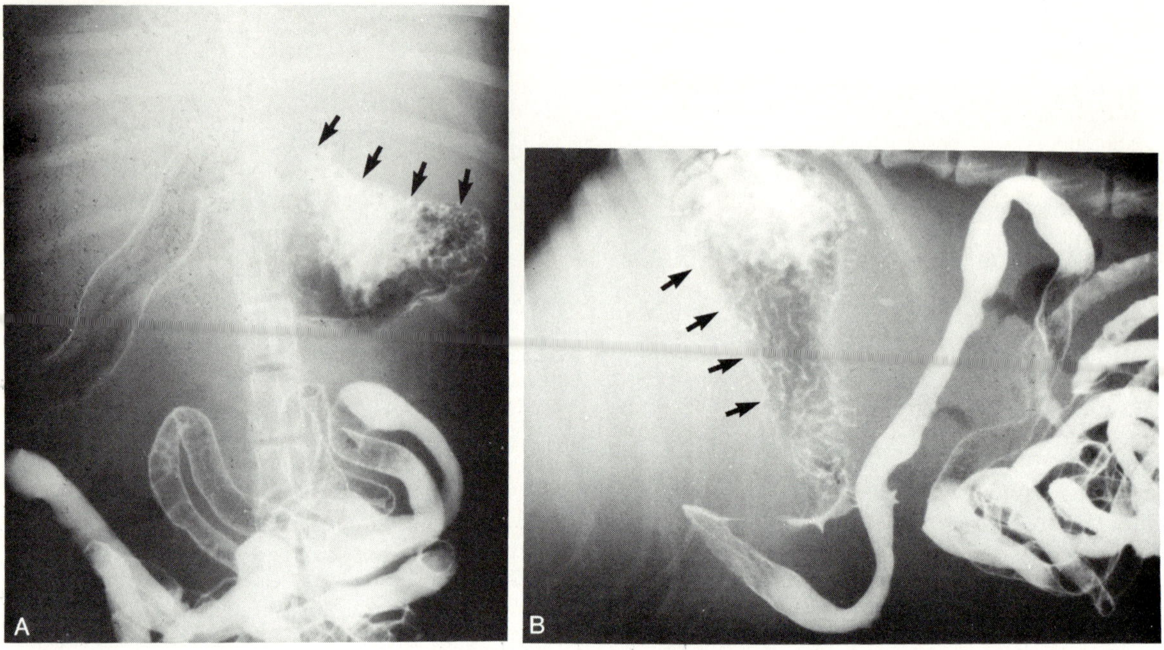

Figure 14–119. Fluid in the abdomen and a lack of fat made it impossible to determine the limits of the abdominal organs in this animal with lymphosarcoma. A barium upper gastrointestinal series outlined the gastrointestinal tract; it indicated that there was massive hepatomegaly and splenomegaly. The opacified gastrointestinal tract showed the typical displacements of symmetrical hepatomegaly. Note also that there is a concave cranial border to the stomach *(arrows)* on both the ventrodorsal *(A)* and lateral *(B)* views where the enlarged liver is pressing against and deforming it.

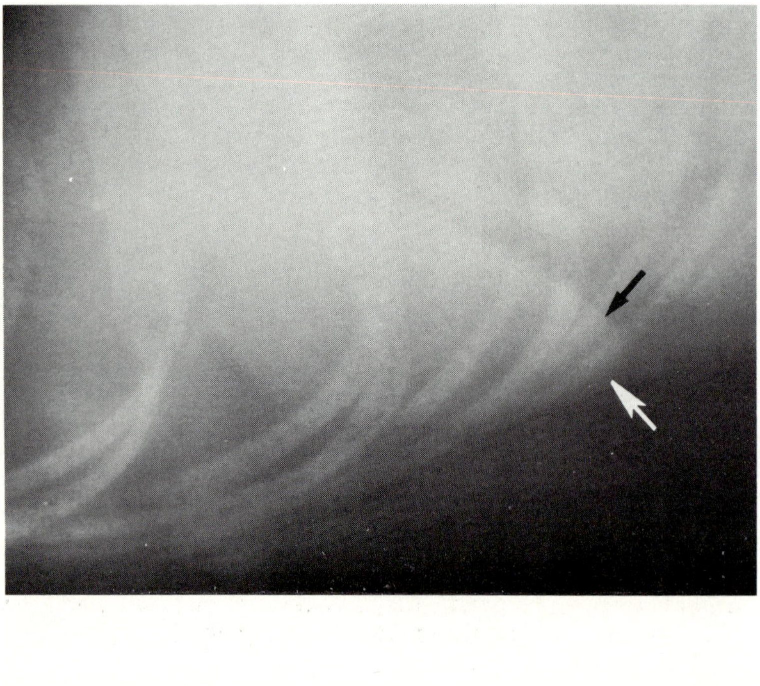

Figure 14–120. Rounding of the caudoventral margin of the liver *(arrows)* may be the only radiographic sign of disease in mild cases of enlargement such as that seen in cases of toxic or viral hepatitis.

not present in the liver. Clinical pathological evidence of altered liver function in animals with known or suspected neoplastic metastasis should be considered suspicious for the presence of liver metastasis, even though no radiographic abnormalities are recognized and altered liver function due to liver metastasis does not usually occur until the tumor burden within the organ is quite high.[34, 75, 88]

Metabolic abnormalities may result in symmetrical enlargement of the liver. They usually exhibit elevation of the liver enzyme levels in association with moderate to marked enlargement of the liver shadow on radiographs. The enlargement usually results from parenchymal deposition of abnormally large quantities of metabolic products such as glycogen, fat, and amyloid. These metabolites may or may not normally be present in the liver in small quantities. Paradoxically, these animals may have few if any signs referable to the liver, or the major clinical problem may be liver dysfunction.[34, 38, 94] Successful medical treatment of the disorder may result in regression of the liver enlargement. The metabolic abnormalities most commonly causing liver enlargement in small animals are Cushing's syndrome and diabetes mellitus (Fig. 14–121).[94]

Right heart insufficiency is another common cause of symmetrical liver enlargement (Fig. 14–122). The degree of enlargement is usually mild to moderate and may be obscured by ascites.[29, 71] Enlargement of the liver in an animal with known right heart disease might be anticipated; however, when clinical signs referable to the liver are present, the liver should be closely examined for evidence of another abnormality superimposed over the enlargement caused by the cardiac dysfunction.

Lymphosarcoma is one of the most common forms of neoplasia in the cat, and although less frequently seen it is not rare in dogs (Figs. 14–123 and 14–124). The parenchymal form of the disease may cause enlargement of the internal organs without a peripheral lymphadenopathy, especially in cats. The classic radiographic triad is symmetrical enlargement of the kidneys, spleen, and liver. Enlargement of any of the organs in the triad, particularly the spleen, is possible without enlargement of the others. Renal enlargement is probably more common in cats than in dogs. Symmetrical liver enlargement in a cat should be regarded as suspicious of lymphosarcoma (Figs. 14–124). Feline lymphosarcoma is not the only cause of symmetrical liver enlargement in the cat, but it is one that should always be considered because of the many forms that the disease may take. Although lymphosarcoma is not as common in dogs as it is in cats, it should also be considered when symmetrical

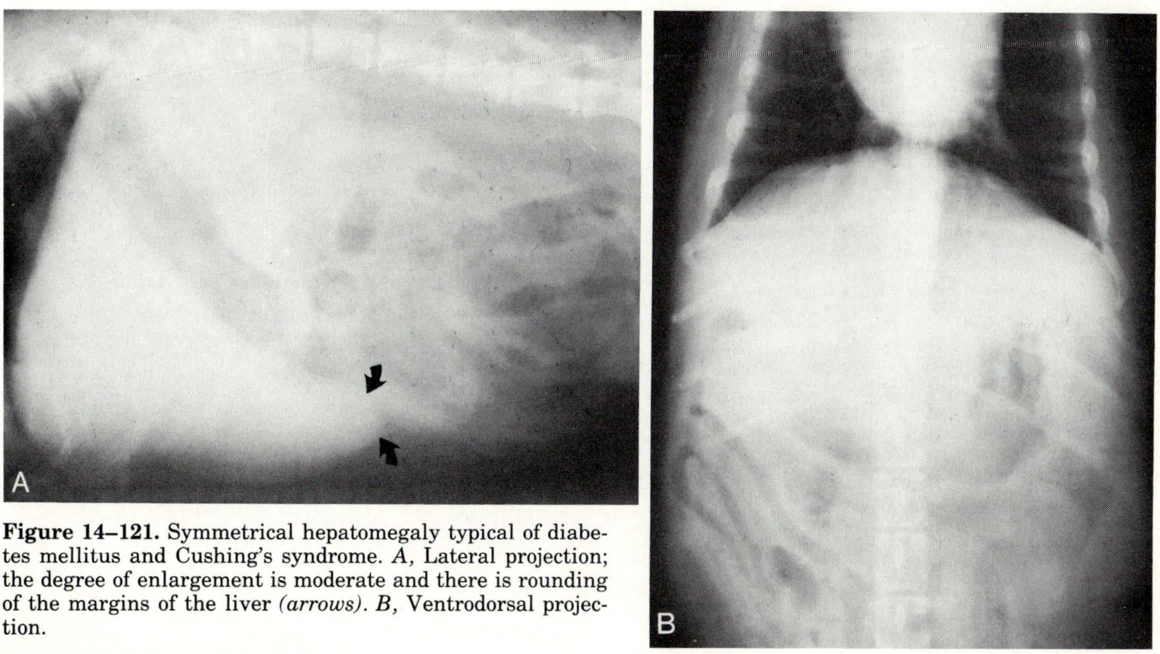

Figure 14–121. Symmetrical hepatomegaly typical of diabetes mellitus and Cushing's syndrome. *A,* Lateral projection; the degree of enlargement is moderate and there is rounding of the margins of the liver *(arrows)*. *B,* Ventrodorsal projection.

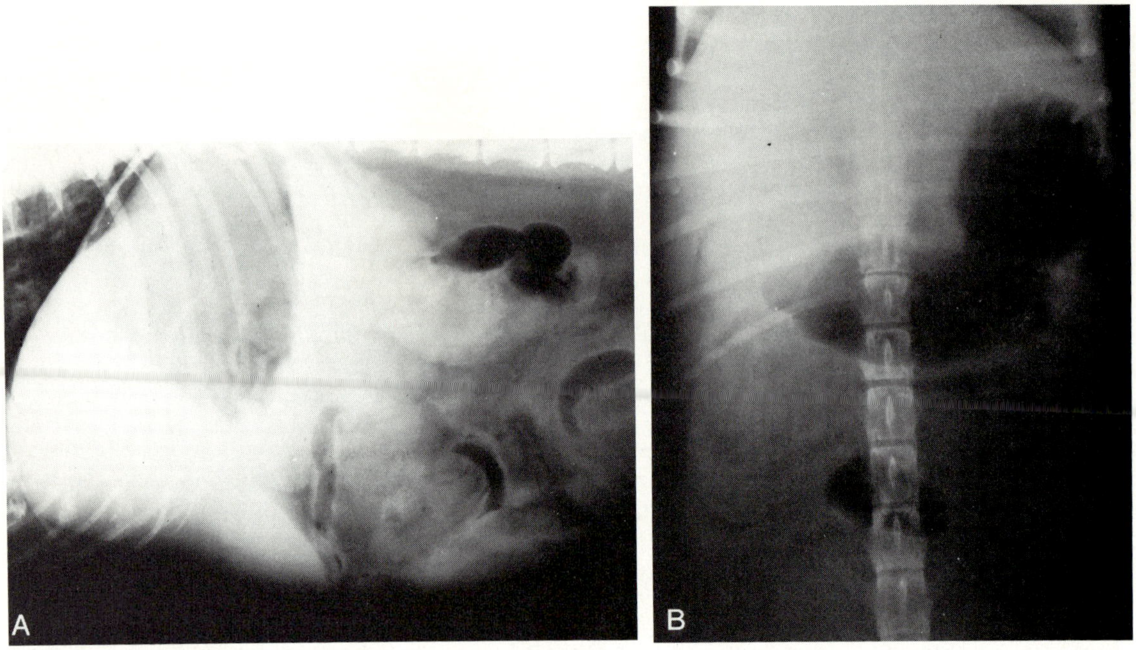

Figure 14–122. Mild to moderate symmetrical enlargement of the liver due to chronic passive congestion secondary to tricuspid insufficiency. Note the rounded caudoventral margin of the liver and the mild caudodorsal displacement of the stomach on the lateral view *(A)*. The ventrodorsal view *(B)* indicates caudal and leftward displacement of the stomach. The stomach is displaced somewhat to the left because most of the liver is on the right.

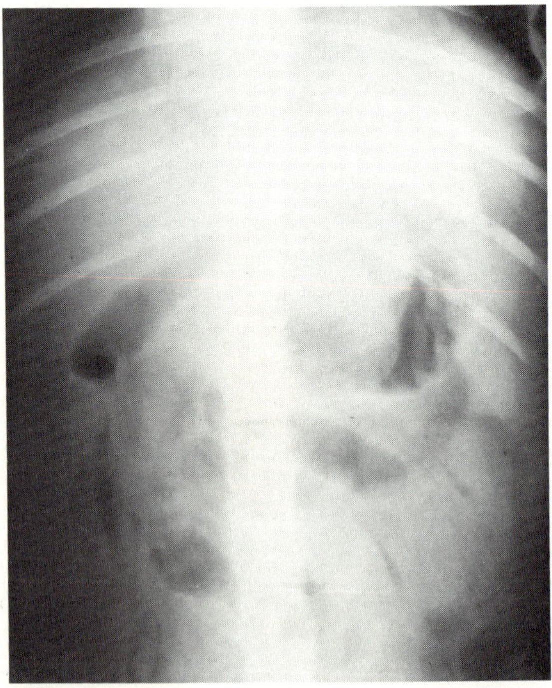

Figure 14–123. Symmetrical enlargement of the liver caused by infiltration of the liver with lymphosarcoma. The stomach is displaced caudally along with the duodenum. Both are displaced medially by the markedly enlarged right and left lateral lobes of the liver dissecting between them and the body wall.

hepatomegaly is present, especially when accompanied by splenomegaly or renomegaly.[1]

Liver enlargement associated with infectious disease is usually symmetrical unless abscesses develop. Viral, bacterial, and fungal diseases all have been described as causes of hepatomegaly, and the degree of enlargement may vary from slight to tremendous.[34, 35, 49] One infectious disease that causes rather remarkable hepatomegaly is histoplasmosis (Fig. 14–125). The liver enlargement is the symmetrical enlargement typically seen with other systemic diseases and may or may not be associated with the thoracic lesions usually seen with histoplasmosis. Also, the animal may exhibit signs of the enteric form of the disease with or without radiographic evidence of thoracic or hepatic involvement. The radiographic findings on an upper GI series are often suggestive of infiltrative bowel disease. The diagnosis can often be established by examination of a colonic scraping, eliminating the need for an operative biopsy, although this is not always the case.

Fatty infiltration can result in marked enlargement of the liver (Fig. 14–126). The fatty infiltration may be the result of a

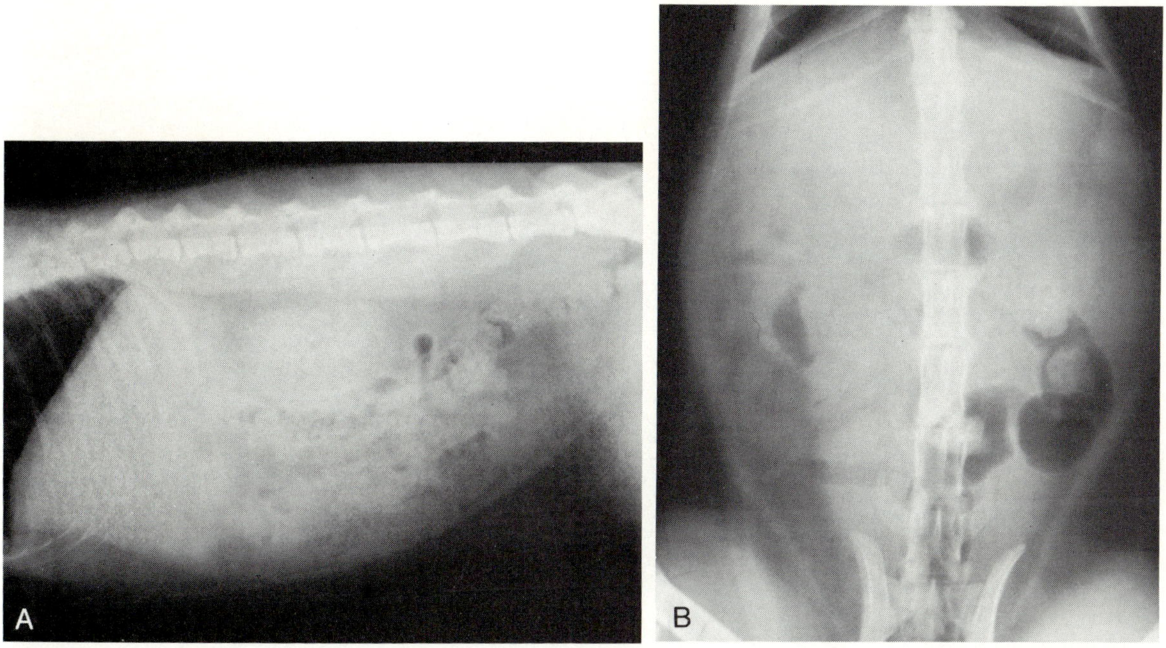

Figure 14–124. Uniform and symmetrical enlargement of the kidneys, spleen and liver due to feline lymphoma: *A*, lateral view; *B*, ventrodorsal view. The degree of enlargement of each of the organs involved is not marked but is definitely present. This is the classical triad of organ enlargement that is very suggestive of the abdominal parenchymal form of this disease.

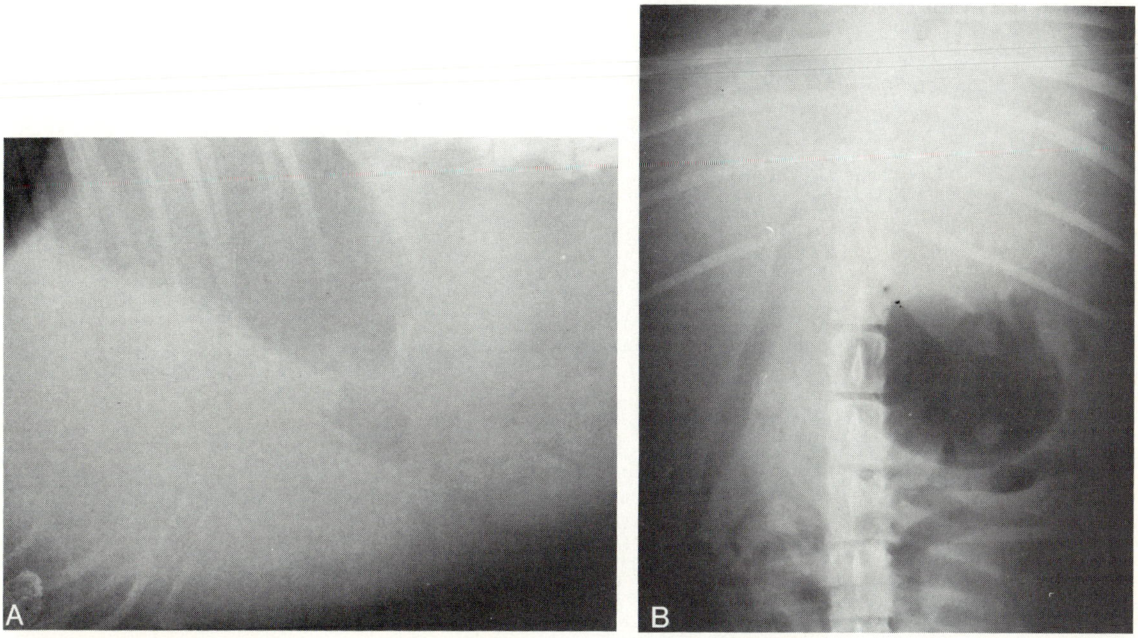

Figure 14–125. Histoplasmosis: *A*, lateral view; *B*, ventrodorsal view. There is tremendous symmetrical hepatomegaly caused by this deep-seated mycosis. Note the extreme caudal displacement of the duodenum. The right lateral liver lobe reaches further caudal than does the left.

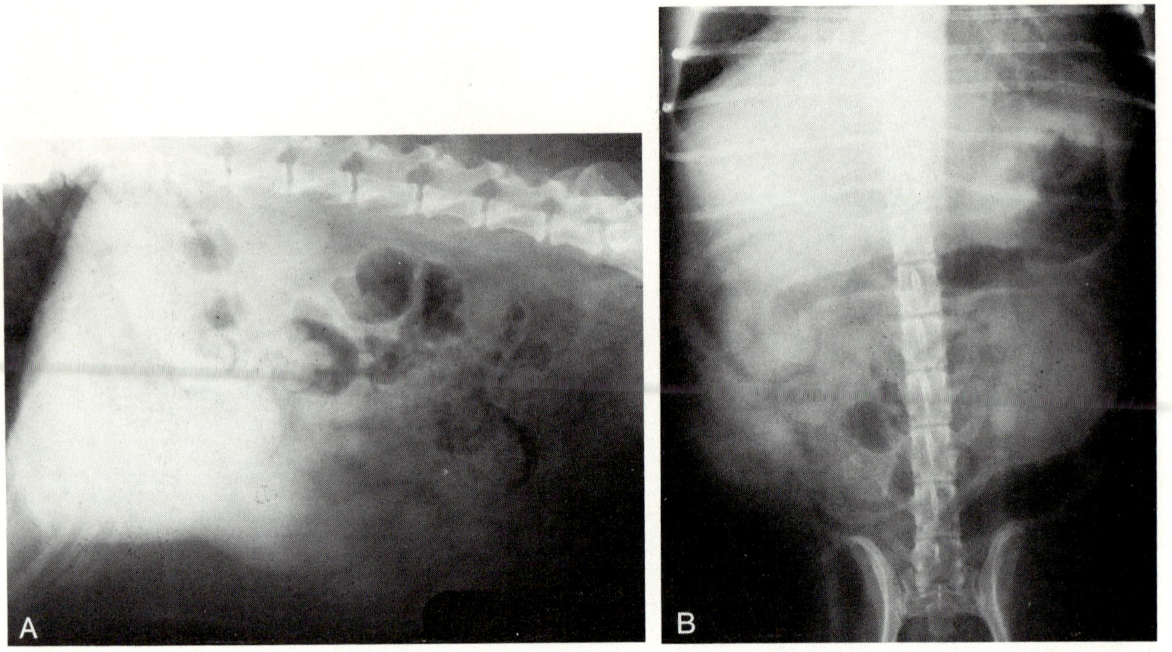

Figure 14–126. Fatty infiltration into the liver: *A,* lateral view; *B,* ventrodorsal view. The liver is symmetrically enlarged, causing caudal displacement of the organs in the cranial abdomen. The stomach is also dorsally displaced. Note the large amount of fat in the abdomen, especially in the falciform ligament.

metabolic disorder or, more commonly, obesity of the patient. As has been previously stated, the degree of liver enlargement may not be proportionate to the obesity of the animal. Dogs seem to show more of a tendency to deposit fat in the liver than do cats. Even when extremely obese, cats seldom show significant radiographic evidence of liver enlargement unless another primary or inciting disease process is present (Fig. 14–127). One example is fatty liver disease in cats. In this syndrome, markedly obese

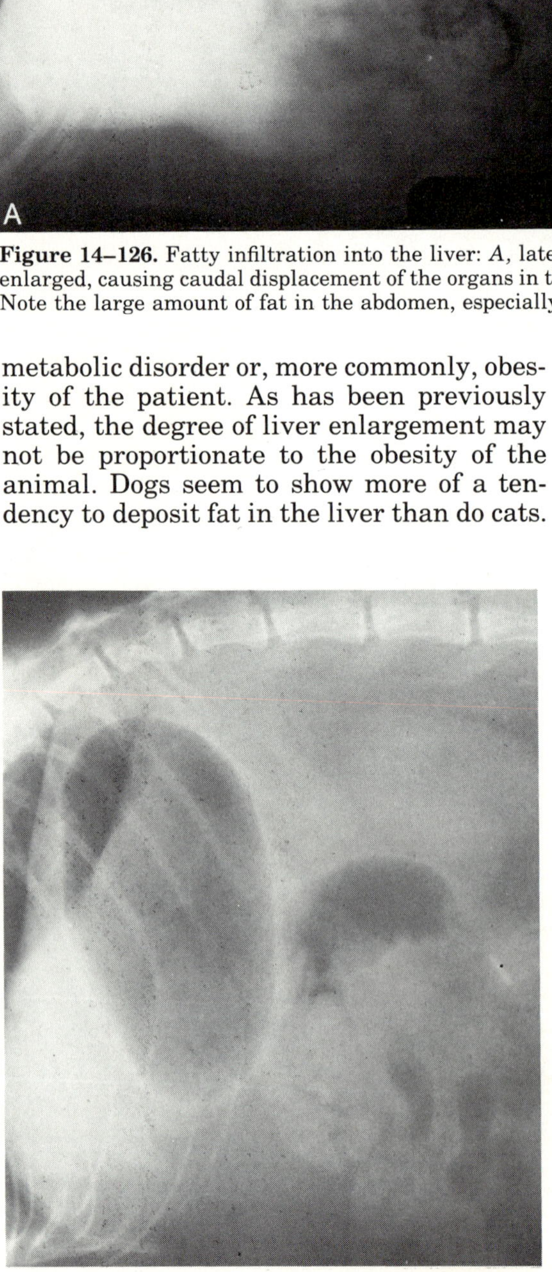

Figure 14–127. Normal obese cat. This animal is very fat; note the extremely large accumulations of fat in the falciform ligament and the perirenal space. The liver does not show any evidence of enlargement, such as is usually seen in obese dogs.

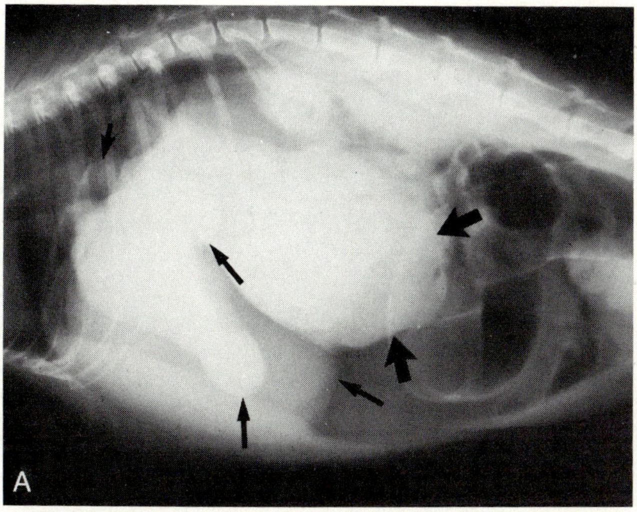

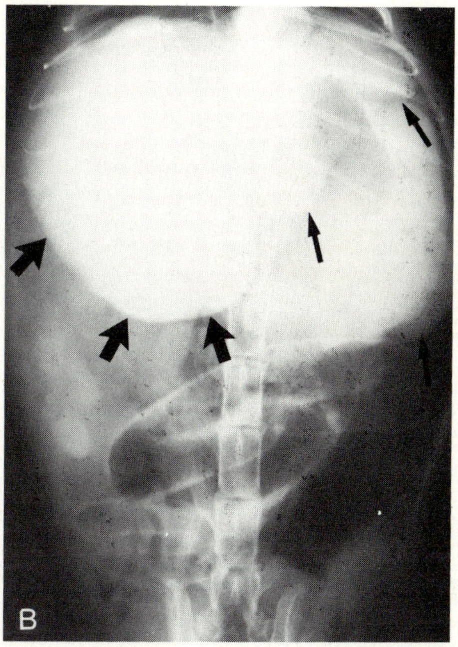

Figure 14–128. Lateral *(A)* and ventrodorsal *(B)* pneumoperitoneograms showing distortion of the normal shape of multiple liver lobes by an intrahepatic bile duct carcinoma. Note the generalized enlargement and rounding of the right lateral lobe *(large arrows)* and the irregular, knobby appearance of the other liver lobes *(small arrows)*. The tumor may well have arisen in the right lateral lobe and metastasized intrahepatically to the other lobes. The marked dorsal displacement of the stomach, accentuated by the pneumoperitoneum, was clearly evident on the survey film examination (not shown).

animals suffer from an anorexia-induced hepatopathy in which the starvation stimulates the deposition of fat in the liver. While the liver disease is probably secondary, it perpetuates the anorexia and often results in the death of the animal.[9]

The direct signs of asymmetrical liver enlargement are somewhat different than those seen with symmetrical enlargement. Although the liver still extends farther caudally than normal, there is generally more distortion of the shape than with symmetrical enlargement. The liver margin may be much rounder than normal or the entire shape of the affected lobe may be distorted, making it irregular and difficult to recognize (Fig. 14–128).[78]

The indirect signs have many different manifestations depending on the portion of the liver affected. Enlargement of the right medial and quadrate lobe will result in caudal and dorsal displacement of the body of the stomach (Figs. 14–129 and 14–149). The displacement may actually be more dorsal than caudal. One may also be able to detect a concavity in the cranial wall of the stomach produced by the tumor pressing on the stomach wall. Enlargement of the right lateral lobe of the liver causes dorsal and medial displacement of the proximal ascending and descending duodenum and the pylorus (Fig. 14–130). Enlargement of the caudate lobe results in caudal displacement of the right kidney (Fig. 14–131) and possible ventrocaudal displacement of the pylorus. Left medial lobe enlargement displaces the entire stomach caudally but will not necessarily displace the proximal ascending loop of the duodenum. It may also push the spleen caudally and laterally (Fig. 14–132). Enlargement of the left lateral lobe will displace the spleen, fundus of the stomach, and transverse loop of the colon caudodorsally and/or medially (Fig. 14–133).[77]

The degree of enlargement and the type of process causing the enlargement affect the kind of displacement seen. As a mass becomes larger it displaces other parts of the liver and eventually causes displacements characteristic of these lobes as well. Very large tumors often cause radiographic signs so complex that it is impossible to determine which lobe was affected first. Highly invasive processes that affect more than one lobe also often cause complex displacements even though the masses may

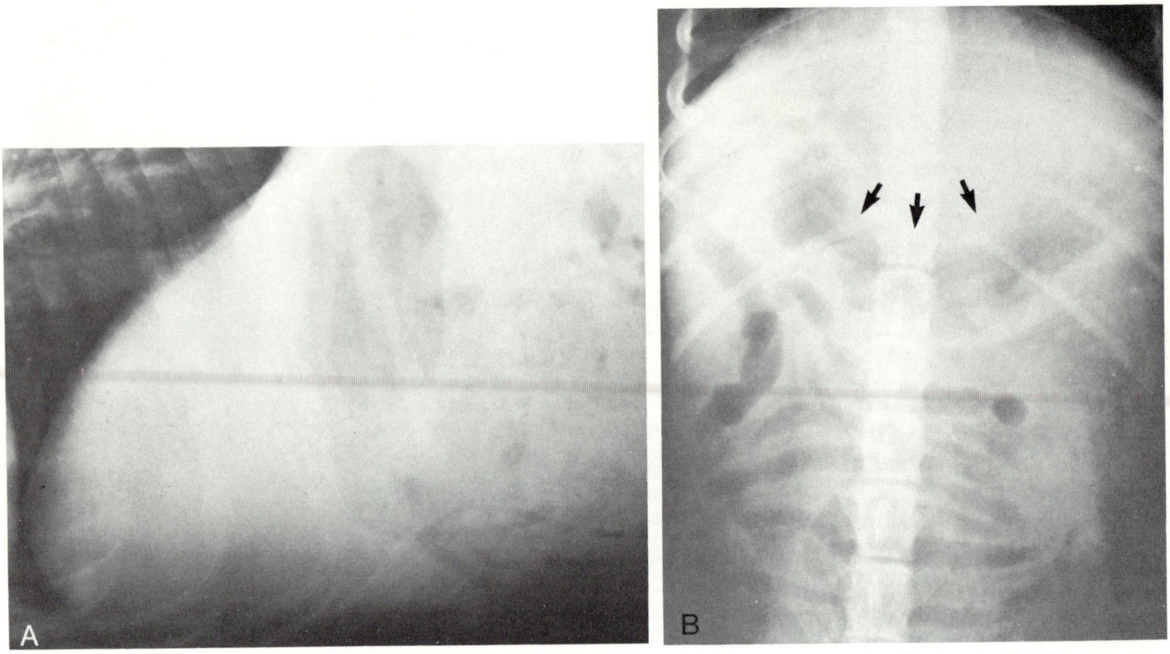

Figure 14–129. Quadrate or right medial liver lobe mass. The stomach appears to be displaced slightly dorsally and caudally on the lateral projection *(A)*, and there is only mild direct evidence of liver enlargement. However, the ventrodorsal view *(B)* indicates caudal displacement of the body of the stomach *(arrows)* that was not apparent on the lateral projection.

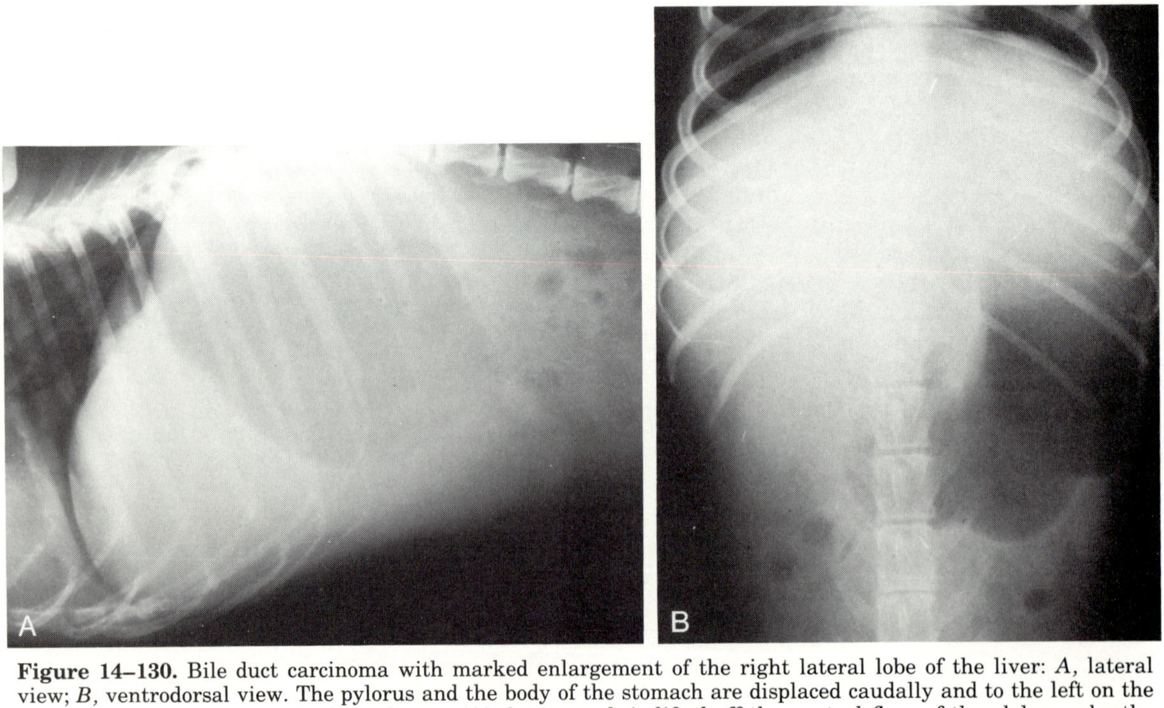

Figure 14–130. Bile duct carcinoma with marked enlargement of the right lateral lobe of the liver: *A*, lateral view; *B*, ventrodorsal view. The pylorus and the body of the stomach are displaced caudally and to the left on the ventrodorsal view *(B)*. On the lateral view *(A)* the stomach is lifted off the ventral floor of the abdomen by the large liver mass that is forcing its way along the floor of the abdomen. The fundus of the stomach is only mildly displaced caudally, indicating that there is much less involvement of the left liver lobes than of the right. The moderate dilatation of the stomach with gas and air is probably indicative of a partial outflow obstruction as a result of the tumor.

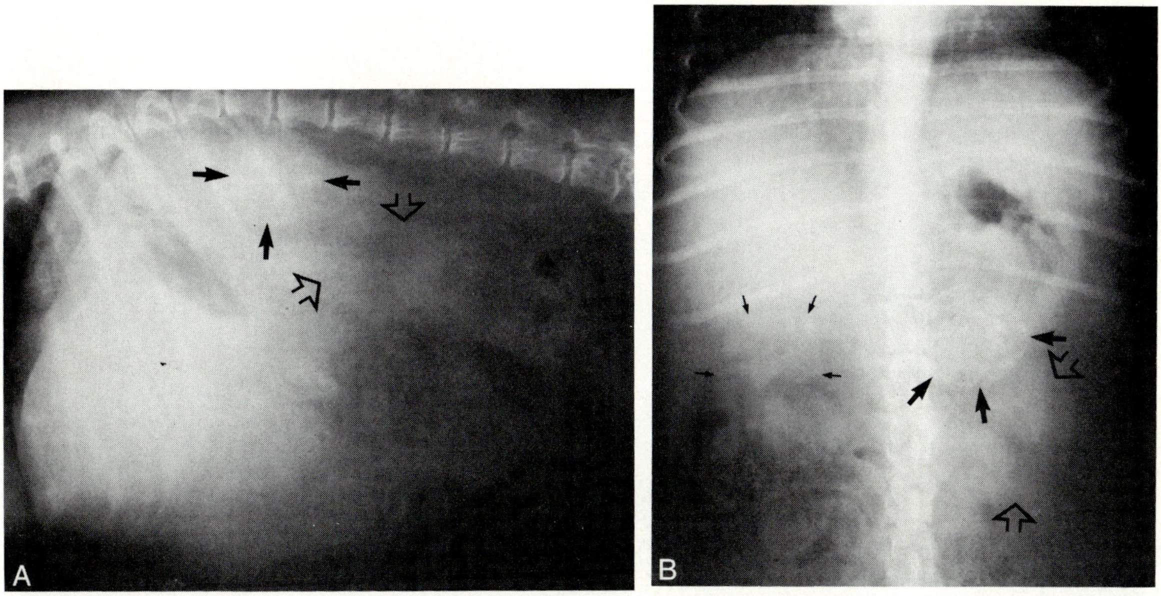

Figure 14–131. Metastatic adrenal adenocarcinoma: *A,* lateral view; *B,* ventrodorsal view. A large, calcified adrenal neoplasm *(large black arrows)* has metastasized to several lobes of the liver. There is distortion of several lobes of the liver and a complex pattern of organ displacements including dorsocaudal displacement of the stomach, small intestines, and transverse colon; and caudal displacement of both kidneys. The right kidney is displaced caudally *(small arrows)* due to enlargement of the caudate lobe of the liver. The caudal displacement of the left kidney *(open arrows)* is primarily due to the presence of the large adrenal tumor.

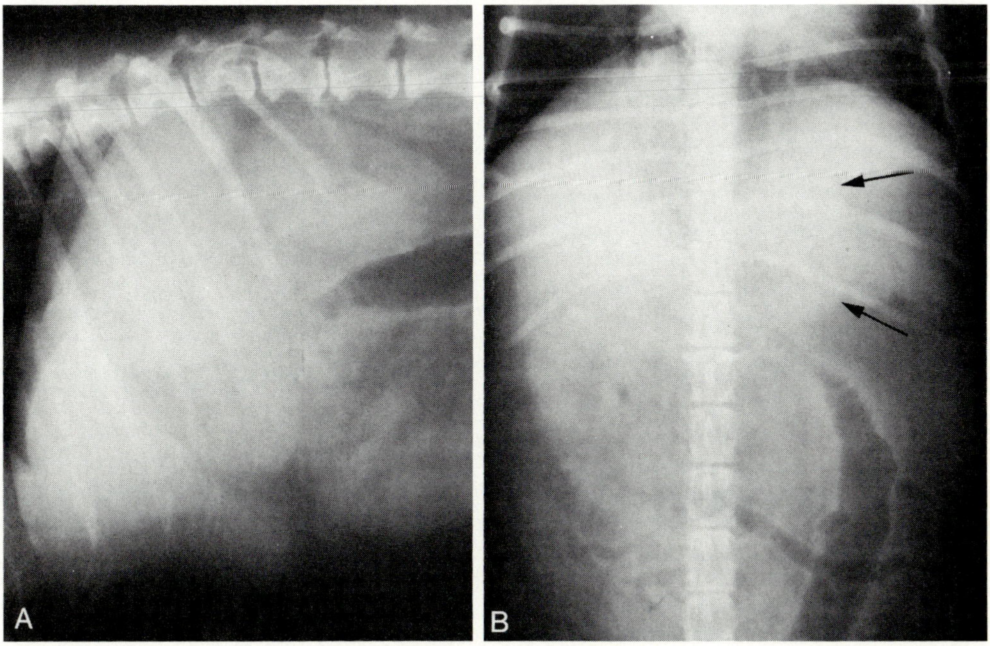

Figure 14–132. Caudal and slight medial displacement of the fundus of the stomach due to a left-sided liver tumor: *A,* lateral view; *B* ventrodorsal view. On this study it appears that the enlargement of the liver is principally in the left medial lobe of the liver. The stomach is displaced caudally and medially *(arrows, B)* without apparent extension of the liver along the lateral body wall such as would usually be observed in enlargement of the left lateral lobe (see Fig. 14–133).

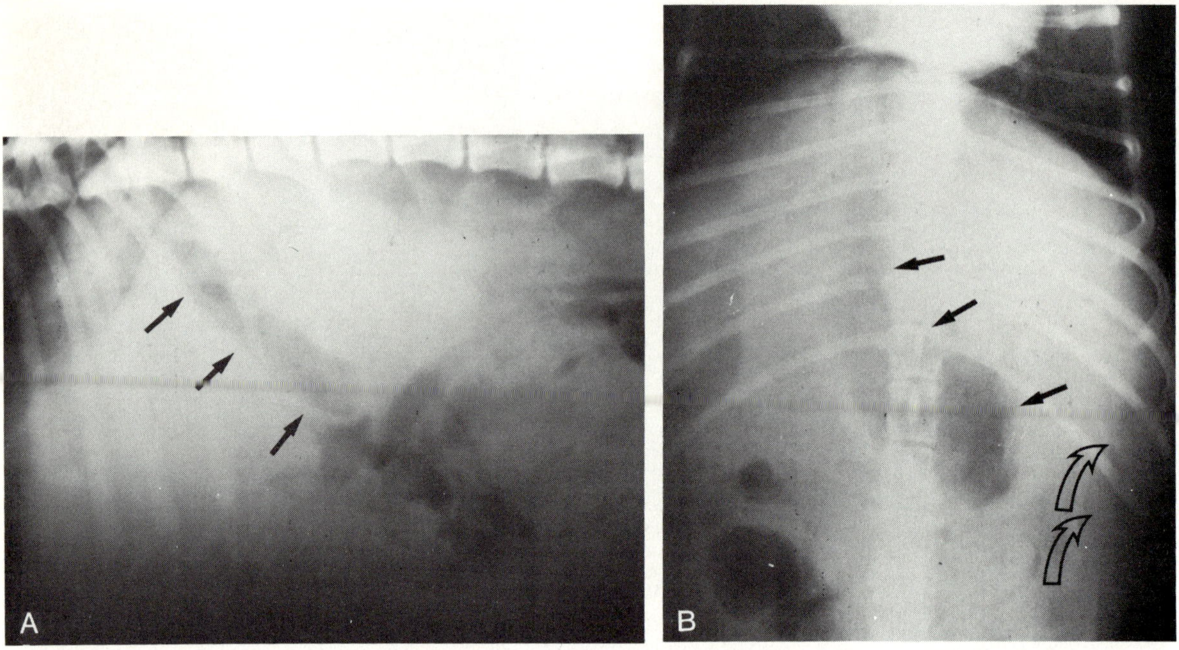

Figure 14–133. Lateral *(A)* and ventrodorsal *(B)* views of large hepatocellular carcinoma in the left lateral and medial lobes of the liver, which is displacing the stomach *(black arrows)* caudally, dorsally, and medially. The spleen is also displaced caudally and laterally *(open arrows, B)*.

not be excessively large. It may not be possible in all cases to determine exactly which lobes of the liver are involved by the disease process, but the radiographs should provide a reasonable idea of the magnitude and origin of the problem.

Asymmetrical enlargement of the liver is usually due to a disease process intrinsic to the liver.[71] Primary neoplasia, nodular hyperplasia, abscessation, and cyst formation are the most important causes diagnostically of asymmetrical liver enlargement; neoplasia is the most frequently observed cause.[29, 35, 51, 62, 78] Metastatic neoplasia may occasionally cause asymmetrical rather than symmetrical enlargement of the liver if only one or a few large metastatic nodules are present rather than many small ones.

Primary neoplasia of the liver usually affects predominantly one lobe of the liver, but tumors that are quite large or arise from more than one lobe may produce multiple lobar enlargements. Hepatocellular carcinoma and bile duct adenocarcinoma are examples of hepatic neoplasias that often have multiple lobe involvement.[75, 90, 91] Rarely, quadrate lobe hepatomas or histiocytomas may be pedunculated and slide under the stomach, producing a cranial and dorsal displacement of the stomach (Fig. 14–134).

Abscesses and hepatic cysts, whether single or multiple, are much less common causes of liver enlargement. Hepatic cysts cause few, if any, clinical signs unless they become infected or physically interfere with liver function.[84] Abscesses usually cause severe clinical signs and may rupture, causing a generalized peritonitis.[51] The presence of a circumscribed accumulation of gas definitely within the liver that is not associated with the gallbladder is highly suspicious of a cavitated liver abscess. The gas usually arises from gas-forming bacteria trapped within the lesion. These bacteria may secondarily infect a hematoma or neoplasm in the liver that has produced anoxic areas within the liver by its injury of the blood vessels. These secondary invading bacteria are normally found within the liver and probably originate from the GI tract. They do not normally cause problems as they are rapidly phagocytized by the reticuloendothelial cells of the liver.[34] Abscesses and cysts may occur in any lobe of the liver in small animals and do not have any predilection for specific lobes as in some other species.

DECREASED LIVER SIZE

Decreased liver size is usually symmetrical. In unusual cases of nonsymmetrical liver cirrhosis or in the case of surgical

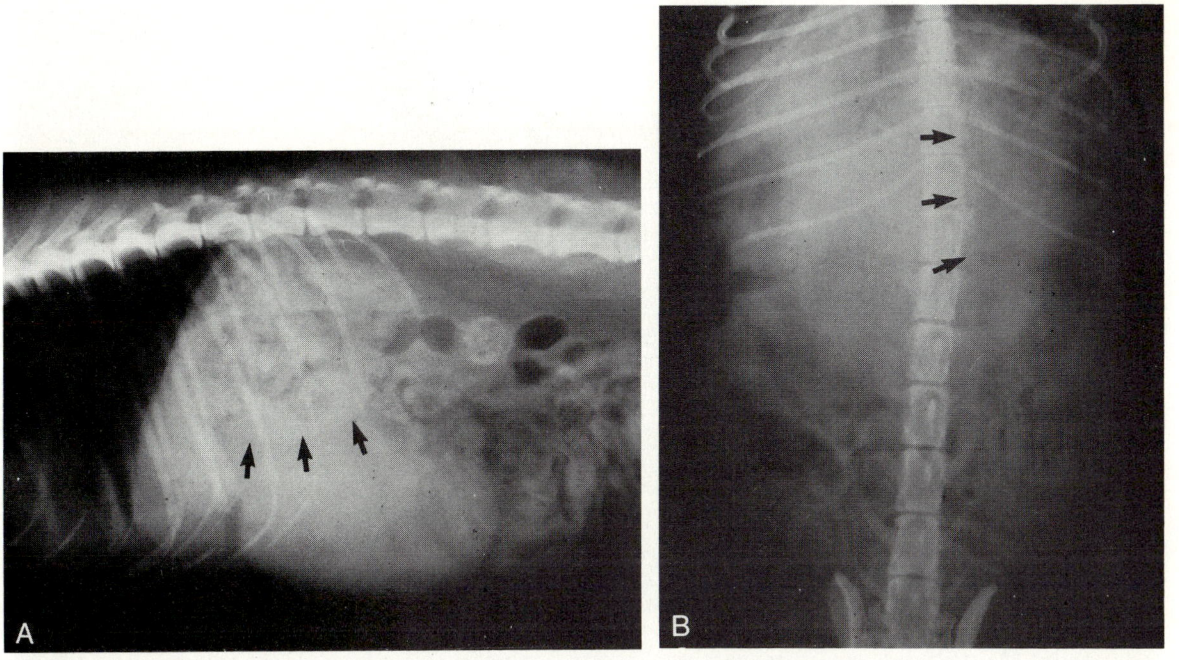

Figure 14–134. Lateral *(A)* and ventrodorsal *(B)* views of large pedunculated tumor of the liver, which has slipped caudally under the body of the stomach. This large, well-circumscribed mass is displacing the stomach *(arrows)* dorsally, cranially, and to the left, much as one would expect a mass in the spleen to do. The transverse colon is also displaced dorsally and to the left.

removal, only a portion of the liver may be reduced in size. A more common cause of an apparent decrease in size of one part of the liver is encountered in diaphragmatic hernias where only a portion of the liver is displaced into the thorax. Recognition of the diaphragmatic hernia explains the apparent reduction in the liver mass (Fig. 14–135).

Decreased liver size has essentially the opposite radiographic effect as increased size. As the mass of the liver shrinks, the adjacent organs occupy the space, resulting in the rest of the abdominal organs being shifted cranially in location. This effect is best appreciated in the stomach. The long axis of the stomach as seen on the lateral view will have a marked cranial angulation, with the gastric axis often approximately paralleling the diaphragm. The stomach will also appear closer to the diaphragm than normal. This may be most noticeable on the right side of the abdomen, where the pylorus is displaced cranially (Fig. 14–136).[71, 90, 91]

When the liver appears smaller than normal, care must be taken to assess all of the signs of a small liver on both views. Large variation in the conformation of the canine abdomen may result in a liver that will appear small if only the angle of the long axis of the stomach is considered. This is particularly true in deep-chested breeds (Fig. 14–109). There is very little variation in the conformation of the abdomen in the feline population; however, care must be taken not to underestimate the size of the liver in cats owing to the slightly more intrathoracic position of the stomach in the cat.

Decreased liver size has two basic causes: Failure of liver tissue to develop fully and a pathological shrinkage of the liver secondary to massive parenchymal necrosis and scarring. Failure of proper development is secondary to congenital defects that cause decreased flow of portal blood to the liver. Since many of the primary functions of the liver are associated with the processing of portal blood, a reduction in portal blood flow removes the stimulus for the liver to grow to its normal size. The most commonly described of these defects is persistence of the fetal blood flow pattern through the liver (Figs. 14–137 and 14–138). Blood returning to the fetus from the placenta bypasses the liver by flowing from the umbilical vein to the caudal vena cava via the ductus venosus. The portal blood also bypasses the liver by

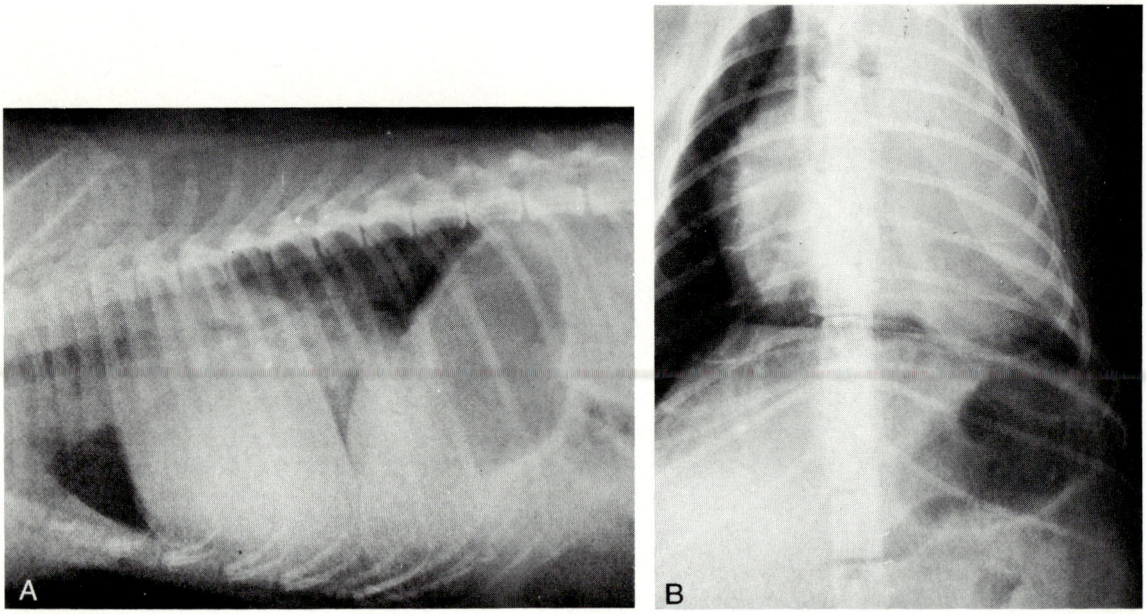

Figure 14–135. Diaphragmatic hernia. The hernia is not readily recognizable on the lateral view *(A)*, and it appears that the stomach is positioned much closer to the diaphragm than normal. Using only this one view for assessment, it would be possible to make the incorrect diagnosis of decreased liver size. The ventrodorsal view *(B)*, however, makes it clear that the real problem is a diaphragmatic hernia. Most of the left side of the liver is within the thorax.

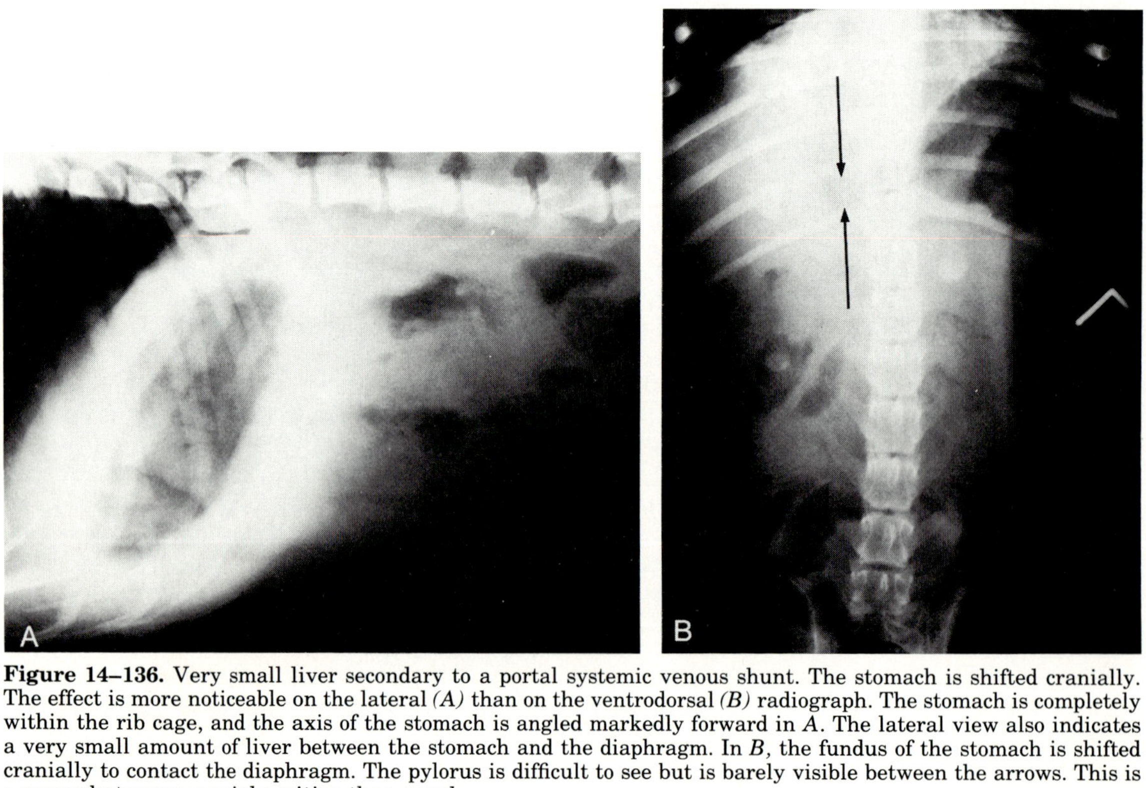

Figure 14–136. Very small liver secondary to a portal systemic venous shunt. The stomach is shifted cranially. The effect is more noticeable on the lateral *(A)* than on the ventrodorsal *(B)* radiograph. The stomach is completely within the rib cage, and the axis of the stomach is angled markedly forward in *A*. The lateral view also indicates a very small amount of liver between the stomach and the diaphragm. In *B*, the fundus of the stomach is shifted cranially to contact the diaphragm. The pylorus is difficult to see but is barely visible between the arrows. This is a somewhat more cranial position than usual.

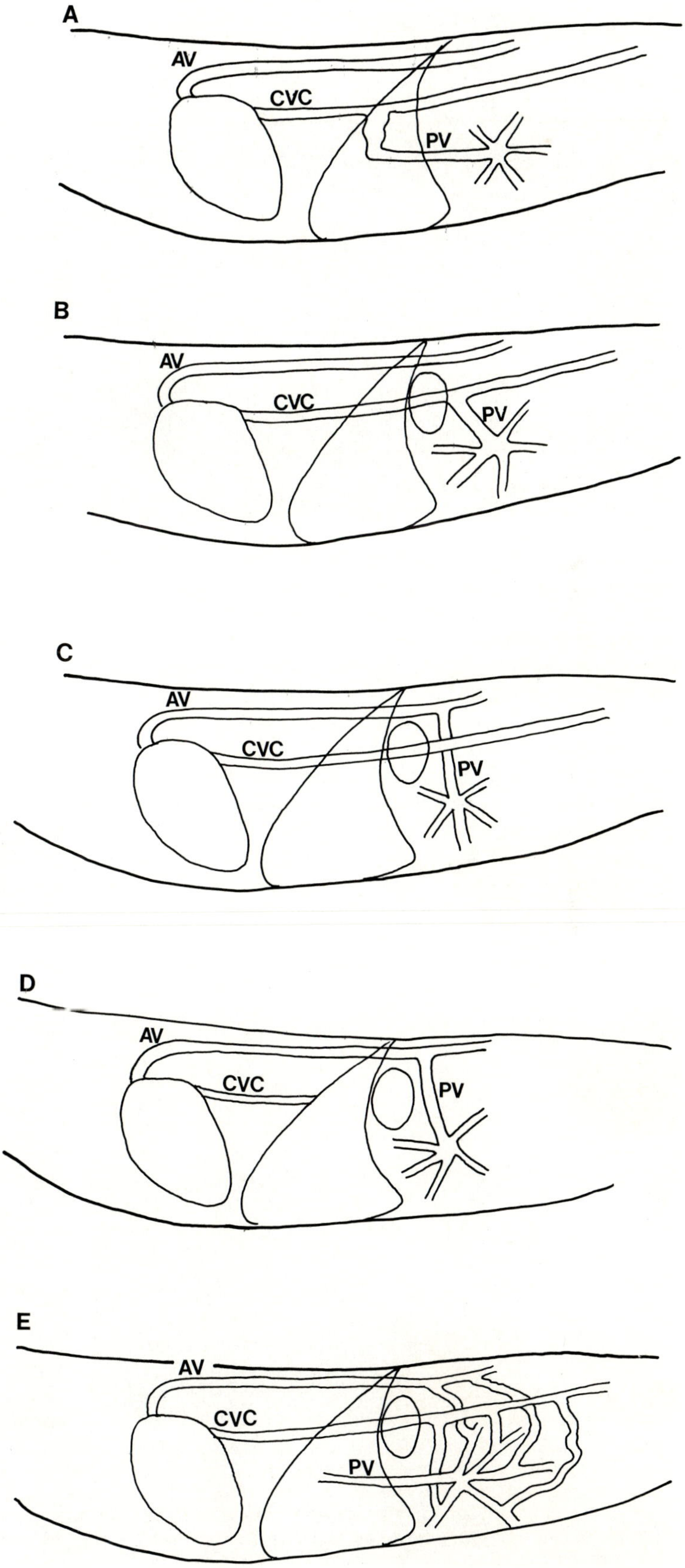

Figure 14–137. Schematic representation of various types of portal systemic venous anastomoses. *A,* Patent ductus venosus (intrahepatic portal-systemic venous shunt); *B,* prehepatic portal-caudal vena cava venous shunt; *C,* portal-azygos venous shunt; *D,* portal-caudal vena cava–azygos venous shunt (aplasia of the prehepatic caudal vena cava); *E,* multiple acquired portal-caudal vena cava and/or azygos venous shunts (portal venous hypertension with hepatofugal flow). AV, azygos vein; CVC, caudal vena cava; PV, portal vein.

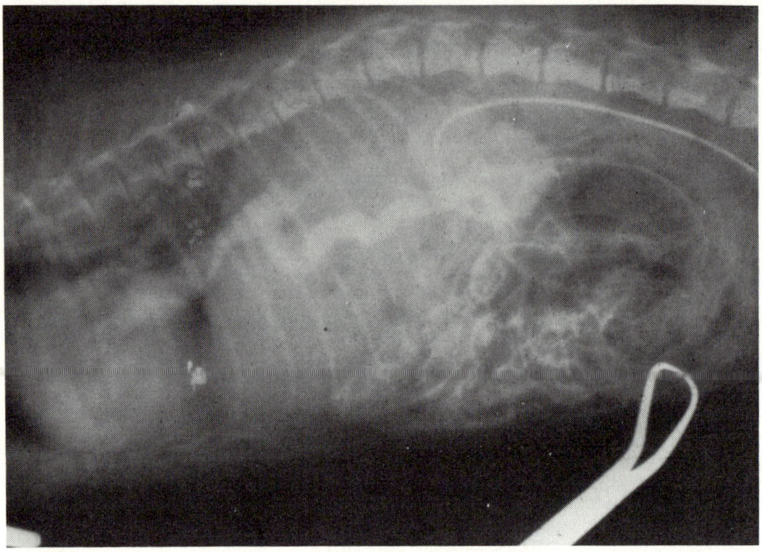

Figure 14–138. Patent ductus venosus (intrahepatic portal systemic venous shunt). This cranial mesenteric arteriogram shows that the blood is effectively bypassing the liver by going directly from the portal vein to the caudal vena cava by way of the open ductus venosus, which normally closes shortly after birth. The catheter is placed in the cranial mesenteric artery and the injection of the contrast medium is made at that point. The portal vein is opacified during the venous drainage phase of the study. Note that the entire venous drainage of the intestinal tract is visible.

empyting into the terminal part of the umbilical vein. When the umbilical vein becomes nonfunctional at birth the ductus venosus normally closes, forcing the portal blood to flow into the liver sinusoids where it is collected and carried to the systemic circulation by the hepatic veins. Failure of the ductus venosus to close results in direct flow of the portal blood into the caudal vena cava, bypassing the liver.[7, 8, 21, 50, 91, 98]

There are several other more complex vascular anomalies. They all consist of an abnormal communication between the portal vein and the caudal vena cava or azygos vein (Figs. 14–137, 14–139, and 14–140).[7, 8, 21, 50, 91, 98] Since the pressure required to force the blood through the liver is slightly higher than the pressure in the systemic central venous system, the majority of the blood bypasses the liver. Rarely the portal vein may be completely absent, resulting in severe deprivation of the liver. In these instances the only blood from the digestive system reaching the liver is that from the stomach and the proximal duodenum. Such complex anatomical abnormalities may not be amenable to surgical correction and must therefore be identified before correction of a

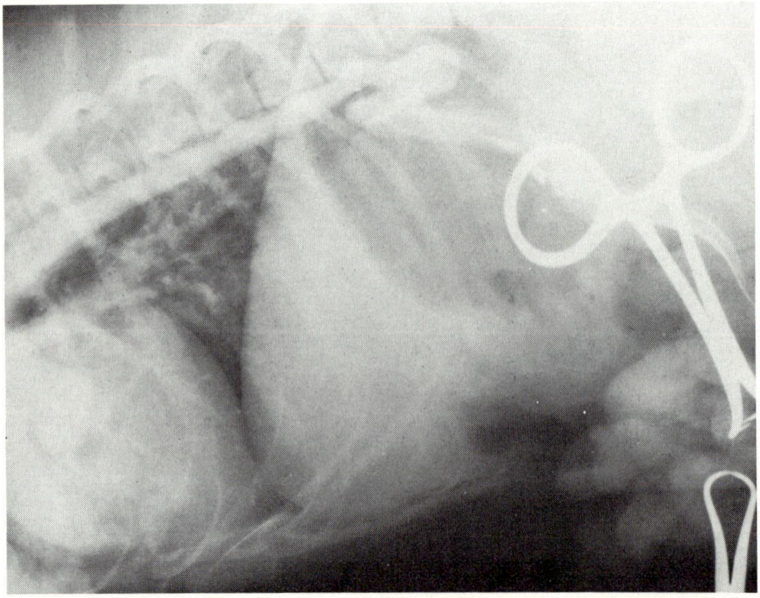

Figure 14–139. Portal-azygos venous shunt. This operative mesenteric venogram shows that the contrast medium is flowing directly from the mesenteric venous bed into the azygos vein, and from there into the right atrium. Animals with this anomaly may also have atresia of the caudal vena cava caudal to the liver, or the shunt may completely bypass the caudal vena cava.

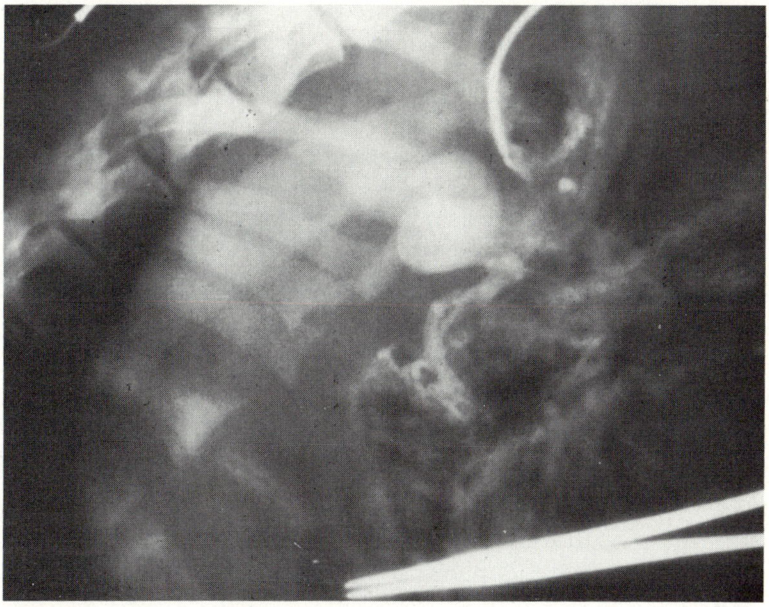

Figure 14–140. Cranial mesenteric artery angiogram demonstrating the presence of prehepatic portal-caudal vena cava venous shunt. The blood is flowing directly from the portal vein into the caudal vena cava well before either vein reaches the liver. There may be either no communication of the mesenteric portal flow to the liver or only a hypoplastic channel to the liver that carries a very small amount of flow. The signs of the syndrome may not be as severe in the latter case.

portal systemic venous shunt can be contemplated.

Loss of normal liver parenchyma due to necrosis may be the end result of several diseases. When loss of liver cells occurs, this space is filled in by fibrous connective tissue (cirrhosis), which usually results in contracture and a decrease in liver size. Infectious, metabolic, autoimmune, toxic, endocrine, and biliary diseases have all been incriminated as causes of liver cirrhosis.[21] As fibrosis advances there is a progressive loss of the vascular spaces in the liver, which increases the blood flow resistance. The increased resistance eventually reaches a point at which elevation in portal blood pressure occurs. As the portal pressure continues to increase, collateral channels leading from the portal to the systemic circulation open to relieve the pressure, resulting in the shunting of blood around the liver. This may explain why some animals with severe cirrhosis do not develop ascites. The effect is the same as if a large congenital shunt were present and the portal blood is shunted away from what functional liver remains (Figs. 14–137 and 14–141).

Animals with acquired shunts differ in

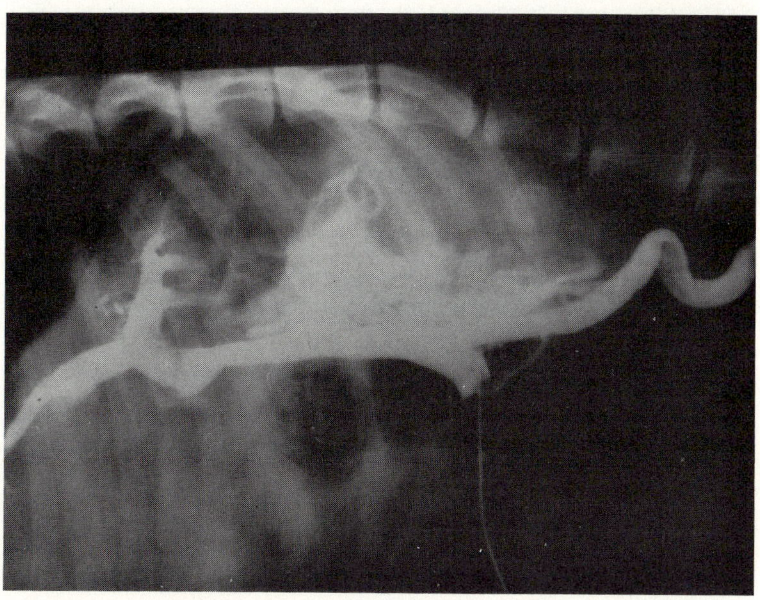

Figure 14–141. Multiple acquired portal systemic venous shunts. Note the dilatation of the intrahepatic branches of the portal vein, the multiple small venous radicles caudal to the stomach, and the hepatofugal flow of the blood caudally through a relatively large shunt channel from the point of injection. This animal had severe cirrhosis of the liver, which caused the portal hypertension.

two important ways from those with congenital shunts: they have advanced irreversible liver damage, and the shunts are multiple. These two factors preclude surgical correction of the animal's presenting problem because it is impossible to correct the basic underlying problem.[73, 91, 99] Since cirrhosis is not found only in old animals, age cannot be used to accurately determine whether a clinically suspected portal-systemic shunt is congenital or acquired; therefore, positive identification of an acquired shunt prior to surgery is imperative.

A portal systemic shunt can be suspected on the basis of presenting signs, blood chemistry values, and survey radiographs.[3, 7, 8, 21, 27, 41, 50, 57, 76, 86, 98, 99] Definitive diagnosis is dependent on the performance of liver biopsies and special radiographic procedures designed to evaluate the portal vascular system.[8, 26, 28, 90, 91] Three procedures of major importance will be described and are summarized in Table 14–2.

Cranial mesenteric arteriography is the injection of a radiopaque contrast material into the cranial mesenteric artery (Figs. 14–138 and 14–140). The pattern of blood flow is then followed by taking serial films at one-second intervals following the injection. The time the film sequence covers is dependent on the subjective evaluation of the circulation time observed under fluoroscopy during a test injection but usually ranges from 10 to 25 seconds. If a large venous shunt is present, it will be seen as a single, large vein bypassing the liver during the venous drainage portion of the study. The multiple smaller channels present in acquired shunts may be more difficult to see but are usually detectable.[82, 91]

Mesenteric arteriography has several advantages. It permits study of virtually the entire portal circulation, both arterial and venous, with a single injection. Repositioning of the catheter in the celiac artery allows study of the hepatic arteries for evidence of hepatic hypertension and evaluation of drainage from the splenic vein. Mesenteric arteriography is also the least invasive technique for visualization of the portal circulation. These attributes make it a safe and relatively quick technique for detecting and defining portal-systemic venous shunts. There are, however, some disadvantages. The technique requires fluoroscopic guidance for placement of the catheter, which should only be done by persons practiced in the selective placement of arterial catheters. The other disadvantage is a direct result of the arterial injection of the contrast material. Because the contrast becomes somewhat diluted with blood as it passes through the circulation, the degree of opacification achieved in the venous circulation is not as great as with the direct venous injection techniques. This is not usually a problem when a single large shunt is present, but it may make detection of multiple very small shunt channels difficult.[91]

Operative mesenteric venography and

Table 14–2. PORTAL CIRCULATION CONTRAST STUDIES

	Cranial Mesenteric Arteriography	Operative Mesenteric Venography	Splenoportography
Site	Cranial mesenteric artery	Any mesenteric vein	Hilus of spleen
Dose*	1.0–1.5 ml/kg	5–15 ml	5–15 ml
Virtues	Less anesthesia required	Densely opacifies portal vein	Densely opacifies portal vein
	Opacifies entire mesenteric artery circulatory bed	Requires no special equipment	Requires no special equipment
	Permits same study on celiac arterial and venous bed	Study easy to evaluate	Study easy to evaluate
Problems	Requires fluoroscope and special catheters	Requires deep general anesthesia	Requires deep general anesthesia
	Training in catheter placement needed	Requires a laparotomy	Requires laparotomy or endoscopy
	Interpretation may be difficult	Does not evaluate all of portal drainage system	Does not evaluate mesenteric venous drainage pathway
	Complete study requires many films (10 to 14)	Danger of vascular damage to small intestine	Danger of lacerating the spleen
		Vascular supply of liver not seen	Vascular supply of liver not seen

*Renografin 76, E. R. Squibb & Sons, Inc., Princeton, NJ.

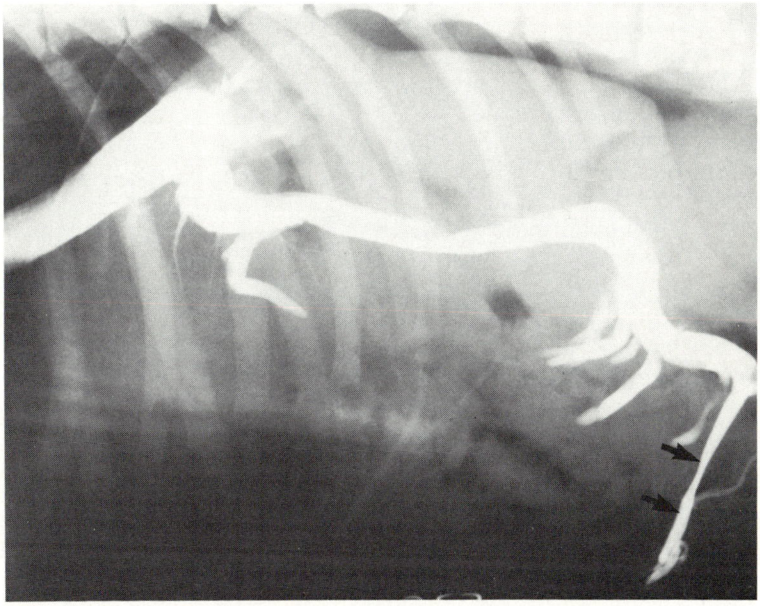

Figure 14–142. Operative mesenteric venography. The bowel is exposed by a ventral midline incision and a loop of bowel exteriorized. A catheter is placed in one branch of the mesenteric vein *(arrows)* and the contrast agent injected. The contrast medium flows directly from the portal vein into the caudal vena cava through a large intrahepatic venous shunt. This method provides very clear visualization of the flow from the point of injection to the caudal vena cava. Note that there is very minimal filling of the small intrahepatic branches of the portal vein.

splenoportography are the other two methods used to evaluate for the presence of portal-systemic venous shunts (Figs. 14–142 and 14–143). These studies involve the injection of radiopaque contrast materials directly into the venous tributaries of the portal vein. The injection is made into one of the mesenteric veins in mesenteric venography. In splenoportography, the injection is actually made into the parenchyma of the spleen at the hilus. Both techniques require that films be taken from the time of the injection at one-second intervals for ten exposures, in order to follow the blood flow back to the heart. The major advantages of these two procedures are that they require no special equipment and that they provide a much more intense opacification of the venous drainage from the point of injection to the heart. The major disadvantages are the requirement for celiotomy to expose the bowel or spleen for injection of the contrast

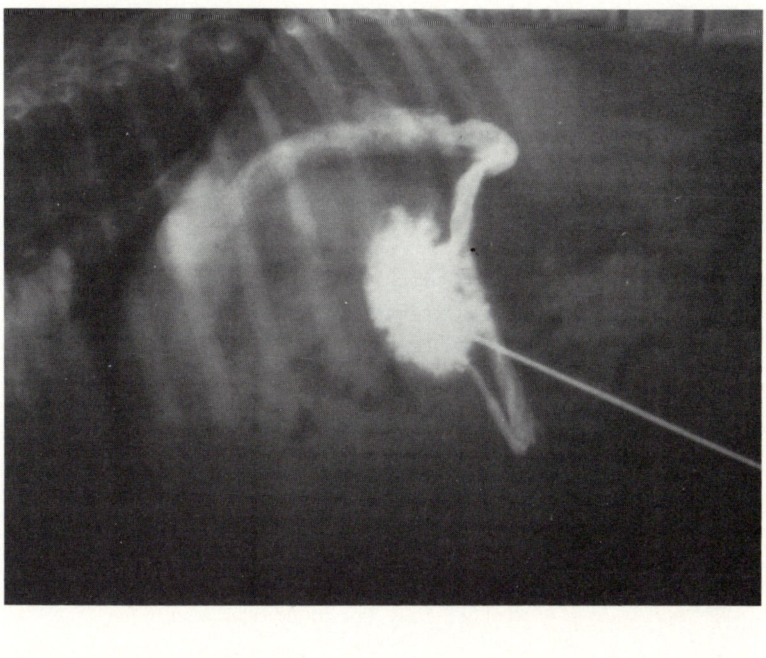

Figure 14–143. Splenoportogram. An endoscope is used to visualize the spleen, and a long, narrow needle is placed within the pulp of the spleen near the hilus. Forcible injection of contrast agent through the needle results in rapid drainage of the material into the splenic vein and then into the portal vein, which shows that the blood is flowing directly into the caudal vena cava through a large intrahepatic shunt. As in Figure 14–142, the opacification of the venous drainage from the point of injection to the caudal vena cava is well defined and the shunt is clearly seen. In this case, however, the drainage from the celiac circulatory bed is being studied.

media and the fact that it is impossible to study the entire vasculature of the gastrointestinal tract or the celiac axis.[8, 28, 91]

The normal portal circulation time (the time required for blood to travel from the cranial mesenteric artery to the intrahepatic portal veins) is approximately eight seconds.[42] This is a much shorter time than the time periods over which films are taken. The reason for the protracted filming sequences is that the flow of blood through the portal system may be slowed by the conditions causing portal systemic shunts. A marked delay in transit time is most often present in animals with acquired shunts secondary to hepatic fibrosis.[42, 91] These animals almost invariably have multiple small shunts rather than a single large one as is the case with congenital shunts. Patients with patent ductus venosus may or may not have an abnormally rapid transit time owing to the fact that the blood bypasses the liver and goes directly to the heart. In any case, animals with portal systemic venous shunts often have alterations in the rate of blood drainage from the portal system as well as an anatomical abnormality.

Gallbladder

The gallbladder is usually not distinguishable as a separate radiographic shadow from the liver in the normal animal. It is positioned adjacent to the diaphragm and between the right medial and quadrate liver lobes in the dog. In cats, it lies within a fossa of the right medial lobe. The gallbladder is therefore part of the liver shadow in both species.[16, 55, 69] Because of this, even major diseases of the gallbladder and its ducts may not be recognized on radiographs until the diseases are quite advanced.

The abnormal gallbladder may present (1) as an area of increased density, (2) as an area of decreased density, (3) or as a mass or mass effect arising from the right ventral region of the liver (asymmetrical enlargement of the liver shadow). Each of these presentations represents different disease processes and will be considered separately.[71]

Increased density of the gallbladder area may be caused by calculi. Cholelithiasis and choledocholithiasis are commonly seen in man but seldom encountered as a clinical problem in the dog and are very rarely recognized in cats. Choleliths are usually of mixed origin, being composed of bile pigments, calcium salts, cholesterol and bilirubin, but may also be composed purely of a single material. Only those choleliths that contain significant amounts of calcium will be radiographically detectable. Choleliths that are radiodense may be irregularly calcified if they are of mixed nature. They may be solid or stippled or form rings around radiolucent cores. A large percentage of choleliths have little or no calcium in them.[71, 72, 81] Many choleliths may therefore be missed on routine radiographs. An animal showing signs of obstructive biliary disease without radiographic evidence of choleliths cannot be judged free of cholelithiasis. Since rupture of the gallbladder can be a fatal sequelae to blockage of the common bile duct by a cholelith, such animals should have biliary system contrast studies performed to completely rule out this problem (Fig. 14–144).[62]

Recognition of a radiodensity in the area of the gallbladder is not always diagnostic of cholelithiasis. Since gastrointestinal tract foreign bodies are much more common than radiopaque choleliths and because the small bowel may be superimposed over the region of the gallbladder, it is advisable to confirm the position and extent of the gastrointestinal (GI) tract. A positive contrast upper GI series is recommended as the best way to rule out a foreign body. Even if a foreign body is ruled out, the possibility of a calcified cyst within the liver parenchyma still exists (Fig. 14–145); thus, a calcified choledocolith can be confirmed only after a contrast cholecystogram is performed.

Decreased density in the gallbladder is the result of gas accumulation in either the gallbladder lumen or wall. The gas may or may not extend into the biliary tree or common bile duct. Emphysematous cholecystitis is a rare but very severe disease that usually causes severe clinical disease. The origin of emphysematous cholecystitis is thought to be gas-forming bacterial infection of the gallbladder, although reflux of gas from the intestinal tract into the gallbladder probably should also be considered as a potential source of the gas. An accumulation of air in the biliary tree has also been observed following the iatrogenic introduction of air into the liver during an attempted abdominal paracentesis.

Radiographically, gas in the gallbladder

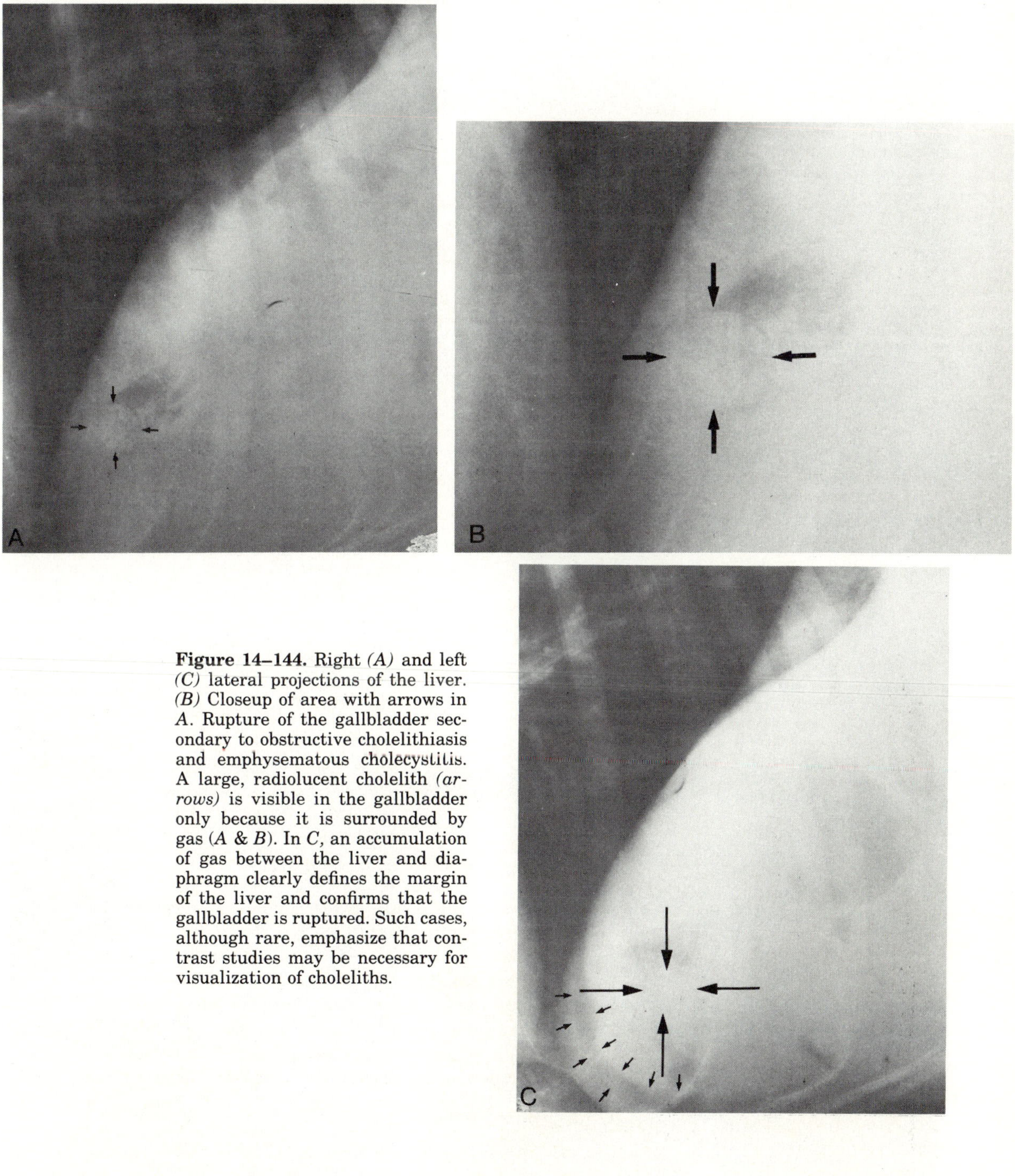

Figure 14–144. Right *(A)* and left *(C)* lateral projections of the liver. *(B)* Closeup of area with arrows in *A*. Rupture of the gallbladder secondary to obstructive cholelithiasis and emphysematous cholecystitis. A large, radiolucent cholelith *(arrows)* is visible in the gallbladder only because it is surrounded by gas (*A* & *B*). In *C*, an accumulation of gas between the liver and diaphragm clearly defines the margin of the liver and confirms that the gallbladder is ruptured. Such cases, although rare, emphasize that contrast studies may be necessary for visualization of choleliths.

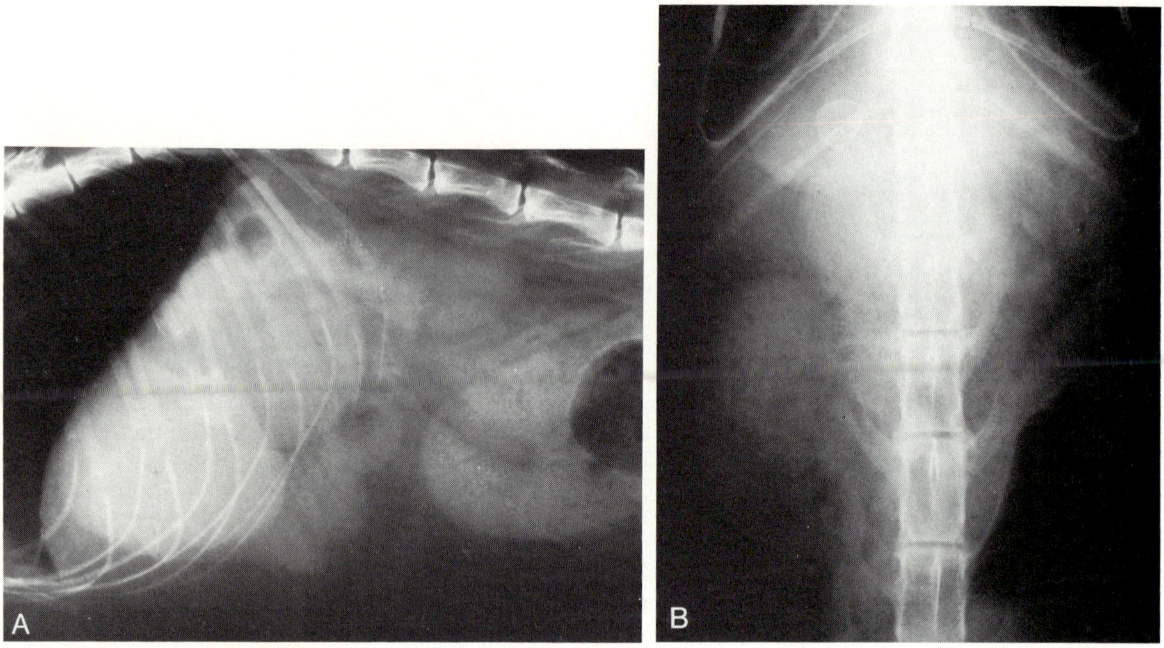

Figure 14–145. Lateral *(A)* and ventrodorsal *(B)* radiographs of a small calcified intrahepatic cyst. On the ventrodorsal view *(B)* the cyst is in the area of the gallbladder, but on the lateral view *(A)* it is too far dorsal and therefore must lie within the liver parenchyma. Other than the position, the appearance of this cyst is identical to that of a composite cholelith.

appears as a radiolucency in the area of the gallbladder (Fig. 14–146). The shape of the gallbladder may be very irregular in cholecystitis, especially if the organ is only partly distended or severely scarred.[79] Shape is therefore not reliable as an identifying criteria, particularly if the gas is confined to the wall of the gallbladder. Positive identi-

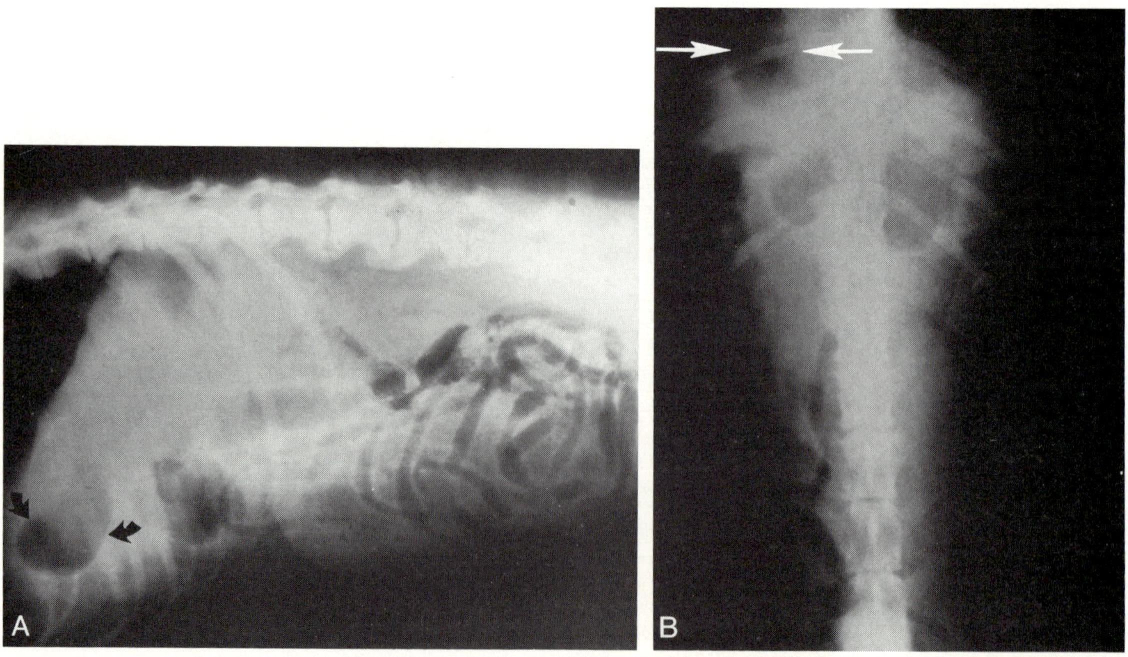

Figure 14–146. Lateral *(A)* and ventrodorsal *(B)* views of emphysematous cholecystitis. There is a large accumulation of gas in the area of the gallbladder *(arrows)*. The shape of the gas density is highly suggestive of the gallbladder; however, a distended loop of bowel cannot be ruled out on the basis of these survey films alone.

fication of the gastrointestinal tract is mandatory. The fact that the gas is not in a loop of small bowel trapped in this area should be confirmed by an upper gastrointestinal series (Fig. 14–147). A cavitated and gas-filled liver abscess should also be considered in the differential diagnosis and may be differentiated on the basis of clinical signs and clinical pathologic data.[34, 51] Confirmation of gas within the gallbladder allows a diagnosis of emphysematous cholecystitis.

A mass or mass effect arising from the region of the gallbladder may not directly involve the gallbladder. Masses in the quadrate lobe of the liver may be indistinguishable from masses originating in the biliary tract. Because of this, it is impossible to state with absolute certainty that a mass is arising from the gallbladder or biliary tree on the basis of survey radiographs alone.

The gallbladder may actually distend sufficiently to be seen as an ovoid mass projecting caudal to the liver on the lateral view (Fig. 14–148). This usually occurs only with blockage of the common bile duct; however, in rare instances it will be seen without such blockage. Although obstructive cholelithiasis is relatively rare in the dog and cat, obstruction of the bile duct by extramural diseases such as pancreatitis and liver or intestinal neoplasia may occur.[54, 81] In such cases the first evidence of clinical disease may be related to the biliary obstruction. The large, round mass of the engorged gallbladder may be the only radiographic evidence visible on plain films. The presence of such a mass along with clinical pathological evidence of obstructive icterus should narrow down the possible diagnosis to diseases such as choledcholithiasis, primary or secondary neoplasia, and chronic pancreatitis, all of which could cause obstruction of the common bile duct.

Neoplasia of the gallbladder and major hepatic ducts will most commonly present as a nondescript mass displacing the body of the stomach caudally, to the left and somewhat dorsally. The duodenum will also be displaced caudally and perhaps somewhat laterally depending on the exact origin of the tumor. Infiltration of the bowel or gastric wall may result in an abnormal configuration of the wall; that is, the wall may radiographically appear concave in outline or fixed in position on multiple sequential films or fluoroscopic examination (Fig. 14–149). Such changes may be observed on a plain film study but should be confirmed by performing a positive-contrast upper gastrointestinal series, with emphasis on the

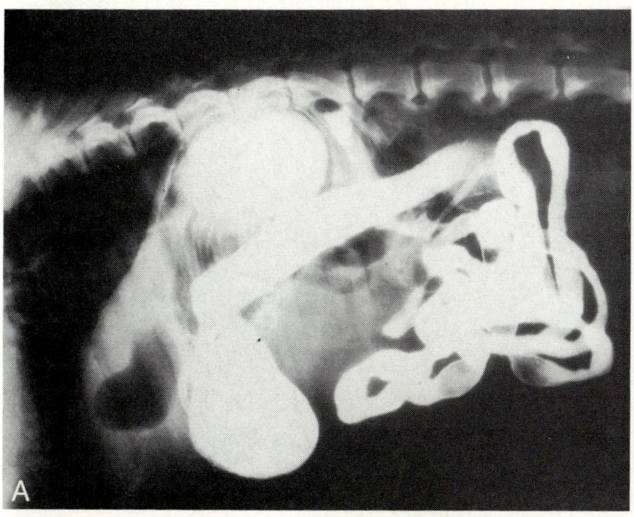

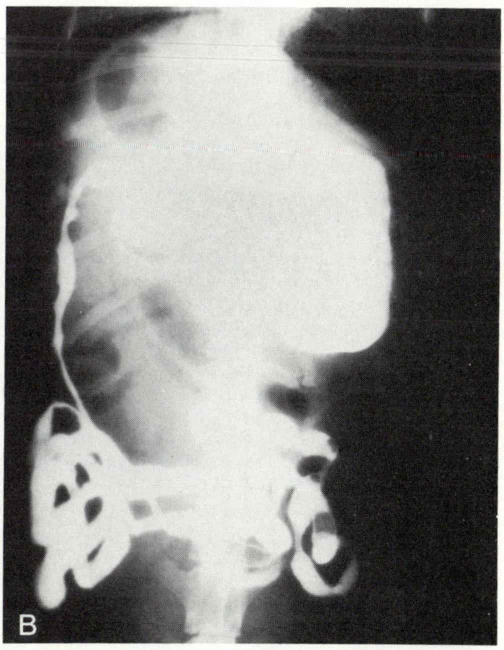

Figure 14–147. Lateral *(A)* and ventrodorsal *(B)* views in upper gastrointestinal contrast series (same dog as in Figure 14–146). The stomach, duodenum, and jejunum are clearly outlined with barium sulfate. It is now obvious that the large gas density in the cranial abdomen is not associated with the bowel; its position within the liver shadow and in the area of the gallbladder makes emphysema of the gallbladder the most likely diagnosis.

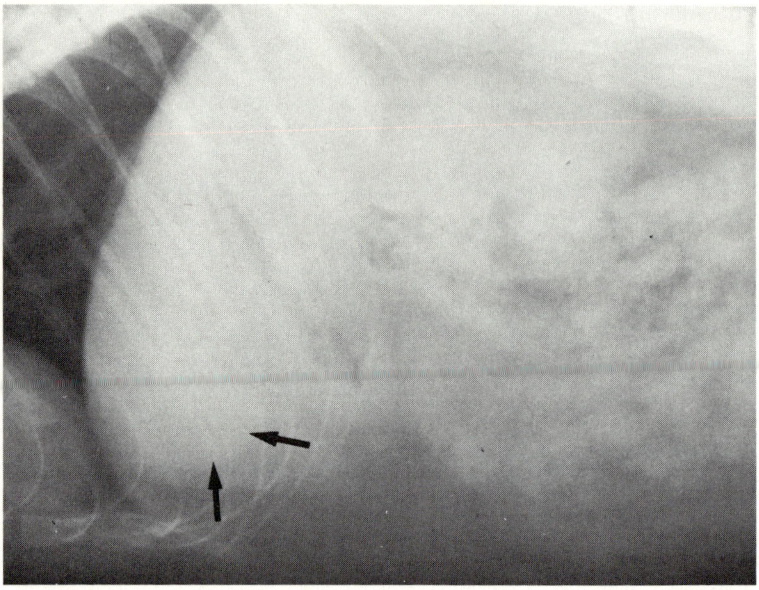

Figure 14–148. Marked engorgement of the gallbladder has increased its size and density so that it can be seen as a distinct portion of the liver shadow on the lateral view *(arrows)*. Although this is an unusual occurrence, which is usually associated with obstruction of the common bile duct, it is occasionally seen in animals without signs of bile duct obstruction.

stomach and duodenum. Unfortunately, by the time that changes such as these are present, the disease is usually far advanced with little hope of successful treatment.

Recognition of gallbladder and biliary tree diseases other than advanced neoplasia or obstruction requires a contrast study. Positive-contrast cholecystography is the most common contrast procedure performed (Fig. 14–150). It is indicated in any animal with clinical pathological evidence of obstructive icterus, in which the underlying disorder cannot be diagnosed by plain radiographs or clinical pathology studies. Examples include radiolucent choleliths, infection, and extramural disease of the gallbladder, common bile duct, or terminal biliary tree.[81] Cholecystography may be the only means of confirming a diagnosis short of surgical exploration.

Unfortunately, it may be difficult to obtain consistently good results with cholecystography in the dog and cat. Failure to opacify the gallbladder may result from insufficient dosage, inflammation of the gallbladder resulting in reabsorption, failure of

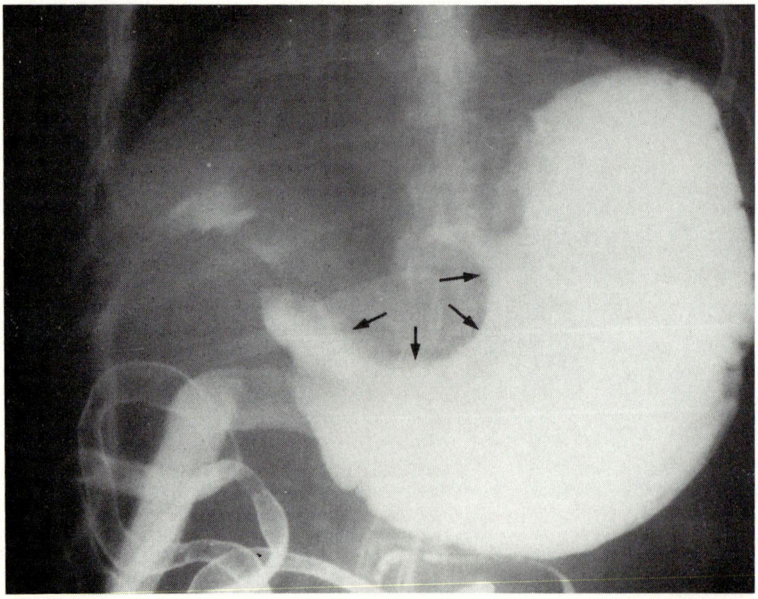

Figure 14–149. Marked concavity of the lesser curvature of the stomach in the region of the cardia with caudolateral displacement of the stomach. In the area surrounding the cardia there is an unusual concavity of the stomach *(arrows)*, which was consistently present on the early films in the series. This is the type of concavity that one would expect to arise from the displacement of the stomach by a mass arising from the area of the gallbladder.

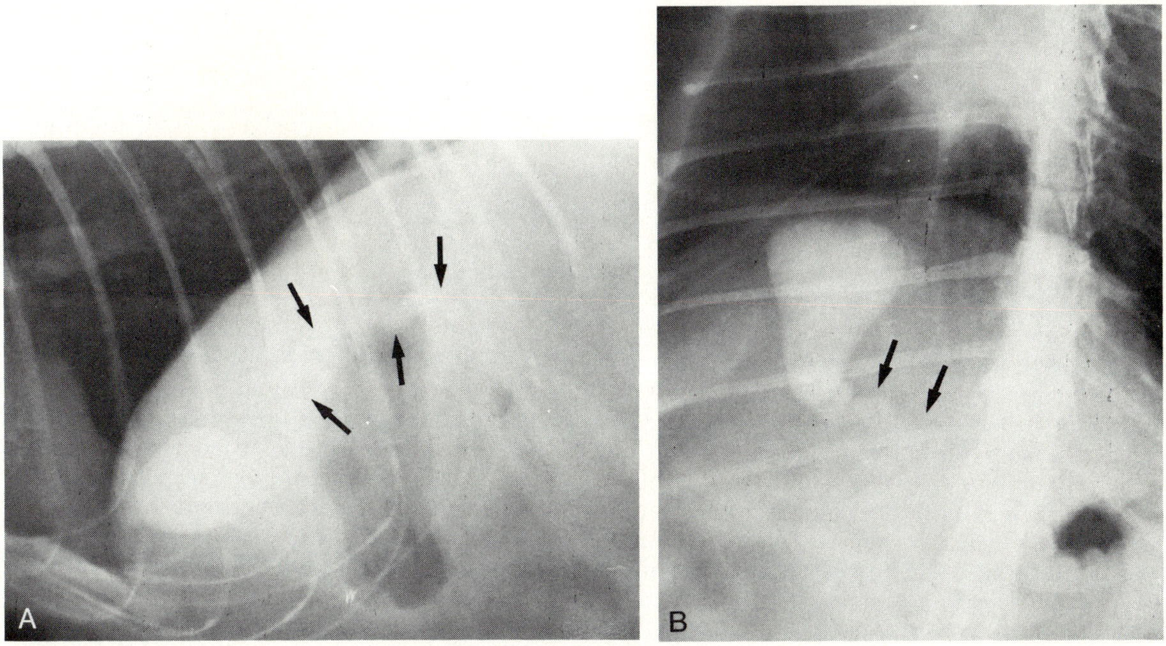

Figure 14–150. Intravenous cholecystography in a cat: lateral *(A)* and ventrodorsal *(B)*. These films, taken approximately 90 minutes after the injection of the contrast agent, clearly delineate the position and size of the gallbladder in this normal cat. The course of the common bile duct *(arrows)* is visible but the degree of delineation is not as good as for the gallbladder proper. It is not possible to see any of the intrahepatic lobar bile ducts; however, if there were an obstruction in one of the lobar ducts or in the common bile duct, the lobar ducts would be quite dilated and therefore visible. The degree of opacification seen in these films is about what should be expected with this technique.

the liver to excrete the contrast medium properly, or failure of the gastrointestinal tract to absorb orally administered contrast media.[6, 48, 71] Close attention to details such as patient preparation, drug administration, and proper filming sequences will substantially reduce the chance of a non-diagnostic study. Although there is some chance of a non-diagnostic study, the study is still among the easiest procedures to perform for the diagnosis of biliary disease. No special equipment other than the contrast agent itself is required and general anesthesia can be avoided in most cases. Table 14–3 de-

Table 14–3. CHOLECYSTOGRAPHY[5, 17, 93]

Contrast Agent	Route	Dose	Time when Films Should be Taken
Dog			
Iodipamide* sodium	IV *slowly*	0.5 ml/kg	60, 90, and 120 minutes after injection
Ipodate Calcium†	Orally	150 mg/kg	12 hours after administration
Iodipamide‡ Meglumine	IV *slowly*	0.2 ml/kg	30, 60, and 90 minutes after injection
Cat			
Ipodate Sodium‖	Orally	150 mg/kg	12 to 14 hours after administration
Iodipamide§ Meglumine	IV *slowly*	0.3 ml/kg	2½ to 5 hours after administration

*Biligrafin Intravenous Forte, Schering AG, Berlin, Germany
†Solu-Biloptin, Schering AG, Berlin, Germany (Oragraphin Calcium, Squibb and Sons, Inc., Princeton, NJ)
‡Cholografin Meglumine, E. R. Squibb & Sons, Inc., Princeton, NJ
‖Biloptin, Schering AG, Berlin, Germany (Oragraphin Sodium, Squibb and Sons, Inc., Princeton, NJ)
§Biligrafin Forte 50%, Schering AG, Berlin, Germany

scribes techniques reported to have been successful in obtaining good results in the dog and cat.

Percutaneous transhepatic cholangiocystography has been recently described.[12, 102] This technique, although somewhat difficult to perform, gives superior visualization of the gallbladder, common bile duct, and occasionally the biliary tree (Fig. 14–151). It consists of percutaneously placing a long needle into one of the hepatic ducts of the gallbladder and injecting a water-soluble radiopaque contrast agent into either the gallbladder or one of the hepatic ducts. This study requires fluoroscopic guidance to confirm the location of the contrast agent in the biliary tree and to monitor the amount of distention of the gallbladder and ducts. While the technique gives superior visualization of the biliary system, the technical difficulties associated with its performance and the problem of general anesthesia in a severely ill patient place it beyond the expertise and facilities of most individuals. Its use should be limited to carefully selected cases in which the diagnosis cannot be determined in any other fashion.

Ultrasound diagnostic procedures have gained rapid acceptance in both human and veterinary medicine (Fig.14–152). Such examinations are safe and easy to perform, require minimal restraint, and are non-invasive. Interpretation is difficult, however, and the equipment required for examinations of the abdominal structure is expensive. Some large referral practices and most teaching centers now offer this diagnostic service to veterinary patients.[18, 30, 53, 63, 64, 65, 79] These studies are much more sensitive in detecting liver and biliary disease than any radiographic examination commonly available to veterinarians. Because of the safety for the patient and the high information gain of the procedure, ultrasonography, if it is available, should be performed prior to radiographic contrast studies.[54] Evaluation of the study must be performed by experienced ultrasonographers to gain the maximum benefit from the study and reduce interpretive errors.

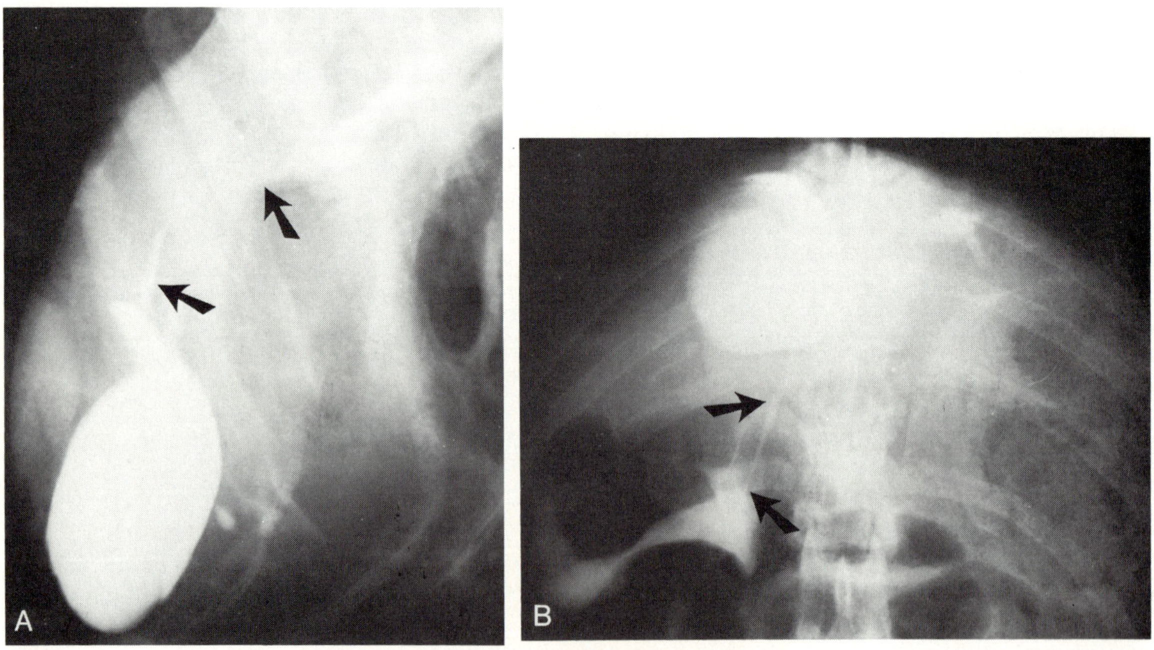

Figure 14–151. Percutaneous transhepatic cholangiocystogram: lateral view *(A)* and ventrodorsal *(B)*. The animal is anesthetized, and a long, thin Chiba needle is inserted on the right side just above the sternum and just caudal to the diaphragm. The needle is then passed forward and slightly dorsally toward the most cranial part of the diaphragmatic curve. Bile can be aspirated when the needle is within the gallbladder. Using this method, the opacification of the gallbladder and common bile duct *(arrows)* is much better than that obtained with intravenous techniques. Since this is an invasive technique that requires some practice to master, it should not be performed unless the animal is a definite surgical candidate in the event of a positive study.

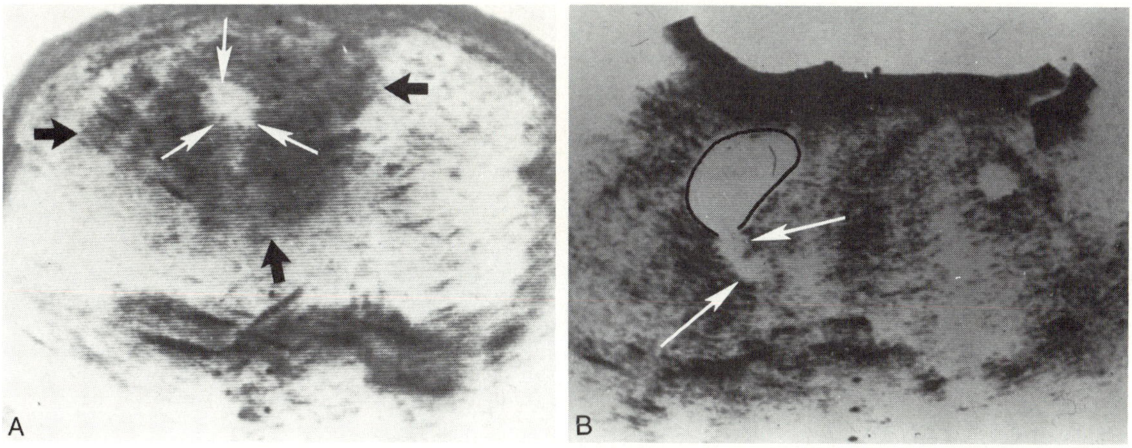

Figure 14–152. Diagnostic ultrasound scans of the liver in two animals with histories indicative of biliary problems. In animal *A*, the gallbladder *(white arrows)* is surrounded by a dark area of intense echos that appear to diffusely infiltrate the surrounding liver *(black arrows)*. These findings and the location of the lesion indicate the presence of an advanced biliary adenocarcinoma. The animal is in dorsal recumbency and the scan is transverse to the body. In animal *B*, the gallbladder *(outline)* and the common bile duct *(arrows)* are grossly distended, indicating a blockage of the common bile duct. The source of the obstruction cannot be seen; only its effect on the biliary tree is visible. The animal is the dorsal recumbency but the orientation of the scan is parasagittal just to the right of the midline.

Pancreas

The pancreas lies along the greater curvature of the body of the stomach and the mesenteric border of the proximal duodenum (Fig. 14–153). It is closely attached to these two organs by mesenteric and omental attachments. The transverse colon usually crosses the abdomen just caudal to the body of the stomach. The pancreas is usually adjacent to the cranial border of the transverse colon, although this relationship is somewhat variable.[55, 71]

On radiographs the pancreas is located partially within the rib cage and near the

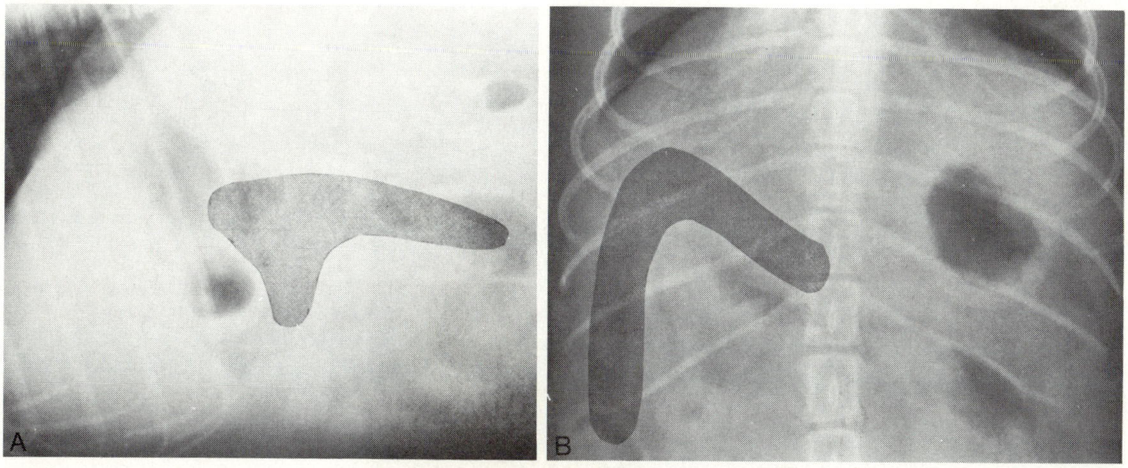

Figure 14–153. Approximate normal limits of the pancreas. The shaded area represents the area where densities attributable to disease of the pancreas can be expected to arise. The complete, true anatomical limits may be different. Note that the shaded area borders the falciform ligament ventrally on the lateral view *(A)*. Loss of detail of the margin of the body of the stomach where it abuts the falciform ligament is one of the earliest radiographic lesion of pancreatitis. On the ventrodorsal projection *(B)* the pancreas lies in the curve of the cranial flexure of the duodenum, and the right and left lobes of the pancreas extend along the duodenum and the greater curvature of the stomach respectively. If the pancreas is significantly enlarged, these are the first portions of the bowel to be displaced.

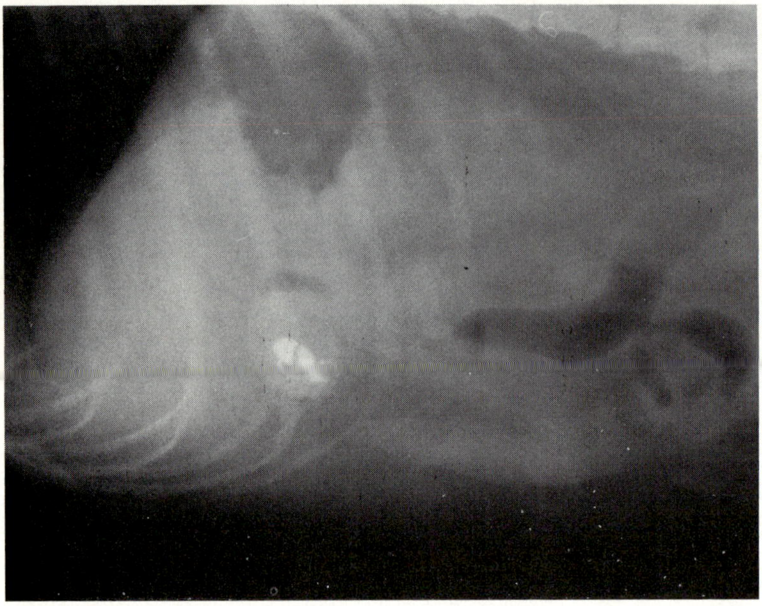

Figure 14–154. Very mild lesions of pancreatitis. There are areas of moderately increased density in the region of the pancreas and over the falciform fat shadow. The detail in the area is still relatively good; however, the caudal wall of the stomach shadow is not as well defined as one might expect when it is compared to the splenic margin. The radiopaque material is contained within the stomach and is not associated with the disease.

right body wall. Because it is a solid, water-dense organ, the pancreas is rarely visible as a distinct entity. The only exception to this rule is the rare instance of calcification of the organ or the surrounding tissue secondary to chronic inflammation.[45]

The radiographic signs of pancreatic disease are often subtle. Mild, acute, or transient disease may not cause any radiographic abnormalities.[71, 77, 80] In fact, the evaluation that the abdomen is within normal limits is probably almost as common as are the findings characteristic of pancreatitis. The only radiographic findings of pancreatic disease directly referable to the pancreas itself are a mild to moderate increase in the density of the abdomen in the pancreatic region and a loss of serosal detail in that same area.[45, 71, 77, 97] These are essentially the signs that one would expect to observe in a regional peritonitis of any origin (Figs. 14–154 and 14–155).

Increased density in the area of the pancreas is a difficult finding to determine. On

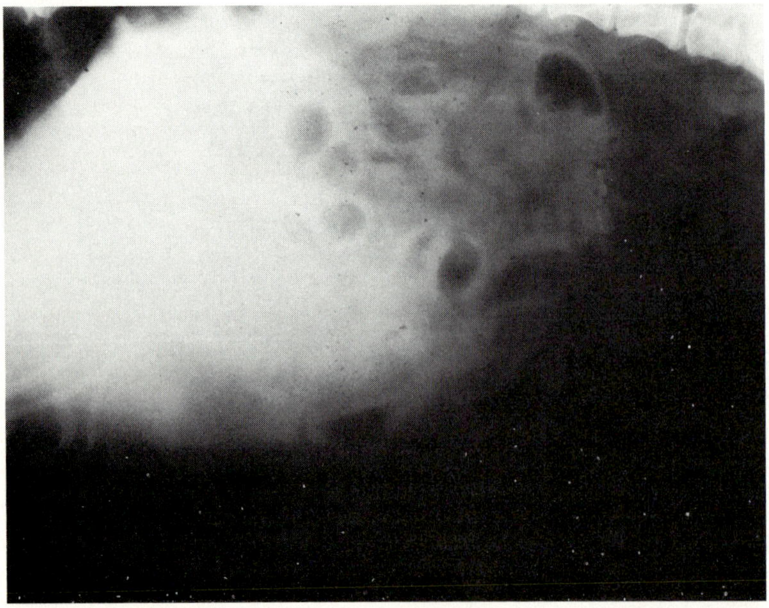

Figure 14–155. Severe lesions of pancreatitis. There is a marked increase in the density of the abdomen in the area of the duodenum, and there is also a regional complete loss of serosal border detail. Note also that the intestinal tract is displaced caudally and dorsally away from the region of the pancreas. This animal died of this disease about eight hours after this film was taken.

the lateral projection the area of the pancreas is just caudal to the body of the stomach. The spleen is often superimposed over the caudal border of the stomach, as is the transverse colon and part of the small bowel. This collection of organs makes this region of the abdomen normally more dense those surrounding it. Recognition of an increased density is a matter of judgment and practice.

The cranial pole of the right kidney, the caudate lobe of the liver, and the spleen are all directly superimposed over the pancreas on the ventral dorsal view. This is also one of the thickest areas of the abdomen, and there is no lung superimposed over the abdomen at this level as there is over the portion of the abdomen cranial to the stomach. As a result of these factors, the pancreatic area is the densest area of the entire abdomen on the ventral dorsal projection. Recognition of abnormal, increased density in this area is thus very difficult.

Loss of detail in the pancreatic area is a more reliable radiographic sign of pancreatic disease than is increased density (Figs. 14–154 and 14–155). Increased density may or may not be associated with a loss of detail; loss of detail is manifested as decreased serosal border sharpness of the stomach and bowel borders in the area just caudal to the body of the stomach and the pylorus. The region of involvement is usually localized unless the disorder is very severe or chronic. To establish that a loss of detail is present, the detail in the pancreatic area must be compared with that present in other areas of the abdomen. The caudal border of the gastric fundus or the caudal margin of the spleen can be compared with the gastric border in the pyloric area. The area of decreased detail is usually rather small, but in some severe cases it may extend to involve the entire abdomen.[45] The margins of the involved area of local peritonitis are irregular and indistinct, which makes recognition difficult unless one is careful to evaluate for this abnormality.

The position and size of the stomach, the transverse colon, and the duodenum can be used to estimate the size of the pancreas.[71] It is usually possible to define the position of the stomach and the transverse colon. Using positive contrast material makes the position of the duodenum obvious.

Lesions in the pancreas have varying effects on the adjacent structures. The type of pathological process and its extent determine whether definable alterations in the position of the adjacent organs can be recognized on radiographs. Mild generalized enlargements of the pancreas or small focal lesions will not cause a sufficient mass effect to be recognized. Large lesions, whether generalized or focal, will cause recognizable displacements. The two anatomical changes most often associated with enlargement of the pancreas are stretching or widening of the cranial duodenal flexure (Fig. 14–156) and separation of the stomach and transverse colon (Fig. 14–157). The latter change is particularly significant if a concave caudal gastric border is also recognized.[45] The presence of a concave caudal border to the stomach is highly suggestive of a physical mass impinging on the wall of the stomach.

Widening of the cranial duodenal flexure may be difficult to assess. The degree to which the flexure is widened is dependent on the severity of the disease. Variations in the position of the stomach and duodenum make the curvature present in the normal duodenum quite variable. The amount of gastric distention present will also markedly affect the acuteness and visibility of the cranial duodenal flexure. All these factors must be taken into account when attempting to determine if an apparent displacement of the duodenum is due to pancreatic disease.

Separation of the transverse colon and gastric shadows is also affected by variability in the position and distention of the stomach. Gastric distention will itself displace the transverse colon caudally. The transverse colon is also freely movable in a dorsoventral direction and may be displaced dorsally instead of caudally. Since this is a position often observed in normal animals without pancreatic disease, no conclusions regarding the size of the pancreas can be drawn in this case unless a visible mass is present.

Indentation of the caudal border of the partially distended stomach is a reliable sign of a mass impinging on the stomach. It does not necessarily indicate, however, that the mass is of pancreatic origin. At least one other sign of pancreatic enlargement should be present to diagnose a pancreatic lesion.

If the disease of the pancreas is focal in one lobe or the hilus it is more difficult to detect radiographically than generalized disease. Diffuse lesions, when radiographi-

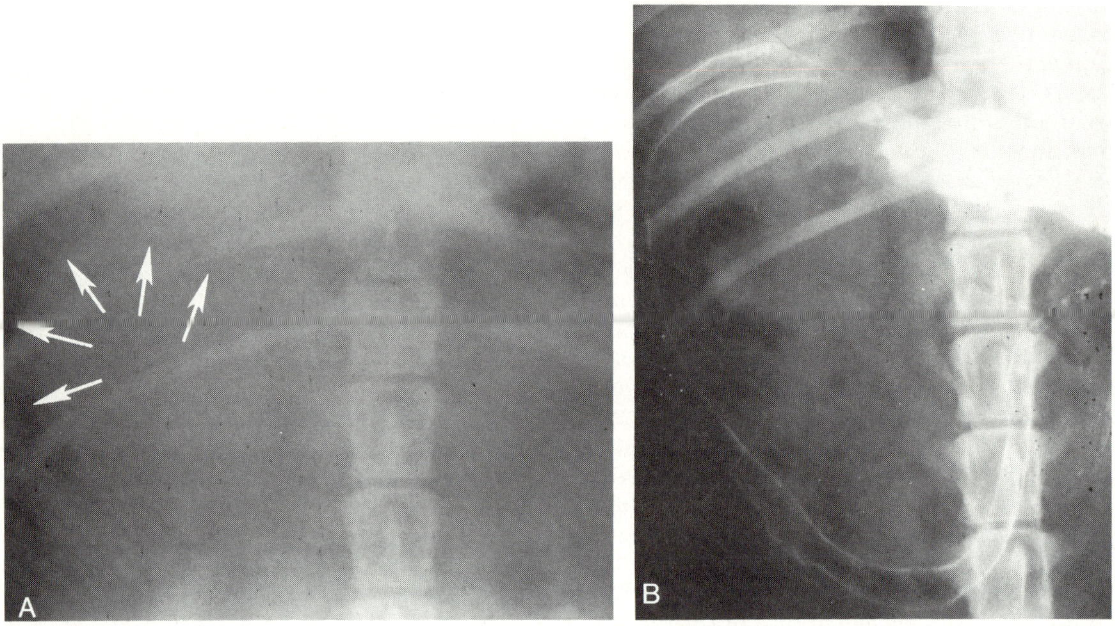

Figure 14–156. Pancreatitis. In *A* there is a large area of homogeneous density in the area of the cranial flexure of the duodenum. The duodenum *(arrows)* is stretched around the perimeter of the homogeneous density and is dilated with gas. The presence of the gas may indicate that there is a regional paralysis of the bowel (sentinel loop) that is secondary to the inflammation in the pancreas. In *B*, after administration of barium sulfate the duodenum is clearly delineated and is stretched over the homogeneous density of the pancreas. The pylorus of the stomach is displaced medially and the descending duodenum is held in position against the lateral body wall by the swollen and inflamed pancreas.

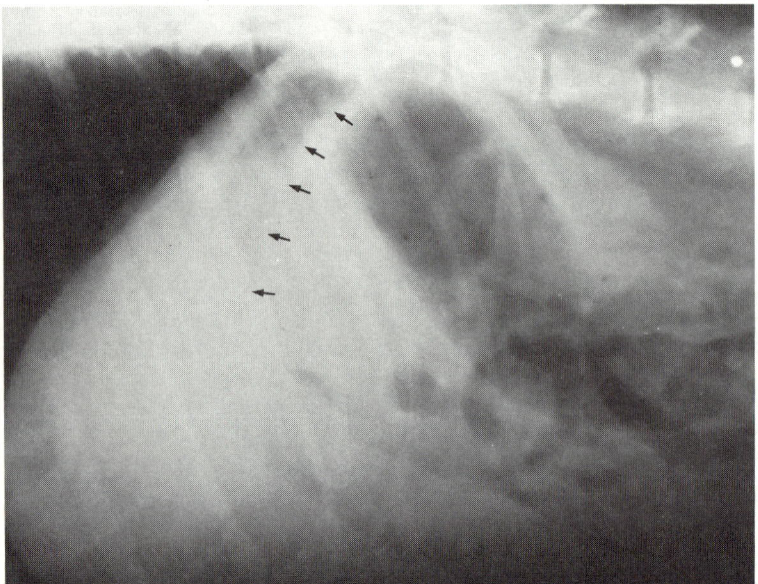

Figure 14–157. Pancreatic mass displacing the stomach. The large, gas-filled transverse colon is displaced caudally away from the caudal border of the stomach *(arrows)*. Note that the caudal border of the stomach is concave in outline, indicating a definite mass impingement on the caudal border of the stomach. A mass in this position causing these displacements with no sign of enlargement of the spleen on either view is highly suspicious of a pancreatic mass. The diagnosis in this case was pancreatic adenocarcinoma (acinar).

cally detectable, may not be distinguishable from lesions of the spleen and liver on the basis of organ displacement alone. In these cases, a diagnosis of pancreatic disease is often made by eliminating all other possibilities. If a diagnosis cannot be established on the basis of plain films, an upper gastrointestinal series should be performed, because bowel structures that play an important role in the diagnosis of pancreatic disease are enhanced by positive-contrast media. Identification of the exact position of the stomach and duodenum is simplified and the contrast coats the mucosal surface of the bowel. In this way ulcerations, constrictions, and other mucosal lesions not seen on plain films are identified. Detection of bowel mucosal lesions may provide insight into the nature of the problem and help to determine the most logical treatment or diagnostic protocol.[71, 78]

Other signs of pancreatic diseae that have been observed include gas in the duodenum, strictures of the duodenum, ulceration and thickening of the wall of the duodenum and pyloric antrum, and fixing of one or more bowel loops in the area of the pancreas by adhesions (Fig. 14–158).[45, 71, 77] These changes are not specific to pancreatic disease, but may be seen with a wide variety of diseases that may or may not involve the pancreas. Because the radiographic lesions of pancreatic disease are so non-specific, a diagnosis should never be based on a single radiographic sign and should always be confirmed by clinical pathology tests.[25, 77, 80, 87]

There is little, if any, difference in the radiographic presentation of neoplasia, inflammation, and abscessation. There may be a slight tendency for widespread involvement of the abdomen with exocrine neoplasia, but this is usually due to late recognition of the disease process. Any of the lesions described may be produced by any disease process of the pancreas or, as in the case of pancreatic atrophy and endocrine neoplasia, there may be no radiographic lesions at all, even though advanced disease is present. If pancreatic disease is suspected on the basis of the case workup (of which radiographs are only a part) and an absolute diagnosis is necessary, a biopsy is probably required.

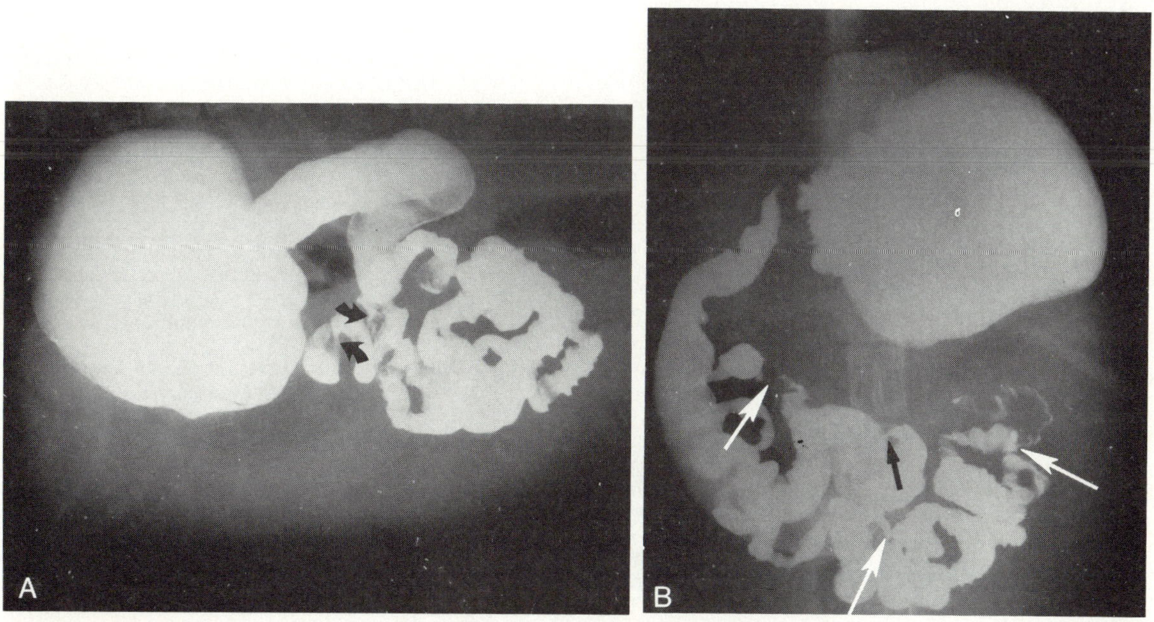

Figure 14–158. Abdominal abscess and granuloma formation of pancreatic origin. This animal, with a history of a chronic gastrointestinal upset, had a very homogeneous abdomen with no serosal detail, indicative of fluid, on the survey film. An upper gastrointestinal series indicated that the bowel was bunched up in the central part of the abdomen and did not move much during the study. The position of the bowel seen on these two films (*A*, lateral view; *B*, ventrodorsal view) remained constant throughout the study. Multiple partial obstructions *(arrows)* with moderately dilated loops of bowel behind them are also present due to fibrous scarring and adhesions. The gastrointestinal transit time and gastric emptying time were moderately increased in this animal as well. Note the large area of homogeneous density between the stomach and the small bowel in *B*. This remained constant throughout the study and represents the main body of the granuloma and what functional pancreas remains.

References

1. Ackerman N, Madewell BR: Thoracic and abdominal radiographic abnormalities in the multicentric form of lymphosarcoma in dogs. J Am Vet Med Assoc 176:36, 1980.
2. Ackerman N, Silverman S: Liver enlargement. Mod Vet Pract 58:949, 1977.
3. Adamsons RJ, Arif S, Babic A, et al: Arterialization of the liver in combination with a portacaval shunt in the dog. Surg Gynecol Obstet. 140:594, 1975.
4. Allan GS, Dixon RT: Cholecystography in the dog: Assessment of radiographic positioning and the use of double contrast examination by visceral and densitometric methods. J Am Vet Radiol Soc 18:177, 1977.
5. Allan GS, Dixon RT: Cholecystography in the dog: The choice of contrast media and optimum dose rates. J Am Vet Radiol Soc 16:98, 1975.
6. Ansell G: Adverse reactions to contrast agents. Invest Radiol 6:374, 1970.
7. Audell L, Jonsson L, Lannek B: Congenital portacaval shunts in the dog: A description of three cases. Zlb Vet Med 21:797, 1974.
8. Barrett RE, Delahunta A, Roenick WJ, et al: Four cases of congenital portacaval shunt in the dog. J Small Anim Pract 17:71, 1976.
9. Barsanti JA, Jones BD, Spano JS, Taylor HW: Prolonged anorexia associated with hepatic lipidosis in three cats. Feline Pract 7:52, 1977.
10. Brodey RS: Alimentary tract neoplasms in the cat: A clinicopathologic survey of 46 cases. Am J Vet Res 27:74–80, 1966.
11. Brodey RS: The biological behavior of canine oral and pharyngeal neoplasms. J Small Anim Pract 11:45–53, 1970.
12. Buonocore E: Transhepatic percutaneous cholangiography. Radiol Clin North Am, Vol. 14 no. 3, 1976, p. 527.
13. Burk RL, Johnson GF: Enphysematous Cholecystitis in the nondiabetic dog: Three case histories. Vet Radiol, Vol. 21 no. 6, 1980, p. 142.
14. Burns MG, Kelly AB, Hornoff WJ, Howerth EW: Pulmonary artery thrombosis in three dogs with hyperadrenocorticism. J Am Vet Med Assoc 178:388, 1981.
15. Campbell TM, Lording PM, Wrigley RH, LaVelle RB: Portal vein anomaly and hepatic encephalopathy in three dogs. Aust Vet J 56:593, 1980.
16. Carlisle CH: Radiographic anatomy of the cat gallbladder. Vet Radiol 18:170, 1977.
17. Carlisle CH: A comparison of techniques for cholecystography in the cat. Vet Radiol 6:173, 1977.
18. Cartee RE: Diagnostic real time ultrasonography of the liver of the dog and cat. J Am Anim Hosp Assoc 17:731, 1981.
19. Chandna IS, Nigam JM: Radiographic evaluation of abdominal disorders in canines. Indian Vet J 57:632, 1980.
20. Cooperberg P, Golding RH: Advances in ultrasonography of the gallbladdder and biliary tract. Radiol Clin North Am 20:611, 1982.
21. Cornelius LM, Thrall DE, Halliwell WH, et al: Anomalous portosystemic anastomoses associated with chronic hepatic insufficiency in six young dogs. J Am Vet Med Assoc 167:220, 1975.
22. Cotter S: Oral pharyngeal neoplasms in the cat. J Am Anim Hosp Assoc 17:917–920, 1981.
23. Craig TM, Smallwood JE, Knauer KW, McGrath JP: *Hepatozoon canis* infection in dogs: Clinical, radiographic, and hematologic findings. J Am Vet Med Assoc 173:967, 1978.
24. Evans SM, Laufer I: Double contrast gastrography in the normal dog. Vet Radiol 22:2–9, 1981.
25. Feldman EC: Diseases of the endocrine pancreas. *In* Ettinger SJ (ed), *Textbook of Veterinary Internal Medicine,* 2nd ed, W. B. Saunders Company, Philadelphia, 1615–1649, 1983.
26. Feldman EC, Ettinger SJ: Percutaneous transthoracic liver biopsy in the dog: A review of 75 cases. J Am Anim Hosp Assoc 13:17, 1977.
27. Fischer JE, Funovics JM, Aguirre A, et al: The role of plasma amino acids in hepatic encephalopathy. Surgery 78:276, 1975.
28. Foster JH, Conkle DM, Crane JM, Burko H: Splenoportography: An assessment of its value and risk. Ann Surg 179:773, 1974.
29. Gibbs C: Radiological features of liver disorders in dogs and cats. *In* Grunsell CS, Hill FW (eds), *Veterinary Annual, 21st ed,* Scientechnica, Bristol, UK, 239–250, 1981.
30. Goldberg HI, Sheft DJ: Abnormalities in small intestine contour and caliber—a working classification. Radiol Clin North Am 14:461–475, 1976.
31. Gomez JA: The gastrointestinal contrast study: Methods and interpretation. Vet Clin North Am 4:805–842, 1974.
32. Gorman NT, McCarthy T, Owen LN: Clearance of Technetium 99m-labeled sulfur colloid particles from the blood in normal dogs and in dogs with hepatic granulomata. J Vet Res 41:613, 1980.
33. Guffy MS: Esophageal disorders. *In* Ettinger SJ (ed), *Textbook of Veterinary Internal Medicine,* W. B. Saunders Company, Philadelphia, 1098–1124, 1975.
34. Hardy RM: Diseases of the liver. *In* Ettinger SJ (ed), *Textbook of Veterinary Internal Medicine,* 2nd ed, W. B. Saunders Company, Philadelphia, 1372–1429, 1983.
35. Hargis AM, Thomassen RW: Hepatic abscesses in beagle puppies. Lab Anim Sci 30:689, 1980.
36. Harvey CE: Sialography in the dog. J Am Vet Radiol Soc 10:18–27, 1969.
37. Harvey CE, O'Brien JA: Disorders of the oropharynx and salivary glands. *In* Ettinger SJ (ed), *Textbook of Veterinary Internal Medicine,* W. B. Saunders Company, Philadelphia, 1068–1097, 1975.
38. Haskins ME, Jezyk PF, Desnick RJ, Patterson DF: Of human disease: Mucopolysaccharidosis I. Comp Pathol Bull 13:3, 1981.
39. Hettwer KJ, Folsom TC: The normal sialogram. Oral Surg 26:790, 1960.
40. Hooft J, Mattheeuws D, Van Bree P: Radiology of deciduous teeth resorption and definitive teeth eruption in the dog. J Small Anim Pract 20: 175–180, 1979.
41. Horak W, Gangi A, Funovics J, Grabner G: Effect of portacaval shunt and arterialization of the liver on bile acid metabolism. Gastroenterol 69:338, 1975.
42. Hornoff WJ, Suter PF: The use of prostaglandin E_1 and tolazoline to improve cranial mesenteric arterial portography in the dog. Veterinary Radiol 20:15, 1979.
43. Itoh Z, Takahashi I: Periodic contractions of the canine gallbladder during the interdigestive state. Am J Physiol 240:G183, 1981.

44. Kealy JK: *Diagnostic Radiology of the Dog and Cat.* W. B. Saunders Company, Philadelphia, 1979.
45. Kleine LJ, Hornbuckle WE: Acute pancreatitis: The radiographic findings in 182 dogs. J Am Vet Radiol Soc 19:102, 1978.
46. Kneller SK: Radiographic interpretation of the gastric dilatation-volvulus complex in the dog. J Am Anim Hosp Assoc 12:154–157, 1976.
47. Koblick RD, Hornoff WJ, Breznock EM: Use of quantitative hepatic scintigraphy to evaluate spontaneous portosystemic shunts in 12 dogs. Veterinary Radiol 24:232–239, 1983.
48. Lasser EC, Lang JH: Contrast-protein interactions. Invest Radiol 5:446, 1970.
49. Liu S, Weitzman I, Johnson GG: Canine tuberculosis. J Am Vet Med Assoc 177:164, 1980.
50. Lohse CL, Selcer RR, Suter PF: Hepatoencephalopathy associated with situs inversus of abdominal organs and vascular anomalies in a dog. J Am Vet Med Assoc 168:681, 1976.
51. Lord PF, Carb A, Halliwell WH, Preuter JC: Emphysematous hepatic abscess associated with trauma, necrotic hepatic nodular hyperplasia and adenoma in a dog: A case history. Vet Radiol 23:46, 1982.
52. Lord PF, Wilkins RJ: Emphysema of the gallbladder in a diabetic dog. J Am Vet Radiol Soc 13:49, 1972.
53. Marchal G, Van de Voorde P, Van Dooren W, et al: Ultrasonic appearance of the filled and contracted normal gallbladder. Clin Ultrasound 8:439, 1980.
54. Menuck L, Amberg J: The bile ducts. Radiol Clin North Am 14:499, 1976.
55. Miller ME: The digestive system and abdomen. *In* Miller ME, Christensen GC, Evans HE, *Anatomy of the Dog,* W. B. Saunders Company, Philadelphia, 645–712, 1964.
56. Miller ME, Christensen GC, Evans HE: *Anatomy of the Dog,* W. B. Saunders Company, Philadelphia, 1964.
57. Millikan WJ, Smith RB III, Khatra B, et al: Effect of portacaval shunt on hepatic Krebs-Henseleit enzymes in dogs. Surg Forum 25:248–250, 1974.
58. Morgan JP, Silverman S: *Techniques of Veterinary Radiography,* 3rd ed, Veterinary Radiology Assoc, Davis, CA, 1982.
59. Morgan JP: *Radiology in Veterinary Orthopedics.* Lea & Febiger, Philadelphia, 1972.
60. Moulton JE: *Tumors in Domestic Animals,* 2nd ed, University of California Press, Berkeley, 1978.
61. Naus MJA, Jones BR: Cholelithiasis and choledocholithiasis in a cat. NZ Vet J 26:160, 1978.
62. North DC: Sudden death in a dog associated with cholelithiasis. Vet Record 102:203, 1977.
63. Nyland TG, Park RD: Hepatic ultrasonography in the dog. Vet Radiol 24:74, 1983.
64. Nyland TG, Gillette NA: Sonographic evaluation of experimental bile duct ligation in the dog. Vet Radiol 23:252, 1982.
65. Nyland TG, Park RD, Lattimer JC, et al: Gray scale ultrasonography of the canine abdomen. Vet Radiol 22:220, 1981.
66. O'Brien JA, Harvey CE, Tucker JA: The larynx of the dog: Its normal radiographic anatomy. J Am Vet Radiol Soc 10:38, 1969.
67. O'Brien TR: *Radiographic Diagnosis of Abdominal Disorders in the Dog and Cat: Radiographic Interpretation, Clinical Signs, Pathophysiology,* W. B. Saunders Company, Philadelphia, 1978.
68. O'Brien TR, Morgan JP, Lebel JL: Pseudoulcers in the duodenum of the dog. J Am Vet Med Assoc 155:713–716, 1969.
69. O'Brien TR: Normal radiographic anatomy of the abdomen. *In* O'Brien TR (ed), *Radiographic Diagnosis of Abdominal Disorders in the Dog and Cat, Radiographic Interpretation, Clinical Signs, Pathophysiology,* W. B. Saunders Company, Philadelphia, 9–47, 1978.
70. O'Brien TR: Abdominal masses. *In* O'Brien TR (ed), *Radiographic Diagnosis of Abdominal Disorders in the Dog and Cat: Radiographic Interpretation, Clinical Signs, Pathophysiology,* W. B. Saunders Company, Philadelphia, 85–109, 1978.
71. O'Brien TR: Liver, spleen and pancreas. *In* O'Brien TR (ed), *Radiographic Diagnosis of Abdominal Disorders in the Dog and Cat: Radiographic Interpretation, Clinical Signs, Pathophysiology,* W. B. Saunders Company, Philadelphia, 396–480, 1978.
72. Okin RE: Canine gallbladder disease. Canine Pract 9:43, 1982.
73. Odievre M, Chaumont P, Montagne JP, Alagile D: Anomalies of the intrahepatic portal venous system in congenital hepatic fibrosis. Radiology 122:427, 1977.
74. Owens JM: *Radiographic Interpretation for the Small Animal Clinician.* Ralston Purina Co., St. Louis, MO, 134–171, 1982.
75. Patnaik AK, Hurvitz AI, Lieberman PH: Canine hepatic neoplasms: A clinicopathologic study. Vet Pathol 17:553, 1980.
76. Reichle RM, Reichle FA: Effect of portacaval shunt and acute hepatic ischemia on brain and liver serotonin and catecholamines. Surg Forum 26:413, 1975.
77. Rogers WA: Diseases of the exocrine pancreas. *In* Ettinger SJ (ed), *Textbook of Veterinary Internal Medicine,* 2nd ed, W. B. Saunders Company, Philadelphia, 1372–1429, 1983.
78. Root CR: Abdominal masses: The radiographic differential diagnosis. J Am Vet Radiol Soc 15:26, 1974.
79. Sanders RC: The significance of sonographic gallbladder wall thickening. J Clin Ultrasound 8:143, 1980.
80. Schaer M: A clinicopathologic survey of acute pancreatitis in 30 dogs and 5 cats. J Am Anim Hosp Assoc 15:681, 1979.
81. Schall WD, Griener TP: Diseases of the gallbladder. *In* Ettinger SJ (ed), *Textbook of Veterinary Internal Medicine,* 2nd ed, W. B. Saunders Company, Philadelphia, 1456–1459, 1983.
82. Schmidt S, Suter PF: Angiography of the hepatic and portal venous system in the dog and cat: An investigative method. Vet Radiol 21:57, 1980.
83. Schuylz MD, Weisberger D: Sialography, its value in diagnosis of swelling about the salivary glands. Oral Surg 1:233, 1948.
84. Smith HA, Jones TC, Hunt RD: The liver. *In* Smith HA, et al (eds), *Veterinary Pathology,* 4th ed, Lea & Febiger, Philadelphia, 1221–1236, 1972.
85. Squire LF: *Fundamentals of Radiology.* 3rd ed, Harvard University Press, Cambridge, MA, 175, 1982.
86. Starzl TE, Porter KA, Watanabe K, Putnam CW: Effects of insulin, glucagon, and insulin/glucagon infusions on liver morphology and cell division after complete portacaval shunt in dogs. Lancet 1:821–825, 1976.

87. Stradley RP, Stern RJ, Hienhold NB: A method for the simultaneous evaluation of exocrine pancreatic function and intestinal absorptive function in dogs. Am J Vet Res 40:1201, 1979.
88. Strombeck DR: Clinicopathologic features of primary and metastatic neoplastic disease of the liver in dogs. J Am Vet Med Assoc 173:267, 1978.
89. Suter P, Watrous B: Oropharyngeal dysphagias in the dog: A cinefluorographic analysis of experimentally induced and spontaneously occurring swallowing disorders. Vet Radiol 21:24–39, 1980.
90. Suter PF: Radiographic diagnosis of liver disease in dogs and cats. Vet Clin North Am 12:153, 1982.
91. Suter PF: Portal vein anomalies in the dog: Their angiographic diagnosis. J Am Vet Radiol Soc 16:81, 1975.
92. Ticer JW: *Radiographic Technique in Veterinary Practice,* 2nd ed, W. B. Saunders Company, Philadelphia, 1984.
93. Ticer JW: Abdomen (Pneumoperitonography; Cholecystography). *In* Ticer JW (ed), *Radiographic Technique in Veterinary Practice,* 2nd ed, W. B. Saunders Company, Philadelphia, 312–335, 1984.
94. Ticer JW: Roentgen signs of endocrine disease. Vet Clin North Am 7:465, 1977.
95. Thrall DE: *In* Strombeck DR (ed), *Small Animal Gastroenterology.* Stonegate Publishing Co., Davis, CA, 61–76, 1979.
96. Toddroff RJ, Brodey RS: Oral and pharyngeal neoplasia in the dog: A retrospective survey of 361 cases. J Am Vet Med Assoc 175:567–571, 1979.
97. Troy GC, Roenigk WJ: Clinical and radiographic findings in a dog with acute necrotizing pancreatitis. Southwest Vet 33:119, 1980.
98. Troy GC: Hepatic encephalopathy in a dog with a patent ductus venosus. Southwest Vet 32:15, 1979.
99. Vulgamott JC: Hepatic encephalopathy associated with acquired portacaval shunt in a dog. J Am Vet Med Assoc 175:724, 1979.
100. Watrous BJ, Suter PF: Oropharyngeal dysphagias in the dog: A cinefluorographic analysis of experimentally induced and spontaneously occurring swallowing disorders. Vet Radiol 24:11–24, 1983.
101. Williams JL: Obstruction of the small intestine. Radiol Clin North Am 2:21–31, 1964.
102. Wrigley RH, Reuter RE: Percutaneous cholecystography in normal dogs. Vet Radiol 23:239, 1982.
103. Zontine WJ: Dental radiographic technique and interpretation. Vet Clin North Am 4:741, 1974.
104. Zontine WJ: Canine dental radiology: Radiographic technique, development, and anatomy of the teeth. J Am Vet Radiol Soc 16:75, 1975.
105. Zontine WJ: Effects of chemical restraint drugs on the passage of barium sulfate through the stomach and duodenum of dogs. J Am Vet Med Assoc 152:878–884, 1973.

CHAPTER

15

Gastrointestinal Parasitism in the Dog and Cat

ROBERT M. CORWIN
SARA E. GREEN

In recent years, gastrointestinal parasitism in dogs and cats has become an increasingly more important diagnostic consideration for the veterinarian. This development stems from an awareness that the regional distribution of some parasites has expanded naturally by the sylvatic route *(Echinococcus multilocularis)* and by the travel and relocation of pets within countries and even between countries so that "exotic" parasites have been introduced into formerly nonendemic areas. Also, the increased recognition of zoonotic transmission and of the threat to public health have bestowed upon the veterinarian the responsibility to educate the clients and the general public about the identification and control of parasites.

Helminth and protozoan parasites are discussed in this chapter according to the alimentary compartment in which they are principally located (Table 15–1). These parasites usually occupy very specific niches in the gut, although some may have migratory stages in extraintestinal tissues. Some are of such common occurrence in the dog and cat *(Toxocara)* that the veterinarian must routinely consider them in making a differential diagnosis and must routinely treat for their removal even when the infection is not apparent. The necessity for routine treatment is especially important in younger animals in which perinatal infection may transpire.

Transmission of these parasites may be accomplished by fecal passage of helminth eggs and protozoan cysts followed by direct oral introduction of larvated eggs (ascarids, trichurids), ensheathed larvae (hookworms), or sporulated cysts (coccidia); by skin penetration of infective larvae *(Strongyloides)*; or by ingestion of paratenic hosts or biological intermediate hosts, which harbor infective larvae (ascarids, spirurids) or cysts *(Sarcocystis)*. Alternatively, even more direct transmission may result from passage of larvae from mother to fetus *(Toxocara)* or to neonate while nursing *(Ancylostoma)*. Knowledge of these specific routes and of alternate ones is important for understanding the epidemiology and control of parasites.

Clinical signs related to parasitism may range from the overt symptoms, such as bloody, tarry stools in pups with hookworm disease, to a generalized unthriftiness. Diagnostically, detection of eggs or cysts in the stool may provide an answer to a clinical problem; however, eggs and cysts are not always passed because of prepatent infection or sporadic release. Therefore, the age of the patient and its history, e.g., taking immunosuppressive drugs, must be considered. Pathology due to parasitism may be caused by tissue trauma, (e.g., larval migration or bloodsucking), by release of allergens, or by the degree of host response; some of these host responses are still to be characterized.

During the 1970's and to date, several new anthelmintics, showing greater efficacy and safety than anthelmintics developed earlier, have become available for veterinary use. Some are broad in spectrum of

Table 15–1. PARASITE SPECIES BY ALIMENTARY COMPARTMENT

		Dog	Cat
Esophagus and Stomach			
Nematodes	*Spirocerca lupi*	Yes	Yes
	Physaloptera spp.	Yes	Yes
	Ollulanus tricuspis	No	Yes
Small Intestine			
Nematodes	*Toxocara canis*	Yes	No
	Toxocara cati	No	Yes
	Toxascaris leonina	Yes	Yes
	Ancylostoma caninum	Yes	No
	Ancylostoma braziliense	Yes	Yes
	Uncinaria stenocephala	Yes	Yes
	Ancylostoma tubaeforme	No	Yes
	Strongyloides stercoralis (S. canis, S. felis)	Yes	Yes
	Capillaria putorii	No	Yes
Cestodes	*Taenia pisiformis*	Yes	Rare
	Taenia hydatigena	Yes	Rare
	Taenia ovis	Yes	No
	Taenia (Multiceps) multiceps	Yes	No
	Taenia (Multiceps) serialis	Yes	No
	Taenia (Hydatigera) taeniaeformis	No	Yes
	Echinococcus granulosus	Yes	No
	Echinococcus multilocularis	Yes	Yes
	Dipylidium caninum	Yes	Yes
	Mesocestoides spp.	Yes	Yes
	Diphyllobothrium latum	Yes	Yes
	Spirometra mansonoides	No	Yes
Trematodes	*Alaria* spp.	Yes	Yes
	Nanophyetus salmincola	Yes	No
Protozoa	*Isospora* spp.	Yes	Yes
	Sarcocystis spp.	Yes	Yes
	Toxoplasma gondii	No	Yes
	Besnoitia spp.	No	Yes
	Hammondia spp.	Yes	Yes
	Giardia spp.	Yes	Yes
Cecum and colon			
Nematodes	*Trichuris vulpis*	Yes	No
	Trichuris campanula	No	Yes
	Strongyloides tumefaciens	No	Yes
Protozoa	*Balantidium coli*	Yes	No
	Entamoeba histolytica	Yes	Rare
Liver and Pancreas			
Trematodes	*Eurytrema procyonis*	No	Yes
	Platynosomum sp.	No	Yes
	Amphimerus sp.	No	Yes

activity, a few even having larvicidal properties; other anthelmintics are purposefully narrow in spectrum. Formulations have also improved. On the other hand, development of antiprotozoal compounds has lagged, presenting a serious problem for practitioners. Better therapeutic drugs for control of coccidia and *Giardia* must be researched and provided. Antiparasitic compounds are discussed in the text and are listed in Table 15–2. Programs for control of parasites to restrict transmission and subsequently decrease parasite numbers are described in the text.

Parasites Of The Esophagus And Stomach

SPIROCERCA

Spirocerca lupi, the "esophageal worm," is a spirurid nematode found in domestic dogs and in wild canids such as the coyote,[54, 57] the red and the gray fox,[57] and the wolf.[11] There have been a few reports of *Spirocerca lupi* in cats, including the bobcat[57] and cheetah.[75] Geographic distribution is usually in warmer regions, al-

Table 15–2. ANTIPARASITIC DRUGS FOR DOGS AND CATS

Drug (Trade Name & Manufacturer)	Dosage	Indications	Comments
Diethylcarbamazine (several manufacturers)	20–500 mg/kg until eggs are no longer seen	*Spirocerca* in dogs, cats	A substituted piperazine, which may also be effective against ascarids; contraindicated for use in animals with microfilaremias
Disophenol (D.N.P. Parenteral, American Cyanamid Co., Princeton, NJ.)	10 mg/kg SC	Hookworms, *Spirocerca* in dogs, cats	3× dose recommended may be fatal; contraindicated for overheated animals or for animals with respiratory problems; do not use in poorly ventilated rooms; can use for nursing young; may cause lens opacity.
Fenbendazole (Panacur, American Hoechst Corp., Somerville, NJ.)	50 mg/kg/day for 3 successive days	Hookworms, ascarids, whipworms, *Taenia* tapeworms, *Eurytrema*	Approved for use in dogs only—granular formulation. Single dose at 150 mg/kg not effective; no known contraindications
Oxfendazole (Benzelmin, Diamond Laboratories, Inc., Des Moines, IA.)	Probably same as for fenbendazole	Same as for fenbendazole	Approved for use in horses only; probably same as for fenbendazole
Pyrantel pamoate (Nemex, Pfizer Laboratories, New York, NY.)	0.5 ml suspension per lb (5 mg/kg) orally or in food	Principally hookworms, ascarids in dogs, cats, possibly *Physaloptera*	All age dogs including nursing pups; no known contraindications
Dichlorvos (Task, Task Tablets, E.R. Squibb, Princeton, NJ.)	Dog: 27–33 mg/kg Puppy, cat: 11 mg/kg	Hookworms, ascarids, whipworms	Split dose BID for debilitated animals; contraindicated for heartworm infections, liver, or kidney disease; do not use with other cholinesterase inhibitors
Mebendazole (Telmintic Powder, Pitman-Moore, Inc., Washington Crossing, NJ.)	22 mg/kg in food daily for 3 days (nematodes) or 5 days (taeniids)	Hookworms, ascarids, whipworms, taeniid tapeworms; not *Dipylidium*	Approved for use in dogs, not cats (although efficacious at 22 mg/kg for 3 days); occasional hepatic necrosis, incoordination, emesis with overdose
Piperazine salts (several manufacturers)	45–65 mg base/kg; max. 150 mg for pups weighing <2.5 kg and for cats and kittens	Ascarids in dogs, cats	Only 50–100 per cent efficacy against ascarids; no contraindications except chronic liver or kidney disease
Thenium closylate (Canopar, Jensen-Salsbery Laboratories, Kansas City, MO.)	2 doses, 8 hrs apart, each dose by wt. level: 2–5 lb 1/2 tab; 5–10 lb, 1 tab; >10 lb, 2 tabs	Hookworms, ascarids	Dogs post weaning, 1st dose before AM feeding, feed between 1st and 2nd dose; No milk or fatty foods
Butamisole HCl (Styquin Injectable, American Cyanamid Co., Princeton, NJ.)	2.4 mg/kg SC	Hookworms, whipworms	4× dose lethal; contraindicated for heartworm-positive or debilitated dogs
Febantel (Rintal Paste, Haver-Lockhart Laboratories, Shawnee, KS.)	15 mg/kg for 3 consecutive days; administered as 3.5 per cent paste	Ascarids, hookworms, whipworms, *Taenia* tapeworms	No effect on mature heartworms
Sodium hypochlorite (several manufacturers)	Spray or mop area with 1 per cent solution	Treatment of premises for hookworm larvae and coccidian oocysts	
DDVP (VIP, Pet Chemicals, Inc., Miami Springs, FL.)	100 gal water + 32 oz concentrate treats 4000 sq ft, 50 gal water + 16 oz concentrate treats 2000 sq ft, 25 gal water + 8 oz concentrate treats 1000 sq ft, 15 gal water + 4 oz concentrate treats 600 sq ft	Treatment of premises for hookworm larvae	
Thiabendazole (Omnizole 43 per cent Wormer Paste, Merck Sharp & Dohme AGVET, Rahway, NJ.)	100–150 mg/kg daily for 3 days	*Strongyloides* in dogs	Some emesis; repeat treatment monthly if needed; not approved for dogs

Table continued on following page

Table 15–2. ANTIPARASITIC DRUGS FOR DOGS AND CATS *Continued*

Drug (Trade Name & Manufacturer)	Dosage	Indications	Comments
Dithiazinine iodide (Dizan Powder or Tablets, Med-Tech, Inc., Elwood, KS.)	22 mg/kg SID for 3–5 days, for 7 days, for 10–12 days	Ascarids, hookworms, whipworms, *Strongyloides* 3–5 days—ascarids 7 days—hookworms, whipworms 10–12 days—*Strongyloides*	Contraindicated in reduced renal function; may cause emesis, nausea, blue-green diarrhea; depression
Levamisole (Tramisol, Ripercol, American Cyanamid, Co., Princeton, NJ. Levasole, Pitman-Moore, Inc. Washington Crossing, NJ.)	2 doses, 7.5 mg/kg at a 2 week interval, 1st dose split, 2nd dose single	*Capillaria putorrii* in cats	Not approved for use in cats
Niclosamide (Yomesan Tablets, Haver-Lockhart Laboratories, Shawnee, KS.)	100–157 mg/kg orally dog, cat	80 per cent *Taenia*; 18–56 per cent *Dipylidium*	Heavy mucus interferes with scolex elimination
Bunamidine HCl (Scolaban Tablets, Jensen-Salsbery Laboratories, Kansas City, MO.)	25–50 mg/kg on empty stomach; Feed light meal 3 hrs later	100 per cent *Taenia;* 56–90 per cent *Dipylidium;* 86–100 per cent *Echinococcus*	Occasional idiosyncratic reaction; do not use with butamisole
Praziquantel (Droncit Injectable or Tablets, Haver-Lockhart Laboratories, Shawnee, KS.)	Injection SC or IM; Dog: 5 mg/kg; Cat: 11 mg/kg (1–3 lb), 22 mg/kg (3–11 lb), 34 mg/kg (>11 lb); Tablets. Cat: ≤4 lb, 1/2 tablet; 5–11 lb, 1 tablet; >11 lb, 1½ tablets; Dog: ≤516, ½ tablets; 6–10 lb, 1 tablet; 11–15 lb, 1½ tablets; 16–30 lb, 2 tablets; 31–45 lb, 3 tablets; 46–60 lb, 4 tablets; >60 lb, 5 tablets	*Taenia, Echinococcus, Dipylidium, Platynosomum*	Tapeworms only, even cestode larvae in intermediate hosts; pain at injection site
Drocarbil (arecoline-acetarsol, Nemural Tablets, Winthrop Laboratories, New York, NY.)	4–6 mg/kg orally after light feeding; dog, cat	50 per cent *Taenia, Dipylidium;* 75 per cent *Echinococcus*	May cause severe vomition, diarrhea
Sulfadimethoxine (Albon, Roche Laboratories, Nutley, NJ. Bactrovet, Pitman-Moore Inc., Washington Crossing NJ.)	55 mg/kg daily for 10–20 days (may be divided BID)	Coccidia	Folic acid inhibitor, effective late in coccidia cycle (2nd schizogonic stage)
Sulfadiazine with trimethoprim (Tribrissen Tablets, Jensen-Salsbery Laboratories, Kansas City, MO)	30–60 mg/kg daily for 6 days	Coccidia	Same as for sulfadimethoxine
Pyrimethamine (Daraprim, Burroughs Wellcome Co., Kansas City, MO.)	0.5–1.0 mg/kg for 4–6 days	Clinical coccidiosis	See reference 25
Amprolium (Corid, Amprol, Merck Sharp & Dohme AGVET, Rahway, NJ.)	100 mg 20 per cent powder daily for 7–12 days in food; 1 oz 10 per cent sol/gal water	Coccidia	Thiamine antagonist; not approved for use in dogs; 1.25 ml 20 per cent powder in food for 4 pups
Metronidazole (Flagyl, Searle Laboratories, Chicago, IL.)	25 mg/kg per os BID for 5 consecutive days; (400 to 800 mg/kg TID for 5 days for *Entamoeba*)	*Giardia* *Balantidium* *Entamoeba*	Cessation of diarrhea within 72 hours of initiation of treatment
Glycobiarsol (Milibis-V, Winthrop Laboratories, New York, NY.)	220 mg/kg daily for 5 days	Whipworms, *Giardia*	110 mg/kg daily for 10 days in debilitated dogs
Quinacrine HCl (Atabrine, Winthrop Laboratories, New York, NY.)	Large breeds: 200 mg/animal TID for 1 day then BID for 6 days, PO or IM Small breeds: 100 mg/animal BID for 1 day, then SID for 6 days, PO or IM Puppies: 50 mg/animal BID for 6 days PO or IM	*Giardia*	Cholinesterase inhibitor; may cause vomiting; a single oral dose of 300 mg/kg or 110 mg/kg for 15–27 days is lethal; not approved for veterinary use
Ivermectin (Merck Sharp & Dohme AGVET, Rahway, NJ.)	Still investigational for the dog. It has shown excellent efficacy for hookworms, ascarids, and whipworms, but has not been effective for tapeworms, flukes or protozoa.		

*Data from references 59 and 60.

though reports have shown this organism to occur in Kansas[54] and in the Yukon Territory of Canada.[11]

Life Cycle

Spirocercosis is primarily an infection of the esophagus and thoracic aorta, although ectopic sites of infection have been described. Adult worms are found coiled, usually in pairs, in granulomatous lesions. Eggs are thick-shelled, ovoid, larvated, and relatively small (35 × 12 μ). Larval development is in arthropods, especially coprophagous beetles, and is probably followed by encystment in paratenic hosts such as lizards, birds including poultry, and small mammals. After the intermediate or paratenic host has been ingested, larvae migrate from the stomach, through the gastroepiploic and celiac arteries to the juxtaposition of the aorta and esophagus. Ectopic sites of infection include the lungs, bronchi, trachea, lymphatic system, thoracic and abdominal cavities, stomach, urinary bladder, kidneys,[2] and rectum.[28]

Pathogenesis

Granulomatous lesions form around larvae in the affected organs; the principal sites of infection are the esophagus and the thoracic aorta just posterior to the aortic arch. Aneurysms and thrombi may form in the aorta, with the threat of imminent hemorrhage.[55] Stenosis of the esophagus results from protrusion of granulomas into the lumen. Neoplasias of the esophagus, such as fibrosarcomas and osteosarcomas, apparently are induced by *Spirocerca* infections, and metastases are common.[4, 40] There has also been a report of *S. lupi* locating in the lung and participating in the development of a fibrosarcoma there.[69] These space-occupying lesions may be responsible for hypertrophic pulmonary osteopathy.[9] A deforming spondylitis of the caudal thoracic vertebrae has been reported.[55]

Clinical Signs

Clinical signs include anorexia, persistent regurgitation followed by weakness and emaciation, dyspnea, anemia, hemorrhagic shock, thickening of the cortex of the long bones (but not of the joints), paraplegia, and convulsions.[55, 75] Death is a sequela of some of these problems.

Diagnosis

Diagnosis is based on clinical signs and the appearance of eggs in emesis or feces. Direct preparations should be made, since eggs do not float well in concentrated sugar or salt solutions. On radiographic examination, a dense mass that involves the caudal esophagus may be seen on a chest film. Contrast radiography with barium salts helps to delineate the mass. Esophagoscopy or gastroscopy could also be useful.[55] At necropsy, aortic lesions are considered pathognomonic.[3]

Treatment

Treatment has included use of diethylcarbamazine* (20 to 500 mg/kg until no eggs are seen).[55] Disophenol† (10 mg/kg SC) reportedly has shown some effectiveness.[13] Fenbendazole‡ or compounds still under investigation for dogs and cats, such as oxfendazole§ might be employed, since they apparently are absorbed readily and have been found effective against larvae in extraintestinal tissues.

Prevention

Clients in endemic areas should be warned of the potential danger of feeding scraps of poultry, and rabbits, and wild game to dogs and cats.

PHYSALOPTERA

Physaloptera spp. are spirurid nematodes that occur throughout the United States, although they are probably more common in the southern regions.

Life Cycle

Physaloptera rara has been found in the stomachs of dogs and coyotes, and both *P. rara* and *P. felidis* have been found in the stomachs and duodenums of cats. *Physaloptera praeputialis* has also been reported in the stomachs of the dog and cat. *Physaloptera* appear rather stout-bodied, measure about 2 cm in length, and may be mistaken

---

*Diethylcarbamazine, several manufacturers.

†D.N.P. Parenteral, American Cyanamid Co., Princeton, NJ.

‡Panacur, American Hoechst Corp., Somerville, NJ.

§Benzelmin, Diamond Laboratories, Inc., Des Moines, IA.

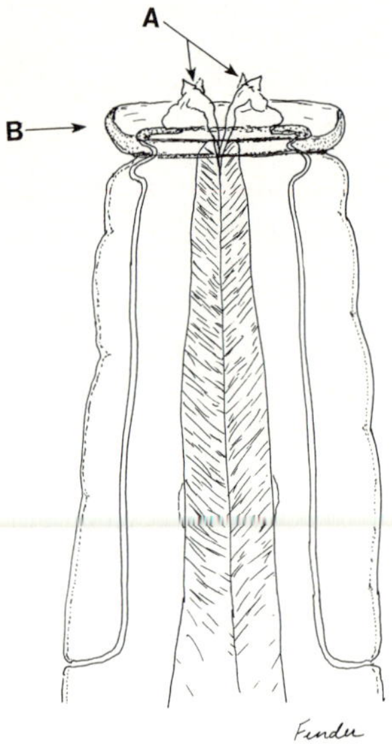

Figure 15–1. *Physaloptera*, adult, a spirurid nematode found in the stomach of dogs and cats. Anterior end with two lips *(A)* at oral opening and a cuticular collar *(B)*.

for small ascarids. Microscopic examination shows two lips at the oral opening rather than the three fleshy ones found on ascarids, and a cuticular cervical collar is present, but there are no cervical alae (Fig. 15–1).

Eggs are in feces or may be seen in vomitus. They measure 50 × 30 μ and are larvated. Dichromate solutions are recommended for flotation.[78] Crickets and cockroaches are true intermediate hosts; frogs, mice, and rattlesnakes, but not chickens, are possibly paratenic hosts.[56] These spirurid nematodes do not migrate, although they do invade the mucosa.

Pathogenesis

Tissue trauma is associated with bite wounds and ingestion of blood. Wounds may continue to bleed after the worm has moved to another site, and the mucosa often is inflamed and ulcerated.

Clinical Signs

The authors have observed acute gastritis with only one or a few worms present. Recurring bouts of vomition have been observed with mucoid and possibly blood-tinged emesis, perhaps with the offending worm in the emesis. This infection should certainly be considered as part of a differential diagnosis when gastritis is observed.

Diagnosis

The appearance of larvated eggs as described previously will confirm a diagnosis when recurring gastritis has been observed.

Treatment

Pyrantel pamoate* (5 mg/kg) has been shown to be efficacious against *Physaloptera*.[74]

Prevention

There are no practical means of preventing *Physaloptera* infection.

OLLULANUS

Ollulanus tricuspis is a tiny trichostrongylid nematode found in the stomach of cats. In the United States it has been reported only in New Jersey[47] and in the state of Washington.[35]

Life Cycle

Morphologically, adults measure about 1 mm in length, with the anterior end coiled. The posterior end of the adult females and of the larval stages has three cusps (Fig. 15–2), whereas the male has a copulatory bursa. The life cycle of *Ollulanus tricuspis* differs from that of other gastrointestinal nematodes in that the female is viviparous and deposits ensheathed third stage larvae. In stomach contents of infected cats, third and fourth stage larvae and adults have been observed. Apparently these worms cycle in the stomach so that several generations are present. The probable vehicle of transmission is vomitus containing the third stage larvae.

Pathogenesis and Clinical Signs

This parasite causes small gastric erosions, and the resulting gastritis induces vomition.

Diagnosis

Finding third or fourth stage larvae or adult *Ollulanus* in the vomitus confirms a diagnosis.

---

*Nemex, Pfizer Laboratories, New York, NY.

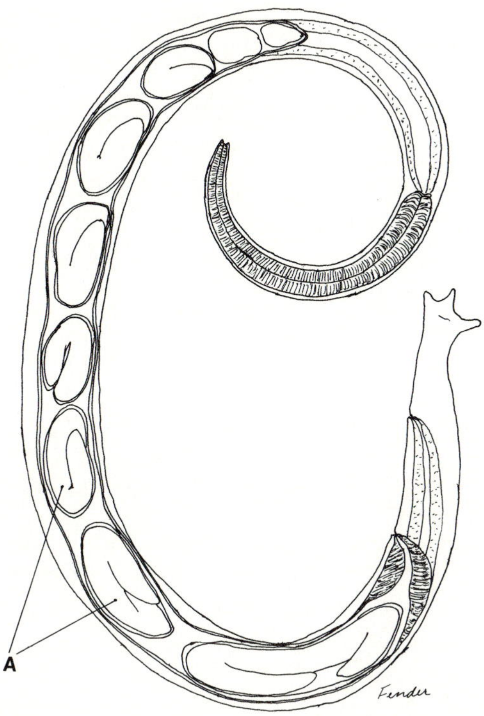

Figure 15–2. *Ollulanus tricuspis*, adult female, a trichostrongylid nematode found in the stomach of cats. Anterior end *(top)* coiled, posterior end with three cusps (male has copulatory bursa). Note developing larvae *(A)* (ensheathed L_3 deposited).

Treatment

Claims have not been made for activity against *Ollulanus*.

Prevention

No means of preventing *Ollulanus* infection is known.

Parasites Of The Small Intestine

TOXOCARA, TOXASCARIS

Species of ascarids found in dogs and cats include *Toxocara canis* and *Toxocara cati (T. mystax)*, respectively, and *Toxascaris leonina* in both. Mature *Toxocara* infections are found most often in pups and kittens, whereas *Toxascaris* infections are usually seen in weaned dogs and cats. Ascarids are cosmopolitan in geographic distribution.

Life Cycle

Ascarids of the dog and cat are commonly referred to as large roundworms or as arrowhead worms. They are relatively long (up to 18 cm) and robust. Inflatable, paired cervical alae produce the arrowhead, which is especially notable in *T. cati* (Fig. 15–3). Males are coiled posteriorly and are smaller than females. The tail of male *Toxocara* has a finger-like projection, whereas that of *T. leonina* does not (Fig. 15–4). The small intestine is the principal site of infection.

There are some marked differences in the life cycles of each of these three ascarid species. *Toxocara* infections can be transmitted in many ways. First, *Toxocara canis* is transmitted from bitch to fetal pups by the migration of larvae from somatic tissues (larvae had been in a state of arrested development) through the placenta and into the liver of the fetus by way of the umbilical vessels. Larvae can be found in the liver and lungs at birth and in the small intestine at 2 to 6 days of age.[64] This transfer probably

Figure 15–3. *Toxascaris leonina, Toxocara cati,* and *Toxocara canis (left to right)*. Anterior ends of adults with inflatable, paired cervical alae producing the arrowhead appearance, especially for *T. cati.*

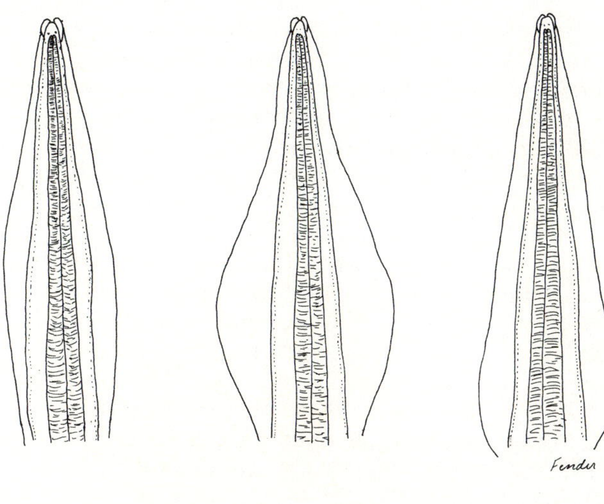

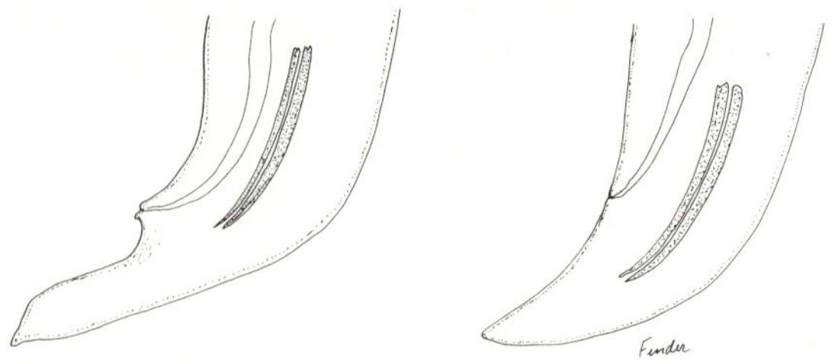

Figure 15–4. *Toxocara canis (left)* and *Toxascaris leonina (right)*. Posterior ends of adult males; that of *T. canis* has a finger-like projection.

accounts for infection rates approaching 100 per cent. Second, larvae have been found in the milk of a bitch on day 22 postpartum.[72] Third, pups also become infected by ingestion of larvated eggs; larvae then burrow into the wall of the small intestine and migrate through the liver, right heart, lungs, respiratory tract, and anterior alimentary tract to the small intestine. By 3 months of age, pups are fairly resistant to migration via the tracheal route.[34] Those larvae that penetrate the wall of the small intestine eventually stop developing when they reach somatic tissue. Fourth, paratenic hosts such as rodents and birds also may be sources of infection, especially in older dogs. Migration of larvae is restricted then to the mucosa of the small intestine, with maturation occurring *in situ*. Fifth, bitches may re-establish infections by coprophagy of puppy stools, with some somatic migration because of a weakened immune status.

Toxocara cati larvae apparently do not migrate across the placenta, but they may employ transmammary passage.[68, 73] These larvae migrate by the liver-heart-lungs route, and immature worms reside briefly on the stomach mucosa. Paratenic hosts (earthworms, cockroaches, birds, and rodents) may be quite important, since older cats frequently are infected.

Dogs and cats that have had the opportunity to feed on rodents may be infected with *T. leonina* because this organism makes extensive use of intermediate hosts in which larvae molt from the second to the third stage. Migration of larvae is restricted to the mucosa of the small intestine.

Pathogenesis

Pathogenesis is associated with larval migration and with the accumulation of large numbers of worms in the small intestine. Clinical disease is seen most often in pups and kittens. Granulomatous and fibrotic lesions develop in the hepatic parenchyma following larval migration, with eosinophils being attracted by secretory-excretory larval antigenic substances. A similar response may occur in the lungs, causing an interstitial pneumonia.

Clinical Signs

Interstitial pneumonia may appear clinically as a puppy cough. Distention and possible impaction of the small intestine result from heavy infection. The worms may produce a colicky pain, malabsorption, and possibly blood loss. Heavily infected young animals become pot-bellied and spraddle-legged, have stunted growth, and have a mucoid diarrhea. Death may result from obstruction or perforation of the small intestine.

Diagnosis

Clinical signs and the age and eating habits of the host are strongly suggestive for diagnosis. Patent infections are represented by eggs and even worms in the feces.

1. *Toxocara canis* have spherical eggs with pitted outer shells. A dark zygote fills the egg's interior. The eggs are 80 to 85 μ in diameter.

2. *Toxocara cati* produce similar eggs that measure 70 μ in diameter.

3. *Toxascaris leonina* eggs are smooth-shelled and ovoid, with a light zygote that does not fill the egg's interior. These eggs measure 85 × 45 μ.

Eggs are demonstrated readily by a flotation technique.

Treatment

Young pups and nursing bitches should be treated at 2, 4, 6, and 8 weeks after birth. Effective anthelmintics include pyrantel pamoate, fenbendazole, dichlorvos,* mebendazole† and salts of piperazine‡. Of the currently available drugs only fenbendazole is effective against migrating larvae.[14]

---

*Task, E. R. Squibb, Princeton, NJ.
†Telmintic Powder, Pitman-Moore, Inc., Washington Crossing, NJ.
‡Piperazine salts, several manufacturers.

Prevention

The mode of transmission from the reservoir bitch, the role of paratenic hosts, and the resistance of ascarid eggs make prevention very difficult. The veterinarian has the responsibility to educate clients, especially those with pups whelped at home.

Public Health Significance

Ascarids are very prolific egg layers; mature *T. canis* females shed 200,000 eggs daily, and *T. cati* females shed 2 to 4 times that number.[42] These eggs are very resistant to environmental stress and may survive in the soil for several years. Of particular concern is the frequency with which the eggs are being found at highway rest areas and in sandboxes.[12] The larvated egg is the infective stage and is potentially transmissible to many animal species, including humans. In dogs more than 4 weeks old and in accidental hosts, larvae follow a somatic route and may become dormant in numerous tissues. This condition is termed visceral larval migrans (VLM).

Both *T. canis* and *T. cati* larvae are potentially responsible for VLM in humans and for a second form of the disease referred to as ocular larval migrans (OLM). The public health significance of VLM and OLM has received much attention and has been reviewed extensively.[31, 46, 62, 79] The age range at greatest risk for VLM is from 1 to 6 years; VLM in this group is usually associated with geophagia, a form of pica. Hence, soil contamination rather than handling of pups and kittens is more important in transmission. Beaver reported children with geophagia who had livers with 300 *T. canis* larvae/g of tissue and brain tissue with 3 to 5 larvae/g.[8] Usually the infection is considered a benign self-limiting one because most infected persons ingest few larvae. Clinical manifestations are dependent on the number of larvated eggs ingested, the frequency of infection, the distribution of larvae, and the intensity of the host's immunological response. Visceral larval migrans is manifested by abdominal pain, diarrhea, wheezing, coughing, and possibly an urticaria or even skin ulcerations. Fatalities have resulted from larval invasion of the brain or myocardium. Diagnostic signs include fever, leukocytosis, persistent eosinophilia of over 80 per cent, hypergammaglobulinemia, and hepatomegaly.

Ocular larval migrans is typically a solitary granulomatous lesion located in close proximity to the optic disc and macula. There have also been reports of circumscribed inflammatory granulomas in the peripheral portion of the retina.[79] Children with OLM rarely have a history of pica and probably have ingested only a few eggs. The immunological response therefore could be considered mild and could allow for unrestrained larval migration. Once in the eye, a single larva can incite a marked local inflammatory response. This condition is important in a differential diagnosis that would include retinoblastoma, a malignancy that requires enucleation of the eye. Although OLM is most likely a transitory disease, enucleation has also been performed because of serious damage to the eye, such as retinal detachment.

A serological diagnostic test called ELISA (enzyme-linked immunosorbent assay), which uses *T. canis* embryonated egg extract, has been developed. Serological surveys and an evaluation of findings have shown 30 per cent of sera tested to have VLM, and 37 per cent of all pediatric retinal cases tested in one Atlanta practice revealed OLM.[46]

ANCYLOSTOMA UNCINARIA

Species of hookworms that infect dogs and cats include *Ancylostoma caninum* in dogs, *Ancylostoma tubaeforme* in cats, and *Ancylostoma braziliense* and *Uncinaria stenocephala* in both. The first two species seem to be cosmopolitan in distribution, whereas *A. braziliense* is found in warmer regions and *Uncinaria* in colder.

Life Cycle

Adult hookworms are relatively small, the largest being 15 mm in length. Oral openings are armed with teeth *(Ancylostoma)* or cutting plates *(Uncinaria)*, and males possess an umbrella-shaped copulatory bursa at their posterior ends.

Morulated, ovoid eggs (60×40 μ) are passed onto the soil, where free-living larvae hatch and develop into an infective stage; this development is enhanced by moisture and warm temperatures. The routes of infection and migration are species dependent. The oral route of infection is followed by *A. caninum, A. tubaeforme,* and *U. stenoce-*

phala, with migration restricted to the intestinal mucosa.[23] Skin penetration is the route used by *A. braziliense*, with migration via the lungs, and a return to the small intestine. Neonatal infections of *A. caninum* also occur, with larvae moving from sequestered sites into the mammary glands and then being ingested with milk. Transmammary transmission occurs during the first 3 weeks of life,[71] but transplacental transmission is not as common (98.9 per cent vs 1.1 per cent).[70] Paratenic hosts are used by any of these species, with migration restricted to the intestinal mucosa.[48]

Pathogenesis and Clinical Signs

Clinical signs may appear as early as 10 days postpartum (prepatent infection). The signs may be related to blood loss and malabsorption with destruction of villi and sloughing of mucosa caused by *A. caninum* and *A. tubaeforme*. Pups and kittens appear depressed, colicky, and weakened, with pale mucous membranes, peripheral edema, and loose, black, mucoid but scanty feces. Heavy burdens of *A. caninum* and *A. tubaeforme* kill their young hosts. Conversely, *A. braziliense* and *Uncinaria* are not bloodsuckers but may cause loss of plasma proteins; they are not considered serious pathogens.[53] The severity of hookworm disease in dogs depends on age and immunity of the host and the species of hookworm. *Ancylostoma braziliense* and *U. stenocephala* infections are rarely fatal.[52] Dermatitis and pneumonitis are associated with skin penetration of *A. braziliense* infective larvae.

Diagnosis

Diagnosis is presumptive and is based upon clinical signs and the age of the patient if infections are acute and prepatent. The diagnosis is confirmed if eggs are present in the feces. Female hookworms are prolific egg producers; however, larvae can undergo arrested development in the wall of the intestine, surviving for several months and remaining unresponsive to drug therapy.[43] This phenomenon invalidates negative results of fecal examinations, and the larvae serve as a source for later patent infections.

Treatment

Treatment is symptomatic when infections are acute. Anthelmintics such as disophenol, pyrantel pamoate, dichlorvos, mebendazole, thenium closylate,* butamisole,† and febantel‡ can be given; attention should be paid to contraindications for these drugs. Repeat treatment in 2 to 4 weeks should remove populations established by emerging larvae.

Prevention

If previous litters have died from hookworm disease, the veterinarian should recommend that their dam not be used in a breeding program. Paratenic hosts again should be considered as possible reservoirs. Surfaces of runs could be treated with sodium hypochlorite§ or DDVP dichorvos‖ to kill free-living and infective larvae.

Public Health Significance

Cutaneous larval migrans (CLM) is associated with *A. braziliense* infective larvae, which in humans is restricted to the epidermis.[42]

STRONGYLOIDES

Strongyloides stercoralis (S. canis or *S. felis*) infection occurs in dogs, cats, and primates, including humans. The species that infects humans has been transmitted experimentally to dogs and cats, although there are apparently differences in the strains. Natural infections in dogs occur worldwide and are common in the United States. Reports of *S. stercoralis* infections in cats are limited to the Far East, although another species, *S. tumefaciens*, has been found in the large intestines of cats in Gulf Coast states.[51]

Life Cycle

Strongyloides stercoralis, the threadworm, is found in the mucosa of the small intestine. Eggs of *S. stercoralis* are larvated and thin-shelled, measuring 60 × 30 μ. Larvae of *Strongyloides* measure about 300 μ in

---

*Canopar, Jensen-Salsbery Laboratories, Kansas City, MO.

†Styquin Injectable, American Cyanamid Co., Princeton, NJ.

‡Rintal Paste, Haver-Lockhart Laboratories, Shawnee, KS.

§Sodium hypochlorite, several manufacturers.

‖VIP, Pet Chemicals, Inc., Miami Springs, FL.

length and develop either directly to infective larvae (homogonic cyle) or to males and females that live freely on soil (heterogonic cycle) and later produce infective larvae. Infective larvae are about 600 μ long, and have a maximum width of 16 μ, are not ensheathed, have a filariform esophagus extending about 40 per cent of the body length, and have a trifid tail.[26] These larvae may penetrate the skin or may be ingested. Although it has not been proven, circumstantial evidence is quite suggestive of transmammary transmission of *S. stercoralis*. Larvae that enter through the skin are carried in the blood to the lungs and then migrate via the trachea and esophagus through the stomach to the small intestine, where they mature in 1½ to 2 weeks. Larvae that are ingested apparently develop directly in the small intestine without migration. Parthenogenetic females of *S. stercoralis* locate in the mucosa of the small intestine.

Pathogenesis and Clinical Signs

A dermatitis associated with skin penetration of *S. stercoralis* larvae in dogs is manifested as an erythema with intense pruritus. Bronchopneumonia results from the migration of *S. stercoralis* through the lungs. Burrowing of the organism in the mucosa of the small intestine induces inflammation with necrosis and sloughing, which occurs in moderate to heavy infections. A mucoid or profuse watery diarrhea, dehydration, and even death may result. Infections of clinical significance occur more commonly in young animals. Older dogs apparently develop an immunity to all but light infections and serve as carriers.

A *S. stercoralis*-like infection has been reported in a 6-month-old Boston terrier with intractable diarrhea, coughing, hemorrhagic pododermatitis, and mild mucopurulent oculonasal discharge. Larvated and nonlarvated eggs 80 × 35 μ and first stage larvae were found in the feces, which were watery and fetid. Culture of the stool showed third stage larvae and adults resembling *S. stercoralis*.[50]

Diagnosis

Routine examination of feces from infected animals usually reveals larvae rather than eggs, and the larvae will be overlooked unless a direct mount is prepared. To differentiate larvae of *Strongyloides*, hookworms, and lungworms passed in the stool[26] or obtained from rectal stool samples, the feces may be incubated at room temperature for 24 hours.[78] The third stage larvae of *Strongyloides* will not be ensheathed; the absence of a sheath is best detected by addition of iodine to the sample.

Treatment

Thiabendazole* (100 to 150 mg/kg for 3 days) and dithiazinine iodide† (22 mg/kg SID for 10 to 12 days) have successfully eliminated infections, although infections may disappear spontaneously. Other benzimidazole carbamates (e.g., fenbendazole) should also be effective. Anti-inflammatory ointments might be applied topically for skin lesions.

Prevention

Since free-living generations may exist in warm, moist soil or bedding, litter after litter of pups may become infected. Clean, dry quarters with exposure to sunlight are recommended. Rigorous, frequent sanitation is necessary owing to the rapid development of the larvae, which are passed in stools, to the infective stage.

Public Health Significance

In one case, *S. stercoralis* was transmitted from dogs to a laboratory worker who suffered enteritis, diarrhea, and prostration. Larvae were then experimentally transmitted back to dogs from the human patient.[27]

CAPILLARIA

Capillaria putorii is a small trichurid nematode reported in the gastric mucus of cats in Iowa. The parasite is probably a resident of the small intestine because there was evidence of intestinal reflux into the stomach in all patients in which the organism was observed.[32]

Life Cycle

The adults measure 2.5 to 7.4 mm.[32] The life cycle of *Capillaria* is unknown.

---

*Omnizole 43% Wormer Paste, Merck Sharp & Dohme AGVET, Rahway, NJ.

†Dizan, Med-Tech, Inc., Elwood, KS.

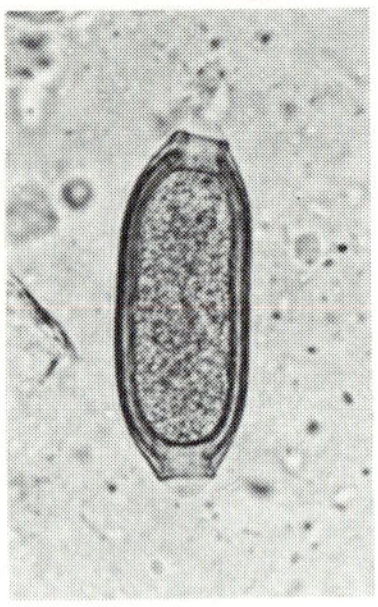

C. putorii

Figure 15–5. Egg of *Capillaria putorii.* (Reprinted with permission from Georgi JR: *Parasitology for Veterinarians*, 4th ed. W.B. Saunders Company, Philadelphia, 242, 1985.)

Pathogenesis and Clinical Signs

Pathogenicity is unknown. No clinical signs or histological lesions were seen in the Iowa cats.[32]

Diagnosis

The eggs are found in the feces. They are smaller than those of *Capillaria aerophila* (a parasite of the lungs), measuring 57 to 66 × 21 to 28 μ[32], are parallel-sided and have bipolar plugs. The egg pictured in Figure 15–5 is a typical egg of *C. putorii*.[26, 32]

Treatment

Eggs disappeared from the feces after a cat had been treated with levamisole* (2 doses, 7.5 mg/kg at a 2-week interval, with the first dose split into two given 12 hours apart and the second dose given as a single treatment.[32]

CESTODES

Several species of cestodes (tapeworms) may parasitize dogs and cats, including taeniid (*Taenia* and *Echinococcus* spp.) and nontaeniid *(Dipylidium)* cyclophyllideans, pseudophyllideans *(Diphyllobothrium* and *Spirometra*), and an intermediate group *(Mesocestoides)*. A very common species in both dogs and cats is *Dipylidium caninum*. *Taenia pisiformis* in dogs and *Taenia (Hydatigera) taeniaeformis* in cats are also common. Other *Taenia* spp. that are also found in dogs, use livestock as intermediate hosts. *Echinococcus granulosus* parasitizes dogs used for sheep herding in western and southwestern states, and *Echinococcus multilocularis* originally was reported in Arctic foxes, but more recently it has been reported in dogs and cats in the north central states.[58] *Diphyllobothrium* has been reported in dogs and cats in the Great Lakes area, and *Spirometra* has been observed in cats in the southwestern and eastern United States. *Mesocestoides* spp. have been reported in dogs.[77]

Life Cycle

The segmented adult cyclophyllidean tapeworm attaches to the mucosa of the small intestine using circular suckers and circlets of rostellar hooks on the scolex as holdfast organs. Terminal proglottids or segments, laden with eggs, are shed in the feces and carried outside the host. The proglottids also crawl from the rectum onto the perianal skin and then fall to the ground. Clients with infected pets become disturbed by the sight of a chain of segments hanging from the anus or surrounding hair or of a segment crawling across a fresh stool.

The mean prepatent period for *T. taeniaeformis* in cats was reported to be 47 days (34 to 80 days) and the mean patent period was 17 months (7 to 34 months). Proglottids that were shed contained 0 to 12,180 eggs; more than 60 per cent had fewer than 500 eggs, making this species less prolific than *T. ovis* and *T. hydatigena* in the dog. The mean daily proglottid output was four.[76]

Eggs are released as the segments dry and rupture. Eggs of the taeniid are spherical, 35 μ in diameter, and are thick-shelled, and occur singly, whereas those of *Dipylidium* are round to ovoid, 55 μ in diameter, and thin-shelled, and may occur in clusters. Eggs contain embryos with six hooks (hexacanth). Taeniid eggs may be ingested by herbivores (ruminants, rabbits) or by rodents; in the stomach, embryos hatch and then actively migrate to the wall of the small intestine and, by way of the portal venous route, to the liver. Each cyst (cysticercus) is vesicular and shows development of a single scolex. In order for dogs and cats to become infected, they must ingest mature cysts that are infecting the liver or viscera of the parasite's intermediate host. In contrast, *D. caninum* eggs are ingested by lar-

*Tramisol, American Cyanamid Co., Princeton, NJ. Ripercol, American Cyanamid Co., Princeton, NJ. Levasole, Pitman-Moore, Inc., Washington Crossing, NJ.

vae of the common dog and cat flea, *Ctenocephalides*. Development of a nonvesicular cyst (cysticercoid) takes place in the flea larva, and the cyst is infective upon maturation of the flea. Infection of the dog and cat depends upon ingestion of fleas.

The segmented adult pseudophyllidean tapeworm *(Diphyllobothrium, Spirometra)* attaches to the mucosa of the small intestine using longitudinal grooves (bothria). The gravid proglottids are not shed in the feces. Instead eggs are discharged from the uterine pore. When segments are shed they are senile and are usually shed in chains rather than singly. The eggs have an operculum and measure 70 × 45 μ. The life cycle of pseudophyllidean worms involves at least two intermediate hosts, a small crustacean (copepod) and a fish. The infective form in the fish is the larval plerocercoid.

Mesocestoides corti is able to multiply asexually by division of the scolex or of the proglottids.[20] *M. corti* and other species of the genus also have a rather complex life cycle. Eggs containing hexacanth embryos measuring 23 × 18 μ[77] are ingested by arthropods, and then birds or rodents serve as intermediate hosts. Parasitic ascites, caused by larval cestodes, presumably tetrathyridia of *Mesocestoides*, has been described in the dog. Highly pleomorphic (elongate to spherical) vesicles were described. Tetrathyridia may penetrate the abdominal cavity and liver, where they multiply by lateral budding or by multiple fission.[33]

Pathogenesis and Clinical Signs

Little clinical disease occurs with tapeworm infections, although abdominal discomfort, diarrhea, and flatulence may be associated with heavy infection. Apparently, movement of the hooks of the scolex and activity of many tapeworms cause some small foci of catarrhal inflammation and granulocytic infiltration. "Scooting" may be due to a perianal pruritus caused by the sticking of segments to the skin, but more often it is caused by inflamed and impacted anal sacs. The appearance of these worms causes esthetic discomfort to the client.

Diagnosis

Diagnosis most often is made by finding tapeworm segments in dog or cat feces. Crushing or macerating the segment in water on a microscope slide frees the eggs and allows for specific diagnosis of *Taenia* or *Dipylidium*. Unfortunately, *Echinococcus* eggs are identical to those of *Taenia*. Taeniid eggs may be seen on flotation, whereas, *Diphyllobothrium, Spirometra*, and *Mesocestoides* eggs do not float well.

Treatment

Cestocidal compounds now available include fenbendazole, mebendazole, niclosamide,* bunamidine hydrochloride,† praziquantel,‡ and drocarbil,§ an arecoline salt. Mebendazole and niclosamide are effective for removal of taeniids but not *Dipylidium*; bunamidine and praziquantel are effective against both taeniids and *Dipylidium*. Praziquantel has also been reported safe for use in cats and 5½-week-old kittens.[63] Arecoline compounds cause violent purgation, and can therefore be dangerous to the patient, and they may not remove the attached scolex, thus allowing for development of a new chain of segments.

Prevention

Control of the parasite includes not feeding dogs meat scraps and offal of rabbits, sheep, and fish. Because cats are instinctive hunters, attempts to prevent feline taeniid infections are impractical. Elimination of fleas by treatment of the dog or cat and of the premises is important in control of *Dipylidium*.

Public Health Significance

Tapeworms can also be of significance to the public health, especially *E. granulosus* hydatid and *E. multilocularis* alveolar or multilocular cysts, and *Spirometra* as an elongate larval form called a sparganum. Adult *Mesocestoides*[29, 30] and *Dipylidium caninum* have been found in children. The segmented form of *Diphyllobothrium* is probably more common in humans than in

---

*Yomesan Tablets, Haver-Lockhart Laboratories, Shawnee, KS.

†Scolaban Tablets, Jensen-Salsbery Laboratories, Kansas City, MO.

‡Droncit, Haver-Lockhart Laboratories, Shawnee, KS.

§Nemural Tablets, Winthrop Laboratories, New York, NY.

dogs and cats, because it is acquired from poorly cooked fish.

TREMATODES

Intestinal flukes seem to have specific geographical distribution, although modern transportation allows for ready dissemination of infected animals from these regions. Life cycles of trematodes are often complex, with snails as intermediate hosts and possibly encystment on vegetation or in the soft tissues of vertebrate or invertebrate second intermediate hosts. *Alaria* and *Nanophyetus* are two common examples. *Alaria* is considered common in dogs and cats in North America.

Alaria

Life Cycle.

Eggs of *Alaria* are large, brownish yellow, and operculated. Rodents that eat frogs, the natural second intermediate host, may serve as paratenic hosts. Adults 2.5 to 4.0 mm long attach by suckers to the mucosa of the small intestine.

Clinical Signs.

Infections are usually asymptomatic.[78]

Nanophyetus salmincola

Nanophyetus salmincola is endemic in the Columbia River valley of the Pacific Northwest.

Life Cycle

Encysted larvae (metacercariae) are found in salmonid fish. Adult flukes are quite small (1.5 mm), are found in the small intestines of dogs, coyotes, raccoons, mink, and lynx, and serve as vectors for a rickettsial pathogen, *Neorickettsia helminthoeca*, the cause of "salmon poisoning."

Clinical Signs

Nanophyetus alone usually is asymptomatic. The presence of *Neorickettsia* produces "salmon poisoning" manifested as fever, hemorrhagic enteritis, and enlargement of lymph nodes. This condition is often fatal.

Diagnosis

Diagnosis of fluke infection may be made by finding the operculated eggs, which measure 116 × 80 μ in *Alaria* or 85 × 42 μ in *Nanophyetus*, in the stool. Flotation fluids may cause collapse of fluke eggs, so that sedimentation techniques may be necessary.[78]

Treatment

Fenbendazole has good effect against some fluke infections although there has not been a report of its specific activity against *Alaria* or *Nanophyetus*. Broad-spectrum antibiotics are used for treatment of "salmon poisoning."

Prevention

Avoidance of second intermediate hosts is necessary to prevent infection.

COCCIDIA

The taxonomy of coccidia of dogs and cats has undergone great change, with many more species being recognized in recent years. The coccidia of dogs include: *Isospora canis, I. ohioensis, I. burrowsi, Hammondia heydorni*, and eight species of *Sarcocystis*. Those of cats include: *Isospora felis, I. rivolta, Besnoitia* spp., *Toxoplasma gondii, Hammondia hammondi*, and at least eight *Sarcocystis* spp.

Life Cycle

The enteroepithelial life cycle of all coccidia except for *Sarcocystis* includes schizogony followed by gametogony with oocyst formation (Fig. 15–6). *Sarcocystis* has only gametogony, with this stage found in the lamina propria. Oocysts sporulate to eight sporozoites; this stage divides in half in *Sarcocystis*. Dimensions of the cysts of various species are presented in Table 15–3. Oocysts are shed for 1 to 2 weeks in great numbers and are infective in 2 to 4 days; the intestinal infection can be reactivated and oocysts can be shed again.[18]

Oocysts that are unsporulated when passed in dog feces are larger than 20 μ (*Isospora* spp.) or are 12 × 11 μ (*H. heydorni*). Sporocysts of *Sarcocystis* are passed in a sporulated state (four sporozoites) and are about 15 × 10 μ. Unsporulated oocysts passed in cat stools may be larger than 20 μ (*Isospora* spp.) or less than 20 μ (*Besnoitia* spp., *Toxoplasma*, and *H. hammondi*). It is important to remember that oocysts sporu-

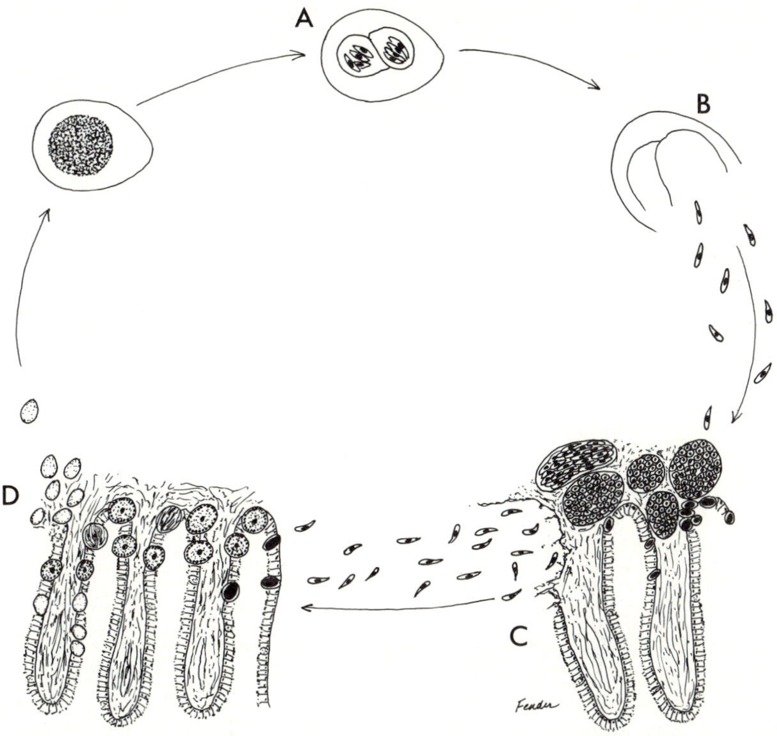

Figure 15–6. The enteroepithelial cycle for the coccidia (*Isospora* and *Hammondia* for the dog, and *Isospora, Besnoitia, Toxoplasma,* and *Hammondia* for the cat). Sporulation outside the host *(A)*, release of sporozoites *(B)*, schizogony with merozoite production and release *(C)*, and gametogony with oocyst production and release *(D)*. (*Sarcocystis* spp. of dogs and cats have gametogony only in the intestine; sporulation occurs in the host.)

late within 12 to 24 hours following passage and that therefore older stool samples will contain sporulated oocysts.[17, 18] Sporocysts of *Sarcocystis* spp. in cats are sporulated when passed and measure 12 × 10 μ.

Transmission of *Isospora* spp. occurs by ingestion of sporulated oocysts or of natural intermediate hosts (small rodents). The other coccidia species listed have intermediate hosts, so carnivorism and ingestion of tissue cysts is the most likely mode of transmission. *Sarcocystis* species have rather specific intermediate hosts and life cycles (e.g, *S. cruzi* has a dog-beef cycle). *Toxoplasma*, on the other hand, has only members of the cat family as definitive hosts but uses many species of mammals and birds as intermediate hosts. Congenital transmission is also possible for *Toxoplasma* in its intermediate hosts, but not in cats (Fig. 15–7).[17, 18]

Release of sporozoites in the gut of the intermediate host results in extraintestinal infections. Schizogony of *Sarcocystis*, for example, may occur in endothelial cells of the vasculature and is known as tachyzoite formation. The rapid proliferative process of tachyzoite formation occurs in vascular sites such as the glomeruli. Tissue cysts with slower proliferation result in bradyzoites, which are infective for dogs or cats. Coyotes probably serve as an important reservoir (definitive) host for infection of sheep and cattle (Fig. 15–8).[1, 16, 22] Raccoons, red foxes, wolves, and dogs serve as definitive hosts

Table 15–3. OOCYSTS AND SPOROCYSTS OF THE COCCIDIAN SPECIES IN DOGS AND CATS

Organism	Host	Size μ	Description
Isospora canis	Dog	≃ 35 × 30 μ	Unsporulated oocyst
Isospora ohioensis	Dog	≃ 25 × 20 μ	Unsporulated oocyst
Isospora burrowsi	Dog	17–22 × 16–19	Unsporulated oocyst
Hammondia heydorni	Dog	12 × 11 μ	Unsporulated oocyst
Sarcocystis spp.	Dog	≃ 15 × 10 μ	Sporulated sporocyst
Isospora felis	Cat	40 × 30 μ	Unsporulated oocyst
Isospora rivolta	Cat	25 × 20 μ	Unsporulated oocyst
Besnoitia spp.	Cat	15 × 12 μ	Sporulated oocyst
Toxoplasma gondii	Cat	12 × 12 μ	Unsporulated oocyst
Hammondia hammondi	Cat	12 × 12 μ	Unsporulated oocyst
Sarcocystis spp.	Cat	12 × 10 μ	Sporulated sporocyst

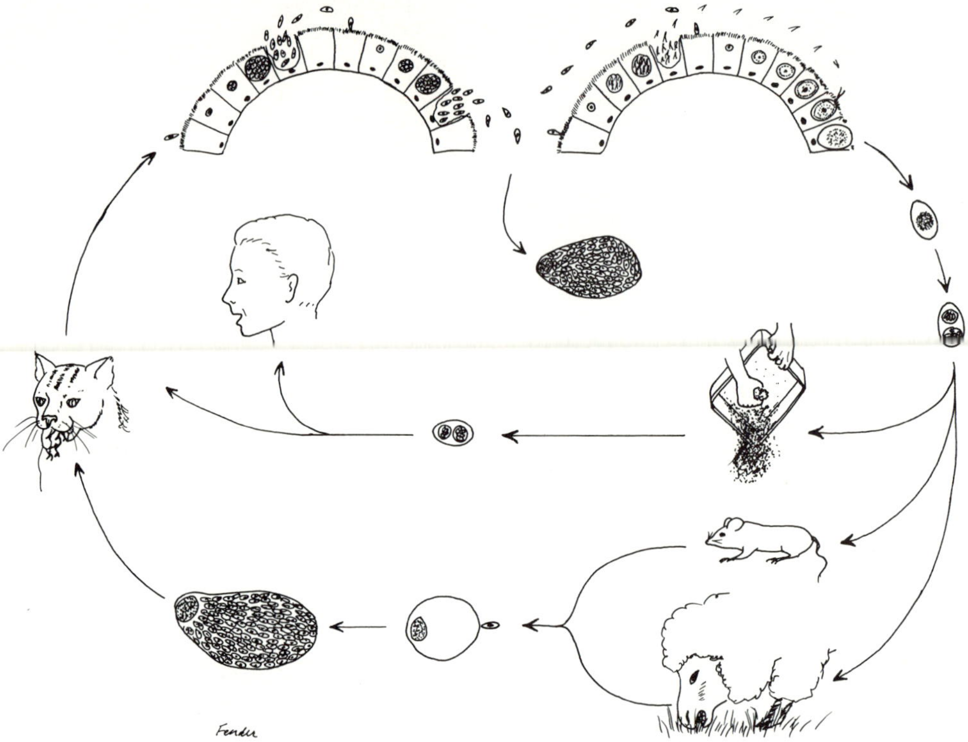

Figure 15–7. Life cycle of *Toxoplasma gondii.* The cat serves as the definitive host. Infection is ingestion of sporulated oocysts or by predation. Schizogony and gametogony occur as an enteroepithelial cycle in the cat with release of oocysts. Rodents, herbivores such as sheep, and humans may become infected, but these serve as intermediate hosts, with schizogony taking place in vascular sites and then in various other tissues of many organs. Humans also may become infected by eating poorly cooked pork or lamb. Congenital transmission is common in the intermediate host.

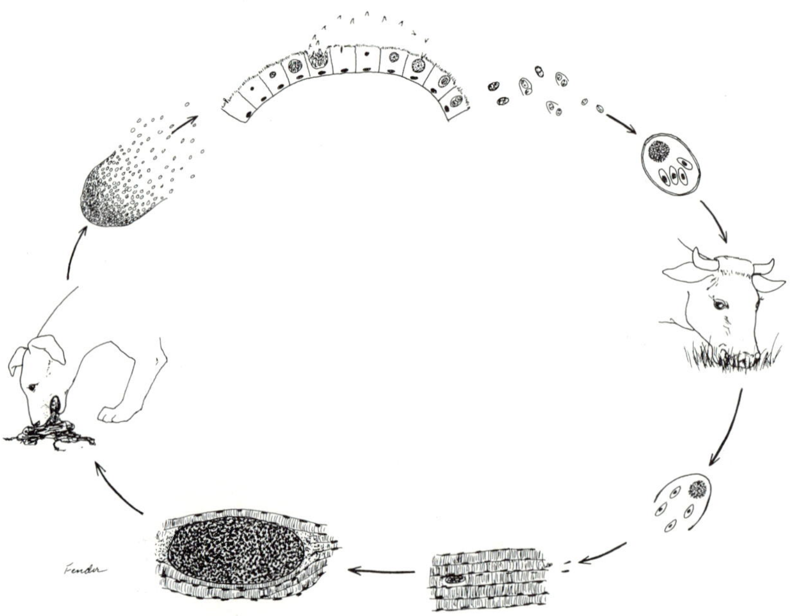

Figure 15–8. Life cycle of *Sarcocystis cruzi*, a dog-cattle cycle. Dogs become infected by eating infected viscera, including muscle, containing tachyzoites or, especially, bradyzoites. Only gametogony occurs in the intestine of the dog. Sporulated sporocysts are passed by the dog; cattle become infected by ingestion of feces-contaminated herbage.

for *S. suicanis* in swine.[7] Exposure to coccidia apparently induces a short-term immunity that is recharged by re-exposure. Thus, older animals usually are partially immune and may serve as asymptomatic carriers.

Pathogenesis and Clinical Signs

Coccidial infections usually are well tolerated by dogs and cats, although clinical coccidiosis can be quite serious in pups and kittens. An enteroepithelial cycle is common for all coccidia, with multiplication by schizogony occurring within the epithelial cells lining the intestine. Most coccidia of dogs and cats invade cells at the villous tip, causing little disease. The more pathogenic species invade subepithelial tissues and induce an inflammatory response.[15] Clinical infections may show diarrhea and dehydration with copious fluid, mucoid, and often bloody feces. Conditions of high-density housing as in kennels and catteries may lead to outbreaks of coccidiosis, as may the stress of weaning, travel, and exposure to cold.

Diagnosis

Diagnosis is based upon finding oocysts or sporocysts in the feces. A direct wet mount is best for finding these stages in the life cycle. Identification of species depends on exact measurements and on sporulation. (Note that *Toxoplasma* and *Sarcocystis* cysts are similar in size, and that *Toxoplasma* oocysts are unsporulated.) The number of oocysts found may not reflect the intensity of infection, since immunity may depress oocyst production. The finding of oocysts in mucoid stools or together with clinical signs would provide a confirmative diagnosis, but oocysts alone do not warrant a diagnosis of clinical disease.

Testing of the serum and feces of cats for *Toxoplasma* is generally not recommended. Serum may not yield positive results for several weeks after the oocysts are shed. A positive test result often represents a past exposure rather than a current infection because there has not been sufficient time for antibody to develop. Fecal examinations of cats are usually not practical because cats shed oocysts for such a short time and specific identification is difficult.[65] A confirmative diagnosis can be made by animal inoculation.[19]

Treatment

Treatment with sulfadimethoxine,* sulfadiazine,† or triple sulfonamides (60 mg/kg) combined with pyrimethamine‡ (0.5 to 1.0 mg/kg) for 4 to 6 days or for as long as oocysts appear is recommended for clinical coccidiosis.[25] Fluid and electrolyte therapy may be necessary. Amprolium§ in the feed or water aids in preventing coccidiosis but may cause anorexia, diarrhea, and nervous signs and may produce a clinical thiamine deficiency.

Prevention

Overcrowding and other stresses, especially weaning, may induce clinical outbreaks of coccidiosis in kennels and catteries. Contaminated water supplies and food, sewage lines that back up, and poor sanitation contribute significantly to the accumulation of oocysts. Correction of these factors and exposure of the area to sunlight or other ultraviolet light sources should decrease or prevent oocyst accumulation. Routine treatment of premises with high pressure hot water or with a sodium hypochlorite solution is advisable. For prevention of *Sarcocystis* infections, feeding raw meat of herbivores should be avoided or discouraged.

Oocysts of *Toxoplasma* are killed by heating at 60°C or possibly by freezing at −20°C. The animals should not be fed raw meat. Outdoor cats should be prevented from moving indoors and, conversely, indoor cats should be prevented from straying outdoors. Litter boxes should be emptied daily, although this task should be avoided by pregnant women.

Public Health Significance

Only domestic cats and other Felidae are known to be definitive hosts for *Toxoplasma* (i.e., the cat's intestinal mucosa is infected with the asexual and sexual stages of the parasite) but cats seldom appear ill.[19, 25, 65] Oocysts may be shed in great numbers in the feces for approximately 2 weeks, and

---

*Albon, Roche Laboratories, Nutley, NJ. Bactrovet, Pitman-Moore, Inc., Washington Crossing, NJ.

†Tribrissen Tablets, Jensen-Salsbery Laboratories, Kansas City, MO.

‡Daraprim, Burroughs Wellcome Co., Kansas City, MO.

§Corid, Merck Sharp & Dohme AGVET, Rahway, NJ. Amprol, Merck Sharp & Dohme AGVET, Rahway, NJ.

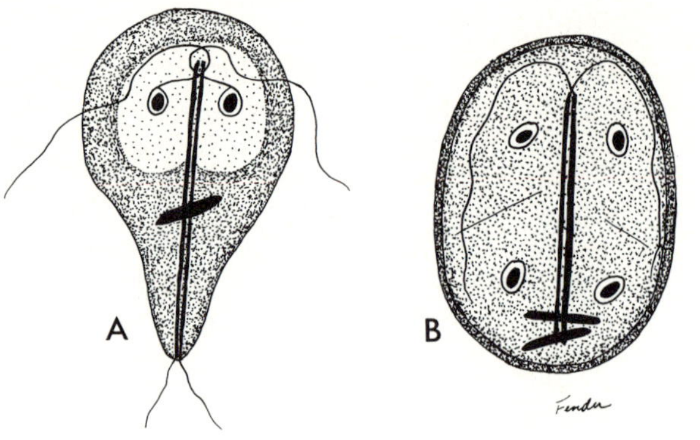

Figure 15–9. *Giardia*, a flagellated protozoan found on the mucosal epithelium of the small intestine, primarily in dogs. *A*, The motile trophozoite (15 × 10 μ). *B*, The encysted stage (12 × 9 μ).

are infective in 2 to 4 days. Humans could be infected by oocysts in cat feces or by the consumption of poorly cooked infected meat (pork or lamb). Extraintestinal infections have been found in brain, heart, muscle, eyes, and lymph nodes.

Of special importance are the infections that occur for the first time in women who are pregnant. Although the fetus is at risk throughout pregnancy, most fetuses who are clinically affected acquire the infection during the first trimester; the greatest number of fetuses are infected during the third trimester, but few have clinical manifestations.[65] Retinochoroiditis is often a sequela of congenital infection. There appears to be no risk to the fetus in women who are seropositive for *Toxoplasma* prior to pregnancy.

Clinical signs of acquired infections in adults include lymphadenopathy, malaise, and fever. Often this infection is mistaken for infectious mononucleosis. Immunosuppressed or debilitated patients are at risk for complications such as encephalitis, myocarditis, and pneumonitis.[65]

GIARDIA

Giardia canis is common in dogs but *G. cati* is rarely seen.

Life Cycle

Trophozoites, which are binucleated, flagellated, and about 15 × 10 μ, usually attach to the mucosal epithelium by a ventral sucking disc (Fig. 15–9). This motile form is passed occasionally in formed stools, but it most often appears in diarrheic feces. Cysts are ovoid but may appear crescent-shaped in flotation fluids, measure 12 × 9 μ, and are found in the formed feces of carrier animals.[66] Thus, the life cycle is direct, with the cyst being the stage of transmission.

Pathogenesis and Clinical Signs

Giardiosis is primarily a disease of young dogs. It is considered a malabsorption syndrome because of the attachment of organisms to the brush border and to the large number of organisms that result from proliferation.

The overwhelming population of *Giardia* could be related to an alteration in physiology and flora of the small intestine. The stress of harboring other parasites or of weaning may cause an infection to become clinical. On clinical examination, pups may have a soft, light-colored, mucoid diarrhea with an oatmeal texture and may be dehydrated. Adult dogs are more likely to show a voluminous frothy stool. Some dogs may have bowel movements of this nature for years before diagnosis is made and treatment is given. Occasionally, blood is seen in the feces in both acute and chronic diarrheas. Often, the glistening, greasy appearance of the feces is due to fat malabsorption.[5]

Diagnosis

The presence of cysts in formed stools indicates only that the patient is a carrier. If trophozoites are found in mucoid to frothy feces, a confirmative diagnosis of giardiosis can be made. Finding trophozoites is best accomplished by making a direct wet mount in a warm saline solution from fresh, unrefrigerated samples. The key to detection is the movement of the trophozoites, which is much like that of a falling leaf.

Treatment

Metronidazole,* glycobiarsol,† and quinacrine hydrochloride‡ have produced good

*Flagyl, Searle Laboratories, Chicago, IL.
†Milibis-V, Winthrop Laboratories, New York, NY.
‡Atabrine, Winthrop Laboratories, New York, NY.

results in the treatment of giardiasis. A high-protein diet should be given to pups.

Prevention

Water supplies, especially in kennels or in crowded, possibly unsanitary quarters, should be tested for *Giardia* cysts. The supply or delivery system should be examined to reduce contamination.

Public Health Significance

Giardia poses a public health problem, also. Although little has been reported on transmission between dogs and humans, it is known that wildlife, such as beavers, can serve as reservoirs, with contaminated water supplies allowing transmission.[41]

Parasites Of The Cecum And Colon

TRICHURIS

Whipworm infections are quite common in dogs but are infrequently seen in cats.[36, 37, 39, 78]

Life Cycle

Trichuris vulpis is found in the cecum and the adjoining portion of the colon in the dog, and *Trichuris campanula* is found in the colon of the cat. The adult measures 5.0 to 7.5 cm in length, including a thin anterior end that is buried in the mucosa (perhaps less than 2 cm is visible when the organism is viewed from the lumen). Eggs larvate on the soil but do not hatch. They are quite resistant to environmental stress and may build up on soil, especially on runs in kennels. The larvated egg is the infective form, and it hatches in the stomach or small intestine. Migration is limited to the gut wall, with the prepatent periods of 70 to 90 days for *T. vulpis* and 62 days for *T. campanula*.[37] Hence, patent infection may not be seen until the pup is at least in its fourth month or the kitten is in its third month.

Pathogenesis and Clinical Signs

Lesions are punctiform owing to the burrowing of *Trichuris* into the mucosa, with ulceration and blood loss likely. Infected dogs may appear unthrifty, lose weight, and pass a bloody, mucoid stool.

Diagnosis

Whipworm eggs are easily identified, being barrel-shaped with bipolar plugs, brown to pale yellow, and measuring 70 to 90 × 30 to 40 μ. Capillarid eggs passed in cat feces may be confused with trichurid eggs, but the former are smaller and have a yellow to green tint, reduced bipolar plugs, and a rough outer shell membrane.

Treatment

Mebendazole, fenbendazole, dichlorvos, butamisole, febantel, and glycobiarsol are quite effective in the removal of adult whipworms. With clinical cases, supportive therapy is needed.

Prevention

Control measures are much the same as those used against ascarids. The runs should be exposed to sunlight, feces should be removed daily, and optimum nutrition should be supplied.

Public Health Significance

Human infection with *Trichuris vulpis* has been reported,[44, 45] but it probably is of little significance.

STRONGYLOIDES

Strongyloides tumefaciens has been reported in cats in Louisiana, Florida, and Texas.[51]

Life Cycle

Strongyloides tumefaciens is found within adenomatous lesions in the wall of the colon. The eggs are larvated and measure 120 × 65 μ. Little is known about this organism's life cycle outside the host, but presumably transmission is similar to that of *S. stercoralis (S. felis)*.

Pathogenesis and Clinical Signs

Small nodules (2 to 3 mm in diameter) representing encapsulated adenomatous proliferations have been described beneath the muscularis mucosa.[51] Sections of adult reproductively active females may be seen on microscopic examination. Infections may cause a chronic colitis with diarrhea and dehydration. Death may follow a wasting-type disease.

Diagnosis

Clinical signs and the presence of large, larvated eggs in stool samples should be diagnostic.

Treatment and Prevention

Methods of treating and preventing *Strongyloides tumefaciens* infections are unknown, but perhaps those measures used for *S. stercoralis* should be considered.

Public Health Significance

No danger to public health is known, although *S. stercoralis* has been reported to be of significance.[26, 27]

BALANTIDIUM

Balantidium coli may infect several host species, including the dog and humans, although the pig is considered the natural host. The organism has worldwide distribution and is quite common in temperate climates.

Life Cycle

This parasite is a ciliated protozoan of 150 μ in diameter, and it actively moves over the mucosal surface of the cecum. Internally, a crescent-shaped sausage-like nucleus may be seen. *Balantidium coli* may invade the mucosa causing ulcers in which large numbers of organisms may be found. Multiplication is by binary fission. These active trophozoites may form a cyst membrane, and cysts of 50 μ may then be passed with the stool. Fecal contamination of food, water, and other fomites and coprophagy allow for transmission. Excystment leads to new infective populations.

Pathogenesis and Clinical Signs

Inflammation and ulceration of the gut may result from *B. coli* infection with secondary bacterial infection possible. The authors' experience has been with dogs living on or near swine farms. The clinical condition is manifested by tenesmus and a bloody liquid diarrhea. There are periods of remission, but clinical recurrence is common, perhaps owing to reinfection.

Diagnosis

The appearance of cysts in formed stools or of cysts and actively motile ciliates in bloody to watery stools as well as knowledge of the habits and habitat of the patient are diagnostic.

Treatment

Metronidazole is the drug of choice for treating *B. coli* infections.

Prevention

Dogs should be prevented from roaming onto hog lots to help control the spread of infection.

Public Health Significance

Balantidium coli is readily transmitted to humans and may have a serious clinical effect.

ENTAMOEBA

Amebiasis, caused by *Entamoeba histolytica*, is an infection of several animal species, including humans, other primates, dogs, cats, rats, and swine. It is worldwide in distribution, being found in all climates, although it is more prevalent in the tropics and subtropics.[38]

Life Cycle

Entamoeba histolytica is an ameboid protozoan found on or within the walls of the cecum and colon. It has an active trophozoite of 10 to 60 μ, which moves by sudden extension of pseudopodia, tongue-like cytoplasmic processes. There is a single nucleus of 4 to 7 μ in diameter, with a distinct central endosome of 0.5 μ in diameter that is surrounded by a clear zone or halo. Food vacuoles may contain erythrocytes that are in the process of being digested.

Trophozoites multiply by binary fission, but only in the host. A cyst is produced by trophozoite division and expulsion of food particles. These cysts are spherical, are 5 to 20 μ in diameter, and have one to four nuclei. Only the forms with four nuclei are viable and capable of producing a new infection. These organisms are quite resistant to environmental stresses and are transmitted by water or food contamination. Infections in the dog are probably acquired from human contact.

Pathogensis

Large trophozoite forms penetrate the gut epithelium, probably by release of proteolytic enzymes.[49] Amebae then multiply forming small colonies, which then penetrate deeper tissues. In the submucosa, they spread laterally, undermining the mucosa and producing a flask-shaped ulcer. Extension and coalescence of ulcers allow for bacterial invasion. Systemic invasion may occur, especially with involvement of the liver, including abscess formation. The lungs and brain may also be involved.

Clinical Signs

In the dog, *Entamoeba* infection is chiefly localized in the cecum and is usually considered asymptomatic.[67]

Diagnosis

The appearance of quadrinucleate cysts in the feces is confirmative for infection. Dysentery may occur, and in areas where human *Entamoeba histolytica* infection is endemic; the presence of dysentery in dogs may suggest such an infection.

Treatment

Metronidazole is the drug of choice. A dose of 400 mg TID should be given for five days for asymptomatic cases and 800 mg TID for 5 days should be administered for acute cases.

Prevention

Good sanitation, including proper sewage disposal and avoidance of fecal contamination of food and water, will prevent *Entamoeba histolytica* infection.

Public Health Significance

Amebic infections should be considered infections of humans and of other primates, with dogs (and possibly cats) secondarily involved.

Parasites Of The Liver And Pancreas

EURYTREMA, PLATYNOSOMUM, AND *AMPHIMERUS*

The *Eurytrema, Platynosomum* and *Amphimerus* species of flukes are harbored in the bile and pancreatic ducts of cats. *Eurytrema procyonis* has the raccoon as its natural host but has also been reported in the red and gray fox. This organism probably gains access to the pancreatic duct from the duodenum, and it may also infect bile ducts.[10] Minor nodularity and fibrosis to severe atrophy of the pancreas have been described. Secretory tests have indicated severe impairment of pancreatic exocrine function, although infected cats appear healthy. Obstruction is a likely reason for disease because of the number of flukes present.[24] Eggs are relatively small (50 × 35 μ). Fenbendazole has been found to be successful for removal of this infection.[60]

Platynosomum is a parasite endemic in wet tropical and subtropical areas, although it has been observed in northern parts of the United States. Infected cats apparently have originated from southern Florida or Louisiana. Eggs of this fluke are operculate and measure 42 × 28 μ. The snail and then lizards or toads act as intermediate hosts. Biliary ducts of cats are infected. Progressive debilitation is commonly reported, usually in older cats that may have depressed immunocompetence.[6] Praziquantel (20 mg/kg PO) has been shown to reduce the number of eggs markedly.[21]

Amphimerus usually occurs in southern regions, but it has been reported in the central and northern sections of the United States.[78] Little is known of the life cycle. *Amphimerus* is found in the bile ducts and occasionally the pancreatic ducts, and it may cause severe chronic inflammatory changes.

References

1. Arthur RG, Post G: Coccidia of the coyotes in eastern Colorado. J Wildl Dis 13:97, 1977.
2. Babero BB, Fawzi AH, Al-Dabagh MA: Zoonoses in Iraq. Further studies on spirocerciasis. Br Vet J 121:183, 1965.
3. Bailey WS: *Spirocerca*-associated esophageal sarcomas (letter). J Am Vet Med Assoc 175:148, 1979.
4. Bailey WS: *Spirocerca lupi*: A continuing inquiry. J Parasitol 58:3, 1972.

5. Barlough JE: Canine giardiasis: A review. J Small Anim Pract 20:613, 1979.
6. Barriga OO, Caputo CA, Weisbrode SE: Liver flukes *(Platynosomum concinnum)* in an Ohio cat. J Am Vet Med Assoc 179:901, 1981.
7. Barrows PL, Smith HM Jr, Prestwood AK, Brown J: Prevalence and distribution of *Sarcocystis* spp among wild swine of southeastern United States. J Am Vet Med Assoc 179:1117, 1981.
8. Beaver PC: Zoonoses, with particular reference to parasites of veterinary importance. *In* Soulsby EJL (ed): *Biology of Parasites.* Academic Press, New York, 215, 1966.
9. Brodey RS: Hypertrophic osteoarthropathy in the dog: A clinicopathologic survey of 60 cases. J Am Vet Med Assoc 159:1242, 1971.
10. Burrows RB, Lillis WG: *Eurytrema procyonis* Denton, 1942 (Trematoda: Dicrocoeliidae). From the domestic cat. J Parasitol 48:810, 1960.
11. Choquett LPE, Gibson GG, Kuyt E, Pearson AM: Helminths of wolves, *Canis lupus* L., in the Yukon and Northwest territories. Can J Zool 51:1087, 1973.
12. Dada BJ, Lindquist WD: Studies on flotation techniques for the recovery of helminth eggs from soil and the prevalence of eggs of *Toxocara* spp in some Kansas public places. J Am Vet Med Assoc 174:1208, 1979.
13. Darne A, Webb JL: The treatment of ankylostomiasis and of spirocercosis in dogs by the new compound, 2,6-diiodo-4-nitro-phenol. Vet Rec 76:171, 1964.
14. Dubey JP: Effect of fenbendazole on *Toxocara canis* larvae in tissues of infected dogs. Am J Vet Res 40:698, 1979.
15. Dubey JP: Pathogenicity of *Isospora ohioensis* infection in dogs. J Am Vet Med Assoc 173:192, 1978.
16. Dubey JP, Fayer R, Seesee FM: *Sarcocystis* in feces of coyotes from Montana: Prevalence and experimental transmission to sheep and cattle. J Am Vet Med Assoc 173:1167, 1978.
17. Dubey JP, Weisbrode SE, Rogers WA: Canine coccidiosis attributed to an *Isospora ohioensis*–like organism: A case report. J Am Vet Med Assoc 173:185, 1978
18. Dubey JP: A review of *Sarcocystis* of domestic animals and of other coccidia of cats and dogs. J Am Vet Med Assoc 169:1061, 1976.
19. Dubey JP: Diagnosis of feline toxoplasmosis. Feline Pract 3:14, 1973.
20. Eckert J, von Brand T, Voge M: Asexual multiplication of *Mesocestoides corti* (Cestoda) in the intestine of dogs and skunks. J Parasitol 55:241, 1969.
21. Evans JW, Green PE: Preliminary evaluation of four anthelmintics against the cat liver fluke, *Platynosomum concinnum.* Aust Vet J 54:454, 1978.
22. Fayer R, Johnson AJ: *Sarcocystis fusiformis* infection in the coyote *(Canis latrans).* J Infect Dis 131:189, 1975.
23. Foster AO, Cross S: The direct development of hookworm after oral infection. Am J Trop Med Hyg 14:565, 1934.
24. Fox JN, Mosley JG, Volger GA, et al.: Pancreatic function in cats with pancreatic fluke infection. J Am Vet Med Assoc 178:58, 1981.
25. Frenkel JK: Common questions on toxoplasmosis: Veterinary, medical, and public health considerations. Vet Med (Small Anim Clin) 77:1188, 1982.
26. Georgi JR: *Parasitology for Veterinarians* 4th ed. W. B. Saunders Company, Philadelphia, 242, 1985.
27. Georgi JR, Sprinkle CL: A case of human strongyloidosis apparently contracted from asymptomatic colony dogs. Am J Trop Med Hyg 24:71, 1974.
28. Georgi ME, Han H, Hartrick DW: *Spirocerca lupi* (Rudolfi, 1809) nodule in the rectum of a dog from Connecticut. Cornell Vet 70:43, 1980.
29. Gleason NN, Kornblum R, Walzer P: *Mesocestoides* (Cestoda) in a child in New Jersey treated with niclosamide (Yomesan). Am J Trop Med Hyg 22:757, 1973.
30. Gleason NN, Healy GR: Report of a case of *Mesocestoides* (Cestoda) in a child in Missouri. J Parasitol 53:83, 1967.
31. Glickman LT, Schantz PM, Cypess RH: Canine and human toxocariasis: Review of transmission, pathogenesis, and clinical disease. J Am Vet Med Assoc 175:1265, 1979.
32. Greve JH, Kung FY: *Capillaria putorii* in domestic cats in Iowa. J Am Vet Med Assoc 183:511, 1983.
33. Greve JH, Hanson RL, McGill LD: Treatment of parasitic ascites in a dog. J Am Vet Med Assoc 174:828, 1979.
34. Greve JH: Age resistance to *Toxocara canis* in ascarid-free dogs. Am J Vet Res 32:1185, 1971.
35. Hargis AM, Prieur DJ, Wescott RB: A gastric nematode *(Ollulanus tricuspis)* in cats in the Pacific Northwest. J Am Vet Med Assoc 178:475, 1981.
36. Hass DK: Feline whipworms do exist. Feline Pract 8:31, 1978.
37. Hass DK, Meisels LS: *Trichuris campanula* infection in a domestic cat from Miami, Florida. Am J Vet Res 39:1553, 1978.
38. Hoare CA: Amoebic infections in animals. Vet Rev Annot 5:91, 1959.
39. Holmes PR, Kelly JD: Occurrence of the genus *Trichuris* in the domestic cat. Aust Vet J 48:535, 1972.
40. Ivoghli B: Esophageal sarcomas associated with canine spirocercosis. Vet Med (Small Anim Clin) 73:47, 1978.
41. Jakubowski W, Hoff JC (eds): *Waterborne Transmission of Giardiasis.* Proceedings of a Symposium. Springfield, Virginia, National Technical Information Service, 1979.
42. Kelly JD, Ng BKY, Whitlock HV: Helminth parasites of dogs and cats. Aust Vet Practitioner 6:89, 1976.
43. Kelly JD, Thompson HG, Chow DCM, Whitlock HV: Arrested development of larval *Ancylostoma caninum* in the gastrointestinal tract. NZ Vet J 24:93, 1976.
44. Kenney M, Yermakov V: Infection of man with *Trichuris vulpis*, the whipworm of dogs. Am J Trop Med Hyg 29:1205, 1980.
45. Kenney M, Eveland LK: Infection of man with *Trichuris vulpis*, the whipworm of dogs. Am J Clin Pathol 69:199, 1978.
46. Kornblatt AN, Schantz PM: Veterinary and public health considerations in canine roundworm control: A survey of practicing veterinarians. J Am Vet Med Assoc 177:1212, 1980.
47. Lillis WG: Helminth survey of dogs and cats in New Jersey. J Parasitol 53:1082, 1967.
48. Little MD: Observations on the possible role of insects as paratenic hosts for *Ancylostoma caninum.* J Parasitol 47:263, 1961.

49. Maegraith BG: Pathogenesis and pathogenic mechanisms in protozoal disease with special references to amoebiasis and malaria. *In* Garnham PCC, Pierce AE, Roitt I (eds): *Immunity to Protozoa.* Oxford, Blackwell Scientific Publications, 1963, pp. 48–65.
50. Malone JB, Breitschwerdt EB, Little MD, et al.: *Strongyloides stercoralis*–like infection in a dog. J Am Vet Med Assoc 176:130, 1980.
51. Malone JB, Butterfield AB, Williams JC, Stuart BS, Travasos H: *Strongyloides tumefaciens* in cats. J Am Vet Med Assoc 171:278, 1977.
52. Miller TA: The diagnosis of hookworm disease. Mod Vet Pract 55:706, 1974.
53. Miller TA: Pathogenesis and immunity in hookworm infection. Trans R Soc Trop Med Hyg 62:473, 1968.
54. Morrison EE, Gier HT: Parasitic infection of *Filaroides osleri, Capillaria aerophila* and *Spirocerca lupi* in coyotes from the southwestern United States. J Wildl Dis 15:557, 1979.
55. Ndiritu CG, Al-Sadi HI: Pathogenesis and lesions of canine spirocercosis. Mod Vet Pract 57:924, 1976.
56. Olsen JL: Life history of *Physaloptera rara* (Hall and Wigdor, 1918) in definitive, intermediate and paratenic hosts. Dissertation Abstracts International 32B:6744, 1972.
57. Pence DB, Stone JE: Visceral lesions in wild carnivores naturally infected with *Spirocerca lupi.* Vet Pathol 15:322, 1978.
58. Polley L: Visceral larva migrans and alveolar hydatid disease. Vet Clin North Am 8:353, 1978.
59. Roberson EL: Chemotherapy of parasitic diseases. *In* Jones LM, Booth NH, McDonald LE (eds): *Veterinary Pharmacology and Therapeutics,* 4th ed. Iowa State University Press, Ames, 967, 1977.
60. Roudebush P, Schmidt DA: Fenbendazole for treatment of pancreatic fluke infection in a cat. J Am Vet Med Assoc 180:545, 1982.
61. Roudebush P: A practical guide to the chemotherapy of small animal intestinal parasites. Canine Pract 7:67, 1980.
62. Schantz PM, Glickman LT: Canine and human toxocariasis: The public health problem and the veterinarian's role in prevention. J Am Vet Med Assoc 175:1270, 1979.
63. Schmidl JA, McCurdy HD, Mozier JO, Kruckenberg SM: Summary of safety evaluations for praziquantel in cats. Vet Med (Small Anim Clin) 77:771, 1982.
64. Scothorn MW, Koutz FR, Groves HF: Prenatal *Toxocara canis* infection in pups. J Am Vet Med Assoc 146:45, 1965.
65. Sikes RK: Toxoplasmosis. J Am Vet Med Assoc 180:857, 1982.
66. Simmons J, Passon TJ Jr: Diagnosis of *Giardia canis*, the elusive parasite. Vet Med (Small Anim Clin) 76:55, 1981.
67. Soulsby EJL: *Helminths, Arthropods and Protozoa of Domesticated Animals*, 7th ed. Lea & Febiger, Philadelphia, 583, 1982.
68. Sprent JFA: The life history of development of *Toxocara cati* (Schrank 1788) in the domestic cat. Parasitology 46:54, 1956.
69. Stephens LC, Gleiser CA, Jardine JH: Primary pulmonary fibrosarcoma associated with *Spirocerca lupi* infection in a dog with hypertrophic pulmonary osteoarthropathy. J Am Vet Med Assoc 182:496, 1983.
70. Stone WM: The transmission, prevalence and control of milk-borne hookworm infection in young puppies. Bull Ga Acad Sci 31:70, 1973.
71. Stone WM, Girardeau MH: Transmammary passage of *Ancylostoma caninum* larvae in dogs. J Parasitol 54:426, 1968.
72. Stone WM, Girardeau MH: Transmammary passage of infective-stage nematode larvae. Vet Med (Small Anim Clin) 62:252, 1967.
73. Swerczek TW, Nielsen SW, Helmboldt CF: Transmammary passage of *Toxocara cati* in the cat. Am J Vet Res 32:89, 1971.
74. Todd AC, Crowley BS Jr, School P, Conway DP: Critical tests with pyrantel pamoate against internal parasites in dogs in Wisconsin. Vet Med (Small Anim Clin) 70:93, 1975.
75. Wandera JG: Further observations on canine spirocercosis in Kenya. Vet Rec 99:348, 1976.
76. Williams JF, Shearer AM: Longevity and productivity of *Taenia taeniaeformis* in cats. Am J Vet Res 42:2182, 1981.
77. Williams JR, Westheimer J, Banman WR: *Mesocestoides* infection in the dog. J Am Vet Med Assoc 166:996, 1975.
78. Williams JF, Zajac A: *Diagnosis of Gastrointestinal Parasitism in Dogs and Cats.* Ralston Purina Company, St. Louis, 1980.
79. Zinkahm WH: Viscera larva migrans. A review and reassessment indicating two forms of clinical expressions: Visceral and ocular. Am J Dis Child 132:627, 1978.

Index

Note: Page numbers in *italics* refer to illustrations. Page numbers followed by (t) refer to tables.